W9-ARG-864

Clinical Obesity in Adults and Children

Clinical Obesity in Adults and Children

EDITED BY

PETER G. KOPELMAN
Professor of Clinical Medicine
Vice-Principal
Barts and The London
Queen Mary's School of Medicine and Dentistry
London
UK

IAN D. CATERSON
Boden Professor of Human Nutrition
Human Nutrition Unit
University of Sydney
Sydney, NSW
Australia

WILLIAM H. DIETZ
Director
Division of Nutrition and Physical Activity
Centers for Disease Control and Prevention
Atlanta, GA
USA

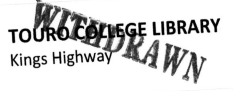
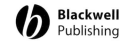
Blackwell
Publishing

© 2005 by Blackwell Publishing Ltd

Blackwell Publishing, Inc., 350 Main Street, Malden, Massachusetts 02148-5020, USA
Blackwell Publishing Ltd, 9600 Garsington Road, Oxford OX4 2DQ, UK
Blackwell Publishing Asia Pty Ltd, 550 Swanston Street, Carlton, Victoria 3053, Australia

First published 1998
Reprinted 1998
Second edition 2005

Library of Congress Cataloging-in-Publication Data on order

ISBN-13: 978-1-4051-1672-5
ISBN-10: 1-4051-1672-2

A catalogue record for this title is available from the British Library

Set in 9 on 12 pt Palatino/Frutiger by SNP Best-set Typesetter Ltd., Hong Kong
Printed and bound in India by Gopsons Papers Ltd., Noida, India

Commissioning Editor: Alison Brown
Development Editor: Mirjana Misina
Production Controller: Kate Charman

For further information on Blackwell Publishing, visit our website:
http://www.blackwellpublishing.com

Contents

Preface to the Second Edition, x

Part 1: Obesity

1 Epidemiology—definition and classification of obesity, 3
2 Measuring body composition in adults and children, 12
3 Social consequences of obesity, 29
4 Obesity and culture, 46

Part 2: Biology of obesity

5 Energy balance and body weight homeostasis, 67
6 Genes and obesity, 81
7 Fetal and infant origins of obesity, 93
8 Metabolic fuels and obesity: carbohydrate and lipid metabolism in skeletal muscle and adipose tissue, 102
9 Energy and macronutrient needs in relation to substrate handling in obesity, 123
10 Biology of obesity: eating behaviour, 137
11 Energy expenditure in humans: the influence of activity, diet and the sympathetic nervous system, 149

Part 3: Obesity and disease

12 Obesity and dyslipidaemia: importance of body fat distribution, 163
13 Obesity and disease: insulin resistance, diabetes, metabolic syndrome and polycystic ovary syndrome, 184
14 Obesity and disease: hormones and obesity, 198

Part 4: Childhood obesity

15 Childhood obesity: definition, classification and assessment, 215
16 Childhood obesity: consequences and physical and psychosocial complications, 231

Part 5: Adult obesity

17 Adult obesity: metabolic syndrome, diabetes and non-alcoholic steatohepatitis, 251
18 Cardiovascular consequences of obesity, 269
19 Adult obesity: fertility, 281
20 Obstructive sleep apnoea, 296

Part 6: Management

21 An overview of obesity management, 319
22 Dietary management of obesity: eating plans, 327
23 Behavioural treatment of obesity: achievements and challenges, 350
24 Exercise and obesity, 363
25 Management of obesity: pharmacotherapy, 380
26 The management of obesity: surgery, 394
27 Weight loss maintenance, 407
28 Educating and training health-care professionals, 421

Part 7: Environmental and policy approaches

29 Obesity in Asian populations, 431
30 Environmental and policy approaches: alternative methods, 443
31 A comprehensive approach to obesity prevention, 456

Index, 473

Contributors

Sarah E. Anderson
MS Friedman School of Nutrition Science and Policy
Tufts University
Boston, Massachusetts
USA

Richard L. Atkinson
Director
Obetech Obesity Research Center
Richmond, VA
USA

Mary Barker
Metabolic Programming Group
MRC Environmental Epidemiological Unit
Southampton General Hospital
Southampton
UK

Colin Bell
School of Exercise and Nutrition Sciences
Deakin University Waterfront Campus
Geelong, VIC
Australia

Ellen E. Blaak
Associate Professor of Human Biology
University of Maastricht
Maastricht
The Netherlands

John E. Blundell
BioPsychology Group
Institute of Psychological Sciences
University of Leeds
Leeds
UK

Kelly D. Brownell
Department of Psychology
Yale University
New Haven, Conneticut
USA

Ian D. Caterson
Boden Professor of Human Nutrition
Human Nutrition Unit
University of Sydney
Sydney, NSW
Australia

Vicki L. Clark
Department of Psychology
Rutgers, The State University of New Jersey
Piscataway, NJ
USA

Pippa Craig
Department of Medical Education
Faculty of Medicine
Edward Ford Building
University of Sydney
Sydney
Australia

Jean-Pierre Després
Professor
Quebec Heart Institute
Laval Hospital Research Center
Quebec City
Canada

Shivani Dewan
Clinical Research Registrar
Clinical Sciences Centre
University Hospital Aintree
Liverpool
UK

William H. Dietz
Director
Division of Nutrition and Physical Activity
Centers for Disease Control and Prevention
Atlanta, GA
USA

John B. Dixon
Centre for Obesity Research and Education
Monash University Medical School
The Alfred Hospital
Melbourne
Australia

Abdul G. Dulloo
Lecturer and Research Staff
Department of Medicine/Physiology
Fribourg
Switzerland

Garry Egger
Director
Centre for Health Promotion and Research
Sydney, NSW
Australia
and
Adjunct Professor of Exercise and Nutrition
Deakin University
Melbourne
Australia

Kristina Elfhag
Obesity Unit
Karolinska University Hospital
Stockholm
Sweden

I. Sadaf Farooqi
Department of Clinical Biochemistry
Addenbrooke's Hospital
Cambridge
UK

Hamid R. Farshchi
School of Biomedical Sciences
University of Nottingham
Queen's Medical Centre
Nottingham

Graham Finlayson
BioPsychology Group
Institute of Psychological Sciences
University of Leeds
Leeds
UK

Janet Franklin
Dietitian
Metabolism and Obesity Services
Royal Prince Alfred Hospital
Camperdown
Sydney, NSW
Australia

Stephen Franks
Department of Reproductive Science and Medicine
Institute of Reproductive and Developmental Biology
Imperial College of Science, Technology and Medicine
Hammersmith Hospital
London
UK

Keith N. Frayn
Professor of Human Metabolism
University of Oxford
Oxford Centre for Diabetes, Endocrinology and Metabolism
Churchill Hospital
Oxford
UK

Timothy Gill
Co-Director
NSW Centre for Public Health Nutrition
Human Nutrition Unit
University of Sydney
Sydney, NSW
Australia

Ronald R. Grunstein
Associate Professor
Centre for Respiratory Failure and Sleep Disorders
Department of Respiratory Medicine
Royal Prince Alfred Hospital
Sydney, NSW
Australia

Jason C.G. Halford
Lecturer in Ingestive Behaviour
Associate Director Kissileff Laboratory
Department of Psychology
University of Liverpool
Liverpool
UK

Kathryn E. Henderson
Department of Psychology
Yale University
New Haven, CT
USA

W. Philip T. James
Honorary Professor
London School of Hygiene and Tropical Medicine
and
Chairman
International Obesity Task Force
London
UK

Susan Jebb
Head of Nutrition and Health Research
Elsie Widdowson Laboratory
Human Nutrition Research
Cambridge
UK

Peter G. Kopelman
Professor of Clinical Medicine
Vice-Principal

Barts and The London
Queen Mary's School of Medicine and Dentistry
London
UK

Jasmine Leonce
Clinical Research Fellow
Metabolic Medicine and Obstetrics
St Mary's Hospital
London
UK

Ian A. Macdonald
Professor
School of Biomedical Sciences
University of Nottingham
Queen's Medical Centre
Nottingham
UK

Aviva Must
Professor
Department of Family Medicine and Community Health
School of Medicine
Tufts University
Boston, MA
USA

Paul E. O'Brien
Professor
Centre for Obesity Research and Education
Monash University Medical School
The Alfred Hospital
Melbourne
Australia

David I.W. Phillips
Metabolic Programming Group
MRC Environmental Epidemiological Unit
Southampton General Hospital
Southampton
UK

Jonathan Pinkney
University of Liverpool Division of Metabolic Medicine
Clinical Sciences Centre
University Hospital Aintree
Liverpool
UK

Joseph Proietto
Professor of Medicine
Department of Medicine
University of Melbourne
Repatriation Hospital
Austin Health
Australia

Rebecca M. Puhl
Department of Psychology
Yale University
New Haven, CT
USA

Stephen Robinson
Consultant Physician and Senior Lecturer
Unit of Metabolic Medicine
St Mary's Hospital
London
UK

Stephan Rössner
Professor
Obesity Unit
Huddinge University Hospital
Stockholm
Sweden

Wim H.M. Saris
Department of Human Biology
Nutrition and Toxicology Research
Institute Maastricht
Faculty of Health Sciences
Maastricht University
Maastricht
The Netherlands

Jacob C. Seidell
Professor of Nutrition and Health
Faculty of Earth and Life Science
Free University of Amsterdam
Amsterdam
The Netherlands

Kate Steinbeck
Associate Professor
Endocrinology and Adolescent Medicine
Royal Prince Alfred Hospital
Camperdown
Australia

Carolyn Summerbell
Professor of Human Nutrition
School of Health and Social Care
University of Teesside
Middlesborough
UK

Boyd Swinburn
School of Exercise and Nutrition Sciences
Deakin University
Burwood, VIC
Australia

Moira A. Taylor
School of Biomedical Sciences
Queen's Medical Centre
Nottingham
UK

André Tchernof
Molecular onology and Endocrinology Research Centre
Department of Nutrition
Quebec City
Canada

Anne Thorburn
Research Manager
St Vincent's Institute of Medical Research
Melbourne
Australia

Marleen A. van Baak
Department of Human Biology
Nutrition and Toxicology Research Institute Maastricht
Faculty of Health Sciences
Maastricht University
Maastricht
The Netherlands

Thomas A. Wadden
Department of Psychiatry
University of Pennsylvania
School of Medicine
Philadelphia
USA

Jonathan Wells
MRC Childhood Nutrition Research Centre
Institute of Child Health
London
UK

John Wilding
Reader in Medicine
Clinical Sciences Centre
University Hospital Aintree
Liverpool
UK

Ian Wilcox
Clinical Associate Professor
Department of Medicine (Central School)
University of Sydney
Sydney, NSW
Australia

Brendon J. Yee
Centre for Respiratory Failure and Sleep Disorders
Department of Respiratory Medicine
Royal Prince Alfred Hospital
Sydney, NSW
Australia

Preface to the Second Edition

Clinical Obesity originated from the previous editors' perception of a need for a textbook emphasizing obesity as a disease entity by reviewing the more clinical and practical aspects of the condition, and addressing its scientific basis. The continuing advances in our knowledge about obesity, and its related conditions, have reinforced this need and provided justification for a second edition. We believe that the original objectives for the book have been achieved with Clinical Obesity proving very relevant to clinicians, and postgraduate and undergraduate medical students, as well as being valuable to newcomers to the research area. We anticipate that readers will find the information in this new edition up-to-date and easily accessible with the choice of chapter headings facilitating cross-reference between sections.

We have broadened the topics covered and the number of authors contributing in this second edition. We have been fortunate in attracting contributors from around the globe to reflect the worldwide scientific and clinical interest as well as the international concerns about obesity. The book is divided into seven sections to address important issues: Obesity; Biology of Obesity; Obesity and disease; Childhood obesity; Adult obesity; Management and Environmental and policy approaches. The final section identifies and discusses environmental and policy approaches in acknowledgement of the critical importance of effective prevention strategies to protect future generations.

We observed in the first edition that obesity research and management had reached a watershed. Although considerable scientific advances have occurred during the intervening seven years, the challenges remain just as great. There has been even greater recognition of the health consequences of excessive weight but, disappointingly, there remains little clarity across the world in the way that this should be tackled at a governmental level. We consider that the second edition of Clinical Obesity will provide a timely review of current knowledge and, using scientific and clinical evidence, make predictions about future directions—essential information for all with an interest in obesity. We remain indebted to Mike Stock, the co-editor of the first edition, for his enormous contribution to the understanding of obesity. His untimely death robbed the scientific community of an inspiring and engaging leader. Nevertheless, his enthusiasm and commitment lives on within the pages of this book—we dedicate the second edition of Clinical Obesity to his memory.

Peter G. Kopelman
Ian D. Caterson
William H. Dietz

Obesity

1

Epidemiology — definition and classification of obesity

Jacob C. Seidell

How to measure obesity, 3

How to measure fat distribution, 4

Who is obese?, 5

Prevalence of obesity in Europe and the USA, 6

Causes of time trends in obesity, 7

Impact of obesity and associated diseases on morbidity and mortality, 8

Conclusions, 10

References, 10

Obesity is generally defined as a body mass index (BMI) of 30 kg/m^2 and higher. Overweight is defined as a BMI between 25 and 30 kg/m^2. The prevalence varies considerably between countries and between regions within countries. It is estimated that more than one-half of adults aged 35–65 years who are living in Europe are either overweight or obese. Overweight is more common among men than among women, but obesity is more common among women. The prevalence of obesity in Europe is probably in the order of 10–20% in men and 15–25% in women. The prevalence of obesity seems to be increasing in most European countries that have reliable data on time trends. In most European countries, obesity is usually inversely associated with socioeconomic status, particularly among women. New classifications of overweight may be based on cut-off points for simple anthropometric measures which reflect both total adiposity and abdominal fatness.

Overweight and obesity are associated with increased mortality and morbidity. Together, they may account for as many as 15–30% of deaths from coronary heart disease (CHD) and 65–75% of new cases of type 2 diabetes mellitus. In addition, overweight and obesity are associated with an increased risk of disabling conditions such as arthritis, respiratory insufficiency and sleep apnoea, and impaired quality of life in general.

How to measure obesity

When we speak about the prevalence of obesity in populations, we actually mean the fraction of people who have an excess storage of body fat. In adult men of average weight, the percentage body fat is in the order of 15–20%. In women, this percentage is higher (about 25–30%). Because differences in weight among individuals are only partly due to variations in body fat, many people object to the use of weight or indices based on height and weight (such as the BMI) to discriminate between overweight and normal-weight people. There are always examples that illustrate the inappropriate use of BMI, such as an identical BMI in a young male body-builder and a middle-aged obese woman. The facts are, however, that despite these obvious extremes there is a very good correlation between BMI (weight divided by height squared) and the percentage of body fat in large populations. Deurenberg *et al.* (1991) established that one can quite accurately estimate the body fat percentage in adults with the following equation:

$$\text{Body fat per cent} = 1.2\,(\text{BMI}) + 0.23\,(\text{age}) - 10.8\,(\text{gender}) - 5.4$$

About 80% of the variation in body fat between (Dutch) individuals could be explained by this formula. The standard error of estimate was about 4%. In this equation, the value for gender is 1 for men and zero for women. It follows that for a given height and weight the body fat percentage is about 10% higher in women than in men. In addition, people get fatter when they get older, even when their body weights are stable. The good correlation between BMI and fat percentage implies that in populations BMI can be used to classify people in terms of excess body fat. In practice, people or populations are usually classified on the basis not of body fat percentage but of BMI. Usually, the same cut-off points are applied for men and women and for different age groups. This is done because

Table 1.1 Classification of overweight by cut-off points of the body mass index (WHO, 1995).

Body mass index (kg/m²)	WHO classification	Popular description
< 18.0	Underweight	Thin
18.5–24.9	–	'Healthy', 'normal' or 'acceptable' weight
25.0–29.9	Grade 1 overweight	Overweight
30.0–39.9	Grade 2 overweight	Obesity
≥ 40.0	Grade 3 overweight	Morbid obesity

the relationships between BMI and mortality are similar (i.e. the relative mortality associated with obesity is similar in men and women; in most age groups the absolute mortality is much lower). The same relative risk and lower absolute risk associated with overweight and obesity among women compared with men implies that women can probably tolerate body fat better than men. The reason could be that in women excess body fat is usually distributed as subcutaneous fat and mainly peripherally (thighs, buttocks, breasts), whereas in men there is a relative excess of body fat stored in the abdominal cavity and as abdominal subcutaneous fat. It has been suggested that optimal BMI (i.e. the BMI associated with lowest relative risk) increases with age (Andres, 1985). The reasons why older people seem to tolerate an excess body fat better than younger people are manifold and range from selective survival to decreased lipolysis of adipose tissue in older people.

Table 1.1 shows the classification of degrees of overweight as measured by BMI (WHO, 1995). These cut-off points apply to both men and women, and to all adult age groups. There are limitations in the interpretation of BMI in very old subjects, as well as in certain ethnic groups with deviating body proportions (e.g. in populations in which stunted growth is common, in those who have relatively short leg length compared with sitting height).

How to measure fat distribution

Since the pioneering work of Jean Vague in the 1940s, it has slowly become accepted that different body morphology or types of fat distribution are independently related to the health risks associated with obesity (Vague, 1956). Jean Vague's brachiofemoral–adipomuscular ratio, as an index of fat distribution, was based on ratios of skinfolds and circumferences of the arms and thighs, whereas more recent indices have been designed specifically to be good predictors of intra-abdominal fat.

The most popular among all measures is the waist–hip circumference ratio. The simplest of these measures is the waist circumference, which has been suggested to predict intra-abdominal fat at least as accurately as the waist–hip ratio

(Pouliot *et al.*, 1994) and to predict levels of cardiovascular risk factors and disease as well as BMI and waist–hip ratio (Han *et al.*, 1995). It has also been suggested that waist circumference could possibly be categorized to replace classifications based on BMI and the waist–hip circumference ratio (Lean *et al.*, 1995).

More complex measures, such as the sagittal abdominal diameter, the ratio of waist–thigh circumference, the ratio of waist–height or the conicity index, have also been proposed to perform even better than waist circumference for one or more of these purposes. However, the differences among these measures are small and the use of ratios may complicate the interpretation of associations with disease and their consequences for public health measures. For instance, the waist–height ratio may be a better predictor of morbidity because the waist measurement is positively associated with disease and because height, for reasons unrelated to body composition or fat distribution, is inversely associated with disease.

Replacing BMI and waist–hip ratio with simple cut-off points that are optimal for each sex, age group, population and relationship with specific diseases may, however, be too simple. Still, as suggested by Lean *et al.* (1995), some cut-off points may be of guidance in interpreting values of waist circumference for adults (Table 1.2). Other cut-off points, based on classification of subjects on a 'critical level' of intra-abdominal fat, have been proposed by investigators from Quebec (Lemieux *et al.*, 1996).

Table 1.2 Sex-specific cut-off points for waist circumference.

	Level 1 ('alerting zone')	Level 2 ('action level')
Men	≥ 94 cm (~37 inches)	≥ 102 cm (~40 inches)
Women	≥ 80 cm (~32 inches)	≥ 88 cm (~35 inches)

Level 1 was initially based on replacing the classification of overweight (BMI ≥ 25 kg/m²) in combination with high waist–hip ratio (WHR ≥ 0.95 in men and ≥ 0.80 in women). Level 2 was based on classification of obesity (BMI ≥ 30 kg/m²) in combination with high waist–hip ratio.

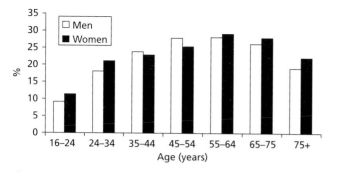

Fig. 1.1 Prevalence of obesity (BMI > 30 kg/m²) in men and women by age (Health Survey for England, 2002; http://www.publications.doh.gov.uk/public/summary.htm).

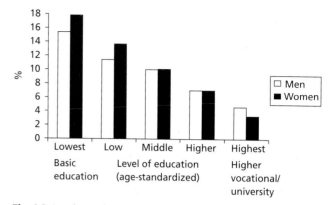

Fig. 1.2 Prevalence of obesity in Dutch adults in the period 1993–97 by highest level of completed education (adapted from Visscher *et al.*, 2002).

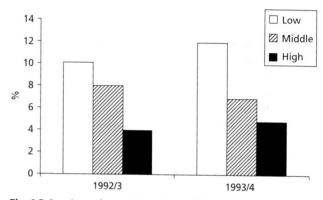

Fig. 1.3 Prevalence of overweight in Dutch children by the level of parental education.

Who is obese?

Very little is known about the factors that may explain the large differences between populations in the distributions of BMI (see next section). Obviously, overweight in individuals in any population is the result of a long-term positive energy balance. Just to say that overweight is characterized by physical inactivity or ingestion of large quantities of food is an oversimplification. Several epidemiological studies have shown that the following factors are associated with overweight in the population:

- Demographic factors:
  - *Age* (increasing with age at least up until age 50–60 years in men and women). Figure 1.1 shows the relationship between age and prevalence of obesity in the United Kingdom (UK, Health Survey for England, 2002).
  - *Gender.* Women have generally higher prevalences of obesity compared with men, especially when older than 50 years of age.
  - *Ethnicity.* Large variations between ethnic groups are not explained by socioeconomic status that is measured by level of education and/or income.
- Sociocultural factors:
  - *Educational level and income.* In industrialized countries the prevalence is higher among those with lower education and/or income. Figure 1.2 illustrates the inverse association between the level of education and the prevalence of obesity in adults in the Netherlands. Similarly, Fig. 1.3 shows the prevalence of overweight in children by the level of education of their parents.
  - *Marital status* (usually increasing after marriage).
- Biological factors:
  - *Parity.* It has been claimed that BMI increases with increasing number of children, but recent evidence suggests that this contribution is, on average, likely to be small and less than 1 kg per pregnancy. Many study designs confound the changes in weight with ageing and changes in weight with parity (Williamson *et al.*, 1994).

- Behavioural factors:
  - *Dietary intake.* Although it is clear that nutrition is of critical importance in establishing a positive energy balance, research on this topic has not been easy to interpret because of confounding (and increased) under-reporting with increasing degrees of obesity. Another reason may be that only small deviations in energy balance are necessary to yield large differences in body weight in the long term. The methodological errors in determining energy intake may be too large to allow detection of the nutritional determinants of obesity. In particular, the fat percentage of the diet has been proposed to be associated with higher prevalence of obesity, although also on this topic the epidemiological evidence may be flawed or biased (Seidell, 1997a).
  - *Smoking.* Smoking lowers body weight and cessation of smoking increases body weight. The associations between smoking and obesity may, however, vary considerably among populations (Molarius *et al.*, 1997).
  - *Alcohol consumption.* The effect of alcohol consumption is unclear in most populations; moderate alcohol consumption is sometimes associated with higher BMI (Prentice, 1995).

– *Physical activity*. Those who remain or become inactive are usually heavier then those who are physically active. Similar limitations apply as for the interpretation of the evidence of nutritional determinants of obesity: methodological problems such as confounding and biased reporting as well as measurement error make it difficult to interpret the literature.

Prevalence of obesity in Europe and the USA

Obesity, defined as a BMI of greater than 30 kg/m^2, is a common condition in Europe and the USA (Seidell and Rissanen, 2004). In the USA there are two important sources of data on the prevalence of obesity. One is the Behavioural Risk Factor Surveillance System (BRFSS), which is based on an annual survey by telephone in random representative samples of the population in the USA (Mokdad *et al.*, 2003). Figure 1.4 shows the time trends of the prevalence of obesity in adult men and women (the two lower lines). The other set of data comes from the National Health and Nutrition Examination Survey (NHANES), which is also based on random representative samples of the US population, but here weight and height are measured in people attending a health examination (Flegal *et al.*, 2002). Figure 1.4 shows that the estimates of the prevalence of obesity are considerably higher, and that the prevalence of obesity is higher in women than in men (not seen in the BRFSS). Although the slopes of the time trends are similar in both studies, this illustrates how difficult it is to assess the true prevalence of obesity. Because of likely under-reporting of weight with increasing obesity, it is likely that the data of NHANES give a more valid estimate of the true prevalence than those based on the self-reported weights and heights in the telephone survey. In Europe, only the UK can provide us with truly nationally representative annual estimates of the prevalence of obesity. Figure 1.5 shows the long-term trends in the UK. These data suggest that in about one-quarter of a century the prevalence of obesity has increased fourfold (UK, Health Survey for England, 2002).

In order to make a comparison possible among countries, it is necessary to compare population-based data on measured height and weight in which identical protocols for measurement were applied and which were collected in the same period. The most comprehensive data on the prevalence of obesity in Europe are from the WHO MONICA study (Molarius *et al.*, 2000). The majority of these data were collected between 1983 and 1986 and a third survey was performed approximately 10 years later. The populations are not necessarily representative of the countries in which they are located.

Tables 1.3 and 1.4 show the increases in the prevalence of obesity in men and women aged 35–64 years in several centres participating in the WHO MONICA project (Molarius *et al.*, 2000). It is clear that there is a rapid increase in the prevalence of obesity in most centres from countries in the European Union, particularly in men. The prevalence of obesity in men and women in European countries in the EU region (Table 1.3) is similar, with a women–men prevalence ratio of 1.07 (range 0.56–1.29). In Central and Eastern European countries (Table 1.4) the prevalence is generally much higher in women than in men (average women–men prevalence ratio 2.03; range: 1.27–2.87).

In centres from countries in Central and Eastern Europe, the prevalence of obesity in women may have stabilized or even slightly decreased, but still these prevalences remain among the highest in Europe. A study by Molarius *et al.* (2000) showed that the social class differences in the prevalence of obesity are increasing with time. Obesity becomes increasingly a lower-class problem in Europe. Table 1.5 shows the high prevalence of obesity in the Baltic states and in some republics in Eastern Europe.

Another systematic examination of the prevalence of obesity across Europe comes from the European Prospective Investigation into Nutrition and Cancer (EPIC) (Haftenberger *et al.*, 2002), which showed that in men and women aged 50–64 years the prevalence of obesity varied from 8% to 40% in men and from 5% to 53% in women, with high prevalences (over 25%) in the centres from Spain, Greece and Italy. In women, the lowest prevalences were seen in France.

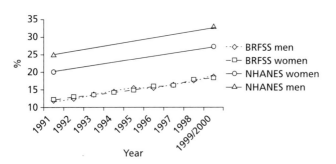

Fig. 1.4 Prevalence of obesity in adult US men and women in the Behavioural Risk Factor Surveillance System (BRFSS) and the National Health and Nutrition Examination Survey (NHANES).

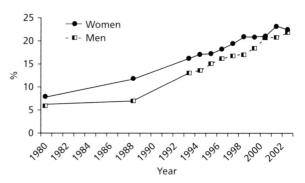

Fig. 1.5 Prevalence of obesity in adult men and women in the United Kingdom (Health Surveys for England).

Table 1.3 Prevalence of obesity (age-standardized percentage with BMI ≥ 30 kg/m²) in centres in EU countries (plus Switzerland and Iceland) participating in the first round of the MONICA study (May 1979 to February 1989) and the third round (June 1989 to November 1996).

Country (centre)	Men		Women		Sex ratio third round, women–men
	First round	Third round	First round	Third round	
Belgium (Ghent)	9	10	11	11	1.10
Denmark (Glostrup)	11	13	10	12	0.92
Finland (north Karelia)	17	22	23	24	1.09
Finland (Kuopio)	18	24	20	25	1.04
Finland (Turku/Loimaa)	19	22	17	19	0.86
France (Toulouse)	9	13	11	10	0.77
France (Lille)	13	17	17	22	1.29
Germany (Augsburg, urban)	18	18	15	21	1.17
Germany (Augsburg, rural)	20	24	22	23	0.96
Iceland (Iceland)	12	17	14	18	1.06
Italy (area Brianza)	11	14	15	18	1.29
Italy (Friuli)	15	17	18	19	1.12
Spain (Catalonia)	10	16	23	25	1.56
Sweden (North)	11	14	14	14	1.00
Switzerland (Vaud/Fribourg)	12	16	12	9	0.56
Switzerland (Ticino)	19	13	14	16	1.23
UK (Belfast)	11	13	14	16	1.23
UK (Glasgow)	11	23	16	23	1.00
Mean	*13.7*	*17.0*	*16.4*	*18.8*	*1.07*

Adapted from Molarius *et al.* (2000).

Table 1.4 Prevalence of obesity (age-standardized percentage with BMI ≥ 30 kg/m²) in centres in countries in Central and Eastern Europe participating in the first round of the MONICA study (May 1979 to February 1989) and the third round (June 1989 to November 1996).

Country (centre)	Men		Women		Sex ratio third round, women–men
	First round	Third round	First round	Third round	
Poland (Warsaw)	18	22	26	28	1.27
Poland (Tarnobrzeg)	13	15	32	37	2.47
Russia (Moscow)	14	8	33	21	2.63
Russia (Novosibirsk)	13	15	43	43	2.87
Czech Republic (rural CZE)	22	22	32	29	1.32
Yugoslavia (Novi Sad)	18	17	30	27	1.59
Mean	*16.3*	*16.5*	*32.7*	*30.8*	*2.03*

Adapted from Molarius *et al.* (2000).

Causes of time trends in obesity

Diminished physical activity, high-fat diets and inadequate adjustments of energy intakes to the diminished energy requirements are likely to be major determinants of the observed changes. Prentice and Jebb (1995) have proposed that, on a population level, limited physical activity may be more important than energy or fat consumption in explaining the time trends of obesity in the UK. Their analyses were based on aspects of physical activity (such as number of hours spent watching television) and household consumption survey data. Although such data may be indicative, such analyses may also be biased. In particular, energy and fat consumption are under-reported with increasing degrees of overweight (Seidell, 1997a).

Changes in smoking behaviour may also contribute to changes in body weight on a population level. Data from the USA showed that, although smoking cessation could explain some of the increase in the prevalence of overweight, smoking cessation alone could not account for the major portion of the increase (Flegal *et al.*, 1995). In other studies it was also shown

Table 1.5 Overweight (BMI 25–29.9 kg/m^2) and obesity (BMI ≥ 30 kg/m^2) levels in the Baltic states.

Country	Year of survey	Sample size	Overweight (%)		Obese (%)	
			Men	Women	Men	Women
Estonia	1997	1154	32.0	23.9	9.9	6.0
Latvia	1997	2292	41.0	33.0	9.5	17.4
Lithuania	1997	2096	41.9	32.7	11.4	18.3
Lithuania*	2000	2195	45.6	31.6	16.9	23.4
Kazakhstan*	1995	3538	–	21.8	–	16.7
Uzbekistan*	1996	4077	–	16.3	–	5.4

Adapted from Pomerleau *et al.* (2000).

*'Finbalt' study based on self-reported height and weight (Janina Petkeviciene, personal communication).

that the increase in the obesity prevalence might be independent of smoking status (Boyle *et al.*, 1994; Wolk and Rössner, 1995).

Epidemiological methods that can be used to assess energy intake and energy expenditure may be subject to bias but, in addition, they also have a considerable ratio of within-subject to between-subject variation. It should be noted that only small changes in energy balance are needed to increase average BMI by one unit. Depending on the distribution of BMI in the population, this may greatly increase the prevalence of obesity. These small changes in energy balance may not be detectable by epidemiological measures of energy expenditure and intake.

It was previously shown (Seidell, 1997b) that dramatic increases in the prevalence of obesity in the Netherlands (about 37% in men and 18% in women over a period of 10 years) can be the consequence of relatively minor changes in average body weight. If height had remained constant, an average weight increase of slightly less than 1 kg over 10 years could have pushed the prevalence of obesity upwards as much as was observed. This could reflect only minute changes in energy balance on a daily basis. Experimentally, overfeeding with about 7000 kcal will result in a weight gain of, on average, about 1 kg. If we neglect all metabolic adaptations to overfeeding and increases in body weight, we can calculate that a constant positive energy balance of about 2 kcal per day may be sufficient to increase the average body weights of individuals by about 1 kg in 10 years. This results in a substantial increase in the prevalence of obesity. It is clear that such small persistent changes in energy balance are not detectable by existing methods for measuring energy expenditure and energy intake in populations.

In the Netherlands, data from two identical nutrition surveys performed in 1987–88 and 1993 suggested that energy intake decreased from 2329 kcal per day (9746 kJ) in 1987–88 to 2216 kcal per day (9278 kJ) in 1993 (Voorlichtingsbureau voor de Voeding, 1993). This reduction of about 113 kcal per day was attributable to a decrease in fat consumption (protein intake increased and carbohydrate and alcohol consumption remained constant). Smoking behaviour had changed,

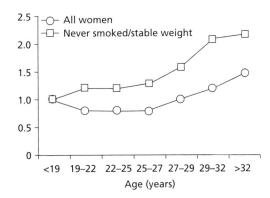

Fig. 1.6 Relation between BMI and relative risk of all-cause mortality in US women (adapted from Manson *et al.*, 1995). Upper line: women who never smoked and had stable body weight. Lower line: all women. Adjusted for age, smoking, menopausal status, oral contraceptive and post-menopausal hormone use, parental history of myocardial infarction, alcohol, saturated fat intake and physical activity.

particularly in men, since the 1970s, but in the 1980s no further decrease was observed. This may imply that daily energy expenditure has decreased during the same period by the same order of magnitude. It is not uncommon in societies that are in a phase of 'post-modernization' to see simultaneous improvement in dietary intakes (reduction in fat and energy) and increases in the prevalence of obesity (Seidell, 1997a).

Impact of obesity and associated diseases on morbidity and mortality

Body mass index is probably linearly related to increased mortality in men and women. In many studies a U- or J-shaped association between BMI and mortality was observed (Troiano *et al.*, 1996), but some recent large studies have suggested that much of the increased mortality at low BMI is due to smoking and smoking-related disease as well as other clinical disorders causing weight loss (Lee *et al.*, 1993; Manson *et al.*, 1995; Jousilahti *et al.*, 1996; Seidell *et al.*, 1996). Figure 1.6 shows the

Table 1.6 Relative impact of overweight and obesity on CHD mortality in three recent large prospective studies in men and women.

| | Jousilahti *et al.* (1996) | | Willett *et al.* (1995) | Seidell *et al.* (1996) | |
	Men	Women	Women	Men	Women
n	7740	8373	115 818	23 306	25 540
Follow-up (years)	15	15	14	12	12
Age at baseline (years)	30–59	30–59	30–55	30–54	30–54
Subjects with BMI ≥ 25 kg/m^2 (%)	58	58	28	40	30
Relative risk BMI ≥ 25 vs. BMI < 25 kg/m^2	1.3	1.5	2.2	1.7	2.3
PAR (BMI ≥ 25 kg/m^2) (%)	15	22	25	20	28
Subjects with BMI ≥ 30 kg/m^2 (%)	11	20	11	4	6
Relative risk BMI ≥ 30 vs. BMI < 30 kg/m^2	1.4	1.3	2.6	2.5	2.3
PAR (BMI ≥ 30 kg/m^2) (%)	4	6	15	6	8

*Fatal and non-fatal coronary heart disease combined.
PAR, population-attributable risk fraction.

Table 1.7 Relative impact of overweight and obesity on diabetes mellitus in some recent large prospective studies in men and women.

	Women (Colditz *et al.*, 1995)	Men (Chan *et al.*, 1994)
n	114 281	51 529
Follow-up (years)	14	5
Age at baseline (years)	30–55	40–75
Subjects with BMI ≥ 25 kg/m^2 (%)	35	50
Relative risk BMI ≥ 25 vs. BMI < 25 kg/m^2	10.3	4.6
PAR (BMI ≥ 25 kg/m^2) (%)	77	64
% Subjects with BMI ≥ 30 kg/m^2	8	7
Relative risk BMI ≥ 30 vs. BMI < 30 kg/m^2	10.6	8.3
PAR (BMI ≥ 30 kg/m^2)	44	33

effect of weight instability, smoking and early mortality on the shape of the association between BMI and total mortality in US women (Manson *et al.*, 1995). It is clear that the U-shaped curve has disappeared after exclusion of women who were ill, had unstable weights or died early. The figure only shows the relative mortality risks. The absolute mortality rates in the women who were non-smokers and had stable weights were much lower than the mortality rates in the total group.

Obesity is related to diabetes mellitus and CHD in men and women. In addition, increasing degrees of overweight are associated with an increased incidence of arthritis of hands and knees, gall bladder disease, sleep apnoea and certain types of cancer (breast cancer and endometrial cancer in women, colon cancer in men). In Tables 1.6 and 1.7 the relative impact of overweight (BMI ≥ 25 kg/m^2) and obesity (BMI ≥ 30 kg/m^2) is calculated for CHD (Willett *et al.*, 1995; Jousilahti *et al.*, 1996; Seidell *et al.*, 1996) and diabetes mellitus (Chan *et al.*, 1994; Colditz *et al.*, 1995). From studies performed in Finland, the USA and the Netherlands it can be shown that BMI in the range of 25–30 kg/m^2 is responsible for the major part of the impact of overweight on CHD mortality. If, in these populations, BMI had remained less than 25 kg/m^2 in all individuals, about 15–30% of all deaths from CHD could theoretically have been

prevented. It will be difficult to determine the impact of the increased prevalence of obesity on CHD mortality because CHD mortality rates have been steadily decreasing in most affluent countries since the 1970s because of better hypertension control, cholesterol lowering, smoking cessation and improved diagnosis and treatment of patients.

The impact of obesity on diabetes mellitus is much larger than the impact on CHD. If these figures are correct, and if BMI remained less than 25 kg/m^2 in all subjects, then about 64% of cases of type 2 diabetes mellitus in men and 77% of cases in women could theoretically have been prevented. It is clear that an epidemic of obesity will be closely followed by an epidemic of type 2 diabetes mellitus (Seidell, 2000).

The impact of the increase in other diseases, such as breast cancer and cerebrovascular disease, may not be noticeable for the next few decades because an increased prevalence of obesity among young adults may not be reflected in an increase in these diseases until these individuals reach their 70s. There are no sensitive monitoring systems for other health consequences such as arthritis, and it will be difficult to directly observe the consequences of an increased proportion of obese subjects in society. Because intervention studies aimed at changing body weights in the general population have been quite unsuccessful (Williamson, 1996), more attention should be given to the prevention of obesity. For these and other reasons, the World Health Organization launched a Task Force on Obesity (James, 1996; Woodman, 1996). Action should be directed not only to food habits of the general population but also against sedentary habits. Specific subgroups such as people who stop smoking, women who are pregnant and those with a family history of obesity and type 2 diabetes mellitus should be targeted separately. Issues of safety, town planning and education are all of great importance and should not be limited to ministries of public health alone.

Conclusions

Overweight and obesity are common in Europe and the USA, and the prevalence seems to be increasing in most countries where reliable data are available. Obesity is associated with increased mortality and incidence of CHD and diabetes mellitus. Although the relative risks for moderate overweight and also the morbidity and mortality risks are usually only slightly elevated, moderate overweight is a major contributor to the total burden of disease associated with increased body weights because of its very high prevalence. Targets to reduce the prevalence of obesity to acceptable levels will not be reached in most countries (Russel *et al.*, 1995; Smith, 1996). International guidelines for the treatment and, in particular, the prevention of obesity are urgently needed (Woodman, 1996). They should be aimed at high-risk groups for weight gain. These include not only those people who have a genetic predisposition for weight gain and obesity but also those who change their lifestyle (e.g. those who stop smoking or those who reduce their physical activity) and, perhaps, women who become pregnant. Special targets should be developed to reach specific socioeconomic and ethnic groups that have a high prevalence of obesity. Efforts to prevent excessive weight gain in children and adolescents should be balanced against the possibility of inducing unnecessary dieting behaviour and eating disorders in girls.

Promoting physical activity is a priority in this context, and attention should be focused not only on more participation in sports clubs but also on stimulating normal outdoor activities such as walking and cycling and the discouragement of 'sedentary behaviour'. International guidelines such as those prepared by the International Task Force on Obesity (Woodman, 1996) can only be implemented when sufficient input and commitment are obtained from governments and health professionals.

References

Andres, R. (1985) Mortality and obesity: the rationale for age-group specific weight–height tables. In: Andres R., Bierman E.L. and Hazzard W.R. eds. *Principles of Geriatric Medicine*. New York: McGraw Hill, 311–318.

Boyle, C.A., Dobson, A.J., Egger, G. and Magnus, P. (1994) Can the increasing weight of Australians be explained by the decreasing prevalence of cigarette smoking? *International Journal of Obesity* **18**, 55–60.

Chan, J.M., Rimm, E.B., Colditz, G.A., Stampfer, M.J. and Willett, W.C. (1994) Obesity, fat distribution, and weight gain as risk factors for clinical diabetes in men. *Diabetes Care* **17**, 961–969.

Colditz, G.A., Willett, W.C., Rotnitzky, A. and Manson, J.E. (1995) Weight gain as a risk factor for clinical diabetes mellitus in women. *Annals of Internal Medicine* **122**, 481–486.

Department of Health (1993) *The Health of the Nation: One Year on . . . a Report on the Progress of the Health of the Nation*. Department of Health. London: HSMO.

Deurenberg, P., Weststrate, J.A. and Seidell, J.C. (1991) Body mass index as a measure of body fatness: age- and sex- specific prediction formulas. *British Journal of Nutrition* **65**, 105–114.

Flegal, K.M., Troiano, R.P., Pamuk, E.R., Kuczmarski, R.J. and Campbell, S.M. (1995) The influence of smoking cessation on the prevalence of overweight in the United States. *New England Journal of Medicine* **333**, 1165–1170.

Flegal, K.M., Carrol, M.D., Ogden, C.L. and Johnson, C.L. (2002) Prevalence and trends in obesity among US adults, 1999–2000. *Journal of the American Medical Association* **288**, 1723–1727.

Haftenberger, M., Lahmann, P., Panico, S., Gonzales, C., Seidell, J.C., Boeing, H., Giurdanella, M.C., Krogh, V., Bueno de Mesquita, H.B., Peeters, P.H., Skeie, G., Hjartaker, A., Rodriguez, M., Quiros, J.R., Berglund, G., Janert, U., Khaw, K.T., Spencer, E.A., Overvad, K., Tjonneland, A., Clavel-Chapelon, F., Tehard, B., Miller, A.B., Klipstein-Grobush, K., Benetou, V., Kiriazi, G., Riboli, E. and Slimani, N. (2002) Overweight, obesity, and body fat distribution in individuals aged 50- to 64 year-old participants in the European Prospective Investigation into Cancer and Nutrition (EPIC). *Public Health Nutrition* **5**, 1147–1162.

Han, T.S., van Leer, E.M., Seidell, J.C. and Lean, M.E.J. (1995) Waist circumference action levels in the identification of cardiovascular risk factors: prevalence study in a random sample. *British Medical Journal* **311**, 1401–1405.

James, W.P.T. (1996) The International Obesity Task Force: obesity at the World Health Organization. *Nutrition, Metabolism and Cardiovascular Disease* **6** (Suppl.), 12–13.

Jousilahti, P., Tuomilehto, J., Vartiainen, E., Pekkanen, J. and Puska, P. (1996) Body weight, cardiovascular risk factors, and coronary mortality: 15 year follow-up of middle-aged men and women in eastern Finland. *Circulation* **93**, 1372–1379.

Lean, M.E.J., Han, T.S. and Morrison, C.E. (1995) Waist circumference indicates the need for weight measurement. *British Medical Journal* **311**, 158–161.

Lee, I-M., Manson, J.E., Hennekens, C.H. and Paffenbarger, R.S. (1993) Body weight and mortality: a 27 year follow-up of middle-aged men. *Journal of the American Medical Association* **270**, 2823–2828.

Lemieux, S., Prudhomme, D., Bouchard, C., Tremblay, A. and Despres, J-P. (1996) A single threshold value of waist girth identifies normal-weight and overweight subjects with excess visceral adipose tissue. *American Journal of Clinical Nutrition* **64**, 685–693.

Manson, J.E., Willett, W.C., Tanpfer, M.J., Colditz, G.A., Hunter, D.J., Hankinson, S.E., Hennekens, C.H. and Speizer, F.D. (1995) Body weight and mortality among women. *New England Journal of Medicine* **333**, 677–685.

Mokdad, A.H., Ford, E.S., Bowman, B.A., Dietz, W.H., Vinicor, F., Bales, V.S. and Marks, J.S. (2003) Prevalence of obesity, diabetes, and obesity-related health risk factors, 2001. *Journal of the American Medical Association* **289**, 76–79.

Molarius, A., Seidell, J.C., Kuulasmaa, K., Dobson, A. and Sans, S. (1997) Smoking and body weight: WHO MONICA Project. *Journal of Epidemiology and Community Health* **51**, 252–260.

Molarius, A., Seidell, J.C., Sans, S., Tuomilehto, J. and Kuulasmaa, K. (2000) Educational levels and relative body weight and changes in their association over 10 years—an international perspective from the WHO MONICA Project. *American Journal of Public Health* **90**, 1260–1268.

Pomerleau, J., Pudule, I., Grinberga, D., Kadziauskiene, K., Abaravicius, A., Bartkeviciute, R., Vaask, S., Robertson, A., and McKee, M. (2000) Patterns of body weight in the Baltic republics. *Public Health Nutrition* **3**, 3–10.

Pouliot, M.C., Despres, J.P., Lemieux, S.L., Moorjani, S., Bouchard, C., Tremblay, A., Nadeau, A. and Lupien, P.J. (1994) Waist circumference and abdominal sagittal diameter: best simple anthropometric indexes of abdominal visceral adipose tissue accumulation and related cardiovascular risk in men and women. *American Journal of Cardiology* **73**, 460–468.

Prentice, A.M. (1995) Alcohol and obesity. *International Journal of Obesity* **19** (Suppl. 5), S44–S50.

Prentice, A.M. and Jebb, S.A. (1995) Obesity in Britain: gluttony or sloth? *British Medical Journal* **311**, 437–439.

Russel, C.M., Williamson, D.F. and Byers, T. (1995) Can the year 2000 objective for reducing overweight in the United States be reached? A simulation study of the required changes in body weight. *International Journal of Obesity* **19**, 149–153.

Seidell, J.C. (1997a) Dietary fat and obesity: an epidemiological perspective. *American Journal of Clinical Nutrition* **67** (Suppl. 3), 546S–550S.

Seidell, J.C. (1997b) Time trends in obesity: an epidemiological perspective. *Hormone and Metabolic Research* **29**, 155–158.

Seidell, J.C. (2000) Obesity, insulin resistance and diabetes—a world-wide epidemic. *British Journal of Nutrition* **83** (Suppl. 1): S5–S8.

Seidell, J.C., and Rissanen A. (2004) Global prevalence of obesity and time trends. In: Bray G.A. and Bouchard C. eds. *Handbook of Obesity. Etiology and Pathophysiology*, 2nd edn. New York: Dekker, 93–107.

Seidell, J.C., Verschuren, W.M.M., van Leer, E.M. and Kromhout, D. (1996) Overweight, underweight, and mortality: a prospective study of 48287 men and women. *Archives of Internal Medicine* **156**, 958–963.

Smith, S.J.L. (1996) Britain is failing to meet targets on reducing obesity. *British Medical Journal* **312**, 1440.

Troiano, R.P., Frongillo, E.A., Sobal, J. and Levitsky, D.A. (1996) The relationship between body weight and mortality: a quantitative analysis of combined information from existing studies. *International Journal of Obesity* **20**, 63–75.

United Kingdom Health Survey for England: http://www.publications.doh.gov.uk/stats/trends1.htm (accessed 15 March 2004).

Vague, J. (1956) The degree of masculine differentiation of obesity—a factor determining predisposition to diabetes, atherosclerosis, gout and uric calculus. *American Journal of Clinical Nutrition* **4**, 20–34.

Visscher, T.L.S, Kromhout, D. and Seidell, J.C. (2002) Long-term and recent time trends in the prevalence of obesity among Dutch men and women. *International Journal of Obesity* **26**, 1218–1224.

Voorlichtingsbureau voor de Voeding (1993) *Zo eet Nederland 1992: Resultaten van de Voedselconsumptiepeiling 1992*. Den Haag.

Willamson, D.F. (1996) The effectiveness of community-based health education trials for the control of obesity. In: Angel A., Anderson, H., Bouchard, C., Lau, D., Leiter, L., Mendelson, R. eds. *Progress in Obesity Research 7*. London: John Libbey, 331–335.

Williamson, D.F., Madans, J., Pamuk, E., Flegal, K.M., Kendrick, J.S. and Serdula, M.K. (1994) A prospective study of childbearing and 10-year weight gain in US white women 25 to 40 years of age. *International Journal of Obesity* **18**, 561–569.

Willlett, W.C., Manson, J.E., Stampfer, M.J., Colditz, G.A., Rosner, B., Speizer, F.E. and Hennekens, C.H. (1995) Weight, weight change, and coronary heart disease in women. Risk within the 'normal' range. *Journal of the American Medical Association* **273**, 461–465.

WHO Expert Committee (1995) *Physical Status: the Use and Interpretation of Anthropometry*. WHO Technical Report Series no. 854. Geneva: WHO.

Wolk, A. and Rössner, S. (1995) Effects of smoking and physical activity on body weight: developments in Sweden between 1980 and 1989. *Journal of Internal Medicine* **237**, 287–291.

Woodman, R. (1996) WHO launches initiative against obesity. *Lancet* **347**, 751.

Measuring body composition in adults and children

Susan Jebb and Jonathan Wells

Introduction, 12

Limitations of the body mass index, 12

Measurement of gross body composition in adults, 13
   Reference methods, 13
   Multicompartment models, 15
   Prediction techniques, 16

Special considerations in children, 18
Fat distribution, 19
Applications of body composition analysis, 21

Conclusions, 24

References, 24

Introduction

Weight is a crude measure of the body's energy reserves, yet it is without doubt the most common method by which obesity is documented. It is also used as a proxy for the successful reduction of fat stores during obesity treatment programmes. More specific measurements of body fat have been commonplace in specialized research laboratories since the 1950s, but they have gradually advanced from the laboratory into the clinic. This is due in part to a growing awareness of the imprecision of body weight as an index of adiposity and, in parallel, the development of other techniques that are suitable for use in clinical practice. There has also been a rise in interest in fat distribution, with the focus on visceral fat as a site of particular metabolic importance. This chapter reviews those methods most relevant to the study of obesity in adults and children, including those with morbid obesity. It provides some practical examples of their application in the context of research and clinical practice.

Limitations of the body mass index

It is salutary to begin by considering some of the errors inherent in the use of body mass index (BMI) as a measure of fatness. First, although weight and height can be measured precisely (Fuller *et al.*, 1991), self-reported measures are biased towards an underestimation of BMI, as there is a tendency to overestimate height and underestimate weight. Second, it gives no in-

dication of the composition of 'excess' weight. Correlation of BMI with other specific measures of fat mass has led to a number of prediction equations to transform BMI into an estimate of fat mass (e.g. Webster *et al.*, 1984). However, this procedure offers little or no further advantage and the absolute estimate of fat mass varies with the prediction equation employed (Elia, 1992).

BMI serves a useful purpose in population assessments, such as surveillance programmes, to document trends in obesity, health inequalities within a population or for international comparisons. But in the context of obesity management a cautious practitioner will always interpret the BMI in the light of a clinical impression that may reveal alternative explanations for apparently high BMIs. Decreases in adult stature, such as those due to kyphosis, and increases in body weight due to oedema or enhanced muscularity will all tend to increase BMI and will be interpreted as implying an elevated body fat mass. Although the BMI may generally rank groups of individuals in order of fatness, considerable absolute errors are apparent in individual patients. In addition there are certain situations in which BMI can be misleading. These include changes in composition with age, racial differences, effects of exercise and weight loss. These limitations have been reviewed in detail elsewhere (Jebb and Prentice, 2001). However, changes in composition with age provide a useful illustration of the general principle.

Ageing is accompanied by a progressive increase in the proportion of fat relative to lean tissue. Thus, even weight-stable patients will become proportionally fatter as they get older. Figure 2.1 shows data from a classic study by Cohn (1987). In a

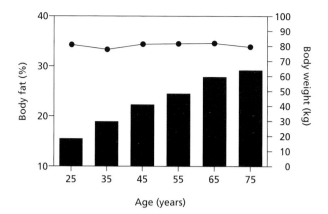

Fig. 2.1 Age-related increase in body fat for healthy men at constant BMI. Line shows body weight. Solid bars show body fat (reproduced from Jebb, S.A. and Prentice A.M. (2001) *Present Knowledge in Nutrition*, 8th edn).

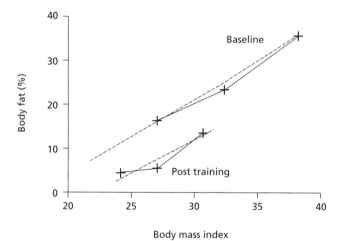

Fig. 2.2 Changes in the lean–fat ratio during physical training. Solid lines show actual data and dotted lines shows regression lines pre and post intervention (reproduced from Jebb, S.A. and Prentice A.M. (2001) *Present Knowledge in Nutrition*, 8th edn).

typical 25-year-old man the proportion of fat would be expected to increase from 15% (12 kg) to 29% (23 kg) by the age of 75 years, even if his weight remained stable. The commonly observed increase in BMI with age, reflecting increases in weight, implies an increase in fatness, but underestimates the true extent of the underlying adiposity.

Inferring changes in body composition in adults based on BMI during periods of weight loss is simply a more complex version of changes in weight, as height may be assumed to remain constant. In most situations, fat loss is proportional to weight loss, but for patients who adopt higher levels of physical activity or specific exercise programmes, BMI can underrepresent the true fat loss. Figure 2.2 shows data from obese male military recruits during a 5-month supervised programme of physical activity and analysed according to three

initial BMI groups (group 1 = 25–29.9, group 2 = 30–34.9, group 3 = >35 kg/m^2) (Sum *et al.*, 1994). Weight loss in the groups was 8.6, 15.7 and 22.0 kg respectively. However, there was an even sharper decrease in body fat, and subjects moved away from the initial relationship between BMI and fatness across the entire group and onto a new regression line, with a much lower intercept, indicating a substantial improvement in the lean–fat ratio.

An important use of the BMI in obesity research has been the recognition of the links to adverse health outcomes. However, it is increasingly evident that waist circumference shows similar and sometimes stronger associations with metabolic diseases. As there is increasing evidence that it is adipose tissue per se that lies at the heart of obesity-related disease, it is logical to suppose that a more specific measure of fatness, either in the whole body or at key sites, for example intra-abdominal or intramuscular fat, will be of greater clinical significance.

Measurement of gross body composition in adults

Reference methods

The classical methods to measure body composition are based on a two-compartment model, in which the body is assumed to be composed of fat and fat-free tissue alone, with fat-free mass (FFM) being the difference between body weight and fat mass. This is therefore a very heterogeneous compartment comprising bone mineral, water, protein, glycogen and other minor constituents. However, data from direct cadaver analysis suggest that the composition of FFM is relatively constant with respect to its density, proportion of water and potassium concentration (Widdowson and Dickerson, 1964). This yields the three classical reference methods to measure body composition: total body water, total body potassium and body density. Today, total body potassium is rarely used to measure body composition and will not be considered further (see instead Lukaski, 1987). In contrast, dual-energy X-ray absorptiometry (DXA) is increasingly widely used, especially in clinical studies to measure bone, fat and fat-free soft tissue (a three-compartment model). These methods may be used individually or combined into more complex multicompartment models which seek to overcome some of the inherent limitations of individual techniques.

Body density

Assuming that the density of fat and fat-free mass (FFM) is known, the proportion of each constituent may be calculated from measurements of body density. Typically, fat is assumed to have a density of 0.9 kg/L and FFM 1.1 kg/L (Siri, 1956), thus:

% fat = 4.95/d − 4.50 × 100

Density (*d*) is calculated as body mass/volume. Traditionally, the measurement of body volume requires complete submergence underwater. Volume is measured either directly by water displacement or calculated as the difference between the weight of the subject underwater and in air. In either case, a correction must be made for the volume of air in the lungs and in the gut. This system is unsuitable for very young children and many others find the procedure difficult and frightening. Most underwater weighing systems are unable to accommodate patients with morbid obesity. A good alternative, based on similar principles, is to use an air displacement technique to measure body volume (Dempster and Aitkens, 1995). The subject is enclosed in a small chamber, composed of two compartments divided by an oscillating diaphragm, and sinusoidal volume perturbations lead to complementary pressure fluctuations in the two compartments. The pressure and volume changes produced in the outer chamber by the presence of the subject allow the volume of the subject to be calculated. This commercial system, Bodpod™, shows excellent agreement with classical underwater weighing, with improved reproducibility and enhanced patient acceptability (McCrory *et al.*, 1995). There are reports of measurements using this equipment in subjects with a BMI of > 70 kg/m² (Das *et al.*, 2003).

Body density can be measured with a high degree of precision and accuracy, but the principal scientific limitation of this method is the error incurred by the assumption of a known density of FFM. The impact on measurements of body density of the variability in FFM has been analysed extensively at a cellular level (Wang *et al.*, 2002), but it is apparent that deviations in body density occur primarily because of changes in hydration or the proportion of bone mineral. One study of obese women (BMI > 30 kg/m²) found that the density of FFM was 1.104 ± 0.006 kg/L (range 1.093–1.117 kg/L) (Fuller *et al.*, 1994), compared with the reference value of 1.1 kg/L. This difference is likely to be exaggerated in patients with morbid obesity and there may be added errors in the measurement of major weight changes, which may be accompanied by systematic changes in the hydration of FFM.

Total body water

Assuming that fat is anhydrous and that FFM contains a known proportion of water, it is possible to estimate FFM from measurements of total body water, and fat can be calculated by difference from body weight. Today, the tracer of choice must be stable, non-radioactive and mix freely with all body-water compartments. In practice, deuterium or oxygen-18 is most commonly used, with the former favoured as it is several-fold cheaper. The isotope can be administered orally or intravenously and a sample of body water, usually saliva, urine or plasma, collected before dosing and after equilibration of the isotope.

The measurement of the isotope in body water is more complex, although some commercial laboratories offer an analyti-

cal service. Both deuterium and oxygen-18 can be measured by mass spectrometry, but a technique to measure deuterium using infrared spectrophotometry has also been described (Jennings *et al.*, 1995). The precision is analogous to that obtained by mass spectrometry, although a much larger dose is recommended, approximately 0.5 g of deuterium per kilogram of body weight. Nonetheless, this procedure is within the capability of most basic laboratories, whereas mass spectrometry is generally confined to specialist centres.

This method is practically feasible in almost all subjects, including babies and young children, and the methodological precision is 1–2% (Coward *et al.*, 1988). However, the critical issue in the accuracy of the technique relates to the hydration fraction of FFM, which changes with growth and development (see below). There are further problems in obese people. A study in healthy non-obese individuals showed a mean of 73.8% with a range of 69.4–78.4% (Fuller *et al.*, 1992). For a 90-kg subject with 50 L of body water, this will give rise to a range in body fat of 18–26 kg. In obese subjects, there may be a systematic increase in the hydration of fat-free tissue (Deurenberg *et al.*, 1989a) and, in addition, many obese people suffer from oedema, so it is difficult to accurately estimate the true hydration fraction of FFM in any given circumstance. A recent study in very obese subjects (BMI = 48.7 ± 8.8 kg/m²) showed that the measured hydration of FFM (using a multicompartment model) was significantly higher than the reference value (0.756 vs. 0.738, *P* < 0.001) (Das *et al.*, 2003).

There may also be particular problems in estimating short-term changes in composition using this technique. For example, the loss of water, in association with glycogen during the early phase of weight loss, will be interpreted as a loss of 1.37 kg of lean tissue for each kilogram of water that is lost. In the longer term, there may be changes in hydration due to decreases in oedema and a generalized trend towards the 'reference' hydration status. However, studies suggest that these changes are very variable between subjects and this confounds accurate measurements of changes in composition with total body water measurements alone.

Dual energy X-ray absorptiometry

Dual energy X-ray absorptiometry (DXA) is widely used for the measurement of bone mineral and soft tissue (Jebb, 1997). Soft-tissue composition is measured in a whole-body scan, which takes between 5 and 30 min, depending on the particular machine. Figure 2.3 illustrates the types of data obtained from such scans. The body is scanned in a rectilinear manner, using two low-dose X-rays at different energies, typically 70 and 140 keV. The effective dose equivalent is similar to a day's background radiation and this low dose makes the procedure suitable for all types of subjects, including babies and children, although it remains prudent not to scan pregnant women. It is also acceptable to make longitudinal measurements in individual subjects. DXA is one of the very few techniques to

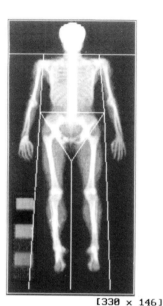

```
Comment:                        Comparison
I.D.:                         Sex:    F
S.S.#:          - -      Ethnic:
                   Height: 163.00 cm
Scan Code:  SAJ  Weight:  48.00 kg
BirthDate: 08/29/64       Age:   28
Physician:
Image not for diagnostic use
  TBAR227
  F.S.   68.00%   0(10.00)%
  Head assumes 17.0% brain fat
  LBM 73.2% water
Region     Fat     Lean+BMC   % Fat
         (grams)   (grams)    (%)
-------  -------   --------   -----
  L Arm    543.8    1639.1    24.9
  R Arm    712.1    1696.9    29.6
  Trunk   2235.4   19618.9    10.2
  L Leg   2168.4    6457.0    25.1
  R Leg   2341.5    6747.3    25.8
 SubTot   8001.2   36159.2    18.1
  Head     650.1    3536.8    15.5
 TOTAL    8651.3   39695.9    17.9
```

[330 × 146]
Hologic QDR-1000/W (S/N 971 P)
Enhanced Whole Body V5.61P

HOLOGIC

Fig. 2.3 DXA scan of a woman with a BMI of 33 kg/m².

bridge the gap between body composition analysis in the laboratory and the clinic. Although the capital costs are high (approximately £70 000), DXA machines are now available in many medium/large hospitals and the running costs are modest. A wider group of researchers than ever before now has access to relatively sophisticated body composition analysis and this is likely to increase the applications of this methodology in clinical studies.

Unfortunately, there are a number of difficulties in the measurement of obese subjects. First, subjects frequently exceed the maximum load of the machine. Second, the scanning area is relatively small (approximately 190×60 cm) and inadequate for most obese subjects. A method has been described for half-body scans in obese subjects (Tataranni and Ravussin, 1995) but this is not ideal as patients inevitably feel embarrassed by the cumbersome procedure. Third, there are concerns that there may be a confounding effect of tissue thickness on the measured fat mass. This has been clearly demonstrated in *in vitro* systems, although the physiological significance is unclear (Tothill *et al.*, 1994a; Jebb *et al.*, 1995). At present, DXA systems are therefore unsuitable for use in patients with morbid obesity.

One of the greatest advantages of DXA is the excellent precision of the measurement. The coefficient of variation for body fat mass is approximately 2%, which in theory makes it particularly suitable for the measurement of relatively small changes in composition (Tothill *et al.*, 1994b). However, Koyama *et al.* (1990) have compared changes in lean tissue mass measured by DXA with nitrogen balance studies in three obese women, studied over two periods of treatment with a very low-energy diet (1.8 MJ per day). Although there was a correlation between the changes in lean tissue measured by

the two methods ($r = 0.40$, $P < 0.05$), there was considerable individual variability, which the investigators attribute to the effect of changes in hydration on the DXA-measured loss of lean tissue.

Multicompartment models

In recent years, it has become increasingly apparent that the inaccuracies of the classical reference methods relate to the limitations of the two-compartment model rather than errors in the measurement of the physical properties of the body. This has led to the development of more sophisticated models of the body in which some of the components of FFM are measured independently. For *in vivo* measurements, a three- or four-compartment model is most widely used, although more complex models have also been described (Heymsfield *et al.*, 1997).

In 1961, Siri proposed the simultaneous measurement of body water and body density to yield a three-compartment model (fat, water and dry fat-free tissue) (Siri, 1961). However, this takes no account of bone mineral. Murgatroyd and Coward (1989) proposed that for the measurement of short-term changes in body composition bone mineral could reasonably be assumed to remain constant, and they derived a model to measure changes in fat and protein, which was also based on total body water and density measurements. A comparison of these indirect techniques to measure changes in fat mass compared with fat balance studies demonstrated the improved precision of this approach (Jebb *et al.*, 1993).

The development of DXA systems to measure whole-body bone mineral content has facilitated the measurement of bone as an additional compartment. Four-compartment models now combine measurements of bone mineral by DXA, and water by deuterium dilution, and hence allow the calculation of the true density of the FFM. In this way, the remaining compartment can be divided into fat and protein on the basis of body density. Glycogen is included as part of the protein compartment as it has a very similar density to protein. Theoretically, this is one of the most accurate methods to assess body composition *in vivo* (Fuller *et al.*, 1992). The propagated measurement error is 0.75 kg of fat in 'reference man' (Snyder *et al.*, 1975). The method has not yet been widely applied, which perhaps reflects the practical limitations of the multitude of techniques that may be particularly difficult in obese subjects.

Using this method, it is possible to calculate the true hydration and density of fat-free tissue and this has served to highlight the limitations of measurements of body density or total body water alone (Jebb and Elia, 1995). A study of body composition in morbidly obese subjects (BMI = 48.7 ± 8.8) using a three-compartment model has confirmed the abnormally high hydration fraction of fat-free tissue, relative to 'reference man' (0.756 vs. 0.738). Interestingly, after weight loss (–44.7 ± 14.6 kg) there was no significant difference. The ratio of extracellular water (measured using a bromide dilution technique) to intracellular water (TBW–ECW) also increased with an increasing proportion of body fat in the pre- and post-weight loss stage (Das *et al.*, 2003). These changes are illustrated in Fig. 2.4 and emphasize the need for multicompartment models to accurately measure changes in body composition in morbidly obese subjects and in those undergoing weight loss.

Multicompartment models can act as accurate reference methods for absolute measures of body composition as they do not carry the errors of traditional two-compartment models with respect to the assumed composition of FFM. A number of studies have used the four-compartment model to determine the accuracy of other simpler techniques (for example Friedl *et al.*, 1992; Fuller *et al.*, 1992; Guo *et al.*, 1992; Bergsma-Kadijk *et al.*, 1996; Forslund *et al.*, 1996).

Prediction techniques

Anthropometry

The measurement of skinfold thicknesses at a number of sites has been used for many years to estimate body fat stores. Subcutaneous fat is measured using callipers that exert a standard pressure, and it is assumed that the thickness of subcutaneous fat at the selected sites is representative, and that there is a known relationship between subcutaneous fat and total fat mass, after allowing for gender differences and changes with age. The most commonly used method involves measurements at four sites: triceps, biceps, subscapula and suprailiac. After log transformation of the data, there is a linear relationship between the sum of the skinfold thickness at these sites and body density, which is age and gender specific (Durnin and Womersley, 1974). Thus, skinfold thickness measurements can be used to predict body density and hence body fat is calculated according to Siri's equation. Different prediction equations are needed for children and for specific racial groups. There has been little validation of the technique in obese subjects.

It will be apparent that this technique combines the error associated with the prediction of body density with the uncertainties regarding the density of FFM, inherent to the density method. Nonetheless, measurements made by a single observer can give good agreement with reference methods and may be more accurate than other prediction techniques (Fuller *et al.*, 1992). Measurements of changes in body fat by skinfold thicknesses may be less reliable than the absolute estimates of fat mass. This is partly because of the measurement error on the pre- and post-weight loss assessments, and also because changes in subcutaneous fat may not fully represent the changes in total body composition.

However, one of the greatest drawbacks to this method is the poor reproducibility of the technique between different observers. The coefficient of variation (CV) for measurements made in six non-obese individuals by six experienced observers was 11%, 16%, 13% and 18% for triceps, biceps, subscapula and suprailiac, respectively, although when summed and translated into an estimate of body fat the CV was only 4.6% (Fuller *et al.*, 1991). In obese people, there are specific problems; some patients may be too large for the jaws of the calipers and it is more difficult to locate the correct anatomical site than in lean individuals. Large subcutaneous fat deposits tend to be very compressible and so the measured thickness will vary with the time taken to make the measurement, which may impair the precision even further. Oedema can lead to an

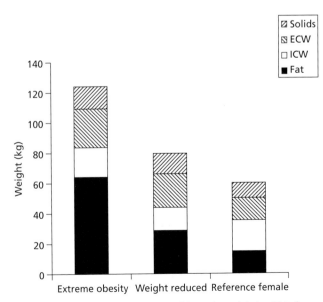

Fig. 2.4 Changes in body composition with massive weight loss (data from Das *et al.*, 2003).

overestimation of body fat, partly because the thickness of the skinfold may be increased, but also because of the increased body weight. Finally, this measurement can be very distressing to some obese patients as it makes such a direct measure of their overt fat stores.

Bioelectrical impedance

This method rests on the principle that fat is a poor conductor of an applied current, whereas fat-free tissue, with its water and electrolyte content, is a good conductor. A small current is passed through the body to measure the body impedance, which is proportional to the conducting volume, i.e. body water (Hoffer *et al.*, 1969). Impedance represents the sum of the resistive and reactive components of the body; some machines measure only resistance, but, as the reactive component in the human body is extremely small, the difference between impedance and resistance is usually insignificant. At high frequencies, typically 50 kHz, the current is able to overcome the capacitance of cell membranes and to fully penetrate the cells, giving a measure of total body water, whereas at low frequencies, for example 1 kHz, it cannot enter the cells and hence measures only extracellular water. Although machines operating at a single high frequency are the most common, an increasing number are able to operate at a number of different frequencies to assess extracellular water too (Tagliabue *et al.*, 1996). These bioelectrical impedance analysis (BIA) measurements of body water are then converted into estimates of body fat and FFM, assuming a standard hydration fraction as for measurements of total body water (TBW) using isotope dilution methods. Traditionally, impedance was measured using a tetrapolar system with electrodes placed on the hand and foot. A new generation of equipment measures impedance from foot to foot.

Prediction equations to convert the measured impedance into an estimate of body composition have been developed by comparison with isotope dilution studies. Although there is a good relationship between the measured impedance and TBW (with correction for height, as a proxy for conductor length), the standard error of the estimate is typically about 2 L. This reflects the complex geometry of the body, which cannot be adequately described using the model of a simple cylinder. Furthermore, it is then necessary to assume the hydration fraction of fat-free tissue (as for the isotope dilution measurements of body water) to extrapolate to soft-tissue composition. Thus, it is important to ensure that subjects are normally hydrated as increases in body water, for example oedema, will be interpreted as an expansion of lean tissue mass and hence body fat will be underestimated. In patients with clinically abnormal hydration, a multifrequency technique will be more useful as it allows the calculation of intracellular water from the difference between total and extracellular volumes, and hence a more accurate measure of the true soft-tissue composition can be made (Maizeish *et al.*, 1995). Abnormalities in the

hydration fraction contribute to errors in the absolute measurement of body composition by BIA in obese subjects. Some studies have shown better agreement between impedance and reference methods in obese subjects following a period of weight loss than at baseline (Van der Kooy *et al.*, 1992; Webber *et al.*, 1994), suggesting that some feature of the obese body composition may be directly contributing to the observed error, such as the expansion of the extracellular water space (Deurenberg *et al.*, 1989b). However, others have found the inter-individual variability to be greater after a period of weight loss, presumably reflecting differences in the composition of tissue lost (Das *et al.*, 2003).

There is a host of commercial impedance machines available. The cost is generally related to the associated software, which may also make predictions of basal metabolic rate, total energy expenditure etc., based on additional measures of weight, height, gender, physical activity etc., which are inserted into the programme. The absolute accuracy of impedance depends on the prediction equation employed (Elia, 1992). The plethora of different population-specific prediction equations has tended to undermine confidence in the BIA technique and no prediction equation has gained widespread acceptance. However, this may change with the publication of new data taken from several laboratories specializing in body composition analysis in the USA, which represents a very comprehensive validation study (Sun *et al.*, 2003) and has already been applied to examine body composition in NHANES III (Chumlea *et al.*, 2002). However, these equations will not be applicable to the foot-to-foot systems and separate validation is required. Despite measuring only a proportion of the total body, with appropriate prediction equations foot-to-foot machines have been shown to offer similar accuracy relative to reference methods as traditional tetrapolar devices (Jebb *et al.*, 2000).

In the study of obesity, the measurement of changes in composition may be at least as important as the absolute measurement of fatness. In the short term, measurements of change in composition with BIA will be undermined by acute changes in hydration. This has been documented in a study in which volunteers consumed a very low-energy diet for 2 days and lost 1.3 ± 0.5 kg (Deurenberg *et al.*, 1989c). This weight loss is likely to be almost entirely composed of water and glycogen (fat-free mass), with only minimal losses of body fat. Whole-body density measurements showed a decrease in fat-free mass of 1.2 ± 0.8 kg, but losses measured by impedance were only 0.5 ± 0.8 kg, implying that 0.8 kg of fat had also been lost. However, over a longer period of time the changes in glycogen become small in relation to the loss of body fat and the validity of this method improves considerably.

Overall, BIA, especially using foot-to-foot systems that make simultaneous measurements of weight and fatness, is a useful method for use in epidemiological surveys and routine clinical practice. It offers better estimates of body fat than BMI alone (Das *et al.*, 2003). It is more precise and has less observer error than skinfold thicknesses (Fuller *et al.*, 1991), and for obese subjects it offers practical advantages.

Special considerations in children

The measurement of body composition in children presents additional difficulties over and above those already encountered in adults: first, children undergo chemical maturation between birth and adulthood, influencing the theoretical assumptions through which physical measurements are converted into body composition values. Second, the collection of physical data is made harder by the greater vulnerability of children, either because some methods are daunting or frightening, or simply because younger subjects may find it difficult to satisfy protocols that involve keeping still. A third related problem is that some techniques were originally designed for adults, and are less successful at accommodating the physical differences between adults and children.

Over the last decade, most practical problems have been addressed, and there are now a number of techniques that can be used to obtain physical data satisfactorily in children. However, the problem of chemical maturation has yet to be addressed in detail, and at present the best data are obtained through a comprehensive but exhaustive approach that minimizes the need for theoretical assumptions.

Chemical maturation

The chemical immaturity of the newborn has been recognized for decades, following direct chemical analyses of stillbirths, and is notable for the high water content and incomplete mineralization compared with adults (Friis-Hansen, 1957). For obvious ethical reasons, cadaver analyses of healthy children have not been undertaken, and the detailed chemical descriptions of adult and neonatal composition are not complemented by intermediary data. Such data are now being obtained by more indirect methods.

Along with the higher TBW content, neonates also differ in the distribution of water between intracellular and extracellular spaces (Friis-Hansen, 1957). Extracellular water contains a lower concentration of solids at birth, and is high in relation to intracellular water because of the proportion of immature cells. Reflecting the higher water content of the FFM, both the protein and mineral contents are reduced (Fomon *et al.*, 1982).

As yet, there is inadequate information as to whether the changes in these properties occur in linear fashion, or whether the developmental patterns are more variable in early life. Only recently have multicomponent models been applied to infants and children, allowing the collection of data in subjects *in vivo*.

In 1982, a paper describing the 'reference child' was published, attempting to describe the changes in body composition between birth and 10 years (Fomon *et al.*, 1982). Actual data were available from several studies for birth, 6 months and 9 years (boys) or 10 years (girls); these data were combined and smoothed on to the National Centre for Health Statistics (NCHS) growth standards. It appears that skinfold data throughout childhood were also used in the calculations. The authors cautioned that their data were provisional, and that the greatest uncertainty concerned the absence of data on TBW, total body calcium and total body potassium at most ages, as well as the problems of converting the physical data on some of these properties into chemical equivalents. Despite this caution, the reference child has been widely used to interpret the data from numerous body composition methods, due to the lack of any viable alternative. In particular, the dataset presents reference values for the hydration, potassium content and density of FFM, thereby allowing the calculation of body composition values from hydrometry, potassium counting and densitometry.

The main limitations of the reference child, in addition to possible inappropriate assumptions, are that it extends only to 10 years, and provides only the average value for each property, with no estimation of between-child variability. A further report (Haschke, 1989) described the reference adolescent in similar fashion, but this article was not published in the mainstream literature and is not widely known. The model of the reference child was revised by Lohman (1989), who made modifications intended to incorporate linear changes in hydration and mineralization throughout childhood and adolescence. These modifications slightly increased the hydration of FFM in both sexes, and increased the density of FFM in girls.

Over the last two decades, reports of multicomponent measurements of children's body composition have begun to emerge, thus providing the opportunity to test the validity of the reference child. Measurements of the hydration of FFM have been relatively consistent with the reference values, both in infancy and childhood (Roemmich *et al.*, 1997; Wells *et al.*, 1999; Butte *et al.*, 2000), although more recent data suggest that actual values are slightly lower, especially in girls (J.C.K. Wells, unpublished). The variability of hydration has also been investigated, and calculated to be ± 1.5% (Wells *et al.*, 1999), similar to the variability reported in adults (Fuller *et al.*, 1992).

The density of FFM appears to be less consistent, particularly in younger children. The variability of this property also appears to be greater than that of hydration, indicating that hydrometry may be a more reliable two-component technique than densitometry. Few data are available for evaluating total body potassium (Burmeister 1961; Forbes 1986; Lohman 1986) but a recent study suggests that the reference values for the potassium content of fat-free tissue in younger children may be misleading (J.C.K. Wells, unpublished).

The lack of comprehensive data on the chemical composition, and physical properties, of the FFM therefore represents a major limitation in measuring children's body composition. A further complication is that obesity appears to alter the composition of the fat-free tissue by increasing mineralization (Goulding *et al.*, 2000) and water content (Battistini *et al.*, 1995).

Physical measurements

A number of techniques described previously are now readily applicable to children, including isotope dilution, DXA and whole-body plethysmography. Used in combination, these techniques provide accurate and precise measurements of gross composition and the constituents of the FFM. Used as simple two-component models, however, all have limitations.

Isotope dilution presents no practical difficulties in healthy children, but presents two potential problems in obese people. First, equilibration of the isotope in the body water pool has been found to require longer, with a 5-hour period recommended on the basis of detailed studies (J.C.K. Wells, unpublished). Second, FFM hydration is higher in obese compared with non-obese children (J.C.K. Wells, unpublished), due in part to the expansion of extracellular water (Battistini *et al.*, 1995).

Plethysmography, using Bodpod™ instrumentation, is easy to undertake in children aged 5 years and over. It has higher precision than the underwater weighing that it has almost invariably replaced, although precision does worsen at lower volumes (Collins and McCarthy, 2003). Validation studies in children aged 8 years or over have suggested that when biases in comparison with other techniques are found, they are small and clinically unimportant (Dewit *et al.*, 2000; Lockner *et al.*, 2000; Demerath *et al.*, 2002). Validation studies are more difficult to undertake in younger children. When plethysmography was used to calculate hydration of FFM in a three-component model in children aged 5–7 years, no bias was found in comparison to hydration values taken from the literature (Wells *et al.*, 2003). However, it is important to use child-specific equations for the prediction of lung volume if actual measurements (difficult for younger children) are not undertaken (Wells *et al.*, 2003).

The conversion of body density into body composition data requires data for the density of FFM. Recent studies in which this property has been measured suggest that the reference values are inaccurate and that they underestimate the bone mineral content of FFM in younger age groups (Wells *et al.*, 1999; 2003). The density of FFM also appears to be significantly reduced in obese children, due to the higher water content.

Dual-energy X-ray absorptiometry has been adopted by some as a gold standard method in children (Bray *et al.*, 2001), although evaluations against multicomponent models have cast serious doubt on the validity of this approach (Wells *et al.*, 1999; Wong *et al.*, 2002). The general limitations of the technique have been discussed above; however, it should be noted that there are two problems particular to children. First, accuracy is influenced by tissue depth, hence some manufacturers have provided size-specific software versions. Second, because of the continuing process of chemical maturation during childhood, the attenuation thresholds at which lean tissue is distinguished from bone are not constant and require modification in relation to age. The technique may also be influenced by hydration. It is not clear how well the manufacturers' adaptations resolve the underlying problems, and instrumentation also differs in the extent to which the various issues have been addressed. At the present time, the high precision of DXA in children does not appear to be matched by equivalent accuracy (Wong *et al.*, 2002).

BIA has been popular in children's studies due to the ease with which measurements can be undertaken. The main problem arises from age-related variability in body proportions. Most validation studies have encompassed a wide age range so that the empirical relationship between height-adjusted impedance and TBW is confounded by variability in the differential length of limb and torso segments (Fuller *et al.*, 2002). The standard error with which BIA predicts TBW is no better than that obtained if the predictors are merely weight and height (Wells *et al.*, 1999). The relationship between impedance and body water is also population specific, so that alternative equations are required in obese people, although even here they become biased once the obese children lose weight. However, new developments such as segmental or vector analyses may eventually overcome some of these limitations.

The most accurate approach at present is to use a multi-component model, thereby avoiding the need to assume constancy of the FFM. Although this may seem intensive, the three-component model is now within the capabilities of many research centres and a few hospitals. Requiring measurements of body weight, TBW and whole-body volume, it can be undertaken using Bodpod™ instrumentation and isotope dilution with the samples analysed using either mass spectrometers or the cheaper option, spectrophotometry. The four-component model is theoretically more accurate than the three-component model and, by adding in a measurement of bone mineral mass, provides information on the protein–mineral ratio. However, the present discrepancy between manufacturers in mineral mass values (Tothill *et al.*, 1994a,b) hinders comparisons between studies using different instrumentation.

Fat distribution

Computerized tomography and magnetic resonance

Imaging techniques have taken an anatomical approach to body composition analysis. Computerized tomography (CT) and magnetic resonance imaging (MRI) allow the examination of the composition of the body by tissue, organ or region (Van der Kooy and Seidell, 1993). CT is an X-ray-based technique, whereas for MRI the subject is placed in a strong magnetic field and irradiated with radiofrequency pulses. The signal intensity is determined by the concentration and relaxation properties of water and fat in the tissues being studied. Adipose tissue has a much shorter relaxation time than other tissues and can be accurately identified. In both cases it is possible to measure total body composition by interpolating between

(a)   (b)

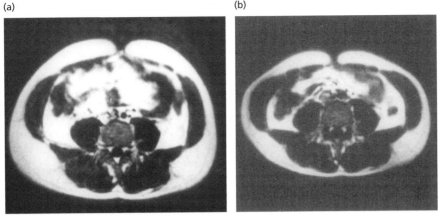

Fig. 2.5 Abdominal MRI scan before (a) and after 10% weight loss (b).

sequential slices; however, this is rarely the most appropriate method to measure whole-body composition because of the limited availability of machines, cost, analysis time and, in the case of CT, a significant radiation exposure of up to 5 mSv. In obese patients these measurements present practical problems as many patients may exceed the capacity of the machines.

However, it is more realistic to use these techniques to provide a direct measure of fat mass at specific sites of the body. CT and MRI have both been used to measure fat distribution, typically in the abdominal or intra-abdominal region. A particular advantage of these techniques is that it is also possible to discriminate between omental, mesenteric and retroperitoneal fat depots that may be associated with independent metabolic effects, and a precise classification system for the adipose tissue depots has been proposed (Shen *et al.*, 2003). The absolute accuracy of the methods has been tested by comparison with sections from cadavers with correlation coefficients for adipose tissue volumes of greater than 0.9 (Van der Kooy and Seidell, 1993). The two methods do give different absolute values for abdominal fat mass, although the ranking of subjects is similar by each method (Seidell *et al.*, 1990). Figure 2.5 shows an abdominal MRI scan, in which subcutaneous and intra-abdominal fat is clearly visible and substantially reduced following a period of weight loss.

Ideally, visceral fat volume is calculated from multiple scans across the abdomen. This gives maximum precision but increased measurement time and, in the case of CT, increased exposure to ionizing radiation (approximately 25–50 mSv per slice) (Kvist *et al.*, 1986). There is, however, a good correlation between the fat area measured in a single CT slice at the level of L4 to L5 with total visceral fat volume ($r > 0.95$) (Kvist *et al.*, 1986), and the precision is estimated to be 1.9% for subcutaneous fat area and 3.9% for visceral fat (Thaete *et al.*, 1995).

Imaging techniques can also be used to examine the size of specific organs. For example, one study has demonstrated that in morbidly obese women with liver steatosis there was an association between visceral fat accumulation and hepatomegaly. Following a period of acute weight loss after bariatric surgery, there was a significant reduction in liver volume (Busetto *et al.*, 2002).

Other developments in this area include the use of magnetic resonance spectroscopy (MRS) to measure very specific body compartments. This includes the measurement of liver glycogen using ^{13}C-NMR (Taylor *et al.*, 1996) and ^{1}H-MRS to measure intracellular triglyceride in skeletal muscle (Savage *et al.*, 2003).

Dual energy X-ray absorptiometry

In addition to the measurement of gross body composition by DXA, it is possible to analyse specific regions of the body, for example arms, legs and trunk, with a coefficient of variation of approximately 5% for the measurement of fat mass (Jebb, 1997). This can give a very crude guide to fat distribution. Absolute measurements of regional body composition in obese and normal-weight subjects by DXA show significant increases in fat in the whole body, arms, legs and trunk in obese subjects relative to lean control subjects, although as a percentage of body weight the regional distribution of fat was not significantly different (Wajchenberg *et al.*, 1995). However, in obese subjects the cramped nature of the scanning position makes regional divisions difficult or even impossible.

It is also possible define a specific abdominal site, usually between L2 and L4, to measure the total fat mass in this region, including both the intra-abdominal and subcutaneous fat deposits, with a coefficient of variation of approximately 3% (Schlemmer *et al.*, 1990; Svendsen *et al.*, 1993a). If subcutaneous fat around the abdomen is estimated from simple anthropometric measures of the sagittal diameter and abdominal skinfold thickness, it is possible to estimate intra-abdominal fat (Svendsen *et al.*, 1993a; Jensen *et al.*, 1995; Treuth *et al.*, 1995). Although the correlation of abdominal fat measured by CT vs. DXA is good ($r = 0.9$) the standard error of the estimate (SEE) is 7% and this increases to 15% for the estimation of intra-abdominal fat in a construct that includes DXA, waist–hip ratio and trunk skinfold thicknesses (Svendsen *et al.*, 1993b). DXA has also been used to estimate skeletal muscle mass (Kim *et al.*, 2002).

Anthropometry

Measurements of body dimensions can be used to give a rough estimate of body shape and it is generally concluded that increasing size reflects increasing fat mass. Skinfold thicknesses, circumferences and, more recently, abdominal diameters have all been used to define increasing abdominal fatness. None of these anthropometric measurements alone can distinguish between visceral and subcutaneous abdominal fat, but they do correlate with risk factors for diabetes and cardiovascular disease, and they are advocated as suitable proxy measures for public health initiatives.

The interpretation of these proxys in terms of absolute measurements varies: a waist–hip ratio of 0.95 in men and 0.80 in women is usually deemed to be indicative of central obesity (National Academy of Sciences, 1991), whereas a waist circumference in excess of 89 cm in women and 102 cm in men has been suggested to identify individuals requiring anti-obesity interventions (Lean *et al.*, 1995). In practice, these cut-offs are artificial definitions, but the underlying concept of waist circumference as a proxy measure of health risks is now well established. The waist–hip ratio has been widely used as a proxy measure of visceral fat, based on studies that have compared the ratio with CT-measured visceral fat (Ashwell *et al.*, 1985). However, the waist–hip ratio predicts less than one-half of the variance in visceral adipose tissue in men and even less in women (Seidell *et al.*, 1987) and after adjustments for total body fat and age there is not always a significant independent association with visceral fat (Seidell *et al.*, 1988). However, one of the strengths of this type of measurement is that the coefficient of variation for body circumferences is less than 2% (Bray *et al.*, 1990) and the validity of self-reported measures is good (Kushi *et al.*, 1988).

The measurement of sagittal diameter as an index of abdominal fat is based on the premise that the accumulation of visceral fat will lead to increases in the sagittal diameter in a supine subject, whereas increases in subcutaneous adipose tissue will reduce sagittal diameter due to the effects of gravity (Sjostrom, 1991). Correlations between the visceral fat area measured by CT or MRI and sagittal diameters range from 0.46 to 0.96 (Van der Kooy and Seidell, 1993). The relationship can be improved by adjusting for the thickness of the abdominal subcutaneous fat layer; however, the poorest correlations are seen in obese subjects in whom subcutaneous fat skinfold thicknesses may be particularly difficult to obtain.

The measurement of skinfold thicknesses represents an attempt to make a direct measure of fat mass at a particular site (Mueller and Stallones, 1981). A variety of skinfold thickness ratios has been proposed to reflect central vs. peripheral fat distribution such as the trunk-to-extremity skinfold ratio [(suprailiac + subscapula + abdominal)/(medial calf + triceps + biceps)] (Rice *et al.*, 1995). These measurements are limited by the same practical drawbacks associated with the prediction of total fat by this method, including inter- and intra-observer variability and the difficulties in actually measuring the thicknesses in obese individuals. However, this approach has been widely used in population-based studies of the genetic component of obesity and fat distribution (e.g. Bouchard *et al.*, 1988; Comuzzie *et al.*, 1994; Rice *et al.*, 1995).

The issues in relation to the measurement of fat distribution in children are similar, although the interpretation is more complex. There are marked changes in fat distribution with growth and development, especially associated with puberty, and it is necessary to have a clear picture of the 'normal' changes in boys and girls in order to identify 'abnormal' patterns of fat distribution. However, as the prevalence of obesity in children increases there is a pressing need to understand the long-term health risks, and measurements of fat distribution are likely to become increasingly important. Already it has been shown that the secular increase in waist circumference is proportionally greater than the increase in BMI, suggesting preferential accumulation of fat in the abdomen (McCarthy *et al.*, 2003).

Bioelectrical impedance

An important advance in BIA has been the development of techniques to measure 'segmental' impedance using electrodes based only on the hands and feet (Organ *et al.*, 1994). Validation studies to measure regional body composition and muscle mass are still limited, but promising, in both adults (Elia *et al.*, 2002) and children (Fuller *et al.*, 2002).

Applications of body composition analysis

Categorization of obesity

In clinical practice, techniques to measure gross body composition may be used to identify obese patients or to monitor the effect of anti-obesity interventions. In practice, patients requiring treatment are almost always identified on the basis of BMI, possibly with additional measurements of waist circumference or the presence of obesity-related co-morbidity. Specific measurements of body composition may also be made at an initial consultation if they form part of a baseline measure for the evaluation of subsequent progress.

The situation in children is more complex because of the way in which BMI changes in age. Unlike in adults, a single cut-off for the diagnosis of overweight and obesity is not sufficient. Clinicians have used a variety of different definitions; however, recently the approach has become considerably more standardized. The publication of BMI SD scores throughout childhood represented the first step, allowing age-specific cut-offs to follow a common rationale (Cole *et al.*, 1995). Second, the data from several countries have been com-

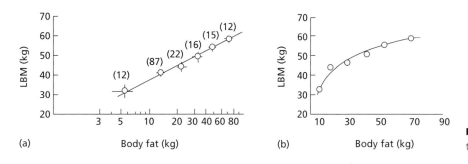

Fig. 2.6 Relationship between fat and lean tissue in women of different body weight.

bined and used to calculate the values that would correspond at each age to the adult cut-offs for overweight and obesity (Cole *et al.*, 2000). These new international cut-offs allow informative comparison between populations, although it should be noted that ethnic differences in the relationship between BMI and fatness that are apparent in adults appear also to apply to children (Deurenberg *et al.*, 2003). Appropriate cut-offs for use in clinical practice are less well defined because of poor understanding of the clinical significance of BMI at specific ages and the tracking of body weight. Children falling above the 85th or 95th centile are often classified as overweight or obese, respectively, but upward centile crossing, identified from sequential measures, is probably more important than any single measurement.

BMI remains central to the categorization of childhood obesity due to the ease with which it can be measured both in the clinic and in population research. Nevertheless, it is important to recognize its limitations. First, BMI reflects variability in FFM as well as in fatness, and there is a twofold range of variation in fatness for a given BMI value (Wells, 2000). Second, BMI appears not to maintain a constant relationship with fatness over time. Several studies have shown that in recent decades children have increased in total and central fatness for a given BMI value, whereas the contribution of lean mass to BMI has declined (Flegal, 1993; Moreno *et al.*, 2001; Wells *et al.*, 2002a). This may be due to the added effect of declines in physical activity, such that the stimulation of lean mass deposition is decreased at the same time as the deposition of fatness is enhanced.

If fat is of interest rather than BMI, then there are as yet no reliable centile data for fat mass or its percentage of weight. Raw skinfold data may be expressed as SD scores, either relative to the data of Tanner and Whitehouse collected in 1966–67 (Davies *et al.*, 1993), or relative to more recent data in infancy (Paul *et al.*, 1998). Due to the association of fatness with size, a particular problem due to the growth of children between measurements, we have argued previously that the most informative manner for data expression is an index adjusting fat mass for height (Wells, 2001; Wells *et al.*, 2002b), as currently being adopted for adults (Kyle *et al.*, 2003).

More research is required in this area, especially given the increasing prevalence of obesity in children and the need to

ensure that weight management programmes do not lead to inappropriate perturbations of healthy growth and development. This requires a clear understanding of changes in body composition during childhood and adolescence and the ability to make measurements with accuracy in both lean and obese individuals.

Obesity management

In clinical practice it is theoretically attractive to use measurements of body fat to define obesity in individual patients, but this rarely occurs because of the relative ease of diagnosis based on BMI, waist circumference or clinical judgement. However, body composition analysis is a useful tool to monitor changes in body fat or its distribution as a consequence of anti-obesity interventions, and is assumed to provide a useful outcome measure before long-term consequences are apparent in morbidity or mortality.

In both adults and children, measurements of body composition have provided the basis for much of our understanding of the physiology of weight loss under different circumstances. Forbes (1987) has undertaken a comprehensive analysis of body composition data, covering a range of body weight, using a variety of two-compartment methods. This demonstrates that there is a curvilinear relationship between body fat and lean tissue, which becomes linear on log transformation (Fig. 2.6). This implies that as weight is gained there is an increase in the relative proportion of fat to lean tissue; as weight is lost, the reverse must be true if the post-obese subject is to achieve a body composition similar to that of the never-obese individual of similar weight. Thus, the appropriate composition of tissue lost will depend in part upon the initial fat mass of the subject. Nonetheless, the general estimate of 25:75% lean–fat tissue lost will be appropriate for severely obese patients.

There is considerable interest in the factors that may affect the composition of weight loss, particularly the extent of the energy deficit and the effect of exercise. A combined analysis from a number of studies, using a variety of two-compartment methods to measure changes in body composition, suggests that the greater the energy deficit the greater the losses of lean tissue (Prentice *et al.*, 1991). This is consistent with classical nitrogen balance studies and a clinical trial that demonstrated greater losses of nitrogen on a very low-energy diet than a 3.3 MJ per day diet (Garrow *et al.*, 1989). However, there is not universal agreement; a complex analysis using *in vitro* neutron activation analysis (IVNAA) shows the loss of lean tissue on a very low-energy diet to be only $78 \pm 8.0\%$ (range 68.1–89.6%) (Ryde *et al.*, 1993).

The macronutrient composition of the diet may also influence the relative proportion of fat and FFM that is lost. Most of the studies that have considered the effect of high-protein diets have been based on nitrogen balance. The classic work of Calloway and Spector (1954) suggests that if energy intake is kept constant nitrogen balance can be improved by increasing the nitrogen intake, although there is little improvement at intakes in excess of 6–7 g per day. Hoffer *et al.* (1984) showed a significant improvement in nitrogen balance when dietary nitrogen was increased from 7 to 13.6 g per day with energy intakes of 2–2.3 MJ per day, but a number of other studies in subjects receiving very low-energy diets (< 3.3 MJ per day) have shown no further improvement in nitrogen balance with intakes in excess of 6–10 g of nitrogen per day (de Haven *et al.*, 1980; Yang *et al.*, 1981; Hendler and Bonde, 1988). Under isoenergetic conditions, differences in the proportion of fat and carbohydrate do not appear to alter the composition of weight loss (Golay *et al.*, 1996).

There is good evidence that the addition of exercise to an energy-restricted diet may minimize the loss of lean tissue. A meta-analysis including measurements made by a variety of two-compartment methods showed that although weight loss was not significantly different in diet-only (DO) and diet-plus exercise (DE) groups, the loss of fat-free tissue was approximately halved in both men and women following the addition of exercise (Ballor and Poehlman, 1994). A study in which changes were measured using MRI has confirmed these findings. In total, 24 women participated in a randomized study of DO vs. DE regimens. Mean weight loss was similar in both groups (DO = -10.0 ± 4.0 kg; DE = -11.7 ± 3.0 kg), but the DE group lost more fat than the DO group (-11.3 ± 3.8 vs. -8.3 ± 3.6 l; $P < 0.05$). Lean tissue and skeletal muscle mass were preserved in the DE group but reduced in the DO group ($P < 0.01$) (Ross *et al.*, 1995).

A limited number of studies have measured changes in regional body composition during weight loss (Fig. 2.6). The study of Hendler *et al.* (1995) demonstrated that in subjects who lost a mean of 24.5 kg to reach ideal body weight there was a decrease of 66% in intra-abdominal fat, 56% in subcutaneous fat at the waist and 51% in subcutaneous fat at the hip, such that the intra-abdominal fat area and hip subcutaneous fat area were reduced to that seen in never-obese individuals at IBW, although the waist subcutaneous fat area remained significantly elevated. It is not yet clear whether these differences in composition in the reduced-obese individuals have any impact on subsequent health risks. Measurements made over a period of weight loss (-12.9 ± 3.3 kg) followed by regain have

shown no difference in the sites of deposition following a weight cycle compared with baseline values (Van der Kooy *et al.*, 1993).

In larger groups of obese subjects anthropometric measurements may be sufficient to identify the changes in fat distribution. For example, in a group of 20 men and 38 women who lost -12.2 ± 3.5 kg and -10.2 ± 3.5 kg, respectively (11.5% body weight for each group), MRI-assessed visceral fat decreased by 40.5 ± 17.1 and $31.7 \pm 16.4\%$ in men and women, whereas waist circumference decreased by 11% and 8% respectively. There was a significant correlation between changes measured by the two methods ($r = 0.66$, $P < 0.001$), such that a 1-cm reduction in waist circumference corresponded with a 5-cm^2 (3.5%) reduction in visceral adipose tissue.

Assessing the health risks of obesity

In epidemiological research, the emphasis is on ranking subjects appropriately rather than accurate individual assessments, and most studies have relied on BMI as a substitute for measurements of body composition. However, there is growing interest in the relationship between body composition/fat distribution and health risks. First, it has been shown that there are differential associations with all-cause mortality for BMI and measures of adiposity (Allison *et al.*, 2002), second, the role of adipose tissue in the pathogenesis of obesity-related disease is more clearly defined and, finally, there has been a marked increase in the availability of, and confidence in, techniques for the measurement of body fat. For these purposes, methods to measure body composition must be simple and rapid to perform. In general, they need to be widely applicable, without introducing systematic errors in specific subgroups of the population. The inclusion of measures of body fat by BIA in NHANES represents an important step and has provided clear evidence of the relationship between fatness and risks of the metabolic syndrome in a large and representative population sample (Zhu *et al.*, 2003). Measurements of fat distribution based on simple anthropometry have also been widely used to assess health risks in a population. In prospective studies, waist circumference is an important predictor of the risk of developing diabetes (Carey *et al.*, 1997).

Fundamental research in obesity

In vivo measurements of body composition have been less widely used in more fundamental research into obesity, although they have been crucial to the development and testing of some fundamental physiological concepts. Here, the accuracy and precision of the measurement of body composition is paramount and sophisticated research methodologies are usually employed.

For example, although it has been apparent for many years that obesity is characterized by an excess of body fat, we now recognize that obese individuals also have increases in other

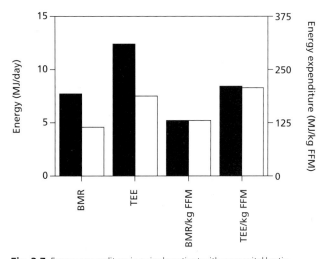

Fig. 2.7 Energy expenditure in a single patient with congenital leptin deficiency (solid bars) relative to an age-matched reference child (open bars) (reproduced from Jebb, S.A. and Prentice A.M. (2001) *Present Knowledge in Nutrition*, 8th edn).

tissues. FFM is enlarged, including both skeletal muscle and visceral organs, and bone mineral mass is increased. Together, they explain the increased energy requirements of obese individuals relative to their lean counterparts and they emphasize that accurate measurements of body composition are necessary to make comparisons of energy expenditure data between lean and obese individuals. Similarly, measurements of basal metabolic rate in patients with Prader–Willi syndrome imply a reduced energy expenditure relative to age-matched non-affected control subjects but, when adjusted for differences in body composition, no residual effect of the disease is reported (Schoeller *et al.*, 1988). This implies that the defect is in the control of nutrient partitioning rather than cellular oxidation. Conversely, Fig. 2.7 shows that the basal and total energy expenditure of patients with congenital leptin deficiency is high in absolute terms, but when adjusted for body composition it is directly similar to an age-matched reference child, thus providing no evidence in humans of any defect in energy expenditure associated with this mutation in the leptin gene (Farooqi *et al.*, 1999).

In recent years, measurements of gross body composition and fat distribution have been used in the phenotyping of patients with specific gene defects known to affect body weight and/or nutrient partitioning (Farooqi *et al.*, 1999; Savage *et al.*, 2003). For example, patients with dominant-negative mutations in the nuclear receptor peroxisome proliferator-activated receptor-γ have a total body fat content (measured by DXA) that is substantially lower than that which is predicted from their BMI. Adipose tissue distribution was measured using MRI and showed a striking paucity of subcutaneous limb and buttock fat, consistent with a partial lipodystrophy. This could not be identified from simple anthropometric indices as both visceral and subcutaneous adipose tissues were

well preserved and thus subjects had relatively 'normal' waist circumference for their BMI (Savage *et al.*, 2003).

Conclusions

Body composition measurements form an integral part of obesity research both in the laboratory and in the clinic. Methods that have been developed and tested in the laboratory are increasingly making their way into the clinic. This progression is partly a consequence of a simplification of the methodology, but it also reflects the recognition of their importance in the clinical management of patients.

Obesity is not a condition of excess weight but of excess body fat, which in turn contributes to the comorbidity of the disease. The site of fat deposition may be particularly important in this respect, but to fully understand the complex interaction more data are needed in which direct measures of fat distribution are combined with accurate measurements of total body fat, including the effect of other confounding factors such as smoking, alcohol consumption and inactivity. Understanding this relationship will ultimately allow a more accurate assessment of the patients at greatest risk and hence help to target limited treatment resources most effectively.

However, we already know that successful obesity treatment must reduce total and abdominal fat. In the clinic, measurements of changes in composition in individual patients provide a valuable method to monitor the efficacy of treatment interventions and to design treatment programmes that maximize the loss of fat tissue. The key issue is to select a method with the necessary accuracy and precision yet which is suited to the practical difficulties encountered in routine clinical practice.

The use of body composition methods in nutrition research is advancing rapidly. This has been stimulated by the development of widely applicable BIA prediction equations for use in epidemiological studies, and the increasing availability of more sophisticated and yet practical techniques to measure body composition in individuals in clinical/research centres using air displacement or DXA. Future analysis using even more sophisticated multicompartment analyses of gross body composition and MRI to assess fat distribution will undoubtedly continue to refine many of the concepts in obesity research, and underpin the evolution of appropriate treatment programmes.

References

Allison, D.B., Zhu, S.K., Plankey, M., Faith, M.S. and Heo, M. (2002) Differential association of body mass index and adiposity with all cause mortality among men in the first and second National Health and Nutrition Examination Surveys (NHANES I and NHANES II) follow-up studies. *International Journal of Obesity* **26**, 410–416.

Ashwell, M., Cole, T. and Dixon, A. (1985) Obesity: new insights into the anthropometric classification of fat distribution shown by computed tomography. *British Medical Journal* 290, 1692–1694.

Ballor, D. and Poehlman, E. (1994) Exercise-training enhances fat-free mass preservation during diet-induced weight loss: a meta-analytical finding. *International Journal of Obesity* 18, 35–40.

Battistini, N., Virgili, F., Severi, S., Brambilla, P., Manzoni, P., Beccaria, L. and Chiumello, G. (1995) Relative expansion of extracellular water in obese vs. normal children. *Journal of Applied Physiology* 79, 94–96.

Bergsma-Kadijk, J., Baumeister, B. and Deurenberg, P. (1996) Measurement of body fat in young and elderly women: comparison between a four-compartment model and widely used reference methods. *British Journal of Nutrition* 75, 649–657.

Bouchard, C., Perusse, L., Leblanc, C., Tremblay, A. and Theriault, G. (1988) Inheritance of the amount and distribution of human body fat. *International Journal of Obesity* 12, 205–215.

Bray, G., Greenway, F. and Molitch, M. (1990) Use of anthropometric measures to assess weight loss. *American Journal of Clinical Nutrition* 31, 769–773.

Bray, G.A., DeLany, J.P., Harsha, D.W., Volaufova, J. and Champagne, C.C. (2001) Evaluation of body fat in fatter and leaner 10-year-old African American and white children: the Baton Rouge Children's Study. *American Journal of Clinical Nutrition*; 73, 687–702.

Burmeister, W. (1961) Potassium-40 content as a basis for the calculation of body cell mass in man. *Science* 148, 1336–1337.

Busetto, L., Tregnaghi, A., De Marchi, F., Segato, G., Foletto, M., Sergi, G., Favretti, F., Lise, M. and Enzi, G. (2002) Liver volume and visceral obesity in women with hepatic steatosis undergoing gastric banding. *Obesity Research* 10, 408–411.

Butte, N.F., Hopkinson, J.M., Wong, W.W., O'Brian Smith, E. and Ellis, K.J. (2000) Body composition during the first 2 years of life: an updated reference. *Paediatric Research* 47, 578–585.

Calloway, D. and Spector, H. (1954) Nitrogen balance as related to calorie and protein intake in active young men. *American Journal of Clinical Nutrition* 2, 405–412.

Carey, V.J., Walters, E.E., Colditz, G.A., Solomon, C.G., Willett, W.C., Rosner, B.A., Speizer, F.E. and Manson, J.E. (1997) Body fat distribution and risk of non-insulin-dependant diabetes mellitus in women. The Nurses Health Study. *American Journal of Epidemiology* 145, 614–619.

Chumlea, W.C., Guo, S.S., Kuczmarski, R.J., Flegal, K.M., Johnson, C.L., Heymsfield, S.B., Lukaski, H.C., Friedl, K. and Hubbard, V.S. (2002) Body composition estimates from NHANES III bioelectrical impedance data. *International Journal of Obesity* 26, 1596–1609.

Cohn, S.H. (1987) New concepts of body composition. In: Ellis K.J., Yasumura S., Morgan W.D. eds. *In Vivo Body Composition Studies*. New York: Plenum Press, 1–14.

Cole, T.J., Freeman, J.V. and Preece, M.A. (1995) Body mass index reference curves for the UK, 1990. *Archives of Diseases in Childhood* 73, 25–29.

Cole, T.J., Bellizzi, M.C., Flegal, K.M. and Dietz, W.H. (2000) Establishing a standard definition for child overweight and obesity worldwide: international survey. *British Medical Journal* 320: 1240–1243.

Collins, A.L. and McCarthy, H.D. (2003) Evaluation of factors determining the precision of body composition measurements by air displacement plethysmography. *European Journal of Clinical Nutrition* 57, 770–776.

Comuzzie, A., Blangero, J., Mahaney, M., Mitchell, B., Stern, M. and MacCluer, J. (1994) Genetic and environmental correlations among skinfold measures. *International Journal of Obesity* 18, 413–418.

Coward, W.A, Parkinson, S.A. and Murgatroyd, P. (1988) Body composition measurements for nutrition research. *Nutrition Research Reviews* 1, 115–124.

Das, S.K., Roberts, S.B., Kehaayias, J.J., Wang, J., Hsu, L.K.G., Shikora, S.A., Saltzman, E. and McCrory, M.A. (2003) *American Journal of Physiology Endocrinology and Metabolism* 284: E1080–E1088.

Davies, P.S., Day, J.M. and Cole, T.J. (1993) Converting Tanner-Whitehouse reference tricep and subscapular skinfold measurements to standard deviation scores. *European Journal of Clinical Nutrition* 47, 559–566.

Demerath, E.W., Guo, S.S., Chumlea, W.C., Towne, B., Roche, A.F. and Siervogel, R.M. (2002) Comparison of percent body fat estimates using air displacement plethysmography and hydrodensitometry in adults and children. *International Journal of Obesity* 26, 389–397.

Dempster, P. and Aitkens, S. (1995) A new air displacement method for the determination of human body composition. *Medicine and Science in Sports and Exercise* 27, 1692–1697.

Deurenberg, P., Van der Kooy, K., Leenen, R. and Schouter, F.J. (1989a) Body impedance is largely dependent on the intra- and extra-cellular water distribution. *European Journal of Clinical Nutrition* 43, 845–853.

Deurenberg, P., Leenen, R., Van der Kooy, K. and Hautvast, J. (1989b) In obese subjects the body fat percentage calculated with Siri's formula is an overestimation. *European Journal of Clinical Nutrition* 43, 569–575.

Deurenberg, P., Westrate, J. and Van der Kooy, K. (1989c) Body composition changes assessed by bioelectrical impedance measurements. *American Journal of Clinical Nutrition* 49, 401–403.

Deurenberg, P., Deurenberg-Yap, M., Foo, L.F., Schmidt, G. and Wang, J. (2003) Differences in body composition between Singapore Chinese, Beijing Chinese and Dutch children. *European Journal of Clinical Nutrition* 57, 405–409.

Dewit, O., Fuller, N.J., Fewtrell, M.S., Elia, M. and Wells, J.C. (2000) Whole body air displacement plethysmography compared with hydrodensitometry for body composition analysis. *Archives of Diseases in Childhood* 82, 159–164.

Durnin, J. and Womersley, J. (1974) Body fat assessed from total body density and its estimation from skinfold thickness measurement in 481 men and women aged 16 to 72 years. *British Journal of Nutrition* 32, 77–97.

Elia, M. (1992) Body composition analysis: an evaluation of 2 component models, multicomponent models and bedside techniques. *Clinical Nutrition* 11, 114–127.

Elia, M., Fuller, N.J., Hardingtoam, C.R., Graves, M., Screaton, N. and Dixon, A.K. (2002) Modelling leg sections by bioelectrical impedance analysis, dual energy X-ray absorptiometry and anthropometry: assessing segmental muscle volume using magnetic resonance imaging as a reference. *Annals of the New York Academy of Science* 904, 298–305.

Farooqi, I.S., Jebb, S.A., Langmack, G., Lawrence, E., Cheetham, C. H., Prentice, A.M., Hughes, I.A., McCamish, M.A. and O'Rahilly, S. (1999) Effects of recombinant leptin therapy in a child with congenital leptin deficiency. *New England Journal of Medicine* 341: 879–884.

Flegal, K.M. (1993) Defining obesity in children and adolescents: epidemiologic approaches. *Critical Reviews of Food Science and Nutrition* **33**, 307–312.

Fomon, S.J., Haschke, F., Ziegler, E.E. and Nelson, S.E. (1982) Body composition of reference children from birth to age 10 years. *American Journal of Clinical Nutrition* **35**, 1169–1175.

Forbes G. (1986) Body composition in adolescence. In: Falkner, F., Tanner, J.M. eds. *Human Growth*, 2. Oxford: Blackwell Scientific, 119–145.

Forbes, G. (1987) Lean body mass-fat interrelationships in humans. *Nutrition Reviews* **45**, 225–231.

Forslund, A., Johansson, A., Sjodin, A., Bryding, G., Ljunghall, S. and Hambraeus, L. (1996) Evaluation of modified multicompartment models to calculate body composition in healthy males. *American Journal of Clinical Nutrition* **63**, 856–862.

Friedl, K., de Luca, J., Marchitelli, L. and Vogel, J. (1992) Reliability of body fat estimations from a four-compartment model by using density, body water and bone mineral measurements. *American Journal of Clinical Nutrition* **55**, 964–970.

Friis-Hansen, B. (1957) Changes in body water compartments during growth. *Acta Paediatrica* **110**, 1–68.

Fuller, N., Jebb, S.A., Goldberg, G., Pullicino, E., Adams, C., Cole, T. and Elia, M. (1991) Inter-observer variability in the measurement of body composition. *European Journal of Clinical Nutrition* **45**, 43–49.

Fuller, N.J, Jebb, S.A., Laskey, M., Coward, W. and Elia, M. (1992) Four component model for the assessment of body composition in humans: comparison with alternative methods and evaluation of the density and hydration of fat free mass. *Clinical Science* **82**, 687–693.

Fuller, N., Sawyer, M. and Elia, M. (1994) Comparative evaluation of body composition methods and predictions, and calculation of density and hydration fraction of fat-free mass, in obese women. *International Journal of Obesity* **18**, 503–512.

Fuller, N.J., Fewtrell, M.S., Dewit, O., Elia, M. and Wells, J.C. (2002) Segmental bioelectrical impedance analysis in children aged 8–12 years: 1. The assessment of whole-body composition. *International Journal of Obesity* **26**, 684–691.

Garrow, J., Webster, J., Pearson, M., Pacy, P. and Harpin, G. (1989) Inpatient-outpatient randomised comparison of Cambridge diet versus milk in 17 obese women over 24 weeks. *International Journal of Obesity* **13**, 521–529.

Golay, A., Allaz, A., Morel, Y., Tonnac, N.D., Tankova, S. and Reaven, G. (1996) Similar weight loss with low or high carbohydrate diets. *American Journal of Clinical Nutrition* **63**, 174–178.

Goulding, A., Taylor, R.W., Jones, I.E. McAuley, K.A., Manning, P.J. and Williams, S.M. (2000) Overweight and obese children have low bone mass and area for their weight. *International Journal of Obesity* **24**, 627–632.

Guo, S., Chumlea, W., Wu, X., Wellens, R., Siervogel, R. and Roche, A. (1992) A comparison of body composition models. In: Ellis K. and Eastmann J. eds. *Human Body Composition: In Vivo Methods, Models and Assessment*. New York: Plenum Press, 27–30.

Haschke, F. (1989) Body composition during adolescence. In: '*Body Composition in Infants and Children*', 98th Ross Conference on Pediatric Research. Columbus, OH: Ross Laboratories, 76–83.

de Haven, J., Sherwin, R., Hendler, R. and Felig, P. (1980) Nitrogen and sodium balance and sympathetic venous-system activity in obese subjects treated with a low calorie protein or mixed diet. *New England Journal of Medicine* **302**, 477–482.

Hendler, R. and Bonde, A. (1988) Very-low-calorie diets with high and low protein content: impact on triiodothyronine, energy expenditure and nitrogen balance. *American Journal of Clinical Nutrition* **48**, 1239–1247.

Hendler, R., Welle, S., Scott, M., Barnard, R. and Amatruda, J. (1995) The effects of weight reduction to ideal body weight on body fat distribution. *Metabolism* **44**, 1413–1416.

Heymsfield, S., Wang, Z., Baumgartner, R. and Ross, R. (1997) Human body composition: advances in models and methods. *Annual Review of Nutrition* **17**, 527–558.

Hoffer, E., Meador, C. and Simpson, D. (1969) Correlation of whole-body impedance with total body water volume. *Journal of Applied Physiology* **27**, 531–534.

Hoffer, L., Bistrian, B., Young, V., Blackburn, G. and Matthews, D. (1984) Metabolic effects of very low calorie weight reducing diets. *Journal of Clinical Investigation* **73**, 750–758.

Jebb, S.A. (1997) Measurement of soft tissue composition by dual energy X-ray absorptiometry. *British Journal of Nutrition* **77**, 151–163.

Jebb, S.A. and Elia, M. (1995) Multicompartment models in health and disease. In: Davies, P. and Cole, T. eds. *Body Composition Techniques in Health and Disease*. Cambridge: Cambridge University Press, 240–254.

Jebb, S.A. and Prentice, A.M. (2001) Lessons from body composition analysis. In: *Present Knowledge in Nutrition*. Washington: International Life Sciences Institute Press, 13–21.

Jebb, S.A., Murgatroyd, P., Goldberg, G., Prentice, A.M. and Coward, W.A. (1993) *In vivo* measurement of changes in body composition: description of methods and their validation against 12-d continuous whole-body calorimetry. *American Journal of Clinical Nutrition* **58**, 455–462.

Jebb, S.A., Goldberg, G., Jennings, G. and Elia, M. (1995) Dual energy X-ray absorptiometry measurements of body composition: effects of depth and tissue thickness, including comparisons with direct analysis. *Clinical Science* **88**, 319–324.

Jebb, S. A., Cole, T.J., Doman, D., Murgatroyd, P.R. and Prentice, A.M. (2000) Evaluation of the novel Tanita body-fat analyser to measure body composition by comparison with a four-compartment model. *British Journal of Nutrition* **83**: 115–122.

Jennings, G., Bluck, L., Chowings, C., Podesta, D. and Elia, M. (1995) Evaluation of an infra-red method for the determination of total body water in a clinical context. *Clinical Nutrition* **14** (Suppl.), 53.

Jensen, M., Kanaley, J., Reed, J. and Sheedy, P. (1995) Measurement of abdominal and visceral fat with computed tomography and dual energy X-ray absorptiometry. *American Journal of Clincal Nutrition* **61**, 274–278.

Kim, J., Wang, Z.M., Heymsfield, S.B., Baumgartner, R.N. and Gallagher, D. (2002) Total-body skeletal muscle mass: estimation by a new dual-energy X-ray absorptiometry method. *American Journal of Clinical Nutrition* **76**, 378–383.

Koyama, H., Nishizawa, Y., Yamashita, N., Furumitsu, Y., Hagiwara, S., Ochi, H. and Morii, H. (1990) Measurement of composition changes using dual photon absorptiometry in obese patients undergoing semi-starvation. *Metabolism* **39**, 302–306.

Kushi, L., Kaye, S., Folsom, A.R., Soler, J.T. and Prineas, R.J. (1988) Accuracy and reliability of self-measurement of body girths. *American Journal of Epidemiology* **128**, 740–748.

Kvist, H., Sjostrom, L. and Tylen, U. (1986) Adipose tissue volume determinations in women by computed tomography. *International Journal of Obesity* **10**, 53–67.

Kyle, U.G., Schhutz, Y., Dupertuis, Y.M. and Pichard, C. (2003) Body composition interpretation: contributions of the fat-free mass index and the body fat mass index. *Nutrition* **19**, 597–604.

Lean, M., Han, T. and Morrison, C. (1995) Waist circumference as a measure for indicating need for weight management. *British Medical Journal* **311**, 158–161.

Lockner, D.W., Heyward, V.H., Baumgartner, R.N. and Jenkins, K.A. (2000) Comparison of air-displacement plethysmography, hydrodensitometry, and dual X-ray absorptiometry for assessing body composition of children 10 to 18 years of age. *Annals of the New York Academy of Sciences* **904**, 72–78.

Lohman, T.G. (1986) Applicability of body composition techniques and constants for children and youths. *Exercise Sport and Science Reviews* **14**, 325–357.

Lohman, T.G. (1989) Assessment of body composition in children. *Paediatric Exercise Science* **1**, 19–30.

Lukaski, H. (1987) Methods for the assessment of human body composition: traditional and new. *American Journal of Clinical Nutrition* **46**, 537–556.

McCarthy, D., Ellis, S.M. and Cole, T.J. (2003) Central overweight and obesity in British youth aged 11–16 years: cross sectional surveys of waist circumference. *British Medical Journal* **22**, 326 (7390): 624.

McCrory, M., Gomez, T., Bernauer, E. and Mole, P. (1995) Evaluation of a new air displacement plethysmograph for measuring human body composition. *Medicine and Science in Sports and Exercise* **27**, 1686–1691.

Moreno, L.A., Fleta, J., Sarria, A., Rodriguez, G., Gil, C. and Bueno, M. (2001) Secular changes in body fat patterning in children and adolescents of Zaragoza (Spain), 1980–1995. *International Journal of Obesity* **25**, 1656–1660.

Mueller, W. and Stallones, L. (1981) Anatomical distribution of subcutaneous fat: skinfold site choice and construction of indices. *Human Biology* **53**, 321–335.

Murgatroyd, P. and Coward, W.A. (1989) An improved method for estimating changes in whole-body fat and protein mass in man. *British Journal of Nutrition* **62**, 311–314.

National Academy of Sciences (1991) *Diet and Health*. Washington DC: National Academy of Sciences Press.

Organ, L.W., Bradham, G.B., Gorem, D.T. and Lozier, S.L. (1994) Segmental bioelectrical impedance analysis: theory and application of a new technique. *Journal of Applied Physiology* **77**, 98–112.

Paul, A.A., Cole, T.J., Ahmed, E.A. and Whitehead, R.G. (1998) The need for revised standards for skinfold thickness in infancy. *Archives of Diseases in Childhood* **78**, 354–358.

Prentice, A.M., Goldberg, G., Jebb, S.A., Black, A., Murgatroyd, P. and Diaz, E. (1991) Physiological response to slimming. *Proceedings of the Nutrition Society* **50**, 441–458.

Rice, T., Bouchard, C., Perusse, L. and Rao, D. (1995) Familial clustering of multiple measures of adiposity and fat distribution in the Quebec family study: a trivariate analysis of percent body fat, body mass index and trunk-to-extremity skinfold ratio. *International Journal of Obesity* **19**, 902–908.

Roemmich, J.N., Clark, P.A., Weltman, A. and Rogol, A.D. (1997) Alterations in growth and body composition during puberty. I. Comparing multicompartmental body composition models. *Journal of Applied Physiology* **83**, 927–935.

Ross, R., Pedwell, H. and Rissanen, J. (1995) Effects of energy restriction on skeletal muscle and adipose tissue in women as measured by magnetic resonance imaging. *American Journal of Clinical Nutrition* **61**, 1179–1185.

Ryde, S., Saunders, N., Birks, J., Alirr, P., Thomas, D., Morgan, W., Evans, C., Al-Zeibak, S., Dutton, J. and Sivyer, A. (1993) The effects of VLCD on body composition. In: Kreitzman S., Howard A. eds. *The Swansea Trial*. London: Smith-Gordon.

Savage, D.B., Tan, G.D., Acerini, C.L., Jebb, S.A., Agostini, M., Gurnell, M., Williams, R.L., Umpleby, A.M., Thomas, E.L., Bell, J.D., Dixon, A.K., Dunne, F., Boiani, R., Cinti, S., Vidal-Puig, A., Karpe, F., Chatterjee, V.K. and O'Rahilly, S. (2003) Human metabolic syndrome resulting from dominant-negative mutations in the nuclear receptor peroxisome proliferator-activated receptor-γ. *Diabetes* **52**, 910–917.

Schlemmer, A., Hassager, C., Haaarbo, J. and Christiansen, C. (1990) Direct measurement of abdominal fat by dual photon absorptiometry. *International Journal of Obesity* **14**, 603–611.

Schoeller, D.A., Levitsky, L.L., Bandini, L.G., Dietz, W.W. and Walczak, A. (1988) Energy expenditure and body composition in Prader–Willi syndrome. *Metabolism* **37**: 115–120.

Seidell, J., Oosterlee, A., Thijssen, M., Burema, J., Deurenberg, P., Hautvast, J. and Ruijs, J. (1987) Assessment of intra-abdominal and subcutaneous abdominal fat: relation between anthropometry and computed tomography. *American Journal of Clinical Nutrition* **45**, 7–13.

Seidell, J., Oosterlee, A. and Deurenberg, P. (1988) Abdominal fat depots measured with computed tomography: effects of degree of obesity, sex and age. *European Journal of Clinical Nutrition* **42**, 805–815.

Seidell, J., Bakker, C. and Van der Kooy, K.(1990) Imaging techniques for measuring adipose tissue distribution—a comparison between computed tomography and 1.5-T magnetic resonance. *American Journal of Clinical Nutrition* **51**, 953–957.

Shen, W., Wang, Z., Punyanita, M., Lei, J., Sinav, A., Kral, J.G., Imielinska, C., Ross, R. and Heymsfield, S.B. (2003) Adipose tissue quantification by imaging methods: a proposed classification. *Obesity Research* **11**, 5–16.

Siri, W. (1956) *The Gross Composition of the Body*. New York: Academic Press.

Siri, W. (1961) *Body Composition from Fluid Spaces and Density: a Combined Analysis of Methods*. Washington DC: National Academy of Sciences – National Research Council.

Sjostrom, L. (1991) A computer-tomography based multi-compartment body composition technique and anthropometric predictions of lean body mass, total and subcutaneous adipose tissue. *International Journal of Obesity* **15**, 19–30.

Snyder, W., Cook, M., Nasset, E., Karhausen, L., Parry-Howells, G. and Tipton, I. (1975) *Report of the Task Force on Reference Man*. Oxford: Pergamon Press.

Sum, C.F., Wang, K.W., Choo, D.C.A., Tan, C.E., Fok, A.C.K. and Tan, E.H. (1994) The effect of a 5-month supervised program of physical activity on anthropometric indices, fat-free mass and resting energy expenditure in obese male military recruits. *Metabolism* **43**, 1148–1152.

Sun, S.S., Chumlea, W.C., Heymsfield, S.B., Lukaski, H.C., Schoeller, D., Friedl, K., Kuczmarski, R.J., Flegal, K.M., Johnson, C.L. and Hubbard, V.S. (2003) Development of bioelectrical impedance analysis prediction equations for body composition with the use of a multicomponent model for use in epidemiologic surveys. *American Journal of Clinical Nutrition* **77**, 331–340.

Svendsen, O., Hassager, C., Bergmann, I. and Christiansen, C. (1993a) Measurement of abdominal and intra-abdominal fat in post-menopausal women by dual energy X-ray absorptiometry and anthropometry: comparison with computerised tomography. *International Journal of Obesity* **17**, 45–51.

Svendsen, O., Haarbo, J., Hassager, C. and Christiansen, C. (1993b) Accuracy of measurements of body composition by dual energy X-ray absorptiometry *in vivo*. *American Journal of Clinical Nutrition* **57**, 605–608.

Tagliabue, A., Cena, H. and Deurenberg, P. (1996) Comparative study of the relationship between multi-frequency impedance and body water compartments in two European populations. *British Journal of Nutrition* **75**, 11–19.

Tataranni, P. and Ravussin, E. (1995) Use of dual energy X-ray absorptiometry in obese individuals. *American Journal of Clinical Nutrition* **62**, 730–734.

Taylor, R., Magusson, I., Rothman, D. L., Cline, G. W., Caumo, A., Cobelli, C. and Shulman, G.I. (1996) Direct assessment of liver glycogen storage by ^{13}C nuclear magnetic resonance spectroscopy and regulation of glucose homeostasis after a mixed meal in normal subjects. *Journal of Clinical Investigation* **97**, 125–132.

Thaete, F., Colberg, S., Burke, T. and Kelley, D. (1995) Reproducibility of computed tomography measurement of visceral adipose tissue area. *International Journal of Obesity* **19**, 464–467.

Tothill, P., Avenell, A., Love, J. and Reid, D. (1994a) Comparisons between Hologic, Lunar and Norland dual energy X-ray absorptiometers and other techniques used for whole-body soft tissue measurements. *European Journal of Clinical Nutrition* **48**, 781–794.

Tothill, P., Avenell, A. and Reid, D. (1994b) Precision and accuracy of measurements of whole-body bone mineral: comparisons between Hologic, Lunar and Norland dual energy X-ray absorptiometers. *Britiish Journal of Radiology* **67**, 1210–1217.

Treuth, M., Hunter, G. and Kebes-Szabo, T. (1995) Estimating intraabdominal adipose tissue in women by dual energy X-ray absorptiometry. *American Journal of Clinical Nutrition* **62**, 527–532.

Van der Kooy, K. and Seidell, J. (1993) Techniques for the measurement of visceral fat: a practical guide. *International Journal of Obesity* **17**, 187–196.

Van der Kooy, K., Leenen, R., Deurenberg, P., Seidell, J., Westerterp, K. and Hautvast, J. (1992) Changes in fat-free mass in obese subjects after weight loss: a comparison of body composition measures. *International Journal of Obesity* **16**, 675–683.

Van der Kooy, K., Leenen, R., Seidell, J., Deurenberg, P. and Hautvast, J. (1993) Effect of a weight cycle on visceral fat accumulation. *American Journal of Clinical Nutrition* **58**, 853–857.

Wajchenberg, B., Bosco, A., Marone, M., Levin, S., Rocha, M., Lerario, A., Nery, M., Goldman, J. and Liberman, B. (1995) Estimation of body fat and lean tissue distribution by dual energy X-ray absorptiometry and abdominal body fat evaluation by computed tomography in Cushing's disease. *Journal of Endocrinology and Metabolism* **80**, 2791–2794.

Wang, Z., Heshka, S., Wang, J., Wielopolski, L. and Heymsfield, S.B. (2002) Magnitude and variation of fat-free mass density: a cellular-level body composition modelling study. *American Journal of Physiology Endocrinology and Metabolism* **284**, E267–E273.

Webber, J., Donaldson, M., Allison, S. and Macdonald, I. (1994) A comparison of skinfold thickness, body mass index, bioelectrical impedance analysis and dual energy X-ray absorptiometry in assessing body composition in obese subjects before and after weight loss. *Clinical Nutrition* **13**, 177–182.

Webster, J., Hesp, R. and Garrow, J. (1984) The composition of excess weight in obese women estimated by body density, total body water and total body potassium. *Human Nutrition: Clinical Nutrition* **38C**, 299–306.

Wells, J.C.K. (2000) A Hattori chart analysis of body mass index in infants and children. *International Journal of Obesity* **24**, 325–329.

Wells, J.C.K. (2001) A critique of the expression of paediatric body composition data. *Archives of Diseases in Childhood* **85**, 67–72.

Wells, J.C.K., Fuller, N.J., Dewit, O., Fewtrell, M.S., Elia, M. and Cole, T.J. (1999) Four-component model of body composition in children: density and hydration of fat-free mass and comparison with simpler models. *American Journal of Clinical Nutrition* **69**, 904–912.

Wells, J.C.K., Coward, W.A., Cole, T.J. and Davies, P.S.W. (2002a) The contribution of fat and fat-free tissue to body mass index in contemporary children and the reference child. *International Journal of Obesity* **26**: 1323–1328.

Wells, J.C.K., Cole, T.J. and ALSPAC study team. (2002b) Adjustment of fat-free mass and fat mass for height in children aged 8 years. *International Journal of Obesity* **26**, 947–952.

Wells, J.C.K., Fuller, N.J., Wright, A., Fewtrell, M.S. and Cole, T.J. (2003) Evaluation of air-displacement plethysmography in children aged 5–7 years using a three-component model of body composition. *British Journal of Nutrition* **90**, 699–707.

Widdowson, E. and Dickerson, J. (1964) Chemical composition of the body. In: Comar, C., Bronner, F. eds. *Mineral Metabolism. An Advanced Treatise*. New York: Academic Press, 2–210.

Wong, W.W., Hergenroeder, A.C., Stuff, J.E., Butte, N.F., Smith, E.O. and Ellis, K.J. (2002) Evaluating body fat in girls and female adolescents: advantages and disadvantages of dual-energy X-ray absorptiometry. *American Journal of Clinical Nutrition* **76**, 384–389.

Yang, M., Barbosa-Saldivar, J., Pi-Sunyer, X. and Itallie, T.V. (1981) Metabolic effect of substituting carbohydrate for protein in a low-calorie diet: a prolonged study in obese individuals. *International Journal of Obesity* **5**, 231–236.

Zhu, S., Wang, Z., Shen, W., Heymsfield, S.B. and Heshka, S. (2003) Percentage body fat ranges associated with metabolic syndrome risk: results based on third National Health and Nutrition Examination Survey (1988–1994). *American Journal of Clinical Nutrition* **78**, 228–235.

3 Social consequences of obesity

Rebecca M. Puhl, Kathryn E. Henderson and Kelly D. Brownell

Social consequences of obesity, 29
    Employment, 29
    Health care, 30
    Education and IQ, 31
    Socioeconomic status, 32
    Interpersonal relationships, 32
    Psychological outcome
    variables, 33

Reasons for social disadvantages of
obesity, 34

Evidence of bias and stigma
against obese persons, 34

Why does weight stigma occur?, 37
    How can bias be reduced?, 37

Clinical implications, 38
    Assisting patients in managing
    stigma experiences, 38
    Reducing stigma in health-care
    professionals, 39

Improving the environment for
obese patients, 39

Conclusions, 39

References, 40

When I was a child, I was sick and absent from school one day. The teacher taking attendance came across my name and said 'She must have stayed home to eat'. The other kids told me about this the next day.

> words from a person seeking treatment for obesity

I remember one incident when I was in the 6th grade and my teacher was looking at my latest handwriting assignment and she announced to the whole class that my handwriting was just like me—'fat and squatty' . . . The pain and humiliation aimed at you as an innocent child never leaves you!

> words from a woman recalling stigma experiences

At no other time in history has there been such a need to prevent obesity and to lessen its impact on health and well-being. As the focus on the obesity epidemic has intensified, most often neglected are the social consequences of being obese, which are serious and pervasive. Obese individuals are highly stigmatized in our society, with bias and discrimination being common outcomes. With one-half of the American population being overweight, the number of people potentially faced with stigmatization is significant.

This chapter describes social consequences of obesity, which range from inequities in employment, social disadvantages in education and health care and lower socioeconomic status to negative experiences in interpersonal relationships, social isolation, lower self-esteem and even suicide. Following a review of the literature, we examine the reasons why obese people face social disadvantages, address how societal bias and negative attitudes can be reduced and provide recom-mendations for health-care professionals working with obese patients.

Social consequences of obesity

Research exists on the association between obesity and a variety of social variables. Obese people face social consequences in multiple domains of living, placing numerous obstacles in everyday life and threatening well-being and, in all likelihood, impairing health.

Employment

There is increasing evidence of economic disadvantages for obese employees, most notably through lower wages of obese employees for the same job performed by non-obese counter-parts. A study of over 2000 women and men (aged 18 years and older) reported that obesity lowered wage growth rates by al-most 6% in 1982–85 (Loh, 1993). More recent research indicates that the wage penalty faced by obese employees is persistent over the first two decades of employees' careers, and ranges from 1.4% to 4.5%, after controlling for socioeconomic and familial variables (Baum and Ford, in press).

Both obese men and women face wage-related obstacles, but are affected differently by wage penalties. An analysis from the National Longitudinal Survey Youth Cohort exam-ined earnings in over 8000 men and women aged 18–25 years, which indicated that obese women earned 12% less than their non-obese female counterparts (Register and Williams, 1990). This study parallels other investigations that show the economic penalty of obesity is greater for women. For example, longitudinal research examined data of 12 686 workers (50% female) and found that the obesity wage penalty was greater for obese women (6.2%) than for obese men (2.6%) (Baum and Ford, in press). The effect of ethnicity on wages for obese women has been documented in studies of labour market outcomes, which reported that body weight lowered wages for white women, but not for Hispanic or black women (Cawley, 2000). Among white women, a weight increase of two standard deviations (approximately 65 lb) decreased their pay by 7%, which is equivalent to 3 years of work experience.

Economic consequences are also evident from research showing that fewer obese employees are hired in high-level positions. Data on earnings of 7000 men and women from the National Longitudinal Survey of Youth showed that obese women are more likely than thinner women to hold low-paying jobs (Pagan and Davila, 1997). Obese men are similarly under-represented and paid less than non-obese men in managerial and professional occupations, and are over-represented in transportation occupations, suggesting that obese men engage in occupational sorting to counteract a wage penalty (Pagan and Davila, 1997).

Finally, it appears that obese employees face inequitable treatment with respect to benefits and termination of employment. A self-report study of 445 obese workers found that 26% of individuals who were 50% or more above ideal weight were denied benefits such as health insurance because of their weight, and 17% reported being fired or pressured to resign because of their weight (Rothblum et al., 1990).

Legal case findings indicate that employment termination against obese persons due to weight does exist and that it occurs in a variety of employment positions that are not necessarily compromised by body weight. Recent wrongful termination cases have been filed by obese employees who were city labourers (Civil Service Commission v. Pennsylvania Human Relations Commission, 1991; Perroni, 1996), state troopers (Frisk, 1996; Smaw v. Virginia Department of State Police, 1994), teachers (Nedder v. Rivier College, 1995) and office managers (Gimello v. Agency Rent-A-Car Systems, Inc., 1991), many of whom had been commended for good job performance or maintained excellent employment records. Several of these cases also involved suspended work without pay or demotion until the obese employee lost weight.

The existence of legal cases does not prove that weight discrimination is widespread, but does show that many perceive their obesity to be the reason for unfair treatment. Additional work is needed to determine the prevalence of wrongful termination and the consequences of wage penalties on the health and well-being of obese employees.

Health care

Obtaining needed health care is critical for obese people whose weight places them at a heightened risk for numerous diseases. Research has demonstrated highly variable obesity management practices among physicians and reluctance of obese patients to seek necessary health-care services, both of which may contribute to the health consequences associated with obesity.

One study involved over 1200 physicians (representing specialties of family practice, internal medicine, gynaecology, endocrinology, cardiology and orthopaedics) completing self-report surveys concerning their care of obese patients. The physicians recognized the health risks of obesity and perceived many of their patients to be overweight, but did not undertake adequate intervention and were unlikely to formally refer a client to a weight loss programme (Kristeller and Hoerr, 1997). Only 18% of physicians reported that they would discuss weight management with overweight patients and 42% addressed the issue with mildly obese patients. A similar self-report study of 318 physicians showed that although the majority felt obligated to treat their obese patients, 23% of physicians did not recommend treatment to any of their obese patients, and 47% said that counselling patients about weight loss was inconvenient (Price et al., 1987a). This parallels an investigation of a population-based sample of over 12 000 obese adults, where only 42% of participants were advised to lose weight by health-care professionals (Galuska et al., 1999).

Other research suggests that physicians may be ambivalent about their role in treating obesity. In a sample of 211 primary care physicians, only 33% reported being centrally responsible for managing their patient's obesity, and physicians indicated that insufficient time, lack of medical training and problems of reimbursement were difficulties in managing obesity effectively (Pratt et al., 1997). Another study of attitudes and practices among 752 general practitioners in weight management found that physicians reported positive views about their roles in managing obesity, but underutilized practices that promoted lifestyle changes in patients, described weight management as professionally unrewarding and reported their most common frustrations in treating obesity to be poor patient compliance and motivation (Campbell et al., 2000).

Some obese patients perceive these practices to be inadequate. In one study, when obese patients were surveyed about their experiences with physicians, most were generally satisfied with their care for general health, but were significantly less satisfied with the care they received for their obesity (Wadden et al., 2000).

Questionable weight management practices could lead obese persons to be hesitant to seek health care. Several studies have documented delays in seeking medical care by obese women. One self-report study of 310 hospital-employed women found that body mass index (BMI) was significantly related to appointment cancellations (Olson et al., 1994). In particular, 12% of women indicated that they delayed or cancelled physician appointments owing to weight concerns, 55% of those with a BMI over 35 delayed or cancelled visits because they knew they would be weighed, and of the 33% of women who had discussed weight with their physicians, discussions were described as negative. The most common response for delaying appointments was embarrassment about weight.

Other self-report data of more than 6000 women obtained in the 1992 National Health Interview Survey reported that increased BMI was associated with decreased preventive health-care services (Fontaine *et al.*, 1998). Obese women were more likely than non-obese women to delay breast examinations, gynaecological examinations and Papanicoloau smears, despite an increase in physician visits as BMI increased (Fontaine *et al.*, 1998). A similar study was conducted to determine the influence of obesity on the frequency of pelvic examinations (Adams *et al.*, 1993). Anonymous responses of 290 women showed that reluctance to have examinations increased with body weight, with very overweight women being significantly less likely to report annual pelvic examinations than thinner women.

Although the reasons for underutilization of health-care services among obese women have not been specified, the positive association between BMI and frequency of physician visits, coupled with questionable obesity management practices reported by some physicians, indicates a need to look closer at the quality of health-care services received by obese patients.

Education and IQ

There is no extensive work on the educational consequences of being obese, but what does exist suggests that obesity may prevent individuals from achieving the same educational goals as their normal-weight counterparts. Most of the work in this area has examined educational attainment among college students. Canning and Mayer (1966) examined high school records and college applications of 2506 high school students and found that obese students were significantly less likely than non-obese peers to be accepted to college, despite having equivalent application rates and academic performance. Moreover, only 31% of obese women were accepted compared with 41% of obese men. Unfortunately, these college admission data are dated and it is necessary to determine the extent to which discriminatory practices now occur.

In an attempt to determine the reasons for the lower college acceptance of obese females, Crandall (1991) assessed weight, financial aid and college income in a sample of 833 undergraduate students. It was found that normal-weight students received more family financial support for college than overweight students, who depended more on financial aid and jobs; this effect was especially pronounced for women. Differences in family support remained, despite controlling for parental education, income, ethnicity and family size.

There have also been cases of obese students who were dismissed from college because of their weight. One case reached the US Supreme Court; this involved an obese nursing student

who was dismissed 1 year before obtaining her nursing degree for failing to lose weight (Weiler and Helms, 1993). Although the school did not object to the student's obesity at her admission, she was later asked to sign a contract agreeing that she could remain in her programme if she lost 2 lb (approximately 1 kg) per week; 1 year later she was dismissed from the school for her inability to lose weight (Weiler and Helms, 1993).

Some research has pointed to an association between obesity and lower intelligence, suggesting that obese individuals may be at an intellectual disadvantage compared with non-obese persons. One study documented lower performance IQ scores among severely obese children (using the Weschler Intelligence Scale for Children—revised) compared with non-obese control subjects (Li, 1995). However, differences in measures of intelligence did not hold up for children with lesser degrees of obesity. A second study prospectively assessed BMI and school difficulties (including learning difficulties, scholastic proficiency, special educational needs and speech or hearing difficulties) among 987 individuals when they were children in the third grade and then again when 20 years old. Children who had learning difficulties, poorer scholastic proficiency or special educational needs were more likely to be obese as young adults (Lissau and Sorensen, 1993). These findings parallel earlier work that documented inverse relationships between obesity and IQ performance measures (Kreze *et al.*, 1974; Sorensen and Sonne-Holm, 1985). Most recently, a prospective study examined a community-based sample of 1423 adults from the Framingham Heart Study and found lower cognitive performance on tests of learning and memory among obese men only (Elias *et al.*, 2003).

Studies outside of the USA have reported similar associations between intelligence performance scores and obesity. A Danish study of over 26 000 adults reported intelligence test scores and educational levels to be highest among individuals who were below the median BMI (Teasdale *et al.*, 1992). An examination of a British cohort of over 12 000 children showed that men and women who had been obese at 16 years of age had significantly fewer years of education than non-obese peers, and obese women demonstrated lower performance on maths and reading tests than non-obese counterparts at ages 7, 11 and 16 years (Sargent and Blanchflower, 1994). Two Chinese studies have also documented differences in intelligence test scores among obese and non-obese children (Lu *et al.*, 1996; Li *et al.*, 1998).

The majority of studies conducted in this area have been correlational, so there should be caution in interpreting these findings. There is insufficient evidence to conclude that obese individuals are at an intellectual disadvantage compared with non-obese persons, and there are many extraneous variables (such as social class) that could be responsible for poorer educational attainment in some obese individuals. At the same time, one could speculate that the correlations obtained in these studies do, in fact, reflect poorer intellectual functioning by obese people, resulting from a potential common genetic or environmental link. For example, it is possible that obesity occurs first, followed by stigma, which negatively affects educational attainment in different ways (such as poorer treatment by teachers, lower expectations by parents, poor self-esteem, etc.). Alternatively, poor intellectual performance could initially occur, creating stress or low self-esteem in some children, which gets soothed by eating and leads to increased weight. Additional research in this area is clearly warranted to determine the direction of this complex relationship and to rule out the influence of extraneous variables.

Socioeconomic status

Numerous studies now show that obesity is more prevalent among lower socioeconomic groups. Sobal and Stunkard's (1989) important review of 144 published studies on this topic demonstrated that individuals of lower socioeconomic status are at a higher risk of being obese across all industrialized nations. In addition, this pattern was more consistent for obese women than men.

Studies conducted since this review demonstrate similar findings. For example, research examining socioeconomic status (SES) and adolescent health using 15 483 adolescent and parent surveys (with separate measures of income, education and occupation) revealed that SES indicators were consistently and linearly related to obesity (Goodman, 1999). This relationship remained despite controlling for factors such as race and number of parents in the home.

A longitudinal study examined obesity and SES in a random sample of over 10 000 adolescents who were followed for 7 years, which established that women who had been overweight in adolescence completed less education, were less likely to be married and had lower incomes and higher rates of poverty than those who had not been overweight (Gortmaker *et al.*, 1993). Men who were overweight in adolescence were also less likely to be married. These results suggest that the socioeconomic consequences are more severe for obese women.

In a recent study of 15 061 respondents to the 1996 Health Survey for England, lower educational attainment and lower socioeconomic status were associated with a higher risk of obesity in both men and women (Wardle *et al.*, 2002). Lower occupational status among women was associated with increased risk of obesity independent of SES, but this was not the case for men. The authors highlighted the finding that education was significantly associated with obesity independent of income and occupation, suggesting that education interventions target lower SES groups of obese individuals.

Despite these consistent findings across multiple studies and the knowledge that the relationship between obesity and SES is bidirectional (Stunkard and Sorensen, 1993), other factors (such as heredity, health-related behaviours, access to health care) common to both of these characteristics make it difficult to determine causality and they highlight the complexity of this relationship. It is also important to note the variability in how SES has been measured in existing studies, which ranges from several indicators such as income, education and occupation to single measures or scales, all of which may have differentially affected the strength of associations reported. Researchers are now beginning to examine components of SES (such as employment, housing, migration status and family unit) separately in order to determine whether these factors predict the relationship between SES and obesity differently (Ball *et al.*, 2002). What remains clear, however, is that socioeconomic consequences create real challenges for obese individuals who are already faced with stigma. It is crucial for research to address both the biological and social factors that relate to economic disadvantages in this population.

Interpersonal relationships

Obese individuals may have negative relationship experiences with peers, family and romantic partners. Additionally, others often perceive obese individuals as less desirable candidates for any of these roles. Here we review the research addressing both perspectives.

Peer relationships

Miller and colleagues (1990) used blind observers to rate heavy and thin women conversing by telephone. The heavy woman was rated more negatively, leading the researchers to conclude that obesity may place limitations on opportunities for social skill acquisition. Snyder and Haugen (1994; 1995) tested this hypothesis by having male subjects holding a phone conversation with a woman; subjects were first shown a photograph of either a thin or large woman, and told that this was the woman they would be speaking to. Men who were told they were speaking with a large woman rated her less positively than men who were told they were speaking with a thin woman. Furthermore, blind raters actually rated the supposed 'large' female conversation partner less positively, even though these raters knew nothing about how she had been presented to the male subjects, suggesting that the female conversation partner began to fulfill the men's communicated expectations of her. Other research suggests that people believe obese people to be unpopular and to have few friends (Harris *et al.*, 1982; Harris and Smith, 1983).

Some research indicates that obese individuals believe their weight has interfered in their participation in social activities (Bullen *et al.*, 1963; Tiggemann and Rothblum, 1988). However, Miller and colleagues (1995) found that larger and thinner women did not differ in self-reported and corroborative report of social support, size of social networks, social skills or socially based self-esteem. Other studies support this finding of no difference in popularity with peers (Sallade, 1973; Jarvie *et al.*, 1983).

Family relationships

Sarlio-Lahteenkorva (2001) studied a large population-based sample and found in women a relationship between obesity and lack of close friends outside the family; however, these women did not report greater feelings of loneliness and were not less likely to be living with a partner. Schumaker and colleagues (1985), however, found that obese women did report greater loneliness than their thinner counterparts; this finding did not hold for the men.

Romantic partnerships

Many obese individuals experience difficulty in the area of romantic partnerships. Some data suggest that obese individuals are less likely to attract a marital partner (Kallen and Doughty, 1984), are older when they marry (Gortmaker *et al.*, 1993) and marry those deemed 'less desirable' partners (Garn *et al.*, 1989a,b). Others have found no association between obesity and marital status in women, and even a positive relationship between BMI and marital status in men (Sobal *et al.*, 1992).

Harris and colleagues (1991) studied attitudes towards obesity in college students and found that for white women, weight was negatively associated with likelihood and frequency of dating, and white men were more likely to have refused to date a woman because of her weight than were African-American men. Sitton and Blanchard (1995) found that fewer men responded to a personal advertisement in which the woman was identified as obese than to an advertisement in which she disclosed having a history of drug problems. Harris (1990) studied a sample of college students and found that larger individuals were rated as less attractive, having lower self-esteem, less likely to be dating, and deserving of heavier and less attractive partners. Regan (1996) found that subjects rated obese women as less sexually attractive, skilled, warm and responsive, and less likely to experience sexual desire than normal-weight women; this difference did not hold when the target stimulus was a man.

For those who do marry, the data on marital quality are mixed. Felitti (1993) reported that clinical patients undergoing obesity treatment were more likely to experience marital break-ups than control subjects, and Margolin and White (1987) reported an association between weight gain in women and marital problems. However, both Cohen and colleagues (1991) and Sobal and colleagues (1995) found little support for the hypothesis that obese people experience poorer quality marriages. In fact, obese women reported less marital unhappiness, and both men and women who gained weight during marriage were happier. Obese men did report more marital problems than their non-obese counterparts.

In summary, negative stereotypes about the relationship skills and desirability of obese individuals clearly abound. Some research supports the contention that obese individuals do, indeed, experience negative outcomes in the interpersonal domain, whereas other research finds that they fare similarly to their normal-weight counterparts. The subgroup most impacted by the negative stereotypes appears to be white women. Given the prevalence of negative stereotypes, it is remarkable that obese people fare as well as they do interpersonally.

Psychological outcome variables

A large body of research exists on the psychological status of obese people as a group. The main variables of interest have been general psychopathology, depression, self-esteem and risk of suicide.

Psychopathology

The data on psychopathology in obese individuals are mixed, with most focused on depression. Early studies actually indicated lower levels of depression and anxiety in some obese demographic groups, giving rise to what became known as the 'jolly fat' person hypothesis (Simon, 1963; Silverstone, 1968; Crisp and McGuiness, 1975; Kittel *et al.*, 1978; Crisp *et al.*, 1980; Stewart and Brook, 1983; Palinkas *et al.*, 1996). Other researchers have found no such relationship (Moore *et al.*, 1962; Hallstrom and Noppa, 1981; Hayes, 1986; Faubel, 1989). Still others report small to moderate relationships between weight and depression across a variety of samples, including women in the NHANES dataset (Istvan *et al.*, 1992), college women (Homer and Utermohlen, 1993) and other large national US samples (Carpenter *et al.*, 2000; Roberts *et al.*, 2000). The relationship appears to be moderated not only by gender (it is stronger in women) but also by education: Ross (1994) found the relationship to hold only for the subset of higher educated individuals.

In their review of this literature, Friedman and Brownell (1995) found little consistent evidence that obese individuals as a group suffer greater psychopathology than their thinner counterparts. However, they argue that specific subpopulations may be more vulnerable, most notably binge eaters, obesity treatment-seeking populations and certain social strata groups (Black *et al.*, 1992; Goldsmith *et al.*, 1992; Fitzgibbon *et al.*, 1993; Kuehnel and Wadden, 1994; Telch and Agras, 1994; Musante *et al.*, 1998).

One criticism of this literature is the use of cross-sectional data. Roberts and colleagues (2002) reported findings from a large prospective study of adults over the age of 50 years. Cross-sectionally, obese individuals were more likely to report poorer perceived mental health, less optimism, greater life dissatisfaction and greater depression. Longitudinally, obesity predicted risk for subsequent depression, pessimism and unhappiness 5 years later, even when controlling for baseline mental health problems. Faith and colleagues (2002) reviewed this literature and concluded that the relationship between obesity and depression will probably prove to be a complex pattern of mediated and moderated relationships.

One sobering finding from a large US population-based sample is that BMI is associated with suicidal ideation in women, and with both suicide attempts and suicidal ideation in men (Carpenter *et al.*, 2000). There is clearly some connection between the experience of overweight and engaging in extreme and desperate behaviours.

Self-esteem

Miller and Downey (1999) published a meta-analysis of the relationship between weight and self-esteem. They found a moderate relationship that was stronger for women, individuals of higher SES, those of non-minority status and those seeking treatment. This relationship does not hold across all studies (e.g. Sarwer *et al.*, 1998). As with obesity and depression, obesity and self-esteem appear more strongly related in certain subpopulations, such as binge eaters and treatment-seeking populations (Miller *et al.*, 1999). It also appears to be moderated by body esteem.

Body esteem

Body esteem has been of interest both as a variable in its own right and, more recently, as a moderator and/or mediator of the relationships between weight and other psychological variables, such as depression and global self-esteem. The relationship between body dissatisfaction and overweight is well established (Cash *et al.*, 1986; Rosen, 1996; Sarwer *et al.*, 1998). Friedman and colleagues (2002) found further that body satisfaction mediated both weight/depression and weight/self-esteem relationships.

Quality of life

There exist some data exploring a more general quality of life in obese individuals. Higher weight is related to decreases in quality of life (Kolotkin *et al.*, 1995; Sarlio-Lahteenkorva *et al.*, 1995; Fontaine, *et al.*, 1996).

In summary, the data on psychosocial outcomes in obese people are mixed. However, much of the data are cross-sectional, thus we have information only on associations rather than causal relationships. It is not clear whether obesity produces these outcomes, whether these psychological variables are involved in the onset and/or maintenance of obesity, or whether the relationship is a complex one involving a broader array of variables. Prospective data are scant and this is a necessary future direction to explore. The findings of greater distress in obese populations are of great concern and a worthwhile target of intervention.

Reasons for social disadvantages of obesity

The widespread social consequences of obesity might be attributed to different causes. One possible explanation is that obese people perform poorly in life activities, such as employment or education, because of deficits in intellectual, interpersonal or work-related skills; there has been little research to address this issue. A more plausible explanation seems that obese people are treated as if they are deficient because of weight stigma, which gets enacted in prejudice, bias and discrimination. There is now substantial research support for this explanation, which consistently illustrates that obese people face negative attitudes and stigma in major life domains such as employment, health care and education. It is also likely that obese people are subject to self-fulfilling prophesies, with which they internalize society's negative views and then act in ways to be consistent with stereotypes.

Evidence of bias and stigma against obese persons

Documentation of weight stigma began several decades ago (Allon, 1982) and has had a resurgence in recent years (see review by Puhl and Brownell, 2001). One main focus has been employment bias. Experimental research shows that overweight people may face biased hiring decisions even before they confront a job interview. This research typically asks participants to evaluate a fictional applicant's qualifications for a job, in which the employee's weight has been manipulated (through written vignettes, videos, photographs or computer morphing). Participants consistently evaluate overweight applicants more negatively and rate them less likely to be hired than average-weight employees, despite having identical qualifications (Decker, 1987; Klassen *et al.*, 1993; Bellizzi and Hasty, 1998). This bias may be especially salient in jobs such as sales positions, in which obese people are perceived to be inappropriate for face-to-face interactions (Rothblum *et al.*, 1988; Everett, 1990; Jasper and Klassen, 1990; Pingitoire *et al.*, 1994).

Negative stereotypes of obese employees are abundant and may be one explanation for inequities in wages, promotions and employment termination. Over two decades ago, Larkin and Pines (1979) documented beliefs that obese workers are less neat, productive, ambitious, disciplined and determined than non-obese employees. More recent studies indicate that this pattern has worsened and that people perceive overweight employees to be sloppy, lazy, less competent, poor role models, lacking in self-discipline, disagreeable, unattractive, unsuccessful and emotionally unstable compared with average-weight employees or job applicants (Paul and Townsend, 1995; Roehling, 1999; Polinko and Popovich, 2001). Other work reveals perceptions that obese workers have low supervisory potential, and poor personal hygiene and professional appearance (Rothblum *et al.*, 1988). Despite no evidence for such negative stereotypes, obese employees remain vulnerable to negative evaluations because of their weight. Interestingly, some research shows that obese job applicants who acknowledge their stigma in an interview are evaluated more negatively than those who do not mention their weight (Hebl and Kleck, 2002).

Health care is another area in which weight stigma is prevalent and in which numerous health-care professionals are perpetrators of bias. As mentioned earlier, negative attitudes have been reported by physicians, psychologists, nurses and medical students (Maddox and Liederman, 1969; Price *et al.*, 1987a; Maroney and Golub, 1992; Wiese *et al.*, 1992; Davis-Coelho *et al.*, 2000). Even health-care professionals who specialize in obesity are not immune to this bias (Teachman and Brownell, 2001; Schwartz *et al.*, 2003). These beliefs are typically acknowledged in anonymous self-report studies, in which health-care providers perceive obese patients to be unsuccessful, unpleasant, unintelligent, dishonest, lacking in self-control, overindulgent, weak-willed and lazy (Maddox and Liederman, 1969; Blumberg and Mellis, 1980; Klein *et al.*, 1982; Price *et al.*, 1987a; Maroney and Golub, 1992). One study of registered nurse (RN) graduate female nurses (*n* = 107) reported that 24% of nurses agreed that caring for an obese patient repulsed them, and 12% reported that they preferred not to even touch an obese patient (Bagley *et al.*, 1989). Considering the utmost importance of health care for obese individuals, who face numerous risks of disease, this study is especially alarming. Other work indicates the presence of illusory correlations in medical settings in which people overestimate the likelihood that obese patients are non-compliant with their physician's advice, despite there being no data to suggest that this relationship exists (Madey and Ondrus, 1999).

Beliefs about the causes of obesity may play a role in widespread negative attitudes towards obese patients. For example, one study of attitudes among 52 health-care professionals specializing in nutrition found that 88% reported that obesity was a form of compensation for lack of love or attention, and 70% attributed the cause of obesity to emotional problems (Maiman *et al.*, 1979). Other work has highlighted assumptions among nurses that obesity can be prevented by self-control (Maroney and Golub, 1992), and that patient non-compliance explains failure at weight loss (Hoppe and Ogden, 1997).

The possibility that biased attitudes influence the quality of care provided to obese patients is very real. In addition to the studies reviewed already, which point to delayed seeking of care by obese patients and questionable treatment practices by physicians, experimental research shows that mental health professionals more frequently assign negative attributes, more severe psychological symptoms and more pathology to obese patients than to average-weight clients (Young and Powell, 1985; Hassel *et al.*, 2001). Other empirical work found that obesity affected treatment planning by psychologists, who assigned a worse prognosis to overweight patients than non-obese patients, and who were more likely to assign 'increasing sexual satisfaction' as a treatment goal for overweight patients despite no indication of sexual difficulties (Davis-

Coelho *et al.*, 2000). The need for increased research in this area to directly assess whether negative attitudes affect the quality of health care for obese patients is clearly warranted.

Reasons for poorer educational attainment among obese students can also be traced to stigma. Although less empirical work has been conducted in educational settings, it appears that educators may also be communicating negative anti-fat attitudes that may affect perceptions of performance among obese students. One self-report study of 115 junior and senior high school teachers and school health-care workers indicated that these educators perceived obesity to be primarily under individual control; 20% agreed that obese persons are untidy; 19% perceived them to be more emotional; 17% believed them to be less likely to succeed at work; and 27% agreed they were more likely to have family problems (Neumark-Sztainer *et al.*, 1999). In addition, 46% agreed that obese persons are undesirable marriage partners for non-obese people, and 28% agreed that becoming obese is one of the worst things that could happen to a person. A study of over 200 elementary school principals' beliefs about contributing causes of obesity similarly indicated that 59% attributed this to lack of self-control, 57% to psychological problems and 47% to lack of parental concern (Price *et al.*, 1987b).

Parental biases may also affect educational outcomes for obese students. Crandall (1995) examined this among over 3000 high school seniors who completed questionnaires about their weight, college aspirations, financial support, grades and parental political attitudes. Overweight students were under-represented in those who attended college, with overweight women being least likely to receive financial support from their families. Politically conservative attitudes of parents predicted who paid for college, in which BMI of students was positively associated to parents whose attitudes were characterized by values of self-discipline and the tendency to perceive people as responsible for their own fate. Thus, parents with these ideological attributions may be more likely to blame their obese children for their weight.

Taken together, a strong argument can be made for the existence of weight stigma and the pervasiveness of negative attitudes in multiple areas of living for obese people. Anti-fat attitudes remain so socially acceptable that we need to go no further than our own living rooms to observe negative stereotypes of obese people who are portrayed so disapprovingly on television (Greenberg *et al.*, 2003). Unfortunately, those images reflect reality for an increasing population of obese people who are confronted with unfounded stereotypes and resulting social denigration on a daily basis.

Obese children: special consideration

Obesity is increasing rapidly in children and adolescents (Flegal *et al.*, 1998; WHO, 1998), thus an increasing number of young people are susceptible to the social consequences of obesity. Although many of the sequelae experienced by children are consistent with those observed in adults, we believe that the particularly vulnerable nature of childhood and adolescence warrants special attention to this issue in children.

Negative stereotypes of obesity in children

Numerous studies have documented the pervasive nature of children's negative attitudes towards obese people in general and obese children specifically. Richardson and colleagues (1961) were the first to demonstrate that children dislike heavier children more than they dislike those with a variety of other stigmatizing conditions, such as physical disabilities or disfigurements. Young children have described overweight individuals as lazy, sloppy, dirty, ugly and stupid, both in early studies (Caskey and Felker, 1971; Lerner and Korn, 1972; Staffieri, 1972; Kilpatrich and Sanders, 1978) and more recent research (Strauss *et al.*, 1985; DeJong and Kleck, 1986; Goldfried and Chrisler, 1995; Wardle *et al.*, 1995; Kraig and Keel, 2001; Latner and Stunkard, 2003).

Negative attitudes towards obese children begin early. Hill and Silver (1995) and Counts and colleagues (1986) have documented the existence of negative obese stereotypes in 9- and 8-year-olds, respectively, whereas others have observed negative attitudes towards overweight in children as young as 3 (Brylinsky and Moore, 1994; Cramer and Steinwert, 1998). In a study of children in grades 4–6, these negative attitudes persisted in both boys and girls across the three grades, regardless of the child's own weight (Tiggemann and Anesbury, 2000). These attitudes appear to persist even in the face of explanations of the uncontrollability of the target child's obesity, explanations originally designed to reduce negative attitudes towards the children (Bell and Morgan, 2000).

Peer harassment and rejection at school

At school, obese children and adolescents suffer harassment and rejection that is directly related to their weight and can be subjected to merciless teasing (Neumark-Sztainer *et al.*, 2002). Pierce and Wardle (1997) reported on 32 clinically overweight 9- to 11-year-olds. These children detailed experiences of unrelenting bullying and verbal abuse from classmates, children in their neighbourhoods and siblings at home. Neumark-Sztainer and colleagues (1998) described the experiences of 55 obese adolescent girls. The girls detailed teasing, jokes and derogatory names, as well as rejection by peers and siblings. For instance, friends would not want to be seen with the obese child, and siblings denied being related to the child. Incidents occurred most frequently at home and at school. It is hardly surprising that obese adolescents—and girls in particular—would encounter difficulties in social interaction (Sobal, 1984).

Given the enduring negative effects of childhood weight-related teasing on women's body image (Grilo *et al.*, 1994), and the role body image plays in the relationship between obesity and psychological distress, the relentless teasing suffered by obese children and adolescents is of great concern. Weight-related teasing is also associated with disordered eating (Fabian and Thompson, 1989; Thompson *et al.*, 1995; Neumark-Sztainer *et al.*, 2002), adding a further route through which psychopathology may potentially develop in these children.

Adults stigmatizing children

Obese children are stigmatized not only by their peers, but by adults as well, including their own parents. The potential impact here is great, as one might imagine, but relatively little research has been carried out. Pierce and Wardle (1993) found that girls who thought that their parents perceived them as overweight had lower self-esteem. No differences in either communication with parents or perceived support from parents were found by Valtolina and Marta (1998) between obese and non-obese adolescents, thus it is likely that some parents buffer their children from society's anti-fat messages, whereas others contribute to the stigma.

Psychological sequelae of obesity in children

Numerous authors have reported increased risk for general psychosocial problems and distress in obese children and adolescents, and girls in particular (Banis, *et al.*, 1988; Dietz, 1998; Mellin *et al.*, 2002). Erickson and colleagues (2000) found that BMI was moderately associated with depressive symptoms in elementary school girls, but not in boys; however, Wadden and colleagues (1989) found no such relationship in their sample of adolescent girls. Sheslow and colleagues (1993) found depressive symptoms to be greater only in those obese children with lower self-esteem, indicating the need to explore moderating variables, as is the case in the adult literature.

General self-esteem and the more specific body esteem have also been studied. French and colleagues (1995) reviewed the literature and concluded that there are modest relationships in children and adolescents between obesity and self-esteem and between obesity and body esteem, although the literature has methodological limitations, including small sample sizes, a focus on clinical populations only and inconsistency in measures across studies. Some have found that obese children and adolescents report lower levels of self-worth or self-esteem (Sallade, 1973; Martin *et al.*, 1988; Braet *et al.*, 1997). Pierce and Wardle (1993; 1997) also found evidence of this relationship, but found it to be moderated by internal vs. external causal attributions for the overweight. Other data do not support the self-esteem/weight relationship (Mendelson and White, 1982; Wadden *et al.*, 1984; Strauss *et al.*, 1985; Kaplan and Wadden, 1986).

As in the adult literature, the data on body esteem and obesity are more consistent. There appears to be a solid moderate negative relationship between body esteem and weight in both adolescent and pre-adolescent girls (Hendry and Gillies, 1978; Mendelson and White, 1982; 1985; Wadden *et al.*, 1989;

Mendelson *et al.*, 1996; Phillips and Hill, 1998; Stradmeijer *et al.*, 2000). In the Phillips and Hill study, heavier girls suffered decreased physical appearance esteem, but were just as popular as their thinner counterparts and were not at risk for decreased global self-esteem. These findings highlight the importance of distinguishing between different domains of self-esteem. Pesa and colleagues (2000) presented data to support the hypothesis that the relationship between weight and self-esteem may, in fact, be driven by body esteem. Israel and Ivanova (2002) studied children aged 8–14 and found that self-esteem in domains other than physical appearance acted as a protective factor for overall self-esteem in overweight children. These findings imply potential inroads for reducing the effects of the stigma of obesity in children.

Schwimmer and colleagues (2003) assessed health-related quality of life (QOL) in a small sample of obese children and adolescents presenting for obesity treatment. They found QOL in the severely obese to be lower than in normal-weight children, and on a par with children diagnosed with cancer—a startling and sad finding. Even more disturbing are the growing number of anecdotal accounts of obese children and adolescents committing suicide following years of teasing and harassment about their weight (Lederer, 1997; Solovay, 1999).

In summary, the data on obese children indicate that their peers have negative attitudes towards obesity, that they can be subjected to harassment both at school and in their homes and neighbourhoods, that they experience poor body esteem and may be at greater risk for depression and low global self-esteem. In extreme cases, stigmatizing experiences may lead to self-harm and even suicidal behaviours.

Why does weight stigma occur?

Although bias against obese people is well established, the reasons for weight stigma have received less attention (Puhl and Brownell, 2003). The primary theoretical model used to explain weight stigma comes from attribution theory. This research, conducted primarily by Crandall and colleagues, highlights perceptions of controllability and causality when making judgements about social groups, and suggests that when we encounter a person with a stigmatized trait, we search for its cause and form our reactions to the person using this causal information (Crandall, 1994; Crandall and Cohen, 1994; Crandall and Martinez, 1996).

One trigger for negative weight attitudes is the common belief that obese people are to blame for their fatness. Crandall and colleagues propose that negative attitudes towards obese people result from particular attributional tendencies of blame (Crandall, 1994; Crandall and Schiffhauer, 1998). Specifically, traditional conservative North American values of self-determination and individualism provide a foundation for weight stigma through beliefs that people get what they deserve, and that the fates of others are due to internal, control-

lable factors (Crandall and Martinez, 1996). These values are similar to Protestant work ethic values that also highlight internal control and self-discipline, within which the condition of another person's life, including weight, is attributed to internal, controllable causes (Crandall and Cohen, 1994; Crandall and Schiffhauer, 1998).

Consistent with this theory, research suggests that stigma is more likely to occur when individuals perceive obese people to be responsible for their weight because of controllable factors, such as laziness, overeating or low self-discipline (Weiner *et al.*, 1988; Rodin *et al.*, 1989; Crandall and Moriarty, 1995; Menec and Perry, 1998; Crandall, 2000). Some studies also demonstrate that obese people are less likely to be denigrated when explanations are provided to show that their obesity is beyond personal control (e.g. due to a thyroid condition) compared with when controllable causes (like overeating) are perceived to be responsible (DeJong, 1980; 1993; Weiner *et al.*, 1988; Menec and Perry, 1998).

These attribution components are associated with variations in weight attitudes across different cultures. Crandall and colleagues (2001) compared attributions towards obese people across six countries, and showed that stigma was best predicted by perceptions that people are responsible for life outcomes as well as cultural values that place a negative emphasis on fatness. Together, these factors significantly predicted negative attitudes towards obesity, where individualistic countries of Australia, Poland and the USA demonstrated more negative attitudes towards obese people than did the collectivist countries of India, Turkey and Venezuela. Overall, these studies indicate that the attribution model of weight stigma is useful in explaining why obese people in particular are perceived to have specific negative traits, and highlights perceptions of responsibility and personal control over weight, which lead to blame.

How can bias be reduced?

Although attribution research provides insight into the origins of obesity stigma, few studies have used this theory to reduce stigma. Only a handful of published studies have addressed attributions of controllability and causality of obesity in direct attempts to improve attitudes. One study improved attitudes towards obese people by providing information to participants about biological, genetic and noncontrollable causes of obesity (Crandall, 1994). However, two more recent studies found that providing explanations for obesity outside of one's personal control did not lead to attitude change (Bell and Morgan, 2000; Teachman *et al.*, 2003). Thus, attribution theory may ultimately play a stronger role in explaining weight stigma than reducing this bias, and it is important to examine other stigma reduction methods.

Concerning the little empirical work that has attempted to alter negative attitudes using other methods, many questions remain unanswered. A school-based intervention improved weight tolerance among elementary students through a curriculum designed to promote size acceptance (Irving, 2000), although children's attitudes were not directly assessed, making it difficult to determine whether actual changes occurred. Negative attitudes were also reduced in a study of medical students following an intervention that used videos of obese people, role-play exercises and written materials about the causes of obesity (Wiese *et al.*, 1992). One-year follow-up results indicated that students had fewer negative stereotypes compared with their pre-intervention attitudes, but outcome measures did not differentiate between the methods that were responsible for attitude changes.

Studies designed to evoke empathy towards obese people have also produced discouraging findings. This research instructed participants to read stories about weight discrimination or watch empathic videos of obese women, neither of which changed negative associations about obese people (Gapinski *et al.*, 2003; Teachman *et al.*, 2003). Another study was unable to improve negative attitudes among medical staff by increasing their direct interpersonal contact with obese patients (Blumberg and Mellis, 1980). There is extensive research support for the effectiveness of increased interpersonal contact on attitude change (see review by Pettigrew and Tropp, 2000), but certain types of stigmas, such as obesity, may resist these strategies.

On a more optimistic note, our own series of experimental studies has begun to demonstrate support for a social consensus approach to changing attitudes towards obese people. Social consensus theory has been used in stigma reduction research with racial stereotypes, and has successfully improved reported attitudes towards ethnic minorities (Stangor *et al.*, 2001). This framework proposes that stereotypes are a function of perceptions that a person has of other people's stereotypical beliefs. We conducted three studies in which students completed self-report measures of attitudes towards obese people prior to and following manipulated feedback depicting the attitudes of other students.

In our first experiment ($n = 60$), university students who received favourable consensus feedback (that others held more favourable beliefs about obese people than they did) reported significantly less negative attitudes and more positive attitudes towards obese persons compared with their reported attitudes prior to feedback (Puhl *et al.*, 2003). In addition, these students changed their reported beliefs about the causes of obesity following favourable consensus feedback that causes of obesity were due to factors outside, rather than within, personal control. In a second study with university students ($n = 55$), participants were more likely to improve their reported attitudes about obese people if they learned about favourable attitudes about obese people from an in-group source to which they belonged (Ivy League students) compared with an out-group source (community college students).

Our third study ($n = 200$) involved five experimental conditions comparing the social consensus approach to other methods of stigma reduction, such as providing information to students about the causes of obesity. Participants' perceptions of others' attitudes again significantly affected their own reported attitudes and their beliefs about the causes of obesity. Providing information about the uncontrollable causes of obesity and fabricated scientific evidence about traits that are commonly perceived to be characteristic of obese people also changed attitudes. However, our findings indicate that providing information about the causes of obesity is not necessary to improve attitudes, and that perceptions of others' attitudes about obese people significantly affect reported attitudes towards obese individuals and beliefs about the causes of obesity.

In summary, the relatively scarce research in this area provides too few clues about how to overcome negative attitudes towards obese people. There is clearly a need for additional work to identify factors that are important in stigma reduction for this population. Our experiments suggest that a social consensus framework is relevant to weight stigma, and propose that addressing perceived normative beliefs about obese people will be useful in future work that aims to improve attitudes towards obese people.

Clinical implications

A startling array of social consequences associated with obesity has been documented. It is easy to imagine that these consequences would affect the well-being, overall life-functioning and a variety of treatment outcomes for obese people. Indeed, there are data to suggest that stigma experiences may affect a patient's willingness to even seek treatment (Fontaine and Bartlett, 2000). Given that obese individuals are at increased risk for a wide variety of medical problems, facilitating their participation in preventive services and treatment is paramount.

We argue strongly that those who work with obese patients address the issue of weight bias with staff and colleagues. In our clinical work, we use a three-tiered approach: helping patients manage stigma experiences and reduce internalized negative stereotypes of obesity; helping health-care providers recognize and take steps to reduce their own weight bias; and improving the physical and social environment of care settings in which we see obese patients.

Assisting patients in managing stigma experiences

Here we have two goals: to encourage patients to address experiences of stigma in the world, and to help them identify their own weight bias and make changes in how they treat themselves. We use a cognitive–behavioural model for changing weight-related thoughts and behaviours, and first provide patients with tools for self-assessment. We have them identify ways in which they have limited their lives based on how they feel about their weight or size (Robinson and Bacon, 1989; 1996). We then present an educational segment, during which we share stigmatizing experiences of others to help clients feel less isolated in their experience, and provide evidence of the pervasiveness of weight stigma (Puhl and Brownell, 2001). We discuss the complex picture of the aetiology and maintenance of obesity to help reduce feelings of self-blame. We encourage patients to monitor weight-related thoughts and behaviours, identify areas in which they would like to see change and set clear goals for easing restrictions that they have placed on themselves owing to their weight, or goals for changing destructive thought patterns. Finally, we encourage patients to become advocates for themselves. We have them identify situations in which they have been penalized because of their weight. We have them analyse and evaluate their handling of the situation, identify a preferred strategy, identify and solve barriers to the new strategy, then script and role-play the new scenario. Our clinical experience with this protocol has demonstrated it to be an emotional and activating intervention.

Reducing stigma in health-care professionals

Our approach to reducing weight bias in health-care professionals runs parallel to our recommendations for obese individuals themselves. Again, we take a cognitive–behavioural approach, employing self-assessment, education and self-monitoring/behaviour-change goals. The purpose of each segment is similar to that for the patient, except that a main goal of education is to evoke empathy for the stigma experiences of obese patients. Honest self-examination of one's weight bias is critical to working effectively and empathically with obese patients.

Improving the environment for obese patients

Improving the environment includes consideration of both the physical and interpersonal environment in which patients are seen. Access to the building and all rooms should include doorways of adequate width for obese patients. Bathrooms should be easily negotiated by larger patients. Waiting rooms should contain sturdy, armless chairs from which an obese individual can rise easily. Doctors' practices should house wide examination tables, larger blood pressure cuffs and gowns of adequate size. Waiting rooms should contain 'obesity-friendly' reading materials, that is publications other than fashion magazines in which ultra-thin models are featured. If patients are to be weighed, the scale should be out of view of the waiting room, and nurses or assistants taking weight should be instructed *not* to provide commentary on the patient's weight; rather, to execute the task in a matter-of-fact fashion.

With respect to creating a facilitative interpersonal environ-

ment, we encourage health-care providers to make an effort to focus on improvements in health and fitness rather than focusing only on weight lost. In addition, noting and commenting on characteristics of the patient that are *not* related to his or her obesity goes a long way in establishing a positive relationship. For example, what does the patient do for a living? How many children does he or she have? Although this recommendation would be appropriate in dealing with most patients, it is especially critical for obese patients for whom health care can easily become an aversive and shaming experience.

Conclusions

Social consequences of obesity are very real and occur in multiple areas affecting the health and well-being of obese individuals. Stigma and bias appear to underlie and create numerous social disadvantages faced by obese people, which may have origins in cultural values of thinness and attributions about the perceived causes and controllability of obesity.

Although there is sufficient research to conclude that social consequences of obesity are significant and far reaching, many key questions remain unanswered in our understanding of how obesity is related to different social variables, the ways in which stigma emerges and how to establish the most effective means to temper society's negative attitudes. Table 3.1 presents our recommendations for research on weight stigma, which will begin to address these unanswered questions.

Taken together, we believe there are several important directions that are necessary to take in order for the field to advance:
1 Psychosocial and health consequences of stigma must be clarified. The impact of bias and discrimination on public health could be considerable, and research is needed to determine the effects of social disadvantages on both psychological and physical health of obese people.
2 The psychological and social origins of weight stigma need to be better understood. Attribution theory is helpful in explaining the origins of obesity stigma and offers substantial contributions to existing knowledge. However, a comprehensive theory of obesity stigma requires not only identification of origins of weight bias, but explanations for why stigma is elicited by obese body types and for the association between certain negative traits and obesity, and needs to provide effective means for reducing bias. Existing theories do not yet meet these criteria, and additional research is needed to test and compare the applicability of different theoretical models of bias to weight stigma.
3 More research should focus on the development, testing and implementation of stigma reduction interventions. The lack of research in this area and the mixed findings indicate the need to integrate theories and to find new conceptual approaches to improve negative attitudes towards obese people. Attribution and social consensus perspectives provide promising avenues for research, and both require further test-

Table 3.1 Recommendations for research needs on weight stigma.

Psychosocial and health consequences of obesity
Determine the direction of association between obesity and psychosocial variables
Clarify more complex relationships between obesity and psychosocial variables
Determine impact of social disadvantages on physical health indices
Explore the relationship between stigma and physical health indices
Examine the mechanisms by which stigma may affect health
Identify subpopulations of obese people who are at greater risk of both psychological and physical health consequences

Understanding the origins of weight stigma
Test the applicability of existing theoretical models of bias in explaining weight stigma
Integrate models for explaining weight stigma
Compare different theories to determine the most effective model(s) to explain stigma
Determine which theories can guide stigma reduction strategies

Reducing weight bias
Identify approaches that can integrate different conceptual models in an effort to reduce weight bias
Create developmentally appropriate models for reducing weight bias in children and adolescents
Integrate models of stigma reduction with existing clinical stigma intervention tools
Determine whether stigma reduction interventions can lead to behavioural changes (not just attitude changes) as well as long-term changes in attitudes/behaviours
Identify how interventions should be implemented with different populations (e.g. in health-care settings, employment settings, etc.)

Clinical research needs
Test proposed interventions for helping obese adults and children cope with stigma
Test proposed interventions for reducing stigmatizing behaviours in health-care professionals
Identify potential protective factors in reducing the impact of stigma on obese individuals
Test the effects of proposed coping interventions on both psychological and physical health indices, in both adults and children
Incorporate proposed stigma coping interventions into more traditional obesity treatment trials
Implement and test larger scale interventions aimed at reducing stigma and stigmatizing behaviours in schools

ing to determine whether attitude change resulting from these methods translates into less biased behaviours towards obese individuals.

4 Clinical tools must be identified and tested to provide health-care professionals with strategies to help obese patients to cope with stigma. Clinical trials that include components to address stigma as part of treatment for obese patients need to be studied. Educational programmes aimed at increasing diversity and reducing bias must also be tested to offer parents and teachers ways of helping obese children confront prejudice.

Any national obesity research agenda must address these important social issues. Clinicians, obesity researchers and health-care professionals have a responsibility to improve the well-being of obese adults and children, which requires us to address not only physical, but emotional, social and psychological indices of health.

References

Adams, C.H., Smith, N.J., Wilbur, D.C. and Grady, K.E. (1993) The relationship of obesity to the frequency of pelvic examinations: Do physician and patient attitudes make a difference? *Women and Health* **20**, 45–57.

Allon, N. (1982) The stigma of overweight in everyday life. In: Woldman B.B. ed. *Psychological Aspects of Obesity*. New York: Van Nostrand Reinhold, 130–174.

Bagley, C.R., Conklin, D.N., Isherwood, R.T., Pechiulis, D.R. and Watson, L.A. (1989) Attitudes of nurses toward obesity and obese patients. *Perceptual and Motor Skills* **68**, 954.

Ball, K., Mishra, G. and Crawford, D. (2002) Which aspects of socioeconomic status are related to obesity among men and women? *International Journal of Obesity* **26**, 559–565.

Banis, H.T., Varni, J.W., Wallander, J.L. *et al.* (1988) Psychological and social adjustment of obese children and their families. *Child Care Health Development* **14**, 157–173.

Baum, C.L. and Ford, W.F. (in press) The wage effects of obesity: A longitudinal study. *Health Economics.*

Bell, S.K. and Morgan, S.B. (2000) Children's attitudes and behavioral intentions toward a peer presented as obese: Does a medical explanation for the obesity make a difference? *Journal of Pediatric Psychology* **25**, 137–145.

Bellizzi, J.A. and Hasty, R.W. (1998) Territory assignment decisions and supervising unethical selling behavior: The effects of obesity and gender as moderated by job-related factors. *Journal of Personal Selling and Sales Management,* **XVIII**, 35–49.

Black, D.S., Goldstein, R.B. and Mason, E.E. (1992) Prevalence of mental disorder in 88 morbidly obese bariatric clinic patients. *American Journal of Psychiatry* **149**, 227–234.

Blumberg, P. and Mellis, L.P. (1980) Medical students' attitudes toward the obese and morbidly obese. *International Journal of Eating Disorders* pp. 169–175.

Braet, C., Mervielde, I. and Vandereycken, W. (1997) Psychological aspects of childhood obesity. *Journal of Pediatric Psychology* **22**, 59–71.

Brylinsky, J.A. and Moore, J.C. (1994) The identification of body build stereotypes in young children. *Journal of Research in Personality* **28**, 170–181.

Bullen, B.A., Monello, L.F., Cohen, H. and Mayer, J. (1963) Attitudes toward physical activity, food, and family in obese and nonobese adolescent girls. *American Journal of Clinical Nutrition* **12**, 1–11.

Campbell, K., Engle, H., Timperio, A., Cooper, C. and Crawford, D. (2000) Obesity management: Australian general practitioners' attitudes and practices. *Obesity Research* **8**, 459–466.

Canning, H. and Mayer, J. (1966) Obesity—its possible effect on college acceptance. *New England Journal of Medicine* **275**, 1172–1174.

Carpenter, K.M., Hasin, D.S., Allison, D.B. and Faith, M.S. (2000) Relationships between obesity and DSM-IV major depressive disorder, suicide ideation, and suicide attempts: results from a general population study. *American Journal of Public Health* **90**, 251–257.

Cash, T.F., Winstead, B.W. and Janda, L.H. (1986) The great American shape-up: body image survey report. *Psychology Today* **20**, 30–37.

Caskey, S.R. and Felker, D.W. (1971) Social stereotyping of female body image by elementary school age girls. *Research Quarterly* **42**, 251–255.

Cawley, J. (2000) *Body Weight and Women's Labor Market Outcomes.* NBER Working Papers, 7841, National Bureau of Economic Research.

Civil Service Commission v Pennsylvania Human Relations Commission, 591 A. 2d (Pa. 1991).

Cohen, S., Schwartz, J.E., Bromet, E.J. and Parkinson, D.K. (1991) Mental health, stress, and poor health behaviors in two community samples. *Preventive Medicine* **20**, 306–315.

Counts, C.R., Jones, C., Frame, C.L., Jarvie, G.J. and Strauss, C.C. (1986) The perception of obesity by normal-weight versus obese school-age children. *Child Psychiatry and Human Development* **17**, 113–120.

Cramer, P. and Steinwert, T. (1998) Thin is good, fat is bad: how early does it begin? *Journal of Applied Developmental Psychology* **19**, 429–451.

Crandall, C.S. (1991) Do heavy-weight students have more difficulty paying for college? *Personality and Social Psychology Bulletin* **17**, 606–611.

Crandall, C.S. (1994) Prejudice against fat people: Ideology and self-interest. *Journal of Personality and Social Psychology* **66**, 882–894.

Crandall, C. S. (1995) Do parents discriminate against their heavyweight daughters? *Personality and Social Psychology Bulletin* **21**, 724–735.

Crandall, C.S. (2000) Ideology and lay theories of stigma: The justification of stigmatization. In: Heatherton, T.F., Kleck, R.E., Hebl, M.R. and Hull J.G. eds. *The Social Psychology of Stigma.* New York: The Guilford Press, 126–152.

Crandall, C.S. and Cohen, C. (1994) The personality of the stigmatizer: Cultural world view, conventionalism, and self-esteem. *Journal of Research in Personality* **28**, 461–480.

Crandall, C. S. and Moriarty, D. (1995) Physical illness stigma and social rejection. *British Journal of Social Psychology* **34**, 67–83.

Crandall, C.S. and Martinez, R. (1996) Culture, ideology, and antifat attitudes. *Personality and Social Psychology Bulletin* **22**, 1165–1176.

Crandall, C.S. and Schiffhauer, K.L. (1998) Anti-fat prejudice: Beliefs, values, and American culture. *Obesity Research* **6**, 458–460.

Crandall, C.S., D'Anello, S., Sakalli, N., Lazarus, E., Wieczorkowska, G. and Feather, N.T. (2001) An attribution-value model of prejudice: Anti-fat attitudes in six nations. *Personality and Social Psychology Bulletin* **27**, 30–37.

Crisp, A.H. and McGuiness, B. (1975) Jolly fat: Relation between obesity and psychoneurosis in the general population. *British Medical Journal* **1**, 7–9.

Crisp, A.H., Queenan, M., Sittampaln, Y. and Harris, G. (1980) 'Jolly fat' revisited. *Journal of Psychosomatic Research* **24**, 233–241.

Davis-Coelho, K., Waltz, J. and Davis-Coelho, B. (2000) Awareness and prevention of bias against fat clients in psychotherapy. *Professional Psychology: Research and Practice* **31**, 682–684.

Decker, W.H. (1987) Attributions based on managers' self-presentation, sex, and weight. *Psychological Reports* **61**, 175–181.

DeJong, W. (1980) The stigma of obesity: The consequences of naïve assumptions concerning the causes of physical deviance. *Journal of Health and Social Behavior* **21**, 75–87.

DeJong, W. (1993) Obesity as a characterological stigma: The issue of responsibility and judgments of task performance. *Psychological Reports* **73**, 963–970.

DeJong, W. and Kleck, R.E. (1986) The social psychological effects of overweight. In: Herman, C.P., Zanna, M.P. and Higgins, E.T. eds. *Physical Appearance, Stigma, and Social Behavior: The Ontario Symposium*, 3. Hillsdale, NJ: Lawrence Erlbaum, 65–88.

Dietz, W.H. (1998) Health consequences of obesity in youth: childhood predictors of adult disease. *Pediatrics* **101**, 518–525.

Elias, M.F., Elias, P.K., Wolf, P.A. and D'Agostino, R.B. (2003) Lower cognitive function in the presence of obesity and hypertension: The Framingham heart study. *International Journal of Obesity* **27**, 260–280.

Erickson, S.J., Robinson, T.N., Haydel, K.F. and Killen, J.D. (2000) Are overweight children unhappy?: Body mass index, depressive symptoms, and overweight concerns in elementary school children [comment]. *Archives of Pediatrics and Adolescent Medicine* **154**, 931–935.

Everett, M. (1990) Let an overweight person call on your best customers? Fat chance. *Sales Marketing Management* **142**, 66–70.

Fabian, L.J. and Thompson, J.K. (1989) Body image and eating disturbance in young females. *International Journal of Eating Disorders* **8**, 63–74.

Faith, M.S., Matz, P.E. and Jorge, M.A. (2002) Obesity-depression associations in the population. *Journal of Psychosomatic Research* **53**, 935–942.

Faubel, M. (1989) Body image and depression in women with early and late onset obesity. *Journal of Psychology* **12**, 385–395.

Felitti V. J. (1993) Childhood sexual abuse, depression, and family dysfunction in adult obese patients: a case control study. *Southern Medical Journal* **86**, 732–736.

Fitzgibbon, M.L., Stolley, M.R. and Kirschenbaum, D.S. (1993) Obese people who seek treatment have different characteristics than those who do not seek treatment. *Health Psychology* **12**, 346–353.

Flegal, K.M., Carroll, M. D., Kuczmarski, R.J. and Johnson, C. L. (1998) Overweight and obesity in the United States: Prevalence and trends, 1960–1994. *International Journal of Obesity* **22**, 39–47.

Fontaine, K.R. and Bartlett, S.J. (2000) Access and use of medical care among obese persons. *Obesity Research* **8**, 403–406.

Fontaine, K.R., Cheskin, L. J. and Barofsky, I. (1996) Health-related quality of life in obese persons seeking treatment. *Journal of Family Practice* **43**, 265–270.

Fontaine, K.R., Faith, M.S., Allison, D.B. and Cheskin, L.J. (1998) Body weight and health care among women in the general population. *Archives of Family Medicine* **7**, 381–384.

French, S.A., Story, M. and Perry, C.L. (1995) Self-esteem and obesity in children and adolescents: a literature review. *Obesity Research* **3**, 479–490.

Friedman, K.E., Reichmann, S.K., Costanzo, P.R. and Musante, G.J. (2002) Body image partially mediates the relationship between obesity and psychological distress. *Obesity Research* **10**, 33–41.

Friedman, M. A. and Brownell, K. D. (1995) Psychological correlates of obesity: Moving to the next research generation *Psychological Bulletin*, **117**, 3–20.

Frisk, A.M. (1996) Obesity as a disability: An actual or perceived problem? *Army Lawyer* pp. 3–19.

Galuska, D.A., Will, J.C., Serdula, M.K. and Ford, E.S. (1999) Are health care professionals advising obese patients to lose weight? *Journal of the American Medical Association* **282**, 1576–1578.

Gapinski, K.D., Schwartz, M.B. and Brownell, K.D. (2003) A media approach to changing antifat attitudes and behavior. Manuscript submitted for publication.

Garn, S., Sullivan, T.V. and Hawthorne, V.M. (1989a) The education of one spouse and the fatness of the other spouse. *American Journal of Human Biology* **1**, 233–238.

Garn, S., Sullivan, T.V. and Hawthorne, V.M. (1989b) Educational level, fatness, and fatness differences between husbands and wives. *American Journal of Clinical Nutrition* **50**, 740–745.

Gimello v Agency Rent-A-Car Systems, Inc., 594 A 2d 264 (N.J. Super Ct. A Div. 1991).

Goldfried, A. and Chrisler, J.C. (1995) Body stereotyping and stigmatization of obese persons by first graders. *Perceptual and Motor Skills* **81**, 909–910.

Goldsmith, S.J., Anger-Friedfeld, K., Beren, S., Rudoph, D., Boeck, M. and Aronne, L. (1992) Psychiatric illness in patients presenting for obesity treatment. *International Journal of Eating Disorders* **12**, 63–71.

Goodman, E. (1999) The role of socioeconomic status gradients in explaining differences in US adolescents' health. *American Journal of Public Health* **89**, 1522–1528.

Gortmaker, S.L., Must, A., Perrin, J.M., Sobol, A.M. and Dietz, W.H. (1993) Social and economic consequences of overweight and young adulthood. *New England Journal of Medicine* **329**, 1008–1012.

Greenberg, B.S., Eastin, M., Hofschire, L., Lachlan, K. and Brownell, K.D. (2003) Portrayals of overweight and obese individuals on commercial television. *American Journal of Public Health* **93**, 1342–1348.

Grilo, C.M., Wilfley, D.E., Brownell, K.D. and Rodin, J. (1994) Teasing, body image, and self-esteem in a clinical sample of obese women. *Addictive Behaviors* **19**, 443–450.

Hallstrom, T. and Noppa, H. (1981) Obesity in women in relation to mental illness, social factors, and personality traits. *Journal of Psychosomatic Research* **25**, 75–82.

Harris, M.B. (1990) Is love seen as different for the obese? *Journal of Applied Social Psychology*, **20**, 1209–1224.

Harris, M.B. and Smith, S.D. (1983) The relationships of age, sex, ethnicity, and weight to stereotypes of obesity and self-perception. *International Journal of Obesity* **7**, 361–371.

Harris, M.B., Harris, R.J. and Bochner, S. (1982) Fat, four-eyed, and female: Stereotypes of obesity, glasses, and gender. *Journal of Applied Social Psychology* **12**, 503–516.

Harris, M.B., Walters, L. C. and Waschull, S. (1991) Gender and ethnic differences in obesity-related behaviors and attitudes in a college sample. *Journal of Applied Social Psychology* **21**, 1545–1566.

Hassel, T.D., Amici, C.J. Thurston, N.S. and Gorsuch, R. L. (2001) Client weight as a barrier to non-biased clinical judgment. *Journal of Psychology and Christianity* **20**, 145–161.

Hayes, C.E. (1986) Body and mind: The effect of exercise, overweight, and physical health on psychological well-being. *Journal of Health and Social Behavior* **27**, 387–400.

Hebl, M.R. and Kleck, R.E. (2002) Acknowledging one's stigma in the interview setting: Effective strategy or liability? *Journal of Applied Social Psychology* **32**, 223–249.

Hendry, L. B. and Gillies, P. (1978) Body type, body esteem, school, and leisure: A study of overweight, average, and underweight adolescents. *Journal of Youth and Adolescence* **7**, 181–195.

Hill, A.J. and Silver, E.K. (1995) Fat, friendless and unhealthy: 9-year old children's perception of body shape stereotypes. *International Journal of Obesity* **19**, 423–430.

Homer, T.N. and Utermohlen, V. (1993) A multivariate analysis of psychological factors related to body mass index and eating preoccupation in female college students. *Journal of the American College of Nutrition* **12**, 459–465.

Hoppe, R. and Ogden, J. (1997) Practice nurses' beliefs about obesity and weight related interventions in primary care. *International Journal of Obesity* **21**, 141–146.

Irving, L.M. (2000) Promoting size acceptance in elementary school children: The EDAP puppet program. *Eating Disorders: Treatment and Prevention* **8**, 221–232.

Israel, A.C. and Ivanova, M.Y. (2002) Global and dimensional self-esteem in preadolescent and early adolescent children who are overweight: age and gender differences. *International Journal of Eating Disorders* **31**, 424–429.

Istvan, J., Zavela, K. and Weidner, G. (1992) Body weight and psychological distress in NHANES I. *International Journal of Obesity* **19**, 999–1003.

Jarvie, G.J., Lahey, B., Graziano, W. and Framer, E. (1983) Childhood obesity and social stigma: what we know and what we don't know. *Developmental Review* **3**, 237–273.

Jasper, C.R. and Klassen, M.L. (1990) Perceptions of salespersons' appearance and evaluation of job performance. *Perceptual and Motor Skills* **71**, 563–566.

Kallen, D. and Doughty, A. (1984) The relationship of weight, the self perception of weight, and self esteem with courtship behavior. *Marriage and Family Review*, **7**, 93–114.

Kaplan, K. and Wadden, T. (1986) Childhood obesity and self-esteem. *Journal of Pediatrics* **109**, 367–370.

Kilpatrich, S.W. and Sanders, D.M. (1978) Body image stereotypes: a developmental comparison. *Journal of General Psychiatry* **132**, 87–95.

Kittel, F., Rustin, R.M., Dramaiz, M., Debacker, G. and Kornitzer, M. (1978) Psycho-socio- biological correlates of moderate overweight in an industrial population. *Journal of Psychsomatic Research* **22**, 145–158.

Klassen, M.L., Jasper, C.R., Harris, R.J. (1993) The role of physical appearance in managerial decisions. *Journal of Business Psychology* **8**, 181–198.

Klein, D., Najman, J., Kohrman, A.F. and Munro, C. (1982) Patient characteristics that elicit negative responses from family physicians. *Journal of Family Practice* **14**, 881–888.

Kolotkin, R.L., Head, S., Hamilton, M. and Tse, C.K. (1995) Assessing impact of weight on quality of life. *Obesity Research* **3**, 49–56.

Kraig, K.A. and Keel, P.K. (2001) Weight-based stigmatization in children. *International Journal of Obesity* **25**, 1661–1666.

Kreze, A., Zelina, M., Juhas, J. and Garbara, M. (1974) Relationship between intelligence and prevalence of obesity. *Human Biology* **46**, 109–113.

Kristeller, J.L. and Hoerr, R.A. (1997) Physician attitudes toward managing obesity: Differences among six specialty groups. *Preventive Medicine* **26**, 542–549.

Kuehnel, R.H. and Wadden, T.A. (1994) Binge eating disorder, weight cycling, and psychopathology. *International Journal of Eating Disorders* **26**, 205–210.

Larkin, J. C. and Pines, H. A. (1979) No fat persons need apply: Experimental studies of the overweight stereotype and hiring preference. *Sociology of Work and Occupations* **6**, 312–327.

Latner, J.D. and Stunkard, A.J. (2003) Getting worse: The stigmatization of obese children. *Obesity Research* **11**, 452–456.

Lederer, E.M. (1997) Teenager takes overdose after years of 'fatty' taunts. London: Associated Press, 1 October 1997.

Lerner, R.M. and Korn, S.J. (1972) The development of body-build stereotypes in males. *Child Development* **43**, 908–920.

Li, X. (1995) A study of intelligence and personality in children with simple obesity. *International Journal of Obesity and Related Metabolic Disorders* **19**, 355–357.

Li, B., Yang, G., Yu, H. and Huang, G. (1998) Intelligent difference between children with simple obesity and malnutrition. *Chinese Mental Health Journal* **12**, 353–354.

Lissau, I. and Sorensen, T.I. (1993) School difficulties in childhood and risk of overweight and obesity in young adulthood: A ten year prospective population study. *International Journal of Obesity and Related Metabolic Disorders* **17**, 169–175.

Loh, E.S. (1993) The economic effects of physical appearance. *Social Science Quarterly* **74**, 420–437.

Lu, B., Wang, G., Xu, P. and Liang, S. (1996) Social competence, intelligence, and behavioral problems in obese children. *Chinese Mental Health Journal* **10**, 11–12.

Maddox, G. L. and Liederman, V. (1969) Overweight as a social disability with medical implications. *Journal of Medical Education* **44**, 214–220.

Madey, S. F, and Ondrus, S. A.(1999) Illusory correlations in perceptions of obese and hypertensive patients' noncooperative behaviors. *Journal of Applied Social Psychology* **29**, 1200–1217.

Maiman, L.A., Wang, V.L., Becker, M.H., Finlay, J. and Simonson, M. (1979) Attitudes toward obesity and the obese among professionals. *Journal of the American Dietetic Association* **74**, 331–336.

Margolin, L. and White, L. (1987) The continuing role of physical attractiveness in marriage. *Journal of Marriage and the Family* **49**, 21–27.

Maroney, D. and Golub, S. (1992) Nurses' attitudes toward obese persons and certain ethnic groups. *Perceptual and Motor Skills* **75**, 387–391.

Martin, S., Housley, K., McCoy, H. *et al.* (1988) Self-esteem of adolescent girls as related to weight. *Perceptual and Motor Skills* **67**, 879–884.

Mellin, A.E., Neumark-Sztainer, D., Story, M., Ireland, M. and Resnick, M.D. (2002) Unhealthy behaviors and psychosocial difficulties among overweight adolescents: the potential impact of familial factors. *Journal of Adolescent Health* **31**, 145–153.

Mendelson, B.K. and White, D.R. (1982) Relation between body-esteem and self-esteem of obese and normal children. *Perceptual and Motor Skills* **54**, 899–905.

Mendelson, B.K. and White, D.R. (1985) Development of self-body-esteem in overweight youngsters. *Developmental Psychology* **21**, 90–96.

Mendelson, B.K., White, D.R. and Mendelson, M.J. (1996) Self-esteem and body esteem: effects of gender, age, and weight. *Journal of Applied Developmental Psychology* **17**, 321–346.

Menec, V.H. and Perry, R.P. (1998) Reactions to stigmas among Canadian students: Testing an attributional-affect-help judgement model. *Journal of Social Psychology* **138**, 443–454.

Miller, C.T. and Downey, K.T. (1999) A meta-analysis of heavyweight and self-esteem. *Personality and Social Psychology Review* **3**, 68–84.

Miller, C.T., Rothblum, E.D., Barbour, L., Brand, P.A. and Felicio, D. (1990) Social interactions of obese and non-obese women. *Journal of Personality* **58**, 365–380.

Miller, C.T., Rothblum, E.D., Brand, P.A. and Felicio, D. (1995) Do obese women have poorer social relationships than nonobese women? Reports by self, friends, and co-workers. *Journal of Personality* **63**, 65–85.

Miller, P. M., Watkins, J.A., Sargent, R.G. and Rickert, E.J. (1999) Self-efficacy in overweight individuals with binge eating disorder. *Obesity Research* **7**, 552–555.

Moore, M.E., Stunkard, A.J. and Strole, L. (1962) Obesity, social class, and mental illness. *Journal of the American Medical Association* **181**, 138–142.

Musante, G.J., Costanzo, P.R. and Friedman, K.E. (1998) The co-morbidity of depression and eating dysregulation processes in a diet-seeking obese population: a matter of gender specificity. *International Journal of Eating Disorders* **23**, 65–75.

Nedder v Rivier College, 908 F. Su 66 (D. N. H. 1995).

Neumark-Sztainer, D., Story, M. and Faibisch, L. (1998) Perceived stigmatization among overweight African-American and Caucasian adolescent girls. *Journal of Adolescent Health* **23**, 264–270.

Neumark-Sztainer, D., Story, M. and Harris T. (1999) Beliefs and attitudes about obesity among teachers and school health care providers working with adolescents. *Journal of Nutrition Education* **31**, 3–9.

Neumark-Sztainer, D., Falkner, N., Story, M., Perry, C., Hannan, P.J. and Mulert, S. (2002) Weight-teasing among adolescents: correlations with weight status and disordered eating behaviors. *International Journal of Obesity* **26**, 123–131.

Olson, C.L., Schumaker, H.D. and Yawn, B.P. (1994) Overweight women delay medical care. *Archives of Family Medicine* **3**, 888–892.

Pagan, J.A. and Davila, A. (1997) Obesity, occupational attainment, and earnings. *Social Science Quarterly* **78**, 756–770.

Palinkas, L.A., Wingard, D.L. and Barrett-Connor, E. (1996) Depressive symptoms in overweight and obese older adults: A test of the 'jolly fat' hypothesis. *Journal of Psychosomatic Research* **40**, 59–66.

Paul, R.J. and Townsend, J.B. (1995) Shape up or ship out? Employment discrimination against the overweight. *Employee Responsibilities and Rights Journal* **8**, 133–145.

Perroni, P.J. (1996) Cook v. Rhode Island, Department of Mental Health, Retardation, and Hospitals: The First Circuit tips the scales of justice to protect the overweight. *New England Law Review* **30**, 993–1018.

Pesa, J.A., Syre, T. R. and Jones, E. (2000) Psychosocial differences associated with body weight among female adolescents: the importance of body image. *Journal of Adolescent Health* **26**, 330–337.

Pettigrew, T.F, and Tropp, L. R. (2000) Does intergroup contact reduce prejudice: Recent meta-analytic findings. In: Oskamp, S. ed. *Reducing Prejudice and Discrimination. 'The Claremont Symposium on Applied Social Psychology'*. NJ: Lawrence Erlbaum Associates, 93–114.

Phillips, R.G. and Hill, A.J. (1998) Fat, plain, but not friendless: self-esteem and peer acceptance of obese pre-adolescent girls. *International Journal of Obesity* **22**, 287–293.

Pierce, J.W. and Wardle, J. (1993) Self-esteem, parental appraisal and body size in children. *Journal of Child Psychology and Psychiatry* **34**, 1125–1136.

Pierce, J.W. and Wardle, J. (1997) Cause and effect beliefs and self-esteem of overweight children. *Journal of Child Psychology and Psychiatry* **38**, 645–650.

Pingitoire, R., Dugoni, R., Tindale, S. and Spring, B. (1994) Bias against overweight job applicants in a simulated employment interview. *Journal of Applied Psychology* **79**, 909–917.

Polinko, N.K. and Popovich, P.M. (2001) Evil thoughts but angelic actions: Responses to overweight job applicants. *Journal of Applied Social Psychology* **31**, 905–924.

Pratt, C.A, Nosiri, U.I. and Pratt, C.B. (1997) Michigan physicians' perceptions of their role in managing obesity. *Perceptual and Motor Skills* **84**, 848–850.

Price, J.H., Desmond, S.M., Krol, R.A., Snyder, F.F. and O'Connell, J.K. (1987a) Family practice physicians' beliefs, attitudes, and practices regarding obesity. *American Journal of Preventive Medicine* **3**, 339–345.

Price J. H., Desmond, S.M. and Stelzer, C.M. (1987b) Elementary school principals' perceptions of childhood obesity. *Journal of School Health* **57**, 367–370.

Puhl, R. and Brownell, K.D. (2001) Obesity, bias, and discrimination. *Obesity Research* **9**, 788–805.

Puhl, R. and Brownell, K.D. (2003) Ways of coping with obesity stigma: Review and conceptual analysis. *Eating Behaviors* **4**, 53–78.

Puhl R., Schwartz, M.B. and Brownell, K.D. (2003) Impact of perceived consensus on stereotypes about obese people: New avenues for stigma reduction. Unpublished research.

Regan, P.C. (1996) Sexual outcasts: the perceived impact of body weight and gender on sexuality. *Journal of Applied Social Psychology* **26**, 1803–1815.

Register, C.A. and Williams, D.R. (1990) Wage effects of obesity among young workers. *Social Science Quarterly* **71**, 130–141.

Richardson, S.A., Goodman, N., Hastorf, A.H. and Dornbusch, S.M. (1961) Cultural uniformity in reaction to physical disabilities. *American Sociological Review*, 241–247.

Roberts, R.E., Kaplan, G.A., Shema, S.J. and Strawbridge, W.J. (2000) Are the obese at greater risk of depression? *American Journal of Epidemiology* **152**, 163–170.

Roberts, R.E., Strawbridge, W.J., Deleger, S. and Kaplan, G.A. (2002) Are the fat more jolly? *Annals of Behavior Medicine* **24**, 169–180.

Robinson, B.E. and Bacon, J.G. (1989) *REACT Scale*. White Bear Lake, MN: Robinson and Bacon.

Robinson, B.E. and Bacon, J.G. (1996) The 'If only I were thin..'

treatment program: Decreasing the stigmatizing effects of fatness. *Professional Psychology: Research and Practice* **27**, 175–183.

Rodin, M., Price, J., Sanchez, F. and McElliot, S. (1989) Derogation, exclusion, and unfair treatment of persons with social flaws: Controllability of stigma and the attribution of prejudice. *Personality and Social Psychology Bulletin* **15**, 439–451.

Roehling, M. V. (1999) Weight-based discrimination in employment: Psychological and legal aspects. *Personnel Psychology* **52**, 969–1017.

Rosen, J.C. (1996) Improving body image in obesity. In: Thompson J.K. ed. *Body Image, Eating Disorders, and Obesity*. Washington, DC: American Psychological Association, 425–440.

Ross, C. (1994) Overweight and depression. *Journal of Health and Social Behavior* **35**, 63–79.

Rothblum, E.D., Miller, C.T. and Garbutt, B. (1988) Stereotypes of obese female job applicants. *International Journal of Eating Disorders* **7**, 277–283.

Rothblum, E.D., Brand, P.A., Miller, C.T. and Oetjen, H.A. (1990) The relationship between obesity, employment discrimination, and employment-related victimization. *Journal of Vocational Behavior* **37**, 251–266.

Sallade, J. (1973) A comparison of the psychological adjustment of obese vs. non-obese children. *Journal of Psychosomatic Research* **17**, 89–96.

Sargent, J.D. and Blanchflower, D.G. (1994) Obesity and stature in adolescence and earnings in young adulthood. Analysis of a British birth cohort. *Archives of Pediatrics and Adolescent Medicine* **148**, 681–687.

Sarlio-Lahteenkorva, S. (2001) Weight loss and quality of life among obese people. *Social Indicators Research* **54**, 329–354.

Sarlio-Lahteenkorva, S., Stunkard, A. and Rissanen, A. (1995) Psychosocial factors and quality of life in obesity. *International Journal of Obesity* **19** (Suppl. 6), s1–s5.

Sarwer, D.B., Wadden, T.A. and Foster, G.D. (1998) Assessment of body image dissatisfaction in obese women: specificity, severity, and clinical significance. *Journal of Consulting and Clinical Psychology* **66**, 651–654.

Schumaker, J.F., Krejci, R.C., Small, L. and Sargent, R.G. (1985) Experience of loneliness by obese individuals. *Psychological Reports* **57**, 1147–1154.

Schwartz, M.B., O'Neal, H., Brownell, K.D., Blair, S.N. and Billington, C. (2003) Weight bias among health professionals specializing in obesity. *Obesity Research* **11**, 1033–1039.

Schwimmer, J.B, Burwinkle, T.M. and Varni, J.W. (2003) Health-related quality of life of severely obese children and adolescents. *Journal of the American Medical Association* **289**, 1813–1819.

Sheslow, D., Hassink, S., Wallace, W. and DeLancey, E. (1993) The relationship between self- esteem and depression in obese children. *Annals of the New York Academy of Sciences* **699**, 289–291.

Silverstone, J.T. (1968) Psychological aspects of obesity. *Proceedings of the Royal Society of Medicine* **61**, 371.

Simon, R. I. (1963) Obesity and depressive equivalent. *Journal of the American Medical Association* **183**, 208–210.

Sitton, S. and Blanchard, S. (1995) Men's preferences in romantic partners: obesity vs addiction. *Psychological Reports* **77**, 1185–1186.

Smaw v Virginia Department of State Police, 862 F. Su 1469 (E.D. Va. 1994).

Snyder, M. and Haugen, J.A. (1994) Why does behavioral confirmation occur? A functional perspective on the role of the perceiver. *Journal of Experimental Social Psychology* **30**, 218–246.

Snyder, M. and Haugen, J.A. (1995) Why does behavioral confirmation occur? A functional perspective on the role of the target. *Personality and Social Psychology Bulletin* **21**, 963–974.

Sobal, J. (1984) Group dieting, the stigma of obesity, and overweight adolescents: contributions of Natalie Allon in the sociology of obesity. *Marriage and Family Review* **7**, 9–20.

Sobal, J. and Stunkard, A.J. (1989) Socioeconomic status and obesity: A review of the literature. *Psychological Bulletin* **105**, 260–275.

Sobal, J., Rauschenbach, B.S. and Frongillo, Jr, E.A. (1992) Marital status, fatness and obesity. *Social Science and Medicine* **35**, 915–923.

Sobal, J., Rauschenbach, B.S. and Frongillo, Jr, E.A. (1995) Obesity and marital quality: Analysis of weight, marital unhappiness, and marital problems in a U.S. national sample. *Journal of Family Issues* **16**, 746–764.

Solovay, S. (1999) Fat doesn't kill, fat hatred does. *Fat!So?* **2**, 19.

Sorensen, T.I. and Sonne-Holm, S. (1985) Intelligence test performance in obesity in relation to educational attainment and parental social class. *Journal of Biosocial Science* **17**, 379–387.

Staffieri, J.R. (1972) Body build and behavioral expectancies in young females. *Developmental Psychology* **6**, 125–127.

Stangor, C., Sechrist, G.B. and Jost, J.T. (2001) Changing beliefs by providing consensus information. *Personality and Social Psychology Bulletin* **27**, 486–496.

Stewart, A. and Brook, R.H. (1983) Effects of being overweight. *American Journal of Public Health* **73**, 171–178.

Stradmeijer, M., Bosch, J., Koops, W. and Seidell, J. (2000) Family functioning and psychosocial adjustment in overweight youngsters. *International Journal of Eating Disorders* **27**, 110–114.

Strauss, C.C., Smith, K., Frame, C. and Forehand, R. (1985) Personal and interpersonal characteristics associated with childhood obesity. *Journal of Pediatric Psychology* **10**, 337–343.

Stunkard, A.J. and Sorensen, T.I. (1993) Obesity and socioeconomic status: A complex relation. *New England Journal of Medicine* **329**, 1036–1037.

Teachman, B.A. and Brownell, K.D. (2001) Implicit anti-fat bias among health professionals: Is anyone immune? *International Journal of Obesity* **25**, 1525–1531.

Teachman, B.A., Gapinski, K.D, Brownell, K.D, Rawlins, M. and Jeyaram, S. (2003) Demonstrations of implicit anti-fat bias: The impact of providing causal information and evoking empathy. *Health Psychology* **22**, 68–78.

Teasdale, T.W., Sorensen, T.I. and Stunkard, A.J. (1992) Intelligence and educational level in relation to body mass index of adults. *Human Biology* **64**, 99–106.

Telch, C.F. and Agras, W.S. (1994) Obesity, binge eating and psychopathology: are they related? *International Journal of Eating Disorders* **15**, 53–61.

Thompson, J.K., Coovert, M.D., Richards, K.J., Johnson, S. and Cattarin, J. (1995) Development of body image, eating disturbance, and general psychological functioning in female adolescents: covariance structure modeling and longitudinal investigations. *International Journal of Eating Disorders* **18**, 221–236.

Tiggemann, M. and Anesbury, T. (2000) Negative stereotyping of obesity in children: the role of controllability beliefs. *Journal of Applied Social Psychology* **25**, 137–145.

Tiggemann, M. and Rothblum, E.D. (1988) Gender differences in social consequences of perceived overweight in the United States and Australia. *Sex Roles* **18**, 75–86.

Valtolina, G. G. and Marta, E. (1998) Family relations and psychosocial risk in families with an obese adolescent. *Psychological Reports* **83**, 251–260.

Wadden, T.A., Foster, G.D. and Brownell, K.D. (1984) Self-concept in obese and normal-weight children. *Journal of Consulting and Clinical Psychology* **52**, 1104–1105.

Wadden, T.A., Foster, G.D., Stunkard, A.J. and Linowitz, J.R. (1989) Dissatisfaction with weight and figure in obese girls but not depression. *International Journal of Obesity* **13**, 89–97.

Wadden, T.A., Anderson, D.A., Foster, G.D., Bennett, A., Steinberg, C. and Sarwer, D.B. (2000) Obese women's perceptions of their physicians' weight management attitudes and practices. *Archives of Family Medicine* **9**, 854–860.

Wardle, J., Volz, C. and Golding, C. (1995) Social variation in attitudes to obesity in children. *International Journal of Obesity* **19**, 562–569.

Wardle, J., Waller, J. and Jarvis, M.J. (2002) Sex differences in the association of socioeconomic status with obesity. *American Journal of Public Health* **92**, 1299–1304.

Weiler, K. and Helms, L.B. (1993) Responsibilities of nursing education: The lessons of Russell v Salve Regina. *Journal of Professional Nursing* **9**, 131–138.

Weiner, B., Perry, R. and Magnusson, J. (1988) An attributional analysis of reactions to stigmas. *Journal of Personality and Social Psychology* **55**, 738–748.

Wiese, H.J., Wilson, J.F., Jones, R.A. and Neises, M. (1992) Obesity stigma reduction in medical students. *International Journal of Obesity* **16**, 859–868.

WHO (1998) *Obesity: Preventing and Managing the Global Epidemic.* Geneva, Switzerland: World Health Organization.

Young, L.M. and Powell, B. (1985) The effects of obesity on the clinical judgments of mental health professionals. *Journal of Health and Social Behavior* **26**, 233–246.

Obesity and culture

Pippa Craig

Definitions of culture, 46

Time, culture and obesity, 47
    Evolution of human culture and
    obesity, 47
    Evolution of fat storage and fat
    distribution, 48

Place, culture and obesity, 48
    Differences between societies, 49
    Differences within societies, 52

Culture and obesity in Western
societies in the twentieth
century, 55

Obesity as a social and cultural
issue, 59
    Resistance to the normalizing
    process, 59
    Body maintenance, health and
    fitness, 60

A renewed social and
environmental orientation on
obesity, 60
Cultural competence, 60
Obesity and culture in the twenty-
first century, 60

Acknowledgements, 61

References, 61

Obesity is a popular topic, and a search of the medical and sociological databases reveals a profusion of books and articles on obesity and culture. Medical texts focus on obesity and are concerned with differing prevalence, perceptions, preferences and dissatisfaction among various cultural groups, and the consequences, complications and management of obesity. In contrast the sociological literature concentrates primarily on culture, with some descriptive and comparative studies, and historical and ecological exposés. These discuss the reverence for obesity in a number of traditional societies, the social significance of obesity in Western culture, the culture of thinness and dieting, contextual factors contributing to the stigma of obesity, the growing interest in the 'social body' and the 'medicalization' of obesity.

These different foci are not altogether unexpected as 'obesity' is a medically defined term, whereas 'culture' falls within the sphere of influence of social scientists. It also reflects the philosophical divide between the body and the mind, and between biological and social science, that has influenced Western thought for several centuries.

Definitions of culture

There is no generally accepted definition of 'culture'. The history of the concept of culture can be traced from antiquity, and the meaning has changed over time. Definitions included tradition, rules, ideas and values, learning, habit, patterning or organization, product or artefact, ideas and symbols (Kroeber, 1963). Although culture as 'civilization' was favoured by

British and German anthropologists and Americans focused more on 'customs', the term 'culture' has become widely accepted and understood. The essence of both these broad definitions is that culture is *learned*.

Cultures are largely ways of thinking, feeling and believing, and consist of a body of learned behaviours that shape ways of thinking and doing from generation to generation (Kluckhohn, 1949). Culture refers to distinctive ways of life that are designed to maintain a group and provide a template for how to respond to the environment and to other people. An important characteristic in the context of this chapter is that culture influences human interactions and expectations. Culture interacts with biology, and biological functioning is modified by cultural norms, whether these manifest as products (such as clothing, body adornment) or processes (ways of doing or reacting).

Although many aspects of culture are explicit, many are implicit. No single individual within a culture knows the whole cultural 'map' of the particular group to which they belong. Each culture has 'universals, alternatives and specialties'; it is also composed of many overlapping subcultures that may be defined on the basis of region, economic status, occupation or subgroup membership (Kroeber, 1963). Although to an outsider an activity performed in one culture might resemble that performed in another, each may be executed for entirely different reasons.

Obesity and culture are inter-related in a non-random way (Brown and Krick, 2001) and the relationship will be explored in this chapter. Obesity did not occur early in human existence, and an evolutionary perspective on obesity and culture will outline how the cultural environment has shaped the body over time. Various aspects of the surroundings in which humans find themselves influence levels of obesity, and at any point in time obesity prevalence differs between and within social and ethnic groups to an extent that cannot be fully explained by genetic variation. Obesity is largely concentrated in the most affluent and stratified societies (Brown and Krick, 2001), and those that are undergoing cultural change towards a more affluent, developed or 'Westernized' lifestyle commonly demonstrate rapid increases in obesity. At the same time, the ways in which those in Westernised societies respond to large bodies is consistent with Western philosophical thought, and thus the cultural context influences ways of thinking and feeling about obesity and being obese.

Time, culture and obesity

Evolution of human culture and obesity

Both food and economy have played pivotal roles in the aetiology of obesity (Brown and Krick, 2001). An environment dominated by abundant variety available in supermarkets and fast-food outlets makes a stark contrast with one where food acquisition for survival was the focus of attention for a whole society. This transition from using only what was required from the environment to survive to the present-day excess and overwhelming choice has shaped how human body size and shape and human culture have evolved over time.

In order to understand this transition, anthropologists have used an evolutionary perspective to show how both genetic and cultural predispositions have contributed to the aetiology of obesity (Brown and Konner, 1998). It has been proposed that those with a genetic predisposition for obesity were selected because of their greater likelihood to survive and then those with the fatter bodies became the culturally preferred symbol of social prestige and good health (Brown and Konner, 1998).

For most of human history, food was acquired by means of hunting and gathering. Cultural evidence from archaeological remains of early human activities and ethnographic exploration of the social organization and cultural traditions of the few remaining hunter–gatherers suggest that they lived in small semi-nomadic groups. They enjoyed high-quality diets, and food was equitably distributed between group members (Brown, 1992). Humans who relied upon hunting and gathering ate a vastly different diet, based on uncultivated plants and wild game, and lived a highly active lifestyle. There are no reported cases of obesity in remaining hunter–gatherer groups (Brown and Krick, 2001) and there is no evidence of obesity from archaeology, but as traditional societies adopt a 'Western' lifestyle, whether by migration or

acculturation, levels of obesity increase dramatically (Eaton *et al.*, 1998).

Domestication of plants and animals and development of food preservation techniques occurred with the introduction of agriculture approximately 12 000 years ago (Lev-Ran, 2001). Although it is generally believed that hunter–gatherers were frequently hungry while the agriculturalist enjoyed a stable food supply supplemented by stored reserves for times of need, ethnographic and archaeological evidence suggests the opposite (Cassidy, 1980). Instead, hunter–gatherers were comparatively healthy, needing to forage for food only every few days, whereas ancient agriculturalists and modern peasant villagers had relatively shorter lives, higher infant mortality, shorter stature and more infections, and suffered higher levels of tooth decay (Cassidy, 1980; Brown and Konner, 1998). With settlement, obtaining food became less efficient, cereal monoculture reduced food variety, and in bad seasons crop failures led to general food shortages, resulting in dietary deficiencies (Brown and Konner, 1998; Lev-Ran, 2001). Given these problems the question as to why such settlement ever took place has been raised, and various hypotheses have been suggested. One plausible explanation is that the impetus was cultural; only settlement allowed the development of more culturally complex societies (Cassidy, 1980).

Following the industrial revolution, a rapid increase in cultural complexity occurred, allowing the emergence of social stratification. Stratified societies enabled the ruling elites to overcome the succession of 'feasts and famines' experienced by their ancestors and ensured continuity of access to food in times of scarcity. Although today obesity is not just a disease of civilization, it most commonly occurs in economically modernized, socially stratified societies that have sufficient affluence and surplus food to allow even the poor to become obese (Brown and Krick, 2001). An intriguing phenomenon demonstrated repeatedly by studies of cultural change is that, given the opportunity, traditional populations readily abandon their healthier diet for a Western one (Brown and Konner, 1998).

It has been proposed that our hunter–gatherer ancestors consumed the diet for which they were originally adapted (high-protein, lower fat, limited carbohydrate diet, with no cereal grains, dairy products or refined foods), and that present chronic disease patterns can be explained by the 'discordance' between human genes and modern lifestyle (Eaton *et al.*, 1998; Lev-Ran, 2001). These diseases are then the result of an interaction of genetically controlled metabolism and biocultural influences; lifestyle and culture have moved ahead in leaps and bounds from a hunter–gatherer nomadic tradition to a modern way of life, outpacing genetic adaptation (Eaton *et al.*, 1998).

Studies of the Westernization process among Native American populations have attempted to identify what occurs during acculturation to trigger the massive increase in obesity and chronic diseases. The different disease co-occurrence patterns in populations at different stages of acculturation implicate environmental factors (Weiss, 1990), with the dietary transition process identified as the critical factor producing upper body obesity. The addition of new, predominantly carbohydrate foods to traditional staples, rather than displacement of the staples, was identified as the key acculturation factor causing obesity (Szathmary, 1990). However, different modernization patterns occur in other groups undergoing rapid rural–urban transitions and these also result in increased obesity. In China, for instance, higher income urban populations consume more fat, sweet foods and animal protein, while reducing carbohydrate and fibre (Popkin, 2001). In all cases, the decreased physical activity accompanying modernization also contributed to increasing obesity rates. The way in which these changes have influenced cultural perceptions and preferences of body size will be discussed later in this chapter.

Humans have undergone various cultural modifications over thousands of years to adapt to the environment in which they found themselves, resulting in vastly different eating and activity patterns and social structures. Adjustment to the environment can be explained as culturally driven, as human groups explored and found ways of survival unique to their circumstances. The present-day widespread acculturation to Western lifestyles is the antithesis to this adaptation. Instead, this process represents a convergence from an infinite variety of lifestyles that are uniquely suited to a myriad of particular situations to a norm that may not be well suited to the human body at all.

Evolution of fat storage and fat distribution

The 'thrifty genotype' hypothesis proposed 40 years ago in relation to type 2 diabetes was recently modified by its author to include genes for obesity and hypertension, referred to as 'civilization syndromes' (Neel, 1999) and characterized by their familial nature and slow onset. Obesity is the result of incremental changes over a long period of time (often starting early in life), and the complex interplay of genetic and environmental factors. As there is no evidence for a strong ethnic predisposition for obesity among native populations pursuing a traditional lifestyle, increased prevalence must predominantly reflect lifestyle changes or 'culture engineering' (Neel, 1999).

The accumulation of lower body fat is a human female characteristic (Lev-Ran, 2001), developed in response to a need to carry the infant while still foraging to meet the energy demands of lactation. Lower body fat can be mobilized during pregnancy and lactation (Lev-Ran, 2001), although some surplus generally remains, resulting in incremental weight gain with each childbearing cycle (Rossner, 1999). Lower body fat is positively related to fertility (Norgan, 1997) and has become a characteristic sign of female beauty in the majority of human societies (Brown and Konner, 1998).

All animals, including humans, favour storage of the more metabolically active but more pathological upper body fat, given optimal conditions for so doing. Famines occurred regularly throughout most of human history (Lev-Ran, 2001) and storage of excess energy for these lean times, whether as food stores or body fat stores, was essential for survival. Large body size was possible among the affluent only and became a conspicuous marker of prosperity in societies based on social hierarchy with overconsumption in times of plenty being the social norm (Brown, 1992; Pollock, 1995). Among the more egalitarian societies formal rituals developed to ensure that there was a more equitable food distribution among members.

This brief anthropological and evolutionary perspective on obesity shows how cultural and societal development can explain the increase in obesity over time (Brown and Konner, 1998). Throughout human evolution cultural changes have occurred far more rapidly than genetic adaptation and obesity finds its genesis in this mismatch (Eaton *et al.*, 1998). Although humans store fat centrally when the situation favours positive energy balance, the female lower body fat has evolved to ensure survival of the human race. Thus plumpness, particularly peripheral plumpness in women, can be seen as a quite rational cultural preference supporting a biological norm. Economic factors were also important in the aetiology of obesity, with the increasing prevalence of obesity accompanying growing cultural complexity and social stratification. As affluence and abundance became widespread, so did obesity. Within this environment a uniquely human creation, culture, has been crucial in shaping human bodies.

Place, culture and obesity

It has been estimated that approximately one-half of the contribution to fatness and fat distribution is genetic, but it is the environment that determines whether obesity is realized (Weinsier *et al.*, 1998; Lev-Ran, 2001). Although environment implies physical circumstances, it can also include the social and cultural context in which people live. Numerous social and cultural factors impinge on a whole society and sometimes in differing ways on subgroups within that society. Even though some of these factors may be explicit, many are implicit and unable to be explained by rational means. If a perceived normative way of acting and/or reacting is reinforced in a number of different ways, it will be strengthened and becomes characteristic of the group. Many descriptive studies exist of such characteristic norms and beliefs in relation to obesity between and within societies, and attempts to explain them. One area for study has been the impact of the process of change in relation to how social gradients and Westernization shape obesity prevalence and beliefs, practices and preferences.

Differences between societies

Desirable body size in developed and developing societies

Populations, when conceived of as cultural groups, differ in their concept of desirable body size. Although obesity is considered a disease and is socially stigmatized in Western cultures (Cahnman, 1968), for other groups large body size signifies health and beauty (Brown and Konner, 1987; Messer, 1989). These differences relate to the core value system of the particular society, with body sizes and shapes sending powerful cultural messages (Ritenbaugh, 1991).

The discourse on body size and culture has been the concern of anthropologists and sociologists. Despite evidence of the impact of socioeconomic variables and disease states on body size and shape these body parameters can, to a limited extent, be manipulated either upwards or downwards in response to perceived cultural values, ideals or myths (Ritenbaugh, 1991). Clothing, footwear and headwear can enhance body height, and body breadths and protusions can be emphasized or minimized by ornamentation or reshaping with restrictive or additional items of clothing.

Large body sizes are still, on the whole, preferred in developing countries, with plumpness favoured in women (Cassidy, 1991). The Human Relation Area Files, founded at Yale University in 1949, is a central dataset of information on 127 cultures studied by ethnographers and historians which is now web based (eHRAF). Less than one-half of those represented in the database (between 30% and 49%, depending on sources) include data on characteristics of ideal body type. Of the records containing this information, none preferred extreme obesity but 81% preferred plumpness or moderate fat levels with only 19% preferring thinness in women (Brown and Konner, 1987; Anderson *et al.*, 1992). For those few societies with specific details peripheral fatness was preferred, in particular large hips and legs (Brown and Konner, 1987). The Human Relation Area Files made even fewer references to male body preferences (Brown and Konner, 1987).

Preference for bigness

Why do people want to be big? Physical bigness can reflect ability to survive, and can symbolize abundance, fertility, success and wealth (Cassidy, 1991). 'Big' can be interpreted in different ways and mean taller, more muscular or fatter.

Tallness is a symbol of power and dominance (Messer, 1989; Cassidy, 1991). 'Big men' are cultural institutions in both New Guinea and West Africa, with the size of tribal leaders reflecting their success and status (Brown and Konner, 1987). The majority of US presidents (34 out of the first 36) were taller than the average American man at the time that they were incumbent (Cassidy, 1991). Despite Napoleon's traditional portrayal as a short man, at 163 cm he was unusually tall for a Corsican and the average height for a man in northern France

at the time (Cassidy, 1991). Although Australia's current prime minister is shorter than average, he has been more than compensated for by some statuesque predecessors (such as Malcolm Fraser and Gough Whitlam measuring 193 cm). Wives are seldom taller than their spouses, and boys are expected to be taller than girls.

Differences in size between leaders and their subjects are in many instances indicators of differences in nutrition and health status (Cook, 1886; Cassidy, 1991). When early European explorers found Polynesian chiefs to be 'almost without exception' taller and heavier than their subjects they at first assumed them to be from a different race. It was only later that they determined the difference to be due to 'different treatment in infancy, (and) superior and regular diet' (Cook, 1886).

The few societies registered in the Human Relation Area Files with information on preferred size and shape of men predominantly reported a preference for muscular physique and moderate to tall stature (Brown and Konner, 1987). There is some evidence for a trend towards a more muscular cultural ideal in Western societies over the past 25 years (Leit *et al.*, 2001). Asian men are generally slighter than Caucasians, but also preferred larger, more muscular bodies (Lee *et al.*, 1996; Craig, 1999; Davis and Katzman, 1999).

Plumpness appears to be admired in women in the context of food scarcity (Brown and Konner, 1987; Cassidy, 1991), and is thought to signify the increased likelihood of fertility and reproductive success (Norgan, 1997). A plump woman reflects well on her male provider (Brown and Konner, 1987; Cassidy, 1991). Certain notable powerful women throughout history (such as Queen Victoria of England, Queen Salote of Tonga) were large in either height or breadth. Even today in Western countries where thinness is revered, larger women in powerful positions may retain their body size, or having lost weight regain it, conscious of the change in power relations with weight loss (Cassidy, 1991).

Large, even fat, bodies have traditionally been a positive attribute in the Pacific (Pollock, 1995), although attitudes are undergoing some change with Western influence (Craig *et al.*, 1996). The physical context in which Polynesians lived, with the constant threat of hurricanes and famines, influenced perceptions of beauty; chiefs and their families in particular were admired for being large. Cooperation in the production and distribution of food was a feature of Polynesian society and a rational response to an erratic food supply (Wright St-Clair, 1980). People ate irregularly and consumed large feasts when food was available. These feasts were organized by the chiefs as demonstrations of conspicuous generosity and a means of gaining prestige, but also reinforced communal attachment (Graves and Graves, 1978). Ritual feasting continues in the Pacific region now with greater regularity in the context of a regular food supply; in Polynesia, weekly feasting accompanies the Sunday church services in now predominantly Christian societies.

Traditional Nauruan fattening practices were realized in the fat female body, demonstrating the value of food as a symbol of well-being and social pride. A young woman of rank was secluded for up to 6 months following her first menses, during which time she was not expected to work and was provided with large amounts of food by her relatives. Similarly, a pregnant woman remained in her hut during pregnancy to conserve her energy. A wide network of relatives was expected to assist with food provision in exchange for reciprocal support. These patterns of reciprocity and cultural reverence for plumpness served to maintain the society at the most vulnerable times in the Nauruan woman's life (Pollock, 1995). Ritual fattening was also practised in Polynesian societies, and has been reported among Tahitians and Cook Island Maori (Buck, 1932; Pollock, 1995).

Examples of preference for fatness in men are rare but do exist. Sumo wrestling in Japan has a 2000-year-old history. With a body mass index (BMI) of around 45 kg/m^2, top-league *Sekitori* provide a striking contrast to the slight physique of the average Japanese male (Hattori, 1995).

The Massa of West Africa participate in the practice of *guru*, with the purpose of making men plump or obese. *Guru* can take the form of collective fattening where groups of men live with the cattle herd, drink large quantities of milk and are preferentially fed by the villagers, or can occur as individual fattening sessions. The esteemed male body shape is one with a protruding stomach and full figure, with smooth shiny skin (DeGarine, 1995). Energy balance studies of nine lean young Massa men found that they gained a substantial amount of weight (a mean of 17 kg, 64–75% as fat) in 2 months (Pasquet *et al.*, 1992).

Preference for smallness

Most non-Western peoples generally value large body size, particularly at certain life stages. A slim appearance reported in a number of anthropological studies was most likely the result of inadequate food supply and associated malnutrition than from food avoidance or increased energy expenditure (Messer, 1989). In a classic study, Audrey Richards described how the Bemba in southern Africa, who preferred plumpness, adjusted for the 'hunger months' by minimizing all physical activity (Richards, 1961). Cultural response by the Kalahari San to regular seasonal weight loss due to food shortages included limiting physical activity, resting more, relocating or activating trade networks (Lee and De Vore, 1976). Systematic underfeeding of children, instigated only from absolute necessity in response to inadequate food supply and at great cost to the children, was reported among some groups in Africa and India (Messer, 1989).

Slenderness is nonetheless admired by a number of South-Eastern, South Asian and North African societies, in which austerity, self-denial and control of appetite form part of the moral tradition for women (Messer, 1989), possibly as a cultural adaptation to long experience with an inadequate food supply. Prescribed abstemiousness in response to chronic food shortages has been described among the Gurage of Ethiopia. Although gorging at festivals was accepted and expected, the Gurage ate in moderation at other times to preserve supplies; constant overeating was considered a measure of bad upbringing (Messer, 1989).

Western cultures prefer slimness but not necessary small stature in women, and Western medical culture values 'small' body fat levels (Messer, 1989), requiring the female body to lengthen and narrow in order to conform. Although lengthening is consistent with secular trends (Gerver *et al.*, 1994), narrowing is more problematic. Weight concerns and dieting behaviour in young Canadian university students were influenced more by the deviation of their skeletal structure (frame size measured with bone callipers) from the ideal than by their degree of adiposity (measured with skinfolds) (Davis *et al.*, 1993).

Cultural predictors of ideal female body shape

Anderson and colleagues (1992) conducted a detailed analysis of the 62 cultures for which information was available in the Human Relations Area Files to provide the 'ultimate explanation' for the differing cross-cultural ideals of female body shape. There have been a number of hypotheses developed to explain the source of attitudes towards female body size and shape (summarized in Table 4.1) and these were used to generate variables used in the analysis. The first variable related to the amount of nutritional stress experienced and tested whether female fat served a biological function to preserve and ensure reproduction when food supply was unreliable (*food security* hypothesis), or whether small bodies were adapted to chronic food shortages (*small but healthy* hypothesis). Latitude was used as an indicator of *climate* to test the observation that those residing in cold climates were relatively fatter than those who lived in hot climates. *Male preference* for fatness assumed that fatness was a sign of fertility and likely reproductive success. The *adaptive reproductive suppression* hypothesis was developed to explain the dieting phenomenon in Western countries. Thinner standards, associated with stress, occurred when sexual activity was encouraged but premarital sex and illegitimacy were punished.

The age gap between menarche and marriage and public awareness of menarche were also indicators of *adaptive reproductive suppression*. The *battle of the sexes* variable included indicators for relative male dominance and aggressiveness, value of female life and freedom to control sexual lives, with male-dominant societies preferring plumper women. Existence of *fraternal interest groups*, in which men consolidated their political position at the expense of women doing so, assumed preference for plump standards and high fertility rates. The *Kirche, Kuche, Kinder* hypothesis associated female fatness with reproduction and childrearing, and was measured by the value of female economic activity (Anderson *et al.*, 1992).

Table 4.1 Hypotheses and indicators of cross-cultural body size preference in women.

Hypothesis name	Hypothesis description	Indicators	Condition for plump body preference	Support for hypothesis
Food security	Female fat ensures survival when food supply unreliable or variable	Level of nutritional stress	Food supply unreliable or variable	Supported*
Small but healthy	Small body size an adaptation to chronic food shortage	Level of nutritional stress	Food supply reliable	No
Climate	Female fat relatively higher in cold climates	Latitude	Greater distance from the equator	Supported*
Male preference	Female fat increases probability of ovulation and pregnancy success	Male domination	Male dominated	Not strongly supported
Adaptive reproductive suppression	Female fat regulates initiation and maintenance of ovulation. Social stressfulness of adolescent sexuality (low if adolescent sexuality and pregnancy tolerated)	(1) Composite of: † Protection from male sexual advances Frequency of premarital sex Consequences of premarital pregnancy Attitude towards premarital sex (2) Composite of: † Adolescent sexual expression Adolescent sexual behaviour Age gap between menarche and marriage Public awareness of menarche	Low stress: Chaperoned Common No bad consequences Expected and/or approved Low stress: Not encouraged Tolerated Small Publicized	Supported*
Battle of the sexes	Socially dominant sex imposes preference (female fatness preferred by males)	Male domination Male aggressiveness Value of female life Freedom to choose potential partner Control over marital and sexual lives	Male dominated Marked emphasis Low value Higher for males Stricter for females	Supported*
Fraternal interest groups	Menstrual taboos and segregation of women consolidate male group	Group size Strength of group Menstrual taboos	Large Strong Restrictions on menstruating females	Not supported
Kirche, Küche, Kinder	Trade-off for females between reproductive and economic activity	Value of female economic activity	Low value (childrearing and home-making the priority)	Supported* Some support*

Source: Anderson et al. (1992).
*Significant predictors.
†Some of the components of a composite measure can be 'or' combinations; others are 'and' combinations; others are 'and/or'. For example, a low-stress situation for an adolescent girl would be one (1) when she's chaperoned, or (2) when sexual activity is tolerated and no bad consequences occur if she gets pregnant. (J. Anderson, personal communication).

Attitudes towards fatness were found to relate to the reliability of the food supply, climate, the relative social dominance of women, the value placed on women's work and likely consequences of the expression of female adolescent sexuality. Male-dominated cultural groups experiencing food insecurity located in colder climates, with low adolescent stress and investing in the female reproductive and home-making role preferred plump women (Anderson *et al.*, 1992). This study indicates some potentially alterable cultural parameters that are likely to result in modifications to body preferences.

Differences within societies

Social factors and obesity

The Midtown Manhattan study, a seminal work from the 1960s, first raised the profile of social factors and obesity (Goldblatt *et al.*, 1965) and has generated a number of subsequent studies. This study found that the prevalence of obesity fell as socioeconomic status rose and with increasing length of time that a migrant family had been in the US particularly for women. Furthermore, upwardly mobile females were less obese than those who were moved down the social scale. Trends, although similar for men, were less marked (Goldblatt *et al.*, 1965). In a longitudinal British study, women from non-manual classes who moved up the social scale were more dissatisfied with their weight than women of the same BMI from manual classes. Similarly, downwardly mobile women were more satisfied with their appearance than those who remained in the non-manual classes. It appeared that the level of educational qualifications was more important than occupationally defined social class in explaining body dissatisfaction (McLaren and Kuh, 2004).

A major review of socioeconomic status and obesity confirmed the strong inverse relationship between obesity and socioeconomic status in women from developed societies but found the opposite to be true in developing countries (Sobal and Stunkard, 1989). The relationship was the same for men and children as for women in developing, but inconsistent for those in developed societies. The direct relationship between obesity and socioeconomic status in developing societies was attributed to lower dietary intake and higher energy output among those of low status. The unique relationship among women in developed societies was attributed to cultural norms of thinness and dietary restraint, and the use of more available leisure time for exercising and 'appearance investment' by higher status women (Sobal and Stunkard, 1989; McLaren and Kuh, 2004). A positive relationship between socioeconomic position and height (Komlos and Kriwy, 2002; Turrell, 2002) may also contribute to lower BMI. Those in the highest social class were taller, and the upwardly mobile were taller than those in the class they had left (Power *et al.*, 2002). More recent US research suggests that ethnicity may explain some of the inconsistencies in men. Although a reverse association between socioeconomic status and obesity was found in both Caucasian women and men, the relationship was positive in African and Mexican Americans (Zhang and Wang, 2004).

Obesity and poverty

Social and cultural factors play a significant role in the apparently anomalous relationship between obesity and poverty, particularly among women. Although extreme poverty is associated with undernutrition, the pattern of obesity common in developed countries is gradually spreading to those countries that are experiencing demographic and epidemiological transition. Prevalence of obesity is increasing in urban areas of Latin America and the Caribbean (Pena and Bacallao, 2000; Filozof *et al.*, 2001). A significant trend for higher rates of obesity with increasing deprivation among children has been reported in southern England (Kinra *et al.*, 2000) and in the US (Alaimo *et al.*, 2001; Matherson *et al.*, 2002).

The process of urbanization results in reduced physical activity and increased consumption of an energy-dense diet, as food becomes more available and inappropriate aspects of the Western lifestyles are adopted (Pena and Bacallao, 2000; Caballero, 2001; Filozof *et al.*, 2001). The poor people face a conflict between their capacity to provide and the ideal cultural images with which they are constantly bombarded but which are beyond their means (Pena and Bacallao, 2002). Foods purchased by those on limited incomes included fatty meats and processed carbohydrates that 'fill' may not 'nourish' but whereas fresh fruit and vegetables do not satiate and remain relatively expensive (Aguirre, 2000; Wrigley *et al.*, 2002). A study among the poorest in Argentina found that processed, mass-produced, energy-dense foods with high fat and sugar content and Western appeal were being targeted to those with low purchasing power (Aguirre, 2000).

There is some evidence that urbanization has different gender effects on energy expenditure of the poor. Women's role was defined as home based and engaging in limited physical activity, whereas men were more likely to work outside the home and participate in sporting activities (Aguirre, 2000).

Women of high socioeconomic status voluntarily restrict their food intake; the body of the upper income woman is valued for its slimness. The poor woman's body needs to be strong to work, to nurture others or just to survive (Olson, 1999; Aguirre, 2000; Townsend *et al.*, 2001). It was not acceptable for overweight disadvantaged African women from Cape Town, who were familiar with food insecurity, to voluntarily regulate intake when food was available (Mvo *et al.*, 1999). For these women, weight gain reflected marital harmony and well-being, and plumpness in their children indicated that they had sufficient food to eat (Mvo *et al.*, 1999). Mothers of overweight low-income pre-school children from Cincinnati, Ohio, described their children as 'solid' or 'big boned', attributing their size to familial predisposition (Jain *et al.*, 2001).

Having a child with a good appetite was their highest priority; only when obesity resulted in inactivity or low self-esteem did it become a problem that warranted attention. To further complicate the picture, cross-national comparison of childhood obesity shows significant variation across countries with different levels of socioeconomic development. In Russia, rural children and adolescents and low- and high-income adolescents (as opposed to those in the middle income range) were at increased risk of obesity; in China, urban, high-income children and adolescents were more at risk, while the inverse relationship between socioeconomic status and obesity was confirmed in USA adolescents (Wang, 2001). Not only does this suggest the importance of considering socioeconomic factors, but different ethnic groups may respond differently to interventions targeting obesity (Zhang and Wang, 2004).

Ethnic differences

Numerous studies have shown that perceptions and preferences of body size differ among ethnic groups. These studies confirmed slim cultural preference, widespread body size dissatisfaction and the likelihood for body size overestimation among Caucasians compared with other groups, including African Americans, Caribbeans, Hispanics, First-Nation Canadians, South Asians, Ugandan Africans and Polynesians (Furnham and Alibhai, 1983; Dawson, 1988; Furnham and Baguma, 1994; Wilkinson *et al.*, 1994; Craig *et al.*, 1996; Gittelsohn *et al.*, 1996; Mossavar-Rahmani *et al.*, 1996; Altabe, 1998; Craig, 1999; Bush *et al.*, 2001). In the few instances when no ethnic differences were found, perceptions and preferences may have been influenced by the cultural values of the adopted country (Miller and Pumariega, 2001).

Views and expectations of children's body sizes reflected those of adults. African-American children were reported to have different attitudes to weight, body size and attractiveness, and to accept larger body proportions than Caucasian Americans (Miller and Pumariega, 2001; Ricciardelli and McCabe, 2001). Young migrants readily adopted a preoccupation with dieting and other weight-related concerns. Despite being lighter, British South-Asian girls reported similar dieting levels to British Caucasian girls (Hill and Bhatti, 1995). US boys were less concerned with body image than girls, but many still reported dissatisfaction with their bodies (Ricciardelli and McCabe, 2001). Although most girls wanted to be thinner, many boys wanted a bigger, more muscular physique (Cohane and Pope, 2001).

A study conducted among Tongans in Tonga, Chinese in Singapore and Caucasians in Australia was able to quantify these differences in terms of BMI. For women, the most attractive size for Tongans was 25.4 kg/m^2, for Australians 20.5 kg/m^2 and for the Chinese in Singapore 19.1 kg/m^2. Tongan men considered 28.7 kg/m^2, Australian men 23.5 kg/m^2 and Chinese men 26.3 kg/m^2 to be the most attractive body size (Fig. 4.1). Tongan women were the most accurate in

Table 4.2 Measured, perceived and preferred body sizes of Tongan, Australian Caucasian and Singaporean Chinese women and men.

	Body size (BMI, kg/m^2)		
	Tongans	**Australians**	**Chinese**
Women	*n* = 299	*n* = 261	*n* = 153
Measured	32.6	25.6	23.1
Perceived	31.1	27.9	25.3
Preferred	24.6	21.3	20.7
Men	*n* = 243	*n* = 220	*n* = 57
Measured	30.4	26.3	24.1
Perceived	32.1	27.5	28.8
Preferred	29.4	24.4	26.3

Source: Craig (1999).

estimating their present body size; Australian and Chinese women overestimated (Table 4.2). Tongan and Australian men slightly overestimated, whereas the Chinese substantially overestimated their own body size. Women from all three ethnic groups chose significantly lower preferred own body sizes (Table 4.2). The Tongans and Caucasian Australian men also chose slightly smaller preferred sizes, but the Chinese men preferred to be larger (Craig, 1999; Craig *et al.*, 2001) (Table 4.2).

These findings confirmed the Polynesian preference for larger body sizes than Caucasians (Wilkinson *et al.*, 1994; Craig *et al.*, 1996; Brewis *et al.*, 1998), although these preferences change with increasing Westernization; the more Westernized Cook Island Maori women preferred smaller ideal body sizes (Craig *et al.*, 1996). Oriental Asian female preferences were also reported to be smaller (Altabe, 1998; Sharps *et al.*, 2001), whereas men preferred larger sizes than did Caucasians (Sharps *et al.*, 2001).

The process of Westernization

The invasiveness of Western social and cultural influences on body size has been confirmed by comparing similar subjects in different settings. Western Samoan women living in New Zealand (Brewis *et al.*, 1998), more acculturated First-Nation (Gittelsohn *et al.*, 1996) and Inuit Canadians (Young, 1996) and South Asians from Kenya and India living in Britain preferred smaller female body sizes than did those remaining at home (Furnham and Alibhai, 1983; Bush *et al.*, 2001).

This was also verified by Mexicans moving to live in the USA. In Mexico, women weighed more than men. With migration to the US, Mexican women weighed less whereas Mexican men weighed more as they advanced up the social strata, reflecting their adopted culture despite a complete reversal of body size norms. The changed association of socioeconomic status with weight could not be explained by biological and genetic means, but only by social and cultural changes (Ross and Mirowsky, 1983).

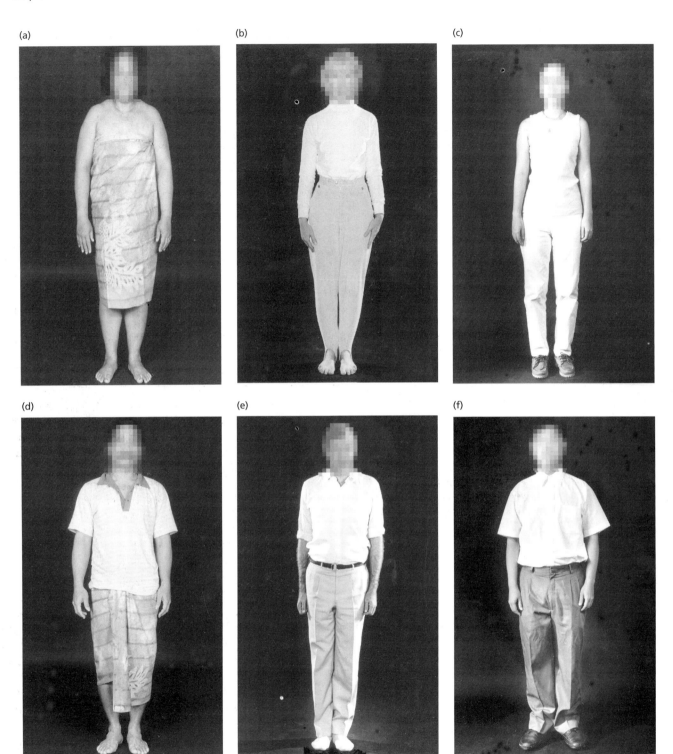

Fig. 4.1 Attractive body sizes selected by Tongans, Australian Caucasians and Singaporean Chinese women and men. (a) Tongan woman (25.4 kg/m^2); (b) Australian woman (20.5 kg/m^2); (c) Chinese woman (19.1 kg/m^2); (d) Tongan man (28.7 kg/m^2); (e) Australian man (23.5 kg/m^2); (f) Chinese man (26.3 kg/m^2).

A number of large sample studies provide further evidence for the influence of cultural norms on body size. Differences between African-American and Caucasian-American women and men from the US National Health Examination and National Health and Nutrition (NHANE) national surveys suggested that there may be cultural set points and norms of acceptable body size determined by ethnicity, gender, age and socioeconomic status (Flegal *et al.*, 1988). Hodge and Zimmet (1994) attributed their observations that ethnicity and poverty were independent predictors of obesity in women in the USA and Australia to different attitudes to obesity. Both ethnicity and socioeconomic status were shown to predict obesity in Caucasian Americans and African Americans (Woodward, 2001).

The Polynesian response to modernization has been explored in various Samoan populations at differing stages of Westernization, showing sex-specific interactions between modernity and obesity. Traditionally, men and women had clearly defined roles with men being more physically active than women. With Western influence, men were the first to become wage-earners, often engaging in relatively labour-intensive work that provided some compensation for their changed diet. Further modernization resulted in adopting occupations with reduced energy expenditure and concomitant weight gain. Activity levels of women were reduced with initial modernization. Food intake changed as the tasks usually allotted to men (growing and harvesting garden staples and cooking them in the earth oven) were replaced with Western foods such as tinned meat and fish with rice, which women were permitted to cook on stoves. Women took up lower activity employment with further modernization. Thus, due to the traditional division of labour, women were likely to develop obesity earlier in the modernization process than men (Bindon, 1995).

Thus, accepted cultural norms can shape both the perceptions and preferences of body size and actual body size within cultural groups and subgroups. There is also convincing evidence that Westernization changes these cultural norms towards the norm of slimness, particularly in women.

Culture and obesity in Western societies in the twentieth century

The changing cultural context and emergence of the slim ideal

During the twentieth century, significant changes have occurred in the perception of the ideal woman in Western culture and in the cultural reactions to body fatness. Slimness became a virtue in the 1920s and received increasing emphasis from the 1950s onwards. The frequently cited study by Garner and colleagues provided evidence of American acceptance of gradually diminishing female dimensions between 1959 and 1978, documented by Miss America pageant winners and *Playboy* centrefolds (Garner *et al.*, 1980). Follow-up studies confirmed the continued trend over subsequent years (Morris *et al.*, 1989; Wiseman *et al.*, 1992; Tovee *et al.*, 1997; Voracek and Fisher, 2002). These changes are summarized in Table 4.3. At the same time, male *Playgirl* centrefold models between 1973 and 1997 became increasingly muscular (Leit *et al.*, 2001), evidence of change in the male cultural ideal.

As the socially approved Western feminine figure became more and more cylindrical, female peripheral fatness, the naturally occurring component of female bodies preferred in the majority of traditional societies, became increasingly disparaged. Women have been expected to remain sexual (but not too sexual), to reproduce and nurture (but not overnurture themselves) and to succeed in a masculine world (McKinley, 1999). The ideal woman has become increasingly distant from the average woman, with the result that the majority of Western women are dissatisfied with their weight (Rodin *et al.*, 1985). It is considered 'normal' for women to be vigilant about their weight, with chronic dietary restraint being an accepted way of life (Way, 1995; McKinley, 1999). Dieting is widespread among adolescents, and girls learn from an early age that they will be judged by their appearance. The widely quoted 'a woman can never be too rich or too thin', attributed to Wallis Simpson, typifies Western culture (Way, 1995). The female body is socially constructed as an object, and slimness has become so internalized as to appear natural (McKinley, 1999). Fat people are seen as morally bad, with the fat person held responsible for his or her condition (Sobal, 1995). Women themselves perpetuate the system by condemning their overweight peers (Way, 1995; Germov and Williams, 1999).

The social/biological body divide

Medical understanding of the body is premised upon the concept of the body as a machine, separate from the soul; a division attributed to the philosophy of Descartes (Turner, 1982). The physical body became the concern of biological sciences, and the mind and emotions fell under the rubric of social sciences, thus creating the dichotomies of nature–culture or body–mind. It was not until the second half of the twentieth century that social scientists began to consider social aspects of the body, recognizing the perceived opposition between nature and culture as a product of Western thought. After all, cultures are assemblages of individuals with both minds and body coexisting in the one organism (Lock, 1993). The way a body is presented by an individual can signify belonging to, or, alternatively rejection of, a particular society or cultural group. When considered as a social entity, the body is not seen as stable, universal, and similar regardless of its setting, but as culturally contextualized (Lock, 1993).

Control and surveillance of the body

In his exploration of dieting, Bryan Turner (1982) draws a

Table 4.3 Changes in preferred body size and shape for Western women: 1950s to 2000.

	Playboy centrefolds			Miss America pageant contestants		Fashion models	
Year	1959–78*	1979–88†	1953–2001‡	1959–78*	1979–88†	1967–87§	1997¶
Number	240	120	577			256	300
Weight	No change	No change	No change	Decreased $r = -0.83$ ($P < 0.001$)	Decreased, $r = 0.77$ ($P < 0.01$)		
Height	Mean = 1.66 m increased $r = 0.22$ ($P < 0.01$)		Increased, $r = 0.36$ ($P < 0.001$)			Increased $F = 17.02$ ($P < 0.001$)	Mean = 1.77 m
Weight–height	Decreased, $r = -0.22$ ($P < 0.001$)						
BMI			Decreased, $r = -0.46$ ($P < 0.001$)		Decreased, $r = -0.46$ ($P < 0.001$)		17.6 kg/m²
Waist	Increased, $r = 0.41$ ($P < 0.001$)		Increased $r = 0.27$ ($P < 0.001$)			Increased, $F = 3.36$ ($P < 0.002$)	
Hips	Decreased, $r = -0.12$ ($P < 0.05$)		Decreased $r = -0.29$ ($P < 0.001$)		Decreased, $r = -0.87$ ($P = 0.01$)	No change	
Compared with population mean or standards	Population weight gain = 0.14 kg/year	In total, 69% had weight more than 15% below expected population weight–height		Different from population mean $t = 6.20$ ($P < 0.001$), pre-1970: 87.6% of mean; post 1970: 84.6% of mean	In total, 60% had weight more than 15% below expected population weight–height		Average population height = 1.66 m Average population BMI = 21.9 kg/m²

*Garner et al. (1980).
†Wiseman et al. (1992).
‡Voracek and Fisher (2002).
§Morris et al. (1989).
¶Tovee et al. (1997).

parallel between the strong morality of religious constraint and the medical dietary regimen, both of which focus on disciplining the body. Abstemiousness is consistent with the biological basis of civilized society, as is metaphor of the body as a machine amenable to scientific control. Modern medical dieting probably began in the seventeenth century with Cheyne, a Scottish doctor who attributed all major illnesses to eating habits. Excessively obese himself, he succeeded in trimming his own size and then proposed a system of dietary management for the London elite as a remedy for the diseases of civilization (Turner, 1982).

The French philosopher Foucault has profoundly influenced anthropological representations of the body, particularly the concept of surveillance over that which is institutionalized within a culture (Lock, 1993). This concept of surveillance and control has been applied to the preoccupation of American females with dieting and slimness (Nichter and Nichter, 1991). Although the efforts to control body size taken out of context appear to be both an ideology and paradox, they can be understood as part of American culture, characterized by a continuous cycling of control and release (puritanism and hedonism). The body becomes both the object of punishment and the site of pleasure, the Protestant ethic espousing hard work and control (self-control, dietary restraint, regular exercise) and in turn permitting reward or indulgence (such as sweet or fatty foods). Within the system, the individual is called upon to balance these oppositions to maintain a culturally acceptable weight, creating yet another dichotomy between the forces of good (slimness) and evil (fatness) (Nichter and Nichter, 1991).

The supportive cultural context for the slim ideal

The pursuit of slimness by dietary restraint tempered by indulgence is a culturally acceptable way of thinking and behaving in Western societies. It is sustained because it is consistent with and reinforced by norms, values and interests within the wider cultural context. Although it has been claimed that Western culture today places undue emphasis on the aesthetics of the human body (Cash and Roy, 1999), every culture has a concept of what is beautiful. What is unprecedented is the persistent diminution of the ideal body, concurrent with relentless enlargement of the actual body. Also unprecedented is how ubiquitous is the presentation of the contrast. The slim ideal is splashed across the pages of magazines and papers, appears in movies and on television, billboards, the side of buses, and is presented as a purchasable commodity, particularly for women (Featherstone, 1991; Cash and Roy, 1999), whereas obesity is obvious all around.

These norms and values are reinforced by many vested interests in the 'business of thinness'. The corporate dieting industry, the fitness industry, manufacturers of diet products, women's clothing and cosmetics, women's beauty magazines and cosmetic surgeons all benefit from perpetuation of a slim

ideology (Way, 1995). It has been estimated that in the USA alone, the dieting industry grosses in the order of $35 billion, cosmetics industry $20 billion, and cosmetic surgeons $300 million per annum (Way, 1995). The majority of people purchasing weight loss products and attending weight loss centres are women, adding support for concern with weight and thinness as a cultural phenomenon (Way, 1995). The preference for thinness in women can also be related to the value placed on youth and the changing role of women with the greater participation in the workforce coinciding with lower acceptance of the more rounded maternal image preferred in the past.

Present understanding of and approaches towards obesity and eating disorders are socially constructed and reflect the shared values, beliefs and practices of Western culture. Slimness as control over one's body, and the converse, obesity as lack of control, fits well with modern Western perceptions of control and release (Nichter and Nichter, 1991) and religiomoral management of the body (Turner, 1991). There are shared meanings of obesity; it is a serious health problem and costly in both economic and personal terms. It is widely held that obesity is self-induced and amenable to change by personal sacrifice. The previously mentioned cross-cultural study on the predictors of ideal female body shape suggested one way to engender a healthier approach to obesity and eating disorders: by broadening the present unrealistic cultural preferences and expectations of female body size to one that is more within the realm of the possible for more women (Anderson *et al.*, 1992).

Cultural influences on medical definitions of obesity

From a sociocultural perspective, the downwards trend in recommended weight for women in the USA demonstrated the influence of the culturally defined desire for thinness on the medical definition of obesity. Ritenbaugh (1982) traced the steady decline in recommended female weight (and more recently men) through various revisions of recommended weight–height tables between 1943 and 1980. At the same time, evidence was mounting that larger body size was a health risk for young and middle-aged adults, particularly men, but not necessarily women (Ritenbaugh, 1982).

Defining the limits of obesity remains controversial. Studies have repeatedly illustrated that 'normal' weight is perceived by many to be the socially desirable ideal, well below medically recommended normal weight. Achieving this 'normal' is unlikely, and may be unnecessary, given the health benefits of moderate weight reduction in obese people (Sobal, 1995). The reduction of the cut-off point for 'ideal' healthy weight ranges, from 27 to 25 kg/m^2 in 1994 (American Institute of Nutrition, 1994), increased the number of overweight and obese people in the USA by 29 million (Kettle, 1998), and dramatically raised the profile of obesity as a cause for concern. Application of an international uniform standard for healthy weight ranges to the global diversity of body types has been questioned from both the slight and the more robust extreme of the body size spectrum (Deurenberg and Yap, 2004).

The medicalization of obesity

The 'medicalization' of obesity during the twentieth century has been investigated by a number of social scientists (Sobal, 1995; Chang and Christakis, 2002). Despite much evidence for obesity as a major health problem, there may have been some selective use of scientific data supporting the risks of obesity at the expense of data portraying less clear evidence of risk (Cogan, 1999). Underutilized data show some potential health benefits of moderate obesity, the negative consequences of dieting, the failure of restrictive dieting to produce long-term weight loss, the psychological toll of weight regain and the potential health risks of weight fluctuation. The economic costs of obesity have been well publicized, but seldom the cost of the pursuit of thinness. The importance of changing other risk factors such as physical fitness, the role of genetics and biology in determining body weight and the evidence that obese people do not necessarily consume substantially more food than the non-obese are not part of the core beliefs surrounding cultural knowledge about obesity. The stigma of being obese is firmly placed among the cultural values in Western societies and perceptions of obesity as multifarious do not fit well with these values (Cogan, 1999).

Although obesity has been claimed as unhealthy for centuries, the medicalization of obesity really began in the 1950s, growing dramatically during the 1960s and 1970s (Sobal, 1995). Obesity was slotted into several medical models, within which it was considered as a genetic, endocrine, environmental, personality or addictive disorder, resulting in multiple medical strategies involving many health professionals in its treatment. Obesity became classified as a disease in the International Classification of Diseases in 1990 (Sobal, 1995).

The medicalization of obesity occurred slowly, as the concept changed within the medical framework. Chang and Christakis documented these developments through their analysis of entries in Cecil's *Textbook of Medicine* between 1927 and 2000 (Chang and Christakis, 2002). During this time, obesity was transformed from a moral deviance and the responsibility of the fat individual to a disease with reduced individual responsibility, thus providing a rationale for therapeutic intervention. As a consequence the importance of structural conditions (sociocultural, environmental and material context) was diminished, as individual factors (lifestyle, personal, behavioural) became the focus of explanation, diagnosis and intervention. Even the mass public health campaigns promoting healthy lifestyles in the 1970s and 1980s directed action towards changes in individual behaviour, minimizing the significance of the broader sociocultural and environmental constraints (Chang and Christakis, 2002).

Within the wider society, the moral overtones surrounding obesity remain, with obese people still considered largely responsible for their own condition. Technological or psychobehavioural interventions by medical or health professionals engage only a small proportion of the obese population in the developed world (Sobal, 1995) and even fewer in those societies undergoing rapid transition. The so-called self-help weight loss organizations, with membership in the millions, have collectively become a 30-billion-dollar weight loss industry. Although established by non-medical groups, many of these apply a medical model that legitimizes the need for external assistance in achieving weight loss (Sobal, 1995).

More recently, a different theoretical paradigm has emerged, which acknowledges the importance of the environment in promoting and perpetuating obesity (Eggar and Swinburn, 1997; Hill and Peters, 1998; Nestle and Jacobson, 2000). However, the recent emphasis on genetic factors runs counter to this approach, and has drawn some attention away from the social and structural context back to the individual body, away from obesity as a social concern and back to obesity as an illness.

The cultural and social context for medicalized obesity

The medicalization of obesity involved the conceptual transfer of perceived control and supervision of solutions to the biomedical model. This change neither necessarily nor solely depended on actions of medical personnel, but was facilitated by consistency with other cultural norms and activities within the wider society (Williams and Calnan, 1996; Chang and Christakis, 2002).

The ideology of systems of surveillance and control focused on the body (Williams and Calnan, 1996). The subordination of desire to reason tempered by religious moral authority, and transferred to secular institutions such as the medical profession, as well as widescale dieting, were all concordant with capitalist ideology so central to twentieth-century Western societies (Chang and Christakis, 2002). At the same time, there was a growing tendency towards measuring and categorizing (whether by insurance companies, physical anthropologists, anthropometrists, elite sporting bodies or scientific researchers).

Powerful groups benefit from obesity as a medical problem, the most obvious being the health-care, pharmaceutical and fitness industries. More broadly, medicalization increased dependence on other industries producing various consumer goods compatible with this form of social control and associated with individual treatment of obesity. Medicalized obesity thus formed a part of the wider system of disciplinary techniques, or the 'technologies of power' that regulated and normalized the population (Williams and Calnan, 1996).

Within the wider Western cultural context, there are a multitude of subcultures, whose perception of their own risks associated with obesity is bound up with their cultural beliefs,

Table 4.4 Moral, medical and sociopolitical paradigms of obesity.

Paradigm characteristics	Moral	Medical	Sociopolitical
Paradigm reach	Wide	Medium	Small and select
Perception of body fat	Bad, sinful, ugly	Promotes illness	A fact
Perception of fat person	Weak	Have an illness which is beyond	A member of society
	Lacks willpower	individual's control	
Relationship with society	Seen as a burden on society	Society a source of harm through ready	Confrontational
		access to excess calories	
Responsibility for fat condition	Personal blame	Condition of illness	None
		Neutral but not value free	
Language	Fat, corpulent, plump	Obese, adipose, overweight	Large, ample, of size
Eating	Gluttony, gorging	Acoria, polyphagia, hyperorexia	A pleasurable social activity
Activity	Sloth, laziness	Lethargy, listlessness	Neutral
Reaction to fat person	Stigmatization of fatness	Stigma of sickness and disability	Acceptance of large people as normal
	Discrimination	Dependence on medical expertise	
	Disdain		
Legitimizing experts	Religious or traditional	Scientific or clinical	Selected scientists and social scientists
Organizations/industries	Fashion and beauty	Health care	Selected magazines and books
supporting paradigm	Weight loss	Pharmaceutical	
	Sport and activity	Weight loss	Specialized fashions
		Sport and activity	
Solution focus	Dependent on willingness and	Treatment with medical supervision	Change society's attitudes to accept
	determination of the fat person		wider range of body sizes
			Political fat liberation

Sources: Sobal (1995; 1999), Chang and Christakis (2002).

moral values and life circumstances (Williams and Calnan, 1996). At one end of the socioeconomic continuum the perceived risk of obesity may be relative to the standard of a slim trim body and addressed by joining a fitness club, attending a health farm or hiring a personal trainer. Conversely, the primary concern of poor mothers from Ohio and Cape Town may be a child with a good appetite and their own ability to provide a regular supply of food and an occasional treat (Mvo *et al.*, 1999; Jain *et al.*, 2001).

Thus, the pursuit of the thin ideal woman and the change in the meaning of obesity from a moral to a medical issue have been consistent with a number of Western cultural norms and values, supported by many powerful interests.

Obesity as a social and cultural issue

The medicalized approach, with its associated reduction in individual moral responsibility and increased dependence on individualized therapeutic action (Chang and Christakis, 2002) cannot alone address the burgeoning epidemic of obesity. The social science discourses on the body presented here have demonstrated how Western cultural context maintains the slim ideal body and systems for its monitoring, measurement and control. But cultural change is possible, and changes are beginning to occur in the Western conception of obesity.

Some new paradigms include resistance to restrictive acceptable body size, a shift towards a self-care model of body maintenance, renewed orientation to the social and environmental causes of obesity and increasing attention to the concept of cultural competence.

Resistance to the normalizing process

The Western concept of obesity has changed during the twentieth century from a moral to a medical issue, and now there are attempts to 'demedicalize' it to an alternative social issue through the size acceptance movement (Sobal, 1999). Size acceptance developed as a reaction to intolerance of fat people, dissatisfaction with the cultural emphasis on thinness and the widespread promotion of dieting offered as a solution to the problem of obesity. It aims to promote size diversity and tolerance in a size-neutral society (Sobal, 1999). The original and largest size acceptance group is the US National Association to Advance Fat Acceptance (NAAFA), with similar organizations in Canada, Britain, Australia and Sweden (Germov and Williams, 1999; Sobal 1999). NAAFA sees obesity as a political problem rather than a moral or medical one, and emphasizes possible psychological harms of dieting over medical claims of health risk (Sobal, 1995) (Table 4.4). Rather than considering themselves victims, members accept their size and learn to respond to the pressure to conform to the slim ideal (Germov and Williams, 1999). Membership of the organization is however small, mostly female and largely from upper socioeconomic groups.

Body maintenance, health and fitness

Changes in the relationship between modern medicine and the public have been accompanied by growing scepticism concerning the limits of medicinal capabilities and transformation towards self-care (Williams and Calnan, 1996). At the end of the twentieth century, health promotion and fitness focusing on body maintenance have become dominant in Western culture (Featherstone, 1991). Although the obsession with 'keeping to a diet' is diminishing, the change is a conceptual one from an externally defined and imposed diet regimen to self-regulation and self-monitoring of healthy eating (Chapman, 1999). The health promotion and fitness movement still adheres to the 'control and release' metaphor and the imperatives of production and consumption. This change has been interpreted as one in which disciplinary power has moved from institutionalized surveillance to 'technologies of self'' (Foucault, 1988). Obese people are still held responsible for their body status, but the fitness, health food, weight loss and beauty industries are there to assist them in their endeavours to achieve culturally acceptable bodies.

A renewed social and environmental orientation on obesity

At the same time there is growing acceptance that many of today's health risks are located in the environment. The food-processing system has been described as a means for 'value adding' fat, sugar and salt. A wide variety of energy-enhanced foods that exploit the human predilection for sweet and fatty flavours, are available, whereas nutrient-dense low-energy foods remain comparatively expensive. Consumption of fast foods, in ever-increasing portion sizes, is escalating. More labour-saving devices, fewer manual jobs, increasing use of motor vehicles, poor town planning and the perceived danger surrounding outside activity all encourage sedentary behaviour (Nestle and Jacobson, 2000; Brown and Krick, 2001).

The sheer weight provided by the increasing proportion and number of the obese in Western societies has tipped the scales towards greater attention to structural aspects of obesity (Eggar and Swinburn, 1997; Hill and Peters, 1998; Chang and Christakis, 2002). Obesity is the result of the accumulation of small incremental gains in weight and a normal response to an abnormal, or 'obesogenic', environment (Eggar and Swinburn, 1997; Neel, 1999; Hill and Peters, 1998; Brown and Krick, 2001). This new paradigm goes beyond interpreting obesity simply as the moral concern of the individual who fails to measure up to the cultural ideal, or a medical condition amenable to correction by individual lifestyle change. It envisages obesity as environmentally caused and largely preventable (Chang and Christakis, 2002), and suggests a reorientation to the ways in which it is addressed.

Cultural competence

There is a growing literature on cultural competence in the provision of more effective cross-cultural communication (Angel and Thoits, 1987; Cross *et al.*, 1989). Initially, cultural competence involved little more than introducing translation services for individuals from a different cultural background to that of the health-care provider. However, cultural competence is a far broader concept and includes a greater cultural understanding, cultural sensitivity and cultural skill (Burchum, 2002) in relating to any cultural or subcultural group. One purpose of this chapter has been to explore some of the various meanings of obesity within different cultures and subcultures, and to demonstrate that the way obesity is conceived is culture specific. Gaining a cultural understanding of a group with different norms, ideas and values takes time and a complete understanding is never possible (Kroeber, 1963). However, any intervention to address obesity will benefit from considering each individual or group within its own cultural context.

Obesity and culture in the twenty-first century

Morbid obesity continues to increase, as does the collective weight of those in Western countries and countries undergoing transition. Considering the body within its social and environmental context may herald a new focus on the structural and environmental aspects of obesity. A deeper understanding of how the cultural and social context contributes to and supports the 'obesogenic' environment can assist in devising more successful strategies to address obesity as a social issue. The Western cultural environment is one of excess with an abundance of highly processed foods in ever-increasing portion sizes. Strategies that tackle instant gratification and the 'more for less' mindset that is so prominent in modern Western culture may benefit from observing and listening to other cultural groups who have a greater respect for and more sophisticated relationship with food (Messer, 1989).

Any discussion on obesity and culture must attempt to obfuscate the mind–body, nurture–nature divide. The Western approach, grounded in the separation of the body and mind (Turner, 1991; Lock, 1993) has focused on changing the obese body. Although obesity is a characteristic of the body, the body 'is not reducible solely to the biological, nor (is it) able to be considered as a mind/body dichotomy, (but) must be considered as whole' (Berthelot, 1991). Many cultures do not make this separation, as verified by the more realistic preference by developing countries and traditional groups for plumpness in women as a signifier of beauty, health, fertility and happiness. Renewed interest by the social sciences in aspects of the body should result in a greater understanding of the place of the body in Western culture, and can contribute to a greater insight into the ways in which the cultural context influences thinking and feeling about obesity and ways of being obese. Such contextual consideration highlights the inappropriateness of 'colonization' of different cultural groups by a globalized norm of the slim Western ideal.

The ever-diminishing breadth of the ideal female body within Western culture calls for a modicum of realism, particularly in light of the persistent expansion of the actual body. Hillel Schwartz's (1986) 'fat utopia', where fatness is revered, is an improbable scenario. Neither is an obese ideal likely to become the cultural norm despite political action by the size acceptance movement. These may, however, suggest the beginning of a more rational approach to a range of body sizes and shapes as constituting 'normal'. An appreciation and respect for different cultural interpretations of body size, norms and behaviour important to different groups and subgroups can assist a broader understanding of the relationship between culture and obesity. An exploration of some of the existing positive aspects of slight plumpness could begin to redress the current imbalance in information available on obesity (Bradley, 1982).

Once a problem is as prevalent in Western cultures as obesity, it is no longer simply a medical problem but a social one. Strategies to address so prevalent an issue, particularly among those with least control over their circumstances, must consider the social determinants and the cultural context in which it occurs. The process of Westernization involves the addition of aspects of the new while retaining many from the traditional culture (Szathmary, 1990; Bindon, 1995; Popkin, 2001), and is frequently accompanied by a rapid increase in obesity. Continued investigation of this acculturation process may help to identify the critical determinants influencing altered body size. The change from preferred plumpness in developing countries and among the most disadvantaged in Western societies to the preference for thinness occurs first among children and adolescents, who readily adopt the norm of body dissatisfaction (Hill and Bhatti, 1995; Ricciardelli and McCabe, 2001). The stage at which this transformation occurs remains obscure and exploration of this process may contribute to a greater understanding of ways in which cultural contexts support obesity. This has begun in a recent analysis of the National Longitudinal Study of Adolescent Health in the USA. Overweight-related behaviours (less healthy meal patterns, more physical inactivity) were readily adopted by migrant Hispanic adolescents, with concomitant weight gain. Mexican Americans, in whom acculturation appears to follow a different pattern, were an exception (see previous discussion) (Gordon-Larsen *et al.*, 2003).

Forty years ago, Mary Douglas (1966) proposed that individual bodies may reflect the anxieties of the social body. Thus fatness 'may function as a site for social reflection, or social diagnosis, an index of our relation to consumption in advanced consumer capitalism'. The obese society as a whole may signify that the present-day Western capitalist culture itself is in need of remedy to prevent obesity.

Acknowledgements

I would like to thank Ross Hansen for comments on a draft of this chapter, and Christine Lacey for advice and assistance with Fig. 4.1.

References

Aguirre, P. (2000) Socioanthropological aspects of obesity in poverty. In: Pena, M., Bacallao, J. eds. *Obesity and Poverty*. Pan American Health Organisation Scientific Publication No. 576. Washington: Pan American Health Organisation: 11–22.

Alaimo, K., Olson, C.M. and Frongillo, E.A. (2001) Low family income and food insufficiency in relation to overweight in US children: is there a paradox? *Archives of Pediatrics and Adolescent Medicine* **155**, 1161–1167.

Altabe, M. (1998) Ethnicity and body image: quantitative and qualitative analysis. *International Journal of Eating Disorders* **23**, 153–159.

American Institute of Nutrition (1994) Report of the American Institute of Nutrition (AIN) Steering Committee on Healthy Weight. *Journal of Nutrition* **124**, 2240–2243.

Anderson, J.L., Crawford, C.B., Nadeau, J. and Lindberg, T. (1992) Was the Duchess of Windsor right? A cross-cultural review of the socioecology of ideals of female body shape. *Ethology and Sociobiology* **13**, 197–227.

Angel, R., and Thoits, P. (1987) The impact of culture in the cognitive structures of illness. *Culture, Medicine and Psychiatry* **11**, 465–494.

Berthelot, J.M. (1991) Sociological discourse and the body. In: Featherstone, M., Hepworth, M., Turner, B.S. eds. *The Body: Social Process and Cultural Theory*. London: Sage Publications, 390–404.

Bindon, J.R. (1995) Polynesian responses to modernization: overweight and obesity in the South Pacific. In: de Garine, I., Pollock, N.J. eds. *Social Aspects of Obesity*. Luxemburg; Gordon and Breach Publishers, 227–251.

Bradley, P.J. (1982) Is obesity an advantageous adaptation? *International Journal of Obesity* **6**, 43–52.

Brewis, A.A, McGarvey, S.T., Jones, J. and Swinburn, B.A. (1998) Perceptions of body size in Pacific Islanders. *International Journal of Obesity* **22**, 185–189.

Brown, P.J. (1992) The biocultural evolution of obesity: an anthropological view. In: Bjorntorp, P., Brodoff, B.N. eds. *Obesity*. Philadelphia: J.B. Lippincott, 320–329.

Brown, P.J. and Konner, M. (1987) An anthropological perspective on obesity. *Annals of the New York Academy of Sciences* **499**, 29–46.

Brown, P.J. and Konner, M. (1998) An anthropological perspective on obesity. In: Brown, P.J. ed. *Understanding and Applying Medical Anthropology*. Mountainview, CA: Mayfield Publishing, 401–413.

Brown, P.J. and Krick, S.V. (2001) Culture and economy in the etiology of obesity: diet, television and the illusions of personal choice. Working paper 003–01, MARIAL Center, Emory University, Atlanta, GA. Available HTTP: http://www.emory.edu/COLLEGE/MARIAL/pdfs/wp003–01obesity.pdf (April 2003).

Buck, P.H. (1932) *Ethnology of Manahiki and Ragahanga*. Bernice P. Bishop Museum Bulletin 99. Honolulu, HI: B.P. Bishop Museum.

Burchum, J.L. (2002) Cultural competence: an evolutionary process. *Nursing Forum* **37**, 5–15.

Bush, H.M., Williams, R.G.A., Lean, M.E.J. and Anderson, A.S. (2001) Body image and weight consciousness among South Asian, Italian and the general population. *Appetite* **37**, 207–215.

Caballero, B. (2001) Introduction to symposium: obesity in developing countries: biological and ecological factors. *Journal of Nutrition* **131**, 866S–870S.

Cahnman, W.J. (1968) The stigma of obesity. *Sociological Quarterly* **9**, 294–297.

Cash, T.F. and Roy, R.E. (1999) Pounds of flesh. In: Sobal, J., Maurer, D. eds. *Interpreting Weight*. New York: Aldine de Gruyter, 209–228.

Cassidy, C.M. (1980) Nutrition and health in agriculturalists and hunter-gatherers. In: Jerome, N.W., Kandel, R.F., Pelto, H.P. eds. *Nutritional Anthropology: Contemporary Approaches to Diet and Culture*. New York: Redgrave Publishing, 117–145.

Cassidy, C.M. (1991) The good body: when bigger is better. *Medical Anthropology* **13**, 181–213.

Chang, V.W. and Christakis, N.A. (2002) Medical modeling of obesity: the transition from action to experience in a 20th century American medical textbook. *Sociology of Health and Illness* **24**, 151–177.

Chang, V.W. and Christakis, N.A. (2003) Self-perception of weight appropriateness in the United States. *American Journal of Preventive Medicine* **24**, 332–339.

Chapman, G.E. (1999) From 'dieting' to 'healthy eating'. In: Sobal, J., Maurer, D. eds. *Interpreting Weight*. New York: Aldine de Gruyter, 73–87.

Cogan, J.C. (1999) Re-evaluating the weight-centred approach towards health. In: Sobal, J., Maurer, D. eds. *Interpreting Weight*. New York: Aldine de Gruyter, 229–253.

Cohane, G.H. and Pope, H.G. (2001) Body image in boys: a review of the literature. *International Journal of Eating Disorders* **29**, 373–379.

Cook, J. (1886) *Captain Cook's Voyages Round the World* (ed. Anon.). London: Ward, Lock Bowden, 1150 (Appendix).

Craig, P. (1999) Which body size? A cross-cultural study of body composition and body perception. PhD dissertation, University of Sydney, Sydney.

Craig, P.L., Swinburn, B.A., Matenga-Smith, T., Matangi, H. and Vaughan, G. (1996) Do Polynesians still believe that big is beautiful? *New Zealand Medical Journal* **109**, 200–203.

Craig, P., Halavatau, V., Comino, E. and Caterson, I. (2001) Differences in body composition between Tongans and Australians: time to rethink the healthy weight ranges? *International Journal of Obesity* **25**, 1806–1814.

Cross, T., Bazron, B.J., Dennis, K.W. and Isaacs, M.R. (1989) Towards a culturally competent system of care. Vol 1: Monograph on effective services for minority children who are emotionally disturbed. Georgetown University Child Development Centre, CASSP Technical Assistance Center, Washington. In: Chin, J.L. ed. (2000) *Culturally Competent Health Care*. Public Health Reports **115**, 25–33.

Davis, C. and Katzman, M.A. (1999) Chinese men and women in the United States and Hong Kong: body and self-esteem ratings as a prelude to dieting and exercise. *International Journal of Eating Disorders* **23**, 99–102.

Davis, C., Durnin, J.V.G.A., Gurevich, M., Le Maire, A. and Dionne, M. (1993) Body composition correlates of weight dissatisfaction and dietary restraint in young women. *Appetite* **20**, 197–207.

Dawson, D.A. (1988) Ethnic differences in female overweight: data from the 1985 National Health Interview Survey. *American Journal of Public Health* **78**, 1326–1329.

De Garine, I. (1995) Sociocultural aspects of the male fattening sessions among the Massa of Northern Cameroon. In: de Garine, I., Pollock, N.J. eds. *Social Aspects of Obesity*. Luxemburg: Gordon and Breach Publishers, 45–70.

Deurenberg, P. and Deurenberg-Yap, M. (2004) Ethnic and geographical influences on body composition. In: Bray, G.A., Bouchard, C. eds. *Handbook of Obesity: Etiology and Pathophysiology*, 2nd edn. New York: Marcel Dekker, 81–108.

Douglas, M. (1966) *Purity and Danger: an Analysis of Concepts of Pollution and Taboo*. London: Routledge and Kegan Paul. In: Chang, V.W., Christakis, N.A. eds (2002) Medical modelling of obesity: the transition from action to experience in a 20th century American medical textbook. *Sociology of Health and Illness* **24**, 151–177.

Eaton, S.B., Shostak, M. and Konner, M. (1998) Stone agers in the fast lane: chronic degenerative diseases in evolutionary perspective. In: Brown, P.J. ed. *Understanding and Applying Medical Anthropology*. Mountainview, CA: Mayfield Publishing, 21–33.

Eggar, G. and Swinburn, B. (1997) An 'ecological' approach to the obesity pandemic. *British Medical Journal* **315**, 477–80.

eHRAF. Collection of Ethnography. Available HTTP: http://ets.umdl.umich.edu/e/ehrafe (April 2003).

Featherstone, M. (1991) The body in consumer culture. In: Featherstone, M., Hepworth, M., Turner, B.S. eds. *The Body: Social Process and Cultural Theory*. London: Sage Publications, 170–196.

Filozof, C, Gonzalez, C, Sereday, M., Mazza, C. and Braguinsky, J. (2001) Obesity prevalence and trends in Latin-American countries. *Obesity Review* **2**, 99–106.

Flegal, K.M., Harlan, W.R. and Landis, J.R. (1988) Secular trends in body mass index and skinfold thickness with socioeconomic factors in young adult women. *American Journal of Clinical Nutrition* **48**, 535–543.

Foucault, M. (1988) Technologies of self: a seminar with Michel Foucault. Martin, L.H., Gutman, H., Hutton, P.H. (eds) Amherst, MA: University of Massachusetts Press. In: Chang, V.W., Christakis, N.A. (2002) Medical modeling of obesity: the transition from action to experience in a 20th century American medical textbook. *Sociology of Health and Illness* **24** 151–177.

Furnham, A. and Alibhai, N. (1983) Cross-cultural differences in the perception of female body shapes. *Psychological Medicine* **13**, 829–837.

Furnham, A. and Baguma, P. (1994) Cross-cultural differences in the evaluation of male and female body shapes. *International Journal of Eating Disorders* **15**, 81–89.

Garner, D.M., Garfinkel, P.E., Schwartz, E. and Thompson, M. (1980) Cultural expectations of thinness in women. *Psychology Reports* **47**, 483–491.

Germov, J. and Williams, L. (1999) Dieting women. In: Sobal, J., Maurer, D. eds. *Weighty Issues: Fatness and Thinness as Social Problems*. New York: Aldine de Gruyter, 117–132.

Gerver, W.J.M., de Bruin, R. and Drayer, N.M. (1994) A persisting secular trend for body measurement in Dutch children. The Oosterwolde II study. *Acta Paediatrica* **83**, 812–814.

Gittelsohn, J., Harris, S.B., Thorne-Lyman, A.L., Hanley, A.J.G., Barnie A. and Zinman, B. (1996) Body image concepts differ by age and sex in an Ojibway-Cree community in Canada. *Journal of Nutrition* **126**, 2990–3000.

Goldblatt, P.B., Moore, M.E. and Stunkard, A.J. (1965) Social factors in obesity. *Journal of the American Medical Association* **192**, 97–102.

Gordon-Larsen, P., Harris, K.M., Ward, D.S. and Popkin, B.M. (2003) National Longitudinal Study of Adolescent Health. Acculturation and overweight-related behaviors among Hispanic immigrants to the US: the National Longitudinal Study of Adolescent Health. *Social Science and Medicine* **57**, 2023–2034.

Graves, N.B. and Graves, T.D. (1978) The impact of modernization on the personality of a Polynesian people. *Human Organisation* **37**, 115–135.

Hattori, K. (1995) Physique of Sumo wrestlers in relation to some cultural characteristics of Japan. In: de Garine, I., Pollock, N.J. eds. *Social Aspects of Obesity*. Luxemburg: Gordon and Breach Publishers, 31–43.

Hill, A.J. and Bhatti, R. (1995) Body shape perception and dieting in preadolescent British Asian girls—links with eating disorders. *International Journal of Eating Disorders* **17**, 175–183. In: Ricciardelli, L.A., McCabe, M.P. eds (2001) Children's body image concerns and eating disturbance: a review of the literature. *Clinical Psychology Review* **21**, 325–344.

Hill, J.O. and Peters, J.C. (1998) Environmental contributions to the obesity epidemic. *Science* **280**, 1371–1374.

Hodge, A.M. and Zimmet, P.Z. (1994) The epidemiology of obesity. In: Caterson, I.D. ed. *Clinical Endocrinology and Metabolism*, Vol. 8, no. 3. London: Baillière Tindall, 577–599.

Jain, A., Sherman, S.N., Chamberlain, L.A., Carter, Y., Powers, S.W. and Whitaker, R.C. (2001) Why don't low income mothers worry about their preschoolers being overweight? *Pediatrics* **107**, 1138–1146.

Kettle, M. (1998) Fat is a mathematical issue—as 29m Americans find out. *Guardian Weekly*, 14 June 1998, p. 4.

Kinra, S., Nelder, R.P. and Lewendon, G.J. (2000) Deprivation and childhood obesity: a cross sectional study of 20973 children in Plymouth, United Kingdom. *Journal of Epidemiology and Community Health* **54**, 456–460.

Kluckhohn, C. (1949) *Mirror for Man*. New York: McGraw-Hill Book Co., 23.

Komlos, J. and Kriwy, P. (2002) Social status and adult heights in the two Germanies. *Annals of Human Biology* **29**, 641–648.

Kroeber, A.L. (1963) *Culture*. New York: Vintage Books.

Lee, R. and De Vore, I. (1976) *Kalahari Hunter-Gatherers*. Cambridge, MA: Harvard University Press. In: Messer, E. ed. (1989) Small but healthy? Some cultural considerations. *Human Organization* **48** 39–52.

Lee, S., Leung, T., Lee, A.M., Yu, H. and Leung, C.M. (1996) Body dissatisfaction among Chinese undergraduates and its implications for eating disorders in Hong Kong. *International Journal of Eating Disorders* **20**, 77–84.

Leit, R.A., Pope, H.G. and Gray, J.J. (2001) Cultural expectations of muscularity in men: the evolution of Playgirl centerfolds. *International Journal of Eating Disorders* **29**, 90–93.

Lev-Ran, A. (2001) Human obesity: an evolutionary approach to understanding our bulging waistline. *Diabetes/Metabolism Research and Reviews* **17**, 347–362.

Lock, M. (1993) Cultivating the body: anthropology and epistemologies of bodily practice and knowledge. *Annual Review of Anthropology* **22**, 133–155.

McKinley, N.M. (1999) Ideal weight/ideal women. In: Sobal, J., Maurer, D. eds. *Weighty Issues: Fatness and Thinness as Social Problems*. New York: Aldine de Gruyter, 97–115.

McLaren, L. and Kuh, D. (2004) Women's body dissatisfaction, social class, and social mobility. *Social Science and Medicine* **58**, 1575–1584.

Matherson, D.M., Varady, J., Varady, A. and Killen, J.D. (2002) Household food security and nutritional status of Hispanic children in the fifth grade. *American Journal of Clinical Nutrition* **76**, 210–217.

Messer, E. (1989) Small but healthy? Some cultural considerations. *Human Organization* **48**, 39–52.

Miller, M.N. and Pumariega, A.J. (2001) Culture and eating disorders: a historical and cross-cultural review. *Psychiatry* **64**, 93–110.

Morris, A., Cooper, T. and Cooper, P.J. (1989) The changing shape of female fashion models. *International Journal of Eating Disorders* **8**, 593–596.

Mossavar-Rahmani, Y., Pelto, G.H., Ferris, A.M. and Allen, L.H. (1996) Determinants of body size perceptions and dieting behavior in a multiethnic group of hospital staff women. *Journal of the American Dietetic Association* **96**, 252–256.

Mvo, Z., Dick, J. and Steyn, K. (1999) Perceptions of overweight African women about acceptable body size of women and children. *Curationis* **22**, 27–31.

Neel, J.V. (1999) The 'thrifty genotype' in 1998. *Nutrition Reviews* **57**, S2–9.

Nestle, M. and Jacobson, M.F. (2000) Halting the obesity epidemic: a public health policy approach. *Public Health Reports* **115**, 12–24.

Nichter, M. and Nichter, M. (1991) Hype and weight. *Medical Anthropology* **13**, 249–284.

Norgan, N.G. (1997) The beneficial effects of body fat and adipose tissue in humans. *International Journal of Obesity* **21**, 738–746.

Olson, C.M. (1999) Nutrition and health outcomes associated with food insecurity and hunger. *Journal of Nutrition* **192** (2S suppl.), 521S–524S.

Pasquet, P., Brigant, L., Froment, A., Koppert, G.A., Bard, D., de Garine, I. and Apfelbaum, M. (1992) Massive overfeeding and energy balance in men: the Guru Walla model. *American Journal of Clinical Nutrition* **56**, 483–490.

Pena, M. and Bacallao, J. (2000) Obesity and the poor: an emerging problem. In: Pena, M., Bacallao, J. eds. *Obesity and Poverty*. Pan American Health Organisation Scientific Publication No. 576. Washington: Pan American Health Organisation, 3–10.

Pena, M. and Bacallao, J. (2002) Malnutrition and poverty. *Annual Review of Nutrition* **22**, 241–253.

Pollock, N.J. (1995) Social fattening patterns in the Pacific—the positive side of obesity. A Nauru case study. In: de Garine, I., Pollock, N.J. eds. *Social Aspects of Obesity*. Luxemburg: Gordon and Breach Publishers, 87–109.

Popkin, B.M. (2001) Nutrition in transition: the changing global nutrition challenge. *Asia Pacific Journal of Clinical Nutrition* **10**, S13–S18.

Power, C., Manor, O. and Li, L. (2002) Are inequalities in height underestimated by adult social position? Effects of changing social structure and height selection in a cohort study. *British Medical Journal* **325**, 131–134.

Ricciardelli, L.A. and McCabe, M.P. (2001) Children's body image concerns and eating disturbance: a review of the literature. *Clinical Psychology Review* **21**, 325–344.

Richards, A.I. (1961) Land, labour and diet in Northern Rhodesia: an economic study of the Bemba tribe. Available HTTP:

http://ets.umdl.umich.edu/e/ehrafe Richards (Audrey
Isabel, 1899–/Doc. Number: 2, OCM 261, April 2003).

Ritenbaugh, C. (1982) Obesity as a culture-bound syndrome. *Culture, Medicine and Psychiatry* **6**, 347–361.

Ritenbaugh, C. (1991) Body size and shape: a dialogue of culture and biology. *Medical Anthropology* **13**, 173–180.

Rodin, J., Silberstein, L. and Striegel-Moore, R. (1985) Women and weight: a normative discontent. In: Sonderegger, T.B. ed. *Nebraska Symposium on Motivation, Psychology and Gender, 1984*, Vol. 32. Lincoln, NE: University of Nebraska Press, 267–307.

Ross, C.E. and Mirowsky, J. (1983) Social epidemiology of overweight: a substantive and methodological investigation. *Journal of Health and Social Behavior* **24**, 288–298.

Rossner, S. (1999) Physical activity and prevention and treatment of weight gain associated with pregnancy: current evidence and research issues. *Medicine and Science in Sports and Exercise* **31** (Suppl.), S560–S563.

Schwartz, H. (1986) *Never Satisfied*. New York: The Free Press.

Sharps, M.J., Price-Sharps, J.L. and Hanson, J. (2001) Body image preferences in the United States and rural Thailand: an exploratory study. *Journal of Psychology* **135**, 518–526.

Sobal, J. (1995) The medicalization and demedicalization of obesity. In: Maurer, D., Sobal, J. eds. *Eating Agendas: Food and Nutrition as Social Problems*. New York: Aldine de Gruyter, 67–90.

Sobal, J. (1999) The size acceptance movement and the social construction of body weight. In: Sobal, J., Maurer, D. eds. *Weighty Issues: Fatness and Thinness as Social Problems*. New York: Aldine de Gruyter, 231–249.

Sobal, J. and Stunkard, A.J. (1989) Socioeconomic status and obesity: a review of the literature. *Psychological Bulletin* **105**, 260–275.

Szathmary, E.J.E. (1990) Diabetes in Amerindian populations: the Dogrib studies. In: Swedland, A.C., Armelagos, G.J. eds. *Disease in Populations in Transition: Anthropological and Epidemiological Perspectives*. New York: Bergin and Garvey, 75–104.

Tovee, M.J., Mason, S.M., Emery, J.L., McCluskey, S.E. and Cohen-Tovee, E.M. (1997) Supermodels: stick insects or hourglasses? *Lancet* **350**: 1474–1475.

Townsend, M.S., Peerson, J., Love, B., Achterberg, C. and Murphy, S.P. (2001) Food insecurity is positively related to overweight in women. *Journal of Nutrition* **131**, 1738–1745.

Turner, B.S. (1982) The government of the body: medical regimens and the rationalization of diet. *British Journal of Sociology* **33**, 254–269.

Turner, B.S. (1991) The discourse of diet. In: Featherstone, M., Hepworth, M., Turner, B.S. eds. *The Body: Social Process and Cultural Theory*. London: Sage Publications, 157–169.

Turrell, G. (2002) Socioeconomic position and height in early adulthood. *Australia and New Zealand Journal of Public Health* **26**, 468–472.

Voracek, M. and Fisher, M.L. (2002) Shapely centerfolds? Temporal change in body measures: trend analysis. *British Medical Journal* **325**: 1447–1448.

Wang, Y. (2001) Cross-national comparison of childhood obesity: the epidemic and the relationship between obesity and socioeconomic status. *International Epidemiological Association* **30**, 1129–1136.

Way, K. (1995) Never too rich . . . or too thin: the role of stigma in the social construction of anorexia nervosa. In: Maurer, D., Sobal, J. eds. *Eating Agendas: Food and Nutrition as Social Problems*. New York: Aldine de Gruyter, 91–113.

Weinsier, R.L., Hunter, G.R., Heini, A.F., Goran, M.I. and Sell, S.M. (1998) The etiology of obesity: relative contribution of metabolic factors, diet, and physical activity. *American Journal of Medicine* **105**, 145–150.

Weiss, K.M. (1990) Transitional diabetes and gallstones in Amerindian peoples: genes or environment? In: Swedland, A.C., Armelagos, G.J. eds. *Disease in Populations in Transition: Anthropological and Epidemiological Perspectives*. New York: Bergin and Garvey, 105–123.

Wilkinson, J., Ben-Tovim, D.I. and Walker, M.K. (1994) An insight into the personal and cultural significance of weight and shape in large Samoan women. *International Journal of Obesity* **18**, 602–606.

Williams, S.J. and Calnan, M. (1996) The 'limits' of medicalization?: modern medicine and the lay populace in 'late' modernity. *Social Science & Medicine* **42**, 1609–1620.

Wiseman, C.V., Gray, J.J., Mosimann, J.E. and Ahrens, A.H. (1992) Cultural expectations of thinness in women: an update. *International Journal of Eating Disorders* **11**, 85–89.

Woodward, J.R. (2001) An examination of the effects of race and socioeconomic status on health behaviours. *Dissertation Abstracts International* **61** 2934A–2935A.

Wright St-Clair, R.E. (1980) Diet of the Maoris of New Zealand. In: Robson, J.R.K. ed. *Food Ecology and Culture*. New York: Gordon and Breach, 35–45.

Wrigley, N., Warm, D., Margetts, B. and Whelan, A. (2002) Assessing the impact of improved retail access on diet in a 'food desert': a preliminary report. *Urban Studies* **39**, 2061–2082.

Young, T.K. (1996) Sociocultural and behavioural determinants of obesity among Inuit in the Central Canadian Artic. *Social Science & Medicine* **43**, 1665–1671.

Zhang, Q. and Wang, Y. (2004) Socioeconomic inequality of obesity in the United States: do gender, age, and ethnicity matter? *Social Science & Medicine* **58**, 1171–1180.

Biology of obesity

Energy balance and body weight homeostasis

Abdul G. Dulloo

Introduction, 67

Basic concepts and principles in human energetics, 67
    Energy balance and laws of thermodynamics, 67
    Pattern of food intake and energy expenditure, 68
    Components of energy expenditure, 69
    Timescale of energy balance, 71

Control of food intake, 71
    Hunger and satiety, 71

Hunger–satiety control centres in the brain, 72
Hunger–satiety signals from the periphery, 72
Integrated models of food intake control, 74

Autoregulatory adjustments in energy expenditure, 75
    The dynamic equilibrium model, 75
    Role of adaptive thermogenesis, 76

Thermogenesis associated with physical activity, 76
Mechanisms of thermogenesis, 77
Models for body composition regulation via adaptive thermogenesis, 78

Integrating intake and expenditure, 78

References, 79

Introduction

Obesity is often considered to result from the failure of homeostatic mechanisms that regulate body weight during exposure to an environment that favours overeating and/or discourages physical activity. In addressing the issue of 'biology of obesity', it is therefore pertinent to raise the question of whether body weight is indeed a regulated variable. A critical feature of any regulated system is that disturbance of the regulated variable results in compensatory responses that tend to attenuate the disturbance and to restore the system to its 'set' or 'preferred' value. The direct application of this approach to test whether body weight is regulated in human beings is difficult because of ethical and practical reasons, but observations on adults recovering from food shortages during post-war famine or from experimental starvation indicate that a return to normal body weight is eventually achieved (Keys *et al.*, 1950).

Conversely, excess weight gained during experimental overeating or during pregnancy is subsequently lost, and most individuals return to their initial body weight (Garrow, 1974). It is also important to emphasize that a fluctuating body weight is in general the rule, even in adults who apparently maintain a stable body weight over months, years and decades, and that there is in reality no absolute constancy of body weight. Instead, body weight tends to fluctuate or oscillate around a mean constant value, with small to large devia-

tions from a 'set' or 'preferred' value being triggered by events that are seasonal and/or cultural (weekend parties, holiday seasons), psychological (stress, depression, anxiety or emotions) and pathophysiological (ranging from minor health perturbations to more serious disease states). According to Garrow (1974), very short-term day-to-day changes in body weight have a standard deviation of about 0.5% of body weight, whereas longitudinal observations over periods of between 10 and 30 years indicate that individuals experience slow trends and reversal of body weight amounting to between 7% and 20% of mean weight. There is therefore little doubt that regulation of body weight occurs, albeit with varying degrees of precision. How such long-term weight homeostasis is achieved in humans is the focus of this chapter. To address this question, it is first important to underscore the basic concepts and principles about the flux of energy transformations through which body weight is regulated.

Basic concepts and principles in human energetics

Energy balance and laws of thermodynamics

Life exists in a flux of energy transformations that are governed by the *laws of thermodynamics*. According to the *first law*, energy can neither be created nor destroyed but can be transformed only from one form into another. Biological systems,

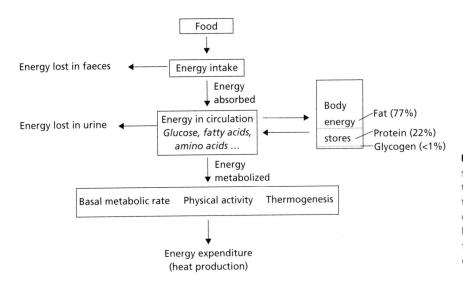

Fig. 5.1 Principles of energy balance, within a schematic framework that depicts the transformation of energy from food to heat through the body. Note that of diets typically consumed in developed countries, the total energy losses in faeces and urine are small (about 5%), so that the metabolizable energy available from these diets is about 95%.

like machines, depend on the transformation of some form of energy in order to perform work. The chemical energy obtained from foods (plant or animal in origin) is used to perform a variety of work, such as in the synthesis of new macromolecules (*chemical work*), in muscular contraction (*mechanical work*) or in the maintenance of ionic gradients across membranes (*electrical work*). The intermediary steps in this flux of energy transformations between food and heat production are illustrated in Fig. 5.1, and are embodied in the following equation:

Energy intake = energy expenditure + Δ energy stores

where energy intake refers to the metabolizable energy intake, i.e. the energy available to perform work after taking into account losses in faeces and urine (see Fig. 5.1).

Thus, if the total energy contained in the body (as fat, protein and glycogen) of a given individual is not altered (i.e. Δ energy stores = 0) then energy expenditure must be equal to energy intake, in keeping with the *first law* of thermodynamics. In this case, the individual is said to be in a *state of energy balance*. If the intake and expenditure of energy are not equal, then a change in body energy content will occur, with *negative energy balance* resulting in the degradation of the body's energy stores (glycogen, fat and protein) or *positive energy balance* resulting in an increase in body energy stores, primarily as fat. The first law of thermodynamics, however, overlooks the possible interrelationships between energy intake and energy expenditure. It does not illustrate that voluntary energy intake may rise with intense physical activity (lumberjacks eat more than clerks), that energy expenditure may increase in response to increased food intake or that both energy intake and energy expenditure can be influenced by changes in body energy stores. It is merely concerned with initial and final states.

The *second law* of thermodynamics, by contrast, makes a subtle distinction between the potential energy of food, useful work and heat. It states that when food is utilized in the body, whether for muscular contraction, synthesis of new tissues or for maintenance of electrolyte equilibrium across membranes, these processes must be accompanied inevitably by a loss of heat. In thermodynamic terms, some energy is degraded, and such heat energy that is no longer available for work is termed 'entropy'. In other words, the conversion of available food energy is not a perfectly efficient process: about 75% of the chemical energy contained in foods may be ultimately dissipated as heat because of the inefficiency of intermediary metabolism in transforming food energy into a form (e.g. adenosine triphosphate, ATP) that can be used for useful work, whether it be the internal work required to maintain structure and function or external physical work (i.e. work performed on the environment). Thus, all the energy used by the body at rest is ultimately lost as heat, and physical (external) work will also be eventually degraded as heat. These theoretical considerations constitute the framework of a biological system in which changes in energy intake and expenditure can oppose changes in energy balance and body weight.

Pattern of food intake and energy expenditure

Humans eat food in a discontinuous mode, and the amount of food eaten can range from zero up to 21 MJ per day in highly active individuals or during acute episodes of hyperphagia. This contrasts with energy expenditure, which is continuous, irrespective of the conditions encountered. This irregularity of food behaviour occurs both within a day and between days, the latter explaining the 2–3 times greater coefficient of variation for energy intake (15–20%) than for energy expenditure (5–8%) (Schutz and Garrow 1996). This also explains the difficulties with which food intake is assessed in order to obtain a representative picture of 'habitual' food (energy) intake. In addition, the wide variety of feeding behaviour makes it tremendously difficult to track adequately both of these factors jeopardizing the interpretation of data on food intake. As many factors can lead to underestimation or overestima-

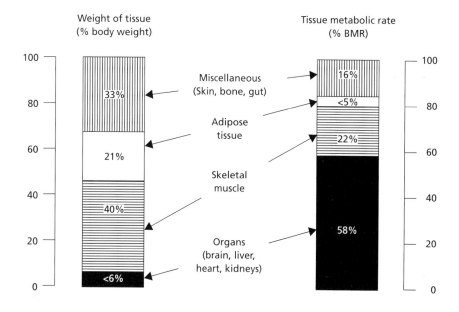

Fig. 5.2 Contribution of organ/tissues to basal metabolic rate (BMR) of a non-obese man (adapted from data of Elia, 1996). Note the disproportionate contribution of organs (< 6% body weight) to BMR (> 50% BMR).

tion of energy intake, and hence leading to a bias in energy balance, it is therefore not surprising that energy requirements are based preferentially on estimates of energy expenditure rather than on energy intake.

Components of energy expenditure

It is customary to consider human energy expenditure as being made up of three components: the energy spent for basal metabolism (or basal metabolic rate), the energy spent on physical activity and the increase in resting energy expenditure in response to a variety of stimuli (including food, cold, stress and drugs). These three components are depicted in Fig. 5.1, and are described below:

Basal metabolic rate

This is the largest component of energy expenditure for most individuals. Typically in developed countries, basal metabolic rate (BMR) accounts for between 60% and 75% of daily energy expenditure (Ravussin and Gautier, 1999). It is measured under standardized conditions—i.e. in an awake subject lying in the supine position, in a state of physical and mental rest in a comfortable warm environment, and in the morning in the post-absorptive state, usually 10–12 h after the last meal. These conditions are referred to as 'basal' as they should reflect the energy needed for the work of vital functions (maintaining electrolyte equilibrium across cell membranes, cell and protein turnover, respiratory and cardiovascular functions, etc.).

By far the most important determinant of BMR is body size, and in particular the fat-free mass of the body, which is influenced by weight, height, age and gender. On average, men have greater fat-free mass and BMR than women, even for the same age, weight and height, and older people have lower fat-free mass and BMR than young adults. Most, but not all, of the differences in BMR among these groups disappear when BMR is expressed as a function of fat-free mass. This is not surprising as fat-free mass contains tissues and organs that have high metabolic activities, such as liver, kidneys, heart, and to a lesser extent the resting muscles. In contrast, the contribution of adipose mass to BMR is small. In a non-obese subject, adipose tissue contributes 3–5% of the total resting energy expenditure, although it represents 20–30% of total body weight (Elia, 1996). The majority of the heat production (about 60%) comes from active organs such as the liver, kidney, heart and brain, although they account for only 5–6% of total body weight (Fig. 5.2). The resting heat production of skeletal muscle per unit mass is 15–40 times lower than that of metabolically active organs, but because of its large size (more than one-half of the total fat-free mass), it makes a significant contribution to total heat production (about 20%).

BMR can vary by up to 10% in individuals of the same age, gender, body weight and fat-free mass, suggesting that genetic factors are also important. Day-to-day intra-individual variability in BMR is low in men (coefficient of variation of 1–3%) but is larger in women because of changes in BMR over the menstrual cycle. In both women and men, BMR is greater than the metabolic rate during sleep by 5–20%, with the difference between BMR and sleeping metabolic rate being explained by the effect of arousal.

Energy expenditure due to physical activity

The energy spent on physical activity depends on the type and intensity of the physical activity and on the time spent in different activities. Physical activity is often considered to be synonymous with 'muscular work', which has a strict definition in physics, i.e. force × distance, during which external work is performed on the environment. During muscular work (muscle contraction), the muscle produces 3–4 times more heat than mechanical energy, so that useful work costs more than muscle work. There is a wide variation in the energy cost of any activity both within and among individuals. The latter variation is due to differences in body size and in the speed and dexterity with which an activity is performed. In order to adjust for differences in body size, the energy cost of physical activities is expressed as multiples of BMR (Durnin, 1991). These generally range from 1–5 for most activities, but can reach values of between 10 and 14 during intense exercise. In terms of daily energy expenditure, physical activity can represent up to 70% of daily energy expenditure in an individual who is involved in heavy manual work or competitive athletics. For most individuals in industrialized societies, however, the contribution of physical activity to daily energy expenditure is relatively small (10–15%). In a hospitalized patient in bed, it is still lower.

Energy expenditure in response to various thermogenic stimuli

This component of energy expenditure—often referred to as 'thermogenesis'—is best described by the various forms in which it can exist. These have been described by Miller (1982) as follows:

1 *Isometric thermogenesis.* This is due to increased muscle tension; no physical work is done in the physical sense. The differences in energy expenditure in a person who is lying, sitting or standing are due mainly to changes in muscle tone.

2 *Dynamic thermogenesis.* The term 'negative work' is used to describe heat production of stretched muscle—with heat again being produced without any work. For example, when someone goes down a ladder, heat production increases but no work is done. In the physical sense of work, contracting muscles produce heat because of their inefficiency, but tensed and stretched muscles are simply thermogenic.

3 *Psychological thermogenesis.* The psychological state may affect energy expenditure, as anxiety, anticipation and stress stimulate adrenaline (or epinephrine) secretion, leading to increased heat production. A twofold difference can be found in the energy cost of sitting at ease and sitting playing chess, a difference that cannot entirely be attributed to muscular movement (Durnin and Passmore, 1972). The best evidence comes from a study on pilots whose energy expenditure increased when they were under air traffic control, with the rise being inversely related to their level of experience (Corey, 1948).

4 *Cold-induced thermogenesis.* Humans rarely need to increase heat production for the purpose of thermal regulation because they are able to seek an equitable environment or wear suitable clothing—i.e. their bodies are generally kept at thermoneutrality. At low temperatures, their resting metabolic rate (and hence heat production) increases. For example, normal-weight women maintained in identical clothing in a calorimeter room adjusted their 24-h heat production by about 7%

when the temperature in the calorimeter room was lowered from 28°C to 22°C (Dauncey, 1981). It is customary to distinguish between two forms of cold-induced thermogenesis—shivering and non-shivering thermogenesis. Shivering is rhythmic muscle contraction, whereas non-shivering thermogenesis is increased heat production not associated with muscle contraction, and is due to increased activity of the sympathetic nervous system (particularly in brown adipose tissue in small mammals). Non-shivering thermogenesis is inversely correlated with body size, age and ambient temperature and has been demonstrated to exist in adult human beings who are chronically exposed to extreme temperatures (Jessen, 1980).

5 *Diet-induced thermogenesis.* Heat production increases following the consumption of a meal, and this thermic effect of food is classically termed 'specific dynamic action'. Heat production also increases on a high plane of nutrition, the so-called 'luxusconsumption'. These two forms of thermogenesis related to food have been regrouped under the term 'diet-induced thermogenesis' or DIT, and are often divided into an *obligatory* component (related to the energy costs of absorption and metabolic processing of nutrients or the energy cost of tissue synthesis during overfeeding) and a *facultative* component, which in part results from the sensory aspects of foods (smell and taste) and in part from stimulation of the sympathetic nervous system.

6 *Drug-induced thermogenesis.* The consumption of caffeine, nicotine and alcohol may form an integral part of daily life for many individuals, and all three 'drugs of everyday life' stimulate thermogenesis (Dulloo, 1993). A cup of coffee (containing 60–80 mg of caffeine) can increase BMR by 5–10% over 1–2 h. Oral intake of 100 mg of caffeine every 2 h during the day or smoking of a packet of 20 cigarettes increases daily energy expenditure by 5% and 15% respectively. Furthermore, the thermogenic effects of nicotine are potentiated by caffeine. The cessation of elevated thermogenesis induced by nicotine, or nicotine and caffeine, may be a factor that contributes to the average weight gain of 7 kg after cessation of smoking.

Alternative compartmentalization of energy expenditure

Another way to look at the components of energy expenditure, proposed by Dulloo and Jacquet (2003) is shown in Fig. 5.3, where energy expenditure is divided into resting and non-resting expenditure, but also into voluntary and involuntary energy expenditure. Resting expenditure comprises all measurements of energy expenditure made at rest—BMR, as well as the thermic effects of food (and other food ingredients or drugs). Non-resting energy expenditure is divided into exercise (voluntary) and low level of involuntary physical activity, which is spontaneous and subconscious. Involuntary activity is often referred to as thermogenesis due to fidgeting or non-exercise activity thermogenesis (NEAT). The potential impor-

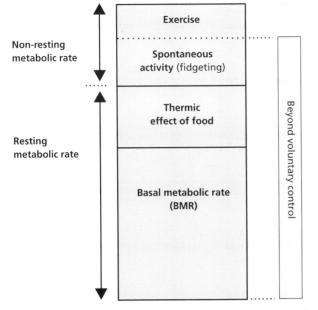

Fig. 5.3 Components of energy expenditure contributing to voluntary and involuntary control of energy expenditure.

tance of variations in this involuntary energy expenditure in body weight regulation is discussed below (in Thermogenesis associated with physical activity).

Timescale of energy balance

As mentioned in the Introduction, there is little doubt that regulation of body weight occurs in human beings (with varying degrees of precision), although the timescale over which it occurs is not clear. In this context, it is important to emphasize the cardinal features of human energy balance and weight regulation:

1 Human beings do not balance energy intake and energy expenditure on a day-to-day basis, nor is positive energy balance one day spontaneously compensated by negative energy balance the next day. Near equality of intake and expenditure most often appears over 1–2 weeks. Longer measurements are difficult to conduct and impractical because of cumulative errors, but there is no doubt that over months and years the total energy intake and expenditure must be very close in any individual whose body weight and body composition have remained relatively constant.

2 This matching of long-term energy intake and energy expenditure must be extremely precise, as a theoretical error of only 1% between input and output of energy, if persistent, will lead to a gain or loss of about 10 kg per decade. This does not occur for most individuals, whose weight remains constant, within a few kilograms, over several decades.

3 Even in adults who apparently maintain a stable body weight over months, years and decades, there is in reality no 'absolute' constancy of body weight. Instead, body weight tends to fluctuate or oscillate around a constant mean value.

Understanding how these short-term deviations in body weight are corrected through changes in energy intake, in energy expenditure, or in both, still remains a challenging issue for human research today. In such a dynamic state, within which weight homeostasis occurs, it is likely that long-term constancy of body weight is achieved through a highly complex network of autoregulatory systems and subsystems through which changes in food intake, body composition and energy expenditure are interlinked.

Control of food intake

Hunger and satiety

Research into the control of energy intake in humans is very difficult, primarily because habitual intake is not easy to measure and also because the intake of foods is altered by the experiments themselves. Because of these difficulties, much of the work carried out in humans has been concerned with short-term hunger and appetite studies, or with short-term satiety and satiation (Blundell *et al.*, 1996; Stubbs 1998).

It is important to differentiate between these terms. Hunger may be defined as a 'demand for calories' (e.g. after starvation), whereas appetite refers to 'a demand for a particular food'. In laboratory animals allowed *ad libitum* access to standard laboratory chow, energy intake is controlled mainly by the sensations of hunger and satiety. If (like human beings) the laboratory rat has access to a variety of palatable foods rather than to a monotonous diet, it may be stimulated to eat something delicious by appetite rather than by hunger. The physiological mechanisms that control energy intake in the rat certainly exist in man. If a person is deprived of food, he becomes hungry, and if he has eaten a lot, he becomes satiated. *Satiation* refers to processes involved in the termination of a meal, and is studied by providing individuals with test meals and measuring the amount consumed when the food is freely available. *Satiety* refers to the inhibition of further intake of a food and meal after eating has ended.

However, lifestyle factors ensure that appetite is a powerful but poorly controlled stimulus to eat even when not hungry because feeding patterns are influenced strongly by psychological, economic and social factors. Even though subjects may feel satiated by one particular food, they will continue to eat when a new food is presented—a phenomenon that is referred to as 'sensory specific satiety'. Conversely, when subjects are presented with a monotonous diet, their intakes are usually low. In many parts of the Third World, the major part of energy intake derives from one staple food, which, together with low fat intakes, constitutes a bland and monotonous diet, so that even when supplies are adequate, obesity is rarely seen. These observations suggest that when the psychosocial incen-

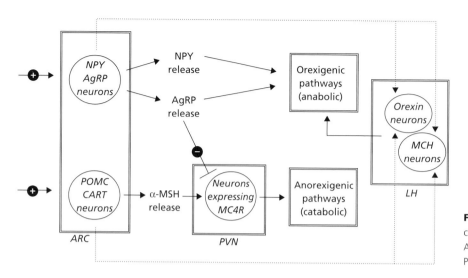

Fig. 5.4 Hypothalamic circuits implicated in the control of food intake (see text for details); ARC = arcuate nucleus; LH = lateral hypothalamus; PVN = paraventricular nucleus.

tives to eat are removed, human beings (like the laboratory rat fed a chow diet) can control food intake quite precisely.

Hunger–satiety control centres in the brain

Much of our understanding about centres in the brain that are involved with the control of food intake derives from studies conducted in laboratory animal models (Hillebrand *et al.*, 2002). As a result of numerous experiments involving ablation, electrical and chemical stimulation of specific areas in the brain, it has been proposed that 'centres' localized in the hypothalamus are involved in the control of feeding behaviour, and in particular in the ventromedial hypothalamic (VMH) region implicated in satiety, the lateral hypothalamic (LH) region implicated in the initiation of feeding, and the paraventricular nucleus (PVN) of the rostral hypothalamus, thought to be important in initiating the cessation of the meal. These 'centres' serve to analyse and integrate afferent signals that are neural (via the vagal nerve) or circulatory (via nutrients and hormones) in origin. Although these centres have received a great deal of attention, it is now apparent that this represents a rather simplistic view because many other hypothalamic and extrahypothalamic areas also play a major role in the control of food intake (Berthoud, 2002).

Nonetheless, the molecular and genetic studies over the past decade have led to major advancements in elucidating the neurochemical basis for the activities of some of these centres (Schwartz *et al.*, 2000; Flier, 2004). In particular, the identification of the two subpopulations of neurons in the arcuate (ARC)–PVN pathway (*NPY/Agouti-related peptide* (*AgRP*) neurons and *proopiomelanocortin* (*POMC*)/*cocaine and cocaine–amphetamine-related transcript* (*CART*) neurons) and the identification of melanin-concentrating hormone (MCH) and orexin in the LH neurons have provided neurochemical insight into the function of these sites (depicted in Fig. 5.4), namely:

1 The *NPY/AgRP* neurons, which coexpress *NPY* (neuropeptide Y) and *AgRP* (Agouti-related peptide), are orexigenic, i.e. their activation stimulates food intake.

2 By contrast, the *POMC/CART* neurons are anorexigenic, i.e. their activation reduces food intake. *POMC* is cleaved into melanocortins, including α-melanocyte stimulating hormone (α-MSH), which exerts anorexigenic action via melanocortin-4 receptors (Mc4r) and, to a lesser extent, via Mc3r. Most arcuate nucleus *POMC* neurons also express *CART*.

3 All of these neurons project to other regions of the hypothalamus, where further signal processing occurs and, in particular, in the LH area to populations of neurons expressing MCH and orexins A and B, all peptides that are orexigenic.

These pathways respond to afferent signals from other hypothalamic/extrahypothalamic regions and from the periphery.

Hunger–satiety signals from the periphery

The sensations of hunger and satiety result from the central integration of numerous signals originating from a variety of peripheral tissues and organs, including the gastrointestinal tract, liver, pancreas and adipose tissue, and perhaps also skeletal muscle. The putative hunger–satiety signalling systems that have generated the most interest are outlined below.

Signals from the gastrointestinal tract

The progression of food through the stomach and small intestine—which can be considered as a short-term nutrient reservoir—initiates a number of sequential peripheral satiety signals that are thought to be important in influencing meal-to-meal feeding responses. Signals from stretch- and mechanoreceptors or from chemoreceptors that respond to the products of digestion (sugars, fatty acids, amino acids and peptides) are transmitted via vagal afferent nerves to the hindbrain, where integration of this visceral output occurs. This provides a pathway whereby the physical and chemical properties of food can have a major role in the short-term regulation of food intake by limiting the size of a single meal (Havel, 2001). These types of signals may also affect energy intake in a subsequent meal. Among endocrine signals from the gut that are believed to exert important influences on food intake are:

1 cholecystokinin (CCK), released from the small intestine into the circulation in response to luminal nutrients, which decreases meal size;

2 peptides that are released postprandially and reduce appetite in humans, including gastric inhibitory peptide (GIP), glucagon-like peptide-1 (GLP-1) and PYY, the peptide YY(3–36); and

3 more recently, the (growth hormone-related peptide) hormone ghrelin, whose concentration increases after food deprivation and decreases in response to the presence of nutrients in the stomach (Tschop *et al.*, 2001).

It is now well established that ghrelin, which is secreted by the stomach, is a powerful stimulator of feeding and can induce obesity when given chronically in rodents (Tschop *et al.*, 2000), through its modulation of *NPY*, *AgRP* and melanocortin systems in the arcuate–PVN axis (Flier, 2004). In contrast, CCK reduces food intake and inhibits gastric emptying through actions on CCKA receptors and afferent vagal information passing to the brainstem regions of the CNS. A physiological role for CCK in the control of meal size is suggested by the obesity seen in rats that have a natural deletion of this gene (Moran, 2000).

Aminostatic or protein-static signals

A link between fluctuations in serum amino acids and food intake was proposed nearly 50 years ago (Mellinkoff *et al.*, 1956), and this topic has more recently been reviewed by Bray (1997). Dietary protein induces satiety in the short term, and consumption of low-protein diets leads to increased appetite for protein-containing foods. Administration of amino acids such as phenylalanine and tryptophan, which are precursors of monoamine neurotransmitters, leads to reduced food intake, and the ratio of plasma tryptophan to other amino acids affects brain serotonin, which is known to have an inhibitory influence on food intake. These observations lead to an *aminostatic* theory, which states that food intake is determined by the level of plasma amino acids, and that this could be related to the regulation of lean body mass, which is known to be rigorously defended against experimental or dietary manipulation. A 'protein-stat' mechanism for the regulation of lean body mass has been proposed by Millward (1995), and draws support from the fact that food intake during growth is known to be dominated by the impetus for lean tissue deposition.

Glucostatic and glycogenostatic signals

A glucostatic theory for the regulation of feeding behaviour was also proposed some 50 years ago (Mayer, 1953). It proposes that there are chemoreceptors in the hypothalamic satiety centre that are sensitive to the arteriovenous difference in glucose or to the availability and utilization of glucose. The arguments in favour of this hypothesis in humans include (a) the small decreases of blood glucose observed prior to spontaneous meal consumption; (b) the suppression of food intake induced by infusion of glucose; and (c) the spontaneous decrease in total energy intake observed when dietary carbohydrate content is increased. These same arguments in support of the glucostatic theory of food intake also form the basis of the proposal of Flatt (1995) that the control of food intake, via the prevention of hypoglycaemia and maintenance of adequate glycogen levels, primarily serves the maintenance of the carbohydrate balance (see Integrated models of food intake control).

Lipostatic and adiposity signals

A lipostatic theory of food intake control, first proposed by Kennedy (1953), postulates that substances released from the fat stores function as satiety signals. This theory is based on a set point control system, with body fat (rather than body weight) acting as the regulated variable and energy intake as the controlled variable. Body fat is thus maintained at a set value, and any deviation from this value is detected by the controller of the system (the hypothalamus) via a circulating metabolite (the error signal) that is related to the size of the fat stores. Having detected such a deviation, the controller elicits compensatory changes in energy intake and hence restores the system to its pre-set or preferred level. The lipostatic hypothesis is perhaps the one that provides the most plausible explanation for long-term regulation of the fat stores. Many experiments support this theory, leading to the suggestion that humans who are predisposed to obesity may have a homeostatic mechanism in which the set point for weight regulation is set at a higher level than in those who are more resistant to obesity. The nature of the various components, such as the set point and feedback signal(s), involved in the lipostatic theory remains unclear.

Leptin and insulin

A major advance came in the mid-1990s following the cloning of the *ob* gene, whose protein product (leptin) is primarily produced by adipocytes, released into the circulation and acts on hypothalamic receptors to induce satiety by inhibiting the orexigenic *NPY/AgRP* neurons and stimulating the anorexigenic *POMC/CART* neurons (Schwartz *et al.*, 2000; Flier, 2004) (Figs 5.4 and 5.5). Rare people with mutations causing complete leptin deficiency, as in the *ob/ob* mice, show marked hyperphagia and severe obesity, which can be reversed by administration of small doses of leptin. Rare people with

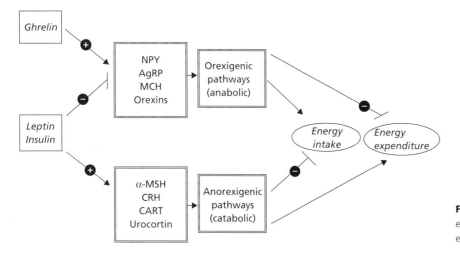

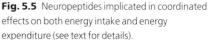

Fig. 5.5 Neuropeptides implicated in coordinated effects on both energy intake and energy expenditure (see text for details).

mutations affecting the leptin receptor mechanism, like the *dbdb* mice, also show hyperphagia and severe obesity, but do not respond to the administration of leptin. In other rare cases of severe childhood onset obesity, single gene defects have been identified for genes which code for proteins that act downstream to the leptin receptor in the hypothalamic neural circuits (Fig. 5.4), in particular for *POMC* and Mc4r. However, in the vast majority of humans, as in laboratory rodents, the blood concentration of leptin is proportional to the adipose mass, and its elevation in obese people has led to the hypothesis that resistance to the action of leptin is a factor in obesity. Because blood leptin concentration varies widely in individuals with the same degree of obesity, the possibility arises that subpopulations might have relative leptin deficiency. Support for this notion can be derived from the fact that relatives of leptin-deficient patients, who are heterozygous for leptin deficiency exhibit modest obesity and leptin levels below that expected for their increased fat mass (Farooqi *et al.*, 2001).

More recently, there has been a resurgence of interest in the role of insulin as an adiposity signal (as it is secreted by the pancreas in proportion to adiposity) in the control of food intake via the CNS. Like leptin, insulin also circulates at levels proportional to body fat content and enters the CNS (in proportion to their plasma level), where it interacts with autonomic circuits that control meal size—including, as indicated in Figs 5.4 and 5.5, via inhibition of *NPY/AgRP* neurons and stimulation of *POMC/CART* neurons (Schwartz *et al.*, 2000). Targeted deletion of the insulin receptor in neurons leads to obesity in mice (Bruning *et al.*, 2000), albeit to a much lesser extent compared with the severe obesity resulting from deletion of leptin receptors from neurons (Cohen *et al.*, 2001).

Although leptin/insulin levels and fat mass are correlated, their rapid fall during starvation and rapid restoration on refeeding suggest that changes in circulating leptin and insulin are independent of the dynamics of acute changes in body fat content. Hence their circulating levels may be a function of changes in the flux of energy intake (coupled with fat

mobilization/storage) rather than a 'lipostatic' signal whose level is altered as a function of the degree of depletion and repletion of the fat stores. Within the context of food intake control based upon the defence of the fat stores, both the feedback signal on food intake and the nature of the set point (if it exists) remain elusive.

Hepatic nutrient metabolism signals

A role for hepatic metabolism in the control of food intake has been advocated in the 1960s (Russek, 1963), and it now appears that a common pathway, leading from nutrient metabolism to ATP production and cell membrane polarity changes, may be involved in the signalling mechanism (Langhans, 1996; Friedman, 1997). The notion that hepatic oxidation of fatty acids plays a role in the control of food intake is based upon studies in rat, mice and man, showing that pharmacological inhibition of fatty acid oxidation leads to an increase in food intake, which, in the rat, has been shown to be attenuated by hepatic branch vagotomy (Langhans, 2003). It would appear therefore that a feeding modulatory signal derived from fatty acid oxidation in abdominal tissues (as in the liver) is conveyed to the brain by vagal afferents. However, in contrast to the stimulatory effect of feeding by inhibition of fatty acid oxidation, the evidence for a suppressive effect of feeding by stimulation of fatty acid oxidation is inconsistent and comparatively weak.

Integrated models of food intake control

These various hunger–satiety signals from the periphery can be integrated in models in which the control of food intake is considered in three phases, but each with a distinct goal:
1 *short-term* (hour to hour) blood glucose homeostasis by dampening episodes of hypoglycaemia or hyperglycaemia;
2 *medium-term* (day-to-day) maintenance of adequate hepatic stores of glycogen that, consistent with Flatt's glycogenostatic

theory (Flatt, 1995), would imply corrective responses to offset deviations from carbohydrate balance during the previous day; and

3 *long-term* (weeks, months or years) maintenance of the body's fat and protein compartments, i.e. fat mass and fat-free mass.

Periods of food deprivation that lead to substantial reductions in body weight are normally followed by increased food intake (hyperphagia). Indeed, the reanalysis of data on food intake and body composition in humans subjected to experimental semistarvation and refeeding in the classic Minnesota Experiment (Keys *et al.*, 1950) suggests that the duration and magnitude of such compensatory hyperphagia is determined by three independent factors:

1 the magnitude of fat loss;
2 the magnitude of fat-free mass loss; and
3 the severity of energy deprivation (Dulloo *et al.*, 1997).

These findings are consistent with the existence of powerful signals that relate food intake to body composition as well as to psychobiological reaction to the state of food deprivation. Conversely, in human overfeeding trials, subjects often report great difficulty in maintaining high levels of food intake over long periods of time, and they spontaneously lose weight over subsequent weeks and months, apparently by eating less (Keys *et al.*, 1950; Garrow, 1974).

According to the model proposed by Flatt (1995), the long-term stability of body weight and body composition requires not only that energy expenditure is equal to energy intake, but also that the composition of the fuel mix that is oxidized follows that which is ingested. As the protein and carbohydrate stores in the body are limited, they tend to be modulated by an autoregulatory process, allowing an increase in their own oxidation in response to an increase in their exogenous supply. In contrast, the stores of fat are not well regulated by fat oxidation, as an increase in dietary fat does not promote its oxidation. Hence (unlike carbohydrate and protein) fat balance is not precisely regulated. The failure to adjust fat oxidation in response to excess intake will contribute to depletion of glycogen stores by increasing carbohydrate oxidation, with consequential negative feedback on total energy intake. In other words, the size of carbohydrate stores exerts negative feedback on total energy intake, so that high-fat diets (containing little carbohydrate) will promote excess energy intake to reach an appropriate level of carbohydrate intake. This energy imbalance would persist until the fat stores build up sufficiently to provide a greater supply for fat oxidation. When the higher fat oxidation matches the higher intake, the individual would then be both in fat balance and in energy balance, but at a higher percentage of body fat. Indeed, obese individuals have a significantly lower respiratory quotient (RQ) than lean people (Schutz, 1995) and hence a greater proportion of their elevated energy expenditure is met by fat oxidation. The interpretation of this concept of nutrient balance is that the control of food intake can be viewed as both glycogenic (short term) and lipostatic (long term), and tends to integrate control of food intake via glycogenostatic and lipostatic signalling. Furthermore, it also explains the role of alcohol in substrate metabolism; alcohol disrupts nutrient balance by sparing fat from oxidation. It may also lead to overconsumption of energy as it is generally consumed in addition to normal food intake.

This nutrient balance theory, which centres upon the need to maintain specific carbohydrate (glycogen) stores as a determinant of appetite, has been challenged by Stubbs (1995); appetite did not increase in people who were fed a very low carbohydrate (high-fat) diet to deplete the glycogen stores, and fat oxidation increased to meet energy needs. Furthermore, in human studies in which fat content was altered from 24% to 47% but the energy density of the diet was maintained constant, there was no evidence of high-fat-induced hyperphagia relative to high-carbohydrate feeding, indicating that the hyperphagia often associated with high-fat diets may not be due to the fat per se, but to the higher energy density (and hence lower volume and weight) that fat contributes to the diet. As Frayn (1995) has argued, it is too simplistic to argue that protein, carbohydrate and fat balance can be considered independently, and that the complex relationships between fat and other constituents of foods in the control of appetite cannot be ignored.

Autoregulatory adjustments in energy expenditure

Whatever mechanisms operate for the control of food intake, however, this control is not by itself sufficient to explain long-term regulation of body weight and body composition. There is ample evidence that autoregulatory adjustments in energy expenditure also play an important role in correcting deviations in body weight and body composition.

The dynamic equilibrium model

There is a built-in stabilizing mechanism in the overall homeostatic system for body weight regulation. As Payne and Dugdale (1977) have illustrated in their mathematical model for weight regulation, any imbalance between energy intake and energy requirements will result in a change in body weight which, in turn, will alter the maintenance energy requirements in a direction that will tend to counter the original imbalance and would hence be stabilizing. There is a built-in negative feedback and the system thus exhibits *dynamic equilibrium*. For example, an increase in body weight will increase metabolic rate, which will then produce a negative energy balance and hence a subsequent decline in body weight.

Similarly, a reduction in body weight would also be automatically corrected as the resulting diminished metabolic rate due to the loss in weight will produce a positive balance and hence a subsequent return towards the 'set' or 'preferred' weight. But in reality, the homeostatic system is much more complex than this simple effect of *mass action*. This is shown in the 'weight-clamping' experiments of Leibel and colleagues (1995), whereby subjects maintaining body weight at 10% above their initial weight showed an increase in daily energy expenditure, even after adjusting for changes in body weight and composition. Similarly, in subjects maintaining weight at 10% below their initial weight, daily energy expenditure was also lower after adjusting for losses in weight and lean tissues.

These compensatory changes in energy expenditure (about 15% above or below predicted values) reflect changes in metabolic efficiency (i.e. thermogenesis) that oppose the maintenance of a body weight that is above or below the 'set' or 'preferred' body weight. There was a large interindividual variability in the ability to readjust energy expenditure in this study, with some individuals showing little or no evidence of altered metabolic efficiency, whereas others showed a marked capacity to decrease or increase energy expenditure through alterations in metabolic efficiency.

Role of adaptive thermogenesis

The most striking feature of virtually all experiments of human overfeeding is the wide range of individual variability in the amount of weight gained per unit of excess energy consumed. These differences in the efficiency of weight gain are mostly attributed to (a) variability in the ability to convert excess calories to heat, i.e. in the large interindividual capacity for diet-induced thermogenesis (DIT), and (b) differences in body composition for the same change in body weight. In his detailed reanalysis of data from some 150 individuals participating in the various 'gluttony experiments' conducted between 1965 and 1999, Stock (1999) argued that at least 40% of these overfed subjects must have exhibited an increase in DIT, albeit to varying degrees. Part of this variation in DIT could be explained by differences in the dietary protein content of the diet, with DIT being more pronounced on unbalanced diets that are low or high in percentage of protein.

But it is also known from overfeeding experiments in identical twins that genes play an important role in the variability in metabolism that underlies susceptibility to weight gain and obesity (Bouchard *et al.*, 1990). Similarly a role for genotype in variability in enhanced metabolic efficiency during weight loss has been suggested from studies in which identical twins underwent slimming therapy on a very low-calorie diet (Hainer *et al.*, 2001). Taken together, these results demonstrate that, in addition to the control of food intake, changes in efficiency of energy utilization (via adaptive thermogenesis) play an important role in the regulation of body weight and body composition, and that the magnitude of adaptive changes in thermogenesis is strongly influenced by the genetic make-up of the individual.

Thermogenesis associated with physical activity

A main cause of controversy about the importance of adaptive thermogenesis in the aetiology of human obesity is the difficulty of identifying which component(s) of energy expenditure could be contributing importantly to the changes in metabolic efficiency, and hence in adaptive thermogenesis. As depicted in Fig. 5.3, the energy expenditure measured in the resting state, whether as basal metabolic rate (BMR) or as thermic effect of food, results in the production of heat (i.e. in thermogenesis). Changes in resting energy expenditure that are not accounted for by changes in body weight and composition reflect changes in metabolic efficiency, and hence in adaptive changes in thermogenesis. By contrast, the heat production from non-resting energy expenditure is more difficult to quantify.

The efficiency of muscular contraction during exercise is low (~25%), but that of spontaneous physical activity (SPA) (including fidgeting, muscle tone and posture maintenance, and other low-level physical activities of everyday life) is even lower as these essentially involuntary (subconscious) activities comprise a larger proportion of isometric work. As the energy actually expended for work on the environment during SPA is very small compared with the total energy spent on such activities, the energy cost associated with SPA is sometimes referred to as movement-associated thermogenesis or SPA-associated thermogenesis. It can also be argued that as SPA is essentially beyond voluntary control (i.e. subconscious), a change in the *level* or *amount* of such involuntary SPA activity in a direction that defends a 'preferred' body weight constitutes autoregulatory mechanisms that contribute to the overall changes in metabolic efficiency. In this context, an increase in the amount of SPA in response to overfeeding, or a decrease during starvation, also constitutes adaptive behavioural changes in thermogenesis.

The importance of SPA-associated thermogenesis in weight regulation is underscored by the findings that even under conditions where subjects are confined to a metabolic chamber, the 24-h energy expenditure attributed to SPA (as assessed by radar systems) was found to vary between 400 and 3000 kJ per day, and to be a predictor of subsequent weight gain. In fact, a main conclusion of early overfeeding experiments (Miller *et al.*, 1967) was that most of the extra heat dissipation in some of the individuals resisting obesity by increased DIT could not be accounted for by an increase in resting metabolic rate, but could be due to an increased energy expenditure associated with simple (low-level) activities of everyday life. This notion has recently gained much support from the findings of Levine *et al.* (1999) that more than 60% of the increase in total daily energy expenditure in response to overfeeding was associated with SPA, and that interindividual variability in energy expenditure associated with SPA—which they referred to as non-exercise activity thermogenesis (NEAT)—was the most significant predictor of the resistance or susceptibility to obesity. It should however be emphasized that NEAT could also include heat production resulting from the impact of physical activity on post-absorptive metabolic rate or postprandial thermogenesis. There is some evidence that relatively low-intensity exercise may potentiate the thermic effect of food, and that the effect of high-intensity exercise on energy expenditure can persist well after the period of the physical activity—this phenomenon is often referred to as post-exercise or post-SPA stimulation of thermogenesis.

Mechanisms of thermogenesis

Ever since studies into mechanisms of DIT started in 1960s, the focus of attention has been on the sympathetic nervous system (SNS) which, via its neurotransmitter noradrenaline (NA), acts upon α- and β-adrenoceptors to influence many body functions ranging from body temperature homeostasis to blood pressure regulation. It is now known that many other hormones play a more permissive or facilitatory role in SNS-mediated thermogenesis, either by altering peripheral adrenergic responsiveness to the thermogenic effects of NA or by acting as peripheral signals for central activation of SNS activity to peripheral tissues. In fact, the interaction of many of the peripheral signals (in Hunger–satiety signals from the periphery) that control feeding behaviour and satiety—via inhibition of NPY/AgRP neurons and stimulation of POMC/CART neurons in the hypothalamus—also results in altered activity of the SNS and thermogenesis (Flier, 2004).

Of particular interest for SNS-mediated thermogenesis is the potential control by NA over biochemical mechanisms, the activation of which leads either to an increased use of ATP (e.g. ion pumping and substrate cycling) or to a high rate of mitochondrial oxidation with poor coupling of ATP synthesis; the net result is an increase in heat production. But it was not until the demonstration that SNS activity in a variety of tissues is increased during overfeeding and decreased during starvation (a state of energy conservation) that the SNS was considered as a potentially pivotal efferent system in the link between diet and thermogenesis (Landsberg *et al.*, 1984). In fact, recent studies in mice lacking genes coding for all three β-adrenoceptors (β_1-AR, β_2-AR and β_3-AR) demonstrate a pivotal role for the SNS in the mediation of DIT (Bachman *et al.*, 2002). In contrast with wild-type mice, which resist obesity by activating DIT during overfeeding, mice lacking β-ARs (or β-less mice) are incapable of increasing thermogenesis and they develop massive obesity despite similar food intake to wild-type control mice. Furthermore, the β-less mice are intolerant to cold exposure, thereby underscoring the overlapping role of SNS via β-AR signalling in the control of heat production in response both to diet and cold.

It was indeed proposed some 20 years ago (Rothwell and Stock, 1979) that these two forms of thermogenesis have a common origin in brown adipose tissue (BAT). The thermogenic activity of BAT, which is abundant in small animals and human infants, is under SNS control and is primarily mediated in brown adipocytes by a mitochondrial protein (UCP) that allows protons to leak back across the inner mitochondrial membrane (Cannon and Nedergaard, 2004). The resulting dissipation of the proton electrochemical gradient (a phenomenon referred to as 'proton leak') allows substrate oxidation to occur without concomitant capture of some of the useful energy via the synthesis of ATP. The net effect during activation of UCP (by cold or diet) is that substrate oxidation is effectively uncoupled from phosphorylation with a resultant increase in heat production.

Although in humans, several lines of evidence are consistent with an important role for SNS in the regulation of thermogenesis (Landsberg *et al.*, 1984; Astrup and Macdonald 1998), the importance of BAT as a site of adaptive thermogenesis in the adult human proved to be elusive. Doubts about the importance and/or recruitability of BAT-UCP or β_3-adrenoceptors in adult human beings (Arch, 2002a) have shifted greater attention to the skeletal muscle, which by its sheer size (30–40% of body weight) and important contribution to daily metabolic rate (> 20% even in 'sedentary' humans) has long been advocated as the major site for adaptive thermogenesis in large mammals.

It was reported in the mid-1990s (Rolfe and Brand, 1996) that the phenomenon of mitochondrial 'proton leak' is not unique to BAT as originally thought, but also exists in tissues other than BAT. The fact that this could contribute as much as 50% of the skeletal muscle heat production at rest prompted the search for uncoupling protein(s) in this tissue. This led to the discoveries of several new members of the 'uncoupling' protein family, particularly two of them, UCP2, UCP3, which have a high sequence homology to BAT-UCP, which was renamed UCP1. Unlike UCP1, which is expressed only in BAT, UCP2 is expressed in all tissues so far examined (including organs involved in immunity or rich in macrophages), whereas UCP3 is expressed predominantly in skeletal muscles and BAT, and, to a lower extent, in white adipose tissue and in the heart.

Although a number of studies have linked polymorphisms of UCP2 and UCP3 with obesity or with low rates of energy expenditure (Walder *et al.*, 1998), there is, however, considerable uncertainty and debate about whether these UCP1 homologues have physiologically relevant uncoupling properties in the context of adaptive thermogenesis and weight homeostasis (Samec *et al.*, 1998; Dulloo and Samec, 2001). In more recent years, the interest about molecular effectors of thermogenesis has focused on the co-activator protein PGC-1, a mediator of cold-induced thermogenesis in brown adipocytes (Puigserver *et al.*, 1998) and whose overexpression in skeletal muscle leads to a change of the muscle from white to red fibre type (Lin *et al.*, 2002). However, as yet there is no published evidence regarding a physiological role for PGC-1 in skeletal muscle thermogenesis and DIT.

From which tissues/organs and by what molecular mechanisms the extra heat due to DIT might be produced still remains a mystery (Dulloo, 2002). Several other tissues and

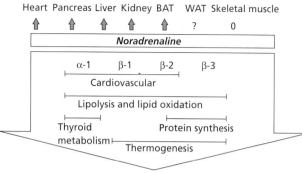

Fig. 5.6 Sympathetic nervous system (SNS) activity in various organs/tissues in response to food. The stippled arrows imply marked increases in SNS activity, as assessed by techniques for measuring 24-h norepinephrine (NA) turnover rates, in rat heart, pancreas, liver, kidney, brown adipose tissue (BAT), white adipose tissue (WAT) and skeletal muscle; the symbols '0' and '?' indicate no significant or unknown changes respectively. Through the release of its neurotransmitter NA, which acts on some or all of various adrenoceptors (α, β_1, β_2 and β_3) present in these tissues/organs, the activated SNS might then coordinate cardiovascular and metabolic events that converge towards increased production of heat—i.e. diet-induced thermogenesis (DIT) (adapted from Dulloo, 2002).

organs (e.g. liver, kidneys, heart, pancreas) are activated by the SNS in response to diet (Fig. 5.6), but whether they contribute to DIT is unknown. As for skeletal muscle, evidence that SNS-mediated thermogenesis occurs in this tissue remains elusive. SNS activity in skeletal muscle of rats is unresponsive to starvation and overfeeding (Dulloo *et al.*, 1988), and in adult humans (where BAT is scarce or quiescent), infusion of NE increases resting metabolic rate, but no detectable increase in thermogenesis occurred in forearm skeletal muscle (Kurpad *et al.*, 1994). Nonetheless, like in rodents, modulation of SNS activity by short-term under- and overnutrition occurs in adult humans, as judged from measurements of NE spillover in blood and urine (Landsberg *et al.*, 1984), and furthermore, a low SNS activity has been shown to be a risk factor for weight gain in Pima Indians (Tataranni *et al.*, 1997).

The central issue of whether in humans the subtle variations in DIT—that over months and years lead to obesity in some but weight maintenance in others—also reside in variations in SNS activity remains to be firmly established, just as the tissue/organ sites and molecular mechanisms that could account for this variability in metabolic efficiency.

Models for body composition regulation via adaptive thermogenesis

Despite major caveats in our understanding of organ sites and molecular mechanisms controlling adaptive thermogenesis, the available evidence, based on studies in the rat and in humans, strongly suggests the existence of two distinct control systems underlying adaptive thermogenesis (Dulloo *et al.*,

2002). One control system is a direct function of energy imbalance and responds rapidly to attenuate the impact of changes in food intake on changes in body weight through alterations in the activity of the SNS; it is suppressed during starvation and increased during overfeeding. The other control system has a much slower time constant as it operates as a feedback loop between the size of the fat stores and thermogenesis (i.e. a lipostatic or adipose-specific control of thermogenesis). Whereas its suppression during weight (and fat) losses is to reduce the overall rate of fuel utilization during starvation, its sustained suppression until body fat is recovered during refeeding is to accelerate the replenishment of the fat stores. Conversely, during periods of excess fat gain, its activation will serve to oppose the maintenance of the excess fat and hence to restore body fat to its 'set' or 'preferred' level.

These autoregulatory control systems, operating through adjustments in heat production or thermogenesis, play a crucial role in attenuating and correcting deviations of body weight from its 'set' or 'preferred' value. The extent to which these adjustments are brought about through adaptive thermogenesis is dependent upon the environment (e.g. diet composition), and is highly variable from one individual to another, largely because of variations in the genetic make-up among individuals. In societies where food is plentiful all year round and physical activity demands are low, the resultant subtle variations among individuals in adaptive thermogenesis can, in dynamic systems and over the long term, be important in determining long-term constancy of body weight in some and in provoking the drift towards obesity in others (Dulloo and Jacquet, 2003).

Integrating intake and expenditure

Modern lifestyle has led to considerable changes in what food is eaten and in the amount of physical activity, within an environment where the precise matching between energy intake and energy expenditure is difficult. Yet, there are many individuals living in the same 'obesogenic' environment who manage to resist obesity. How they achieve energy balance is likely to be importantly determined by highly complex neuroendocrine systems and subsystems, some of which could be integrated in the simple model presented in Fig. 5.7. However, it needs to be pointed out that, despite the advances of the past decade in our understanding of molecular pathways and control systems underlying the regulation of body weight and body composition, the explanation for an accurate regulation of long-term body weight in the face of poor short-term control still remains a challenging issue for human research. When 1attempting to explain the actual responses in energy balance and weight regulation in real life, it is important to recognize that several factors may be operating simultaneously on both sides of the energy balance equation. In order to achieve long-term constancy of body weight, compensatory adjustments

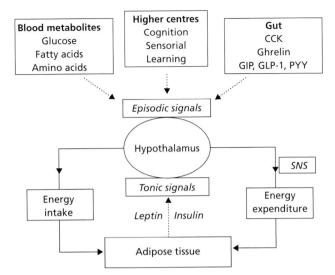

Fig. 5.7 Integrating energy intake and energy expenditure in an overview of energy balance (adapted from Arch, 2002b).

occur in both energy intake and energy expenditure, so that unravelling the importance of one or other is difficult, if not impossible.

Models of body weight regulation have primarily focused on physiologically induced *autoregulatory* adjustments in energy intake and in energy expenditure, i.e. those beyond voluntary control. However, the range of variation in body weight is large enough to be detected consciously and there is certainly some degree of cognitive control. As pointed out by Garrow (1974), a change of several kilograms in body weight can hardly be ignored as clothes that formerly would fit will no longer do so, and there will be conceivable changes in appearance, exercise tolerance and general well-being. When such chronic energy imbalance occurs during adolescent or adult life, it is also corrected by more or less conscious effort when the individual decides—for efficient survival, cultural or health reasons—that the change in body weight is no longer acceptable. In response, they control or attempt to control food intake or energy expenditure via changes in physical activity. In many individuals, the importance of such cognitive (conscious) controls over food intake and energy expenditure can be as important as non-conscious physiological controls in achieving energy balance and weight homeostasis.

References

Arch, J.R.S. (2002a) Beta-3-adrenoceptor agonists: potential pitfalls and progress. *European Journal of Pharmacology* **440**, 99–107.

Arch, J.R.S. (2002b) Lessons in obesity from transgenic animals. *Journal of Endocrinological Investigation* **25**, 867–875.

Astrup, A. and MacDonald, I.A. (1998) Sympathoadrenal system and metabolism. In: Bray, G.A., Bouchard, C. and James, W.P.T. eds. *Handbook of Obesity*. New York: Marcel Dekker, 491–511.

Bachman, E.S., Dhillon, H., Zhang, C.Y., Cinti, S., Bianco, A.C.,

Kobilka, B.K. and Lowell, B.B. (2002) BetaAR signaling required for diet-induced thermogenesis and obesity resistance. *Science* **297**, 843–845.

Berthoud, H.R. (2002) Multiple neural systems controlling food intake and body weight. *Neuroscience Biobehavioural Review* **26**, 393–428.

Blundell, J.E., Lawton, C.L., Cotton, J.R. and Macdiarmid, J.I. (1996) Control of human appetite: implications for the intake of dietary fat. *Annual Review of Nutrition* **16**, 285–319.

Bouchard, C., Tremblay, A., Desprès, J.P., Nadeau, A., Lupien, P.J., Theriault, G., Dussault, J., Moorjani, S., Pinault, S. and Fournier, G. (1990) The response to long-term overfeeding in identical twins. *New England Journal of Medicine* **322**, 1477–1482.

Bray, G.A. (1997) Amino acids, protein and body weight. *Obesity Research* **5**, 373–379.

Bruning, J.C., Gautam, D., Burks, D.J., Gillette, J., Schubert, M., Orban, P.C., Klein, R., Krone, W., Muller-Wieland, D. and Kahn, C.R. (2000) Role of brain insulin receptor in control of body weight and reproduction. *Science* **289**, 2122–2125.

Cannon, B. and Nedergaard, J. (2004) Brown adipose tissue: function and physiological significance. *Physiology Review* **84**, 277–359.

Cohen, P., Zhao, C., Cai, X., Montez, J.M., Rohani, S.C., Feinstein, P., Mombaerts, P. and Friedman, J.M. (2001) Selective deletion of leptin receptor in neurons leads to obesity. *Journal of Clinical Investigation* **108**, 1113–1121.

Corey, E.L. (1948) Pilot metabolism and respiratory activity during varied flight tasks. *Journal of Applied Physiology* **1**, 35–44.

Dauncey, M.J. (1981) Influence of mild cold on 24 hour energy expenditure, resting metabolism and diet-induced thermogenesis. *British Journal of Nutrition* **45**, 257–267.

Dulloo, A.G. (1993) Strategies to counteract readjustments toward lower metabolic rates during obesity management. *Nutrition* **9**, 366–372.

Dulloo, A.G. (2002) A sympathetic defense against obesity. *Science* **297**, 780–781.

Dulloo, A.G. and Samec, S. (2001) Uncoupling proteins: their roles in adaptive thermogenesis and substrate metabolism reconsidered. *British Journal of Nutrition* **86**, 123–139.

Dulloo, A.G. and Jacquet, J. (2003) Adaptive thermogenesis is important in the aetiology of human obesity. *Ninth International Congress of Obesity*. Medeiros-Neto, G., Halpern, A. and Bouchard, C. eds. Hampshire: John Libbey, 708–712.

Dulloo, A.G., Young J.B. and Landsberg, L. (1988) Sympathetic nervous system responses to cold exposure and diet in rat skeletal muscle. *American Journal of Physiology* **255**, E180–E188.

Dulloo, A.G., Jacquet, J. and Girardier, L. (1997) Poststarvation hyperphagia and body fat overshooting in humans: a role for feedback signals from lean and fat tissues. *American Journal of Clinical Nutrition* **65**, 717–723.

Dulloo, A.G., Jacquet, J. and Montani, J.P. (2002) Pathways from weight fluctuations to metabolic diseases: focus on maladaptive thermogenesis during catch-up fat. *International Journal of Obesity* **26** (Suppl. 2), S46–S57.

Durnin, J.V.G.A. (1991) Practical estimates of energy requirements. *Journal of Nutrition* **121**, 1907–1913.

Durnin, J.V.G.A. and Passmore, R. (1972) *Energy, Work and Leisure*. London: Livingstone.

Elia, M. (1996) Fuel of the tissues. In: Garrow, J.S., James, W.P.T. and Ralph, A. eds. *Human Nutrition and Dietetics*, 10th edn. Edinburgh: Churchill Livingstone, 37–59.

Farooqi, I.S., Keogh, J.M., Kamath, S., Jones, S., Gibson, W.T., Trussell, R., Jebb, S.A., Lip, G.Y. and O'Rahilly, S. (2001) Partial leptin deficiency and human obesity. *Nature* **414**, 34–35.

Flatt, J.P. (1995) Diet, lifestyle and weight maintenance. *American Journal of Clinical Nutrition* **62**, 820–836.

Flier, J.F. (2004) Obesity wars: molecular progress confronts an expanding epidemic. *Cell* **116**, 337–350.

Frayn, K.N. (1995) Physiological regulation of macronutrient balance. *International Journal of Obesity* **19** (Suppl. 5), S4–10.

Friedman, M.I. (1997) An energy sensor for control of energy intake. *Proceedings of the Nutrition Society* **56**, 41–50.

Garrow, J.S. (1974) *Energy Balance and Obesity in Man*. Amsterdam: North-Holland Publishing Company.

Hainer, V., Stunkard, A.J., Kunesova, M., Parizkova, J., Stich, V. and Allison, D.B. (2001) A twin study of weight loss and metabolic efficiency. *International Journal of Obesity* **25**, 533–537.

Havel, P.J. (2001) Peripheral signals conveying metabolic information to the brain: short-term and long-term regulation of food intake and energy homeostasis. *Experimental Biological Medicine* **226**, 963–977.

Hillebrand, J.J., de Wied, D. and Adan, R.A. (2002) Neuropeptides, food intake and body weight regulation: a hypothalamic focus. *Peptides* **23**, 2283–2306.

Jessen, K. (1980) An assessment of human regulatory nonshivering thermogenesis. *Acta Anaesthesia Scandinavica* **24**, 138–143.

Kennedy, A.G. (1953) The role of the fat depot in the hypothalamic control of food intake in the rat. *Proceedings of the Royal Society of London Board of Biological Science* **140**, 578–592.

Keys, A., Brozek, J., Hanschel, A., Mickelson, O. and Taylor, H.L. (1950) *The Biology of Human Starvation*. Minneapolis: University of Minnesota Press.

Kurpad, A.V., Khan, K., Calder, A.G. and Elia, M. (1994) Muscle and whole body metabolism after norepinephrine. *American Journal of Physiology* **266**, E877–844.

Landsberg, L., Saville, M.E. and Young, J.B. (1984) The sympathoadrenal system and regulation of thermogenesis. *American Journal of Physiology* **247**, E181–189.

Langhans, W. (1996) Metabolic and glucostatic control of feeding. *Proceedings of the Nutrition Society* **55**, 497–515.

Langhans, W. (2003) Role of the liver in the control of glucose-lipid utilization and body weight. *Current Opinion of Clinical Nutrition and Metabolic Care* **6**, 449–455.

Leibel, R.L., Rosenbaum, M. and Hirsch, J. (1995) Changes in energy expenditure resulting from altered body weight. *New England Journal of Medicine* **332**, 621–628.

Levine, J.A., Eberhardt, N.L. and Jensen, M.D. (1999) Role of nonexercise activity thermogenesis in resistance to fat gain in humans. *Science* **283**, 212–214.

Lin, J., Wu, H., Tarr, P.T., Zhang, C.Y., Wu, Z., Boss, O., Michael, L.F., Puigserver, P., Isotani, E., Olson, E.N., Lowell, B.B., Bassel-Duby, R. and Spiegelman, B.M. (2002) Transcriptional co-activator PGC-1 alpha drives the formation of slow-twitch muscle fibres. *Nature* **418**, 797–801.

Mayer, J. (1953) Glucostatic mechanism of regulation of food intake. *New England Journal of Medicine* **249**, 13–16.

Mellinkoff, S.M., Franklund, M., Bouyle, D. and Greipel, M. (1956) Relationships between serum amino acid concentration and fluctuations in appetite. *Journal of Applied Physiology* **8**, 535–538.

Miller, D.S. (1982) Factors affecting energy expenditure. *Proceedings of the Nutrition Society* **41**, 193–202.

Miller, D.S., Mumford, P. and Stock, M.J. (1967) Gluttony 2. Thermogenesis in overeating man. *American Journal of Clinical Nutrition* **20**, 1223–1229.

Millward, D.J. (1995) A protein-stat mechanism for the regulation of growth and maintenance of the lean body mass. *Nutrition Research Review* **8**, 93–120.

Moran, T.H. (2000) Cholecystokinin and satiety: current perspectives. *Nutrition* **16**, 858–865.

Payne, P.R. and Dugdale, A.E. (1977) Mechanisms for the control of body weight. *Lancet* **I**, 583–586.

Puigserver, P., Wu, Z., Park, C.W., Graves, R., Wright, M. and Spiegelman, B.M. (1998) A cold-inducible coactivator of nuclear receptors linked to adaptive thermogenesis. *Cell* **92**, 829–839.

Ravussin, E. and Gautier, J.F. (1999) Metabolic predictors of weight gain. *International Journal of Obesity* **23** (Suppl. 1), 37–41.

Rolfe, D.F. and Brand, M.D. (1996) Contribution of mitochondrial proton leak to skeletal muscle respiration and to standard metabolic rate. *American Journal of Physiology* **271**, 1380–1389.

Rothwell, N.J. and Stock, M.J. (1979) A role for brown adipose tissue in diet-induced thermogenesis. *Nature* **281**, 31–35.

Russek, M. (1963) An hypothesis on the participation of hepatic glucoreceptors in the control of food intake. *Nature* **197**, 79–80.

Samec, S., Seydoux, J. and Dulloo, A.G. (1998) Role of UCP homologues in skeletal muscles and brown adipose tissue: mediators of thermogenesis or regulators of lipids as fuel substrate? *FASEB J* **12**, 715–724.

Schutz, Y. (1995) Macronutrients and energy balance in obesity. *Metabolism* **44** (Suppl. 3), 7–11.

Schutz, Y. and Garrow, J.S. (1996) Energy and substrate balance, and weight regulation. In: Garrow, J.S., James, W.P.T. and Ralph, A. eds. *Human Nutrition and Dietetics*, 10th edn. Edinburgh: Churchill Livingstone, 137–148.

Schwartz, M.W., Woods, S.C., Porte, D., Seeley, R. and Baskin, D. (2000) Central nervous system control of food intake. *Nature* **404**, 661–671.

Stock, M.J. (1999) Gluttony and thermogenesis revisited. *International Journal of Obesity* **23**, 1105–1117.

Stubbs, F.J. (1995) Macronutrient effects on appetite. *International Journal of Obesity* **19** (Suppl. 5), S11–S19.

Stubbs, R.J. (1998) Appetite, feeding behaviour and energy balance in humans. *Proceedings of the Nutrition Society* **57**, 341–356.

Tataranni, P.A., Young, J.B., Bogardus, C. and Ravussin, E. (1997) A low sympathoadrenal activity is associated with body weight gain and development of central adiposity in Pima Indian men. *Obesity Research*, **5**, 341–347.

Tschop, M., Smiley, D.L. and Heiman, M.L. (2000) Ghrelin induces adiposity in rodents. *Nature* **407**, 908–913.

Tschop, M., Wawarta, R., Riepl, R.L., Friedrich, S., Bidlingmaier, M., Landgraf, R. and Folwaczny, C. (2001) Postprandial decrease of circulating human ghrelin levels. *Journal of Endocrinology Investigation* **24**, RC19–RC21.

Walder, R.L., Norman, R.A., Hanson, R.L., Schrauwen, P., Neverova, M., Jenkinson, C.P., Easlick, J., Warden, C.H., Pecqueur, C., Raimbault, S., Ricquier, D., Silver, M.H., Shuldiner, A.R., Solanes, G., Lowell, B.B., Chung, W.K., Leibel, R.L., Pratley, R. and Ravussin, E. (1998) Association between uncoupling protein polymorphisms (UCP2-UCP3) and energy metabolism/obesity in Pima Indians. *Human Molecular Genetics* **7**, 1431–1435.

6 Genes and obesity

I. Sadaf Farooqi

Introduction, 81

Historical perspective, 81

Gene–environment interactions, 81

Evidence for the heritability of fat
mass, 82
  Adoption studies, 82
  Twin studies, 82

Genetic basis of common
obesity, 83
  Association studies, 83
  Linkage analysis, 83

Pleiotropic obesity syndromes, 83
  Prader–Willi syndrome, 84
  Albright hereditary
  osteodystrophy, 84
  Fragile X syndrome, 84
  Bardet–Biedl syndrome, 85

Molecular mechanisms involved in
energy homeostasis, 85
  Rodent models of obesity, 85
  Leptin–melanocortin
  pathway, 85

Human monogenic obesity
syndromes, 86

Congenital leptin deficiency, 86
Response to leptin therapy, 86
Partial leptin deficiency, 87
Leptin receptor deficiency, 88
Pro-opiomelanocortin
deficiency, 88
Prohormone convertase 1
deficiency, 89

Energy expenditure genes, 89

Perspectives, 90

References, 90

Introduction

Obesity is determined by an interaction between genetic, environmental and behavioural factors acting through the physiological mediators of energy intake and energy expenditure. Body weight is the archetypal polygenic trait, a quantitative phenotype that usually fails to display a mendelian pattern of inheritance because it is influenced by many different regions of the genome. The concept that environmental factors operate on an underlying pool of genes that contribute to obesity susceptibility has important implications for our approach to the prevention and treatment of obesity. If some environmental variables manifest themselves only on certain genotypes, efforts to prevent obesity at a public health level can be focused on recognition and counselling of susceptible individuals. In addition, appreciating the importance of genetic variation as an underlying cause helps to dispel the notion that obesity represents an individual defect in behaviour with no biological basis, and provides a starting point for efforts to identify the genes involved.

Much of the recent excitement about understanding and treating obesity is based on the identification of genes that are responsible for existing murine obesity syndromes, and the subsequent realization that several of these genes uncover fundamental physiological pathways that were unappreciated previously. As the endocrinological, metabolic and behavioural features of monogenic rodent obesities have been well characterized, these then provide considerable insight into the biology that underlies each mutation. In the last 4 years, five single gene defects causing severe human obesity have been identified. Studies of patients with mutations in these molecules have shed light on the physiological role of these molecules in the regulation of body weight in humans.

Historical perspective

Obesity, defined as an excess of body fat, is frequently considered to be a 'modern' disease — a reflection of the excesses of Western urbanized society. However, artefacts dating from the Palaeolithic Stone Age clearly represent subjects with an excess of body fat, and descriptions of obese individuals have emerged in manuscripts and medical texts from many of the ancient civilizations from Mesopotamia to Arabia, from China to India. This historical evidence suggests that, independent of diet and geographical region, throughout history some individuals have harboured the propensity to store excess energy as fat.

Gene–environment interactions

The increase in the prevalence of obesity in the last 30 years suggests the importance of changing environmental factors, in particular the increasing availability of energy-dense high-fat foods and a reduction in physical activity. Further evidence for the critical role of environmental factors in the development of obesity comes from migrant studies and the 'Westernization' of diet and lifestyles in developing countries. A marked change in body mass index (BMI) is frequently witnessed in migrant populations, where subjects with a common genetic heritage live under new and different environmental circumstances. Pima Indians, for example, living in the USA are on average 25 kg heavier than Pima Indians living in Mexico (Kopelman, 2000). A similar trend is seen for Africans living in the USA and Asians living in the UK. Moreover, within some ethnic groups the prevalence of obesity has increased very dramatically, not only among migrants but also among the indigenous population. In fact, the prevalence of obesity is at present more than 60% in Nauruan men and women and also among Polynesians in Western Samoa. This observation suggests that subjects from these ethnic groups may be more susceptible to developing obesity and that environmental factors have varying effects depending upon genetic background.

Evidence for the heritability of fat mass

There is considerable evidence to suggest that like height, weight is a heritable trait. Genetic epidemiological studies in different populations can attribute the underlying phenotypic variance of a trait into genetic and/or environmental sources. Longitudinal data from one of the largest family studies, the Quebec Family Study of over 400 families, suggest a significant cross-trait familial resemblance for parents and their offspring (0.20–0.25) and sibling relationships (0.25–0.35) (Rice *et al.*, 1999). However, in traditional nuclear families, family members generally share both genes and environment to some degree, so it is difficult to assess the contribution of each component.

Adoption studies

Complete adoption studies are useful in separating the common environmental effects, as adoptive parents and their adoptive offspring share only environmental sources of variance, whereas the adoptees and their biological parents share only genetic sources of variance. One of the largest series, based on over 5000 subjects from the Danish adoption register, which contains complete and detailed information on the biological parents, demonstrated a strong relationship between the BMI of adoptees and biological parents across the whole range of body fatness, but no relationship when adoptees were compared with their adoptive parents (Stunkard *et al.*, 1986a). The Danish group have also shown a close correlation between BMI of adoptees and their biological full siblings who were reared separately by the biological parents of the adoptees, and a similar, but weaker relationship with half-siblings (Sorensen *et al.*, 1989).

Twin studies

Traditionally, the most favoured model for separation of the genetic component of variance is based on studies of twins, as monozygotic co-twins share 100% of their genes and dizygotes 50% on average. Heritability estimates the proportion of the total variance attributable to genetic variation under a polygenic model by comparing the similarity of a trait within monozygotic twins with the similarity within dizygotic twins. Heritability is both a function of the number of genes influencing a phenotype and the proportion of phenotypic variation accounted for by each of these genes. The advantage of studies of the heritability of BMI is that age-dependent influences of genes or environmental factors are the same for both twins. Genetic contribution to the BMI has been estimated to be 64–84% (Stunkard *et al.*, 1986b).

The most powerful genetic epidemiological design is the study of monozygotic twins reared apart, which has all the advantages of a twin study, but does not rely on the equal environmental exposure assumption. Correlation of monozygotic twins reared apart is virtually a direct estimate of the heritability, although monozygotic twins do share the intrauterine environment, which may contribute to lasting differences in body mass in later life. Estimates vary from 40–70%, depending on age of separation of twins and the length of follow-up. Longitudinal data from Virginia looking at adult twins and their offspring have reported a heritability of 69% (Maes *et al.*, 1997). Studies of Swedish twins have suggested a heritability of 0.70 for men and 0.66 for women (Stunkard *et al.*, 1990), whereas a heritability of 0.61 was observed in a cohort of UK twins (Price and Gottesman, 1991). In a meta-analysis of results derived from Finnish, Japanese and American archival twins, Allison observed similar correlation (Allison *et al.*, 1996). In addition, Price and colleagues have shown that these correlations did not differ significantly between twins reared apart and twins reared together, and between twins reared apart in relatively more similar (i.e. with relatives) vs. less similar environments (Price and Gottesman, 1991).

Familial resemblance in nutrient intake has been reported in parents and their children (Perusse *et al.*, 1988), although the extent to which this is genetically determined is unclear. Twin data suggest that there are notable genetic influences on the overall intake of nutrients, size and frequency of meals and intake of particular foods. Bouchard and Tremblay (1990) have shown that about 40% of the variance in resting metabolic rate, thermic effect of food and energy cost of low- to moderate-intensity exercise may be explained by inherited characteristics. In addition, significant familial resemblance for level of habitual physical activity has been reported in a large cohort of healthy female twins (Samaras *et al.*, 1999).

Table 6.1 Human pleiotropic obesity syndromes.

Syndrome	Additional clinical features	Locus	Reference
Autosomal dominant			
Ulnar–mammary syndrome	Ulnar defects, delayed puberty, hypoplastic nipples	12q24.1	Bamshad *et al.* (1995)
Autosomal recessive			
Alstom's syndrome	Retinal dystrophy, neurosensory deafness, diabetes	2p13	Collin *et al.* (2002)
Cohen's syndrome	Prominent central incisors, ophthalmopathy, microcephaly	8q22	Tahvanainen *et al.* (1994)
X-linked			
Borjeson–Forssman–Lehmann syndrome	Mental retardation, hypogonadism, large ears	Xq26	Turner *et al.* (1989)
Mehmo's syndrome	Mental retardation, epilepsy, hypogonadism, microcephaly	Xp22.13	Steinmuller *et al.* (1998)
Simpson–Golabi–Behmel, type 2	Craniofacial defects, skeletal and visceral abnormalities	Xp22	Brzustovic *et al.* (1999)
Wilson–Turner syndrome	Mental retardation, tapering fingers, gynaecomastia	Xp21.1	Wilson *et al.* (1991)

Genetic basis of common obesity

Genetic determinants of interindividual variation in obesity and related phenotypes are likely to be multiple and interacting, with most single variants producing only a moderate effect.

Association studies

Genetic association studies assess correlations between genetic variants at a polymorphic site and a phenotype trait of interest. Such variants can either be directly involved in disease predisposition or indirectly involved through linkage disequilibrium with pathogenic variants in close proximity. To date, association studies have largely been restricted to candidate genes, the dysfunction of which might reasonably be expected to result in obesity by virtue of their having putative effects on energy intake, energy expenditure or nutrient partitioning. This strategy has been extensively utilized in obesity genetics but brings with it a number of problems, as many association studies have been underpowered, some grossly so, and there is a publication bias towards the reporting of positive rather than negative associations, which tends to exaggerate the true nature or strength of an association. A comprehensive and updated reference for all association studies in obesity genetics is available in the form of the obesity gene map established by Bouchard and colleagues at The Pennington Biomedical Research Centre (link to http://www.obesite.chaire.ulaval.ca/genemap.html).

Linkage analysis

In linkage analysis, regions of the genome that cosegregate with disease in families are identified. This has been an enormously powerful technique for the identification of gene defects causing monogenic disorders. Its utility in identifying chromosome regions containing susceptibility genes for complex disorders is less certain, given the lack of clear patterns of inheritance and the multiple genetic and environmental influences on complex traits. In a genome-wide scan, linkage analysis is conducted using a series of anonymous polymorphisms, spaced at relatively constant intervals over the entire genome e.g. ~350–370 markers with an average spacing of 10 cM. Genome scans are complicated by the fact that instead of a single test for linkage, one must conduct multiple tests across the entire genome. In light of this, it has been proposed that a logarithm of odds (LOD) score ≥ 3.3 can be taken as strong evidence of linkage, and a LOD score ≥ 1.9 but < 3.3 as evidence suggestive of linkage.

Results from reported genome-wide linkage studies that have examined obesity and/or related intermediate traits have identified several loci that show positive evidence for linkage with a LOD score ≥ 2.6. Genome-wide scans in different ethnic populations have localized major obesity loci on chromosomes 2, 5, 10, 11 and 20 (Clement *et al.*, 2002; Comuzzzie, 2002).

Pleiotropic obesity syndromes

It is well established that obesity runs in families, although the vast majority of cases do not segregate with a clear mendelian pattern of inheritance. There are about 30 mendelian disorders that have obesity as a clinical feature but often associated with mental retardation, dysmorphic features and organ-specific developmental abnormalities (i.e. pleiotropic syndromes). A number of families with these rare pleiotropic obesity syndromes have been studied by linkage analysis and the known chromosomal loci for obesity syndromes are summarized in Table 6.1. For a comprehensive list of syndromes in which obesity is a recognized part of the phenotype, see Online Mendelian Inheritance in Man (OMIM) (www.ncbi.nlm.nih.gov/omim/).

Prader–Willi syndrome

Prader–Willi syndrome (PWS) is the most common syndromal cause of human obesity, with an estimated prevalence of about 1 in 25 000. It is an autosomal dominant disorder and is caused by deletion or disruption of a paternally imprinted gene or genes on the proximal long arm of chromosome 15. The PWS is characterized by diminished fetal activity, obesity, hypotonia, mental retardation, short stature, hypogonadotropic hypogonadism, and small hands and feet (Butler, 1990). The diagnostic criteria arrived at by a consensus group were based on a point system; one point each was allowed for each of five major criteria, such as feeding problems in infancy and failure to thrive, and one-half point each for seven minor criteria, such as hypopigmentation. A minimum of eight and a half points was considered necessary for the clinical diagnosis of PWS (Holm et al., 1993). There is mild prenatal growth retardation, with a mean birth weight of about 6 lb (2.8 kg) at term, hyporeflexia and poor feeding in neonatal life due to diminished swallowing and sucking reflexes; infants often require assisted feeding for about 3 to 4 months. Feeding difficulties generally improve by the age of 6 months. From 12 to 18 months onwards, uncontrollable hyperphagia results in severe obesity, invariably associated with abdominal striae. Diabetes mellitus is not a diagnostic criterion for PWS but it is often found in older PWS patients.

Although hyperphagia is a dominant feature in PWS subjects, the eating behaviour in PWS might be due to decreased satiation as well as increased hunger. One suggested mediator of the obesity phenotype in PWS patients is the novel enteric hormone ghrelin, which is implicated in the regulation of meal-time hunger in rodents and humans, and is also a potent stimulator of growth hormone secretion. Fasting plasma ghrelin levels are 4.5-fold higher in PWS subjects than in equally obese controls and thus may be implicated in the pathogenesis of hyperphagia in these patients (Cummings et al., 2002).

Children with PWS display diminished growth, reduced muscle mass (lean body mass) and increased fat mass—body composition abnormalities resembling those seen in growth hormone (GH) deficiency. Diminished GH responses to various provocative agents, low insulin-like growth factor-I levels and the presence of additional evidence of hypothalamic dysfunction support the presence of true GH deficiency (GHD) in many children with PWS. GH treatment in these children decreases body fat, and increases linear growth, muscle mass, fat oxidation and energy expenditure.

It is clear that the syndrome is caused by lack of the paternal segment 15q11.2–q12, either through deletion of the paternal 'critical' segment or through loss of the entire paternal chromosome 15 with the presence of two maternal homologues (uniparental maternal disomy). The opposite, i.e. maternal deletion or paternal uniparental disomy, causes another characteristic phenotype, the Angelman syndrome. This indicates that both parental chromosomes are differentially imprinted, and that both are necessary for normal embryonic development. Within the 4.5-Mb PWS region in 15q11–q13, several candidate genes include necdin, small nuclear ribonucleoprotein polypeptide N (SNRPN), ring zinc finger 127 polypeptide gene, the MAGE-like 2 gene and the Prader–Willi critical region 1 gene. However, the precise role of these genes and the mechanisms by which they lead to a pleiotropic obesity syndrome remain elusive. DNA methylation can be used as a reliable post-natal diagnostic tool.

Albright hereditary osteodystrophy

Gs is the ubiquitously expressed heterotrimeric G protein that couples receptors to the effector enzyme adenylcyclase, and is required for receptor-stimulated intracellular cAMP generation. Inactivating and activating mutations in the gene encoding G alpha s (GNAS1) are known to be the basis for two well-described contrasting clinical disorders: Albright hereditary osteodystrophy (AHO) and McCune–Albright syndrome (MAS). AHO is an autosomal dominant disorder due to germline mutations in GNAS1 that decrease expression or function of G alpha s protein. Heterozygous loss-of-function mutations lead to AHO, a disease characterized by short stature, obesity, skeletal defects and impaired olfaction. Maternal transmission of GNAS1 mutations leads to AHO plus resistance to several hormones (e.g. parathyroid hormone) that activate Gs in their target tissues (pseudohypoparathyroidism type IA), whereas paternal transmission leads only to the AHO phenotype (pseudopseudohypoparathyroidism). Studies in both mice and humans demonstrate that GNAS1 is imprinted in a tissue-specific manner, being expressed primarily from the maternal allele in some tissues and biallelically expressed in most other tissues, thus multihormone resistance occurs only when Gs (alpha) mutations are inherited maternally (Weinstein et al., 2002).

Fragile X syndrome

Fragile X syndrome is characterized by moderate to severe mental retardation, macro-orchidism, large ears, prominent jaw and high-pitched jocular speech associated with mutations in the FMR1 gene (Kaplan et al., 1994). Expression is variable, with mental retardation being the most common feature. A Prader–Willi-like subphenotype of the Fragile X syndrome has been described. The features are extreme obesity with a full, round face, small, broad hands and feet and regional skin hyperpigmentation. Behavioural characteristics such as hyperkinesis, autistic-like behaviour and apparent speech and language deficits may help point towards the diagnosis of the Fragile X. It has been suggested that a reasonable estimate of frequency is 0.5 per 1000 males.

Bardet–Biedl syndrome

Bardet–Biedl syndrome (BBS) is a rare (prevalence < 1 : 100 000) autosomal recessive disease characterized by obesity, mental retardation, dysmorphic extremities (syndactyly, brachydactyly or polydactyly), retinal dystrophy or pigmentary retinopathy, hypogonadism or hypogenitalism (limited to male patients) and structural abnormalities of the kidney or functional renal impairment. The differential diagnosis includes Biemond's syndrome II (iris coloboma, hypogenitalism, obesity, polydactyly and mental retardation) and Alstrom's syndrome (retinitis pigmentosa, obesity, diabetes mellitus and deafness).

Bardet–Biedl syndrome is a genetically heterogeneous disorder that is now known to map to at least six loci: 11q13 (BBS1), 16q21 (BBS2), 3p13–p12 (BBS3), 15q22.3–q23 (BBS4), 2q31 (BBS5) and 20p12 (BBS6). Although BBS had been originally thought to be a recessive disorder, Katsanis and colleagues (2001) demonstrated that clinical manifestation of some forms of Bardet–Biedl syndrome requires recessive mutations in one out of the six loci plus an additional mutation in a second locus.

The BBS1 gene has recently been identified; however, the protein does not show any significant similarity to any known protein and its function is unknown (Mykytyn *et al.*, 2002). Families with BBS mapping to BBS6 have been found to harbour mutations in MKKS, which has sequence homology to the alpha subunit of a prokaryotic chaperonin in the thermosome *Thermoplasma acidophilum*. Mutations in this gene also cause McKusick–Kaufman syndrome (hydrometrocolpos, post-axial polydactyly and congenital heart defects). In addition, the genes underlying BBS2 and BBS4 have recently been identified. However, they have no significant homology to chaperonins and the functions of these proteins remain unknown.

Molecular mechanisms involved in energy homeostasis

The first description of hypothalamic injury associated with obesity was published by Mohr in 1840 (Mohr, 1840), but remained unsupported until two landmark papers by Babinski in 1901 (Babinski, 1900) and by Frohlich in 1900 (Frohlich, 1901), describing tumours in the region of the hypothalamus that were associated with obesity, gonadal atrophy, decreased vision and short stature. In 1940, Hetherington and Ranson published their first report, demonstrating that electrolytic lesions in rodents involving, but not restricted to, the ventromedial region of the hypothalamus (VMH) were associated with hyperphagia (increased food intake), hyperinsulinaemia and obesity. However, the precise nature of these hypothalamic pathways and the nature of their inputs and outputs was only clarified with the identification and characterization of single gene defects in rodent models of obesity.

Rodent models of obesity

Since the early 1900s, a number of obese inbred strains of mice, both dominant (yellow, *Ay/a*) and recessive (*ob/ob*, *db/db*, *fa/fa*, *tb/tb*), had been studied. In the 1990s, the genes responsible for these syndromes were identified mostly by positional cloning techniques and these observations have given substantial insights into the physiological disturbances that can lead to obesity, the metabolic and endocrine abnormalities associated with the obese phenotype, and the more detailed anatomical and neurochemical pathways that regulate energy intake and energy expenditure (Leibel *et al.*, 1997). These studies provide the basic framework upon which the understanding of the more complex mechanisms in humans can be built.

Leptin–melanocortin pathway

The initial observations in this field were made as a result of positional cloning strategies in two strains of severely obese mice (*ob/ob* and *db/db*). Severely obese *ob/ob* mice were found to harbour mutations in the *ob* gene, resulting in a complete lack of its protein product leptin (Zhang *et al.*, 1994). Administration of recombinant leptin reduced the food intake and body weight of leptin-deficient *ob/ob* mice and corrected all of their neuroendocrine and metabolic abnormalities. The signalling form of the leptin receptor is deleted in *db/db* mice, which are consequently unresponsive to endogenous or exogenous leptin. The identification of these two proteins established the first components of a nutritional feedback loop from adipose tissue to the brain. However, it is considered that the physiological role of leptin in humans and rodents might be to act as a signal for starvation, because as fat mass increases, further rises in leptin have a limited ability to suppress food intake and prevent obesity (Flier, 1998).

Considerable attention has focused on deciphering the hypothalamic pathways that coordinate the behavioural and metabolic effects downstream of leptin. The first-order neuronal targets of leptin action in the brain are anorectic (reducing food intake) proopiomelanocortin (POMC) and orexigenic (increasing food intake) neuropeptide-Y/ Agouti-related protein (NPY/AgRP) neurons in the hypothalamic arcuate nucleus, where the signalling isoform of the leptin receptor is highly expressed (Schwartz *et al.*, 2000). In total, 40% of POMC neurons in the arcuate nucleus express the mRNA for the long form of the leptin receptor, and POMC expression is regulated positively by leptin. POMC is sequentially cleaved by prohormone convertases to yield peptides, including α-melanocyte stimulating hormone (αMSH), which have been shown to play a role in feeding behaviour. There is clear evidence in rodents that α-

MSH acts as a suppressor of feeding behaviour, probably through the melanocortin 4 receptor (Mc4r). In fact, targeted disruption of Mc4r in rodents leads to increased food intake, obesity, severe early hyperinsulinaemia and increased linear growth; heterozygotes have an intermediate phenotype compared with homozygotes and wild-type mice (Huszar *et al.*, 1997).

Human monogenic obesity syndromes

Congenital leptin deficiency

In 1997, we reported two severely obese cousins from a highly consanguineous family of Pakistani origin (Montague *et al.*, 1997). Both children had undetectable levels of serum leptin and were found to be homozygous for a frameshift mutation in the *ob* gene (ΔG133), which resulted in a truncated protein that was not secreted. We have since identified three further affected individuals from two other families who are also homozygous for the same mutation in the leptin gene (Farooqi *et al.*, 2002). All of the families are of Pakistani origin but not known to be related over five generations. A large Turkish family that carries a homozygous missense mutation has also been described (Strobel *et al.*, 1998). All subjects in these families are characterized by severe early-onset obesity and intense hyperphagia (Farooqi *et al.*, 1999; 2002; Ozata *et al.*, 1999). Hyperinsulinaemia and an advanced bone age are also common features. Some of the Turkish subjects are adults with hypogonadotropic hypogonadism (Strobel *et al.*, 1998). Although normal pubertal development did not occur, there was some evidence of a delayed but spontaneous pubertal development in one person (Ozata *et al.*, 1999).

We demonstrated that children with leptin deficiency had profound abnormalities of T-cell number and function (Farooqi *et al.*, 2002), consistent with high rates of childhood infection and a high reported rate of childhood mortality from infection in obese Turkish subjects. Most of these phenotypes closely parallel those seen in murine leptin deficiency. However, there are some phenotypes for which the parallels between human and mouse are not as clear-cut. Thus, although *ob/ob* mice are stunted, it appears that growth retardation is not a feature of human leptin deficiency (Farooqi *et al.*, 2002), although abnormalities of dynamic growth hormone secretion have been reported in one human subject (Ozata *et al.*, 1999). *ob/ob* mice have marked activation of the hypothalamic pituitary adrenal axis, with very elevated corticosterone levels. In humans, abnormalities of cortisol secretion are, if present at all, much more subtle (Farooqi *et al.*, 1999). The contribution of reduced energy expenditure to the obesity of the *ob/ob* mouse is reasonably well established (Trayhurn *et al.*, 1977). In leptin-deficient humans, we found no detectable changes in resting or free-living energy expenditure (Farooqi *et al.*, 1999), although it was not possible to examine how such systems adapted to stressors such as cold. Ozata and colleagues (1999) reported abnormalities of sympathetic nerve function in leptin-deficient humans consistent with defects in the efferent sympathetic limb of thermogenesis.

Response to leptin therapy

Recently, the dramatic and beneficial effects of daily subcutaneous injections of leptin reducing body weight and fat mass in three congenitally leptin-deficient children were reported (Farooqi *et al.*, 2002). Therapy in the other two children has recently commenced and comparably beneficial results have been seen. All children showed a response to initial leptin doses designed to produce plasma leptin levels at only 10% of those predicted by height and weight (i.e. approximately 0.01 mg/kg of lean body mass). The most dramatic example of leptin's effects was with a 3-year-old boy, severely disabled by gross obesity (weight 42 kg), who now weighs 32 kg (75th centile for weight) after 48 months of leptin therapy (Fig. 6.1) (Farooqi *et al.*, 2002).

The major effect of leptin was on appetite, with normalization of hyperphagia. Leptin therapy reduced energy intake during an 18-MJ *ad libitum* test meal by up to 84% (Fig. 6.2a). We were unable to demonstrate a major effect of leptin on basal metabolic rate (BMR) or free-living energy expenditure (Fig. 6.2b), but, as weight loss by other means is associated with a decrease in BMR (Rosenbaum *et al.*, 2002), the fact that energy expenditure did not fall in our leptin-deficient subjects is notable.

The administration of leptin permitted progression of appropriately timed pubertal development in the single child of appropriate age and did not cause early onset of puberty in the younger children (Farooqi *et al.*, 2002) (Fig. 6.3). Free thyroxine and thyroid-stimulating hormone (TSH) levels, although in the normal range before treatment, had consistently increased at the earliest post-treatment time point and subsequently stabilized at this elevated level (Farooqi *et al.*, 2002). These findings are consistent with evidence from animal models, which shows that leptin influences thyrotrophin-releasing hormone (TRH) release from the hypothalamus (Harris *et al.*, 2001) and from studies illustrating the effect of leptin deficiency on TSH pulsatility in humans (Mantzoros *et al.*, 2001).

Throughout the trial of leptin administration, weight loss continued in all subjects, albeit with refractory periods that were overcome by increases in leptin dose. The families in the UK harbour a mutation that leads to a prematurely truncated form of leptin and thus wild-type leptin is a novel antigen to them. Thus, all subjects developed anti-leptin antibodies after ~6 weeks of leptin therapy, which interfered with interpretation of serum leptin levels and, in some cases, were capable of neutralizing leptin in a bioassay. These antibodies are the likely cause of refractory periods that occur during therapy. The fluctuating nature of the antibodies probably reflects the complicating factor that leptin deficiency is itself an immunodeficient state and administration of leptin leads to a change from

(a)

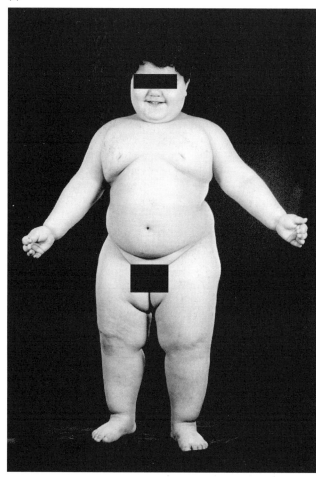

(b)

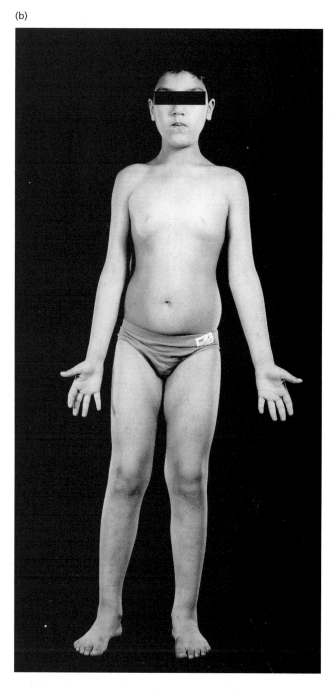

Fig. 6.1 Clinical response to leptin therapy in congenital leptin deficiency.

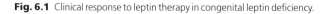

the secretion of predominantly Th$_2$ to Th$_1$ cytokines, which may directly influence antibody production. Thus far, we have been able to regain control of weight loss by increasing the dose of leptin.

Partial leptin deficiency

The major question with respect to the potential therapeutic use of leptin in more common forms of obesity relates to the shape of the leptin dose–response curve. We have clearly shown that at the lower end of plasma leptin levels, raising

leptin levels from undetectable to detectable has profound effects on appetite and weight. Supraphysiological doses (0.1–0.3 mg/kg of body weight) of leptin have been administered to obese subjects for 28 weeks (Heymsfield *et al.*, 1999). On average, subjects lost significant weight, but the extent of weight loss and the variability between subjects has led many to conclude that the leptin resistance of common obesity cannot be usefully overcome by leptin supplementation, at least when administered peripherally. However, on scientific rather than pragmatic grounds, it is of interest that there was a significant effect on weight, suggesting that plasma leptin can

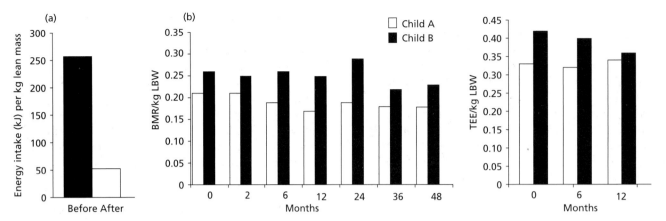

Fig. 6.2 (a) Change in *ad libitum* food intake with leptin therapy in congenital leptin deficiency. (b) Changes in energy expenditure in response to leptin. BMR = basal metabolic rate; TEE = total energy expenditure.

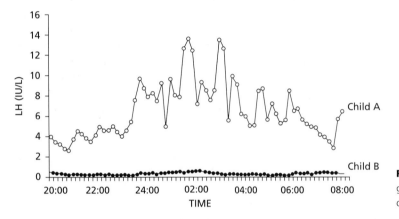

Fig. 6.3 Leptin therapy is associated with pulsatile gonadotrophin secretion at an appropriate developmental age in child A (age 11 years) compared with child B (age 5 years).

continue to have a dose–response effect on energy homeostasis across a wide plasma concentration range. To test this hypothesis, we studied the heterozygous relatives of our leptin-deficient subjects. Serum leptin levels in the heterozygous subjects were found to be significantly lower than expected for percentage body fat and they had a higher prevalence of obesity than seen in a control population of similar age, sex and ethnicity (Farooqi *et al.*, 2001). Additionally, percentage body fat was higher than predicted from their height and weight in the heterozygous subjects compared with control subjects of the same ethnicity. These findings closely parallel those in heterozygous *ob–* and *db/–* mice (Chung *et al.*, 1998). These data provide further support for the possibility that leptin can produce a graded response in terms of body composition across a broad range of plasma concentrations.

Leptin receptor deficiency

A mutation in the leptin receptor has been reported in one consanguineous family (Clement *et al.*, 1998). Affected individuals were homozygous for a mutation that truncates the receptor before the transmembrane domain and the mutated receptor circulates bound to leptin. There are a number of phenotypic similarities with the leptin-deficient subjects. Leptin receptor-deficient subjects were also born of normal birth weight, exhibited rapid weight gain in the first few months of life, with severe hyperphagia and aggressive behaviour when denied food. In contrast, some neuroendocrine features were unique to leptin receptor deficiency. The presence of mild growth retardation in early childhood, with impaired basal and stimulated growth hormone secretion, decreased insulin-like growth factor (IGF)-1 and IGF-BP3 levels and evidence of hypothalamic hypothyroidism in these subjects suggests that loss of the leptin receptor results in a more diverse phenotype than loss of its ligand leptin (Clement *et al.*, 1998).

Pro-opiomelanocortin deficiency

Two unrelated obese German children with homozygous or compound heterozygous mutations in POMC have been reported (Krude *et al.*, 1998). These children were hyperphagic, developing early-onset obesity as a result of impaired melanocortin signalling in the hypothalamus. They presented in neonatal life with adrenal crisis due to isolated adrenocorticotrophic hormone (ACTH) deficiency (POMC is a precursor of ACTH in the pituitary) and had pale skin and red hair due to the lack of MSH function at melanocortin 1 receptors in the skin. A number of groups have identified a heterozygous missense mutation (Arg236Gly) in POMC that disrupts the dibasic amino acid processing site between β-MSH and β-endorphin (Challis *et al.*, 2002). This mutation results in an aberrant β-MSH–β-endorphin fusion peptide that binds to Mc4r, with an affinity identical to that of α- and β-MSH but has a markedly reduced ability to activate the receptor. Thus, this cleavage site mutation in POMC may confer susceptibility to obesity through a novel molecular mechanism (Challis *et al.*, 2002).

Prohormone convertase 1 deficiency

Further evidence for the role of the melanocortin system in the regulation of body weight in humans comes from the description of a 47-year-old woman with severe childhood obesity, abnormal glucose homeostasis, very low plasma insulin but elevated levels of proinsulin, hypogonadotropic hypogonadism and hypocortisolaemia associated with elevated levels of POMC. This subject was found to be a compound heterozygote for mutations in prohormone convertase 1 (PC1), which cleaves prohormones at pairs of basic amino acids, leaving C-terminal basic residues that are then excised by carboxypeptidase E (CPE) (Jackson *et al.*, 1997). We have also recently identified a child with severe, early-onset obesity who was a compound heterozygote for complete loss of function mutations in PC1 (Jackson *et al.*, 2003). Although failure to cleave POMC is a likely mechanism for the obesity in these patients, PC1 cleaves a number of other neuropeptides in the hypothalamus, such as glucagon-like-peptide 1, which may influence feeding behaviour. Intriguingly, this second patient suffered from severe small intestinal absorptive dysfunction as well as the characteristic severe early-onset obesity, impaired prohormone processing and hypocortisolaemia. We hypothesized that the small intestinal dysfunction seen in this patient, and to a lesser extent in the first patient we described, may be the result of a failure of maturation of propeptides within the enteroendocrine cells and nerves that express PC1 throughout the gut. The finding of elevated levels of progastrin and proglucagon provided *in vivo* evidence that, indeed, prohormone processing in enteroendocrine cells was abnormal (Jackson *et al.*, 2003).

Melanocortin 4 receptor deficiency

Heterozygous mutations in Mc4r have been reported to cause a dominantly inherited obesity syndrome in different ethnic groups. In a study of 500 severely obese probands, we found that approximately 5% harboured pathogenic mutations in the Mc4r gene, making this the commonest monogenic cause of obesity thus far described in humans (Farooqi *et al.*, 2003). A small number of homozygotes for Mc4r mutations have been described; however, the heterozygotes in these families do have an intermediate phenotype consistent with a co-dominant mode of inheritance.

Detailed phenotypic studies of patients with Mc4r mutations reveal that this syndrome is characterized by an increase in lean body mass and bone mineral density, increased linear growth throughout childhood, hyperphagia and severe hyperinsulinaemia (Farooqi *et al.*, 2003). These features are similar to those seen in Mc4r knockout mice, suggesting the preservation of the relevant melanocortin pathways between rodents and humans. Of particular note is the finding that the severity of receptor dysfunction seen in *in vitro* assays can predict the amount of food ingested at a test meal by the subject harbouring that particular mutation (Farooqi *et al.*, 2003).

We have studied in detail the signalling properties of many of these mutant receptors and this information should help to advance the understanding of structure–function relationships and potentially provide *in vitro* support for the use of Mc4r agonists in this group of patients (Yeo *et al.*, 2003). Importantly, we have been unable to demonstrate evidence for dominant negativity associated with these mutants, which suggests that *Mc4r* mutations are more likely to result in a phenotype through haploinsufficiency.

Energy expenditure genes

Although several lines of evidence suggest that obesity in humans may be in part determined by reduced energy expenditure, molecular insights into the pathways for energy expenditure have lagged behind those related to altered appetite (Flier and Lowell, 1997). In most well-identified syndromes of obesity in rodents, such as those involving defects in leptin and the melanocortin pathway, obesity results from both increased feeding and decreased energy expenditure, suggesting that the leptin and melanocortin pathways are upstream of effector mechanisms that regulate both appetite and energy expenditure, and thus disruption of these pathways is likely to have subtle effects on energy expenditure in humans too.

One biologically plausible mechanism whereby a defect in energy expenditure could be involved in the pathophysiology of human obesity is through an inability to adapt to positive energy balance. Evidence for this was recently provided by mice with deletion of the three beta receptor subtypes, β1, β2 and β3. When these 'betaless' mice are fed a high-fat diet, they develop severe obesity despite food intake identical to control mice (Bachman *et al.*, 2002). Unlike normal mice, betaless mice are unable to increase energy expenditure in response to a calorifically dense diet.

Another discovery with potential relevance to the regulation of energy expenditure is the identification of the co-activator protein PGC-1, which can induce mitochondrial biogenesis and change the thermogenic state of muscle from white to red fibre type. PGC-1-dependent transcriptional pathways have recently been linked to the pathogenesis of type 2 diabetes in humans, although the precise mechanism through which such effects might occur has not been fully explored *in* vivo (Mootha *et al.,* 2003).

Polymorphisms in candidate genes involved in nutrient partitioning have been studied in a few population-based cohorts in whom extensive and detailed information on diet, physical activity and markers of intermediate metabolism have been measured. The relationship between the Pro12Ala variant in the nuclear receptor peroxisome proliferator-activated receptor-gamma (PPARgamma) and the ratio of dietary polyunsaturated fat to saturated fat (P/S ratio) has been studied, and there is some evidence for a gene–nutrient interaction (Meirhaeghe *et al.*, 1998).

Perspectives

Although monogenic syndromes are rare, an improved understanding of the precise nature of the inherited component of severe obesity has undoubted medical benefits. For individuals at highest risk of the complications of severe obesity, such findings provide a starting point for providing more rational mechanism-based therapies, as has successfully been achieved for congenital leptin deficiency. Thus, in patients with severe obesity, a history of hyperphagia, age of onset and family history should be sought. As congenital leptin deficiency is a treatable condition, it is plausible that all children with features of a recessive disorder should have a serum leptin measurement. Additional features such as hypogonadism, severe hyperinsulinaemia, postprandial hypoglycaemia and developmental delay should be sought as genetic counselling of families with monogenic disorders is important.

For common polygenic obesity, a number of recent advances are likely to make significant contributions to the search for obesity genes, including the completion of a draft of the human genome sequence and the discovery and cataloguing of single nucleotide polymorphisms (SNPs), the most prevalent source of sequence variation throughout the human genome. These efforts promise to enhance our ability to identify risk-conferring genes for complex traits such as obesity. In this way it is hoped that genetics will continue to make a significant contribution to understanding the pathophysiology of obesity, towards the identification of potential drug targets and the development of more rational mechanism-based interventions at both the individual and population levels.

References

Allison, D.B., Kaprio, J., Korkeila, M., Koskenvuo, M., Neale, MC. and Hayakawa K. (1996) The heritability of body mass index among an international sample of monozygotic twins reared apart. *International Journal of Obesity and Related Metabolic Disorders* **20**, 501–506.

Babinski, MJ. (1900) Tumeur du corps pituitaire sans acromegalie et avec de developpement des organes genitaux. *Revue Neurologie* **8**, 531–533.

Bachman, E.S., Dhillon, H., Zhang, C.Y., Cinti, S., Bianco, A.C., Kobilka, B.K. and Lowell, B.B. (2002) betaAR signaling required for diet-induced thermogenesis and obesity resistance. *Science* **297**, 843–845.

Bamshad, M., Krakowiak, P.A., Watkins, W.S., Root, S., Carey, J.C. and Jorde, L.B. (1995) A gene for ulnar-mammary syndrome maps to 12q23-q24.1. *Human Molecular Genetics* **4**, 1973–1977.

Bouchard C. and Tremblay A. (1990) Genetic effects in human energy expenditure components. *International Journal of Obesity* **14** (Suppl. 1), 49–55, discussion 55–58.

Brzustowicz, L.M. F.S., Khan, M.B. and Weksberg, R. (1999) Mapping of a new SGBS locus to chromosome Xp22 in a family with a severe form of Simpson–Golabi–Behmel syndrome. *American Journal of Human Genetics* **65**, 779–783.

Butler, M. (1990) Prader–Willi syndrome: current understanding of cause and diagnosis. *American Journal of Medical Genetics* **35**, 319–332.

Challis, B.G., Pritchard, L.E., Creemers, J.W., Delplanque, J., Keogh, J.M., Luan J., Wareham, N.J., Yeo, G.S., Bhattacharyya, S., Froguel, P., White, A., Farooqi, I.S. and O'Rahilly, S. (2002) A missense mutation disrupting a dibasic prohormone processing site in proopiomelanocortin (POMC) increases susceptibility to early-onset obesity through a novel molecular mechanism. *Human Molecular Genetics* **11**, 1997–2004.

Chung, W.K., Belfi, K., Chua, M., Wiley, J., Mackintosh, R., Nicolson, M., Boozer, C.N. and Leibel, R.L. (1998) Heterozygosity for Lep(ob) or Lep(rdb) affects body composition and leptin homeostasis in adult mice. *American Journal of Physiology* **274,** R985–990.

Clement, K., Vaisse, C., Lahlou, N., Cabrol, S., Pelloux, V., Cassuto, D., Gourmelen, M., Dina, C., Chambaz, J., Lacorte, J.M., Basdevant, A., Bougneres, P., Lebouc, Y., Froguel, P. and Guy-Grand, B. (1998) A mutation in the human leptin receptor gene causes obesity and pituitary dysfunction [see comments]. *Nature* **392**, 398–401.

Clement, K., Boutin, P. and Froguel, P. (2002) Genetics of obesity. *American Journal of Pharmacogenomics* **2**, 177–187.

Collin, G.B., Marshall, J.D., Ikeda, A., So, W.V., Russell-Eggitt, I., Maffei, P., Beck, S., Boerkoel, C.F., Sicolo, N., Martin, M., Nishina, P.M. and Naggert, J.K. (2002) Mutations in ALMS1 cause obesity, type 2 diabetes and neurosensory degeneration in Alstrom syndrome. *Nature Genetics* **31**, 74–78.

Comuzzie, A.G. (2002) The emerging pattern of the genetic contribution to human obesity. *Best Practice Research in Clinical Endocrinology Metabolism* **16**, 611–621.

Cummings, D.E., Clement, K., Purnell, J.Q., Vaisse, C., Foster, K.E., Frayo, R.S., Schwartz, M.W., Basdevant, A. and Weigle, D.S. (2002) Elevated plasma ghrelin levels in Prader–Willi syndrome. *Natural Medicine* **8**, 643–644.

Farooqi, I.S., Jebb, S.A., Langmack, G., Lawrence, E., Cheetham, C.H., Prentice, A.M., Hughes, I.A., McCamish, M.A. and O'Rahilly, S. (1999) Effects of recombinant leptin therapy in a child with congenital leptin deficiency. *New England Journal of Medicine* **34**, 879–884.

Farooqi, IS., Keogh, JM., Kamath, S., Jones, S., Gibson, WT., Trussell,

R., Jebb, S.A., Lip, G.Y. and O'Rahilly, S. (2001) Partial leptin deficiency and human adiposity. *Nature* **414**, 34–35.

Farooqi, I.S., Matarese, G., Lord, G.M., Keogh, J.M., Lawrence, E., Agwu, C., *et al.* (2002) Beneficial effects of leptin on obesity, T cell hyporesponsiveness, and neuroendocrine/metabolic dysfunction of human congenital leptin deficiency. *Journal of Clinical Investigation* **110**, 1093–1103.

Farooqi, I.S., Keogh, J.M., Yeo, G.S., Lank, E.J., Cheetham, T. and O'Rahilly, S. (2003) Clinical spectrum of obesity and mutations in the melanocortin 4 receptor gene. *New England Journal of Medicine* **348**, 1085–1095.

Flier, J.S. (1998) Clinical review 94: What's in a name? In search of leptin's physiologic role. *Journal of Clinical Endocrinology Metabolism* **83**, 1407–1413.

Flier, J.S. and Lowell, B.B. (1997) Obesity research springs a proton leak. *Nature Genetics* **15**, 223–224.

Frohlich, A. (1901) Ein fall von tumor der hypophysis cerebri ohne akromegalie. *Wien Klin Rund* **15**, 883–886.

Harris, M., Aschkenasi, C., Elias, C.F., Chandrankunnel, A., Nillni, E.A., Bjoorbaek, C. *et al.* (2001) Transcriptional regulation of the thyrotropin-releasing hormone gene by leptin and melanocortin signaling. *Journal of Clinical Investigation* **107**(1), 111–120.

Hetherington, A.W. and Ranson, S.W. (1940) Hypothalamic lesions and adiposity in the rat. *Anatomy Record* **78**, 149–172.

Heymsfield, S.B., Greenberg, A.S., Fujioka, K., Dixon, R.M., Kushner, R., Hunt T., Lubina, J.A., Patane, J., Self, B., Hunt, P. and McCamish, M. (1999) Recombinant leptin for weight loss in obese and lean adults: a randomized, controlled, dose-escalation trial. *Journal of the American Medical Association* **282**, 1568–1575.

Holm, V.A., Cassidy, S., Butler, M.G., Hanchett, J.M., Greenswag, L.R., Whitman, B.Y. and Greenberg, F. (1993) Prader–Willi syndrome: consensus diagnostic criteria. *Pediatrics* **91**, 398–402.

Huszar, D., Lynch, C.A., Fairchild-Huntress, V., Dunmore, J.H., Fang, Q., Berkemeier, L.R., Gu, W., Kesterson, R.A., Boston, B.A., Cone, R.D., Smith, F.J., Campfield, L.A., Burn, P. and Lee, F. (1997) Targeted disruption of the melanocortin-4 receptor results in obesity in mice. *Cell* **88**, 131–141.

Jackson, R.S., Creemers, J.W., Ohagi, S., Raffin-Sanson, M.L., Sanders, L., Montague, C.T., Hutton, J.C. and O'Rahilly, S. (1997) Obesity and impaired prohormone processing associated with mutations in the human prohormone convertase 1 gene. *Nature Genetics* 1997, **16**, 303–306.

Jackson, R.S., Creemers, J.W., Farooqi, I.S., Raffin-Sanson, M.L., Varro, A., Dockray, G.J., Holst, J.J., brubaker, P.L., Corvol, P., Polonsky, K.S., Ostrega, D., Becker, K.L., Bertagna, X., Hutton, J.C., White, A., Dattari, M.T., Hussain, K., Middleton, S.J., Nicole, T.M., Milla, P.J., Lindley, K.J. and O'Rahilly, S. (2003) Small-intestinal dysfunction accompanies the complex endocrinopathy of human proprotein convertase 1 deficiency. *Journal of Clinical Investigation* **112**, 1550–1560.

Kaplan, G., Kung, M., McClure, M. and Cronister, A. (1994) Direct mutation analysis of 495 patients for fragile X carrier status/proband diagnosis. *American Journal of Medical Genetics* **51**, 501–502.

Katsanis, N., Lupski, J.R. and Beales, P.L. (2001) Exploring the molecular basis of Bardet–Biedl syndrome. *Human Molecular Genetics* **10**, 2293–2299.

Kopelman, P.G. (2000) Obesity as a medical problem. *Nature* **404**, 635–643.

Krude, H., Biebermann, H., Luck, W., Horn, R., Brabant, G. and Gruters, A. (1998) Severe early-onset obesity: adrenal insufficiency and red hair pigmentation caused by POMC mutations in humans. *Nature Genetics* **19**, 155–157.

Leibel, R.L., Chung, W.K. and Chua, Jr, S.C. (1997) The molecular genetics of rodent single gene obesities. *Journal of Biological Chemistry* **272**, 31937–31940.

Maes, H.H., Neale, M.C. and Eaves, L.J. (1997) Genetic and environmental factors in relative body weight and human adiposity. *Behavioural Genetics* **27**, 325–251.

Mantzoros, C.S., Ozata, M., Negrao, A.B., Suchard, M.A., Ziotopoulou, M., Caglayan S., Elashoff, R.M., Cogswell, R.J., Negro, P., Liberty, V., Wong, M.L., Veldhvis, J., Ozdemir, I.C., Gold, P.W., Flier, J.S. and Licinio, J. (2001) Synchronicity of frequently sampled thyrotropin (TSH) and leptin concentrations in healthy adults and leptin-deficient subjects: evidence for possible partial TSH regulation by leptin in humans. *Journal of Clinical Endocrinology Metabolism* **86**, 3284–3291.

Meirhaeghe, A.F.L., Helbecque, N., Cottel, D., Lebel, P., Dallongeville, J., Deeb, S., Auwerx, J. and Amouyel, P. (1998) A genetic polymorphism of the peroxisome proliferator-activated receptor gamma gene influences plasma leptin levels in obese humans. *Human Molecular Genetics* **7**, 435–440.

Mohr, B. (1840) Hypertrophie der hypophysis cerebri und dadurchbedin* ter druck auf die hirngrundflache, insbesondere auf die Schnerven, das chiasma deselben und den linkseitigen. *Hirnschenkel Wschr Ges Heilk*, **6**, 565–571.

Montague, C.T., Farooqi, I.S., Whitehead, J.P., Soos, M.A., Rau, H., Wareham NJ., Sewter, C.P., Digby, J.E., Mohammed, S.N., Hurst, J.A., Cheetham, C.H., Earley, A.R., Barnett, A.H., Prins, J.B. and O'Rahilly, S. (1997) Congenital leptin deficiency is associated with severe early-onset obesity in humans. *Nature* **387**, 903–908.

Mootha, V.K., Lindgren, C.M., Eriksson, K.F., Subramanian, A., Sihag, S., Lehar, J., Puigserver, P., Carlsson, E., Ridderstrale, M., Laurila, E., Houstis, N., Daly, M.J., Patterson, N., Mesirov, J.P., Golub, T.R., Tamayo, P., Spiegelman, B., Lander, E.S., Hirschhorn, J.N., Altshuler, D. and Groop, L.C. (2003) PGC-1alpha-responsive genes involved in oxidative phosphorylation are coordinately downregulated in human diabetes. *Nature Genetics* **34**, 267–273.

Mykytyn, K.N.D., Searby, C.C., Shastri, M., Yen, H.J., Beck, J.S., Braun, T., Streb, L.M., Cornier, A.S., Cox, G.F., Fulton, A.B., Carmi, R., Luleci, G., Chandrasekharappa, S.C., Collins, F.S., Jacobson, S.G., Heckenlively, J.R., Weleber, R.G., Stone, E.M. and Sheffield, V.C. (2002) Identification of the gene (BBS1) most commonly involved in Bardet–Biedl syndrome, a complex human obesity syndrome. *Nature Genetics* **31**, 435–438.

Ozata, M., Ozdemir, I.C. and Licinio, J. (1999) Human leptin deficiency caused by a missense mutation: multiple endocrine defects, decreased sympathetic tone, and immune system dysfunction indicate new targets for leptin action, greater central than peripheral resistance to the effects of leptin, and spontaneous correction of leptin-mediated defects. *Journal of Clinical Endocrinology Metabolism* **84**: 3686–3695.

Perusse, L., Tremblay, A., Leblanc, C., Cloninger, C.R., Reich, T., Rice, J. and Bouchard, C. (1988) Familial resemblance in energy intake: contribution of genetic and environmental factors. *American Journal of Clinical Nutrition* **47**, 629–635.

Price, R.A. and Gottesman, I.I. (1991) Body fat in identical twins reared apart: roles for genes and environment. *Behavioural Genetics* **21**, 1–7.

Rice, T., Perusse, L., Bouchard, C. and Rao, D.C. (1999) Familial aggregation of body mass index and subcutaneous fat measures in the longitudinal Quebec family study. *Genetic Epidemiology* **16**, 316–334.

Rosenbaum, M., Murphy, E.M., Heymsfield, S.B., Matthews, D.E. and Leibel, R.L. (2002) Low dose leptin administration reverses effects of sustained weight reduction on energy expenditure and circulating concentrations of thyroid hormones. *Journal of Clinical Endocrinology Metabolism* **87**, 2391.

Samaras, K., Kelly, P.J., Chiano, M.N., Spector, T.D. and Campbell, L.V. (1999) Genetic and environmental influences on total-body and central abdominal fat: the effect of physical activity in female twins. *Annals of Internal Medicine* **130**: 873–882.

Schwartz, M.W., Woods, S.C., Porte, Jr, D., Seeley, R.J. and Baskin, D.G. (2000) Central nervous system control of food intake. *Nature* **404**, 661–671.

Sorensen, T.I., Price, R.A., Stunkard, A.J. and Schulsinger, F. (1989) Genetics of obesity in adult adoptees and their biological siblings. *British Medical Journal* **298**, 87–90.

Steinmuller, R., Steinberger, D. and Muller, U. (1998) MEHMO (mental retardation, epileptic seizures, hypogonadism and -genitalism, microcephaly, obesity), a novel syndrome: assignment of disease locus to Xp21.1-p22.13. *European Journal of Human Genetics* **6**, 201–206.

Strobel, A., Issad, T., Camoin, L., Ozata, M. and Strosberg, A.D. (1998) A leptin missense mutation associated with hypogonadism and morbid obesity. *Nature Genetics* **18**, 213–215.

Stunkard, A.J., Sorensen, T.I., Hanis, C., Teasdale, T.W., Chakraborty, R., Schull, W.J. and Schulsinger, F. (1986a) An adoption study of human obesity. *New England Journal of Medicine*, **314**, 193–198.

Stunkard, A.J., Foch, T.T. and Hrubec, Z. (1986b) A twin study of human obesity. *Journal of the American Medical Association* **256**, 51–54.

Stunkard, A.J., Harris, J.R., Pedersen, N.L. and McClearn, G.E. (1990) The body mass index of twins who have been reared apart [see comments]. *New England Journal of Medicine* **322**, 1483–1487.

Tahvanainen, E., Norio, R., Karila, E., Ranta, S., Weissenbach, J., Sistonen, P. and de la Chapelle, A. (1994) Cohen syndrome gene assigned to the long arm of chromosome 8 by linkage analysis. *Nature Genetics* **7**, 201–204.

Trayhurn, P., Thurlby, P.L. and James, W.P.T. (1977) Thermogenic defect in pre-obese *ob/ob* mice. *Nature* **266**, 60–62.

Turner, G., Gedeon, A., Mulley, J., Sutherland, G., Rae, J., Power, K. and Arthur, I. (1989) Borjeson–Forssman–Lehmann syndrome: clinical manifestations and gene localization to Xq26–27. *American Journal of Medical Genetics* **34**, 463–469.

Weinstein LS., Chen M. and Liu J. (2002) Gs(alpha) mutations and imprinting defects in human disease. *Annals of the New York Academy of Science* **968**, 173–197.

Wilson, M., Mulley, J., Gedeon, A., Robinson, H. and Turner, G. (1991) New X-linked syndrome of mental retardation, gynecomastia, and obesity is linked to DXS255. *American Journal of Human Genetics* **40**, 406–413.

Yeo, G.S, Lank, E.J., Farooqi, I.S., Keogh, J., Challis B.G. and O'Rahilly, S. (2003) Mutations in the human melanocortin-4 receptor gene associated with severe familial obesity disrupts receptor function through multiple molecular mechanisms. *Human Molecular Genetics* **12**, 561–574.

Zhang, Y., Proenca, R., Maffei, M., Barone, M., Leopold, L. and Friedman, J.M. (1994) Positional cloning of the mouse obese gene and its human homologue [published erratum appears in Nature 1995 Mar 30, 374(6521): 479]. *Nature* **372**, 425–432.

7

Fetal and infant origins of obesity

Mary Barker and David I. W. Phillips

Introduction, 93

Early growth and adult obesity, 93
  Tracking of obesity throughout
  life, 93
  Size at birth and adult body
  weight, 93
  Childhood growth and adult body
  weight, 95

Identifiable early life factors that lead
to obesity, 96

Maternal nutrition, 96
Social position in early life, 96
Maternal smoking, 96
Nutritional excess during
pregnancy or early infancy, 97
Infant feeding, 97
Early climate, 98

Mechanisms linking early
environmental influences with adult
body weight, 98

Fetal programming of
appetite, 99
Leptin resistance, 99
Hyperinsulinaemia, 99

Conclusion, 99

References, 99

Introduction

Although there is now a large body of evidence that many chronic diseases of adult life, including cardiovascular disease and diabetes, are related to impaired fetal or infant growth (Barker, 1998), much less is known about the early origins of obesity. Yet there is compelling evidence from animal studies that the quantity and distribution of adipose tissue may be set during intrauterine or early post-natal life. A number of recently published human studies now support the findings of these animal studies, and suggest that the early environment should be a focus in the search for the determinants of body weight. This chapter describes the findings from human studies relating anthropometric measurements at birth and during infancy with adult obesity. It also describes observational studies implicating a role for specific early life exposures as a cause of obesity in the offspring. Although this research is still in an early stage, it has enormous public health implications as it may lead to novel strategies for the prevention of obesity.

Early growth and adult obesity

Tracking of obesity throughout life

It has long been known that obese children tend to become obese adults. Longitudinal studies have shown that anthropometric measurements in infancy and early childhood predict body size in later life (Charney et al., 1976) and that body mass index (BMI) in childhood and adolescence 'track' into late middle age (Casey et al., 1992). For example, among 3659 Finnish adults whose body mass indices had been measured at intervals from birth through to late adulthood, those who were obese in later life were much more likely to have been obese as children. In men and women, those who had above average BMI at the age of 7 years were three times more likely to be obese adults (Eriksson et al., 2001). These and other studies support the idea that adult obesity may begin or become 'entrained' during childhood (Dietz, 1996), whereby factors influencing body weight in the early years of life may exert long-lasting effects. However, there are data to suggest that a predisposition to obesity may be initiated even earlier, specifically that body weight regulation may in part be determined *in utero*.

Size at birth and adult body weight

In a series of studies of 1750 men and women born in Hertfordshire, UK, at the beginning of the last century, body weight and height were measured. At the age of 65 years, the mean BMI (BMI = weight/height^2) of the people born weighing 5.5 lb or less was 26 kg/m^2, compared with a mean BMI of 25.5 kg/m^2 in those born weighing between 5.5 and 6.5 lb, and of 27.4 kg/m^2 in those born weighing up to 9.5 lb (Barker and Phillips, 1999). Similar findings were observed in this group with respect to obesity; with obesity defined as a BMI greater than 30 kg/m^2, 15.2% of those in the lowest birth weight group were found to be obese, declining to 11.5% among those who

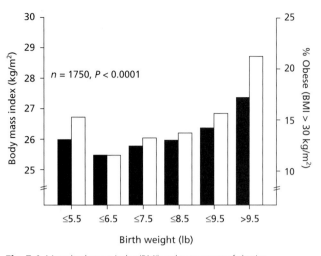

Fig. 7.1 Mean body mass index (BMI) and percentage of obesity (BMI > 30 kg/m²) in 1750 men and women born in Hertfordshire, UK, at the age of 65, according to birth weight, *P* < 0.0001.

weighed 5.5–6.5 lb at birth but rising steeply in the highest birth weight group, among whom 21.2% were found to be obese (Fig. 7.1). These findings parallel previous studies in a variety of populations, including 50-year-old Swedish men (Casey *et al.*, 1992) and 30- to 55-year-old American women (Curhan *et al.*, 1996). The Nurses Health study in the USA found that the odds of being obese as an adult rose from 1.0 in the women weighing between 7 and 8.8 lb at birth to 1.19 in women whose birth weights were between 8.5 and 10 lb, and up to 1.62 in the women who were heaviest at birth (Curhan *et al.*, 1996).

A criticism of the studies relating birth weight to indices of obesity is that few have considered whether this relationship is confounded by other factors, particularly maternal and paternal body size. A recent analysis of the 1958 British birth cohort showed that when adjustment was made for maternal weight, the relationship between birth weight and BMI at age 33 disappeared (Parsons *et al.*, 2001). Father's weight or height, however, had no effect. A further problem with these studies is that they have depended on a definition of obesity based on weight for height as indicated by the BMI. It is known that this may be misleading as individuals with similar BMI values may have very different body composition. Very few studies have so far analysed the relationship between birth weight and body composition, but data so far published suggest that a substantial part of the increased BMI of men and women who were heavy at birth may be due to an increase in muscle and lean body tissue rather than adipose tissue.

This evidence has come from a study of 143 men and women of known birth weight that used dual energy X-ray absorptiometry (DXA) to assess body composition at the age of 70 (Gale *et al.*, 2001). The authors found significant positive associations between birth weight and body mass and lean mass

but no statistically significant relationships between birth weight and whole body fat. In both men and women, 25% of the variation in lean mass was explained by birth weight after adjusting for age, adult height and adult weight.

Recently, we examined 737 men born between 1931 and 1939 who had records of birth weight and weight at 1 year. We measured their heights, weights, skinfold thickness and grip strength; analysis showed that birth weight correlated strongly with measures of height, weight and non-fat mass including muscle mass, but not with any of the measures of adiposity (Aihie Sayer *et al.*, 2003). Higher birth weight in this study therefore described babies born with more muscle and who grew into more muscular adults, rather than babies who were fatter and who became fatter adults. This finding may also explain why several studies have reported that the correlation between birth weight and BMI is stronger in men than in women, men being more muscular than women. Studies in twins have confirmed this finding. In an analysis of twins recruited from the East Flanders Prospective Twin Study (Loos *et al.*, 2002), it was found that the larger twin at birth tended to remain heavier and taller but had more lean mass and less subcutaneous and abdominal fat in adult life. As these associations were seen in both mono- and dizygotic twins, the findings suggest that these effects are independent of genetic influences. These data suggest that the contribution of the heavy baby to adult obesity has been very much overestimated and that it merely reflects the association between parental size, birth weight and subsequent size in adult life.

There is, however, increasing evidence that smaller babies have a genuinely higher risk of obesity as adults. The small amount of data available suggests that babies born small and light tend to have less muscle relative to their weight than do larger babies (Fall *et al.*, 1999). Other work suggests that these small babies are more likely to deposit fat on the central regions of the body as they grow older. This is a pattern of fat distribution found in the insulin resistance syndrome, and associated with an increased risk of diabetes and cardiovascular disease. Elderly men in Hertfordshire who were born small had higher waist circumferences relative to their hip circumferences by comparison with men who were larger at birth (Law *et al.*, 1992). This association was seen after allowing for BMI. However, this interpretation is challenged by a study of Swedish men, which, although demonstrating that low birth weight was associated with higher waist–hip ratios after controlling for BMI (Byberg *et al.*, 2000), went on to show that the higher waist–hip ratios of these lower birth weight men were the result of their smaller hip measurements, and hence did not reflect greater deposition of abdominal fat.

An increasing body of data suggests that low birth weight is more closely associated with truncal fat deposition rather than an increased waist–hip ratio. Young adult Mexicans and non-Hispanic Americans of low birth weight were found to have greater fat deposits on the trunk, as indicated by higher subscapular–triceps skinfold ratios (Valdez *et al.*, 1994). Similarly,

Table 7.1 Mean subscapular–triceps ratio by birth weight in girls aged 14 to 16 years, above and below their median BMI.

Birth weight	BMI (kg/m²)		Total
	Up to 21	Over 21	
Up to 3000 g	0.79 (31)	0.84 (24)	0.81 (55)
Up to 3500 g	0.74 (44)	0.81 (49)	0.76 (93)
Over 3500 g	0.76 (33)	0.77 (35)	0.77 (68)
Total	0.76 (108)	0.80 (108)	0.78 (216)

Numbers of girls in parentheses.

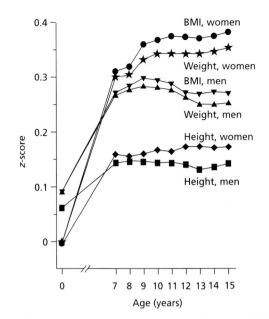

Fig. 7.2 Height, weight and BMI during childhood in 531 men and 715 women who later became obese. (A z-score of 0 corresponds to the mean value in the whole cohort; a z-score of 1 corresponds to a value of 1 SD above the mean.) (From Eriksson, J. *et al.*, 2001.)

7 to 12-year-old American children who were born small tended to have higher subscapular–triceps skinfold ratios (Malina *et al.*, 1996). In both of these groups, these effects were seen across the normal range of birth weight. Being fatter adds to the effect of birth weight on body fat distribution. In 14- to 16-year-old English girls, those who were smallest at birth, but fattest as teenagers, had the highest ratios of subscapular–triceps skinfolds (Table 7.1) (Barker *et al.*, 1997). It has been suggested that at younger ages these measures of truncal obesity may be a better indicator of regional fat distribution than waist–hip ratio. In addition, data from a number of studies of cardiovascular risk suggest that the subscapular–triceps skinfold thickness ratio has an effect that is independent of, and additive to, abdominal adiposity (Haffner *et al.*, 1987).

Childhood growth and adult body weight

It now appears that not only size at birth but also the rate of growth in early childhood has an impact on subsequent levels of obesity. Several studies suggest that faster rates of maturation, including earlier adiposity rebound and puberty, are associated with adult fatness. In the 1958 birth cohort, people who achieved a greater percentage of their adult height by the age of 7 had an increased risk of obesity at age 33 (Parsons *et al.*, 2001).

However, the effect of childhood growth on obesity varied by birth weight such that there was a stronger effect in people who were smallest at birth. Those who were born smallest but who 'caught-up' fastest were most likely to be obese as adults. The idea that rate of growth in childhood can compound the risk of later disease and/or obesity associated with birth size has been explored in a cohort of 3659 men and women born in Helsinki between 1924 and 1933 (Eriksson *et al.*, 2001). In this group, there was a raised risk of obesity in people who were heavier and fatter at birth. However, those who became obese in adult life tended to have faster rates of growth in childhood. Those who were fattest at the age of 7 had a threefold increase in their risk of adult obesity compared with those who were thinnest at 7 years. Figure 7.2 shows that those people who became obese in later life were already taller, heavier and fatter at the age of 7 than average. This is consistent with findings from

the 1958 British birth cohort, and adds weight to the argument that obesity is initiated early in life.

Different patterns of growth in childhood seem also to result in different patterns of body fat distribution. Observations from the study of a cohort born in the UK in one week in 1946 suggest that for any given adult body size, those who were lighter in childhood were more at risk of abdominal obesity (Kuh *et al.*, 2002). Being born relatively small and 'catching up' may also predispose to a more central pattern of body fat distribution. Approximately one-third of the children taking part in the Avon Longitudinal Study of Pregnancy and Childhood have shown clinically significant catch-up growth, here defined as a gain in weight of greater than 0.67 standard deviation (SD) scores between birth and 2 years (Ong *et al.*, 2000). These children were smaller and thinner at birth than other children, but were heavier, taller and had a higher BMI, percentage body fat and waist circumference at the age of 5.

Two studies of children identified as 'stunted' at birth or in infancy have described relationships between poor growth and a more pronounced central pattern of fat distribution in puberty. Walker and colleagues (2001) compared 116 stunted Jamaican children whose height for age was more than two standard deviations below the mean for between 9 and 24 months with 190 non-stunted Jamaican children. They found that the lower birth weight children had higher subscapular–triceps skinfold thickness ratios at age 11, and that the subscapular–triceps skinfold thickness ratio increased more in stunted than in non-stunted children between the ages of 7 and 11 years. Despite remaining relatively lean, the stunted children had more fat on their trunks than their generally fatter peers. This remained the case in the children who had been stunted in early childhood but who had caught up in height by the time they reached 11 years. The authors claim that 'the lower birth weights among the stunted children are in large part responsible for the differences in fat distribution between the stunted and non-stunted children'.

Bénéfice and colleagues (2001) measured the growth of 406 Senegalese girls aged 11–15 years. They found that the girls who were stunted in infancy caught up in body weight and subcutaneous fat mass during puberty but not in height, and that they, like the Jamaican girls, tended to accumulate more subcutaneous fat on their upper bodies, including the trunk and upper arms.

There are strong indications that these patterns of fat distribution track from adolescence into adulthood (van Lenthe, 1996). These findings are of concern because they suggest that to be born small and then to 'catch up' in late childhood confers a higher risk of central obesity and related conditions in adulthood.

Identifiable early life factors that lead to obesity

Maternal nutrition

Human studies suggest that both fetal undernutrition and overnutrition might play a part in the development of adult obesity. Fetal nutrition is not necessarily a direct consequence of maternal dietary intake, as the nutrients a mother consumes are not passed directly on to the growing fetus. Fetal nutrition is dependent on the mother's nutritional reserves, her metabolic and endocrine status, blood flow to the uterus and the functioning of the placenta (Harding 2001). As a consequence, mothers' diet in pregnancy, even following extreme undernutrition, tends only to have small effect on the baby's size at birth. There is evidence that it can nevertheless affect the development of the baby's organs, systems and later body composition.

The most widely known example of the effect of maternal starvation on adult obesity comes from the study of children born to women following the Dutch Winter famine of 1944–45. During the last 6 months of the Second World War, western Holland was blockaded by the occupying German army and large areas were affected by acute famine. At the beginning of the blockade in November 1944, the official ration was 1200 kcal per day falling to 800 by the end of the year and dropping to 580 by February 1945. For pregnant women, the calorie intake fell at times to 700 kcal per day or less than one-third of the recommended daily intake, and less than one-half of the energy intake from rations in liberated Holland. People born following the famine were studied at the age of 19. Although birth weights were not much affected by exposure to the famine, the subjects' body weight in later life was. Levels of

obesity in these people were dependent on the period of their exposure to famine. Those who had been exposed to the famine during the first two trimesters of pregnancy were twice as likely to be obese as those not exposed (Ravelli *et al.*, 1976); those exposed in the last trimester of pregnancy or in early infancy had 40% less chance of being obese at the age of 19.

By the time the men and women exposed to famine *in utero* reached the age of 50, the picture had changed. The men were no longer more obese than other men, but the women conceived in famine were on average 7.9 kg heavier than their unexposed counterparts, had BMIs that were 7.4% higher and waist circumferences 7.4 cm larger (Ravelli *et al.*, 1999). Although these gender differences are unexplained, the authors believe that these data are consistent with the idea that early pregnancy is a critical period in the development of the baby's hypothalamus, and that nutritional deprivation at this time resets the regulation of appetite and growth for life. The Dutch 'Hunger Winter' data provide clear evidence not only that undernutrition in fetal life has far-reaching consequences for body composition throughout life, but also that the timing of nutritional deprivation is critical in determining the precise nature of those consequences.

Social position in early life

There is increasing evidence that social position in early life is a predictor of obesity. In a review of childhood predictors of adult obesity, Parsons and colleagues (1999) found 12 studies that examined the influence of socioeconomic status (SES) on fatness in adulthood between 10 and 55 years after birth. In total, 10 of these studies reported an inverse relationship between obesity and the influence of SES, based on a variety of indicators including parental occupation, parental education and income. In the 1958 birth cohort, the mean BMI in women increased from 23.6 kg/m² among women born into social classes I and II (professional and managerial) to 24.4 kg/m² in women born into social classes IV and V (unskilled manual) backgrounds. In men, the range was from 25.0 to 26.1 kg/m². Social position is clearly an indirect measure of early life environment but these findings suggest that factors related to low SES in early life lead to adult obesity. It is, however, unclear what these factors might be and as yet there is little evidence to support or refute any speculation. Possible explanations include the effects of infant and childhood feeding, the contribution of undernourishment in early life followed by relative overnourishment, emotional deprivation leading to comfort eating later in life or the tendency to conform to the cultural and social norms absorbed during childhood (Power and Parsons, 2000).

Maternal smoking

A study of the 1958 birth cohort suggests that maternal smoking is a factor in the development of obesity. Infants of mothers who smoked in pregnancy were, as expected, lighter at birth than the infants of non-smokers. However, from adolescence they had a higher risk of obesity, which increased with age. By the age of 33, the mean BMI of men born to mothers who smoked was 26.09 kg/m^2 compared with 25.44 kg/m^2 in men born to non-smokers, with similar differences seen in women (25.12 vs. 24.38 kg/m^2) (Power and Jefferis, 2002). Interestingly, this effect of smoking was not reduced by adjustment for birth weight.

Nutritional excess during pregnancy or early infancy

Higher obesity rates in later life have also been associated with nutritional excess in fetal life and in infancy. People who have been exposed to maternal hyperglycaemia during pregnancy are more likely to become obese in adult life. Animal studies have shown that the offspring of rats made hyperglycaemic in the last week of pregnancy by continuous infusion of intravenous glucose are heavier both at birth and during infancy (Proietto and Thorburn, 1994). The human parallel is in studies of the children of women with diabetes during pregnancy. The children were born heavy and macrosomic, which resolved itself by the time they were 1 year old. But their obesity recurred in childhood. At the age of 4 years, these children began to increase in BMI over and above the norm, so that by the age of 14–17 years their mean BMI was 24.6 kg/m^2 compared with 20.9 kg/m^2 in a control group of children. Obesity in these adolescents was associated with excessive insulin secretion *in utero*. This association remained after correcting for mother's weight. It is not simply that heavier, diabetic mothers have heavier children. These findings lead the authors to conclude that obesity in the offspring of diabetic mothers is the result of 'metabolic programming' of the fetus, that is the offspring's glucose–insulin metabolism is permanently altered by its exposure to the metabolic consequences of the mother's diabetes.

A longer term follow-up of children born to diabetic mothers was carried out among the Pima Indians of Arizona (Pettit *et al.*, 1993). In this group, women who were hypoglycaemic in the last two trimesters of pregnancy had heavier babies who remained fatter through childhood and in whom the tendency to fatness persisted into adulthood. Again these effects were independent of mothers' size. In order to disentangle the genetic influences from the effects of intrauterine exposure, a further study was conducted, following up families in which at least one sibling was born after the mother was diagnosed with diabetes (Dabelea *et al.*, 2000). In this group of 183 siblings, those born to a mother with diabetes had a BMI of 2.6 kg/m^2 higher on average than those born to the same mother before she became diabetic. As siblings who are born before or after their mother became diabetic have the same genetic risk of obesity, the difference in BMI has to be attributed to difference in the intrauterine environment.

Infant feeding

There is a continuing debate about the role of infant feeding and its relationship with obesity in later life. The debate centres on the possibility of a protective effect of breast-feeding and studies have produced contradictory findings. A large, recent study of 15 000 children aged 9 to 14 years in the USA found that those who had been only or mostly fed breast milk in the first 6 months of life were less likely to be obese than their peers (Gillman *et al.*, 2001). Those who had been only or mostly breast fed had an odds ratio of 0.78 for being overweight (95% CI 0.66–0.91), after adjusting for age, sex, sexual maturity, energy intake, time spent watching television, physical activity, mother's BMI and other variables reflecting social, economic and lifestyle factors. Being only or mostly breast fed for at least 7 months conferred additional benefits in protecting against obesity over being fed in this way for only 3 months. A recent review of 11 studies examining the prevalence of overweight among children older than 3 years of age found that eight of these studies showed a lower risk of overweight in children who had been breast fed (Dewey, 2003). The three studies that did not find this relationship lacked information on the exclusivity of breast-feeding.

There are, however, major problems with interpreting these studies. Infant feeding formulas have changed over time and it is not clear whether certain formulas are more likely to lead to obesity than others. It is also possible that the earlier introduction of solid foods and their nature may be more important than breast-feeding per se. Finally, much less is known about whether this effect of breast-feeding persists into adulthood. The difficulties of obtaining accurate retrospective data about infant feeding mean there are very few such studies. However, the records kept during the famine in western Holland in the Second World War provide an opportunity for retrospective analysis. The precise timing of the period of famine and the records kept throughout make the 'Hunger Winter' a valuable natural experiment. A group of 625 adults aged 45 to 53 years born in Amsterdam at the time of the famine were traced and examined (Ravelli *et al.*, 2000). The maternity records for these people showed no relationship between method of infant feeding and later life obesity.

The mechanisms underlying the protective effect of breast-feeding are not yet clear. Some have speculated that breast-fed children have greater control of their intake than those who were bottle fed and therefore develop better mechanisms for self-regulating (Gillman *et al.*, 2001). Bottle feeding may promote more parental control over how much and how often the infant eats, a high degree of parental control having been found in older children to undermine intrinsic settings for appetite and satiety (Birch and Fisher, 1998). Alternatively, the protective effect of breast-feeding may originate in the ingestion of hormones and growth factors present in breast milk, which may have a programming effect on the mechanisms maintaining appetite and body weight.

Early climate

Several intriguing studies have demonstrated that environmental temperature around the time of birth may affect long-term fatness; 150 years ago, Bergmann and Bodenheimer (1847) pointed out the tendency for animals living in cooler regions of the world to have a greater body size and shorter extremities than those in warmer regions. Thus, for example, wolves living in arctic conditions, such as the Siberian wolf, are much larger than their warmer cousins, the Indian or Arabian wolf. These differences in morphology, presumably designed to aid heat conservation, have always been considered to be genetic in origin. However, this cannot be the only explanation as some of the differences can be reproduced experimentally by exposing animals to different temperatures in early life.

Several authors have described differences in the physical appearance of piglets raised at different temperatures. Animals raised in the warm appear to be lean and elongated, whereas those raised in the cold, even when they were litter mates of the same body weight, have a rotund appearance, with short limbs and snout, small tail and ears, and more body hair (Ingram and Dauncey, 1986). These differences in morphology are associated with differences in physiology, behaviour, cell structure and cell function. In a recent series of experiments in rats, Young and Shimano (1998) studied fat accumulation in rats reared in a cool environment (18°C) compared with rats raised at 30°C. At 60 days old, the animals were transferred to a common temperature and their growth and development were studied. The rats whose early rearing was in the cooler environment gained more weight and accumulated more fat in abdominal depots than the animals raised at the higher temperature. Interestingly, this response was exacerbated when the rats were given access *ad libitum* to sucrose.

Although the studies described here were carried out in laboratory animals, data are available that suggest that early exposure to cold may increase body weight in humans as well. In humans, thermoregulatory responses to cold or heat are known to be influenced by the temperature of the early environment (Glass *et al.*, 1968; Diamond, 1991). Furthermore, in 1955, Newman and Munro (1955) published their analyses of height and weight from 15 216 young healthy white men drafted in to the US Army between 1946 and 1953. They divided their subjects by state of birth and analysed the relationships between state means for height and weight and the mean state temperature in the months of January and July. The data from their paper is shown in Fig. 7.3. Recruits from the colder states had much higher BMIs than those of their peers.

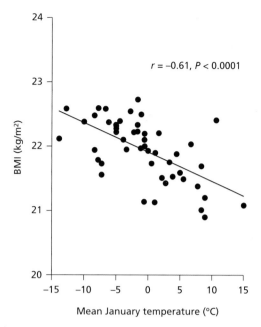

Fig. 7.3 BMI in 15 216 US Army recruits, aged 18–21 years, according to the mean January temperature of the state in which they were born ($r = -0.61$, $P < 0.0001$). (From Newman, R.W. and Munro, E.H., 1955.)

Mechanisms linking early environmental influences with adult body weight

What then are the mechanisms that could link events occurring in very early life with adult body weight? The amount of adipose tissue reflects both the number and average volume of the component adipose cells. Brook (1972) has suggested that the basic complement of adipose cells is determined during a critical period from 30 weeks of gestation to the first year of life. After this period, growth in adipose tissue mass depends on an increase in cell size rather then cell number. Studies of animals exposed to overnutrition during intrauterine and early post-natal life show that they have more numerous adipocytes (Brook, 1972; Aubert *et al.*, 1979). It has therefore been suggested that nutritional abundance in late gestation or infancy—for example, that occurring in the offspring of gestationally diabetic women—may increase adipocyte mass by means of an increase in cell numbers. Recent studies, however, suggest that the number of adipocytes in adult life is not fixed (Prins and O'Rahilly, 1997), but that fat cell acquisition seems to occur throughout life in a process involving the expansion and differentiation of pre-adipocytes. It is more likely that events in early life imprint upon the development of the systems regulating body weight, permanently altering their set point and leading to adult obesity. Although the mechanisms are poorly understood, there is an increasing body of evidence that appetite regulation is programmed during early life and that leptin and insulin resistance is important in this process.

Fetal programming of appetite

Animal work in New Zealand has shown that appetite can be programmed *in utero*. Programming, the science of altered gene expression by exposure to the environment *in utero*, suggests that there may be a route to obesity involving programming of the hypothalamus, and perturbed secretion of leptin and insulin, both hormones related to appetite. Rats born to severely undernourished mothers were born much smaller than control rats, but were found to have greater appetites especially for very high-calorie foods (Vickers *et al.*, 2000; Breier *et al.*, 2001). Their appetites grew as they grew older, and their daily calorie intake remained higher than control groups, even after controlling for body weight. As adult rats, they were shorter but had more body fat than adequately nourished control rats, and had higher blood pressure and markedly increased fasting plasma insulin and leptin concentrations. The overall picture is of animals born smaller and malnourished but with an inappropriately large appetite for high-calorie foods, which, in time, amplifies the metabolic abnormalities shown at birth.

Leptin resistance

Leptin is a polypeptide hormone synthesized in adipocytes, which acts at the level of the hypothalamus to suppress appetite and increase energy expenditure. Many studies show that the plasma concentrations of leptin correlate closely with present-day weight and adiposity, and that this relationship is established early in life, as there are positive associations between the concentrations of leptin in cord blood and adiposity at birth (Ong *et al.*, 1999). Studies of 502 men and women from the Hertfordshire cohort born in the 1920s (Phillips *et al.*, 1999) and of 1462 women born between 1908 and 1930 (Lissner *et al.*, 1999) have shown that, after adjustment for the level of current BMI, people who were small at birth have higher levels of leptin. This suggests that they have a degree of leptin resistance. These inverse relationships have also been described in pigs (Ekert *et al.*, 2000). Further studies have determined that these relationships are established in the first year of life. Growth-retarded newborn infants have lower than normal leptin concentrations at birth; by 12 months of age, they have higher than normal levels (Jaquet *et al.*, 1999).

It also appears that infants with lower plasma leptin concentrations at birth and lower body weight tend to gain weight more rapidly in the first months of post-natal life (Ong *et al.*, 1999), suggesting that it is the increased availability of nutrients post-natally which may be responsible for subsequent obesity. This may be an explanation for the adult studies in the UK (Power and Parsons, 2000) and Finland (Eriksson *et al.*, 2001) showing that catch-up growth is associated with obesity. It is unclear, however, whether the increased availability of nutrients programmes leptin expression through the action of nutrient-sensitive hormones, such as insulin or insulin-like growth factor-1, or whether these are direct effects on the adipocyte.

Hyperinsulinaemia

It has also been proposed that increased concentrations of insulin in early life may reset the systems involved in the regulation of food intake and weight. Plagemann and colleagues (1999) have developed a rodent model of overnutrition in early life, based on reduction of litter size, which increases the milk intake of the pups. These pups gain weight rapidly and become obese in adult life, as well as developing many of the features of the metabolic syndrome. The rats also have a marked increase in galanin-containing neurons in the arcuate nucleus of the hypothalamus. Galanin is a potent stimulator of food intake and it suggests that hyperinsulinaemia in the perinatal period may alter the functional maturation of galanin-containing neurons.

Conclusion

Many Western countries are now facing an epidemic of obesity. Although this affects all ages, the most dramatic increase has been among children. Between 1990 and 2000, in the USA, the number of children who are overweight has more than doubled. This observation suggests that the likely explanation of the obesity epidemic is to be found in the early years of life. The studies summarized in this chapter are tantalizing, as they point towards the fetal or early infant environment as being an important period in the development of lifelong obesity. In particular, the evidence suggests that alterations in the tempo of growth in early childhood are importantly linked with later obesity, and that this time of life, which is often poorly documented in longitudinal studies, should be a focus for future research. This research needs to be linked with appropriate studies in animal models, which will help us understand how early diet and other environmental factors influence the neuroendocrine function of the hypothalamus in determining the set point for appetite throughout life.

References

Aihie Sayer, A., Syddall, H.E., Dennison, E.M., Gilbody, H.J., Duggleby, S.L., Cooper, C., Barker, D.J.P. and Phillips, D.I.W. (2004) Birthweight, weight at 1 year of age, and body composition in older men: findings from the Hertfordshire Cohort Study. *American Journal of Clinical Nutrition* **80**, 199–203.

Aubert, R., Suquet, J.P. and Lemmonier, D. (1979) Long-term morphological and metabolic effects of early under and over nutrition in mice. *Journal of Nutrition* **110**, 649–661.

Barker, D.J.P. (1998) *Mothers, Babies and Health in Later Life*. London: BMJ.

Barker, M. and Phillips, D.I.W. (1999) Early environmental influences on adult body weight. In: Kopelman, P. ed. *Appetite, Obesity and Disorders of Over and Undereating*. London: Royal College of Physicians, 51–61.

Barker, M., Robinson, S., Osmond, C. and Barker, D.J.P. (1997) Birth weight and body fat distribution in adolescent girls. *Archives of Disease in Childhood* **77**, 381–383.

Bénéfice, E., Garnier, D., Simondon, K.B. and Malina, R.M. (2001) Relationship between stunting in infancy and growth and fat distribution during adolescence in Senegalese girls. *European Journal of Clinical Nutrition* **55**, 50–58.

Bergman, A. andBodenheimer, F.S. (eds) (1847) *Problems of Animal Ecology*. Oxford: Oxford University Press, 595.

Birch, L.L. and Fisher, J.O. (1998) Development of eating behaviours among children and adolescents. *Pediatrics* **101**, 539–549.

Breier, B.H., Vickers, M.H., Ikenasio, B.A., Chan, K.Y. andWong, W.P.S. (2001) Fetal programming of appetite and obesity. *Molecular and Cellular Endocrinology* **185**, 73–79.

Brook, C.G. (1972) Evidence for a sensitive period in adipose-cell replication in man. *Lancet* **2**, 624–627.

Byberg, L., McKeigue, P.M., Zethelius, B. and Lithell, H.O. (2000) Birth weight and the insulin resistance syndrome: association of low birth weight with truncal obesity and raised plasminogen activator inhibitor-1 but not with abdominal obesity or plasma lipid disturbances. *Diabetologia* **43**, 54–60.

Casey, V.A., Dwyer, J.T., Coleman, K.A. and Valadian, I. (1992) Body mass index from childhood to middle age: a 50 year follow-up. *American Journal of Clinical Nutrition* **56**, 14–18.

Charney, E., Goodman, H.C., McBride, M., Lyon, B. and Pratt, R. (1976) Childhood antecedents of adult obesity. *New England Journal of Medicine* **295**, 6–9.

Curhan, G.C., Chertow, G.M., Willett, W.C., Spiegelman, D., Colditz, G.A., Manson, J.E., Speizer, F.E. and Stampfer, M.J. (1996) Birth weight and adult hypertension and obesity in women. *Circulation* **94**, 1310–1315.

Dabelea, D., Hanson, R.L., Lindsay, R.S., Pettit, D.J., Imperatore, G., Gabir, M.M., Roumain, J., Bennett, P.H. and Knowler, W.C. (2000) Intrauterine exposure to diabetes conveys risks for Type 2 diabetes and obesity: a study of discordant sibships. *Diabetes* **49**, 2208–2211.

Dewey, K.G. (2003) Is breastfeeding protective against child obesity? *Journal of Human Lactation* **19**, 9–18.

Diamond, J. (1991) Pearl Harbor and the Emperor's physiologists. *Natural History* **12**, 2–7.

Dietz, W.H. (1996) Early influences on body weight regulation. In: Bouchard, C. and Bray, G.A. eds. *Regulation of Body Weight*. Chichester: John Wiley and Sons.

Ekert, J.E., Gatford, K.L., Luxford, B.G., Campbell, R.G. and Owens, P.C. (2000) Leptin expression in offspring is programmed by nutrition in pregnancy. *Journal of Endocrinology* **165**, R6.

Eriksson, J.G., Forsén, T., Tuomilehto, J., Osmond, C. and Barker, D. (2001) Size at birth, childhood growth and obesity in adult life. *International Journal of Obesity* **25**, 735–740.

Fall, C.H.D., Yajnik, C.S., Rao, S., Coyaji, K.J. and Shier, R.P. (1999) The effects of maternal body composition before birth on fetal growth: the Pune Maternal Nutrition and Fetal Growth Study. In: O'Brien, P.M.S., Wheeler, T. and Barker, D.J.P. eds. *Fetal Programming: Influences on Development and Disease in Later Life*. London: RCOG Press, 231–242.

Gale, C.R., Martyn, C.N., Kellingray, S., Eastell, R. and Cooper, C.

(2001) Intrauterine programming of adult body composition. *Journal of Clinical Endocrinology and Metabolism* **86**, 267–272.

Gillman, M.W., Rifas-Shiman, S.L., Camargo, C.A., Berkey, C.S., Frazier, A.L., Rockett, H.R.H., Field, A.E. and Colditz, G.A. (2001) Risk of overweight among adolescents who were breastfed as infants. *Journal of the American Medical Association* **285**, 2461–2467.

Glass, L., Silverman, W.A. and Sinclair, J.C. (1968) Effect of the thermal environment on cold resistance and growth of small infants after the first week of life. *Pediatrics* **41**, 1033–1046.

Haffner, S.M., Stern, M.P., Hazuda, H.P., Pugh, J. and Patterson, J.K. (1987) Do upper-body and centralized adiposity measure different aspects of regional body-fat distribution? Relationship to non-insulin-dependent diabetes mellitus, lipids, and lipoproteins. *Diabetes* **36**, 43–51.

Harding, J. (2001) The nutritional basis of the fetal origins of adult disease. *International Journal of Epidemiology* **30**, 15–23.

Ingram, D.L. and Dauncey, M.J. (1986) Environmental effects on growth and development. In: Buttery, P.J., Haynes, N.B. and Lindsay, D.B. eds. *Control and Manipulation of Animal Growth*. London: Butterworths, 5–20.

Jaquet, D., Leger, J., Tabone, M.D., Czernichow, P. and Levy-Marchal, C. (1999) High serum leptin concentrations during catch-up growth of children born with intrauterine growth retardation. *Journal of Clinical Endocrinology and Metabolism* **84**, 1949–1953.

Kuh, D., Hardy, R., Chaturvedi, N. and Wadsworth, M.E. (2002) Birthweight, childhood growth and abdominal obesity in adult life. *International Journal of Obesity and Related Metabolic Disorders* **26**, 40–47.

Law, C.M., Barker, D.J.P., Osmond, C., Fall, C.H.D. and Simmonds, S.J. (1992) Early growth and abdominal fatness in adult life. *Journal of Epidemiology and Community Health* **46**, 184–186.

van Lenthe, F.J., Kemper, H.C.G., van Mechelen, W. and Twisk, J.W.R. (1996) Development and tracking of central pattern of subcutaneous fat in adolescence and adulthood: the Amsterdam growth and health study. *International Journal of Epidemiology* **25**, 1162–1171.

Lissner, L., Karlsson, C., Lindroos, A.K., Carlsson, B., Carlsson, L. and Bengtsson, C. (1999) Birth weight, adulthood BMI, and subsequent weight gain in relation to leptin levels in Swedish women. *Obesity Research* **7**, 150–154.

Loos, R.J., Beunen, G., Fagard, R., Derom, C. and Vlietinck, R. (2002) Birth weight and body composition in young women: a prospective twin study. *American Journal of Clinical Nutrition* **75**, 676–682.

Malina, R.M., Katzmarzyk, P.T. and Beunen, G. (1996) Birth weight and its relationship to size attained and relative fat distribution at 7 to 12 years of age. *Obesity Research* **4**, 385–390.

Newman, R.W. and Munro, E.H. (1955) The relation of climate and body size in US males. *American Journal of Anthropology* **13**, 1–17.

Ong, K.K.L., Ahmed, M.L., Sherriff, A., Woods, K.A., Watts, A., Golding, J., The Alspac Study Team and Dunger, D.B. (1999) Cord blood leptin is associated with size at birth and predicts infancy weight gain in humans. *Journal of Clinical Endocrinology and Metabolism* **84**, 1145–1148.

Ong, K.K.L., Ahmed, M.L., Emmet, P.M., Preece, M.A. and Dunger, D.B. (2000) Association between postnatal catch-up growth and obesity in childhood: prospective cohort study. *British Medical Journal* **320**, 967–971.

Parsons, T.J., Power, C., Logan, S. and Summerbell, C.D. (1999) Childhood predictors of adult obesity: a systematic review. *International Journal of Obesity* **23**, S1–S107.

Parsons, T.J., Power, C. and Manor, O. (2001) Fetal and early life growth and body mass index from birth to early adulthood in 1958 British cohort: longitudinal study. *British Medical Journal* **323**, 1331–1335.

Pettit, D.J., Nelson, R.G., Saad, M.F., Bennett, P.H. and Knowler, W.C. (1993) Diabetes and obesity in the offspring of Pima Indian women with diabetes during pregnancy. *Diabetes Care* **16**, 310–314.

Phillips, D.I.W., Fall, C.H.D., Cooper, C., Norman, R.J., Robinson, J.S. and Owens, P.C. (1999) Size at birth and plasma leptin concentrations in adult life. *International Journal of Obesity* **23**, 1025–1029.

Plagemann, A., Harder, T., Rake, A., Voits, M., Fink, H., Rohde, U. and Dörner, G. (1999) Perinatal elevation of hypothalamic insulin, acquired malformation of hypothalamic galaninergic neurons, and syndrome X-like alterations in adulthood of neonatally overfed rats. *Brain Research* **836**, 146–155.

Power, C. and Parsons, T. (2000) Nutritional and other influences in childhood as predictors of adult obesity. *Proceedings of the Nutrition Society* **59**, 267–272.

Power, C. and Jefferis, B.J.M.H. (2002) Fetal environment and subsequent obesity: a study of maternal smoking. *International Journal of Epidemiology* **31**, 413–419.

Prins, J.B. and O'Rahilly, S. (1997) Regulation of adipose cell number in man. *Clinical Science* **92**, 3–11.

Proietto, J. and Thorburn, A.W. (1994) Animal models of obesity — theories of aetiology. In: *Baillière's Clinical Endocrinology and Metabolism*. London: Baillière Tindall, 509.

Ravelli, G.P., Stein, Z.A. and Susser, M.W. (1976) Obesity in young men after famine exposure *in utero* and early infancy. *New England Journal of Medicine* **295**, 349–353.

Ravelli, A.C.J., van der Meulen, J.H.P, Osmond, C., Barker, D.J.P. and Bleker, O.P. (1999) Obesity at the age of 50 years in men and women exposed to famine prenatally. *American Journal of Clinical Nutrition* **70**, 811–816.

Ravelli, A.C.J, van der Meulen, J.H.P., Osmond, C., Barker, D.J.P. and Bleker, O.P. (2000) Infant feeding and adult glucose tolerance, lipid profile, blood pressure, and obesity. *Archives of Diseases in Childhood* **82**, 248–252.

Valdez, R., Athens, M.A., Thompson, G.H., Bradshaw, B.S. and Stern, M.P. (1994) Birthweight and adult health outcomes in a biethnic population in the USA. *Diabetologia* **37**, 624–631.

Vickers, M.H., Breier, B.H., Cutfield, W.S., Hofman, P.L. and Gluckman, P.D. (2000) Fetal origins of hyperphagia, obesity, and hypertension and postnatal amplification by hypercaloric nutrition. *American Journal of Physiology Endocrinology and Metabolism* **279**, E83–E87.

Walker, S.P., Gaskin, P.S., Powell, C.A. and Bennett, F.I. (2001) The effects of birth weight and postnatal linear growth retardation on body mass index, fatness and fat distribution in mid and late childhood. *Public Health Nutrition* **5**, 391–396.

Young, J.B. and Shimano, Y. (1998) Effects of rearing temperature on body weight and abdominal fat in male and female rats. *American Journal of Physiology* **274**, R398–R405.

Metabolic fuels and obesity: carbohydrate and lipid metabolism in skeletal muscle and adipose tissue

Keith N. Frayn and Ellen E. Blaak

Metabolic importance of skeletal
muscle and white adipose tissue, 102

Role of skeletal muscle and
adipose tissue in normal daily
energy fluxes, 104

Skeletal muscle, 105
  Routes of ATP synthesis in
  skeletal muscle: outline and
  methodology, 105
  Carbohydrate metabolism in
  skeletal muscle at rest and during
  exercise, 107

Lipid metabolism in skeletal
muscle at rest and during
exercise, 107
Disturbances in skeletal muscle
metabolism and the development
of obesity, 109
Skeletal muscle metabolism in
obesity, 110

White adipose tissue, 111
  Adipose tissue carbohydrate
  metabolism, 111
  Non-esterified fatty acid release
  from adipose tissue, 111

Triacylglycerol clearance by
adipose tissue, 112
Disturbances in adipose tissue
metabolism and the development
of obesity, 113
Adipose tissue metabolism in
obesity, 114

Acknowledgements, 115

References, 115

Metabolic importance of skeletal muscle and white adipose tissue

Skeletal muscle makes up 40% of body weight in 'reference man' and 30% in 'reference woman' (Snyder, 1975). In trained athletes, skeletal muscle may contribute up to 65% of body mass (Spenst *et al.*, 1993). Even at rest, skeletal muscle metabolism plays a major role in whole-body energy fluxes simply by virtue of its bulk. During exercise, the metabolic flux in skeletal muscle may increase enormously and skeletal muscle metabolism dominates whole-body energy fluxes.

Skeletal muscle is the major reservoir of carbohydrate, in the form of glycogen, in the body. A typical liver glycogen content in the fed state is around 100 g, whereas whole-body skeletal muscle contains about 400 g typically, and may contain much more during high-carbohydrate feeding (Acheson *et al.*, 1988). It is therefore evident that skeletal muscle plays a major role in the regulation of the metabolic disposal of carbohydrate in the body. This role is particularly evident in the fed state, when muscle glucose utilization is increased by insulin. However, the role of skeletal muscle in lipid metabolism should not be underestimated. Because of its large mass, skeletal muscle is one of the most important organs in the removal from the bloodstream of non-esterified fatty acids (NEFAs) both at rest and during exercise. It is also an important site of the removal of plasma triacylglycerol (TG).

Skeletal muscle plays an important role in amino acid metabolism. Intracellular concentrations of some amino acids are several-fold greater than those in plasma, and again, by virtue of its mass, skeletal muscle constitutes the largest reservoir of free amino acids in the body (Bergström *et al.*, 1974). Skeletal muscle also contains the largest amount of protein of any single tissue in the body, and although its rate of protein turnover is slower than that of some smaller organs, the absolute rate of turnover is the largest in the body (Daniel *et al.*, 1977).

The oxygen consumption of skeletal muscle at rest, expressed per unit of tissue weight, is not as high as that of some other organs (e.g. liver 60 mL of O_2/min per kilogram wet weight; resting skeletal muscle 4 mL of O_2/min per kilogram wet weight; Frayn, 1992), but once again, because of its mass, it is one of the major consumers of O_2 in the whole body. Variations in skeletal muscle O_2 consumption have been shown to make a major contribution to the between-person variability in resting energy expenditure (Zurlo *et al.*, 1990a). During exercise, the O_2 consumption of skeletal muscle increases enormously; values of 350 mL of O_2/min per kilogram wet weight have been recorded (Rådegran *et al.*, 1999), and under those conditions muscle O_2 consumption dominates that of the body.

In comparison with skeletal muscle, white adipose tissue contributes a smaller proportion of body weight in non-obese subjects: 20% in 'reference man' and 30% in 'reference woman' (Snyder, 1975). However, as a source of NEFA, one of the most important plasma energy-bearing fuels, the contribution of white adipose tissue to whole-body energy fluxes is of major importance. In trained athletes, the proportion of adipose tissue is smaller than in non-athletes (typically 9–12% of body weight in men and women—Björntorp, 1991a), but it still plays a key role in the supply of NEFA to exercising muscle. In obesity, the amount of adipose tissue may, of course, increase enormously. Although this excessive adipose tissue may not be as metabolically active as in lean subjects, by virtue of its mass it exerts powerful influences on whole-body energy fluxes.

The important role of adipose tissue in regulating delivery of NEFA into the plasma is clear, but adipose tissue also plays an important part in the regulation of plasma TG concentrations, in two ways. The rate of NEFA delivery plays a critical role in determining hepatic TG secretion rates. In addition, adipose tissue is a major site of extraction of plasma TG, especially during the postprandial period. In contrast, it is clear that adipose tissue plays only a small role in whole-body glucose disposal (Coppack *et al.*, 1990; Mårin *et al.*, 1992; Virtanen *et al.*, 2001). The importance of white adipose tissue in whole-body amino acid metabolism is not entirely clear, although for some amino acids it may approach that of skeletal muscle (Frayn *et al.*, 1991).

In recent years it has become apparent that adipose tissue also exerts major effects on whole-body energy metabolism through the secretion of a range of peptides and other factors, some of which may act in a local paracrine manner, but some of which undoubtedly act as hormones signalling to the brain, skeletal muscle and other tissues. The best understood is the adipocyte-derived hormone leptin. Leptin deficiency in humans is characterized by widespread metabolic and physiological disturbances, including failure of sexual maturation, many of which are normalized on treatment with recombinant leptin (Farooqi *et al.*, 2002). Another adipocyte-derived peptide that has been intensively studied recently is adiponectin (also known as adipoQ or Acrp30). An interesting feature of adiponectin secretion is that it decreases with increasing adipose tissue mass, the opposite of what happens with leptin (Weyer *et al.*, 2001). It has been suggested that adiponectin has insulin-sensitizing effects in tissues other than adipose (Berg *et al.*, 2001; Yamauchi *et al.*, 2001). Although these novel aspects of adipose tissue function are not the subject of this chapter, they may well complement the better established functions of adipose tissue in energy metabolism. Secretory functions of adipose tissue have been extensively reviewed elsewhere (Mohamed-Ali *et al.*, 1998; Frühbeck *et al.*, 2001; Frayn *et al.*, 2003).

The metabolism of brown adipose tissue is different in most respects from that of white adipose tissue and, as its contribution to whole-body energy fluxes in adult humans is probably small, it will not be covered in this chapter. However, the study of brown adipose tissue led to the elucidation of a potentially very important aspect of energy metabolism in skeletal muscle, white adipose tissue and other tissues. Brown adipose tissue is specialized for the production of heat. This is achieved by the expression of a protein, uncoupling protein 1 (UCP1) or thermogenin, in the inner mitochondrial membrane. UCP1 is a member of the mitochondrial transporter family. It is a proton transporter. The effect is that the proton gradient that is generated by the electron transport chain across the inner mitochondrial membrane, and is normally used for the synthesis of ATP, is instead discharged. Metabolic energy is therefore released as heat. Brown adipose tissue generates most of its heat by oxidation of fatty acids. In 1997, a protein related to UCP1 was discovered, now called UCP2 (Fleury *et al.*, 1997). There is now known to be a family of UCPs (Ricquier and Bouillaud, 2000a). UCP2 is ubiquitously expressed, whereas UCP3 is expressed mainly in skeletal muscle. The possibility has been raised that these UCPs (2 and 3 especially) are involved in uncoupling of oxidative phosphorylation in tissues other than brown adipose tissue, although this has also been much debated (Dulloo and Samec, 2001). UCP3, in particular, could potentially play a major role in energy metabolism because of its expression in skeletal muscle. This will be discussed further in the consideration of skeletal muscle energy metabolism.

Both skeletal muscle and white adipose tissue are distributed in discrete sites throughout the body. These sites are not homogeneous in their metabolic characteristics. Muscles vary in their oxidative capacity, although in humans (as opposed to rodents) all skeletal muscles are of mixed fibre type (Johnson *et al.*, 1973). Clearly, during exercise, there are muscle-specific differences in metabolism, as different muscles are recruited to different extents, and this implies that there is local regulation of skeletal muscle metabolism. In the case of adipose tissue, the differences between depots in their metabolic characteristics may be quite marked and may be relevant to their role in whole-body energy metabolism. These site-specific properties will be discussed later in this chapter and elsewhere in this book (see Chapter 12), but it is important at this stage to note the large body of evidence that links the accumulation of abdominal, and especially intra-abdominal adipose tissue, with adverse metabolic changes in obesity (Björntorp, 1990; Kissebah and Krakower, 1994; Banerji *et al.*, 1995; Abate *et al.*, 1995; Arner, 1997; Couillard *et al.*, 1999). Unfortunately, because the intra-abdominal fat depots are not accessible for direct study, our knowledge of them comes only from *in vitro* studies on the metabolic properties of samples that are removed at operation. Most of the metabolic properties of adipose tissue discussed below are therefore based on studies of subcutaneous adipose tissue, which is accessible for study *in vivo* (Arner and Bülow, 1993; Frayn and Coppack, 2001).

The metabolic pathways of skeletal muscle (Jones and Round, 1990; Henriksson, 1995) and adipose tissue (Crandall and DiGirolamo, 1990; Hollenberg, 1990; Frayn *et al.*, 2003), and their regulation in different states have been discussed in detail elsewhere. The theme of this chapter will be the main fluxes of energy-bearing fuels in these tissues, and their contributions to whole-body energy fluxes. Because the emphasis will be on energy metabolism, we will say little about amino acid and protein metabolism, although its importance should not be minimized. We will outline the normal metabolic contributions of these tissues in the whole body, and then discuss whether alterations in skeletal muscle or adipose tissue metabolism may underlie the development of obesity. As evidence on this question is not strong, we will devote more space to a consideration of the consequences of obesity on skeletal muscle and adipose tissue metabolism, and show how such consequences may lead in turn to many of the adverse metabolic characteristics associated with obesity.

Role of skeletal muscle and adipose tissue in normal daily energy fluxes

On a typical Western diet in which fat provides around 40% of energy, humans eat around 300 g of carbohydrate and 100 g of fat (mainly TG) per day. (Clearly these are round figures, for illustration only.) As we eat most of this in three main meals, a 'typical' meal might contain around 100 g of carbohydrate and 30–40 g of fat.

The free glucose content of the body in the post-absorptive state is around 12 g. (The plasma glucose concentration is 5 mmol/L or about 0.9 g/L, and the extracellular fluid volume is about 20% of body weight or 13 L.) Therefore, at one meal we eat enough glucose to raise the plasma glucose concentration around eightfold. In normal people, however, the rise is more like 60–80% of basal. There are powerful homeostatic mechanisms that minimize the excursions of plasma glucose concentration. These mechanisms include rapid suppression of endogenous hepatic glucose production, together with increased glucose disposal into cells. Skeletal muscle metabolism switches rapidly in the postprandial state from almost complete independence from carbohydrate, to rapid glucose uptake, such that skeletal muscle is undoubtedly the major extrahepatic tissue involved in this coordinated regulation of glucose metabolism. The contribution of white adipose tissue is very small in comparison.

A very similar argument can be made for TG fluxes. The extracellular TG is confined to the plasma volume (in a normal individual, around 3 L at 1 mmol/L or 0.85 g/L; i.e. 2.5–3 g of extracellular TG). We eat enough TG in a typical meal to raise our plasma TG concentration at least 10-fold. Again this does not happen; a typical postprandial excursion in plasma

TG concentration is more like 50–60% of the fasting concentration (Coppack *et al.*, 1990; Summers *et al.*, 1999). This must also imply the existence of coordinated mechanisms for regulating the delivery of endogenous TG to the circulation, and stimulating TG clearance. These have been much less studied than those responsible for glucose homeostasis, particularly the regulation of hepatic TG secretion in the postprandial period (because of the methodological difficulties of such experiments), but it is clear that peripheral tissues are responsible for most of the increased TG clearance in the postprandial period. Among these, skeletal muscle and adipose tissue play major roles.

The role of skeletal muscle appears to be very variable from person to person, and greatest in the highly endurance-trained individual, in whom TG clearance is very rapid (Tsetsonis *et al.*, 1997). It may be much less in the habitually sedentary person. In non-athletes, the role of adipose tissue appears to be larger than that of skeletal muscle, and this may be understood metabolically on the basis that insulin (released in the postprandial period) activates adipose tissue lipoprotein lipase (LPL), the key enzyme in plasma TG clearance. Adipose tissue also plays a key role in overall lipid homeostasis since a major and dramatic effect of meal ingestion is to suppress intra-adipocyte TG hydrolysis and thus the release of NEFA from adipose tissue. The rate of supply of NEFA to the liver is a major determinant of hepatic TG secretion, and reduction in adipose tissue NEFA release is an important component of the suppression of hepatic TG secretion by insulin *in vivo* (Cummings *et al.*, 1995; Lewis *et al.* 1995; Malmström *et al.*, 1998). These considerations have led to the description of adipose tissue as a 'buffer' for the daily influx of dietary fatty acids into the circulation (Frayn, 2002). As dietary fat enters the circulation, adipose tissue TG clearance is increased by insulin, and the release of NEFA is suppressed. By these means, postprandial excursions of 'fatty acids' (TG and NEFA) are minimized, just as the liver and skeletal muscle 'buffer' the daily influx of glucose.

It is important to realize that metabolic regulation in tissues such as skeletal muscle and adipose tissue is not simply a matter of fine-tuning metabolic pathways; even during the normal daily pattern of meal ingestion and fasting overnight, there are major and dramatic switches in the patterns of metabolism and the fluxes through pathways. This is clearly illustrated in Fig. 8.1, which also illustrates one important methodological approach to the investigation of these regulatory mechanisms.

As there can be no doubt that obesity represents a state of disturbed energy fluxes and storage, it is very reasonable to consider that disturbances in these highly regulated pathways of energy metabolism in skeletal muscle and adipose tissue might underlie the development of obesity. It is also easy to imagine that, if such disturbances develop as a result of obesity, they might have widespread and potentially adverse metabolic consequences.

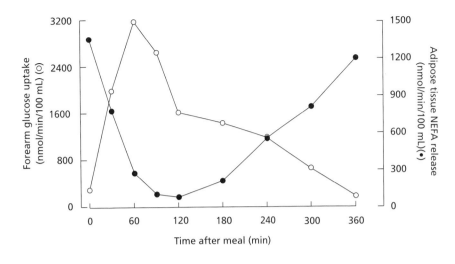

Fig. 8.1 Major metabolic fluxes in skeletal muscle (glucose uptake, ○) and white adipose tissue (NEFA release, ●) in the overnight fasted state, and their responses to ingestion of a mixed meal. Changes of several-fold are observed within 60–90 min of meal ingestion. Fluxes were estimated by selective venous catheterization with measurement of arteriovenous differences and blood flow. Data taken from the studies reported in Coppack *et al.* (1990; 1996) with the addition of further subjects for NEFA release.

Table 8.1 Typical glycogen and triacylglycerol (TG) contents of human skeletal muscle.

	Units	Low-carbohydrate diet	Mixed diet	High-carbohydrate diet	Reference
Glycogen	g/kg wet weight	10	20	30–40	Bergström *et al.* (1967)
	kJ/kg wet weight	170	340	510–680	
Typical whole-body store (assumes 25 kg of muscle)	MJ	4.25	8.5	15	
TG	mmol/kg wet weight	–	15 (range 1–100)	–	Collated from a number of sources: range from Phillips *et al.* (1996)
	kJ/kg wet weight	–	450 (range 30–3000)	–	
Typical whole-body store (assumes 25 kg of muscle)	MJ	–	11	–	

Skeletal muscle

Routes of ATP synthesis in skeletal muscle: outline and methodology

Skeletal muscle is a major site of ATP turnover in the body, especially during exercise. During a marathon run, the mass of ATP turned over in skeletal muscle alone is approximately equal to body mass (Frayn, 2003). Clearly, skeletal muscle has very efficient pathways for regeneration of ATP.

The main sources of free energy for ATP synthesis in skeletal muscle are anaerobic glycolysis and the complete oxidation of both carbohydrate and fatty acids. Amino acid oxidation also plays an important role, especially oxidation of the branched-chain amino acids valine, leucine and isoleucine: in humans, these are largely completely oxidized within skeletal muscle. These substrates arise from the circulation (plasma glucose,

NEFA, TG fatty acids and amino acids), from the intramuscular stores of glycogen and TG and from muscle protein. These sources of substrate are illustrated in Fig. 8.2. Typical muscle contents of glycogen and of TG are difficult to define, as there is considerable variability among muscles, nutritional states and individuals, but some representative figures are collated in Table 8.1.

The relative contributions of extramuscular and intramuscular sources of fuel have been the subject of much research, although there are many methodological difficulties in such studies. For instance, the contribution of intramuscular TG during exercise has been estimated in several studies by sequential biopsy of the muscles involved. The results are not consistent, due in part to the fact that skeletal muscle TG concentrations are extremely variable even from site to site within a single muscle (Frayn, 1980). These studies mostly show the expected decline in muscle TG concentration during exercise (Carlson *et al.*, 1971; Kimber *et al.*, 2003), although one study

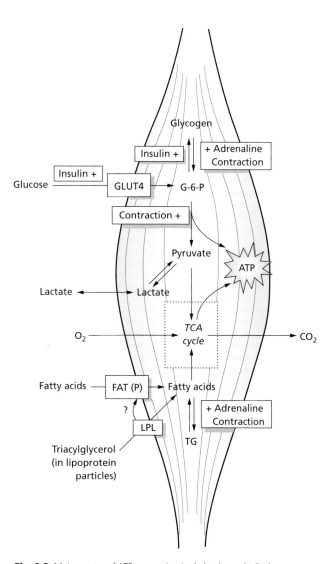

Fig. 8.2 Major routes of ATP generation in skeletal muscle. Each arrow may represent more than one step in a pathway. Glucose uptake is mainly by the insulin-regulatable transporter GLUT4 in the fed state but GLUT1 may play an important role in the fasting state. The contribution of amino acids to oxidative metabolism is not shown for simplicity. 'Contraction' refers to stimulation of muscle contraction, which is coordinated with metabolism via a number of intracellular mediators including intracellular Ca^{2+}. FAT(P) represents a possible fatty acid transporter; G-6-P, glucose-6-phosphate; LPL, lipoprotein lipase; TG, triacylglycerol; TCA cycle, tricarboxylic acid (Krebs) cycle. (Reproduced from Frayn, 2003, with permission.)

using sequential biopsy suggested that muscle TG utilization was most pronounced during the post-exercise period (Kiens and Richter, 1998). This post-exercise decline has not been substantiated in other studies (Kimber *et al.*, 2003).

An alternative approach is to estimate the contribution of plasma NEFA to oxidative metabolism by the infusion of a labelled ^{13}C-NEFA tracer to measure $^{13}CO_2$ production in expired air, whereas whole-body fat oxidation is measured by indirect calorimetry, and the difference is assumed to reflect

oxidation of intramuscular TG fatty acids on the basis that a correction for the incomplete recovery of the ^{13}C-label in expired air is made (acetate recovery factor—Sidossis *et al.*, 1995a). However, this technique does not distinguish intramuscular TG fatty acids from those arising from plasma (lipoprotein) TG. In the last few years, a procedure has been developed for measurement of intramuscular TG (called intramyocellular lipid, IMCL) by magnetic resonance spectroscopy (Boesch *et al.*, 1997). This has been applied to the measurement of muscle TG before and after exercise. Such measurements show the expected duration-dependent decline in IMCL with endurance exercise, although no change with high-intensity exercise (Brechtel *et al.*, 2001). A summary and critical review of the data on intramuscular TG utilization during exercise concluded that this energy store is, indeed, a significant source of fatty acids for oxidation during exercise (Watt *et al.*, 2002).

Muscle biopsy techniques have been more informative on the utilization of muscle glycogen during exercise and a reasonably consistent picture of glycogen depletion during exercise and repletion thereafter has been built up (Coyle, 1995). Muscle glycogen deposition in the resting state after a meal has been studied by the technique of ^{13}C-nuclear magnetic resonance (NMR) spectroscopy (Taylor *et al.*, 1993).

A technique which has provided a great deal of consistent information on skeletal muscle substrate utilization is the 'glucose clamp' (DeFronzo *et al.*, 1979). In this technique, glucose is infused intravenously, usually against a background of insulin infusion at a constant rate to raise the plasma insulin concentration to some predetermined level (hyperinsulinaemic clamp). The rate of glucose infusion is varied as necessary to keep the plasma glucose concentration, measured regularly at the bedside, constant within narrow limits: hence the plasma glucose concentration is 'clamped'. Under these conditions the rate of glucose disappearance from the plasma must equal the rate of glucose entry, which is known (as it is being infused). Any contribution from hepatic glucose release is usually small under these conditions, although it may be estimated by additional infusion of a labelled glucose tracer. The technique therefore provides a means for assessing whole-body glucose utilization at controlled plasma insulin concentrations, and thus gives a measure of whole-body insulin sensitivity: it is usually regarded as providing the 'gold standard' assessment of this parameter.

If indirect calorimetry is performed at the same time, the whole-body rate of carbohydrate oxidation can be assessed. It is usually found that under hyperinsulinaemic conditions glucose oxidation increases and accounts for around 20–30% of the total glucose disposal rate (DeFronzo *et al.*, 1981; Felber *et al.*, 1993). The remainder reflects 'non-oxidative glucose disposal', sometimes called glucose storage, although anaerobic glycolysis will also be included in this portion. This technique may be combined with selective catheterization of the venous drainage of skeletal muscle, usually that of the forearm. This allows the estimation of glucose uptake by a specific muscle, and—making assumptions about the uniformity of the muscle mass—by skeletal muscle in the whole body. Such studies show that the contribution of skeletal muscle in whole-body glucose disposal during hyperinsulinaemia is a major one (70–85%; DeFronzo *et al.*, 1981; Yki-Järvinen *et al.*, 1987). A corollary is that skeletal muscle is the tissue which predominantly 'sets' the insulin sensitivity of glucose metabolism in the whole body.

Carbohydrate metabolism in skeletal muscle at rest and during exercise

It has been known since the forearm venous catheterization experiments of Andres, Zierler and colleagues in the 1950s that the main oxidative fuel of skeletal muscle after an overnight fast at rest must be lipid; the respiratory quotient measured across the forearm is around 0.76 (Baltzan *et al.*, 1962). Plasma glucose disposal by skeletal muscle in that state is therefore small. The rate of anaerobic glycolysis of glucosyl units from both plasma glucose and muscle glycogen also appears to be small: net release of lactate from resting skeletal muscle after an overnight fast is inconsistent, and close to zero (Jackson *et al.*, 1987).

This picture changes rapidly, however, after a meal. In the postprandial state, the increased plasma glucose and insulin concentrations lead to increased glucose uptake by muscle, mainly by the insulin-regulatable glucose transporter GLUT4, and to increased glucose disposal within the muscle cell by coordinated regulation of the pathways of glycogen deposition, glycolysis and pyruvate oxidation. Skeletal muscle rapidly begins to dominate the extrahepatic disposal of glucose in the body. The glucose taken up from the plasma by muscle is either oxidized or stored as glycogen, with some being released as lactate. Measurements made by selective venous catheterization suggest that around 25% (Elia *et al.*, 1988; Kelley *et al.*, 1988; Coppack *et al.*, 1990) to 45% (Jackson *et al.*, 1987) of an oral glucose load (whether given as a pure glucose load or as part of a mixed meal) is disposed of by resting skeletal muscle during the 4- to 6-h postprandial period. Direct measurements of muscle glycogen deposition by ^{13}C-NMR spectroscopy show muscle glycogen content increasing by around 25%; net glycogen deposition in muscle during the 7 h following a mixed meal accounted for around 20% of that ingested (Taylor *et al.*, 1993).

In resting subjects, therefore, the role of skeletal muscle in whole-body carbohydrate metabolism in the fasted state is small, but in the fed state it is extremely important and dominates that of extrahepatic tissues.

During exercise, the situation changes even more dramatically. During light exercise (25% $\dot{V}o_{2\,max}$) there is little mobilization of muscle glycogen, but glucose uptake, oxidation and conversion to lactate are stimulated. In this condition whole-body glucose turnover increases initially by about 50% and it

seems likely that all this increase is directed to skeletal muscle (Romijn *et al.*, 1993). The major point of regulation of increased glucose uptake in this condition is not entirely clear, but muscle vasodilatation with increased glucose delivery may be an important factor. Furthermore, the amount of GLUT4 protein is a primary factor in determining the maximal rate of glucose transport into skeletal muscle. Under normal resting conditions, most of the GLUT4 molecules reside in membrane vesicles inside the muscle cells. In response to insulin or muscle contraction, GLUT4 translocates to the cell membrane, where it inserts to stimulate glucose transport. Plasma insulin concentrations do not change during light exercise. However, rapid changes in GLUT4 mRNA and protein may occur in response to exercise. Increased GLUT4 expression may be mediated by the enzyme AMP-activated kinase, which is activated during exercise and has been demonstrated to increase GLUT4 transcription (Rodnick *et al.*, 1992; Ren *et al.*, 1994; Dohm, 2002). Further research needs to be done on the regulation of muscle GLUT4 expression during exercise.

During heavier exercise (e.g. 65% $\dot{V}o_{2\,max}$), muscle glycogen breakdown is stimulated and glucosyl residues from this source are a major fuel for anaerobic and oxidative metabolism. Plasma glucose utilization is also increased and lactate may thus be recycled via hepatic gluconeogenesis. Whole-body glucose turnover increases to more than three times its resting value after 2 h of exercise at this intensity, and again this is largely taken up by skeletal muscle (Romijn *et al.*, 1993). Whole-body glucose oxidation measured by indirect calorimetry may increase by about 12-fold (Romijn *et al.*, 1993) and most of this must be accounted for by skeletal muscle; at 85% $\dot{V}o_{2\,max}$, glucose oxidation increases about 30-fold. Metabolic and physiological adjustments bringing about this increased carbohydrate oxidation include increased cardiac output and muscle vasodilatation, vastly increasing glucose delivery to working muscle and the coordinated regulation, via changes in intracellular Ca^{2+} and P_i concentrations, of contraction and of glycogenolysis and glycolysis (Crowther *et al.*, 2002; for a review, see Frayn, 2003). During moderate or heavy exercise skeletal muscle is therefore by far the dominant tissue in glucose disposal in the body.

Lipid metabolism in skeletal muscle at rest and during exercise

The size of the intramuscular TG store does not appear to fluctuate greatly during normal daily life, except during exercise. Although it may turn over, it is not therefore a net contributor to muscle fatty acid oxidation at rest. In the overnight fasted state, muscle extracts both NEFA and lipoprotein TG fatty acids from the plasma. As in adipose tissue, the key enzyme in plasma TG extraction is LPL, bound to the skeletal muscle capillary endothelium. This enzyme is more active in oxidative than glycolytic muscles, and it is activated by training. Selective venous catheterization clearly demonstrates that TG extraction does occur (Kiens and Lithell, 1989; Potts *et al.*; 1991). Nevertheless, measurements of plasma TG extraction by muscle are difficult to make and we lack much information on the magnitude and metabolic importance of this process. In contrast, the extraction of plasma NEFA by muscle has been much studied, usually by a combination of tracer infusion and selective venous catheterization (Capaldo *et al.*, 1994). At rest, in the overnight fasted state, NEFA extraction from plasma appears to provide most of the fatty acids required for oxidation. [Whether these fatty acids pass through an intramuscular TG pool before oxidation is not clear: older evidence for such a pathway (Dagenais *et al.*, 1976) has more recently been challenged (Sidossis *et al.*, 1995b).]

Interestingly, a recent study showed that, on a high-fat diet, TG-derived fatty acid oxidation is increased, suggesting that although plasma NEFA remain the main source of fat oxidation, diet composition may affect the contribution of both sources to some extent (Schrauwen *et al.*, 2000). The rate of fatty acid extraction from the plasma by skeletal muscle appears under most circumstances to be limited by their delivery in plasma, i.e. by the product of muscle blood flow and the plasma NEFA concentration (Soop *et al.*, 1988). Additionally, new evidence from *in vitro* and whole animal studies supports the existence of transmembrane transport of NEFA, which is likely to co-exist with passive diffusional uptake. Evidence is also emerging for concerted actions between the membrane and cytoplasmic fatty acid binding proteins (FABPs) that allow for efficient regulation of NEFA transport and metabolism (Glatz and Storch, 2001).

The rate of uptake of fatty acids by skeletal muscle is also a determinant of their oxidation, as the muscle TG pool is of relatively constant size. The oxidation of fatty acids has been proposed to be linked to that of glucosyl units by mechanisms described by Randle and colleagues in the 1960s (summarized in Randle *et al.*, 1963). Within this concept, it has been postulated that products of fatty acid oxidation (acetyl-CoA, cytosolic citrate) exert inhibitory feedback control over the rate of glucose uptake and oxidation via inhibition of phosphofructokinase (a key regulatory enzyme in glycolysis) and pyruvate dehydrogenase. This link has received most attention with respect to the development of insulin resistance and type 2 diabetes mellitus, although there is also evidence for it operating in normal daily life (Piatti *et al.*, 1991). Although there is consistent evidence that increased NEFA concentrations are associated with insulin resistance, there are also studies that argue against the mechanisms proposed by Randle and colleagues. In this respect, an early NEFA-induced decline in glucose-6-phosphate concentration has been reported, suggesting that NEFAs primarily inhibit glucose transport/phosphorylation (Roden *et al.*, 1996; 1999).

Furthermore, contrary to the prediction of the glucose–fatty acid cycle, there are indications that the intracellular availability of glucose (rather than NEFA) may determine the nature of substrate oxidation in human subjects by controlling fatty acid

transport into the mitochondria (Sidossis *et al.*, 1996; Sidossis and Wolfe, 1996). This may occur via the well-known inhibitory effect of malonyl-CoA (formed under conditions of high glucose and insulin) on carnitine palmitoyl transferase-1 (CPT1), a key regulatory enzyme in fatty acid oxidation (Zammit, 1999). However, there is some difficulty with this concept, as muscle malonyl-CoA concentrations either remain constant or tend to fall during exercise (Saha *et al.*, 1994; Odland *et al.*, 1996; Winder and Hardie, 1996).

In the period following a meal, fatty acid utilization by skeletal muscle decreases rapidly as glucose uptake and oxidation become the more important processes. It seems that an important site of control of muscle fatty acid utilization is exerted at the level of NEFA release from adipose tissue, which is rapidly reduced after a meal (Fig. 8.1). Also, there are some recent indications from rat studies that insulin may regulate fatty acid uptake and esterification in the myocyte (Dyck *et al.*, 2001; Luiken *et al.*, 2002), suggesting there may also be direct control of muscle fatty acid uptake in the postprandial state. However, the physiological significance of these findings remains to be determined in man.

During exercise, muscle NEFA utilization increases dramatically. Plasma NEFAs are the major fuel for exercise at low intensity (25% $\dot{V}o_{2\,max}$) (Romijn *et al.*, 1993). At greater intensities of exercise they are also important, but other fuel sources are more important at least for the first 2 h or so. After that, these other sources (e.g. muscle glycogen) are depleted, and the ultra-endurance athlete utilizes almost entirely plasma NEFA as a fuel. Considering the size of the adipose tissue TG store, this seems wholly sensible.

The extraction of plasma TG fatty acids by muscle has been little explored, as mentioned above. Again, although it may not occur at a high rate per unit mass of skeletal muscle, the bulk of skeletal muscle means that its contribution to whole-body plasma TG clearance may be substantial. The expression of skeletal muscle LPL is increased considerably by training (Seip *et al.*, 1995), and training is also associated with a marked improvement in fat tolerance (the increase in plasma TG concentration following a fat load, also called postprandial lipaemia) (Tsetsonis *et al.*, 1997; Herd *et al.*, 1998; Malkova *et al.*, 2000). It has been suggested that plasma TG fatty acids extracted by skeletal muscle serve mainly to replenish the intramuscular TG pool (Oscai *et al.*, 1990). However, on the basis of a recent study in rats, a model has been proposed in which fatty acids from TG mix locally at the capillaries with plasma NEFA, where they would lead to an increase in local NEFA concentration, and hence, NEFA uptake. This suggests that a distinction between TG-derived NEFA and plasma NEFA in metabolic fate within muscle cannot be made (Teusink *et al.*, 2003). Skeletal muscle LPL is suppressed by insulin (Farese *et al.*, 1991), in contrast with adipose tissue, in which LPL is activated by insulin. This suggests that adipose tissue plays a more important role than skeletal muscle in clearance of plasma TG in the postprandial state. This may not be accurate, because the suppression of skeletal muscle LPL by insulin is not very marked, and the bulk of skeletal muscle—particularly in an athlete in whom muscle LPL is particularly active—may give it an equally, or even more important role. The situation probably differs considerably between individuals.

It is generally considered that plasma TG fatty acids make only a small contribution to oxidative fuel metabolism during exercise. This seems to be true for exercise carried out in the fasting state, in which plasma TG is mainly present as very low-density lipoprotein (VLDL)-TG. However, it is possible that the situation is different after a meal containing fat (Griffiths *et al.*, 1994; Henriksson, 1995). Chylomicron-TG is a better substrate for muscle LPL than is VLDL-TG (Potts *et al.*, 1991) and there is some evidence for marked TG clearance from postprandial plasma by exercising muscle (Ruys *et al.*, 1989; Griffiths *et al.*, 1994). In addition, if the marked improvement of fat tolerance evident in highly trained subjects does indeed reflect improved TG clearance by skeletal muscle then this again suggests more than a modest contribution to muscle fatty acid delivery. However, more work is needed in this area.

Disturbances in skeletal muscle metabolism and the development of obesity

In principle, disturbances of a number of aspects of muscle metabolism might impinge upon the development of obesity. As skeletal muscle is such an important site for the ultimate oxidation of energy-bearing substrates, any impairment of muscle oxidative metabolism will lead to the accumulation of body energy stores. Because skeletal muscle O_2 consumption is a major determinant of resting metabolic rate, it has been suggested that differences between individuals in muscle oxidative capacity might play a role in the pathogenesis of obesity (Zurlo *et al.*, 1990a).

In practice, there is some evidence for specific impairments of muscle metabolism in subjects at risk of developing obesity, or in the post-obese (people who were once obese but have now lost weight). The impairment of fatty acid oxidation in skeletal muscle apparent in obese subjects (Blaak *et al.*, 1994a; Colberg *et al.*, 1995) might be a causal factor in the development of obesity but, until there is clear evidence for the direction of cause and effect, it is difficult to interpret such findings. It is interesting, however, that this impairment was not reversed by weight reduction, whereas some other aspects of muscle metabolism were, such as glucose uptake and lactate release (Blaak *et al.*, 1994b). Additionally, post-obese women, when compared with never-obese women, show decrements in postprandial (Raben *et al.*, 1994) and 24-h fat oxidation (Astrup *et al.*, 1994). Also, a high respiratory quotient (i.e. a low ratio of fat to carbohydrate oxidation) has been correlated with weight gain in post-obese women (Froidevaux *et al.*, 1993) and in Pima Indians in Arizona (Zurlo *et al.*, 1990b). These findings may suggest that a lowered capacity to oxidize fat could be primary to the obese state rather than an adaptational response.

One of the marked consequences of obesity (discussed in greater detail below) is the development of insulin resistance. In skeletal muscle, this is evidenced by low rates of glucose uptake during hyperinsulinaemic clamp, and most studies of obesity and of type 2 diabetes mellitus show that the main defect, under these specific conditions, is in glucose storage (i.e. glycogen synthesis) rather than glucose oxidation (Bonora *et al.*, 1993). This finding has been extended by looking at glycogen synthase activation in muscle biopsies and cultured fibroblasts from non-diabetic relatives of subjects with type 2 diabetes. Although glycogen synthase activation in such samples is indeed insulin resistant (Schalin Jantti *et al.* 1992; Wells *et al.*, 1993), it is difficult to know whether this represents cause or effect, as such relatives are themselves already insulin resistant (Schalin Jantti *et al.*, 1992).

It is even more difficult to know whether any such defect in insulin sensitivity could be a cause of obesity. In fact, in prospective studies of weight change over several years, those most at risk of gaining weight are those showing better insulin sensitivity (Swinburn *et al.*, 1991; Hoag *et al.*, 1995). This has been interpreted in terms of insulin resistance tending to favour fat oxidation over that of glucose, and thus helping to maintain a favourable fat balance (Eckel, 1992). Therefore, a change in skeletal muscle predisposing to the development of obesity might be more in the direction of increased sensitivity to insulin. This seems counterintuitive and may be an overinterpretation of prospective data. Against the prospective data, and in favour of insulin resistance in muscle as a primary defect, is the demonstration that transgenic mice with targeted disruption of insulin sensitivity only in skeletal muscle accumulate body fat and display some of the dyslipidaemic characteristics of obesity (Moller *et al.*, 1996).

It is known that in obese subjects postprandial skeletal muscle blood flow is reduced (Baron *et al.*, 1990). Impaired muscle blood flow, either resting, postprandially, during exercise or in all these states might predispose to obesity. As muscle blood flow delivers substrates such as glucose, NEFA and TG to the muscle tissue, defects in muscle blood flow regulation might well have important effects, leading to the development of insulin resistance and the laying down of adipose tissue TG stores. However, as yet there has been no prospective work in this area and it is again difficult to determine whether reduced muscle blood flow causes obesity or whether it occurs as a result of the obese state.

Despite the difficulties of determining cause and effect, it can clearly be seen that a reduction in the oxidative capacity of skeletal muscle, whether due to some intrinsic change within the muscle or simply to lack of muscle mass, will lead to low rates of substrate oxidation, and thereby to a propensity for positive energy storage. This situation is particularly evident in one situation, that of the sedentary individual. The sedentary lifestyle clearly leads to reduction in muscle mass, in muscle capillary density and thus substrate delivery, and in muscle oxidative capacity. Of course, the sedentary lifestyle also leads to positive energy balance simply on the grounds of reduced energy expenditure, but changes in skeletal muscle metabolism might be seen as the internal means by which this is mediated.

One interesting mechanism that could in principle link skeletal muscle metabolism to the development of (or protection from) obesity is uncoupling of respiration. The mitochondrial uncoupling protein UCP3, described earlier, is expressed in skeletal muscle. An attractive hypothesis is that UCP3 might protect against obesity in those in whom it is particularly active by dissipating metabolic energy as heat. However, although UCP3 is able to uncouple mitochondrial respiration from ATP production, mice lacking UCP3 have normal metabolic rates and are not obese (Vidal-Puig *et al.*, 2000). In addition, it was recently shown in humans that a diet-induced upregulation of UCP3 did not affect mitochondrial coupling (Hesselink *et al.*, 2003). Rather, evidence is accumulating that UCP3 is involved in mitochondrial transport of fatty acid anions (Schrauwen *et al.*, 2001). Although the primary function of UCP3 does not seem to be mitochondrial uncoupling, UCP3 could still, as a consequence of its physiological function, affect metabolic rate explaining the observed associations between UCP3 and energy metabolism (Ricquier and Bouillaud, 2000b).

Skeletal muscle metabolism in obesity

The insulin resistance of skeletal muscle in obese subjects was noted in 1961 by Rabinowitz and Zierler (1961), who injected insulin into a brachial artery in obese subjects and noted a diminished stimulation of glucose uptake compared with lean control subjects. The impairment of insulin-stimulated glucose utilization in muscle in obesity is now well recognized (Fig. 8.3). Because of the important role of skeletal muscle in whole-body insulin-mediated glucose disposal outlined earlier, the result is reduced sensitivity to insulin in the whole body. The consequent persistent hyperinsulinaemia may, in turn, lead to downregulation of insulin-stimulated pathways in other tissues including adipose tissue, as discussed later.

One consistent hypothesis for the development of insulin resistance in obesity is that increased delivery of NEFA to the circulation from the expanded adipose tissue mass (discussed in more detail below) reduces the sensitivity of muscle glucose uptake to insulin by substrate competition. This hypothesis has been fully developed elsewhere (Felber *et al.*, 1993). There is also evidence that skeletal muscle in obese subjects has an impaired ability to oxidize fatty acids (Blaak *et al.* 1994a; Colberg *et al.*, 1995), and insulin resistance has been correlated with accumulation of intramuscular triacylglycerol (Falholt *et al.* 1988; Phillips *et al.*, 1996; Forouhi *et al.*, 1999). Obese women accrue more fat in their muscle and this is directly related to the degree of insulin resistance, decreased oxidative capacity and increased anaerobic and glycolytic capacity (Simoneau *et al.*, 1995). There is increasing evidence that it is not increased TG

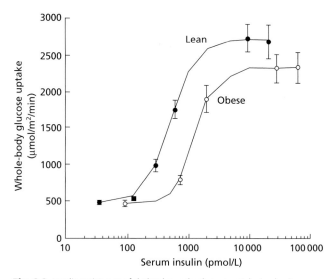

Fig. 8.3 Insulin resistance of skeletal muscle glucose uptake in obesity. Glucose uptake was measured across the leg by femoral venous catheterization and measurement of blood flow, and insulin was infused at increasing rates to construct the dose–response curves. Plasma glucose concentrations were 'clamped' at 5 mmol/L. There is a clear shift to the right of the dose–response curve of glucose uptake against serum insulin concentration in the obese group. (Reproduced from Laakso *et al.*, 1990b, with permission.)

storage per se that causes insulin resistance, but rather other lipid intermediates such as long-chain fatty acyl-CoA and diacylglycerol (Ellis *et al.*, 2000; Itani *et al.*, 2002), which may interfere with insulin signalling, thereby affecting GLUT4 translocation.

The cellular mechanisms for the loss of sensitivity to insulin in obesity have been studied both in humans *in vivo* and in animal models. There has been considerable study in animal models of the cellular and molecular mechanisms that may underlie such a change, but these are outside the scope of this chapter (Kahn and Flier, 2000). In humans, there is a clear impairment of the uptake of glucose across the muscle cell membrane, demonstrated by a number of means (Laakso *et al.*, 1990a; Friedman *et al.*, 1992; Kelley *et al.*, 1996). It has been suggested that there is no deficiency in total cellular content of the insulin-regulatable glucose transporter GLUT4, but its translocation to the cell membrane in response to insulin is defective (Friedman *et al.*, 1992; Kelley *et al.*, 1996). A recent study, using immunohistochemistry combined with morphometry, showed a reduction in the fraction of slow-twitch fibres and a reduction in GLUT4 expression in slow fibres in obese and type 2 diabetic subjects, which may both contribute to skeletal muscle insulin resistance (Gaster *et al.*, 2001). In addition, it has been proposed that a defect in insulin-mediated vasodilatation, potentially an important aspect of the stimulation of glucose uptake by insulin, might be involved. This has been demonstrated both during infusion of insulin (Laakso *et al.* 1990a,b) and during the endogenous hyperinsulinaemia following an oral glucose load (Baron *et al.*, 1990). The cytokine tumour necrosis factor alpha (TNF-α) is overexpressed in adipose tissue in obesity (discussed below), and the same is true of skeletal muscle (Saghizadeh *et al.*, 1996). TNF-α expression (mRNA content) in skeletal muscle was negatively related to whole-body insulin sensitivity (Saghizadeh *et al.*, 1996).

The reduction in glucose uptake, at least during conditions of hyperinsulinaemia, reflects impairment of both oxidative and non-oxidative glucose disposal, the latter being much more affected than the former (Felber *et al.*, 1987; Bonora *et al.*, 1993). In obese subjects, skeletal muscle has reduced oxidative capacity and increased anaerobic and glycolytic capacities (Simoneau *et al.*, 1995; 1999). Skeletal muscle insulin resistance in obesity has been explored in more detail in subjects with type 2 diabetes in addition to obesity, and again it appears that multiple aspects of glucose metabolism are deranged (Kelley *et al.*, 1992).

White adipose tissue

Major metabolic pathways relevant to this chapter in white adipose tissue are outlined in Fig. 8.4.

Adipose tissue carbohydrate metabolism

The uptake of glucose by white adipocytes *in vitro* must be one of the most studied metabolic processes. Unfortunately, there is little evidence that it contributes more than a few per cent to whole-body glucose utilization, and even less that adipose tissue glucose uptake makes a significant contribution to glucose disposal in the postprandial period when it is dwarfed by the contribution of skeletal muscle. Adipocytes have a small store of glycogen, the concentration of which varies with feeding and fasting (Rigden *et al.*, 1990) but, again, this cannot be a major contributor to whole-body carbohydrate economy.

The role of glucose in adipocyte metabolism is twofold. First, glucose metabolism (mainly complete oxidation) seems to be the major route of ATP generation in white adipocytes (Frayn *et al.*, 1995a). In addition, in the postprandial period, glycolysis provides glycerol-3-phosphate, which is needed for esterification of the fatty acids delivered to adipocytes from LPL in the capillaries. It might therefore be expected that adipose tissue glucose uptake would increase at this time, but the proportion of glucose metabolism diverted to glycerol-3-phosphate production, even after a high-fat meal, is only around 20% (Frayn *et al.*, 1994).

Non-esterified fatty acid release from adipose tissue

The rate of release of NEFA from adipose tissue is, as outlined above, the major determinant of the systemic plasma NEFA concentration and thus of the delivery of NEFA to other tissues. As shown in Fig. 8.1, this is a highly regulated process, switching in a short time from its maximal rate in the normal daily pattern to almost zero. These rapid changes in NEFA release reflect regulation of the key enzyme in the hydrolysis of adipocyte TG, the intracellular enzyme hormone-sensitive lipase (HSL) (Fig. 8.4). Regulation of HSL is coordinated (inversely) with regulation of the pathway of fatty acid esterification: when HSL is suppressed by insulin, fatty acid esterification is stimulated and fatty acids are effectively trapped in adipocytes.

Recently, it has been shown in HSL-deficient animals that adipose tissue lipolysis is maintained, although sensitivity to catecholamine stimulation is largely lost (Osuga *et al.*, 2000; Wang *et al.*, 2001). This has led to more detailed investigation of the process of lipolysis. It now seems that there is at least one other TG lipase expressed in adipose tissue, although this other lipase does not have the cholesterol esterase activity that is characteristic of HSL (Okazaki *et al.*, 2002). It has also been

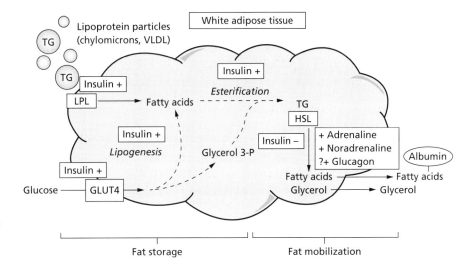

Fig. 8.4 Major routes of fat deposition and mobilization in white adipose tissue. GLUT4, insulin-regulated glucose transporter; HSL, hormone-sensitive lipase; LPL, lipoprotein lipase; TG, triacylglycerol. (Reproduced from Frayn, 2003, with permission).

appreciated that the acute regulation of lipolysis is achieved only in part through reversible phosphorylation of HSL and consequent changes in its enzyme activity. Perilipin is a protein that coats the fat droplet in white adipocytes (Londos *et al.*, 1996). Perilipin, like HSL, is phosphorylated in response to elevation of cellular cyclic AMP (via protein kinase A). Phosphorylation of perilipin causes it to move away from the fat droplet, whereas HSL translocates from a cytoplasmic location onto the surface of the lipid droplet (Clifford *et al.*, 2000).

In normal daily life, it appears that most of the regulation of NEFA delivery from adipose tissue reflects the inhibitory effect of insulin on HSL. HSL is stimulated by agents that raise the cellular cyclic AMP concentration, particularly β-adrenergic agents, and in the longer term by a number of hormones, including growth hormone and cortisol, which may either affect enzyme expression or modify the sensitivity to catecholamines (e.g. by regulation of adrenoceptor expression). In normal subjects fasted overnight, local introduction of propranolol into subcutaneous adipose tissue has no effect on lipolysis, suggesting that adrenergic stimulation of lipolysis is not operative in this state (Arner *et al.*, 1990). Instead the lipolytic 'tone' against which insulin acts may be set by the normal early morning rise in cortisol (Samra *et al.*, 1996a) and perhaps by overnight growth hormone pulses (Cersosimo *et al.*, 1996; Samra *et al.*, 1999).

During exercise, there is a marked increase in NEFA delivery from adipose tissue, and this is undoubtedly mediated primarily by β-adrenergic stimulation (Arner *et al.*, 1990). In sustained high-intensity exercise, it may be reinforced by a slight fall in the plasma insulin concentration, and by secretion of both cortisol and growth hormone (Hodgetts *et al.*, 1991). Despite these changes, the rate of NEFA delivery does not increase in proportion to the intensity of exercise (Romijn *et al.*, 1993). It seems that adipose tissue perfusion during intense exercise may be inadequate to carry away all the fatty acids released in lipolysis (Bülow, 1993). Evidence for this comes from the sudden release of NEFA that is observed when exercise stops (Hodgetts *et al.*, 1991, Romijn *et al.*, 1993); presumably a sudden relief of relative vasoconstriction allows 'flushing out' of NEFAs that have been trapped within the tissue.

Triacylglycerol clearance by adipose tissue

Adipose tissue LPL is least active in the overnight fasted state, but even in that condition there is significant removal of plasma TG. In fact, systemic plasma TG concentrations correlate inversely with adipose tissue TG clearance (Potts *et al.*, 1995), suggesting a role for adipose tissue in 'setting' the fasting plasma TG concentration. Clearly, the rate of hepatic VLDL-TG secretion is also a determinant of plasma TG concentrations, but this in turn is regulated largely by the rate of delivery of NEFA from adipose tissue. TG clearance in skeletal muscle does not relate in such a way to the plasma TG concentration (Potts *et al.*, 1991).

It has been suggested earlier that adipose tissue may play a particularly important role in TG clearance in the postprandial period when its LPL is activated by insulin, and possibly by other hormones including those released from the gut in response to feeding (Oben *et al.*, 1992). Adipose tissue extraction of chylomicron-TG is avid, averaging around 30% of the arterial concentration in a single passage through the tissue (Potts *et al.*, 1991), although we find that this varies considerably from person to person. The quantitative role of adipose tissue in removal of plasma TG in the postprandial period has been estimated by a number of means. Mårin *et al.* (1990) fed a meal containing 120 g of fat labelled with ^{14}C-oleic acid and assessed deposition by sequential adipose tissue biopsies. After 24 h, 60 g of this had been deposited in adipose tissue (in a group who had eaten a carbohydrate-rich breakfast), and the figure increased slowly over the next month. Romanski *et al.* (2000) performed similar studies and found that 24% (in men) to 35% (in women) of an oral fat load had been deposited in subcutaneous adipose tissue after 24 h. Studies with selective venous catheterization suggest that in normal subjects about 35% of the fat load given in a mixed meal is stored in adipose tissue over the subsequent 6 h (Coppack *et al.*, 1990). The magnitude of postprandial lipaemia is inversely related to the LPL activity measured in plasma following injection of heparin, which releases LPL from its endothelial binding sites (Jeppesen *et al.*, 1995), although this does not distinguish between LPL released from different tissues. Defective activation of adipose tissue LPL is associated with increased postprandial lipaemia (Katzel *et al.*, 1994).

It is important to understand differences in the action of LPL in different tissues. In skeletal muscle it appears that the fatty acids released by the action of LPL on plasma TG are quantitatively extracted by the muscle: no net 'overspill' of fatty acids is seen during the postprandial period, for instance, when skeletal muscle LPL is active against chylomicron-TG (Coppack *et al.*, 1990; Evans *et al.*, 2002). The fate of these fatty acids is, as outlined earlier, either esterification to replenish the intramuscular TG pool (ultimately a source for fatty acid oxidation) or direct oxidation. In adipose tissue, plasma TG extraction by LPL provides the source of fatty acids for deposition as intracellular TG, the ultimate energy store of the body. This process must be highly regulated, as the body's fat store is so closely related to whole-body energy balance. It is not therefore surprising to find an additional level of control in adipose tissue. LPL-derived fatty acids in adipose tissue are not all taken up by adipocytes for esterification and storage. A proportion of these appear always to be released into the venous plasma in the form of NEFA (Frayn *et al.*, 1994; Evans *et al.*, 2002).

So far as is known at present, this role of LPL in delivery of NEFA into the plasma is specific to white adipose tissue. However, regulation of the fate of LPL-derived fatty acids is a key process in the regulation of fat storage. In the fasted state there would seem little 'sense' in storage of plasma TG-derived fatty acids, when the adipocyte itself is liberating fatty acids at a high rate into the plasma. Accordingly, in that state there is almost complete release of LPL-derived fatty acids as NEFA into the plasma (Frayn *et al.*, 1994). Adipose tissue LPL in the fasted state acts as a generator of plasma NEFA additional to the intracellular HSL, except that the source of fatty acids is hepatic TG, secreted as VLDL-TG, rather than adipocyte TG. In the postprandial period, however, this changes dramatically with much greater 'capture' of LPL-derived fatty acids for esterification within the adipocytes (although never complete, at least after the relatively normal meals that we have studied) (Frayn *et al.*, 1994; 1995b; Evans *et al.*, 2002).

Regulation of fat storage in white adipose tissue therefore primarily involves regulation of LPL, but the fine-tuning is provided by regulation of the pathway of fatty acid uptake and esterification in adipocytes. The regulation of this pathway is becoming clearer. First, it depends upon simultaneous suppression of HSL activity, generating a concentration gradient so that fatty acids flow into rather than out from adipocytes. It is stimulated in a positive sense by insulin (Frayn *et al.*, 1994) and by the acylation-stimulating protein (ASP). ASP is a potent stimulator of fatty acid esterification in adipocytes (Sniderman *et al.*, 1997). It is produced locally within adipose tissue by the interaction of three components of the alternate complement pathway (D or adipsin, B and C3), themselves secreted from adipocytes, and this interaction is markedly stimulated by the presence of chylomicrons (Maslowska *et al.*, 1997; Scantlebury *et al.*, 1998). Regulation of the fate of LPL-derived fatty acids in adipose tissue is the subject of intense study at present, not least because of the potentially adverse consequences of disturbed regulation of this pathway (Sniderman *et al.*, 1998).

Disturbances in adipose tissue metabolism and the development of obesity

The question has often been posed as to whether alterations in adipose tissue metabolism might lead to a predisposition to obesity. This simple question is extraordinarily difficult to answer, not least because adipose tissue metabolism is so profoundly altered by obesity per se, and potentially by a previous history of obesity, that it is virtually impossible to distinguish cause and effect. Nevertheless, there are some very plausible mechanisms whereby particular characteristics of adipose tissue might predispose to obesity.

The theory, once prevalent, that the number of fat cells is determined in infancy and invariant thereafter, suggests that an overweight child may become an overweight adult because the capacity is there, whereas a lean child could not so easily become obese in adulthood. Attractive as this idea is, there is no evidence for it (Ashwell, 1992): in fact, even octogenarians have adipocyte precursors that can differentiate into mature adipocytes (Hauner *et al.*, 1989).

Much attention has centred upon adipose tissue LPL. The idea that overexpression of LPL might provide a stimulus to fat storage has found some favour, not least because many studies show adipose tissue LPL activity to be increased in established obesity (Eckel, 1989). However, it is again extremely difficult to distinguish cause and effect. Because of the complex regulation of fat storage discussed above, it seems unlikely that overactivity of LPL in itself could cause excessive storage. Adipose tissue seems to have the capacity to regulate the amount of fat it stores independently of LPL capacity. For instance, in human LPL deficiency, adipocytes are normally fat filled (Peeva *et al.*, 1992), and in mice with adipose tissue-specific deficiency of LPL, adipose tissue lipid stores are maintained by upregulation of *de novo* lipogenesis (Weinstock *et al.*, 1997). The possibility that disturbed regulation of other components of the fat-storage system, e.g. of the enzymes of fatty acid esterification or of ASP, could lead to excessive fat deposition has not been explored extensively, although it is known that ASP concentrations are increased in obese subjects (Cianflone *et al.*, 1995).

In healthy groups of obese women, entrapment of LPL-derived fatty acids (fatty acids delivered with a meal) in adipose tissue appears to be increased (Binnert *et al.*, 1998; Kalant *et al.*, 2000). It is difficult to know whether this might be primary, or some form of adaptive response to obesity, or perhaps a feature of subject selection: fatty acid 'trapping' might be most effective in those who are protected from the metabolic complications of obesity. It is clear that insulin has a fat storage-promoting effect. Weight gain is a notable feature in type 1 diabetic subjects intensively treated with insulin (The DCCT Research Group, 1988). It can easily be seen how insulin could promote fat storage through stimulation of adipose tissue LPL and of the esterification pathway. However, this is difficult to reconcile with the demonstration in prospective studies (discussed earlier) that insulin resistance within the normal range is associated with protection against weight gain, as hyperinsulinaemia is a marker for such insulin resistance. It may be that the effect of intensive insulin treatment is mediated more via increased energy intake in response to hypoglycaemia. Alternatively, there may be differences between acute and chronic effects of insulin.

There is some direct evidence for a role of HSL in susceptibility to obesity. Net fat deposition reflects the balance between two processes: fat mobilization and fat storage. If HSL activity is reduced, then there will be an increase in net fat deposition. This possibility was examined by measurement of HSL activity in adipose tissue biopsies in non-obese first-degree relatives of obese subjects (Hellström *et al.*, 1996); it was found that maximal HSL activity was reduced by about 50% in the relatives, compared with control subjects with no immediate family history of obesity. In the more physiological setting of responses *in vivo* to a mixed meal or to insulin infusion, there is evidence that in post-obese women (formerly obese women who have reduced their weight to the normal range, and who are considered to be a model of the genetically 'at risk') the ability of insulin to suppress plasma NEFA concentrations is enhanced (Raben *et al.*, 1994; Toubro *et al.*, 1994). Thus, the tendency towards net fat storage would again be enhanced.

Again, it is possible that blood flow plays a part in the development of obesity. Fasting adipose tissue blood flow is decreased in obese subjects as is the postprandial rise (Coppack *et al.*, 1990; Summers *et al.*, 1996). The mechanism by which reduced blood flow could lead to obesity is not clear and other factors, such as increased ASP production, seem much more likely to predispose to an increase in adipose tissue mass.

In animal models, more direct roles for changes in adipose tissue metabolism may be observed. For instance, in the model of rodent obesity produced by lesion of the ventromedial hypothalamus, adipose tissue metabolism remains normally sensitive to insulin (at least as judged by glucose uptake), whereas muscle metabolism becomes insulin resistant, and fuels are diverted to adipose tissue, where they are stored as TG (Pénicaud *et al.*, 1987). The obese (*ob/ob*) mouse fails to produce the signal molecule leptin in adipose tissue, and as leptin is thought to signal to the hypothalamus both to increase energy expenditure and to decrease food intake, obesity follows (Rohner-Jeanrenaud and Jeanrenaud, 1996). However, it appears that human obesity is characterized more by 'leptin resistance' (elevated plasma leptin concentrations) than by hypoleptinaemia (Considine *et al.*, 1996). Only a very small number of subjects have been described in whom there is complete leptin deficiency (Barsh *et al.*, 2000).

Adipose tissue metabolism in obesity

Obesity involves a disproportionate increase in the amount of adipose tissue relative to other tissues. A notable feature of established obesity is an elevation of the plasma NEFA concentration (Opie and Walfish, 1963). This has been attributed to the increased adipose tissue mass (Flatt, 1972). In fact, NEFA release per unit mass of adipose tissue is reduced in obese compared with lean subjects (Lillioja *et al.*, 1986), and a truer picture is probably that fat mass, responsible for NEFA release, expands more than lean body mass, responsible for NEFA clearance. The reduction in NEFA release per unit mass of adipose tissue may be explained in part by the presence of larger adipocytes, the increased volume representing mainly inert TG in the intracellular droplet. The compensatory fasting hyperinsulinaemia in obesity also downregulates NEFA release from adipose tissue (Campbell *et al.*, 1994). Large adipocytes filled with inert lipid may also explain the reduction in blood flow per unit mass of adipose tissue which is observed in obesity (Coppack *et al.* 1992; Blaak *et al.*, 1995; Summers *et al.*, 1996; Virtanen *et al.*, 2002), although not the failure of 'obese' adipose tissue blood flow to respond to nutrient ingestion (Coppack *et al.*, 1992; Summers *et al.*, 1996; Karpe *et al.*, 2002).

In established obesity, adipose tissue acquires many characteristics that could be described as insulin resistance. HSL is not suppressed normally by insulin (Jensen *et al.*, 1989;

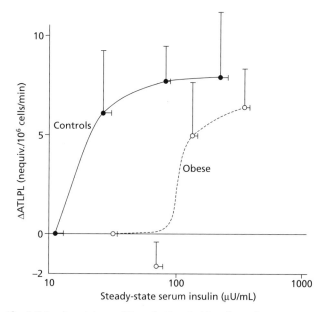

Fig. 8.5 Insulin resistance of the activation of white adipose tissue lipoprotein lipase (LPL) in obesity. Dose–response curves were constructed by infusing insulin at different rates on different occasions for 6 h, and activation of adipose tissue LPL was measured as the difference in LPL activity in biopsies taken before and after insulin infusion. (Reproduced from Eckel, 1987, with permission.)

Coppack *et al.*, 1992), and adipose tissue LPL is not activated normally by insulin (Coppack *et al.*, 1992; Eckel, 1987; Ong and Kern, 1989) (Fig. 8.5). The net effect is that there is a resistance to net fat storage, even in the presence of elevated insulin concentrations (Frayn *et al.*, 1996a). Thus, it has been speculated that insulin resistance is an adaptive phenomenon in obesity, which tends to limit further weight gain (Eckel, 1992). This is probably no different from saying that energy requirements in the whole body increase in obesity (Prentice *et al.*, 1986); thus, larger meals are needed to generate fat storage equivalent to that seen in leaner subjects. Insulin resistance of adipose tissue metabolism might then be seen as the metabolic mechanism for readjustment of body fat content (Frayn *et al.*, 1996a).

There are many reasons, however, for supposing that the 'insulin resistance' of adipose tissue metabolism is a major factor underlying the cardiovascular risk of established obesity (Kissebah *et al.*, 1976; Frayn and Coppack, 1992; Frayn, 1993; Sniderman *et al.*, 1998). Insulin resistance appears to affect multiple metabolic processes in adipose tissue. Of these, the most studied but perhaps least physiologically relevant is glucose transport. In fact, there is divergent evidence for insulin resistance of glucose utilization in adipose tissue *in vivo* in obesity, some studies showing no such effect (Coppack *et al.*, 1996) but others showing impaired glucose utilization (Virtanen *et al.*, 2002).

Other metabolic processes that are responsive to insulin in adipose tissue include suppression of fat mobilization by HSL, activation of LPL and stimulation of the pathway of fatty acid esterification. There is evidence that each of these may become 'insulin resistant' in obesity (reviewed above for HSL and LPL). The net effect may be increased delivery of fatty acids to the circulation, especially in the postprandial period due to failure to entrap fatty acids in adipose tissue (Frayn, 2002). The adverse consequences of inappropriate fatty acid delivery in the postprandial period have been reviewed recently (Frayn *et al.*, 1996b; 1997). In addition, there may be impaired clearance of circulating TG in the postprandial period, due both to failure to activate LPL (Coppack *et al.*, 1992; Potts *et al.*, 1995) and impaired postprandial vasodilatation in adipose tissue (Summers *et al.*, 1996: Virtanen *et al.*, 2002): substrate delivery is an important component of LPL action (Samra *et al.*, 1996b).

Obesity is characterized by widespread insulin resistance, as noted earlier, so that it is reasonable to suggest that some factor associated with increased adipose tissue mass leads to the development of insulin resistance in other tissues. The possible role of excess delivery of NEFA to the circulation has been discussed above. Other candidates have, however, been suggested. An interesting one is the cytokine, TNF-α. TNF-α is expressed in adipose tissue, and its expression is increased in obesity (Hotamisligil *et al.*, 1995). TNF-α is a powerful inducer of insulin resistance in other tissues, including skeletal muscle (Hotamisligil *et al.*, 1994). In animal models of obesity, neutralization of TNF-α with a specific antiserum markedly improves sensitivity to insulin (Hotamisligil *et al.*, 1993). The idea that excessive TNF-α liberation from an expanded adipose tissue mass might explain the widespread insulin resistance of obesity (Hotamisligil and Spiegelman, 1994) is an attractive one, but is not yet proven in humans (Koistinen *et al.*, 2000). Other so-called adipokines have been invoked to explain this link, as discussed earlier in the chapter. Resistin is a peptide secreted from adipose tissue that seems to produce insulin resistance in rodents (Steppan *et al.*, 2001). However, the evidence about resistin has been conflicting even in rodents (Way *et al.*, 2001) and even more so in humans (Savage *et al.*, 2001; Janke *et al.*, 2002; McTernan *et al.*, 2002). This is an interesting and developing area but it is outside our scope.

The quantitative relationship between degree of obesity and insulin resistance is not particularly strong (Bogardus *et al.*, 1985), although it is certainly true that the vast majority of obese people are insulin resistant (Clausen *et al.*, 1996). Some of the variability observed undoubtedly reflects variations in fat distribution: it is clear that visceral or upper body fat distribution is more strongly associated with insulin resistance than lower body fat distribution (Björntorp, 1991b; Kissebah and Krakower, 1994).

There is an ongoing debate on which of the abdominal fat compartments, visceral or subcutaneous, is most strongly associated with insulin resistance (Frayn, 2000). Excess supply of NEFA from visceral fat directly enters the portal circulation and could have several adverse effects on hepatic metabolism, leading to hyperglycaemia and hyperinsulinaemia. Although subcutaneous adipose tissue may be less metabolically active (per unit weight) than visceral adipose tissue, it is a considerably larger mass than the visceral fat compartment, resulting in a large release of NEFA into the systemic circulation (Guo *et al.*, 1999). Abate *et al.* (1995) concluded that subcutaneous truncal fat plays a major role in obesity-related insulin resistance in men, whereas intraperitoneal and retroperitoneal fat have a role of less importance. The impact of type 2 diabetes on insulin sensitivity is much greater than that of obesity (Hollenbeck *et al.*, 1984), although within subjects with type 2 diabetes, the degree of obesity is a major determinant of insulin resistance (Campbell and Carlson, 1993). The latter observation suggests a reason why weight loss can induce marked improvement in glycaemic control in type 2 diabetes (Campbell and Carlson, 1993).

Alterations in adipose tissue metabolism in obesity may therefore have profound effects throughout the body. It can certainly be argued that adipose tissue is a key site of the pathogenesis of the diverse metabolic consequences of obesity.

Acknowledgements

The authors thank Dr Lucinda K. M. Summers, who contributed material to the first edition of this book, some of which has been reutilized in the present chapter. K.N.F. thanks the Wellcome Trust for support of his research work in this area.

References

Abate, N., Garg, A., Peshock, R. M., Stray-Gundersen, J. and Grundy, S. M. (1995) Relationships of generalized and regional adiposity to insulin sensitivity in men. *Journal of Clinical Investigation* **96**, 88–98.

Acheson, K.J., Schutz, Y., Bessard, T., Anantharaman, K., Flatt, J.-P. and Jéquier, E. (1988) Glycogen storage capacity and *de novo* lipogenesis during massive carbohydrate overfeeding in man. *American Journal of Clinical Nutrition* **48**, 240–247.

Arner, P. (1997) Impact of visceral fat. *International Journal of Obesity* **21** (Suppl. 2), S20.

Arner, P. and Bülow, J. (1993) Assessment of adipose tissue metabolism in man: comparison of Fick and microdialysis techniques. *Clinical Science* **85**, 247–256.

Arner, P., Kriegholm, E., Engfeldt, P. and Bolinder, J. (1990) Adrenergic regulation of lipolysis in situ at rest and during exercise. *Journal of Clinical Investigation* **85**, 893–898.

Ashwell, M. (1992) Why do people get fat: is adipose tissue guilty? *Proceedings of the Nutrition Society* **51**, 353–365.

Astrup, A., Buemann, B., Christensen, N.J. and Toubro, S. (1994) Failure to increase lipid oxidation in response to increasing dietary fat content in formerly obese women. *American Journal of Physiology* **266**, E592–E599.

Baltzan, M.A., Andres, R., Cader, G. and Zierler, K.L. (1962)

Heterogeneity of forearm metabolism with special reference to free fatty acids. *Journal of Clinical Investigation* **41**, 116–125.

Banerji, M.A., Buckley, M.C., Chaiken, R.L., Gordon, D., Lebovitz, H.E. and Kral, J.G. (1995) Liver fat, serum triglycerides and visceral adipose tissue in insulin-sensitive and insulin-resistant black men with NIDDM. *International Journal of Obesity* **19**, 846–850.

Baron, A.D., Laakso, M., Brechtel, G., Hoit, B., Watt, C. and Edelman, S.V. (1990) Reduced postprandial skeletal muscle blood flow contributes to glucose intolerance in human obesity. *Journal of Clinical Endocrinology and Metabolism* **70**, 1525–1533.

Barsh, G.S., Farooqi, I.S. and O'Rahilly, S. (2000) Genetics of body-weight regulation. *Nature* **404**, 644–651.

Berg, A.H., Combs, T.P., Du, X., Brownlee, M. and Scherer, P.E. (2001) The adipocyte-secreted protein Acrp30 enhances hepatic insulin action. *Natural Medicine* **7**, 947–953.

Bergström, J., Hermansen, E., Hultman, E. and Saltin, B. (1967) Diet, muscle glycogen and physical performance. *Acta Physiologica Scandinavica* **71**, 140–150.

Bergström, J., Fürst, P., Norée, L.-O. and Vinnars, E. (1974) Intracellular free amino acid concentration in human muscle tissue. *Journal of Applied Physiology* **36**, 693–697.

Binnert, C., Pachiaudi, C., Beylot, M., Hans, D., Vandermander, J., Chantre, P., Riou, J.-P. and Laville, M. (1998) Influence of human obesity on the metabolic fate of dietary long- and medium-chain triacylglycerols. *American Journal of Clinical Nutrition* **67**, 595–601.

Björntorp, P. (1990) 'Portal' adipose tissue as a generator of risk factors for cardiovascular disease and diabetes. *Arteriosclerosis* **10**, 493–496.

Björntorp, P. (1991a) Importance of fat as a support nutrient for energy: metabolism of athletes. *Journal of Sports Science* **9**, 71–76.

Björntorp, P. (1991b) Metabolic implications of body fat distribution. *Diabetes Care* **14**, 1132–1143.

Blaak, E.E., Van Baak, M.A., Kemerink, G.J., Pakbiers, M.T., Heidendal, G.A. and Saris, W.H. (1994a) β-Adrenergic stimulation of energy expenditure and forearm skeletal muscle metabolism in lean and obese men. *American Journal of Physiology* **267**, E306–E315.

Blaak, E.E., Van Baak, M.A., Kemerink, G.J., Pakbiers, M.T., Heidendal, G.A. and Saris, W. H. (1994b) β-Adrenergic stimulation of skeletal muscle metabolism in relation to weight reduction in obese men. *American Journal of Physiology* **267**, E316–E322.

Blaak, E.E., van Baak, M.A., Kemerink, G.J., Pakbiers, M.T.W., Heidendal, G. A.K. and Saris, W.H.M. (1995) β-Adrenergic stimulation and abdominal subcutaneous fat blood flow in lean, obese, and reduced-obese subjects. *Metabolism* **44**, 183–187.

Boesch, C., Slotboom, J., Hoppeler, H. and Kreis, R. (1997) *In vivo* determination of intra-myocellular lipids in human muscle by means of localized 1H-MR-spectroscopy. *Magnetic Resonance Medicine* **37**, 484–493.

Bogardus, C., Lillioja, S., Mott, D.M., Hollenbeck, C. and Reaven, G. (1985) Relationship between degree of obesity and *in vivo* insulin action in man. *American Journal of Physiology* **248**, E286–E291.

Bonora, E., Bonadonna, R.C., Del Prato, S., Gulli, G., Solini, A., Matsuda, M. and DeFronzo, R.A. (1993) *In vivo* glucose metabolism in obese and type II diabetic subjects with or without hypertension. *Diabetes* **42**, 764–772.

Brechtel, K., Niess, A.M., Machann, J., Rett, K., Schick, F., Claussen, C.D., Dickhuth, H.H., Häring, H.U. and Jacob, S. (2001) Utilisation of intramyocellular lipids (IMCLs) during exercise as assessed by proton magnetic resonance spectroscopy (1H-MRS). *Hormone and Metabolic Research* **33**, 63–66.

Bülow, J. (1993) Lipid mobilization and utilization. *Medicine and Sport Science* **38**, 158–185.

Campbell, P.J. and Carlson, M.G. (1993) Impact of obesity on insulin action in NIDDM. *Diabetes* **42**, 405–410.

Campbell, P.J., Carlson, M.G. and Nurjhan, N. (1994) Fat metabolism in human obesity. *American Journal of Physiology* **266**, E600–E605.

Capaldo, B., Napoli, R., Di Marino, L., Guida, R., Pardo, F. and Saccá, L. (1994) Role of insulin and free fatty acid (FFA) availability on regional FFA kinetics in the human forearm. *Journal of Clinical Endocrinology and Metabolism* **79**, 879–882.

Carlson, L.A., Ekelund, L.-G. and Fröberg, S.O. (1971) Concentration of triglycerides, phospholipids and glycogen in skeletal muscle and of free fatty acids and β-hydroxybutyric acid in blood in man in response to exercise. *European Journal of Clinical Investigation* **1**, 248–254.

Cersosimo, E., Danou, F., Persson, M. and Miles, J.M. (1996) Effects of pulsatile delivery of basal growth hormone on lipolysis in humans. *American Journal of Physiology* **271**, E123–E126.

Cianflone, K., Kalant, D., Marliss, E.B., Gougeon, R. and Sniderman, A.D. (1995) Response of plasma ASP to a prolonged fast. *International Journal of Obesity* **19**, 604–609.

Clausen, J.O., Borch-Johnsen, K., Ibsen, H., Bergman, R.N., Hougaard, P., Winther, K. and Pedersen, O. (1996) Insulin sensitivity index, acute insulin response, and glucose effectiveness in a population-based sample of 380 young healthy Caucasians. Analysis of the impact of gender, body fat, physical fitness, and lifestyle factors. *Journal of Clinical Investigation* **98**, 1195–1209.

Clifford, G.M., Londos, C., Kraemer, F.B., Vernon, R.G. and Yeaman, S.J. (2000) Translocation of hormone-sensitive lipase and perilipin upon lipolytic stimulation of rat adipocytes. *Journal of Biological Chemisty* **275**, 5011–5015.

Colberg, S.R., Simoneau, J.-A., Thaete, F.L. and Kelley, D.E. (1995) Skeletal muscle utilization of free fatty acids in women with visceral obesity. *Journal of Clinical Investigation* **95**, 1846–1853.

Considine, R.V., Sinha, M.K., Heiman, M.L., Kriauciunas, A., Stephens, T.W., Nyce, M.R., Ohannesian, J.P., Marco, C.C., McKee, L.J., Bauer, T.L. and Caro, J.F. (1996) Serum immunoreactive-leptin concentrations in normal-weight and obese humans. *New England Journal of Medicine* **334**, 292–295.

Coppack, S.W., Fisher, R.M., Gibbons, G.F., Humphreys, S.M., McDonough, M.J., Potts, J.L. and Frayn, K.N. (1990) Postprandial substrate deposition in human forearm and adipose tissues *in vivo*. *Clinical Science* **79**, 339–348.

Coppack, S.W., Evans, R.D., Fisher, R.M., Frayn, K.N., Gibbons, G.F., Humphreys, S.M., Kirk, M.J., Potts, J.L. and Hockaday, T.D.R. (1992) Adipose tissue metabolism in obesity: lipase action *in vivo* before and after a mixed meal. *Metabolism* **41**, 264–272.

Coppack, S.W., Fisher, R.M., Humphreys, S.M., Clark, M.L., Pointon, J.J. and Frayn, K.N. (1996) Carbohydrate metabolism in insulin resistance: glucose uptake and lactate production by adipose and forearm tissues *in vivo* before and after a mixed meal. *Clinical Science* **90**, 409–415.

Couillard, C., Bergeron, N., Prud'homme, D., Bergeron, J., Tremblay, A., Bouchard, C., Mauriège, P. and Després, J. P. (1999) Gender difference in postprandial lipemia: importance of visceral adipose tissue accumulation. *Arteriosclerosis Thrombosis and Vascular Biology* **19**, 2448–2455.

Coyle, E. F. (1995) Substrate utilization during exercise in active people. *American Journal of Clinical Nutrition* **61**(Suppl.), 968S–979S.

Crandall, D.L. and DiGirolamo, M. (1990) Hemodynamic and metabolic correlates in adipose tissue: pathophysiologic considerations. *FASEB J* **4**, 141–147.

Crowther, G.J., Carey, M.F., Kemper, W.F. and Conley, K.E. (2002) Control of glycolysis in contracting skeletal muscle. I. Turning it on. *American Journal of Physiology* **282**, E67–E73.

Cummings, M.H., Watts, G.F., Umpleby, A.M., Hennessy, T.R., Kelly, J.M., Jackson, N.C. and Sönksen, P.H. (1995) Acute hyperinsulinemia decreases the hepatic secretion of very-low-density lipoprotein apolipoprotein B-100 in NIDDM. *Diabetes* **44**, 1059–1065.

Dagenais, G.R., Tancredi, R.G. and Zierler, K.L. (1976) Free fatty acid oxidation by forearm muscle at rest, and evidence for an intramuscular lipid pool in the human forearm. *Journal of Clinical Investigation* **58**, 421–431.

Daniel, P.M., Pratt, O.E. and Spargo, E. (1977) The metabolic homoeostatic role of muscle and its function as a store of protein. *Lancet* **ii**, 446–448.

DeFronzo, R.A., Tobin, J. and Andres, R. (1979) Glucose clamp technique: a method for quantifying insulin secretion and resistance. *American Journal of Physiology* **237**, E214–E223.

DeFronzo, R.A., Jacot, E., Jequier, E., Maeder, J., Wahren, J. and Felber, J.P. (1981) The effect of insulin on the disposal of intravenous glucose. Results from indirect calorimetry and hepatic and femoral venous catheterization. *Diabetes* **30**, 1000–1007.

Dohm, G.L. (2002) Invited review: Regulation of skeletal muscle GLUT-4 expression by exercise. *Journal of Applied Physiology* **93**, 782–787.

Dulloo, A.G. and Samec, S. (2001) Uncoupling proteins: their roles in adaptive thermogenesis and substrate metabolism reconsidered. *British Journal of Nutrition* **86**, 123–139.

Dyck, D.J., Steinberg, G. and Bonen, A. (2001) Insulin increases FA uptake and esterification but reduces lipid utilization in isolated contracting muscle. *American Journal of Physiology* **281**, E600–E607.

Eckel, R.H. (1987) Adipose tissue lipoprotein lipase. In: Borensztajn, J. ed. *Lipoprotein Lipase*. Chicago: Evener, 79–132.

Eckel, R.H. (1989) Lipoprotein lipase. A multifunctional enzyme relevant to common metabolic diseases. *New England Journal of Medicine* **320**, 1060–1068.

Eckel, R.H. (1992) Insulin resistance: an adaptation for weight maintenance. *Lancet* **340**, 1452–1453.

Elia, M., Folmer, P., Schlatmann, A., Goren, A. and Austin, S. (1988) Carbohydrate, fat, and protein metabolism in muscle and in the whole body after mixed meal ingestion. *Metabolism* **37**, 542–551.

Ellis, B.A., Poynten, A., Lowy, A.J., Furler, S.M., Chisholm, D.J., Kraegen, E.W. and Cooney, G.J. (2000) Long-chain acyl-CoA esters as indicators of lipid metabolism and insulin sensitivity in rat and human muscle. *American Journal of Physiology* **279**, E554–E560.

Evans, K., Burdge, G.C., Wootton, S.A., Clark, M.L. and Frayn, K.N. (2002) Regulation of dietary fatty acid entrapment in subcutaneous adipose tissue and skeletal muscle. *Diabetes* **51**, 2684–2690.

Falholt, K., Jensen, I., Lindkaer Jensen, S., Mortensen, H., Volund, A., Heding, L.G., Petersen, P.N. and Falholt, W. (1988) Carbohydrate and lipid metabolism of skeletal muscle in type 2 diabetic patients. *Diabetic Medicine* **5**, 27–31.

Farese, R.V., Yost, T.J. and Eckel, R.H. (1991) Tissue-specific regulation of lipoprotein lipase activity by insulin/glucose in normal-weight humans. *Metabolism* **40**, 214–216.

Farooqi, I.S., Matarese, G., Lord, G. M., Keogh, J. M., Lawrence, E., Agwu, C., Sanna, V., Jebb, S. A., Perna, F., Fontana, S., Lechler, R.I., DePaoli, A.M. and O'Rahilly, S. (2002) Beneficial effects of leptin on obesity, T cell hyporesponsiveness, and neuroendocrine/metabolic dysfunction of human congenital leptin deficiency. *Journal of Clinical Investigation* **110**, 1093–1103.

Felber, J.-P., Ferrannini, E., Golay, A., Meyer, H.U., Theibaud, D., Curchod, B., Maeder, E., Jequier, E. and DeFronzo, R.A. (1987) Role of lipid oxidation in pathogenesis of insulin resistance of obesity and type II diabetes. *Diabetes* **36**, 1341–1350.

Felber, J.-P., Acheson, K.J. and Tappy, L. (1993) *From Obesity to Diabetes*. Chichester: John Wiley.

Flatt, J.-P. (1972) Role of the increased adipose tissue mass in the apparent insulin insensitivity of obesity. *American Journal of Clinical Nutrition* **25**, 1189–1192.

Fleury, C., Neverova, M., Collins, S., Raimbault, S., Champigny, O., Levi Meyrueis, C., Bouillaud, F., Seldin, M.F., Surwit, R. S., Ricquier, D. and Warden, C.H. (1997) Uncoupling protein-2: a novel gene linked to obesity and hyperinsulinemia. *Nature Genetics* **15**, 269–272.

Forouhi, N.G., Jenkinson, G., Thomas, E.L., Mullick, S., Mierisova, S., Bhonsle, U., McKeigue, P.M. and Bell, J. D. (1999) Relation of triglyceride stores in skeletal muscle cells to central obesity and insulin sensitivity in European and South Asian men. *Diabetologia* **42**, 932–935.

Frayn, K.N. (1980) Skeletal muscle triacylglycerol in the rat: methods for sampling and measurement, and studies of biological variability. *Journal of Lipid Research* **21**, 139–144.

Frayn, K.N. (1992) Studies of human adipose tissue *in vivo*. In: Kinney, J.M. and Tucker, H.N. eds. *Energy Metabolism: Tissue Determinants and Cellular Corollaries*. New York: Raven Press, 267–295.

Frayn, K.N. (1993) Insulin resistance and lipid metabolism. *Current Opinion in Lipidology* **4**, 197–204.

Frayn, K.N. (2000) Visceral fat and insulin resistance: causative or correlative? *British Journal of Nutrition* **83** (Suppl. 1), S71–S77.

Frayn, K.N. (2002) Adipose tissue as a buffer for daily lipid flux. *Diabetologia* **45**, 1201–1210.

Frayn, K.N. (2003) *Metabolic Regulation: A Human Perspective*, 2nd edn. Oxford: Blackwell Publishing.

Frayn, K.N. and Coppack, S.W. (1992) Insulin resistance, adipose tissue and coronary heart disease. *Clinical Science* **82**, 1–8.

Frayn, K. N. and Coppack, S. W. (2001) Assessment of white adipose tissue metabolism by measurement of arteriovenous differences. *Methods in Molecular Biology* **155**, 269–279.

Frayn, K.N., Khan, K., Coppack, S.W. and Elia, M. (1991) Amino acid metabolism in human subcutaneous adipose tissue *in vivo*. *Clinical Science* **80**, 471–474.

Frayn, K.N., Shadid, S., Hamlani, R., Humphreys, S.M., Clark, M.L., Fielding, B.A., Boland, O. and Coppack, S. W. (1994) Regulation of fatty acid movement in human adipose tissue in the postabsorptive-to-postprandial transition. *American Journal of Physiology* **266**, E308–E317.

Frayn, K.N., Humphreys, S.M. and Coppack, S.W. (1995a) Fuel selection in white adipose tissue. *Proceedings of the Nutrition Society* **54**, 177–189.

Frayn, K.N., Coppack, S.W., Fielding, B.A. and Humphreys, S.M. (1995b) Coordinated regulation of hormone-sensitive lipase and lipoprotein lipase in human adipose tissue *in vivo*: implications for the control of fat storage and fat mobilization. *Advances in Enzyme Regulation* **35**, 163–178.

Frayn, K.N., Humphreys, S.M. and Coppack, S.W. (1996a) Net carbon flux across subcutaneous adipose tissue after a standard meal in normal-weight and insulin-resistant obese subjects. *International Journal of Obesity* **20**, 795–800.

Frayn, K.N., Williams, C.M. and Arner, P. (1996b) Are increased plasma non-esterified fatty acid concentrations a risk marker for coronary heart disease and other chronic diseases? *Clinical Science* **90**, 243–253.

Frayn, K.N., Summers, L.K.M. and Fielding, B.A. (1997) Regulation of the plasma non-esterified fatty acid concentration in the postprandial state. *Proceedings of the Nutrition Society* **56**, 713–721.

Frayn, K.N., Karpe, F., Fielding, B.A., Macdonald, I.A. and Coppack, S.W. (2003) Integrative physiology of human adipose tissue. *International Journal of Obesity* **27**, 875–888.

Friedman, J.E., Dohm, G.L., Leggett Frazier, N., Elton, C.W., Tapscott, E.B., Pories, W.P. and Caro, J.F. (1992) Restoration of insulin responsiveness in skeletal muscle of morbidly obese patients after weight loss. Effect on muscle glucose transport and glucose transporter GLUT4. *Journal of Clinical Investigation* **89**, 701–705.

Froidevaux, F., Schutz, Y., Christin, L. and Jéquier, E. (1993) Energy expenditure in obese women before and during weight loss, after refeeding, and in the weight-relapse period. *American Journal of Clinical Nutrition* **57**, 35–42.

Frühbeck, G., Gomez-Ambrosi, J., Muruzabal, F.J. and Burrell, M.A. (2001) The adipocyte: a model for integration of endocrine and metabolic signaling in energy metabolism regulation. *American Journal of Physiology* **280**, E827–E847.

Gaster, M., Staehr, P., Beck-Nielsen, H., Schroder, H.D. and Handberg, A. (2001) GLUT4 is reduced in slow muscle fibers of type 2 diabetic patients: is insulin resistance in type 2 diabetes a slow, type 1 fiber disease? *Diabetes* **50**, 1324–1329.

Glatz, J. F. and Storch, J. (2001) Unravelling the significance of cellular fatty acid-binding proteins. *Current Opinion in Lipidology* **12**, 267–274.

Griffiths, A.J., Humphreys, S.M., Clark, M.L. and Frayn, K.N. (1994) Forearm substrate utilization during exercise after a meal containing both fat and carbohydrate. *Clinical Science* **86**, 169–175.

Guo, Z., Hensrud, D.D., Johnson, C.M. and Jensen, M.D. (1999) Regional postprandial fatty acid metabolism in different obesity phenotypes. *Diabetes* **48**, 1586–1592.

Hauner, H., Entenmann, G., Wabitsch, M., Gaillard, D., Ailhaud, G., Negrel, R. and Pfeiffer, E.F. (1989) Promoting effect of glucocorticoids on the differentiation of human adipocyte precursor cells cultured in a chemically defined medium. *Journal of Clinical Investigation* **84**, 1663–1670.

Hellström, L., Langin, D., Reynisdottir, S., Dauzats, M. and Arner, P. (1996) Adipocyte lipolysis in normal weight subjects with obesity among first-degree relatives. *Diabetologia* **39**, 921–928.

Henriksson, J. (1995) Muscle fuel selection: effect of exercise and training. *Proceedings of the Nutrition Society* **54**, 125–138.

Herd, S.L., Hardman, A.E., Boobis, L.H. and Cairns, C.J. (1998) The effect of 13 weeks of running training followed by 9 d of detraining on postprandial lipaemia. *British Journal of Nutrition* **80**, 57–66.

Hesselink, M.K., Greenhaff, P.L., Constantin-Teodosiu, D., Hultman, E., Saris, W.H., Nieuwlaat, R., Schaart, G., Kornips, E. and Schrauwen, P. (2003) Increased uncoupling protein 3 content does not affect mitochondrial function in human skeletal muscle *in vivo*. *Journal of Clinical Investigation* **111**, 479–486.

Hoag, S., Marshall, J.A., Jones, R.H. and Hamman, R.F. (1995) High fasting insulin levels associated with lower rates of weight gain in persons with normal glucose tolerance: The San Luis Valley Diabetes Study. *International Journal of Obesity* **19**, 175–180.

Hodgetts, V., Coppack, S.W., Frayn, K.N. and Hockaday, T.D.R. (1991) Factors controlling fat mobilization from human subcutaneous adipose tissue during exercise. *Journal of Applied Physiology* **71**, 445–451.

Hollenbeck, C.B., Chen, Y.-I. and Reaven, G.M. (1984) A comparison of the relative effects of obesity and non-insulin-dependent diabetes mellitus on *in vivo* insulin-stimulated glucose utilization. *Diabetes* **33**, 622–626.

Hollenberg, C.H. (1990) Perspectives in adipose tissue physiology. *International Journal of Obesity* **14** Suppl. 3, 135–152.

Hotamisligil, G.S. and Spiegelman, B.M. (1994) Tumor necrosis factor alpha: a key component of the obesity-diabetes link. *Diabetes* **43**, 1271–1278.

Hotamisligil, G.S., Shargill, N.S. and Spiegelman, B.M. (1993) Adipose expression of tumor necrosis factor alpha: direct role in obesity-linked insulin resistance. *Science* **259**, 87–91.

Hotamisligil, G.S., Murray, D.L., Choy, L.N. and Spiegelman, B.M. (1994) Tumor necrosis factor alpha inhibits signaling from the insulin receptor. *Proceedings of the National Academy of Sciences of the USA* **91**, 4854–4858.

Hotamisligil, G.S., Arner, P., Caro, J.F., Atkinson, R.L. and Spiegelman, B.M. (1995) Increased adipose tissue expression of tumor necrosis factor-α in human obesity and insulin resistance. *Journal of Clinical Investigation* **95**, 2409–2415.

Itani, S.I., Ruderman, N.B., Schmieder, F. and Boden, G. (2002) Lipid-induced insulin resistance in human muscle is associated with changes in diacylglycerol, protein kinase C, and IkappaB-alpha. *Diabetes* **51**, 2005–2011.

Jackson, R.A., Hamling, J.B., Sim, B.M., Hawa, M.I., Blix, P.M. and Nabarro, J.D.N. (1987) Peripheral lactate and oxygen metabolism in man: the influence of oral glucose loading. *Metabolism* **36**, 144–150.

Janke, J., Englei, S., Gorzelniak, K., Luft, F.C. and Sharma, A.M. (2002) Resistin gene expression in human adipocytes is not related to insulin resistance. *Obesity Research* **10**, 1–5.

Jensen, M.D., Haymond, M.W., Rizza, R.A., Cryer, P.E. and Miles, J.M. (1989) Influence of body fat distribution on free fatty acid metabolism in obesity. *Journal of Clinical Investigation* **83**, 1168–1173.

Jeppesen, J., Hollenbeck, C.B., Zhou, M.-Y., Coulston, A.M., Jones, C., Chen, Y.-D.I. and Reaven, G.M. (1995) Relation between insulin resistance, hyperinsulinemia, postheparin plasma lipoprotein lipase activity, and postprandial lipemia. *Arteriosclerosis Thrombosis and Vascular Biology* **15**, 320–324.

Johnson, M.A., Polgar, J., Weightman, D. and Appleton, D. (1973) Data on the distribution of fibre types in thirty-six human muscles. An autopsy study. *Journal of Neurological Science* **18**, 111–129.

Jones, D.A. and Round, J.M. (1990) *Skeletal Muscle in Health and Disease. A Textbook of Muscle Physiology*. Manchester: Manchester University Press.

Kahn, B.B. and Flier, J.S. (2000) Obesity and insulin resistance. *Journal of Clinical Investigation* **106**, 473–481.

Kalant, D., Phélis, S., Fielding, B.A., Frayn, K.N., Cianflone, K. and

Sniderman, A.D. (2000) Increased postprandial fatty acid trapping in subcutaneous adipose tissue in obese women. *Journal of Lipid Research* **41**, 1963–1968.

Karpe, F., Fielding, B.A., Ilic, V., Macdonald, I.A., Summers, L.K.M. and Frayn, K.N. (2002) Impaired postprandial adipose tissue blood flow response is related to aspects of insulin sensitivity. *Diabetes* **51**, 2467–2473.

Katzel, L.I., Busby-Whitehead, M.J., Rogus, E.M., Krauss, R.M. and Goldberg, A.P. (1994) Reduced adipose tissue lipoprotein lipase responses, postprandial lipemia, and low high-density lipoprotein-2 subspecies levels in older athletes with silent myocardial ischemia. *Metabolism* **43**, 190–198.

Kelley, D., Mitrakou, A., Marsh, H., Schwenk, F., Benn, J., Sonnenberg, G., Arcangeli, M., Aoki, T., Sorensen, J., Berger, M., Sonksen, P. and Gerich, J. (1988) Skeletal muscle glycolysis, oxidation, and storage of an oral glucose load. *Journal of Clinical Investigation* **81**, 1563–1571.

Kelley, D.E., Mokan, M. and Mandarino, L.J. (1992) Intracellular defects in glucose metabolism in obese patients with NIDDM. *Diabetes* **41**, 698–706.

Kelley, D.E., Mintun, M.A., Watkins, S.C., Simoneau, J.A., Jadali, F., Fredrickson, A., Beattie, J. and Theriault, R. (1996) The effect of non-insulin-dependent diabetes mellitus and obesity on glucose transport and phosphorylation in skeletal muscle. *Journal of Clinical Investigation* **97**, 2705–2713.

Kiens, B. and Lithell, H. (1989) Lipoprotein metabolism influenced by training-induced changes in human skeletal muscle. *Journal of Clinical Investigation* **83**, 558–564.

Kiens, B. and Richter, E.A. (1998) Utilization of skeletal muscle triacylglycerol during postexercise recovery in humans. *American Journal of Physiology* **275**, E332–E337.

Kimber, N.E., Heigenhauser, G.J., Spriet, L.L. and Dyck, D.J. (2003) Skeletal muscle fat and carbohydrate metabolism during recovery from glycogen-depleting exercise in humans. *Journal of Physiology* **548**, 919–927.

Kissebah, A.H. and Krakower, G.R. (1994) Regional adiposity and morbidity. *Physiological Reviews* **74**, 761–811.

Kissebah, A.H., Alfarsi, S., Adams, P.W. and Wynn, V. (1976) Role of insulin resistance in adipose tissue and liver in the pathogenesis of endogenous hypertriglyceridaemia in man. *Diabetologia* **12**, 563–571.

Koistinen, H.A., Bastard, J.P., Dusserre, E., Ebeling, P., Zegari, N., Andreelli, F., Jardel, C., Donner, M., Meyer, L., Moulin, P., Hainque, B., Riou, J.P., Laville, M., Koivisto, V.A. and Vidal, H. (2000) Subcutaneous adipose tissue expression of tumour necrosis factor-α is not associated with whole body insulin resistance in obese nondiabetic or in type-2 diabetic subjects. *European Journal of Clinical Investigation* **30**, 302–310.

Laakso, M., Edelman, S.V., Olefsky, J.M., Brechtel, G., Wallace, P. and Baron, A.D. (1990a) Kinetics of *in vivo* muscle insulin-mediated glucose uptake in human obesity. *Diabetes* **39**, 965–974.

Laakso, M., Edelman, S.V., Brechtel, G. and Baron, A.D. (1990b) Decreased effect of insulin to stimulate skeletal muscle blood flow in obese man. A novel mechanism for insulin resistance. *Journal of Clinical Investigation* **85**, 1844–1852.

Lewis, G.F., Uffelman, K.D., Szeto, L.W., Weller, B. and Steiner, G. (1995) Interaction between free fatty acids and insulin in the acute control of very low density lipoprotein production in humans. *Journal of Clinical Investigation* **95**, 158–166.

Lillioja, S., Foley, J., Bogardus, C., Mott, D. and Howard, B.V. (1986) Free fatty acid metabolism and obesity in man: *in vivo* and *in vitro* comparisons. *Metabolism* **35**, 505–514.

Londos, C., Gruia-Gray, J., Brasaemle, D.L., Rondinone, C. M., Takeda, T., Dwyer, N.K., Barber, T., Kimmel, A.R. and Blanchette Mackie, E. J. (1996) Perilipin: possible roles in structure and metabolism of intracellular neutral lipids in adipocytes and steroidogenic cells. *International Journal of Obesity* **20** (Suppl. 3), S97–S101.

Luiken, J.J., Koonen, D.P., Willems, J., Zorzano, A., Becker, C., Fischer, Y., Tandon, N.N., Van Der Vusse, G.J., Bonen, A. and Glatz, J.F. (2002) Insulin stimulates long-chain fatty acid utilization by rat cardiac myocytes through cellular redistribution of FAT/CD36. *Diabetes* **51**, 3113–3119.

McTernan, C.L., McTernan, P.G., Harte, A.L., Levick, P.L., Barnett, A.H. and Kumar, S. (2002) Resistin, central obesity, and type 2 diabetes. *Lancet* **359**, 46–47.

Malkova, D., Evans, R.D., Frayn, K.N., Humphreys, S.M., Jones, P.R. and Hardman, A.E. (2000) Prior exercise and postprandial substrate extraction across the human leg. *American Journal of Physiology Endocrinology and Metabolism* **279**, E1020–E1028.

Malmström, R., Packard, C.J., Caslake, M., Bedford, D., Stewart, P., Yki-Järvinen, H., Shepherd, J. and Taskinen, M.R. (1998) Effects of insulin and acipimox on VLDL1 and VLDL2 apolipoprotein B production in normal subjects. *Diabetes* **47**, 779–787.

Mårin, P., Rebuffé-Scrive, M. and Björntorp, P. (1990) Uptake of triglyceride fatty acids in adipose tissue *in vivo* in man. *European Journal of Clinical Investigation* **20**, 158–165.

Mårin, P., Högh-Kristiansen, I., Jansson, S., Krotkiewski, M., Holm, G. and Björntorp, P. (1992) Uptake of glucose carbon in muscle glycogen and adipose tissue triglycerides *in vivo* in humans. *American Journal of Physiology* **263**, E473–E480.

Maslowska, M., Scantlebury, T., Germinario, R. and Cianflone, K. (1997) Acute *in vitro* production of acylation stimulating protein in differentiated human adipocytes. *Journal of Lipid Research* **38**, 1–11.

Mohamed-Ali, V., Pinkney, J.H. and Coppack, S. W. (1998) Adipose tissue as an endocrine and paracrine organ. *International Journal of Obesity* **22**, 1145–1158.

Moller, D.E., Chang, P.-Y., Yaspelkis, B.B.I., Flier, J.S., Wallberg-Henriksson, H. and Ivy, J.L. (1996) Transgenic mice with muscle-specific insulin resistance develop increased adiposity, impaired glucose tolerance, and dyslipidemia. *Endocrinology* **137**, 2397–2405.

Oben, J., Elliott, R., Morgan, L., Fletcher, J. and Marks, V. (1992) The role of gut hormones in the adipose tissue metabolism of lean and genetically obese (*ob/ob*) mice. In: Ailhaud, G., Guy-Grand, B., Lafontan, M. and Ricquier, D. eds. *Obesity in Europe 91. Proceedings of the 3rd European Congress on Obesity.* London: Libbey, 269–272.

Odland, L.M., Heigenhauser, G.J., Lopaschuk, G.D. and Spriet, L.L. (1996) Human skeletal muscle malonyl-CoA at rest and during prolonged submaximal exercise. *American Journal of Physiology* **270**, E541–E544.

Okazaki, H., Osuga, J., Tamura, Y., Yahagi, N., Tomita, S., Shionoiri, F., Iizuka, Y., Ohashi, K., Harada, K., Kimura, S., Gotoda, T., Shimano, H., Yamada, N. and Ishibashi, S. (2002) Lipolysis in the absence of hormone-sensitive lipase: evidence for a common mechanism regulating distinct lipases. *Diabetes* **51**, 3368–3375.

Ong, J.M. and Kern, P.A. (1989) Effect of feeding and obesity on lipoprotein lipase activity, immunoreactive protein, and messenger RNA levels in human adipose tissue. *Journal of Clinical Investigation* **84**, 305–311.

Opie, L.H. and Walfish, P.G. (1963) Plasma free fatty acid concentrations in obesity. *New England Journal of Medicine* **268**, 757–760.

Oscai, L.B., Essig, D.A. and Palmer, W.K. (1990) Lipase regulation of muscle triglyceride hydrolysis. *Journal of Applied Physiology* **69**, 1571–1577.

Osuga, J., Ishibashi, S., Oka, T., Yagyu, H., Tozawa, R., Fujimoto, A., Shionoiri, F., Yahagi, N., Kraemer, F. B., Tsutsumi, O. and Yamada, N. (2000) Targeted disruption of hormone-sensitive lipase results in male sterility and adipocyte hypertrophy, but not in obesity. *Proceedings of the National Academy of Sciences of the USA* **97**, 787–792.

Peeva, E., Brun, D.L., Ven Murthy, M.R., Després, J.-P., Normand, T., Gagné, C., Lupien, P.-J. and Julien, P. (1992) Adipose cell size and distribution in familial lipoprotein lipase deficiency. *International Journal of Obesity* **16**, 737–744.

Pénicaud, L., Ferré, P., Terrataz, J., Kinebanyan, M.F., Leturque, A., Doré, E., Girard, J., Jeanrenaud, B. and Picon, L. (1987) Development of obesity in Zucker rats. Early insulin resistance in muscles but normal sensitivity in white adipose tissue. *Diabetes* **36**, 626–631.

Phillips, D.I.W., Caddy, S., Ilic, V., Fielding, B.A., Frayn, K.N., Borthwick, A.C. and Taylor, R. (1996) Intramuscular triglyceride and muscle insulin sensitivity: evidence for a relationship in non-diabetic subjects. *Metabolism* **45**, 947–950.

Piatti, P.M., Monti, L.D., Pacchioni, M., Pontiroli, A.E. and Pozza, G. (1991) Forearm insulin- and non-insulin-mediated glucose uptake and muscle metabolism in man: role of free fatty acids and blood glucose levels. *Metabolism* **40**, 926–933.

Potts, J.L., Fisher, R.M., Humphreys, S.M., Coppack, S.W., Gibbons, G.F. and Frayn, K.N. (1991) Peripheral triacylglycerol extraction in the fasting and post-prandial states. *Clinical Science* **81**, 621–626.

Potts, J.L., Coppack, S.W., Fisher, R.M., Humphreys, S.M., Gibbons, G.F. and Frayn, K.N. (1995) Impaired postprandial clearance of triacylglycerol-rich lipoproteins in adipose tissue in obese subjects. *American Journal of Physiology* **268**, E588–E594.

Prentice, A.M., Black, A.E., Coward, W.A., Davies, H.L., Goldberg, G.R., Murgatroyd, P.R., Ashford, J., Sawyer, M. and Whitehead, R.G. (1986) High levels of energy expenditure in obese women. *British Medical Journal* **292**, 983–987.

Raben, A., Andersen, H.B., Christensen, N.J., Madsen, J., Holst, J.J. and Astrup, A. (1994) Evidence for an abnormal postprandial response to a high-fat meal in women predisposed to obesity. *American Journal of Physiology* **267**, E549–E559.

Rabinowitz, D. and Zierler, K.L. (1961) Forearm metabolism in obesity and its response to intra-arterial insulin. Evidence for adaptive hyperinsulinism. *Lancet* **1**, 690–692.

Rådegran, G., Blomstrand, E. and Saltin, B. (1999) Peak muscle perfusion and oxygen uptake in humans: importance of precise estimates of muscle mass. *Journal of Applied Physiology* **87**, 2375–2380.

Randle, P.J., Garland, P.B., Hales, C.N. and Newsholme, E.A. (1963) The glucose fatty-acid cycle. Its role in insulin sensitivity and the metabolic disturbances of diabetes mellitus. *Lancet* **1**, 785–789.

Ren, J.M., Semenkovich, C.F., Gulve, E.A., Gao, J. and Holloszy, J.O. (1994) Exercise induces rapid increases in GLUT4 expression, glucose transport capacity, and insulin-stimulated glycogen storage in muscle. *Journal of Biological Chemistry* **269**, 14396–14401.

Ricquier, D. and Bouillaud, F. (2000a) The uncoupling protein homologues: UCP1, UCP2, UCP3, StUCP and AtUCP. *Biochemistry Journal* **345**, 161–179.

Ricquier, D. and Bouillaud, F. (2000b) Mitochondrial uncoupling proteins: from mitochondria to the regulation of energy balance. *Journal of Physiology* **529**, 3–10.

Rigden, D.J., Jellyman, A.E., Frayn, K.N. and Coppack, S.W. (1990) Human adipose tissue glycogen levels and responses to carbohydrate feeding. *European Journal of Clinical Nutrition* **44**, 689–692.

Roden, M., Price, T.B., Perseghin, G., Petersen, K.F., Rothman, D.L., Cline, G. W. and Shulman, G.I. (1996) Mechanism of free fatty acid-induced insulin resistance in humans. *Journal of Clinical Investigation* **97**, 2859–2865.

Roden, M., Krssak, M., Stingl, H., Gruber, S., Hofer, A., Furnsinn, C., Moser, E. and Waldhausl, W. (1999) Rapid impairment of skeletal muscle glucose transport/phosphorylation by free fatty acids in humans. *Diabetes* **48**, 358–364.

Rodnick, K.J., Slot, J.W., Studelska, D.R., Hanpeter, D.E., Robinson, L.J., Geuze, H.J. and James, D.E. (1992) Immunocytochemical and biochemical studies of GLUT4 in rat skeletal muscle. *Journal of Biological Chemistry* **267**, 6278–6285.

Rohner-Jeanrenaud, F. and Jeanrenaud, B. (1996) Obesity, leptin and the brain. *New England Journal of Medicine* **334**, 324–325.

Romanski, S.A., Nelson, R.M. and Jensen, M.D. (2000) Meal fatty acid uptake in adipose tissue: gender effects in nonobese humans. *American Journal of Physiology* **279**, E455–E462.

Romijn, J.A., Coyle, E.F., Sidossis, L.S., Gastaldelli, A., Horowitz, J.F., Endert, E. and Wolfe, R. R. (1993) Regulation of endogenous fat and carbohydrate metabolism in relation to exercise intensity and duration. *American Journal of Physiology* **265**, E380–E391.

Ruys, T., Sturgess, I., Shaikh, M., Watts, G.F., Nordestgaard, B.G. and Lewis, B. (1989) Effects of exercise and fat ingestion on high density lipoprotein production by peripheral tissues. *Lancet* **ii**, 1119–1122.

Saghizadeh, M., Ong, J.M., Garvey, W.T., Henry, R.R. and Kern, P.A. (1996) The expression of TNFα by human muscle. Relationship to insulin resistance. *Journal of Clinical Investigation* **97**, 1111–1116.

Saha, A.K., Kurowski, T.G. and Ruderman, N.B. (1994) A malonyl-CoA fuel-sensing mechanism in muscle: effects of insulin, glucose, and denervation. *American Journal of Physiology* **267**, E95–E101.

Samra, J.S., Clark, M.L., Humphreys, S.M., Macdonald, I.A., Matthews, D.R. and Frayn, K.N. (1996a) Effects of morning rise in cortisol concentration on regulation of lipolysis in subcutaneous adipose tissue. *American Journal of Physiology* **271**, E996–E1002.

Samra, J.S., Simpson, E.J., Clark, M.L., Forster, C.D., Humphreys, S.M., Macdonald, I.A. and Frayn, K.N. (1996b) Effects of epinephrine infusion on adipose tissue: interactions between blood flow and lipid metabolism. *American Journal of Physiology* **271**, E834–E839.

Samra, J.S., Clark, M.L., Humphreys, S.M., Macdonald, I.A., Bannister, P.A., Matthews, D.R. and Frayn, K.N. (1999) Suppression of the nocturnal rise in growth hormone reduces subsequent lipolysis in subcutaneous adipose tissue. *European Journal of Clinical Investigation* **29**, 1045–1052.

Savage, D.B., Sewter, C.P., Klenk, E.S., Segal, D.G., Vidal-Puig, A., Considine, R.V. and O'Rahilly, S. (2001) Resistin Fizz3 expression in relation to obesity and peroxisome proliferator-activated receptor-gamma action in humans. *Diabetes* **50**, 2199–2202.

Scantlebury, T., Maslowska, M. and Cianflone, K. (1998) Chylomicron-specific enhancement of acylation stimulating protein and precursor protein C3 production in differentiated human adipocytes. *Journal of Biological Chemistry* **273**, 20903–20909.

Schalin Jantti, C., Harkonen, M. and Groop, L. C. (1992) Impaired activation of glycogen synthase in people at increased risk for developing NIDDM. *Diabetes* **41**, 598–604.

Schrauwen, P., Wagenmakers, A.J., van Marken Lichtenbelt, W.D., Saris, W.H. and Westerterp, K.R. (2000) Increase in fat oxidation on a high-fat diet is accompanied by an increase in triglyceride-derived fatty acid oxidation. *Diabetes* **49**, 640–646.

Schrauwen, P., Saris, W.H. and Hesselink, M.K. (2001) An alternative function for human uncoupling protein 3: protection of mitochondria against accumulation of nonesterified fatty acids inside the mitochondrial matrix. *FASEB Journal* **15**, 2497–2502.

Seip, R.L., Angelopoulos, T.J. and Semenkovich, C.F. (1995) Exercise induces human lipoprotein lipase gene expression in skeletal muscle but not adipose tissue. *American Journal of Physiology* **268**, E229–E236.

Sidossis, L.S. and Wolfe, R.R. (1996) Glucose and insulin-induced inhibition of fatty acid oxidation: the glucose-fatty acid cycle reversed. *American Journal of Physiology* **270**, E733–E738.

Sidossis, L.S., Coggan, A.R., Gastaldelli, A. and Wolfe, R.R. (1995a) A new correction factor for use in tracer estimations of plasma fatty acid oxidation. *American Journal of Physiology* **269**, E649–E656.

Sidossis, L.S., Coggan, A.R., Gastaldelli, A. and Wolfe, R.R. (1995b) Pathway of free fatty acid oxidation in human subjects. Implications for tracer studies. *Journal of Clinical Investigation* **95**, 278–284.

Sidossis, L.S., Stuart, C.A., Shulman, G.I., Lopaschuk, G.D. and Wolfe, R.R. (1996) Glucose plus insulin regulate fat oxidation by controlling the rate of fatty acid entry into the mitochondria. *Journal of Clinical Investigation* **98**, 2244–2250.

Simoneau, J.A., Colberg, S.R., Thaete, F.L. and Kelley, D.E. (1995) Skeletal muscle glycolytic and oxidative enzyme capacities are determinants of insulin sensitivity and muscle composition in obese women. *FASEB Journal* **9**, 273–278.

Simoneau, J.A., Veerkamp, J.H., Turcotte, L.P. and Kelley, D.E. (1999) Markers of capacity to utilize fatty acids in human skeletal muscle: relation to insulin resistance and obesity and effects of weight loss. *FASEB Journal* **13**, 2051–2060.

Sniderman, A.D., Cianflone, K., Summers, L.K.M., Fielding, B.A. and Frayn, K. N. (1997) The acylation-stimulating protein pathway and regulation of postprandial metabolism. *Proceedings of the Nutrition Society* **56**, 703–712.

Sniderman, A.D., Cianflone, K., Arner, P., Summers, L.K.M. and Frayn, K.N. (1998) The adipocyte, fatty acid trapping and atherogenesis. *Arteriosclerosis Thrombosis and Vascular Biology* **18**, 147–151.

Snyder, W.S. (1975) *Report of the Task Force on Reference Man*. Oxford: Pergamon Press for the International Commission on Radiological Protection.

Soop, M., Björkman, O., Cederblad, G., Hagenfeldt, L. and Wahren, J. (1988) Influence of carnitine supplementation on muscle substrate and carnitine metabolism during exercise. *Journal of Applied Physiology* **64**, 2394–2399.

Spenst, L.F., Martin, A.D. and Drinkwater, D.T. (1993) Muscle mass of competitive male athletes. *Journal of Sports Science* **11**, 3–8.

Steppan, C.M., Bailey, S.T., Bhat, S., Brown, E.J., Banerjee, R.R., Wright, C.M., Patel, H.R., Rexford, S.A. and Lazar, M.A. (2001) The hormone resistin links obesity to diabetes. *Nature* **409**, 307–312.

Summers, L.K.M., Samra, J.S., Humphreys, S.M., Morris, R.J. and Frayn, K.N. (1996) Subcutaneous abdominal adipose tissue blood flow: variation within and between subjects and relationship to obesity. *Clinical Science* **91**, 679–683.

Summers, L.K.M., Fielding, B.A., Herd, S.L., Ilic, V., Clark, M.L., Quinlan, P.T. and Frayn, K.N. (1999) Use of structured triacylglycerols containing predominantly stearic and oleic acids to probe early events in metabolic processing of dietary fat. *Journal of Lipid Research* **40**, 1890–1898.

Swinburn, B.A., Nyomba, B.L., Saad, M.F., Zurlo, F., Raz, I., Knowler, W.C., Lillioja, S., Bogardus, C. and Ravussin, E. (1991) Insulin resistance associated with lower rates of weight gain in Pima Indians. *Journal of Clinical Investigation* **88**, 168–173.

Taylor, R., Price, T.B., Katz, L.D., Shulman, R.G. and Shulman, G.I. (1993) Direct measurement of change in muscle glycogen concentration after a mixed meal in normal subjects. *American Journal of Physiology* **265**, E224–E229.

Teusink, B., Voshol, P.J., Dahlmans, V.E., Rensen, P.C., Pijl, H., Romijn, J.A. and Havekes, L.M. (2003) Contribution of fatty acids released from lipolysis of plasma triglycerides to total plasma fatty acid flux and tissue-specific fatty acid uptake. *Diabetes* **52**, 614–620.

The DCCT Research Group (1988) Weight gain associated with intensive therapy in the diabetes control and complications trial. *Diabetes Care* **11**, 567–573.

Toubro, S., Western, P., Bülow, J., Macdonald, I., Raben, A., Christensen, N.J., Madsen, J. and Astrup, A. (1994) Insulin sensitivity in post-obese women. *Clinical Science* **87**, 407–413.

Tsetsonis, N.V., Hardman, A.E. and Mastana, S.S. (1997) Acute effects of exercise on postprandial lipemia: a comparative study in trained and untrained middle-aged women. *American Journal of Clinical Nutrition* **65**, 525–533.

Vidal-Puig, A.J., Grujic, D., Zhang, C.Y., Hagen, T., Boss, O., Ido, Y., Szczepanik, A., Wade, J., Mootha, V., Cortright, R., Muoio, D.M. and Lowell, B.B. (2000) Energy metabolism in uncoupling protein 3 gene knockout mice. *Journal of Biological Chemistry* **275**, 16258–16266.

Virtanen, K.A., Peltoniemi, P., Marjamäki, P., Asola, M., Strindberg, L., Parkkola, R., Huupponen, R., Knuuti, J., Lönnroth, P. and Nuutila, P. (2001) Human adipose tissue glucose uptake determined using [^{18}F]-fluoro-deoxy-glucose ([^{18}F]FDG) and PET in combination with microdialysis. *Diabetologia* **44**, 2171–2179.

Virtanen, K.A., Lönnroth, P., Parkkola, R., Peltoniemi, P., Asola, M., Viljanen, T., Tolvanen, T., Knuuti, J., Rönnemaa, T., Huupponen, R. and Nuutila, P. (2002) Glucose uptake and perfusion in subcutaneous and visceral adipose tissue during insulin stimulation in nonobese and obese humans. *Journal of Clinical Endocrinology and Metabolism* **87**, 3902–3910.

Wang, S.P., Laurin, N., Himms-Hagen, J., Rudnicki, M.A., Levy, E., Robert, M.-F., Pan, L., Oligny, L. and Mitchell, G.A. (2001) The adipose tissue phenotype of hormone-sensitive lipase deficiency in mice. *Obesity Research* **9**, 119–128.

Watt, M.J., Heigenhauser, G.J. and Spriet, L.L. (2002) Intramuscular triacylglycerol utilization in human skeletal muscle during exercise: is there a controversy? *Journal of Applied Physiology* **93**, 1185–1195.

Way, J.M., Görgün, C.Z., Tong, Q., Uysal, K.T., Brown, K.K., Harrington, W.W., Oliver, Jr, W.R., Willson, T.M., Kliewer, S.A. and Hotamisligil, G.S. (2001) Adipose tissue resistin expression is severely suppressed in obesity and stimulated by peroxisome proliferator-activated receptor γ agonists. *Journal of Biological Chemistry* **276**, 25651–25653.

Weinstock, P.H., Levak Frank, S., Hudgins, L.C., Radner, H., Friedman, J.M., Zechner, R. and Breslow, J. L. (1997) Lipoprotein lipase controls fatty acid entry into adipose tissue, but fat mass is preserved by endogenous synthesis in mice deficient in adipose tissue lipoprotein lipase. *Proceedings of the National Academy of Sciences of the USA* **94**, 10261–10266.

Wells, A.M., Sutcliffe, I.C., Johnson, A.B. and Taylor, R. (1993) Abnormal activation of glycogen synthesis in fibroblasts from NIDDM subjects. Evidence for an abnormality specific to glucose metabolism. *Diabetes* **42**, 583–589.

Weyer, C., Funahashi, T., Tanaka, S., Hotta, K., Matsuzawa, Y., Pratley, R.E. and Tataranni, P.A. (2001) Hypoadiponectinemia in obesity and type 2 diabetes: close association with insulin resistance and hyperinsulinemia. *Journal of Clinical Endocrinology and Metabolism* **86**, 1930–1935.

Winder, W.W. and Hardie, D.G. (1996) Inactivation of acetyl-CoA carboxylase and activation of AMP-activated protein kinase in muscle during exercise. *American Journal of Physiology* **270**, E299–E304.

Yamauchi, T., Kamon, J., Waki, H., Terauchi, Y., Kubota, N., Hara, K., Mori, Y., Ide, T., Murakami, K., Tsuboyama-Kasaoka, N., Ezaki, O., Akanuma, Y., Gavrilova, O., Vinson, C., Reitman, M.L., Kagechika, H., Shudo, K., Yoda, M., Nakano, Y., Tobe, K., Nagai, R., Kimura, S., Tomita, M., Froguel, P. and Kadowaki, T. (2001) The fat-derived hormone adiponectin reverses insulin resistance associated with both lipoatrophy and obesity. *Nature Medicine* **7**, 941–946.

Yki-Järvinen, H., Young, A.A., Lamkin, C. and Foley, J.E. (1987) Kinetics of glucose disposal in whole body and across the forearm in man. *Journal of Clinical Investigation* **79**, 1713–1719.

Zammit, V.A. (1999) The malonyl-CoA-long-chain acyl-CoA axis in the maintenance of mammalian cell function. *Biochemical Journal* **343**, 505–515.

Zurlo, F., Larson, K., Bogardus, C. and Ravussin, E. (1990a) Skeletal muscle metabolism is a major determinant of resting energy expenditure. *Journal of Clinical Investigation* **86**, 1423–1427.

Zurlo, F., Lillioja, S., Esposito-Del Puente, A., Nyomba, B.L., Raz, I., Saad, M.F., Swinburn, B.A., Knowler, W.C., Bogardus, C. and Ravussin, E. (1990b) Low ratio of fat to carbohydrate oxidation as predictor of weight gain: study of 24-h RQ. *American Journal of Physiology* **259**, E650–E657.

Energy and macronutrient needs in relation to substrate handling in obesity

W. Philip T. James

Introduction, 123

An evolutionary perspective: the importance of animal protein and essential fatty acids, 123
  Biological evolution in terms of dietary availability, 124
  Fat intakes, 124
  The transformation in food supply and its effects on macronutrient intake, 124
  Sugars, 125
  Fructosans and corn syrups, 125

Energy density and food intake, 125
  The effective normal control of food intake in relation to dietary macronutrients, 126

Dietary factors overwhelming the normal control of food intake, 127

Energy requirements and how to assess them in normal and obese subjects, 128
  Monitor food patterns not energy intake, 128
  Predicting or measuring energy needs as a true index of normal food intakes, 128
  Are obese subjects more metabolically efficient?, 129
  Gender-based differences in metabolic efficiency, 130

Optimum macronutrient intakes, 130

The adjustments in food-intake control with weight gain: implications for weight loss diets, 131
  Prescribing a weight loss diet, 131
  Fats and fatty acids in relation to weight loss regimens, 132
  Carbohydrates, glycaemic index and fructosans, 133
  Protein intakes, 133
  Alcohol, 133
  Salt implications in relation to obesity, 133

Conclusions, 134

References, 134

Introduction

The role of dietary composition in modifying the risk of excess weight gain has become a subject of intense interest since the issue of obesity gained prominence as a new public health problem (WHO, 2000). The major policy implications affect industrial interests and therefore have political implications. The problem of excess weight gain is also of considerable clinical significance. Few doctors know how to handle the distinctions between the nutritional and dietary factors which contribute to managing weight loss and those dietary principles which contribute to the primary prevention of weight gain, or of regain in those patients who have lost weight. Additionally, there is also often confusion about the role of different macronutrients, i.e. fat, carbohydrate, protein and alcohol, and how to cope with new propositions suggesting that particular aspects of dietary composition, affecting either the structure or detailed composition of the macronutrient, influence metabolism or weight management. This chapter provides an overview of these issues, how to assess the energy needs of obese patients and whether obese patients have a particular propensity to metabolize nutrients differently, thereby limit-ing their ability to lose weight and their tendency to weight regain. First, however, it may be helpful to understand why people are eating as they do and how this dietary pattern is different from the foods available during the evolutionary pressures on humans.

An evolutionary perspective: the importance of animal protein and essential fatty acids

There has been some debate about how dietary factors have affected the evolutionary development of human energy needs, and what these imply in terms of the types of food which, ideally, we should eat. Particular interest has been taken in the idea that, as *Homo sapiens* evolved in Africa, early humans moved from a vegetarian existence, seen in other primates, to an omnivorous lifestyle characterized by the need for the hunting of animals as well as the gathering of fruits and roots from the jungle. The food habits of early man have been claimed to be particularly rich in animal protein with a plentiful supply of fruit, leaves and root vegetables (Eaton *et al.*, 1988). Crawford and Marsh (1989) have highlighted the step change in the increased brain size of man compared with other non-human primates and suggested that this induces an intrinsically greater need for the *n*-3 essential fatty acids (EFAs) for brain myelination and development than in other primates and animals (except the dolphin!). The supply of these *n*-3 EFAs was assured by the availability of fish from rivers, thereby directly providing the essential long chain *n*-3 EFAs as well as the appreciable amounts of the precursor *n*-3 fatty acid, linolenic acid. Linolenic acid was in addition found in tree nuts and in the membranes of lean animals, which were also consuming a wider range of linolenic acid-containing plants than those eaten by man.

Crawford emphasized the importance of rivers and the sea coast not only in allowing the ready transport in primitive boats of humans out of Africa, but also in providing a ready source of fish protein enriched with these essential fatty acids. The fish and other meats also provided rich sources of minerals such as zinc and iron needed to ensure effective growth, immunity and haematopoiesis in areas where malaria was rampant. Thus, the movement of tribes down the Nile delta into the Mediterranean and through the Arabian Sea led to the development of the first outstanding civilization between the Tigris and Euphrates (in present-day Iraq), where the family groups benefited from nutrient-rich river deltas ideal for fish and the development of semi-permanent hamlets.

Then, 10 000 years ago, came the discovery of the ability to keep cereal seeds in a dried form for eventual consumption and for planting prior to the next season. This led to the first formal agriculture. Towns and cities were viable because it was now possible to store good sources of energy from cereals on cleared land that could then be intensively cultivated. The body was used to handling the carbohydrates found in fruits and roots but what are traditionally called complex carbohydrate sources of cereal origin were, in evolutionary terms, new major food sources. There seems to have been, over the very few millennia since then, little opportunity for evolutionary pressures on humans to alter markedly their normal processing of nutrients. Famines and long periods of semistarvation have probably been of importance in selecting metabolically efficient humans, preferably of small size, as emphasized by Neel's development of the thrifty genotype hypothesis (Neel *et al.*, 1998) and Prentice's highlighting of the numerous famines over the last 10 000 years (Prentice, 2001). Certainly humans as well as animals have highly effective and duplicated neurohormonal mechanisms that trigger greater food intakes and behavioural responses to food deprivation, but only modest systems for shutting off excess consumption (see later).

Biological evolution in terms of dietary availability

The traditional mammalian and early human diets were very low in fat, with intakes probably of the order of 10% of total energy and most of the dietary fatty acids in unsaturated forms derived from plants, fish and the membranes of other animals. Similarly, sugar intakes were very modest and derived mainly from ripe fruit. Perhaps in keeping with this evolutionary history, humans have specialized taste receptors for sweet, salt and the umami taste which is derived from glutamine and other amino acids found in animal proteins. There is also a great appreciation of the mouth feel and olfactory properties of different fats. Thus, these primeval drives relate to rare and essential dietary features with sugars/sweetness being a surrogate for the drive for energy.

Fat intakes

The traditional Mediterranean, Chinese and Japanese diets consumed until about 50 years ago contained very modest amounts of fat (15–25% energy), although extremely active Cretan shepherds, studied as part of the famous Keys' Seven Country Study (Keys, 1980), had higher intakes from olive oil than was normal in the Mediterranean area at that time (Ferro-Luzzi *et al.*, 2002). Dietary fat has traditionally been seen as a rare commodity that amplifies the quality of the diet because it usually contains volatile fatty acids, and other odours, which are readily sensed by the 300 or more human olfactory receptors and perceived as extremely attractive. In addition, humans (as well as animals) enjoy the 'mouth feel' and melting qualities of fats. This feature is poorly understood and does not seem to relate to specific taste or olfactory receptors, but it is increasingly being studied, for example, by chocolate manufacturers!

The transformation in food supply and its effects on macronutrient intake

Butter was a traditionally expensive food, available only to the rich. With the French invention of margarine in the nineteenth century, with its better keeping qualities, it became possible to obtain cheaper fat. Then, in the twentieth century—particularly after the Second World War—there was a universal governmental initiative, with huge subsidies of agricultural research, buildings and equipment, as well as direct payments for crop and animal production. This led to a remarkable increase in animal protein and crop production and substantial increases in the availability of butter and vegetable oils. These prized commodities could then be eaten even by the poor. Detailed UK and US studies showed the relationship between stunted sick children and their prevailing appalling diets and poverty (Boyd Orr, 1936). Stunting could be remedied if the diet had more animal protein—stunted children then grew. This led to a strategic focus on intensive agricultural production. Thus, as countries became more affluent and went through the so-called 'nutrition transition', there was a marked increase in sugars, fats, oils and animal protein. This 'cheap food' policy allowed even the poor to eat plenty of meat, butter/fats and sugar and thereby obtain the animal protein conducive to their children's growth, as well as plenty of energy from fats and sugars to maintain physical workload.

Unfortunately, this food policy was associated with a huge epidemic of coronary heart disease in the 1940–60s, affecting first the more affluent and agriculturally most innovative countries. Cardiovascular disease and especially coronary heart disease have become the biggest causes of death and disability in the world, and particularly now in developing countries (WHO, 2002). Western countries responded from the 1970s by removing the overt fat from carcasses and manipulating the fatty acid composition of vegetable oils to first lower the saturated and later the trans fatty acid content. However, they maintained the production of less metabolically adverse fats to fill cheap but desirable foods, e.g. fried and baked products. These are sold in huge amounts on the basis of 'consumer choice', with incomprehensible, although compositionally accurate, food labels. Heart disease rates fell as the saturated fatty acid intakes came down (Stephen and Wald, 1990), but obesity and diabetes rates escalated as total fat and sugar intakes went up further (see later). Soon the industrial production of excess beef, fat and oils exceeded the food needs of affluent societies and so were dumped, with huge US, EU and Japanese farming and export subsidies, on the developing world where now coronary heart disease deaths and disability numbers exceed those of the developed world (Ezzati *et al.*, 2002) and obesity rates are escalating (Popkin, 2001).

Sugars

The traditional Mediterranean, Chinese and Japanese diets contained negligible amounts of free sugar, the only sugar coming from the modest amounts in ripened fruits and vegetables. These staple foods of early man were important sources of energy, so perhaps it is not surprising that not only are there specific taste receptors for sweetness, but also that the thresholds for discriminating sweetness fall and the pleasurable appreciation of sweet tastes increases when the body is deprived of energy and sweet sensations. This pleasurable sensation arises from the linking of the primary afferent input from the taste-related neurons to the limbic system, which responds to the development of pleasant tastes. Dried fruits were therefore sought-after commodities; later it was found that sugar cane could be crushed and processed to extract crystallized sugar. In the second half of the twentieth century, sugar beet growing was encouraged in temperate climates, which resulted in a vast multibillion dollar trade in sugar being produced in excess, and marketed as one of the cheapest, as well as universally desirable, commodities. Sugared drinks, including teas, and confectionery have been prized for centuries and the remarkable expansion of the soft drink industry globally is another indication of a manufacturing response to biological drives and commercial opportunities.

Fructosans and corn syrups

The industrial intensification of cereal production became so effective that production exceeded even the huge demand for cattle-lot feeding. It was then discovered that corn could be treated industrially with fermenting enzymes to produce food-quality syrups, rich in fructose and mixtures of varying molecular weight saccharides. These could then be sold in bulk for use in soft drinks and foods instead of using the products for industrial alcohol production or other less profitable enterprises. Thus, corn syrup and fructosan use has escalated remarkably and has been linked observationally to the development of obesity in the US by Bray and others (Bray *et al.*, 2004, in press). Elliott *et al.* (2002) now propose that the marked increase in fructose, as distinct from glucose, intake is particularly conducive to the development of obesity and its comorbidities for a variety of metabolic reasons (see below).

The combination of fats and sweets is an even more powerful and pleasurable stimulant, as Drewnowski (1998) has emphasized. It is little wonder that food manufacturers, responding to taste panels and sales returns, have focused, particularly in the last 20 years, on providing this evolutionarily rare but highly prized sensory mix as a routine in an increasingly varied number of foods made for convenient consumption. They have then gone further and recognized that more can be consumed if, for example, cereal-based products are refined to remove their bulk by disrupting the cellular structure of the cereals and therefore limiting the water bulking nature of the grain. These 'fast food' products are easily consumed but, from a weight management point of view, they are very energy dense, i.e. high in kilocalories per gram of product.

Energy density and food intake

Clearly, fat with its intrinsic energy value of 9 kcal/g is more energy dense than sugars (4 kcal/g), so if both are contained within foods with little bulking water, they can readily be consumed, stimulate pleasurable sensations and yet provide substantial amounts of energy. Prentice and Jebb (2003) have recently provided an excellent summary of the huge variation in the energy density of present-day Western foods and compared them with traditional unrefined cereal-based African (Gambian) foods. Figure 9.1 shows that fats dominate the development of high energy density foods but some high-quality 'Western' products can be produced with similar energy densities to the Gambian foods.

Energy density has an important impact on daily food intake: if volunteers are offered a variety of foods that have had either their fat or their sugar content manipulated then the normal response of adults is to eat the same volume of food as usual, i.e. there is no immediate adaptation in intake to reduce overall consumption when the fat or the sugar content is surreptitiously raised (Stubbs *et al.*, 2001). This means that

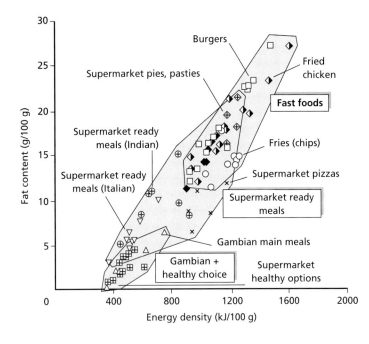

Fig 9.1 Relationship between energy density and fat percentage of energy of different foods. (Reproduced from Prentice, A.M. and Jebb, S.A., 2003, with permission.)

normal adults who are provided (unwittingly) with an array of high-fat foods, providing 60% rather than 20% energy as fat, automatically continue to eat the same volume of food for several days and can accumulate 2 extra days' energy intake, for example 5000 kcal, within 1 week without consciously or subconsciously responding to the higher energy density of the meals. Figure 9.2 provides an integrated graph of studies (Prentice and Jebb, 2003) on the responses during the first 2 weeks to changes in the energy density of the diet and indicates this in terms of the proposed limits for low, medium and high energy density foods suggested by Cameron-Smith and Egger (2003). Clearly, the types of foods that are being consumed at present by many Western populations (see Fig. 9.1) are highly conducive to weight gain, particularly if the individuals are inactive.

The effective normal control of food intake in relation to dietary macronutrients

Animal studies have shown that body weight is remarkably well regulated when animals live under their normal environmental conditions. In rodents, and perhaps in man, there are separate systems for physiologically altering the choice of foods so that animals seek and eat an appropriate combination of foods to meet their needs for both protein and energy. Animal experiments show that the quality of the protein affects intake and that essential amino acids, and an appropriate balance of amino acids in relation to the growing needs of the animal, govern the amount of protein consumed. Protein-rich foods readily lead to satiety and rodents are particularly likely to then search for sugar-rich carbohydrates to meet their energy needs. These two systems are traditionally associated with different neurophysiological mechanisms.

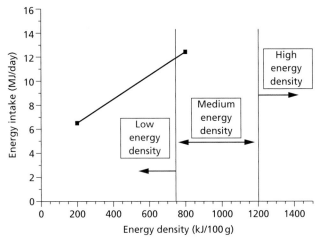

Fig 9.2 The overall medium-term effect of covertly increasing energy density on total energy intake when assessed from different intervention trials. (Adapted from Prentice, A.M. and Jebb, S.A., 2003, with permission.) The limits to low, moderate and high energy density are those proposed by Cameron-Smith and Egger (2003).

Some of these findings seem to apply to humans and, under normal environmental conditions, total energy intake is exceptionally well controlled. Fomon and colleagues (1969) showed that when babies have their milks diluted they will rapidly adjust the volume of milk consumed to maintain their energy intake. Normal adults also respond to intakes, for example a soft drink 30–60 min before a normal meal, but may not compensate fully, particularly if the pre-meal snack or drink contains fat (Cotton *et al.*, 1996). The energy content of the early part of a meal, e.g. a soup, is also unconsciously sensed so that either immediately or over a 3–4 day period people spontaneously alter their intake of the main course to compensate for the physiologically perceived energy content of the early part of that meal. The quick responders alter their main course intake rapidly, whereas the slow responders take up to 4 days to adjust (Booth *et al.*, 1976).

Visual and other taste and olfactory cues are also triggered so that unconsciously a highly coloured or flavoured item on the table, presented with a high-energy soup, automatically leads subsequently to a reduced intake of the main course. Then, if that day's soup is changed to a lower energy content, the visual and/or olfactory cues confuse the short-term regulation of intake and it takes the slow responders a further 3–4 days to readjust, provided that there is a consistent conjunction of the soup's energy content and the colour/taste of say a yoghurt pot on the table (Booth *et al.*, 1976)!

This physiological control of behavioural responses explains why so many clinical studies lead to confusing results without very careful control of the circumstances of testing. Readers may also be familiar with the sudden marked satiety that develops after a weekend of exceptionally large meals. Indeed, the control of energy intake is so effective with rapid, medium- and longer term adjustments that in almost all people energy intake is controlled on a month-by-month basis to within about 1% of body needs. A consistent 2% error will lead within a year to about a 5-kg gain or loss in weight, whereas even in our modern conditions—so conducive to weight gain—the average weight increase of the average man or woman amounts to 0.5–1.0 kg per year—an error of less than 1.5% of energy turnover.

The control of food intake in young women is more complex because they have a menstrual cycle-linked fall in energy intake in the pre-ovulatory stage of the cycle—and a smaller hormonally controlled fall in basal metabolic rate (BMR)—followed by a post-ovulatory rise in intake and BMR. Thus, there is a negative energy balance before ovulation and a positive balance post ovulation in premenopausal women not taking an oral contraceptive (Bisdee *et al.*, 1989). On a month-by-month basis, they remain in balance unless general circumstances lead to their eating more than their energy needs. If women then become pregnant, their post-ovulatory positive energy balance persists so that they accumulate energy, this positive balance being accentuated in most societies by the marked fall in physical activity in the third trimester when the women's BMR related to fetal and uterine metabolism rises. Only when women have to continue their physical activity in late pregnancy does their physiologically controlled intake go up (Durnin, 1987). Yet once breast-feeding starts, the mothers immediately become very hungry as they cope with the extra 750 kcal per day energy demand for breast milk production; some of this energy comes from stored fat.

Traditionally, women on low-fat diets, i.e. 15–20% fat, with little or no added sugars do not gain weight during adult life, as seen in Japanese or Chinese societies. After the menopause, when their menstrual cycling of intake and BMR wanes and then eases, weight gain may occur (Yoshiike *et al.*, 2002). In so-

cieties in which the breast-feeding rate is low, post-pregnancy weight gain is more common, in part because of the failure to reduce the extra body fat physiologically produced in anticipation of breast-feeding.

Genetic factors also influence intake, BMR and exercise patterns (Bouchard *et al.*, 1997), but compensatory intake mechanisms seem better in the young, as shown by the subsequent restitution of body weight in young compared with older overfed adults who had gained weight (Roberts *et al.*, 1995). The control of intake is also normally downregulated with increasing age. The last few decades of progressive mechanization and computerization of the home, transport and work have led to most people in affluent societies becoming sedentary. The secular and age-related fall in food intake of the young active man to the same individual 45 years later has been shown to amount to about 270 kcal per day for each decade of declining activity, with little or no change in the metabolic efficiency of the declining lean body mass (James *et al.*, 1989).

Dietary factors overwhelming the normal control of food intake

Despite this regulatory ability of humans to control their weight, three factors, already highlighted, seem able to bypass or overwhelm the normal control of food intake and thereby induce weight gain: (a) an increase in dietary fat that seems to have less satiety-inducing properties (Astrup, 2001; Bray *et al.*, 2004); (b) raised sugar intakes, particularly if given between meals in drinks (De Castro, 1993; Raben *et al.*, 2002); and (c) a sedentary state.

Inactivity automatically demands that our physiological downregulation of intake is effective even when confronted with societal pressures to take part in social events where meals, often of high density, but of unknown composition, are served. When these, and other foods, are available with visually attractive variety and highly desirable sweet/fat options of high energy density then the habitual amount of food, based on physiological behavioural programming, breaks down.

Cotton *et al.* (1996) showed that an evening meal that is rich in fat is particularly conducive to inducing a positive energy imbalance because the opportunity for short-term physiological compensation by going to sleep overnight and then having a standard breakfast (if consumed at all) is lost. The same calories, however, taken as a large breakfast can lead to physiological adjustments in intake at lunch time and during the rest of the day. Furthermore, substantial amounts of fat or sugars in a single meal—for example, at a weekend—will not entrain a consistent subsequent fall in appetite because the input is episodic. Therefore, having the main meal of the day in the evening and episodic feasting, particularly with high-fat/sugar meals, may circumvent our normal energy balance controlling mechanisms.

The difference in the effective control of intake with age is also seen when people are presented with large portion sizes. Orlet Fisher *et al.* (2003) have shown that babies and very young children do not respond to the presentation of an abnormally large portion of food or drink, whereas older children and adults spontaneously consume more when given larger portions. These greater portion sizes are presented by food marketers as a desirable and economically attractive option so that psychological and social factors, together with marketing pressures, can confuse, and indeed overwhelm, the normal physiological regulation of food intake.

Energy requirements and how to assess them in normal and obese subjects

Monitor food patterns not energy intake

Doctors and dietitians have traditionally assumed that all they have to do to assess energy needs is to ask the individual or patient to recall or write down what he or she has had to eat either the previous day (the 24-h recall method) or over the last week, month or year (dietary history methods). Alternatively, patients can be asked to write down details as they eat their meals and snack, and provide some indication of the quantities eaten over a week or two. The health professional can even go further and specify that they weigh everything to obtain really accurate records. This is time-consuming and difficult if meals are taken out because recipes are unavailable for checking the hidden fat and sugar intakes.

Unfortunately, all of these methods may give extremely inaccurate results, particularly in obese people—the more overweight the subject the greater their underestimation of actual routine energy consumption. The 24-h recall technique, even in good hands, produces on average a 20% underestimate, and dietary histories have to be taken very carefully, for example with food models and urinary checks to assess whether the urinary nitrogen output is consistent with the supposed dietary protein intake (Kipnis *et al.*, 2002). Even the 'gold standard' method of weighing everything unfortunately leads some individuals—particularly weight-conscious women and overweight subjects—to unconsciously reduce their intake as shown by their weight loss during the measurement period. These biases led nutritionists and doctors to believe that obese patients were really existing on 800 kcal per day and yet failing to lose weight when in practice they were consciously or unconsciously failing to register what they were really eating. The fundamental point is that weight loss always occurs (in the absence of occasional water accumulation) when energy intake falls below energy needs.

Food diaries are still, however, exceptionally valuable if doctors can train themselves to be non-judgemental and supportive. This way, patients asked to record both a food diary and the amount of activity they undertake for a week or a month but, who fail to lose weight, will often come to realize their inappropriate patterns of eating. They may have considered these to reflect unusual celebrations when in practice the diary shows them to be routine. They may also be surprised to realize how sedentary they are.

Predicting or measuring energy needs as a true index of normal food intakes

These concepts of inaccurate food records led to the development of a new approach that relies on predicting total food needs. Figure 9.3 shows that a substantial proportion of food needs reflects the demands of the BMR. The BMR is highly reproducible (1–2% variation at most) if measured with great care, and prediction equations based on BMR measurements on over 11 000 adults globally were developed (Schofield *et al.*, 1985), which take account of women's lower BMR for their weight. Women have more fat and less metabolically active lean tissue, otherwise known as fat-free mass (FFM), so their BMR and total energy needs are about 80% of that of men of the same age and weight. The BMR equations also reflect the fall in FFM with age—the FFM itself does not decline in its metabolic rate with age. Figure 9.3 shows how much the energy needs decline with age and how food intake control seems to be permanently reset at a higher level in post-obese people, despite what would have been expected for their weight-related lower energy requirements.

To this BMR can be added about 10% of the total energy intake which, on average, is the cost of digesting, absorbing, storing, processing and oxidizing the energy consumed. This has been called diet-induced thermogenesis (DIT) because it is an inevitable use of dietary energy just to remain in energy balance. Protein intake leads to about 10–20% of its energy being used in its assimilation, whereas the cost of storing fat is very small—about 3–5%. Glucose storage as glycogen costs 5% of the glucose energy consumed but much more is used if synthesized into fat. This fat synthesis is, however, unusual in humans on modest fat intakes because any extra energy is readily stored from the dietary fat component with the dietary carbohydrate being oxidized preferentially to fuel metabolic processes. Thus, overfeeding with fat leads to very small increases in thermogenesis (Dallosso and James, 1984), whereas carbohydrate overfeeding induces a greater metabolic response but with the associated dietary fat then being preferentially stored (Bisdee and James, 1985).

Once the BMR is measured or estimated then it is possible to predict the total amount of energy being used, depending on whether people are engaged in light, moderate or heavy physical activity. To simplify the concepts, the DIT costs are incorporated into the costs of physical activity and express the total energy output as a physical activity level (PAL) that is the ratio of total energy expenditure to the BMR. This concept is now almost universally used because it takes account of the fact that moving around costs more in heavier people. The average PALs can then be estimated for men and women and their total

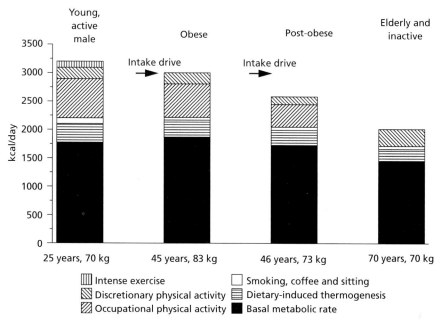

Fig 9.3 The sequence of falling energy needs, weight gain and slimming effects in adult men. Note: The fall in energy needs in young adulthood reflects abandoning sport, having a more sedentary job and giving up smoking (which in addition to boosting the metabolic rate, suppresses appetite). Weight gain induces the buffering rise in BMR. After slimming, the BMR and the cost of everyday activity fall, but habit and probable neurophysiological adaptation keep the drive to eat more than needed for the reduced energy requirements. The widely used physical activity levels (PALs) are multiples of the BMR to give total energy expenditure; light activity PALs for both men and women are 1.4–1.69, moderate activity 1.7–1.99 and heavy activity 2.0–2.4. Activity > 2.4 is very unusual and hard to sustain. The BMRs can be estimated as shown in Table 9.2, based on the original Schofield *et al.* (1985) equations, with more robust data provided to the UK Coma Committee for those > 60 years. BMR in MJ per day can be converted to kcal per day by dividing the kilojoules by 4.182 (1000 kJ = 1 MJ).

energy requirements displayed (Fig. 9.3). All of these values are specified and take account of the subject's age, sex and size. Note that in general the literature shows that women are less physically active than men, so the PAL ranges are crude estimates of the energy needs of men and women of all ages and weights, but of different physical activity levels. The heavy physical activity values are, however, rarely of relevance because this level of exertion is so unusual in most industrialized societies. Multiple studies with doubly labelled D_2 ^{18}O water, the new reference method for the accurate but extremely expensive monitoring of total energy expenditure, have shown that these PAL and BMR estimates are far more accurate than those based on food diaries or history-taking to assess food habits (see Chapter 2).

Are obese subjects more metabolically efficient?

We showed many years ago that the DIT (Shetty *et al.*, 1981) and the metabolic response to the sympathetic nervous system's metabolic drive (Jung *et al.*, 1979) seemed less in both obese and, more importantly, post-obese subjects (i.e. formerly obese individuals) who are now of normal weight and have a family history of obesity. The differences were small and had to be measured with meticulous care. Children of overweight parents were also observed to be both lower in their resting metabolism and less spontaneously active (Griffiths and

Payne, 1976) and members of obese Pima Indian families had a family-associated lower resting metabolic rate and were more prone to subsequent weight gain (Ravussin *et al.*, 1988). Furthermore, Bouchard, in his classic, highly controlled twin overfeeding studies (Bouchard *et al.*, 1990), showed that twin pairs differed greatly in their weight gain but the differences between monozygotic twins were very small.

Given the recognized multiple genetic contributions to the susceptibility of different individuals to weight gain, the issue is whether there are differences in the handling of carbohydrates, fats and protein, which might explain these different susceptibilities as highlighted by Bouchard. There is some evidence that the formerly obese individuals have a lower oxidation rate of fats and therefore oxidize more glucose (Lean and James, 1988) when studied with meticulous care in whole-body calorimeters. These results could have reflected possible longstanding physiological adaptations to the prescribed lower fat intakes for post-obese subjects and not to genetic differences. Many other studies of BMR or DIT have, in practice, failed to pick up differences, but the authors then conclude, incorrectly, that the individual metabolic differences do not exist or are unimportant (James *et al.*, 1987a).

Many years ago, Dugdale and Payne (1971) proposed that if an individual stored more of their energy during the day as protein rather than glycogen or fat then they would automatically be using more dietary energy to synthesize proteins. If they also gained more FFM than fat during weight gain then they would have a greater BMR as well as an enhanced DIT, thereby limiting the further long-term accumulation of energy. Reanalysis (Dulloo *et al.*, 1996) of both the differential weight and FFM losses and regain in the classic Minnesota semistarvation studies (Keys *et al.*, 1950) showed a marked variation in the ratio of energy deposited or lost as protein (this being called the 'p value' for an individual) (see Chapter 5). However, this 'p ratio' is not easily measured, even with the more sophisticated techniques of protein turnover measurement that we introduced for use in humans. Nevertheless, it is clear that there is a limit to the amount of FFM that can be accumulated or lost as protein on normal diets, so the fatter the person, the smaller the 'p ratio' for subsequent further weight gain (Forbes, 1987). If a patient continues to overeat despite pre-existing weight gain then the increment of metabolically active FFM that can then be laid down falls to 15–20%. This in turn means that, as Schutz (1995) showed, even more weight has to be accumulated before sufficient FFM has been gained to burn off the extra kilocalories coming from the excess intake.

If discrepancies of only 0.5–1.0% in energy turnover explain normal weight gain, a metabolic basis for an individual's weight gain could be responsible for their susceptibility to obesity. These interindividual differences are, however, small compared with the more readily measured rates of energy intake and expenditure. As daily food intake varies even more than physical activity, this means that appetite control is exceptionally well controlled. The issue is whether small discrepancies in intake control, or interindividual metabolic differences, dominate in the determination of who gains weight. The societal shifts in weight must, however, be explained by the failure of most people to adapt their intakes perfectly. When young adults stop playing sports this often induces energy imbalance and weight gain. The weight gain in women following the menopause is probably a reflection of the changes in the hormonal control of appetite (see below). Thus, societal, social and personal factors, as well as interindividual differences in metabolism, probably determine why one person rather than another gains weight.

Gender-based differences in metabolic efficiency

We showed that men automatically gain more protein per unit weight increase than women and thereby burn more calories and so gain less weight before again achieving energy balance. This seems to be a reasonable explanation for why in most societies women on average are more obese than men (James and Reeds, 1997). The limits on FFM accumulation also help to explain why there is a remarkable shift in BMI distribution curves in the population so that extreme obesity (BMIs > 40) increases far faster than expected from the average weight gains of the population. The rebalancing or a plateau in weight with an excess intake of only 50–100 kcal per day may take 3–5

years to achieve because of the incremental diurnal effects of energy storage during the day and loss at night (Schutz, 1995). At these extreme weights, with less extra FFM/kg weight gained, about 8000–8500 kcal/kg have been stored rather than the usual 7000–7700 kcal/kg. This amplifies the difficulty of losing weight because in practice a daily deficit of 1000 kcal will still require 2–3 years for many very obese individuals to lose all the excess weight that they had slowly stored over 20–30 years.

Optimum macronutrient intakes

Table 9.1 gives the World Health Organization's recent assessment of nutrient needs for the population. Here the fat intake is set at 15–35%—the latter higher figure assumes there is a substantial amount of physical activity that in practice is unusual. The World Health Organization, from an obesity point of view, had considered 20–25% fat as the upper limit for fat intakes (WHO, 2000). This lower fat limit is also more appropriate for combating hypertension as shown by the DASH trials (Sacks

Table 9.1 Ranges of population nutrient intake goals.

Dietary factor	Goal (% of total energy, unless otherwise stated)
Total fat	15–30%
Saturated fatty acids	< 10%
Polyunsaturated fatty acids (PUFAs)	6–10%
n-6 Polyunsaturated fatty acids	5–8%
n-3 Polyunsaturated fatty acids	1–2%
Trans fatty acids	< 1%
Monounsaturated fatty acids (MUFAs)	By difference*
Total carbohydrate	55–75%†
Free sugars‡	< 10%
Protein	10–15%¶
Cholesterol	< 300 mg per day
Sodium chloride (sodium)§	< 5 g per day (< 2 g per day)
Fruits and vegetables	400 g per day
Total dietary fibre	From foods**
Non-starch polysaccharides (NSP)	From foods**

*This is calculated as: total fat (saturated fatty acids + polyunsaturated fatty acids + trans fatty acids).

†The percentage of total energy available after taking into account the energy consumed as protein and fat, hence the wide range.

‡The term 'free sugars' refers to all monosaccharides and disaccharides added to foods by the manufacturer, cook or consumer, plus sugars naturally present in honey, syrups and fruit juices.

§The suggested range should be seen in the light of the Joint WHO/FAO/UNU Expert Consultation on Protein and Amino Acid Requirements in Human Nutrition, held in Geneva from 9–16 April 2002.

¶Salt should be iodized appropriately. The need to adjust salt iodization, depending on observed sodium intake and surveillance of iodine status of the population, should be recognized (WHO, 2003).

et al., 2001) and even lower intakes were used by Ornish to reverse the poor atheromatous state of patients with pre-existing coronary artery disease (Ornish *et al.*, 1990). Table 9.1 includes a 10% figure for added sugars, which reflects the new concerns about the effects of free sugars, e.g. in sugary drinks, on energy imbalance (Raben *et al.*, 2002).

The report also proposes exercise patterns equivalent to PALs of 1.7–1.8, which demand 60–90 min of daily active walking to help with weight maintenance. This differs from the previous proposal for 30 min five times weekly, which was suggested on the basis of the recognized cardiovascular benefits of some exercise in the current state of exceptionally inactive Americans. Morris's original studies emphasized the importance of some vigorous activity to obtain cardiological fitness to prevent myocardial infarction (Erlichman *et al.*, 2002a,b).

The adjustments in food-intake control with weight gain: implications for weight loss diets

The histograms in Fig. 9.3 illustrate the fact that, as patients gain weight, their BMR and total energy expenditure rise unless they reduce their physical activity (as often happens, seemingly, in response to the handicap of moving their heavier weight around) (Petersen *et al.*, 2004). Nevertheless, overweight and obese patients are usually eating more than people of the same age and height, which seems strange if their long-term food-intake control is working properly. This regulated but higher intake of food seems to suggest an upward readjustment of the apparent 'set point' of appetite control. This is in keeping with careful clinical observation: when obese patients are put on a severely restricted diet one might expect them to simply lose weight without any desire to eat, given their huge energy stores. In reality, they immediately respond as if they are being semistarved!

Thus, as with normal-weight volunteers who are experimentally semistarved, there is a sharp 15% fall in their BMR and an immediate induction of hunger with a natural food-seeking response (Leibel *et al.*, 1995). This implies that, unlike Roberts' studies (Roberts *et al.*, 1995) on acute overfeeding in the young, the pathophysiological adjustment in food-intake control makes it more difficult to lose weight. Indeed, studies of post-obese people showed that they considered themselves as severely restricted in what they could eat years after losing weight, and therefore recorded spuriously low intakes for their measured total expenditure. The much larger groups of formerly obese individuals studied in the US also show a continuing obsessive and conscious control of their food intake and a determination to exercise substantially—dissipating 2000–3000 kcal per week by exercising in an attempt to control their apparent pathophysiological drive to eat more and regain the weight that they had lost (Klern *et al.*, 1997).

Table 9.2 The predicted basal metabolic rates for males and females.

Years	BMR in MJ per day from body weight (W)	
	Male	Female
10–17	0.074 W + 2.754	0.056 W + 2.898
18–29	0.063 W + 2.896	0.062 W + 2.036
30–59	0.048 W + 3.653	0.034 W + 3.538
60–74	0.0499 W + 2.930	0.0386 W + 2.875
75+	0.0350 W + 3.434	0.0410 W + 2.610

These values are based on Schofield *et al.* (1985), which were used by FAO/WHO/UNU in their energy requirement report, but with the > 60-year-old values taken from the UK Department of Health's calculations using substantially greater numbers of BMR values for those > 60 years.

Prescribing a weight loss diet

The implications of these marked differences in energy needs relating to gender, weight, age and physical activity are important clinically. It is inappropriate, given the huge differences in energy needs, to simply put all patients on a calorie-restricted diet with a total intake of, for example 1000 kcal per day—the bigger the person the greater their present intake so on a standard low-calorie diet these very heavy patients will get an intense physiological drive to eat and resist weight loss. This led us to propose (Lean and James, 1986) and then use a deficit diet that provides 500–600 kcal less than their individually estimated energy needs. This deficit diet scheme is now used in most clinical drug trials of weight loss (Finer *et al.*, 2000; James *et al.*, 2000). Figure 9.4 provides graphs to specify the energy intake of patients on an energy-deficit diet, and the appropriate total fat, saturated fat and protein intakes.

It has been shown that, whether patients are placed on a 1000-kcal or a 500-kcal deficit diet, they lose weight at the same rate because, again unconsciously, those on a 1000-kcal deficit adjust their intake to limit their deficit to about 500 kcal (Toplak *et al.*, 2002).

As weight loss occurs, the FFM inevitably declines, so the BMR falls together with the physical activity costs of movement. There are two components contributing to the fall in BMR. The initial fall reflects an increase in the metabolic efficiency of the FFM in response to a reduction in plasma T3 levels and a fall in the adrenergic drive to the BMR-related tissues (Jung *et al.*, 1980). Subsequently, there is a slow progressive fall in BMR as the FFM declines with weight loss (Prentice *et al.*, 1991).

This reduction in energy output minimizes the impact of the energy-deficit diet, so a downwards readjustment in the energy prescription is needed if weight loss is to continue. These deficit diets do not immediately stress the physiological control of food intake and can be expected to lead to 7 × 500 kcal/week = 3500 kcal, which amounts to about a 0.5-kg weekly weight loss. A 10-kg weight loss leads to a

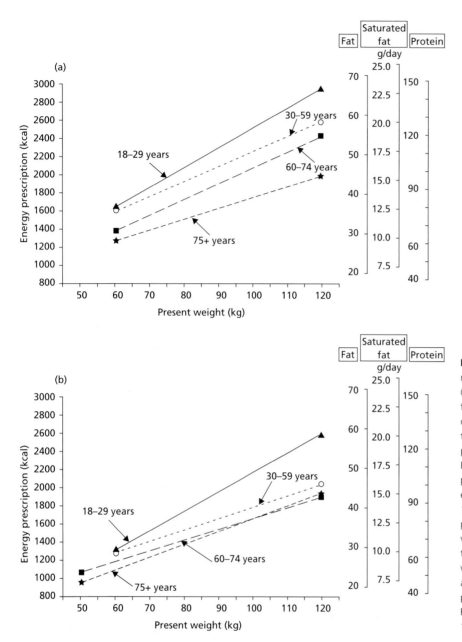

Fig 9.4 Selecting appropriate energy and macronutrient intake with an energy-deficit diet. (a) Men; (b) women. Prescribing appropriate diets for individual needs based on a 600-kcal deficit diet (Lean and James, 1986) that provides 20% total fat, 7% saturated fatty acids and 20% protein. The energy prescription is based on the BMR equations shown in Table 9.2, with the total predicted energy need for weight stability estimated on the basis of light activity with a PAL of 1.4. From these values, 600 kcal are subtracted to provide the prescribed intakes needed (as shown) when there is an energy deficit of 600 kcal. Thus, the overweight or obese patient can be provided with a specific series of menus with the maximum appropriate fat content and with the additional protein needed for individuals in energy deficit. Free sugar intake should be limited to less than 10% of the prescribed energy diet.

permanent fall in energy needs amounting to about 300 kcal per day: a patient then has permanently to eat 300 kcal per day less, or do considerably more exercise, to maintain his or her lower weight plateau. Unfortunately, weight gain is common because patients consider that once they have lost weight they can then return to their previous food and exercise habits.

Fats and fatty acids in relation to weight loss regimens

For several decades, formula diets were advocated for obese patients, based on the concept that severely restricting the carbohydrate intake to below about 60 g per day would induce ketosis and thereby put patients into an anorexic state as they slim. The original 340–350 kcal diets of protein only with minerals and vitamins (e.g. the original Cambridge diet) were then banned because it was considered that they had not been tested adequately for their long-term safety. In any case, a re-analysis of the weight losses showed that, in practice, after 3 months, the patients could not have been keeping to the prescribed diets because they failed to continue to lose weight at the expected rate (James, 1984).

The re-emergence of the Atkins diet also reflects a scheme for inducing ketosis but combines the low carbohydrate intake with the use of an unlimited protein intake to help boost satiety. In the short term, despite the inappropriately high saturated fatty acid composition, the weight loss itself allows a fall in plasma cholesterol and triglycerides (Samaha *et al.*, 2003) but there are, as yet, no studies showing the long-term superiority of the Atkins diet in weight management. It is clear, however, that it is very unwise to maintain a high saturated fatty acid intake over a long period, as this has been proven to increase markedly the risk of cardiovascular disease.

Weight loss is proportional to the lowering of the fat intake (Astrup *et al.*, 2000) providing that total energy intakes do fall—*ad libitum* low-fat diets are less effective. There is also a debate as to whether carbohydrate-rich diets should be modified to include much more monounsaturated fat, for example from olive oil, the new safflower or maize oils, thereby helping to minimize the carbohydrate-induced rise in plasma triglycerides, and a tendency for HDL-cholesterol to fall. Older longer term studies, however, showed that this carbohydrate-induced hypertriglyceridaemia is a short-term effect (Fried and Rao, 2003). These studies underline the importance of not being confused by short-term effects.

Carbohydrates, glycaemic index and fructosans

Many years ago it was emphasized that high fibre-containing diets were needed for optimum colonic function and to minimize the demand for insulin in the post-absorptive state, but confusion arose over the most appropriate way of measuring fibre. The most direct and logical approach is that based on Englyst's methods, as his techniques monitor specific components of cellular carbohydrates. The non-starch polysaccharides are diverse in nature, with pectins and gums having a lipid-lowering effect, whereas the less digestible water cellulose-containing polysaccharides have greater colonic bulking properties (Cummings *et al.*, 1997). Insulin secretion and the induction of insulin resistance depend in part on the rapidity of glucose absorption, which can now be measured as rapidly digestible starches, but Jenkins and colleagues (2002) have developed a crude test for the glycaemic properties of foods (Foster-Powell *et al.*, 2002) and these diets are becoming popular. There is some evidence that a low glycaemic index diet promotes weight loss. It also seems clear that the induction of insulin secretion leads to greater energy storage—as seen for example in the routine weight gain that follows the more intensive treatment of diabetics with insulin itself or sulphonylureas. Low glycaemic, fibre-rich diets are therefore valuable components of diets aimed at minimizing weight gain (Swinburn *et al.*, 2004).

Fructose-rich diets, although not stimulating immediate insulin secretion, are now being invoked as particularly disadvantageous because the fructose eludes the normal glucose-mediated controls on metabolism and perhaps appetite. The fructose is readily absorbed and transported into cells, where triglyceride synthesis is stimulated (Elliott *et al.*, 2002; Bray *et al.*, 2004). Thus, weight management needs to take account of both the total energy intake and the type of fats and carbohydrates in the advised dietary scheme.

Protein intakes

Although the usual diets eaten by mankind contain 10–15% of the dietary energy as protein, there is an increased need for protein once the energy intake is reduced below the maintenance requirements. Thus, a protein intake that amounts to about 1.5 g of protein per kilogram ideal body weight is needed for weight loss diets, and this higher intake not only reduces the loss of lean body mass (Layman *et al.*, 2003), but also helps to enhance satiety as previously noted. Thus, it is useful to have up to 20% protein in weight loss diets.

Alcohol

Alcohol, once ingested, is preferentially metabolized and excess energy taken as alcohol seems to lead to selective fat storage. On this basis, one might expect alcohol intakes to be strongly related to excess weight gain. However, at higher intakes, alcohol induces microsomal oxidation, which then dissipates energy without being linked to ATP turnover and the propensity to weight gain. Thus, heavy drinkers are not necessarily overweight and may even be thin, particularly if the alcohol induces gastritis and other intestinal dysfunctions. In management terms, alcohol has the disadvantage of not only providing additional calories without nutrients, but it can also lead patients to take a more relaxed view of their diet and induce non-compliance with a prescribed weight reduction programme.

Salt implications in relation to obesity

Logically, salt would seem to have nothing to do with obesity and metabolic needs but clinically it can be important for three reasons.

1 It is of physiological significance; as highly salted foods make children and adults thirsty, this amplifies the likelihood in modern circumstances of greater soft drink or other calorie-containing intakes.

2 The propensity of obese patients to hypertension will be amplified if they are on a high salt intake—a common feature because of the obese patient's higher absolute intake.

3 Attempts to treat the associated hypertension with angiotensin-converting enzyme (ACE) inhibitors are thwarted by high-salt diets; thus, clinicians need to consider salt as well as the macronutrient needs of their patients.

Unfortunately, high-salt diets have been sought after for centuries, substantial amounts of salt being used to preserve foods, as well as to enhance or disguise the taste of different prepared and cooked foods. Salt has been derived from either sea water or the discovery of salt sources in pits and mines—this formerly rare commodity was used as a form of payment (the 'salary') by the Romans, with salt as well as spice trails traversing the Andes, the Sahara and Asian trade routes for centuries. Today, manufacturers deliberately keep the salting of foods high, not only to stimulate thirst but to enhance crudely the taste of their products. In most Western societies, 85% of salt comes from purchased foods, not cooking or table salt (James *et al.*, 1987b), so patients need explicit advice on food purchases and the problems associated with high-salt intakes.

Conclusions

It is important to understand how to estimate patients' energy requirements and to recognize the likelihood of their being confused about their energy intake. They will also be constantly bombarded by the marketing of novel diets that are often geared to providing a mechanism for constraining total energy intake by advocating very specific foods, or eating patterns, which, in practice, means that the patients control their intake.

Although the normal protein intake amounts to 10–15% of energy in most normal diets, it is accepted that a higher protein intake (e.g. 20%) not only helps to maintain satiety, but also minimizes the loss of lean tissues when energy intake is below that required to maintain body weight. In practice, low-fat (e.g. 15–20%) diets are appropriate as long as the carbohydrate intake is rich in plant-based, non-starch polysaccharides and that the intake of added sugars is kept to a minimum. The standard use of a minimum of 400 g of vegetables and fruit per day brings additional benefits in terms of both bulking, and the cardiovascular- and cancer-protective properties of these dietary components. Thus, patients who are put on a carefully arranged programme of eating with a low energy density diet may find themselves eating far more in weight terms than they have consumed for many years. The heavier patient may also be able to progressively lose weight on diets that contain 2000–3000 kcal per day, depending upon the degree of overweight of the patient and their estimated energy requirements.

The biggest challenge is to change the microenvironment of the patient. This means that the individual's partner and his or her family need to transfer to a similar type of diet, thereby minimizing the risk of the patient regaining their weight. Additionally, this helps the long-term maintenance of a more appropriate diet conducive to the well-being of both children and adults in the family.

References

Astrup, A. (2001) The role of dietary fat in the prevention and treatment of obesity. Efficacy and safety of low-fat diets. *International Journal of Obesity and Related Metabolic Disorders* **25** (Suppl. 1), S46–50.

Astrup, A., Grunwald, G.K., Melanson, E.L., Saris, W.H. and Hill, J.O. (2000) The role of low-fat diets in body weight control: a meta-analysis of ad libitum dietary intervention studies. *International Journal of Obesity and Related Metabolic Disorders* **12**, 1545–1552.

Bisdee, J.T. and James, W.P.T. (1985) The role of carbohydrate (CHO) in dietary thermogenesis (DT) in man. *International Journal of Obesity* **9** (Suppl. 2), A23.

Bisdee, J.T., James, W.P.T and Shaw, M.A. (1989) Changes in energy expenditure during the menstrual cycle. *British Journal of Nutrition* **61**, 187–199.

Booth, D.A., Lee, M. and Mcaleavey, C.(1976) Acquired sensory control of satiation in man. *British Journal of Psychology* **67**, 137–147.

Bouchard, C., Tremblay, A., Depres, J.P., Nadeau, A., Lupien, P.J., Moorjani, S., Prudhomme, D. and Fournier, G. (1990) The response to long term overfeeding in identical twins. *New England Journal of Medicine* **322**, 1477–1482.

Bouchard, C., Pérusse, L., Rice, T. and Rao, DC. (1997) The genetics of human obesity. In: Bray, G.A., Bouchard, C. and James, W.P.T. eds. *Handbook on Obesity.* New York: Marcel Dekker, 555–571.

Boyd Orr, Lord John. (1936) *Food, Health and Income.* London: Macmillan.

Bray, G.A., Nielsen, S.J. and Popkin, B.M. (2004) Consumption of high-fructose corn syrup in beverages may play a role in the epidemic of obesity. *American Journal of Clinical Nutrition* **79**, 537–543. Erratum in *Am J Clin Nutr* **80**, 1090.

Cameron-Smith, D. and Egger, G. (2003) *Professor Trim's The Ultimate Food Energy Guide.* Crows Nest, NSW, Australia: Allen and Unwin.

Cotton, J.R., Burley, V.J., Weststrate, J.A. and Blundell, J.E. (1996) Fat substitution and food intake: effect of replacing fat with sucrose polyester at lunch or evening meals. *British Journal of Nutrition* **75**, 545–556.

Crawford, M. and Marsh, D. (1989) *The Driving Force: Food, Evolution, and the Future.* London: Manderin Paperbacks.

Cummings, J.H., Roberfroid, M.B., Andersson, H., Barth, C., Ferro-Luzzi, A., Ghoos, Y., Gibney, M., Hermonsen, K., James, W.P.T., Korver, O., Lairon, D., Pascal, G. and Voragen, A.G. (1997) A new look at dietary carbohydrate: chemistry, physiology and health. Paris Carbohydrate Group. *European Journal of Clinical Nutrition* **51**, 417–423.

Dallosso, H.M. and James, W.P.T. (1984) Whole body calorimetry studies in adult men. 1. The effect of fat over-feeding on 24 h energy expenditure. *British Journal of Nutrition* **52**, 49–64.

De Castro, J.M. (1993) The effects of the response to particular foods and beverages on the meal pattern and overall nutrient intake of humans. *Physiological Behaviour* **59**, 179–187.

Drewnowski, A. (1998) Energy density palatability and satiety: implications for weight control. *Nutrition Reviews* **56**, 347–353.

Dugdale, A.E. and Payne, P.R. (1971) Pattern of lean and fat deposition in adults. *Nature* **266**, 349–351.

Dulloo, A.G., Jaquet, J. and Giardier, L. (1996) Autoregulation of body composition during weight recovery in human: the Minnesota Experiment revisited. *International Journal of Obesity* **20**, 393–405.

Durnin, J.V. (1987) Energy requirements of pregnancy: an integration of the longitudinal data from the five-country study. *Lancet* **ii**: 1131–1133.

Eaton, S.B., Shostak, M. and Konner, M. (1988) *The Paleolithic Prescription: A Program of Diet and Exercise and a Design for Living.* New York: Harper & Row.

Elliott, S.S., Keim, N.L., Stern, J.S., Teff, K. and Havel, P.J. (2002) Fructose, weight gain, and the insulin resistance syndrome1–3. *American Journal of Clinical Nutrition* **76**, 911–922.

Erlichman, J., Kerbey, A.L. and James, W.P.T. (2002a) Physical activity and its impact on health outcomes. Paper 1: the impact of physical activity on cardiovascular disease and all-cause mortality: an historical perspective. *Obesity Reviews* **3**, 257–271.

Erlichman, J., Kerbey, A.L. and James, W.P.T. (2002b) Physical activity and its impact on health outcomes. Paper 2: prevention of unhealthy weight gain and obesity by physical activity: an analysis of the evidence. *Obesity Reviews* **3**, 273–287.

Ezzati, M., Lopez, A.D., Rodgers, A., Vander Hoorn, S., Murray, C.J. Comparative Risk Assessment Collaborating Group. (2002) Selected major risk factors and global and regional burden of disease. *Lancet* **360**, 1347–1360.

Ferro-Luzzi, A., James, W.P. and Kafatos, A. (2002) The high-fat Greek diet: a recipe for all? *European Journal of Clinical Nutrition* **56**, 796–809.

Finer, N., James, W.P., Kopelman, P.G., Lean, M.E. and Williams, G. (2000) One-year treatment of obesity: a randomized, double-blind, placebo-controlled, multicentre study of orlistat, a gastrointestinal lipase inhibitor. *International Journal of Obesity and Related Metabolic Disorders* **24**, 306–313.

Fomon, S.J., Filer, L.J., Thomas, L.N., Rogers, R.R. and Proksch, A.M. (1969) Relationship between formula concentration and rate of growth of normal children. *Journal of Nutrition* **98**, 241–254.

Forbes, G.B. (1987) *Human Body Composition: Growth, Ageing, Nutrition and Activity.* New York: Springer-Verlag.

Foster-Powell, K., Holt, S.H. and Brand-Miller, J.C. (2002) International table of glycemic index and glycemic load values: 2002. *American Journal of Clinical Nutrition* **76**(1): 5–56.

Fried, S.K. and Rao, S.P. (2003) Sugars, hypertriglyceridemia, and cardiovascular disease. *American Journal of Clinical Nutrition* **78** (Suppl.), S873–S880.

Griffiths, M. and Payne, P.R. (1976) Energy expenditure in small children of obese and non-obese parents. *Nature* **260**, 698–700.

Griffiths, M., Payne, P.R., Stunkard, A.J., Rivers, J.P.W. and Cox, M. (1990) Metabolic rate and physical development in children at risk of obesity. *Lancet* **336**, 76–78.

James, W.P.T. (1984) Treatment of obesity: the constraints on success. *Clinics in Endocrinology and Metabolism* **13**, 635–663.

James, W.P.T. and Reeds, P.J. (1997) Nutrient partitioning. In: Bray, G.A., Bouchard, C., James, W.P.T. eds. *Handbook on Obesity.* New York: Marcel Dekker, 555–571.

James, W.P.T., Lean, M.E.J. and McNeill, G. (1987a) Dietary recommendations after weight loss: how to avoid relapse of obesity. *American Journal of Clinical Nutrition* **45**, 1135–1141.

James, W.P.T., Ralph, A. and Sanchez-Castillo, C.P. (1987b) The dominance of salt in manufactured food in the sodium intake of affluent societies. *Lancet* **i**, 426–429.

James, W.P.T., Ralph, A. and Ferro-Luzzi, A. (1989) Energy needs of the elderly: a new approach. In: Munro, H.N., Danford, D.E. eds. *Nutrition, Aging, and the Elderly.* New York: Plenum Press, 129–151.

James, W.P.T., Astrup, A., Finer, N., Hilsted, J., Kopelman, P., Rössner, S., Saris, W.H.N. and Van Gaal, L.F. (2000) A two year sibutramine trial of obesity reduction and maintenance (STORM). *Lancet* **356**, 2119–2125.

Jenkins, D.J., Kendall, C.W., Augustin, L.S., Franceschi, S., Hamidi, M., Marchie, A., Jenkins, A.L. and Axelsen, M. (2002) Glycemic index: overview of implications in health and disease. *American Journal of Clinical Nutrition* **76**(1): 266S–273S.

Jung, R.T., Shetty, P.S., James, W.P.T, Barrand, M.A. and Callingham, B.A. (1979) Reduced thermogenesis in obesity. *Nature* **279**, 322–323.

Jung, R.T., Shetty, P.S. and James, W.P.T. (1980) The effect of beta-adrenergic blockade on metabolic rate and peripheral thyroid metabolism in obesity. *European Journal of Clinical Investigation* **10**, 179–182.

Keys, A. (ed.) (1980) *Seven Countries. A Multivariate Analysis of Death and Coronary Heart Disease.* Cambridge, MA: Harvard University Press.

Keys, A., Brozek, J., Henschel, A., Mickelsen, O. and Taylor, H.L. (1950) *The Biology of Human Starvation.* Minnesota: University of Minnesota Press.

Kipnis, V., Midthune, D., Freedman, L., Bingham, S., Day, N.E., Riboli, E., Ferrari, P. and Carroll, R.J. (2002) Bias in dietary-report instruments and its implications for nutritional epidemiology. *Public Health and Nutrition* **5**, 915–923.

Klern, M.L., Wing, R.R., Mcguire, M.T., Seagle, H.M. and Hill, J.O. (1997) A descriptive study of individuals successful at long term maintenance of substantial weight loss. *American Journal of Clinical Nutrition* **66**, 239–246.

Layman, D.K., Boileau, R.A., Erickson, D.J., Painter, J.E., Shiue, H., Sather, C. and Christou, D.D. (2003) A reduced ratio of dietary carbohydrate to protein improves body composition and blood lipid profiles during weight loss in adult women. *Journal of Nutrition* **133**, 411–417.

Lean, M.E.J. and James, W.P.T. (1986) Diabetes: prescription of diabetic diets in the 1980s. *Lancet* **i**, 723–725.

Lean, M.E.J. and James, W.P.T. (1988) Metabolic effects of isoenergetic nutrient exchange over 24 hours in relation to obesity in women. *International Journal of Obesity* **12**, 15–27.

Leibel, R.L., Rosenbaum, M. and Hirsch, J. (1995) Changes in energy expenditure resulting from altered body weight. *New England Journal of Medicine* **332**, 621–628.

Neel, J.V., Weder, A.B. and Julius, S. (1998) Type II diabetes, essential hypertension, and obesity as 'syndromes of impaired genetic homeostasis': the 'thrifty genotype' hypothesis enters the 21st century. *Perspectives in Biological Medicine* **42**, 44–74.

Orlet Fisher, J, Rolls, B.J. and Birch, L.L. (2003) Children's bite size and intake of an entree are greater with large portions than with age-appropriate or self-selected portions. *American Journal of Clinical Nutrition* **77**, 1164–1170.

Ornish, D., Brown, S.E., Scherwitz, L.W., Billings, J.H., Armstrong, W.T., Ports, T.A., McLanahan, S.M., Kirkeeide, R.L., Brand, R.J. and Gould, K.L. (1990) Can lifestyle changes reverse coronary heart disease? The Lifestyle Heart Trial. *Lancet* **336**, 129–133.

Petersen, L., Schnohr, P. and Sorensen, T.I. (2004) Longitudinal study of the long-term relation between physical activity and obesity in adults. *International Journal of Obesity and Related Metabolic Disorders* **28**(1): 105–112.

Popkin, B.M. (2001) The nutrition transition and obesity in the developing world. *Journal of Nutrition* **131**, 871S–873S.

Prentice, A.M. (2001) Fires of life: the struggles of an ancient metabolism in a modern world. *Nutrition Bulletin (British Nutrition Foundation)* **26**, 13–27.

Prentice, A.M. and Jebb, S.A. (2003) Fast foods, energy density and obesity: a possible mechanistic link. *Obesity Reviews* **4**, 187–194.

Prentice, A.M., Goldberg, G.R., Jebb, S.A., Black, A.E., Murgatroyd, P.R. and Diaz, E.O. (1991) Physiological responses to slimming. *Proceedings of the Nutrition Society* **50**, 441–458.

Raben, A., Vasilaras, T.H., Møller, A.C. and Astrup, A. (2002) Sucrose compared with artificial sweeteners: different effects on ad libitum intake and body weight after 10 weeks of supplementation in overweight subjects. *American Journal of Clinical Nutrition* **36**, 721–729.

Ravussin, E., Lilloja, S., Knowler, W.C., Christian, L., Freymond, D. Abbott, W.G.H., Boyce, V. and Howard, B.V. (1988) Reduced rate of energy expenditure as a risk factor for body weight gain. *New England Journal of Medicine* **318**, 467–472.

Roberts, S.B., Fuss, P., Heyman, M.B., Evans, W.J., Tsay, R., Rasmussen, H., Fiatarone M., Cortiella, J., Dallal, G.E. and Young V.R. (1995) Control of food intake in older men. *Journal of the American Medical Association* 30, **272**, 1601–1606. (Erratum in *Journal of the American Medical Association* **273**, 702.)

Sacks, F.M., Svetkey, L.P., Vollmer, W.M., Appel, L.J., Bray, G.A., Harsha, D., Obarzanek, E., Conlin, P.R., Miller, E.R., Simons-Morton, D.G., Karanja, N. and Lin, P.H. (2001) Effects on blood pressure of reduced dietary sodium and the Dietary Approaches to Stop Hypertension (DASH) diet. DASH-Sodium Collaborative Research Group. *New England Journal of Medicine* **344**(1), 3–10.

Samaha, F.F., Iqbal, N., Seshadri, P., Chicano, K.L., Daily, D.A., McGrory, J., Williams, T., Williams, M., Gracely, E.J. and Stern, L. (2003) A low-carbohydrate as compared with a low-fat diet in severe obesity. *New England Journal of Medicine* **348**, 2074–2081.

Schofield, W.N., Schofield, C. and James, W.P.T. (1985) Basal metabolic rate – review and prediction, together with an annotated bibliography of source material. *Human Nutrition Clinical Nutrition* **39C** (Suppl 1.), 1–96.

Schutz, Y. (1995) Macronutrients and energy balance in obesity. *Metabolism* **44**, (Suppl. 3), 7–11.

Shetty, P.S., Jung, R.T., James, W.P.T., Barrand, M.A. and Callingham, B.A. (1981) Postprandial thermogenesis in obesity. *Clinical Science* **60**, 519–525.

Stephen, A.M. and Wald, N.J. (1990) Trends in individual consumption of dietary fat in the United States, 1920–1984. *American Journal of Clinical Nutrition* **52** 457–469.

Stubbs, R.J., Maslan, N. and Whybrow, S. (2001) Carbohydrates, appetite and feeding behaviour in humans. *Journal of Nutrition* **131**, 2775S–2781S.

Swinburn, B.A., Caterson, I., Seidell, J.C. and James, W.P. (2004) Diet, nutrition and the prevention of excess weight gain and obesity. *Public Health and Nutrition* **7**(1A): 123–146.

Toplak, H., Sharma, A.M. and Van-Gaal, L. (2002) Rapid weight loss with orlistat plus diet after 6 months of treatment [abstract 574]. *International Journal of Obesity* **26** (Suppl. 1), S152.

World Health Organization (2002) *World Health Report*. Geneva: WHO.

World Health Organization (2000) *Obesity: Preventing and Managing the Global Epidemic*. WHO Technical Report Series No. 894. Geneva: WHO.

World Health Organization (2003) *Diet, Nutrition and the Prevention of Chronic Diseases. Report of a Joint WHO/FAO Expert Consultation*. WHO Technical Report Series No. 916. Geneva: WHO.

Yoshiike, N., Seino, F., Tajima, S., Arai, Y., Kawano, M., Furuhata, T. and Inoue, S. (2002) Twenty-year changes in the prevalence of overweight in Japanese adults: The National Nutrition Survey 1976–1995. *Obesity Reviews* **3**, 183–190.

10 Biology of obesity: eating behaviour

John E. Blundell, Graham Finlayson and Jason Halford

Eating behaviour and appetite control, 137

Can eating behaviour be controlled for the management of obesity?, 137

Conceptualization of the system controlling eating behaviour, 138

Episodic and tonic signals for appetite control, 139
  Satiety signals and the satiety cascade, 139
  Cholecystokinin, 139
  Glucagon-like peptide (GLP)-1, 140

Peptide YY, 141
Amylin, 141
Satiety cascade peptides, 141
Tonic signals of appetite control: role of leptin, 142

Genetic mutations and appetite control, 142
  Leptin deficiency, 142
  Mutations in the melanocortin system, 143
  Appetite signals: satiety or drive?, 143
  Ghrelin and hunger drive, 144

Homeostatic and hedonic processes of appetite control, 144
  Hunger and pleasure – do they interact?, 144
  Food choice, hedonic response and obesity, 145
  Hedonic responsivity and addiction?, 145

Risk factors for appetite control, 146

Individual variability: resistance and susceptibility to weight gain, 146

References, 147

Eating behaviour and appetite control

Appetite fits into an energy-balance model of weight regulation, but it is not necessary to believe that appetite control is an outcome of the regulation of energy balance. Appetite is separately controlled and is relevant to energy balance, as it modulates the energy intake side of the equation. This happens because appetite includes various aspects of eating patterns, such as the frequency and size of eating episodes (gorging vs. nibbling), choices of high- or low-fat foods, energy density of foods consumed, variety of foods accepted, palatability of the diet and variability in day-to-day intake. All of these features can play a role in encouraging energy intake to exceed energy expenditure, thereby creating a positive energy balance. If this persists then weight gain will ensue. Moreover, there appears to be no unique pattern of eating or forms of energy intake that will exclusively or invariably lead to an excess of energy intake over expenditure.

Nevertheless, some characteristics of the expression of appetite do render individuals vulnerable to overconsumption of food; these characteristics can be regarded as *risk factors*. These risk factors and other modulating features of the expression of appetite will be highlighted by an analysis of how appetite is regulated.

Can eating behaviour be controlled for the management of obesity?

It is widely accepted that body weight control and, by implication, a lack of control arise from an interaction between biology and the environment, particularly the food supply reflected in the nutritional environment. The link between these two domains is eating behaviour and the associated subjective sensations that make up the expression of appetite. It is this eating behaviour that transmits the impact of biological events into the environment, and which also mediates the effects of the nutrient environment on biology. Appetite is not nutrition, rather it is the expression of appetite which allows nutrition to exert an effect on biology and vice versa. Consequently, adjustments in the processes regulating the expression of appetite should have a significant impact on body weight regulation.

Of course, obesity can be managed by direct changes in the environment itself, to enforce an increase in physical activity or to coercively prevent food consumption. Equally, pharmacological or surgical interventions can be made directly in biology to prevent the assimilation of food or to alter the energy balance. In addition, adjustments in the environment and biology have the potential to influence body weight *indirectly* by altering food intake, often by acting on the signals involved in processes regulating appetite.

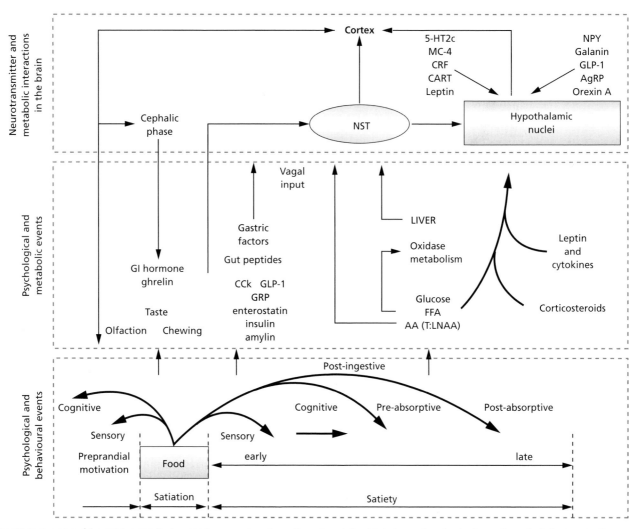

Fig 10.1 A version of the *satiety cascade*, showing the expression of appetite as the relationship between three levels of operations: the behavioural pattern, peripheral physiology and metabolism, and brain activity. PVN, paraventricular nucleus; NST, nucleus of the tractus solitarius; CCK, cholecystokinin; FFA, free fatty acids; T: LNAA, tryptophan: large neutral amino acids (see Blundell, 1991, for detailed diagram).

It should be kept in mind that behaviour is only approximately 30–60% of energy expenditure (depending on the amount of volitional exercise taken and the extent of non-intentional movements or spontaneous activity), but behaviour accounts for 100% of energy intake. As this behaviour is controlled by the voluntary musculature, eating should, in principle, be subject to conscious control. In practice, such control is very difficult to implement.

However, in principle, appetite can be controlled for the management of obesity. We can envisage interventions either in specific foods that influence biology, which in turn adjusts eating behaviour, or through a direct and deliberate cognitive control of behaviour. Alternatively, eating can be influenced via pharmacological or physiological interventions in the mechanisms controlling behaviour. There are many reasons to believe that an adjustment to the expression of appetite is the best chance we have to prevent the persistent surfeit of energy consumed over energy expended, which is characterizing

much of the world's population. At the end of this chapter we should be better informed about the possible strategies for regulating appetite to prevent further escalation of the obesity epidemic.

Conceptualization of the system controlling eating behaviour

It is now accepted that the control of appetite is based on a network of interactions forming part of a psychobiological system. The system can be conceptualized on three levels (Fig. 10.1). These are the levels of psychological events (hunger perception, cravings, hedonic sensations) and behavioural operations (meals, snacks, energy and macronutrient intakes); the level of peripheral physiology and metabolic events; and the level of neurotransmitter and metabolic interactions in the brain (Blundell, 1991). Appetite reflects the synchronous operation of events and processes in the three levels. When appetite is disrupted, as in certain eating disorders, these three levels become desynchronized. Neural events trigger and guide behaviour, but each act of behaviour involves a response in the peripheral physiological system; in turn, these physiological events are translated into brain neurochemical activity. This brain activity represents the strength of motivation to eat and the willingness to refrain from feeding.

The lower part of the psychobiological system (Fig. 10.1) illustrates the appetite cascade which prompts us to consider the events which stimulate eating and which motivate organisms to seek food. It also includes those behavioural actions that actually form the structure of eating, and those processes that follow the termination of eating and which are referred to as post-ingestive or postprandial events.

Even before food touches the mouth, physiological signals are generated by the sight and smell of food. These events constitute the cephalic phase of appetite. Cephalic phase responses are generated in many parts of the gastrointestinal tract; their function is to anticipate the ingestion of food. During and immediately after eating, afferent information provides the major control over appetite. It has been noted that 'afferent information from ingested food acting in the mouth provides primarily positive feedback for eating; that from the stomach and small intestine is primarily negative feedback' (Smith *et al.*, 1990).

Episodic and tonic signals for appetite control

It is useful to distinguish between two types of signals involved in appetite control. Traditionally, a distinction has been drawn between short- and long-term regulation of appetite, but the connotation of episodic and tonic is more appropriate functionally (Halford and Blundell, 2000). Episodic signals are mainly inhibitory (but can be excitatory) and are usually generated by meals or episodes of eating. These signals oscillate in accordance with the pattern of eating, and are intimately associated with the signalling of satiety; they are the counterparts of the short-term signals. Tonic signals arise from tissue stores, including adipose tissue, and exert a tonic pressure on the expression of appetite; they are equivalent to the long-term signals. These two sets of signals—one set responding sharply to changes in behaviour and the other providing a slow modulation—are integrated within complex brain networks that control the overall expression of appetite (Fig. 10.2).

Satiety signals and the satiety cascade

Important episodic signals are the physiological events that are triggered as responses to the ingestion of food and which form the inhibitory processes that first of all stop eating and then prevent the recurrence of eating until another meal is triggered. These physiological responses are termed *satiety signals*, and can be represented by the *satiety cascade*.

Satiation can be regarded as the complex of processes that brings eating to a halt (causes meal termination), whereas *satiety* can be regarded as those events that arise from food consumption and which serve to suppress hunger (the urge to eat) and maintain an inhibition over eating for a particular period of time. This characteristic form of an eating pattern (size of meals, snacks, etc.) is therefore dependent upon the coordinated effects of satiation and satiety, which control the size and frequency of eating episodes (Blundell and Halford, 1994).

Initially, the brain is informed about the amount of food ingested and its nutrient content via sensory input. The gastrointestinal tract is equipped with specialized chemo- and mechanoreceptors that monitor physiological activity and pass information to the brain mainly via the vagus nerve (Mei, 1985). This afferent information constitutes one class of 'satiety signals' and forms part of the preabsorptive control of appetite. It is usual to identify a post-absorptive phase that arises when nutrients have undergone digestion and have crossed the intestinal wall to enter the circulation. These products, which accurately reflect the food consumed, may be metabolized in the peripheral tissues or organs or may enter the brain directly via the circulation. In either case, these products constitute a further class of metabolic satiety signals. Additionally, products of digestion and agents responsible for their metabolism may reach the brain and bind to specific chemoreceptors, influence neurotransmitter synthesis or alter some aspect of neuronal metabolism. In each case, the brain is informed about some component of the metabolic state resulting from food consumption.

It seems likely that chemicals released by gastric stimuli or by food processing in the gastrointestinal tract are involved in the control of appetite (Read, 1990). Many of these chemicals are peptide neurotransmitters, and many peripherally administered peptides cause changes in food consumption (Smith and Gibbs, 1995). At present, a good deal of interest is being shown in these peripheral signals of appetite control and some will be described below.

Cholecystokinin

Much recent research has confirmed the status of cholecystokinin (CCK) as a hormone mediating meal termination (satiation) and possibly early-phase satiety. This can be demonstrated by administering CCK intravenously and measuring changes in food intake and hunger. CCK will reduce meal size and also suppress hunger before the meal; these effects do not depend on the nausea that sometimes accompanies an intravenous infusion (Greenough *et al.*, 1998a,b). Food consumption (mainly protein and fat) stimulates the release of CCK (from duodenal mucosal cells), which in turn activates CCKA-type receptors in the pyloric region of the stomach. This signal is transmitted via afferent fibres of the vagus nerve

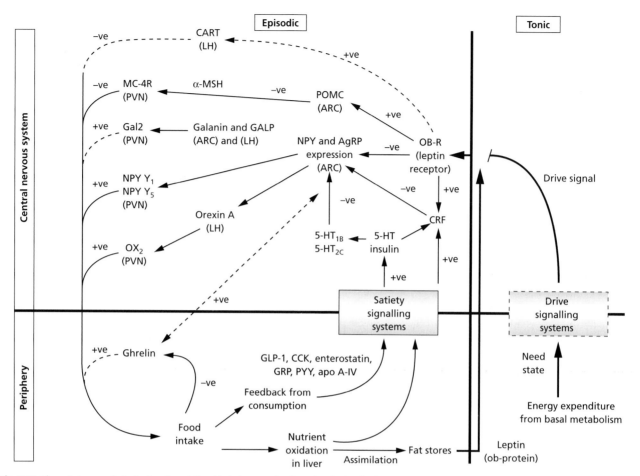

Fig 10.2 The *satiety cascade*, indicating the relationship between episodic and tonic signals of appetite control.

to the nucleus tractus solitarius (NTS) in the brainstem. From here the signal is relayed to the hypothalamic region, where integration with other signals occurs.

Animal data suggest that endogenous CCK release mediates the preabsorptive satiating effect of intestinal fat infusions, and may in turn be critical in regulating the intake of fat (Greenberg *et al.*, 1992). As in rats so in humans—intestinal infusions of fat produce a reduction in food intake and promote satiety (Welch *et al.*, 1985). In humans, the satiety effect of fat infused directly into the duodenum can be blocked by the CCKA receptor antagonist loxiglumide. Fat infusions significantly decrease both food intake and hunger in both male and female volunteers, effects that are reversed by the CCKA antagonist (Lieverse *et al.*, 1994). High-fat breakfasts have been shown to produce both greater feelings of satiety (signified by reduced levels of hunger, desire to eat and prospective consumption) and elevated endogenous plasma CCK levels. Collectively, these studies support the theory that CCK plasma levels are a potent fat (or fatty acid)-stimulated endogenous satiety factor, the effects of which on food intake and feeding behaviour are mediated by CCKA receptors. The CCKA receptor antagonist loxiglumide blocks the effect of CCK-8 on appetite in humans (Gutzwiller *et al.*, 2000), demonstrating

that the appetite-suppressing effect of CCK-8 infusions, such as that of duodenal fat, is mediated by CCKA receptors.

It has also been shown that synthetic CCKA-type agonists suppress food intake in humans. This type of drug has been developed because of its potential as an anti-obesity agent, and it has been necessary to design the chemical structure in order to prolong the duration of action. In one example, the drug was administered by a nasal spray (when taken by mouth the drug was too rapidly metabolized in the stomach).

This drug, known by the number ARL1718, caused a significant reduction in meal size and had a longer duration of action than observed after infusions of CCK itself. These studies, together with those on the peptide hormone itself, do suggest that CCK has the properties of a true satiation signal that contributes to the termination of a meal. The action of CCK certainly acts in concert with other meal-related events, such as gastric distention for example.

Glucagon-like peptide (GLP)-1

Glucagon-like peptide (GLP)-1 is an incretin hormone, released from the gut into the bloodstream in response to intestinal nutrients. Endogenous GLP-1 levels increase following food intake. In lean men, infusions of glucose directly into the gut produce corresponding decreases in appetite and increases in blood GLP-1 (Lavin *et al.*, 1998). Oral carbohydrate induces an endogenous plasma GLP-1 response in lean women (Ranganath *et al.*, 1996). These studies suggest a role for GLP-1 in mediating the effects of carbohydrate (specifically glucose) on appetite.

In healthy men of normal weight, infusions of synthetic human GLP-1 (7–36) during the consumption of a fixed breakfast test meal enhanced ratings of fullness and satiety when compared with the placebo infusion (Flint *et al.*, 1998). During a later *ad libitum* lunch, food intake was also significantly reduced by the earlier GLP-1 infusion. Intravenous GLP-1 dose-dependently reduced spontaneous food intake and adjusted appetite in lean male volunteers. This marked reduction in food intake and enhancement in satiety was also observed in overweight/obese male patients with type 2 diabetes. In obese men, intravenous GLP-1 potently reduced food intake either during or post infusion (Näslund *et al.*, 1998) and, at lower sub-anorectic doses, slowed gastric emptying. Reductions in intake and slowed gastric emptying were accompanied by decreased feelings of hunger, desire to eat and prospective consumption, and a prolonged period of post-meal satiety.

These data demonstrate that exogenous GLP-1 reduces food intake and enhances satiety in humans, both lean and obese. However, it should be kept in mind that the doses of GLP-1 administered are usually higher than the normal values seen in blood after a meal. Consequently, although GLP-1 receptors could be a possible target for anti-obesity drugs, the physiological role of GLP-1 itself in the normal mediation of satiety is still not confirmed. Nonetheless, GLP-1, through its action as an incretin which prompts the release of insulin, will certainly have some indirect role on the pattern of eating behaviour.

Peptide YY

This peptide has received substantial publicity following the publication of a report in 2002. This hormone is similar in structure to the orexigenic neuropeptide NPY (70% amino acid sequence identity), and in the past, peptide YY (PYY) has been regarded, like NPY, as a potent stimulator of food intake. However, in a series of studies in rats, mice and in one human study (all included in one paper), Batterham and colleagues (2002) have demonstrated that peripheral PYY3–36 administration reduces food intake and inhibits weight gain in rodents. These effects on intake and body weight are not observed in transgenic animals that are lacking NPY Y2 receptors (the NPY Y2 receptor knockout), thereby implicating these receptors in mediating the anorectic effects of PYY.

In 12 lean healthy people (male and female), a 90-min PYY3–36 infusion (at levels mimicking a normal physiological response) reduced hunger. Then, 2 h after the infusion, the participants were offered a buffet meal. Food intake was significantly reduced in those who had received the PYY3–36 in-

fusion, and the inhibition over appetite was maintained for the following 12 h. In addition, in a further report, PYY infusions were made in both lean and obese subjects, causing a 30% reduction in the size of a lunch offered after the infusion, and also decreasing the 24-h energy intake by 23% in lean and by 16% in obese people (Batterham *et al.*, 2003). The feeling of hunger was also suppressed for over 3 h following the PYY infusion, as were the plasma levels of ghrelin (see later). Moreover, the natural plasma levels of PYY were lower in obese people than in the lean subjects, and were inversely correlated with the body mass index (BMI). The lower levels of PYY in obese people could mean a weaker satiety signalling through this hormone and therefore a greater possibility of overconsumption. All of these findings are consistent, and together they make a coherent story concerning the role of PYY in appetite control and obesity. But, for the moment, only very few studies have been carried out on humans.

However, it should be noted that there is considerable disagreement about the effect of PYY administered in animals. Rather a large number of researchers have been unable to demonstrate a reduction in food consumption following PYY administration, despite the application of considerable methodological power. These data may point to differences in the action or metabolism of administered PYY between animals and humans, but they have not halted progress towards developing a PYY-based treatment for obesity.

Amylin

Much recent research has also focused on amylin, a pancreatic rather than a gastrointestinal hormone, which also has a potent effect on both food intake and body weight (Reda *et al.*, 2002). Peripheral administration of amylin reduces food intake in mice and rats, and meal size in rats. Chronic or peripheral administration of amylin over a period of 5–10 days produces significant reductions in cumulative food intake, body weight and body mass of rats (Rushing *et al.*, 2001). Amylin administration blocks the hyperphagic effects of NPY (Morris and Nguyen, 2001). Thus, amylin appears to be a component part of the appetite regulation system. The effect of amylin on human food intake, food choice or appetite expression has yet to be assessed fully. However, pramlintide (a human amylin analogue), given to replace deficits in endogenous amylin in people with diabetes, does prevent weight gain and induces a small weight loss in patients over a 1-year period (Ratner *et al.*, 2002).

Satiety cascade peptides

In the overall control of the eating pattern, the sequential release and then deactivation of the peptides described above can account for the evolving biological profile of influence over the sense of hunger and the feeling of fullness (Blundell and Näslund, 1999). The actions of these hormones therefore contribute to the termination of an eating episode (thereby controlling meal size) and subsequently influence the strength and duration of the suppression of eating after a meal. Individual variability in the release and maintenance of the levels of hormones (or the sensitivity of receptors) may determine whether some individuals are prone to snacking between meals or to other forms of opportunistic eating. The overall strength or weakness of the action of these peptides will help to determine whether individuals are resistant or susceptible to weight gain.

Tonic signals of appetite control: role of leptin

One of the classical theories of appetite control has been the notion of a long-term regulation involving a signal that informs the brain about the state of adipose tissue stores. This idea has given rise to the notion of a lipostatic or ponderstatic mechanism (Weigle, 1994). Indeed this is a specific example of a more general class of peripheral appetite (satiety) signals believed to circulate in the blood, reflecting the state of depletion or repletion of energy reserves that directly modulate brain mechanisms. Such substances may include satietin, adipsin, tumour necrosis factor (TNF or cachectin, so named because it is believed to be responsible for cancer-induced anorexia), adiponectin and resistin, together with other substances belonging to the family of agents called cytokines.

In 1994, a landmark scientific event occurred with the discovery and identification of a mouse gene responsible for obesity (Zhang *et al.*, 1994). A mutation of this gene in the *ob/ob* mouse produces a phenotype characterized by the behavioural trait of hyperphagia and the morphological trait of obesity. The gene controls the expression of a protein (the ob protein) by adipose tissue and this protein can be measured in the peripheral circulation. The identification and synthesis of the protein made it possible to evaluate the effects of experimental administration of the protein either peripherally or centrally (Campfield *et al.*, 1995). Because the ob protein caused a reduction in food intake (as well as a possible increase in metabolic energy expenditure) it has been termed 'leptin'. There is some evidence that leptin interacts with NPY, one of the brain's most potent neurochemicals involved in appetite, and with the melanocortin system. Together, these and other neuromodulators are involved in a peripheral–central circuit that links an adipose tissue signal with central appetite mechanisms and metabolic activity.

In this way the protein called leptin probably acts in a similar manner to insulin, which has both central and peripheral actions; for some years it has been proposed that brain insulin represents a body weight signal with the capacity to control appetite.

At the present time the precise relationship between the ob protein and weight regulation has not been determined. However, it is known in animals and humans who are obese that the measured amount of ob protein in the plasma is greater than in lean counterparts. Indeed there is always a very good correlation between the plasma levels of leptin and the degree of bodily fatness (Maffei *et al.*, 1995). Therefore although the ob protein is perfectly positioned to serve as a signal from adipose tissue to the brain, high levels of the protein obviously do not prevent obesity or weight gain. However, the ob protein certainly reflects the amount of adipose tissue in the body. As the specific receptors for the protein (namely the ob receptor) have been identified in the brain (together with the gene responsible for its expression) a defect in body weight regulation could reside at the level of the receptor itself rather than with the ob protein. It is now known that a number of other molecules are linked in a chain to transmit the action of leptin in the brain. These molecules are also involved in the control of food intake, and in some cases a mutation in the gene controlling these molecules is known and is associated with the loss of appetite control and obesity. For example, the MC4-R mutation (melanocortin concentrating hormone receptor 4) leads to an excessive appetite and massive obesity in children, just like leptin deficiency (see below and Chapter 6).

Genetic mutations and appetite control

Leptin deficiency

It seems clear that for the majority of obese people, the ob protein (leptin) system is not a major cause of rapid or massive weight gain. However, for certain individuals very low levels of leptin (or the absence of leptin) do constitute a major risk factor. Recently, a very few individuals have come to light. For example, two young cousins have been studied who displayed marked hyperphagia from a very early age. This hyperphagia took the form of a constant hunger, accompanied by food cravings and a continuous demand for food (Montague *et al.*, 1997). The eldest of the two cousins had reached a body weight of more than 90 kg by the age of 9. Her serum leptin level (like that of the cousin) was very low, and subsequently a mutation in the gene for leptin was revealed. This finding seems to implicate leptin (ob protein) in the control of the drive for food, that is, in the expression of hunger and active food seeking rather than with satiety or the short-term inhibition of eating. Leptin therefore appears to modulate the tonic signal associated with the translation of need into drive; when leptin levels are low or absent then the drive is *unleashed* and results in voracious food seeking (see Fig. 10.2).

The human examples of leptin deficiency due to a genetic mutation are largely consistent with the experimentally demonstrated effects of leptin in animals. One feature is very clear. The cases of human leptin deficiency indicate that the effect of leptin on body weight is exerted entirely through an action on appetite control (energy intake), and not through energy expenditure (see Chapter 6). Leptin deficiency does not involve a defect in metabolic energy expenditure. The human observations are consistent with the removal of a braking action of leptin on appetite control. This phenomenon is quite different from the removal of a single satiety signal, which would lead only to an increase in meal size or a modest increase in meal frequency.

Mutations in the melanocortin system

Histochemical studies have shown the existence of a network of pathways in the brain that use chemicals called melanocortins. These are compounds derived from the precursor proopiomelanocortin (POMC). A significant member of this class is called alpha-melanocyte stimulating hormone (α-MSH). When administered directly into the brain of an experimental animal, α-MSH inhibits food intake and the effect is mediated via the MC4 receptors (Mc4r) in the paraventricular nucleus (PVN). Consistent with these experimental findings are the observations on individuals with mutations in the MC4-R gene who display a form of severe obesity. As the Mc4r is inhibitory for food intake, a mutation that caused a deficiency of these receptors would be expected to remove the inhibition. The phenotype of the Mc4r mutation is characterized by a defect in appetite regulation that manifests as severe hyperphagia, particularly in children. At test meals, carriers of the Mc4r mutation have been shown to eat three times the amount of food of normal-weight children (Farooqi *et al.*, 2003). There is no doubt that people with the Mc4r mutation have abnormal energy intakes and are obese, but the suggestion that they have a tendency to display binge eating disorder (Branson *et al.*, 2003) has been hotly disputed. However, this particular system is clearly implicated in the central system of appetite regulation, and Mc4r mutations represent the single most common monogenic form of obesity.

Appetite signals: satiety or drive?

Of the studies that indicate an increase in appetite, many attribute the effect to a defect in satiety (normal inhibition of eating) or to the loss of some braking action on appetite. That is, inferences about overconsumption tend to favour a disruption of inhibition rather than a stimulation of drive. However, some 50 years ago, there was an equal emphasis on the excitatory or drive features of appetite. This was embodied in Morgan's 'central motive state' and in Stellar's location of this within the hypothalamus (Stellar, 1954). One major issue was to explain what gave animals (and humans) the energy and direction that motivated the seeking of food. These questions are just as relevant today, but the lack of research has prevented much innovative thinking.

In the light of knowledge about the physiology of energy homeostasis, and the utilization of different fuel sources in the body, it is possible to make some proposals. One source of the drive for food arises from the energy used to maintain physiological integrity and behavioural adaptation. Consequently, there is a drive for food generated by energy expenditure. Approximately 60% of total energy expenditure is contributed by the resting metabolic rate (RMR). Consequently, RMR provides a basis for drive and this resonates with the older concept of 'needs translated into drives'. In addition, through adaptation, it can be envisaged that other components of energy expenditure would contribute to the drive for food. The actual signals that help to transmit this energy need into behaviour could be reflected in oxidative pathways of fuel utilization (Friedman and Rawson, 1994), abrupt changes in the availability of glucose in the blood (Campfield *et al.*, 1995) and, eventually, levels of brain neurotransmitters such as NPY, which appear to be linked to metabolic processes. Leptin is also likely to play a role via this system.

In turn, this drive to seek food, arising from a need generated by metabolic processing, is given direction through specific sensory systems associated with smell, but more particularly with taste. It is logical to propose that eating behaviour will be directed to foods having obvious energy value. Of particular relevance to the present situation are the characteristics of sweetness and fattiness of foods. In general, most humans possess a strong liking for the sweet taste of foods and for the fatty texture. Both of these commodities indicate foods that have beneficial (energy yielding) properties.

Accordingly, appetite can be considered as a balance between excitatory and inhibitory processes. The excitatory processes arise from bodily energy needs and constitute a drive for food (which in humans is reflected in the subjective experience of hunger). The most obvious inhibitory processes arise from post-ingestive physiological processing of the consumed food, and these are reflected in the subjective sensation of fullness and a suppression of the feeling of hunger. However, the sensitivity of both the excitatory and inhibitory processes can be modulated by signals arising from the body's energy stores.

It should be noted that the drive system probably functions in order to ensure that energy intake at least matches energy expenditure. This has implications for the maintenance of obesity, as total energy expenditure is proportional to body mass. This means that the drive for food may be strong in obese individuals in order to ensure that a greater volume of energy is ingested to match the raised level of expenditure. At the same time, although there is a process to prevent energy intake falling below expenditure, there does not seem to be a strong process to prevent intake rising above expenditure. Consequently, any intrinsic physiological disturbance that leads to a rise in excitatory (drive) processes or a slight weakening of inhibitory (satiety) signals would allow consumption to drift upwards without generating a compensatory response. For some reason a positive energy balance does not generate an error signal that demands correction. Consequently, the balance between the excitatory and inhibitory processes has implications for body weight regulation and for the induction of obesity.

Ghrelin and hunger drive

Ghrelin is found both in the gut and the brain, the gut being the major source of plasma ghrelin. Endogenous ghrelin levels appear to be responsive to nutritional status; for instance, human plasma ghrelin immunoreactivity increases during fasting and decreases after food intake. Unlike the other peripheral peptides described earlier, ghrelin stimulates rather than inhibits feeding behaviour. Both peripheral and central infusions of ghrelin have been shown to stimulate food intake in rats and mice (Wren *et al.*, 2000). Decreased endogenous ghrelin levels are observed in genetically obese rats and mice, and in dietary-induced obese rats exposed to a high-fat diet (Ariyasu *et al.*, 2002). In lean humans, endogenous plasma ghrelin levels rise markedly before a meal (Cummings *et al.*, 2001) and are suppressed by food intake. In lean healthy volunteers, ghrelin infusions increase food intake, pre-meal hunger and prospective consumption, demonstrating a marked but short-term effect on human appetite (Wren *et al.*, 2001). However, when tested in the laboratory, obese people have a lower level of endogenous ghrelin which is not suppressed by food intake (Tschöp *et al.*, 2001).

For these reasons it has been proposed that ghrelin, linked to the initiation of eating, acts as a compensatory hormone. This means that in obese people and in animals that are made fat experimentally, ghrelin levels would be reduced in an apparent attempt to restore a normal body weight status. Therefore, ghrelin illustrates the characteristics of both an episodic and tonic signal in appetite control. From meal to meal, the oscillations in the ghrelin profile act to initiate and to suppress hunger; over longer periods of time, some factor associated with fat mass applies a general modulation over the profile of ghrelin and therefore, in principle, over the experienced intensity of hunger. This means that when weight is lost, for example following a period of food restriction and weight loss, ghrelin levels would rise and therefore promote the feeling of hunger. This is likely to be one of the signals that makes the loss of body weight so difficult to maintain.

Homeostatic and hedonic processes of appetite control

In the homeostatic approach to appetite control, the emphasis is on processes subserving hunger and fullness in which drives arising from biological needs (see previous section) are balanced by physiological satiety signalling systems. The hedonic component of eating refers to the feeling of pleasure that is associated with eating, and with the concepts of incentive value and reward value of foods. As noted in the previous sections, a physiological substrate for the homeostatic control of eating has become quite well characterized (Figs 10.1 and 10.2) and involves a cluster of peripheral peptides, together with a network of biogenic amines and neuropeptides in the

brain. A biological substrate mediating hedonic processes has also been investigated and includes a largely separate set of brain neurotransmitters, including glutamate, opioids, endocannabinoid and dopamine pathways and the associated receptor systems. Together, these circuits are probably responsible for the biological basis of concepts such as needing, wanting and liking that are associated with the selection and consumption of foods.

One immediate question concerns the degree of independence or separation of these two sets of processes, and therefore of the underlying neural circuits. Another question, equally significant, concerns the extent to which the homeostatic and hedonic components are responsible for the development of weight gain and obesity. Are individuals who are susceptible to weight gain characterized by defects in satiety signalling and chronic high levels of hunger; or are they characterized by an overwhelming hyper-responsivity to the perceived pleasantness of foods?

Researchers have recently attempted to test the independence of the two systems by methodologically separating hedonic response from homeostatic drive. Pharmacological evidence suggests that the substrates are rather separate. For example, in obese subjects, administration of the serotoninergic drug D-fenfluramine (Blundell and Hill, 1987) suppressed the sensation of hunger, but had no effect on the appreciation of the pleasantness of food. Conversely, nalmafene, an opioid agonist, reduced the rated pleasantness of palatable foods, but had no effect on hunger (Yeomans and Wright, 1991).

This double dissociation concept indicates that appreciation of palatability is associated with a specific substrate that can be pharmacologically and, to an extent, methodologically dissected from the substrate mediating hunger (Blundell and Rogers, 1991). However, it is still possible for a functional interaction to occur when the manipulation is made through the natural commodity (selected food), rather than through a more selective artificial manipulation.

Hunger and pleasure—do they interact?

Considering that most studies have repeatedly shown that palatability has a positive effect on intake and meal size would suggest that the palatability of foods is involved in the process of satiation. However, it is less clear whether the palatability of food also has an influence on feelings of hunger and satiety (de Graaf *et al.*, 1999). The possibility of an interaction between palatability and hunger was specifically investigated almost 20 years ago. On separate occasions, subjects consumed a fixed energy meal composed of either highly preferred foods or less preferred equivalent food items (Hill *et al.*, 1984). There was an enhancing effect of palatability (even the sight of a preferred food) on subsequent hunger, which remained high during the meal. However, this fixed meal design did not allow the disclosure of any effect on energy intake. More recently, an overall increase in hunger following consumption of a palatable preload and an equivalent decrease in hunger following a bland preload with corresponding adjustments in *ad libitum* intake were revealed (Yeomans *et al.*, 2001). The authors reported this difference to be irrespective of preload energy or macronutrient content.

Several researchers have examined the effect of food palatability on subsequent satiety. Foods eliciting an enhanced hedonic response appear to promote a more rapid recovery in hunger up to 3 h following consumption than a less palatable preload (Rogers and Blundell, 1990). Moreover, there is evidence that some stimulation of intake occurs over the 24-h period following consumption of optimal-preference sweetened yoghurt preloads (Monneuse *et al.*, 1991). In a more recent study, the effect of food palatability on the degree of energy compensation following preloads has been investigated (Yeomans *et al.*, 2001). The capacity of people to demonstrate compensation is usually regarded as a sign of the sensitivity of the system and indicates good appetite control. However, the presence of a more palatable food prevented compensation. Taken together these studies indicate that the response to the palatability of food does exert an effect on energy intake, and this appears to be mediated via a modulation of hunger. This means that when the homeostatic and hedonic systems are stimulated simultaneously (by food) a synergy occurs that modulates the control of appetite. This process appears to constitute one way through which the hedonic potential of foods could lead to weight gain.

The system does appear to operate asymmetrically; although enhanced hedonic response to foods can augment hunger (and therefore food intake), the presence of strong satiety (developing over the course of a meal) does not downregulate palatability (e.g. Yeomans and Symes, 1999). Indeed it has been documented that subjects in a state of satiety can be induced to prolong their eating by offering them highly palatable foods (Looy *et al.*, 1992). It is also noticeable that the reasons people give for stopping eating emphasize fullness and loss of hunger rather than a decline in the pleasantness of the food (Mook and Votaw, 1992; Zandstra *et al.*, 2000). In other words subjects do not generally perceive the decline in pleasantness to be the most important factor in terminating meals.

Food choice, hedonic response and obesity

In addition to an interaction between palatability and hunger, the perceived pleasantness or hedonic response to foods could also modulate appetite control indirectly by influencing the choice of foods. There is considerable evidence that this is the case. In an experiment in which subjects sampled a range of foods containing varying amounts of fat and rated their sensory preferences, there was a positive relationship between the rated pleasantness of the fat content of the foods and measures of the adiposity of the subjects (Mela and Sacchetti, 1991). The fatter the subjects, the greater was their rated pleasantness

of the fatty foods. More recently, the food choices of monozygotic twins discordant for body weight have been assessed (Rissanen *et al.*, 2002). The twins with the highest degree of fatness displayed a significantly higher preference for fatty foods. If it is assumed that the expression of food preferences is influenced at least in part by the pleasure yielded by the foods then these studies have demonstrated that levels of body fat are associated with a greater rating of pleasantness of fat-containing foods.

Hedonic responsivity and addiction?

In recent times it has been suggested in the media that some people may crave particular foods excessively because they have become addicted to the properties of the foods in a manner analogous to the way in which people become addicted to certain drugs. In fact, it is likely that the reward value of foods and the reward properties of drugs are mediated via the same neural pathways. The pleasure that arises from the taste and consumption of food depends upon the activity of particular neurotransmitter systems (see earlier section). This activity is generated through a natural physiological route, namely the afferent pathways linking gustatory and olfactory sense organs to the brain circuits. Certain addictive drugs can have such powerful rewarding properties (and potent withdrawal effects) because they act directly upon the receptors of the neural circuits with a strength far in excess of that generated by food being eaten. Consequently, there is a huge difference in the potency and quality of the reinforcing sensations generated by food and drugs.

Recent research has explored the link between vulnerability for addiction, its relation to brain dopamine activity and potential of excessive weight gain. Sensitivity to reward (STR), a psychobiological trait reportedly linked to the neurobiology of the mesolimbic dopamine pathway, was used to examine how hedonia, the capacity to experience pleasure, might relate to overconsumption and subsequent weight gain (Davis *et al.*, 2004). Contrary to predictions of a linear relationship between BMI and STR, an inverted-U relationship was revealed with overweight subjects (BMI > 25, < 30) scoring higher than obese and normal-weight subjects. Is it possible that low anhedonia (high STR) promotes a lifestyle of hedonically driven overconsumption, which, over time, downregulates mesolimbic dopamine availability to compensate for its overstimulation?

There is evidence to support this proposition. For example, positron emission tomography (PET) scans of normal-weight healthy subjects eating a favourite meal revealed an increase in dopamine release that correlated with the degree of experienced pleasure. Another study demonstrated that the availability of the dopamine D2 receptor was decreased in obese subjects in proportion to their BMI (Wang *et al.*, 2001).

These studies map onto the idea that there is an optimal level or inverted-U relationship between hedonic predisposition and dopamine activation (Volkow *et al.*, 1999). Subjects who were administered with the dopamine agonist methylphenidate found it either pleasant or unpleasant, depending on their DRD2 receptor levels. Those finding the effects pleasant had significantly lower levels of the dopamine receptor than those who found it unpleasant (Volkow *et al.*, 1999). It can therefore be construed that potent stimuli (including palatable foods) elicit a positive hedonic response through the stimulation of dopamine activity in people who have a tendency towards anhedonia (low pleasure response). However, there is no evidence to date to test the notion that particularly hedonic individuals respond aversively to highly palatable foods. It has been suggested that dopamine activity relating to excessive food consumption might only involve activation of brain reward circuitry within normal limits, with other psychological factors exerting stronger effects (Robinson and Berridge, 2003).

Risk factors for appetite control

Most researchers do not have any trouble accepting the idea that the state of a person's metabolism constitutes a major risk for developing weight gain and becoming obese. However, as obesity develops, metabolic characteristics change so that the state of obesity itself is associated with a different metabolic profile to that accompanying the process of weight gain. This makes it important to do longitudinal studies (while weight is increasing) as well as cross-sectional studies (comparing lean and obese subjects). Recently, Ravussin and Gautier (1999) have drawn attention to this issue and have outlined those metabolic and physiological factors associated with weight gain and with the achievement of obesity.

The tendency to gain weight is associated with a low basal metabolic rate, low-energy cost of physical activity, a low capacity for fat oxidation (relatively high respiratory quotient—RQ), high insulin sensitivity, low sympathetic nervous system activity and a low plasma leptin concentration. In the state of obesity itself, many of these risk factors (or predictors of weight again) are reversed.

Just as certain metabolic variables (risk factors) can lead to a positive energy balance, so we can envisage certain behaviourally mediated processes that themselves constitute the *risk factors* leading to hyperphagia or 'overconsumption' (high-energy intake leading to a positive energy balance). These processes may be patterns of eating behaviour, the sensory or hedonic events that guide behaviour or sensations that accompany or follow eating. For convenience, this cluster of events can be referred to as behavioural risk factors. These events may include a preference for fatty foods, weakened satiation (end-of-meal signals), relatively weak satiety (post-ingestive inhibition over further eating), strong orosensory preferences (e.g. for sweetness combined with fattiness in foods), a binge potential and a high food-induced pleasure re-

sponse. In turn, these events may be subdivided to describe more specific components, leading to a risk of overconsumption (Blundell and Cooling, 2000).

These behavioural risk factors can be regarded as biological dispositions that create a vulnerability for weight gain and which manifest themselves through behavioural acts themselves, or through physiological processes that promote or permit changes in behaviour.

However, such risk factors alone would be unlikely to lead to a positive energy balance in a benign environment, i.e. one in which the food supply and the cultural habits worked against excessive consumption. In most of today's societies, however, the food environment exploits biologically based dispositions and this promotes the achievement of a high-energy intake. This concept is set out in Table 10.1.

Individual variability: resistance and susceptibility to weight gain

The features described in Table 10.1 indicate that it is not the environment alone that is to blame for the epidemic of obesity. Individual traits and characteristics make some people (adults and children) much more likely than others to gain weight and become obese. Some of these traits are associated with physiological processes such as the strength of satiety signalling or the potency of the hedonic response to highly palatable foods; in turn these processes will certainly be linked to allelic variation in particular genes. The picture is complicated, and the polygenic nature of the processes contributing to weight gain will be difficult to elucidate, and even more difficult to convert into management strategies.

Table 10.1 Postulated interactions between behavioural risk factors and the obesogenic environment, which generate a tendency for overconsumption.

Biological vulnerability (behavioural risk factor)
Preference for fatty foods
Weak satiation (end-of-meal signals)
Orosensory responsiveness
Weak post-ingestive satiety
Environmental influence
Abundance of high-fat (high energy density) foods
Large portion size
Availability of highly palatable foods with specific sensory–nutrient combinations
Easy accessibility to foods and presence of potent priming stimuli
Potential for overconsumption
↑ Fat intake
↑ Meal size
↑ Amount eaten
↑ Frequency of eating
↑ Tendency to reinitiate eating

The individual risk factors that confer susceptibility to weight gain may exist not only at the level of specific satiety mechanisms but also at the level of general dispositions, such as the one measured by the disinhibition factor of the Three Factor Eating Questionnaire (TFEQ) (Stunkard and Messick, 1985). The processes underlying a high score on this factor seem to encourage 'opportunistic eating', a tendency that will be exacerbated by many food-related features of the obesogenic environment (Lawton *et al.*, 2004). Just as some individuals are very susceptible to weight gain, others are resistant and can remain lean even consuming a potentially weight-inducing high-fat diet (MacDiarmid *et al.*, 1996).

The logic concerning weight gain can also be applied to weight loss, and there is now clear evidence that in response to the negative energy balance induced by physical activity, some people compensate by increasing food intake so as to resist weight loss, whereas others do not and consequently lose weight (Blundell *et al.*, 2003).

The message from studies on eating behaviour and appetite control is that there exists considerable individual variability underlying the strength of satiety, the willingness to eat and the degree of susceptibility to environmental stimulation; managing the epidemic of obesity is made substantially more difficult (and complicated) by this variability.

References

Ariyasu, H., Takaya, K., Hosoda, H., Iwakura, H., Ebihara, K., Mori, K., Ogawa, Y., Hosoda, K, Akamizu, T., Kojima, M., Kangawa, K. and Nakao, K. (2002) Delayed short-term secretory regulation of ghrelin in obese animals: Evidenced by a specific RIA for the active form of ghrelin. *Endocrinology* **143**, 3341–3350.

Batterham, R.L., Cowley, M.A., Small, C.J., Herzog, H., Dakin, C.L., Wren, A.M., Brynes, A.E., Low, M.J., Ghatel, M.A., Cone, R.D. and Bloom. S.R. (2002) Gut hormone PYY3–36 physiologically inhibits food intake. *Nature* **418**, 650–654.

Batterham, R.L., Cohen, M.A., Ellis, S., Le Roux, C.W., Withers, D.J., Frost, G.S., Ghatei, M.A. and Bloom, S.R. (2003) Inhibition of food intake in obese subjects by peptide YY 3–36. *New England Journal of Medicine* **349**, 941–948.

Blundell, J.E. (1991) Pharmacological approaches to appetite suppression. *Trends in Pharmacological Science* **12**,147–157.

Blundell, J.E. and Hill, A.J. (1987) Serotoninergic modulation of the pattern of eating and the profile of hunger-satiety in humans. *International Journal of Obesity* **11**, 141–153.

Blundell, J.E. and Rogers, P.J. (1991) Hunger, hedonics, and the control of satiation and satiety. In: Friedman, M.I., Tordoff, M.G., Kare, M.R. eds. *Chemical Senses, Appetite and Nutrition*, 4. New York: Marcel Dekker, 127–148.

Blundell, J.E. and Halford, J.C. (1994) Regulation of nutrient supply: the brain and appetite control. *Proceedings of the Nutrition Society* **53**, 407–418.

Blundell, J.E. and Naslund, E. (1999) Invited commentary: Glucagon-like peptide-1, satiety and appetite control. *British Journal of Nutrition* **81**, 259–260.

Blundell, J.E. and Cooling, J. (2000) Routes to obesity: phenotypes, food choices and activity. *British Journal of Nutrition* **83**, S33–S38.

Blundell, J.E., Stubbs, R.J., Hughes, D.A., Whybrow, S. and King, N.A. (2003) Cross talk between physical activity and appetite control: does physical activity stimulate appetite? *Proceedings of the Nutrition Society* **62**, 651–661.

Branson, R., Opotoczna, N., Kral, J.G., Lentes, K.U.,Hoche, M.R. and Horber, F.F. (2003) Binge eating as a major phenotype of melanocortin 4 receptor gene mutation. *New England Journal of Medicine* **348**, 1096–1103.

Campfield, L.S., Smith, F.J., Guiswz, Y., Devos, R. and Burn, P. (1995) Recombinant mouse ob protein: evidence for a peripheral signal linking adiposity and central neural networks. *Science* **269**, 546–549.

Cummings, D.E., Purnell, J.Q., Frayo, R.S., Schmidova, K., Wisse, B.E. and Weigle, D.S. (2001) A pre-prandial rise in plasma ghrelin levels suggests a role in meal initiation in humans. *Diabetes* **50**, 1714–1719.

Davis, C., Strachan, S. and Berkson, M. (2004) Sensitivity to reward: implications for overeating and overweight. *Appetite* **42**,131–138.

Farooqi, I.S., Keogh, J.M.,Yeo, G.S.H., Lank, E.J., Cheetham, T. and O'Rahilly, S. (2003) Clinical spectrum of obesity and mutations in the melanocortin 4 receptor gene. *New England Journal of Medicine* **348**, 1085–1095.

Flint, A., Raben, A., Astrup, A. and Holst, J. (1998) Glucagon like peptide 1 promotes satiety and suppresses energy intake in humans. *Journal of Clinical Investigation* **101**, 515–520.

Friedman, M.I. and Rawson, N.E. (1994) Fuel metabolism and appetite control. In: Fernstrom, J.D., Miller, G.D. eds. *Appetite and Body Weight Regulation*. Boca Raton, FL: CRC Press, 63–76.

de Graaf, C., De Jong, L.S. and Lambers, A.C. (1999) Palatability affects satiation but not satiety. *Physiology and Behaviour* **66**, 681–688.

Greenberg, D., Smith, G.P. and Gibbs, J. (1992) Cholecystokinin and the satiating effect of fat. *Gastroenterology* **102**, 1801–1803.

Greenough, A., Cole, G., Lewis, J., Lockton, A. and Blundell, J. (1998a) Untangling the effects of hunger, anxiety, and nausea on energy intake during intravenous cholecystokinin octapeptide (CCK-8) infusion. *Physiological Behaviour* **65**, 303–310.

Greenough, A., Cole, G., Lewis, J., Lockton, J.A. and Blundell, J.E. (1998b) Intranasal administration of a novel CCK agonist on appetite control in lean men. *International Journal of Obesity* **22** (Suppl.), S16.

Gutzwiller, J.P., Drewe, J., Ketter, S., Hildebrand, P., Krautheim, A. and Beglinger, C. (2000) Interaction between CCK and a preload on food intake is mediated by CCK-A receptors in humans. *American Journal of Physiology* **279**, R189–195.

Halford, J.C.G. and Blundell, J.E. (2000) Differing roles for serotonin and leptin in appetite regulation. *Annals of Medicine* **32**, 222–232.

Hill, A.J.,Magson, L.D. and Blundell, J.E. (1984) Hunger and palatability: tracking ratings of subjective experience before, during and after the consumption of preferred and less preferred food. *Appetite* **5**, 361–371.

Lavin, J.H., Wittert, G.A., Andrews, J., Wishart, J.M., Morris, H.A., Morley, J.E., Horowitz M. and Read N.W. (1998) Interaction of insulin, glucagon-like peptide 1, gastric inhibitory polypeptide, and appetite in response to intraduodenal carbohydrate. *American Journal of Clinical Nutrition* **68**, 591–598.

Lawton, C.L., Croden, F., Alam, R., Golding, C., Whybrow, S., Stubbs, J. and Blundell, J. (2004) Differences between individuals resistant (DIOR) and susceptible (DIOS) to weight gain on a high fat (HF) diet. *International Journal of Obesity* **28** (Suppl.), S218.

Lieverse R.J., Jansen, J.B.M.J., Masclee, A.A.M., Rovati, L.C. and Lamer, C.B.H.W. (1994) Effect of a low dose of intraduodenal fat on satiety in humans: studies using the type A cholecystokinin (CCK) receptor antagonist loxiglumide. *Gut* **35**, 501–505.

Looy, H., Callaghan, S. and Weingarten, H.P. (1992) Hedonic response of sucrose likers and dislikers to other gustatory stimuli. *Physiological Behaviour* **52**, 219–225.

MacDiarmid, J.I., Cade, J.E. and Blundell, J.E. (1996) High and low fat consumers, their macronutrient intake and body mass index: further analysis of the national diet and nutrition survey of British adults. *European Journal of Clinical Nutrition* **50**, 505–512.

Maffei, M., Halaas, J., Ravussin, E., Pratley, R.E., Lee, G.H., Zhang, Y., Fei, H., Kim, S., Lallone, R., Ranganathan, S., Kern, P.A. and Friedman, J.M. (1995) Leptin levels in human and rodent: measurement of plasma leptin and ob RNA in obese and weight reduced subjects. *Nature Medicine* **1**, 1151–1161.

Mei, N. (1985) Intestinal chemosensitivity. *Physiology Review* **65**, 211–237.

Mela, D.J. and Sacchetti, D.A. (1991) Sensory preferences for fats: Relationship with diet and body composition. *American Journal of Clinical Nutrition* **53**, 908–915.

Monneuse, M.O., Bellisle, F. and Louise-Sylverstre, J. (1991) Responses to an intense sweetener in humans: immediate preference and delayed effects on intake. *Physiological Behaviour* **49**, 325–330.

Montague, C.T., Farooqi, I.S., Whitehead, J.P., Soos, M.A., Rau, H., Wareham, N.J., Sewter, C.P., Digby, J.E., Mohammed, S.N., Hurst, J.A., Cheetham, C.H., Earley, A.R., Barnett, A.H., Prins, J.B. and O'Rahilly, S. (1997) Congenital leptin deficiency is associated with severe early onset obesity in humans. *Nature* **387**, 903–908.

Mook, D.G. and Votaw, M.C. (1992) How important is hedonism? Reasons given by college students for ending a meal. *Appetite* **18**, 69–75.

Morris, M.J. and Nguyen, T. (2001) Does neuropeptide Y contribute to the anorectic action of amylin? *Peptides* **22**, 541–546.

Näslund, E., Gutniak, M., Skogar, S., Rössner, S. and Hellström, P.M. (1998) Glucagon-like peptide 1 increases the period of postprandial satiety and slows gastric emptying in obese men. *American Journal of Clinical Nutrition* **68**, 525–530.

Ranganath, L.R., Beety, J.M., Morgan, L.M., Wright, W., Howland, R. and Marks, V. (1996) Attenuated GLP-1 secretion in obesity: cause or consequence? *Gut* **38**, 916–919.

Ratner, R.E., Dickey, R., Fineman, M., Maggs, D.G., Shen, L., Strobel, S.A., Weyer, C. and Kolterman, O.G. (2004) Amylin replacement with pramlintide as an adjunct to insulin therapy improves long-term glycaemic and weight control in Type 1 diabetes mellitas: a 1-year, randomized controlled trial. *Diabetic Medicine* **21**, 1204–1212.

Ravussin, E. and Gautier, J.F. (1999) Metabolic predictors of weight gain. *International Journal of Obesity* **23**, 37–41.

Read, N.W. (1990) Role of gastrointestinal factors in hunger and satiety in man. *Proceedings of the Nutrition Society* **51**, 7–11.

Reda, T.K., Geliebter, A. and Pi-Sunyer, F.X. (2002) Amylin, food intake, and obesity. *Obesity Research* **10**, 1087–1091.

Rissanen, A., Hakala, P., Lissner, L., Matlar, C.E., Koskenvuo, M. and Ronnemaa, T. (2002) Acquired preference especially for dietary fat and obesity: A study of weight-discordant monozygotic twin pairs. *International Journal of Obesity* **26**, 973–977.

Robinson, T.E. and Berridge, K.C. (2003) Addiction. *Annual Review of Psychology* **54**, 25–53.

Rogers, P.J. and Blundell, J.E. (1990) Umami and appetite: effects of monosodium glutamate on hunger and food intake in human subjects. *Physiological Behaviour* **48**, 801–804.

Rushing, P.A., Hagan, M.M., Seeley, R.J., Lutz, T.A., D'Alessio, D.A., Air, E.L. and Woods, S.C. (2001) Inhibition of central amylin signaling increases food intake and body adiposity in rats. *Endocrinology* **142**(1), 5035–5038.

Smith, G.P. and Gibbs, J. (1995) Peripheral physiological determinants of eating and body weight. In: Brownell, K.D., Fairburn, C.G. eds. *Eating Disorders and Obesity: A Comprehensive Handbook.* New York: Guildford Publications, 8–12.

Smith, G.P., Greenberg, D., Corp, E. and Gibbs, J. (1990) Afferent information in the control of eating. In: Bray, G.A., Liss, A.R. eds. *Obesity: Towards a Molecular Approach.* New York: Alan R. Liss, 63–79.

Stellar, E. (1954) The physiology of motivation. *Psychology Review* **61**, 5–22.

Stunkard, A.J. and Messick, S. (1985) The three-factor eating questionnaire to measure dietary restraint, dishinibition, and hunger. *Journal of Psychosomatic Research* **29**, 71–81.

Tschöp, M., Weyer, C., Tataranni, A., Devenarayan, V., Ravussin, E. and Heiman, M.L. (2001) Circulating ghrelin levels are decreased in human obesity. *Diabetes* **50**, 707–709.

Volkow, N.D., Wang, G.J., Fowler, J.S., Logan, J., Gatley, S.J., Gifford, A., Hitzemann, R., Ding, Y.S. and Pappas, N. (1999) Prediction of reinforcing responses to psychostimulants in humans by brain dopamine D2 receptor levels. *American Journal of Psychiatry* **156**, 1440–1443.

Wang, G.J., Volkow, N.D., Logan, J., Pappas, N.R., Wong, C.T., Zhu, W., Netusil, N. and Fowler, J.S. (2001) Brain dopamine and obesity. *Lancet* **357**, 354–357.

Weigle, D. (1994) Appetite and the regulation of body composition. *Journal of the Federal American Society of Experimental Biology* **8**, 302–310.

Welch, I., Saunders, K. and Read, N.W. (1985) Effect of ileal and intravenous infusions of fat emulsions on feeding and satiety in human volunteers. *Gastroenterology* **89**, 1293–1297.

Wren, A.M., Small, C.J., Ward, H.L., Murphy, K.G., Dakin, C.L. Taheri, S., Kennedy, A.R., Roberts, G.H., Morgan, D.G.A., Ghatei, M.A. and Bloom, S.R. (2000) The novel hypothalamic peptide ghrelin stimulates food intake and growth hormone secretion. *Endocrinology* **141**, 4325–4328.

Wren, A.M., Seal, L.J., Cohen, M.A. Brynes, A.E., Frost, G.S., Murphy, K.G., Dhillo, W.S. and Ghatei, M.A. (2001) Ghrelin enhances appetite and increases food intake in humans. *Journal of Clinical Endocrinology and Metabolism* **86**, 5992–5995.

Yeomans, M.R. and Symes, T. (1999) Individual differences in the use of pleasantness and palatability ratings. *Appetite* **32**, 383–394.

Yeomans, M.R. and Wright, P. (1991) Lower pleasantness of palatable foods in nalmefene-treated human volunteers. *Appetite* **16**, 249–259.

Yeomans, M.R., Lee, M.D., Gray, R.W. and French, S.J. (2001) Effects of test-meal palatability on compensatory eating following disguised fat and carbohydrate preloads. *International Journal of Obesity* **25**, 1215–1224.

Zandstra, E.H., de Graaf, C., Mela, D.J. and Van Staveren, W.A. (2000) Short- and long-term effects of changes in pleasantness on food intake. *Appetite* **34**, 253–260.

Zhang, Y., Proenca, R., Maffei, M., Barone, M., Leopold, L. and Friedman, J.M. (1994) Positional cloning of the mouse obese gene and its human homologue. *Nature* **372**, 425–432.

Energy expenditure in humans: the influence of activity, diet and the sympathetic nervous system

Hamid R. Farshchi, Moira A. Taylor and Ian A. Macdonald

Introduction, 149

Energy expenditure: definition,
measurement and components, 149
   Definitions, 149
   Measurements, 149
   Components of energy
   expenditure, 151
   Resting energy expenditure, 152
   Physical activity, 154

Mechanisms and sites of
thermogenesis and the sympathetic
nervous system, 156
   Thermogenic stimuli, 156
   The sympathetic nervous
   system, 156

Obesity and energy expenditure, 157

References, 158

Introduction

This chapter will consider the basic components of whole-body energy metabolism, including the contributions from physical activity and diet, and the potential regulatory role of the sympathetic nervous system. The main part of the chapter will focus on non-obese people, aiming to describe the underlying normal physiology, but the final sections will consider the influence of obesity on energy expenditure.

Energy expenditure: definition, measurement and components

Definitions

The various chemical processes that underlie the functions of the body require the continuous provision of energy. In most cases, this energy is supplied by high-energy bonds within adenosine triphosphate (ATP). ATP availability is maintained by the utilization of the major fuels, glucose and fatty acids. Although in the short term some fuel utilization and ATP production can occur anaerobically (e.g. by the production of lactate from glucose), the capacity and duration of such provision is limited, and for all practical purposes only the oxidation of the fuels to carbon dioxide and water is of importance. Thus, the overall processes involved in the body's energy metabolism can be summarized by first, the oxidation of fuels producing carbon dioxide, water and ATP (with approximately 60% of the food energy being released as heat during the production of ATP) and second, the utilization of the ATP in the chemical processes of the body. Thus, the energy contained within the fuels (originally the food consumed) is first converted to ATP or lost as heat, and subsequently utilized in various metabolic processes (Fig. 11.1). This overall process is referred to as energy expenditure, and represents the utilization of food energy to maintain the functions of the body. The close relationship between energy expenditure and the metabolic processes of the body explains why the term metabolic rate is used synonymously with energy expenditure.

Measurements

Energy expenditure can be measured using either the release of heat or the consumption of oxygen and production of carbon dioxide (as a by-product of the chemical reactions). Direct caloric measurement (i.e. measuring heat released) of whole-body energy expenditure requires complex, expensive equipment (a direct calorimeter) and is only appropriate in closely defined experimental conditions. An alternative, more widely used approach is to assess energy expenditure using indirect calorimetry, calculating energy expenditure from the rates of oxygen use and carbon dioxide production. The advantage of such measurements of respiratory gas exchange is that an assessment can also be made of which fuel (i.e. carbohydrate or fat) is being used as a substrate for energy

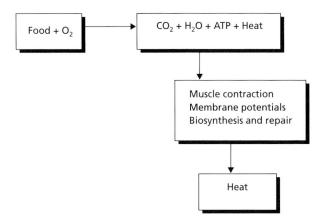

Fig 11.1 Summary of energy exchanges in the body.

Table 11.1 Summary of oxidation of the macronutrients. (Adapted from Frayn and Macdonald, 1997.)

Glucose
1 g of glucose + 0.747 L O_2 = 0.747 L of CO_2 + 0.6 g H_2O + 15.15 kJ
RQ = 1.0
Energy content = 15.15 kJ/g
Energy release = 20.83 kJ/L O_2

Triglyceride
1 g of fat + 2.023 L O_2 = 1.436 L CO_2 + 1.07 g H_2O + 39.63 kJ
RQ = 0.71
Energy content = 39.63 kJ/g
Energy release = 19.59 kJ/L O_2

Protein
1 g of protein + 1.031 L O_2 = 0.859 L CO_2 + 0.403 g H_2O + (urea, ammonia and creatinine) + 19.72 kJ
RQ = 0.833
Energy content = 19.72 kJ/g
Energy release = 19.13 kJ/L O_2

metabolism. The disadvantage of indirect calorimetry is the need for either a respiratory valve and noseclip for exercising subjects or a ventilated canopy for resting subjects. A respiration chamber can be used for both resting and exercising measurements, the complexity and expense being less than for a direct calorimeter. A more extensive account of the principles of indirect calorimetry and methods of measurement can be found in Frayn and Macdonald (1997) and Murgatroyd *et al.* (1993).

An important principle in relation to energy expenditure and substrate utilization relates to the differences in oxygen utilization and energy release for the different macronutrients. Table 11.1 illustrates the major differences, showing the more than twofold difference in energy released per gram of nutrient during the oxidation of fat compared with carbohydrate or protein, and that for the energy expenditure a greater oxygen uptake is needed when using fat as a fuel rather than carbohy-

drate. The other major difference between the substrates is the ratio of carbon dioxide produced to oxygen consumed—the respiratory quotient (RQ). Thus, measurement of respiratory gas exchange enables energy expenditure to be estimated, and the RQ value provides an indication of the principal substrate(s) being utilized.

The traditional approaches of using direct or indirect calorimetry techniques to determine energy expenditure are able to detect minute-by-minute changes in energy expenditure but are of limited use in longer term studies, or for measuring free-living energy expenditure. This problem can be overcome by using the doubly labelled water (DLW) technique (using the non-radioactive isotopes deuterium and oxygen-18) to assess mean daily total energy expenditure over a period of 10–14 days in adults (for a review, see Prentice, 1988 and Chapter 2). This technique is based on the principle that the metabolic processes of the body involve the incorporation of water in a number of reactions. When such reactions occur, the oxygen from the water will end up as carbon dioxide (and be lost from the body in expired air), whereas the hydrogen will end up in water and only be lost in sweat, urine and as respiratory water vapour. The rate of incorporation of water and labelled water into these metabolic pathways is proportional to the rate of whole-body energy metabolism, so a measurement of the differential loss of oxygen and hydrogen labels from an initial, 'doubly labelled' loading dose provides an estimate of the body's rate of carbon dioxide production, and thus oxygen consumption, over the period of measurement (for a more detailed account, see Murgatroyd *et al.*, 1993).

The disadvantages of the DLW method are the availability and cost of the isotope, and the duration of the measurement. The method is unsuitable for detecting short-term differences in energy expenditure. The technique is also unable to determine what fuel mix is being used. The former problems can be overcome with the 'bicarbonate–urea' method (Elia *et al.*, 1995), which produces valid estimates of total energy expenditure over a period for 2–3 days, involving the measurement of carbon-14 appearance in urinary urea. This method is relatively inexpensive, but does involve administering a radioactive substance (admittedly in very small amounts).

Many researchers have attempted to use techniques such as heart rate (HR) monitoring and movement sensing to find cheaper and more feasible ways of measuring energy expenditure. There is a reasonably close relationship between HR and energy expenditure, so records of HR give an estimate of energy expenditure. The optimal method for energy expenditure estimation via HR monitoring is called the FLEX HR method (Spurr *et al.*, 1988). In this method, HR and oxygen uptake ($\dot{V}O_2$) for each person are simultaneously monitored while lying down, sitting, standing and doing exercise. The FLEX HR is determined from the highest HR in the resting state and the lowest HR from light activity. At low levels of energy expenditure (i.e. changes in posture at rest), HR rises more steeply than energy expenditure. Furthermore, HR

Table 11.2 Prediction formulas for resting metabolic rate (kJ/24 h).

Author(s)	Formula*	Population in which formula was developed
Males		
Harris and Benedict	[66 + (13.8 × W) + (5 × H) − (6.8 × A) × 4.18]	Normal weight
Schofield (18–29 years)	[(63 × W) + 2896)]	Normal weight and obese
Schofield (30–59 years)	[(48 × W) + 3653)]	Normal weight and obese
Schofield (18–29 years)	[(63 × W) − (0.42 × H) + 2953]	Normal weight and obese
Schofield (30–59 years)	[(48 × W) − (0.11 × H) + 3670]	Normal weight and obese
Females		
Harris and Benedict	[655 + (9.5 × W) + (1.9 × H) − (4.7 × A) × 4.18]	Normal weight
Schofield (18–29 years)	[(62 × W) + 2036]	Normal weight and obese
Schofield (30–59 years)	[(34 × W) + 3538]	Normal weight and obese
Schofield (18–29 years)	[(57 × W) + (11.84 × H) + 411]	Normal weight and obese
Schofield (30–59 years)	[(34 × W) + (0.06 × H) + 3530]	Normal weight and obese

*W, weight in kilograms; H, height in centimetres; A, age in years.

is affected by factors other than physical activity, such as emotional stress, high temperature and humidity, dehydration and illness in which changes in HR are unrelated to $\dot{V}o_2$ changes.

Motion sensors are mechanical and electronic instruments that are used to estimate energy expenditure by picking up motion or acceleration of a limb or the trunk. This method has been criticized because of inaccuracy. Pedometers rely heavily on individual calibration of stride length. Triaxial monitors are designed to incorporate more planes of measurement. Most devices are inappropriate for use in a swimming pool. Recently, the combination of HR and motion sensors has been used to estimate energy expenditure. The principle is to use a motion sensor as a back-up measure to confirm that elevations in HR are representative of response to physical activity. The preliminary studies showed of this method for energy expenditure estimation to be valid (Rennie *et al.*, 2000). Further investigation in free-living subjects to validate against DLW is necessary.

Predicting resting metabolic rate

Information on resting energy expenditure in conjunction with a multiplier for other components of energy expenditure (see next section) is essential to calculate energy requirements at a population level. There are several prediction formulas for resting metabolic rate (RMR). The most commonly used RMR prediction equations are those of Harris and Benedict (1919) and Schofield (1985) (Table 11.2). The formulas are different in terms of the inclusion of weight, height, age and sex (Harris and Benedict, 1919; Schofield, 1985). These formulas provide a valid estimation of RMR for population-based studies in which measuring RMR is not feasible. However, individual er-

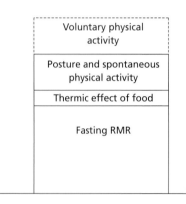

Fig 11.2 Components of daily energy expenditure—the distribution represents a sedentary individual. Broken lines indicate that voluntary activity can be variable, a large amount of voluntary activity will increase the total energy expenditure and reduce the proportional contribution of the other components.

rors make it necessary to measure RMR instead of predicting it in individual studies.

Components of energy expenditure

Whole-body energy expenditure can be separated into a number of components, with the major distinctions being between rest and activity (Fig. 11.2). The actual distribution of total energy expenditure between these two components obviously depends on the level of physical activity. In sedentary non-obese people the energy expended in physical activity accounts for only 20–40% of the total energy expenditure (Ravussin *et al.*, 1986), whereas this proportion can be even less in obese individuals.

Resting energy expenditure

Fasting, resting metabolic rate

In most individuals the major component of total energy expenditure is resting metabolic rate (RMR). The fasting RMR, measured after an overnight fast and a period of at least 30 min of supine rest at a comfortable temperature, is a more appropriate assessment of a person's baseline level of metabolism than trying to determine their basal metabolic rate (BMR), which has stricter measurement criteria. The latter is of little value when considering energy metabolism in relation to obesity and is an expression that should not be used unless the criteria have been strictly met. The fasting RMR includes the expenditure of energy for maintaining membrane potentials, resting cardiorespiratory function, basal rates of turnover of proteins and maintenance of body temperature.

Other factors such as cold, stress and drugs can affect RMR. The main determinants of fasting RMR are body size and composition, in particular the size of the fat-free mass (FFM), which is of course where the metabolic processes occur. Thus, the larger a person is, the greater their fasting RMR will be. Although the size of the FFM is the major determinant of fasting RMR, there may also be an influence of fat mass, age and sex, and these four factors can together account for approximately 80% of the variation in fasting RMR that is seen among individuals (Rising *et al.*, 1994). However, it is clear that FFM is the most important determinant of fasting RMR. Segal and colleagues (1989) showed that in young men (thus, removing influences of age and gender) when differences in FFM were taken into account by analysis of covariance, there was no residual effect of fat mass, even though their subjects had a wide range of fat masses.

In general, fasting RMR is approximately 90 J/kg FFM/min. Thus, someone weighing 75 kg, with a FFM of 63 kg (i.e. 16% fat), will have a fasting RMR of approximately 5.7 kJ/min. Some variation in the metabolic activity of the FFM does occur, as a consequence of differences in the composition of the FFM (Elia, 1992). Thus, a person with a larger proportion of their FFM as muscle will tend to have a lower fasting RMR/kg FFM than someone who had a greater proportion as visceral organs, brain and heart (which have a higher metabolic activity than resting muscle).

Food ingestion

The consumption of food is associated with an increase in energy expenditure and oxygen consumption. This was first observed over 200 years ago by Lavoisier and, since then, has been described by a number of terms. The most appropriate terms for this process are the thermic effect of food (TEF) and dietary (or diet-induced) thermogenesis (DIT). Thermogenesis literally means heat production, and so can be equated with energy expenditure. However, it is most appropriately used to represent conditions in which energy expenditure is stimulated above baseline. The term TEF is most appropriately used when considering the increase in metabolism associated with a single meal, and can be measured in resting subjects using indirect calorimetry with a ventilated canopy. DIT should really be used to describe the longer term effects on total energy expenditure of a given dietary intake (i.e. it is that component of 24-h energy expenditure associated with the amount and composition of the food consumed). Thus, DIT can be reduced during periods of underfeeding, or when consuming a high-fat diet, or increased during overfeeding, especially with a high carbohydrate intake.

The thermic effect of food: potential influencing factors

A major problem when trying to draw conclusions about possible differences in thermogenic responses to different-sized meals is the duration of the responses. Large meals (in excess of 4 MJ) can stimulate energy expenditure for several hours, making it very difficult to determine the total responses. There is some evidence that small meals produce smaller overall thermogenic responses than large meals, but in many cases the conclusions may not be reliable because of inappropriate study designs. For example, Tai and colleagues (1991) compared the thermogenic responses over a 5-h period to a single, 3.1-MJ meal, or to six 0.52-MJ meals eaten at 30-min intervals. The overall thermogenic response over the 5 h was less with the six small meals, but this is likely to be in part due to the intermittent nature of the measurements, and the failure to measure the total response to the multiple small meals. Similarly, Vaz and colleagues (1995) found a smaller thermogenic response over 2 h to three 1.05-MJ meals consumed in the first 60 min than to a single 3.15-MJ meal at the start of the 2 h. However, neither response was maximal by 2 h, and measurements of energy expenditure were only made for 10–12 min in every 30. Thus, it would be unsafe to conclude that for the same total energy intake, a series of small meals is associated with a smaller thermogenic response than a single large meal.

We recently found that an irregular meal frequency for 14 days led to a lower postprandial energy expenditure than with a regular meal frequency in lean (Farshchi *et al.*, 2004) and obese women (Farshchi *et al.*, 2005). Although a comprehensive feeding study is required to investigate the mechanism of this effect, it may have some practical significance as Western populations are increasingly moving away from regular meals, perhaps because of wider availability of ready prepared meals at home and greater opportunity to eat more meals outside the home.

It appears that meal type affects the TEF, with solid food producing a greater response than homogenized liquids with the same nutrient content (Brondel and Le Blanc, 1985). This has been attributed to the solid food being more palatable, producing a hedonistic response that increases the activation of the sympathetic nervous system (SNS). However, although we have confirmed this effect of solid food (compared with a liquid test meal), we did not find an accompanying enhancement of the plasma noradrenaline response (an index of the SNS) to the test meal (Habas and Macdonald, 1998).

It is widely believed that the TEF is greater when consuming a high-carbohydrate meal than after an isoenergetic meal that is high in fat. This is partly based on the demonstrations that administration of glucose (either orally or intravenously) stimulates energy expenditure by the equivalent of 7–10% of the amount of glucose stored (Thiebaud *et al.*, 1983a) but triglyceride infusion only produces an increase in energy expenditure equivalent to 2% of the fat stored (Thiebaud *et al.*, 1983b). However, these effects are not always apparent when food is ingested, as Kinabo and Durnin (1990) found no difference in the TEF over 5 h when meals with 70% carbohydrate or 65% fat were compared.

The types of carbohydrate and fat ingested may also have significant effects on the TEF. Oral ingestion of fructose produces a greater thermogenic response than the same amount of glucose (Tappy *et al.*, 1986), but it is less clear whether similar effects occur when mixed-nutrient test meals are used. Meals containing saturated fat appear to produce a lower TEF than meals containing medium-chain triglyceride (Scalfi *et al.*, 1991). It has been shown that substitution of 6 g of visible fat for fish oil for a period of 3 weeks was accompanied by an increase in fasting energy expenditure and fat oxidation (Couet *et al.*, 1997). It has been known for over 100 years that protein has a larger stimulatory effect on TEF than fat or carbohydrate. How this translates to possible differences in meals with varying protein content remains the subject of investigation. Further work is needed to establish the effect of diet composition on energy expenditure.

Recently, much attention has been focused on the flavanol content of foods and their possible influence on energy expenditure. It was reported that tea consumption can promote fat oxidation and increase 24-h energy expenditure (Dulloo *et al.*, 1999; Rumpler *et al.*, 2001). Admittedly, both studies reported that these promoting effects are related not only to caffeine content, but also to other constituents such as polyphenols, which have a synergistic effect on thermogenesis. Polyphenols may reduce the turnover of noradrenaline, explaining the synergistic impact of these components on energy expenditure.

Diet-induced thermogenesis: effects on total energy expenditure

With normal diets, eaten in sufficient quantities to satisfy energy requirements, the overall stimulation of energy expenditure is equal to 8–10% of the energy intake (Schutz *et al.*, 1984). Thus, an individual with a fasting RMR of 4 kJ/min remaining supine and fasting for 24 h would use 5.76 MJ of energy. In order to maintain energy balance, the individual would require an energy intake equivalent to 110% of this (6.34 MJ) because of the amount of energy expended in DIT. Thus, it should be obvious that a low total energy intake will be associated with a lower DIT, and thus a smaller total energy expenditure. This contributes to the reduction in energy expenditure seen with negative energy balance. However, the adaptation to excess energy intake is controversial. It was reported that an excessive total energy intake can lead to increased DIT and total energy expenditure, especially if carbohydrate is eaten to excess. This implies that the weight gain is lower than expected according to the raised energy intake. On the other hand, other investigations failed to confirm this phenomenon. It was suggested that there is a threshold in cumulative overfeeding which could trigger the facultative thermogenesis to maintain energy balance. However, this is unlikely to occur with the modest degrees of overeating that are likely to contribute to the development of obesity.

Growth

Growth in children involves numerous complex chemical processes that have a substantial energy cost. Protein synthesis and turnover alone account for approximately 25% of fasting RMR in healthy adults. The increased protein deposition occurring during growth has an additional energy cost and contributes to the elevated energy expenditure seen during growth spurts in children.

Cold

There is no doubt that in many animal species (e.g. rats), chronic exposure to the cold is associated with an increase in energy expenditure. During the early stages of cold exposure, energy expenditure increases due to shivering, but in the rat this is soon replaced by non-shivering mechanisms of increased energy expenditure (non-shivering thermogenesis).

Exposure of human beings to the cold will produce an increase in energy expenditure due to shivering. Vigorous shivering can raise energy expenditure at least fourfold above baseline resting values. There is some controversy over the effects of cold exposure on non-shivering energy expenditure in humans. There is some evidence of increased thyroid hormone function and sleeping energy expenditure in non-obese women exposed to mild cold (Lean *et al.*, 1988), which may represent a stimulation of non-shivering thermogenesis. In addition, Bruck and colleagues (1976) showed that 10 days of continued exposure to mild/moderate cold was associated with an increase in fasting, resting energy expenditure. However, this effect was small (10–15%) compared with the effect seen in cold-adapted rodents, and was only observed in those subjects demonstrating adaptation to the cold by a lowering of the core temperature threshold needed to elicit a shivering response.

Hormonal factors

It has been known for several decades that thyroid hormone

administration increases RMR. The effect on the RMR appears after several days of hormonal administration. Hyperthyroid patients have a higher metabolic rate due to the blood T_3 level and may attain 180% of the standard value (Randin *et al.*, 1986). There is no general agreement about the mechanism of thyroid hormone effect, but an increase in the Na,K-ATPase activity in various tissues and in the protein turnover rate are likely contributors.

There is some evidence that menstrual cycle affects RMR in women (Solomon *et al.*, 1982). Solomon and colleagues (1982) reported that RMR decreased at menstruation and fell to its lowest point approximately 1 week before ovulation, subsequently rising until the beginning of the next menstrual period. The variation of RMR measurements over the menstrual cycle may be due to the sex hormone variations over the period. Further investigation is needed to determine the effect of menstrual cycle on RMR variation in women.

Gene polymorphism and energy expenditure

Genetic factors may contribute to the interindividual differences observed in the components of energy expenditure. It has been reported that variations in resting metabolic rate appear to be lower within families than between them, which indicates that resting metabolic rate is at least to some extent genetically determined.

Adrenoceptors have attracted substantial attention as possible genetic factors contributing to energy expenditure regulation. It was reported that a missense mutation in codon 64 of the gene for the β_3-adrenoceptor with a replacement of tryptophan by arginine (Trp64Arg) may be implicated in obesity (Clement *et al.*, 1995; 1996). However, this was not confirmed by others (Gagnon *et al.*, 1996). Studies on the association between the Trp64Arg polymorphism and RMR also showed contradictory results (Clement *et al.*, 1995; Gagnon *et al.*, 1996; Sipilainen *et al.*, 1997).

Uncoupling proteins (UCPs) have also been investigated as factors controlling heat generation at the mitochondrial level, which might affect energy balance, but the results were inconclusive (Ricquier and Bouillaud, 2000). Overall, in light of the emerging importance of gene polymorphisms in energy expenditure regulation, further investigations are required.

Non-exercise activity thermogenesis

Non-exercise activities are the activities of daily living other than exercise and include sitting, standing and fidgeting. Evidence has recently appeared that variation in non-exercise activity thermogenesis (NEAT) may tend to change energy balance and contribute to the physiology of weight change (Levine *et al.*, 2000). NEAT was identified as an effective factor for resisting fat gain in the event of overfeeding. A variety of factors affect NEAT such as occupation, age, genetic background, body composition and seasonal variations. However, determining the true estimate of non-exercise activities is difficult in free-living individuals. The mechanism of NEAT needs further investigations (Levine, 2003).

Table 11.3 Energy costs of physical activities.

Sleeping	4.5
Sitting	5.0
Standing	6.0
Brisk walking (6.4 km/h)	30
Running (8 km/h)	43
Cycling (16 km/h)	30
Swimming (25 rn/min)	28

Values are kJ/min for a non-obese 70-kg individual.

Physical activity

The majority of the population are now so sedentary that physical activity accounts for only approximately 30% of total daily energy expenditure. This has undoubtedly contributed to the increased incidence of obesity in recent years, and low levels of physical activity are also a separate identified risk factor for the occurrence of cardiovascular disease. Thus, increased levels of physical activity are important for promoting health, and as part of the necessary lifestyle strategy needed to reduce the chances of developing obesity. This section will focus on the latter, considering the levels of energy expenditure associated with different types of physical activity, and also assessing the potential effects of regular physical activity on resting energy expenditure and weight control.

At the simplest level, activity-related energy expenditure can be defined as any situation that raises energy expenditure above the resting supine or seated level. Thus, maintaining an upright posture requires a higher energy expenditure than when seated, and the difference is usually 20–50% of the seated value. Any type of activity which is weight bearing (e.g. walking, running, climbing) requires an energy expenditure that is proportional to body weight and speed of movement. By contrast, activities such as swimming, rowing and to some extent cycling are less affected by body weight. Table 11.3 shows approximate energy expenditures for standard activities, although the actual value for any individual is dependent on his or her body weight and how the exercise is performed. One of the effects of learning an activity and performing it regularly is that improvements can be made in the effectiveness (or efficiency) of movements, so that a slightly lower energy expenditure is needed for the same activity. However, this effect is fairly modest, and is unlikely to alter the energy expenditure by more than a few per cent.

Consideration of the values presented in Table 11.3 shows the potential effect of different levels of physical activity on energy expenditure. If a 70-kg individual with an inactive total daily energy expenditure of 9 MJ increased his or her activity levels by walking for 30 min every day at 6.4 km/h, this would require the expenditure of an additional 750 kJ (i.e. 30 kJ/min for exercise—5 kJ/min resting value × 30 min).

Thus, this would increase total daily expenditure by only 8%. Obviously, if the individual walked or ran faster, for longer, uphill or carrying a load, this would increase the energy costs.

Types of physical activity

The simplest distinction that can be made is to separate the types of activity into those that occur as a result of aerobic metabolic pathways, and those that require anaerobic mechanisms of energy release. The latter are the short-duration, high-intensity types of activity, such as sprinting (e.g. running for a bus) or running up the stairs. These types of activity have very high rates of energy expenditure (over 100 kJ/min) but can only be sustained for a few seconds. Thus, the total amount of energy expended is small. In addition, because the immediate energy release is anaerobic (usually with the production of lactate) it takes several minutes to recover from the metabolic disturbances produced. This anaerobic type of activity is of little value in relation to the control of body weight, although it may be of value in relation to developing and maintaining muscle mass.

Aerobic types of physical activity are of much greater importance for total daily energy expenditure, and the prevention and treatment of obesity. When describing an individual's capacity for aerobic activity, the term maximal oxygen uptake ($\dot{V}O_{2\,max}$ is widely used. This is usually expressed as millilitres of O_2 per kilogram of body weight (or sometimes kilogram of FFM) per min and describes the maximum rate that an individual can sustain for at least 1 min. Sedentary individuals with a low $\dot{V}O_{2\,max}$ will usually have values ranging from 30 to 40 mL/kg/min, whereas those accustomed to high levels of physical activity and with a high $\dot{V}O_{2\,max}$ can have values exceeding 60 mL/kg/min. When one considers that a non-obese individual would have a fasting, resting energy expenditure of approximately 75 J/kg/min (equivalent to 3.8 mL/O_2/kg/min) if his or her $\dot{V}O_{2\,max}$ was 35 mL/kg/min the individual would be exhausted when increasing energy expenditure by less than 10-fold above resting.

Physical activity at a large proportion of $\dot{V}O_{2\,max}$ (above 70%) cannot be maintained for long periods of time, except in those who are physically highly trained. However, provided someone becomes accustomed to being active, lower intensities of effort (40–60% $\dot{V}O_{2\,max}$) can be sustained for extensive periods of time (up to several hours). Under these conditions, physical activity can make a substantial contribution to total energy expenditure, especially if the person's $\dot{V}O_{2\,max}$ is reasonably high. For example, a 75-kg individual with a $\dot{V}O_{2\,max}$ of 45 mL/kg/min would consume approximately 300 L of oxygen if exercising at 50% of this maximum for 3 h, which is the equivalent of 6 MJ (1 L of oxygen leading to the release of approximately 20 kJ of energy). If the individual remained at rest for those 3 h, the energy expenditure would have been 1 MJ. Thus, sustained recreational activities such as walking or cycling can be associated with a substantial energy expenditure.

Fuel utilization during activity

It has been known for many years that high-intensity activity requires a continuous supply of carbohydrate to the exercising muscles, whereas lower intensity exercise can be sustained through the oxidation of fatty acids (for a review, see Astrand and Rodahl, 1977). At exercise intensities below 50% of an individual's $\dot{V}O_{2\,max}$, oxidation of fat is the major source of energy, whereas activity above this intensity requires a greater contribution from carbohydrate. Thus, if increased physical activity is to be used as part of a lifestyle strategy to prevent or treat obesity, it is usually of benefit to use lower intensity activities that maximize the rates of fat oxidation. There have been some suggestions that obese individuals are characterized by an alteration in the fibre-type profile within their skeletal muscles, such that they have a reduced capacity for oxidizing fat (Wade *et al.*, 1990), but this is a controversial topic that has not been confirmed by subsequent studies. It is clear that increasing the level of habitual physical activity (training) can improve fat utilization at a given exercise intensity, but as most obese individuals are physically inactive, obesity will reduce the level of fat utilization during activity.

Physical activity and resting energy expenditure

There has been substantial debate for many years as to whether the level of physical activity, or training, can affect resting energy expenditure. It is well established that prolonged, high-intensity exercise can elevate resting energy expenditure for several hours but it is less clear whether regular exercise training, or increased habitual physical activity, has a similar effect. In a cross-sectional study, Broeder and colleagues (1992a) could find no relationship between $\dot{V}O_{2\,max}$ and resting energy expenditure (per kg FFM), although it is interesting to note that the subjects with the lowest $\dot{V}O_{2\,max}$ had the highest percentage body fat content. An associated study from the same authors (Broeder *et al.*, 1992b) could find no effect of 12 weeks of increased physical activity, which increased $\dot{V}O_{2\,max}$ by 10% on resting energy expenditure of young men. However, an interesting observation from this study was that the trained subjects showed small reductions in body fat content, indicative of a slight negative energy balance over the study period. Normally, negative energy balance is associated with a reduction in resting energy expenditure, but the exercise-trained subjects did not show such a reduction. By contrast, Poehlman and colleagues (1991) found a weak relationship between resting energy expenditure and $\dot{V}O_{2\,max}$ in non-obese young women, even when body composition was taken into account.

Physical activity, energy balance and body weight

One argument against the use of increased physical activity as a means of regulating energy balance is that it will stimulate energy intake. However, many studies have now shown that when subjects change from a sedentary lifestyle to moderate degrees of physical activity, there is no increase in energy intake. The study by Broeder and colleagues (1992b) provides an example of this, where 1 h of exercise, 4 days per week for 12 weeks, was not accompanied by any increase in voluntary food intake. Obviously, very high levels of physical activity need to be accompanied by an appropriate energy intake, with a high-carbohydrate diet being of particular importance when high-intensity exercise is performed.

The other benefit of increased physical activity is as an adjunct to dietary modification for weight loss in obesity. Obviously, if increased activity is added to a certain dietary energy deficit then theoretically a greater negative energy balance and more body fat loss should be achieved. However, of greater importance is that the combination of diet and exercise produces a greater loss of body fat (but not FFM) than diet alone (Kempen et al., 1995). Furthermore, Racette and colleagues (1995) showed that increasing physical activity levels improved the ability of obese subjects to comply with a dietary restriction programme.

In addition, physical activity is widely recommended to prevent and treat obesity-related complications such as diabetes and coronary heart disease (CHD). Although the cardiovascular benefits of increased physical activity are likely to be multifactorial, much attention has been focused on the known high-density lipoprotein (HDL) cholesterol-raising effects of regular physical activity. Physical activity can also lower serum triglyceride concentration and favourably influence both low-density lipoprotein and HDL particle sizes. Furthermore, physical activity increases insulin sensitivity and reduces the likelihood of type 2 diabetes developing. Although the beneficial effects of physical activity on lipid and carbohydrate metabolism are modest and variable, they are likely to be specifically important in reducing the morbidity and mortality from CHD on a population level, and may be important in patients with atherogenic dyslipidaemia.

Mechanisms and sites of thermogenesis and the sympathetic nervous system

There are numerous thermogenic mechanisms, including substrate cycling, mitochondrial uncoupling in brown adipose tissue and increased sodium pump activity, the details of which are beyond the scope of this chapter. However, it is worthwhile considering which tissues and organs may be important sites of thermogenesis (i.e. increased resting energy expenditure) in adult humans, and what role the SNS may have in regulating their metabolic activity.

Thermogenic stimuli

It has been known for over 60 years that the catecholamines noradrenaline and adrenaline can stimulate resting energy expenditure in humans (Cori and Buchwald, 1930). The plasma adrenaline threshold for stimulating energy expenditure is just above normal resting adrenaline concentrations (Macdonald et al., 1985), with mild stimuli such as postural change and mental arithmetic being capable of raising the concentrations above this threshold. Maximal stimulation of energy expenditure (25–30% above resting) occurs when adrenaline concentrations rise to 5- to 10-fold above basal. It was originally thought that catecholamine-induced thermogenesis was due to a stimulation of lipolysis in adipose tissue and increased fat oxidation (Steinberg et al., 1964), but it is now clear that at steady state there is a generalized stimulation of metabolism with increased fat and carbohydrate oxidation and little change in RQ. In association with this, it is clear that many tissues of the body are involved in the thermogenic response to catecholamines, with skeletal muscle and the viscera being particularly important (for a review, see Webber and Macdonald, 1993).

It is possible that some of the nutrient-induced thermogenesis discussed earlier is due to a stimulatory effect of catecholamines, as in some circumstances the beta-adrenoceptor antagonist propranolol can reduce the energy expenditure response to glucose (Acheson et al., 1983) or to food (Astrup et al., 1990).

However, it is of interest that not all nutrients produce thermogenic responses in the same tissues or organs. Intravenous infusion of amino acids increases whole-body energy expenditure by 19%, with one-half of the effect occurring in the splanchnic tissues (Aksnes et al., 1995). By contrast, the stimulation of energy expenditure due to oral ingestion of fructose or glucose has no effect on the splanchnic tissues (Brundin and Wahren, 1993).

The sympathetic nervous system

Since the demonstration by Landsberg and Young (1978) of reduction in SNS activity during fasting in rats, there has been great interest in the possibility that altered sympathoadrenal control of metabolism and thermogenesis may contribute to the development of obesity. Furthermore, sympathomimetics, which stimulate energy expenditure, are viewed as of potential therapeutic value for obese individuals. However, review of the literature on the assessment of sympathoadrenal activity in obese people yields conflicting information, with similar numbers of studies showing reduced, unchanged or increased SNS activity in obese people compared with lean subjects (Young and Macdonald, 1992). Interestingly, this review provided clearer evidence of reduced adrenal medullary activity in obese people, and the implications of this for energy expenditure deserve further attention. An extension to this review (Macdonald, 1995) revealed an altered relationship between an index of SNS activity (muscle sympathetic nerve activity) and resting energy expenditure in Pima Indians, indicating that the development of obesity in this group may be associated with a defective SNS influence on metabolism.

Although there is some evidence of a link between SNS activation and the TEF response to a meal, especially in younger but not older subjects (Schwartz *et al.*, 1990), the administration of a beta-adrenoceptor antagonist does not always reduce the TEF response (Nacht *et al.*, 1987). However, we have observed an effect of diet composition on fasting plasma noradrenaline concentrations (an index of SNS activity) and the responses to meal ingestion, such that high-sucrose diets and test meals produce larger responses than high starch or high fat (Raben *et al.*, 1997). In addition, the high-sucrose diet was associated with a greater 24-h energy expenditure than the other two diets. Thus, further studies are needed to examine the influence of diet composition on any SNS effect on energy expenditure.

Some caution is needed when considering the possible use of sympathomimetics to stimulate energy expenditure in obese people because undesirable cardiovascular effects may occur. It is clear that catecholamine stimulation of energy expenditure in humans is mediated by beta-adrenoceptors, with some debate as to the dominant receptor subtype (β_2 or β_3). However, the concern is that any generalized activation of the SNS or release of adrenaline from the adrenal medulla has the potential of producing stimulation of the heart (β_1-adrenoceptors) or of increasing blood pressure due to alpha-adrenoceptor effects causing arterial vasoconstriction. Thus, any pharmacological approach needs to be selective for effects on energy expenditure, in order that undesirable side-effects are avoided.

Obesity and energy expenditure

Given that obesity can only develop as a consequence of a prolonged period of positive energy imbalance, a reduction in energy expenditure can theoretically contribute to weight gain. For many years there was a widely held view that very low resting energy expenditures may be a cause of obesity. However, it is now clear that such low resting energy expenditures only occur in severe hypothyroidism and that this is a negligible cause of obesity. The advent of respiration chamber and DLW techniques for the measurement of 24-h energy expenditure has shown that obese people do not have reduced resting or total energy expenditures compared with non-obese people. In fact, because obese people are larger, with a greater FFM than non-obese people, they usually have a greater total energy expenditure expressed per person (Welle *et al.*, 1992). In weight-stable obese subjects, this higher total energy expenditure is usually accompanied by a fasting resting energy expen-

Table 11.4 Body composition and body energy content.

	Non-obese	Obese
Weight (kg)	70	100
Fat mass (kg)	8.4	35
Fat % body weight	12	35
Fat energy (MJ)	327	1365
FFM (kg)	61.6	65
Glycogen (kg)	1	1
CHO energy (MJ)	16	16
Protein (kg)	15	16
Protein energy (MJ)	255	272
Total energy (MJ)	598	1653
Fat energy as % total	55	83

diture per kilogram of FFM, which is the same as that seen in non-obese subjects.

That the development of obesity requires a prolonged period of positive energy balance is easily demonstrated by considering the amounts of energy involved. Table 11.4 compares the body composition of a non-obese 70-kg individual and a 100-kg obese person. The difference in total body fat (26.6 kg) is equivalent to 1037 MJ of stored energy. If the non-obese person's total energy expenditure was 10 MJ/day, with a positive energy imbalance of +10% of this (1 MJ/day), it would take at least 3 years to increase body weight and fat content to those of the 100-kg person. In reality, most cases of obesity probably develop over a longer period of time, with a smaller daily positive energy imbalance. The increased incidence of obesity in the UK over the past 15 years has occurred at a time when the total energy intake of the population is said to have fallen (Prentice and Jebb, 1995), indicating the important contribution that low energy expenditure is likely to have. Prospective studies in the Pima Indians (a group with a high predisposition to the development of obesity) have shown that in adults a low 24-h energy expenditure is associated with a high weight gain over the next 2 years (Ravussin *et al.*, 1988).

Similar observations have been made in infants (Roberts *et al.*, 1988) and children (Griffiths *et al.*, 1990), although in all cases the lower energy expenditure does not statistically account for more than 40% of the weight gain. Subsequent observations on the Pima Indians showed that in males (but not females), weight gain was associated with a lower energy expenditure that was associated with spontaneous physical activity (Zurlo *et al.*, 1992).

Thus, a low 24-h energy expenditure, due at least in part to low physical activity, is a risk factor for weight gain and the development of obesity. Weight-stable obese people do not have a low energy expenditure, if anything it is elevated, but physical activity makes a smaller contribution to total energy expenditure than in non-obese people. Although there is evidence of reduced TEF responses to meals in obese people, this is probably secondary to their insulin resistance and possibly the insulating effect of the adipose tissue (Brundin *et al.*, 1992). Weight reduction to non-obese values is almost always associated with a normalization of these reduced TEF responses (Bukkens *et al.*, 1991; Tataranni *et al.*, 1994).

References

Acheson, K.J., Jequier, E. and Wahren, J. (1983) Influence of f~-adrenergic blockade on glucose induced thermogenesis in man. *Journal of Clinical Investigation* **72**, 893–902.

Aksnes, A.K., Brundin, T., Hjeltnes, N. and Wahren, J. (1995) Metabolic, thermal and circulatory effects of intravenous infusion of amino acids in tetraplegic patients. *Clinical Physiology* **15**, 377–396.

Astrand, P.O. and Rodahl, K. (1977) *Textbook of Work Physiology*, 2nd edn. New York: McGraw-Hill.

Astrup, A., Christensen, N.J., Simonsen, L. and Bulow, J. (1990) Effects of nutrient intake on sympathoadrenal activity and thermogenic mechanisms. *Journal of Neuroscience Methods* **34**, 187–192.

Broeder, C.E., Burrhus, K.A., Svanevik, L.S. and Wilmore, J.H. (1992a) The effects of aerobic fitness on resting metabolic rate. *American Journal of Clinical Nutrition* **55**, 795–801.

Broeder, C.E., Burrhus, K.A., Svanevik, L.S. and Wilmore, J.H. (1992b) The effects of either high-intensity resistance or endurance training on resting metabolic rate. *American Journal of Clinical Nutrition* **55**, 802–810.

Brondel, I. and Le Blanc, J. (1985) Role of palatability on meal-induced thermogenesis in human subjects. *American Journal of Physiology* **248**, E333–E336.

Bruck, K., Baum, E. and Schwennicke, H.P. (1976) Cold-adaptive modifications in man induced by repeated short-term cold exposures and during a 10-day and night cold exposure. *Pflugers Archives* **363**, 125–133.

Brundin, T. and Wahren, J. (1993) Whole body and splanchnic oxygen consumption and blood flow after oral ingestion of fructose or glucose. *American Journal of Physiology* **264**, E504–E513.

Brundin, T., Thörne, A. and Wahren, J. (1992) Heat leakage across the abdominal wall and meal-induced thermogenesis in normal-weight and obese subjects. *Metabolism* **41**, 49–55.

Bukkens, S.G.F., McNeill, G., Smith, J.S. and Morrison, D.C. (1991) Postprandial thermogenesis in post-obese women and weight matched controls. *International Journal of Obesity* **15**, 147–154.

Clement, K., Vaisse, C., Manning, B.S.J., Basdevant, A., Guy-Grand, B., Ruiz, J., Silver, K.D., Shuldiner, A.R., Froguel, P. and Strosberg, A.D. (1995) Genetic variation in the β3-adrenergic receptor and an increased capacity to gain weight in patients with morbid obesity. *New England Journal of Medicine* **333**, 352–354.

Clement, K., Ruiz, J., Cassard-Doulcier, A., Bouillaud, F., Ricquier, D., Basdevant, A., Guy-Grand, B. and Froguel, P. (1996) Additive effect of A→G (-3826) variant of the uncoupling protein gene and the Trp64Arg mutation of the beta 3-adrenergic receptor gene on weight gain in morbid obesity. *International Journal of Obesity and Related Metabolic Disorders* **20**, 1062–1066.

Cori, C.F. and Buchwald, K.W. (1930) Effect of continuous injection of epinephrine on the carbohydrate metabolism, basal metabolism and vascular system of normal man. *American Journal of Physiology* **95**, 71–78.

Couet, C., Delarue, J., Ritz, P., Antoine, J-M. and Lamisse, F. (1997) Effect of dietary fish oil on body fat mass and basal fat oxidation in healthy adults. *International Journal of Obesity* **21**, 637–643.

Dulloo, A.G., Duret, C., Rohrer, D., Girardier, L., Mensi, N., Fathi, M., Chantre, P. and Vandermander, J. (1999) Efficacy of a green tea extract rich in catechin polyphenols and caffeine in increasing 24-h energy expenditure and fat oxidation in humans. *American Journal of Clinical Nutrition* **70**, 1040–1045.

Elia, M. (1992) Organ and tissue contribution to metabolic rate. In: Kinney, J.M. and Tucker, H.N. eds. *Energy Metabolism: Tissue Determinants and Cellular Corollaries*. New York: Raven Press, 61–79.

Elia, M., Jones, M.G., Jennings, G., Poppitt, S.D., Fuller, N.J., Murgatroyd, P.R. and Jebb, S.A. (1995) Estimating energy expenditure from the specific activity of urine urea during lengthy subcutaneous infusion of NaH^{14}CO$_3$. *American Journal of Physiology* **269**, E172–E182.

Farshchi, H., Taylor, M. and Macdonald, I. (2004) Decreased thermic effect of food after an irregular compared with a regular meal pattern in healthy lean women. *International Journal of Obesity and Related Metabolic Disorders* **28**, 653–660.

Farshchi, H.R., Taylor, M. and Macdonald, I.A. (2005) Beneficial metabolic effects of regular meal frequency on dietary thermogenesis, insulin sensitivity and fasting lipid profiles in healthy obese women. *American Journal of Clinical Nutrition* (in press).

Frayn, K.N. and Macdonald, I.A. (1997) Assessment of substrate and energy metabolism *in vivo*. In: Draznin, B., Pizza, R. eds. *Clinical Research in Diabetes and Obesity*, Vol. 1. Totoura, NJ: Humana Press, 101–124.

Gagnon, J., Mauriege, P., Roy, S., Sjostrom, D., Chagnon, Y.C., Dionne, F.T., Oppert, J-M., Perusse, L., Sjostrom, L. and Bouchard, C. (1996) The Trp64Arg mutation of the beta 3 adrenergic receptor gene has no effect on obesity phenotypes in the Quebec family study and Swedish obese subjects cohorts. *Journal of Clinical Investigation* **98**, 2086–2093.

Griffiths, M., Payne, P.R., Stunkard, A.J., Rivers, J.P.W. and Cox, M. (1990) Metabolic rate and physical development in children at risk of obesity. *Lancet* **336**, 76–77.

Habas, E.M.M.A. and Macdonald, I.A. (1998) Metabolic and cardiovascular responses to a liquid and solid test meal. *British Journal of Nutrition* **79**, 241–247.

Harris, J. and Benedict, F. (1919) *A Biometric Study of Basal Metabolism in Man*. (Publication no. 279). Washington DC: Camegie Institute of Washington, 1–266.

Kempen, K.P.G., Saris, W.H.M. and Westerterp, K.R. (1995) Energy balance during an 8-wk energy restricted diet with and without exercise in obese women. *American Journal of Clinical Nutrition* **62**, 722–729.

Kinabo, J.L. and Durnin, J.V.G.A. (1990) Thermic effect of food in man: effect of meal composition and energy content. *British Journal of Nutrition* **74**, 37–44.

Landsberg, L. and Young, J.B. (1978) Fasting, feeding and the regulation of the sympathetic nervous system. *New England Journal of Medicine* **298**, 1295–1301.

Lean, M.E.J., Murgatroyd, P.R., Rothnie, I., Reid, I.W. and Harvey, R. (1988) Metabolic and thyroid responses to mild cold are abnormal in obese and diabetic women. *Clinical Endocrinology* **28**, 665–673.

Levine, J. (2003) Non-exercise activity thermogenesis. *Proceedings of the Nutrition Society* **62**, 667–679.

Levine, J.A., Schleusner, S.J. and Jensen, M.D. (2000) Energy expenditure of non-exercise activity. *American Journal of Clinical Nutrition* **72**, 1451–1454.

Macdonald, I.A. (1995) Advances in our understanding of the role of the sympathetic nervous system in obesity. *International Journal of Obesity* **19** (Suppl. 7), 52–57.

Macdonald, I.A., Bennett, T. and Fellows, I.W. (1985) Catecholamines and the control of metabolism in man. *Clinical Science* **68**, 613–619.

Murgatroyd, P.R., Shetty, P.S. and Prentice, A.M. (1993) Techniques for the measurement of human energy expenditure: a practical guide. *International Journal of Obesity* **17**, 549–568.

Nacht, C.A., Chnistin, L., Temler, E., Chiolero, R., Jequies E. and Acheson, K. (1987) Thermic effect of food: possible implication of parasympathetic nervous system. *American Journal of Physiology* **253**, E481–E488.

Poehlman, E.T., Viers, H.F. and Detzer, M. (1991) Influence of physical activity and dietary restraint on resting energy expenditure in young, non-obese females. *Canadian Journal of Physiology and Pharmacology* **69**, 320–326.

Prentice, A.M. (1988) Applications of the doubly labelled water ($^2H_2^{18}O$) method in free-living adults. *Proceedings of the Nutrition Society* **47**, 259–268.

Prentice, A.M. and Jebb, S.A. (1995) Obesity in Britain, gluttony or sloth. *British Medical Journal* **311**, 437–439.

Raben, A., Macdonald, I.A. and Astrup, A. (1997) Replacement of dietary fat by sucrose or starch: Effects on 14 days' *ad libitum* energy intake, energy expenditure and body weight in formerly obese and non-obese subjects. *International Journal of Obesity* **21**, 846–859.

Racette, S.B., Schoeller, D.A., Kushner, R.F. and Neil, K.M. (1995) Exercise enhances dietary compliances during moderate energy restriction in obese women. *American Journal of Clinical Nutrition* **62**, 345–349.

Randin, J., Schutz, Y., Scazziga, B., Lemarchand-Beraud, T., Felber, J. and Jequier, E. (1986) Unaltered glucose-induced thermogenesis in Graves' disease. *American Journal of Clinical Nutrition* **43**, 738–744.

Ravussin, E., Lillioja, S., Anderson, T.E., Christin, L. and Bogardus, C. (1986) Determinants of 24-hour energy expenditure in man: methods and results using a respiratory chamber. *Journal of Clinical Investigation* **78**, 1568–1578.

Ravussin, E., Lillioja, S., Knowles, W.C., Christin, L., Freymond, D., Abbott, W., Boyce, V., Howard, B. and Bogardus, C. (1988) Reduced rate of energy expenditure as a risk factor for body weight gain. *New England Journal of Medicine* **318**, 467–472.

Rennie, K., Rowsell, T., Jebb, S., Holburn, D. and Wareham, N. (2000) A combined heart rate and movement sensor: proof of concept and preliminary testing study. *European Journal of Clinical Nutrition*. **54**, 409–414.

Ricquier, D. and Bouillaud, F. (2000) Mitochondrial uncoupling proteins: from mitochondria to the regulation of energy balance. *Journal of Physiology (London)* **529**, 3–10.

Rising, R., Harpei, L.T., Fontvieille, A.M., Ferraro, R.T., Spraul, M. and Ravussin, E. (1994) Determinants of total daily energy expenditure: variability in physical activity. *American Journal of Clinical Nutrition* **59**, 800–804.

Roberts, S.B., Savage, J., Coward, W.A., Chew, B. and Lucas, A. (1988) Energy expenditure and intake in infants born to lean and overweight mothers. *New England Journal of Medicine* **318**, 461–466.

Rumpler, W., Seale, J., Clevidence, B., Judd, J., Wiley, E., Yamamoto, S., Komatsu, T., Sawaki, T., Ishikura, Y. and Hosoda, K. (2001) Oolong tea increases metabolic rate and fat oxidation in men. *Journal of Nutrition* **131**, 2848–2852.

Scalfi, L., Coltorti, A. and Contaldo, F. (1991) Post-prandial thermogenesis in lean and obese subjects after meals supplemented with medium-chain and long-chain triglycerides. *American Journal of Clinical Nutrition* **53**, 1130–1133.

Schofield, W. (1985) Predicting basal metabolic rate, new standard and review of previous work. *Human Nutrition Clinical Nutrition* **39c**, 5–41.

Schutz, Y., Bessard, T. and Jequie, E. (1984) Diet induced thermogenesis measured over a whole day in obese and non-obese women. *American Journal of Clinical Nutrition* **40**, 542–582.

Schwartz, R.S., Jaeger, L.F. and Veith, R.C. (1990) The thermic effect of feeding in older men: the importance of the sympathetic nervous system. *Metabolism* **39**, 733–737.

Segal, K.R., Lacayanga, I., Dunaif, A., Gutin, B. and Pi-Sunyer, F.X. (1989) Impact of body fat mass and percent fat on metabolic rate and thermogenesis in men. *American Journal of Physiology* **256**, E573–E579.

Sipilainen, R., Uusitupa, M., Heikkinen, S., Rissanen, A. and Laakso, M. (1997) Polymorphism of the beta3-adrenergic receptor gene affects basal metabolic rate in obese Finns. *Diabetes* **46**, 77–80.

Solomon, S., Kurzer, M. and Calloway, D. (1982) Menstrual cycle and basal metabolic rate in women. *American Journal of Clinical Nutrition* **36**, 611–616.

Spurr, G., Prentice, A., Murgatroyd, P., Goldberg, G., Reina, J. and Christman, N. (1988) Energy expenditure from minute-by-minute heart-rate recording: comparison with indirect calorimetry. *American Journal of Clinical Nutrition* **48**, 552–559.

Steinberg, D., Nestel, P.I., Buskirk, E.R. and Thompson, R.H. (1964) Calorigenic effect of norepinephrine correlated with plasma free fatty acid turnover and oxidation. *Journal of Clinical Investigation* **43**, 167–176.

Tai, M.M., Cartillo, P. and Pi-Sunyer, F.X. (1991) Meal size and frequency: effect on the thermic effect of food. *American Journal of Clinical Nutrition* **54**, 783–787.

Tappy, L., Randin, J.P., Felber, J.P., Chiolero, Simonson, D.C., Jecquier, E. and Defronzo, R.A. (1986) Comparison of thermogenic effect of fructose and glucose in normal humans. *American Journal of Physiology* **250**, E718–E724.

Tataranni, P.A., Mingrone, G., Greco, A.V., Caradonna, P., Capristo, E., Raguso, C.A., De Gaetano, A., Tacchino, R.M. and Castagneto, M. (1994) Glucose-induced thermogenesis in post-obese women who have undergone biliopancreatic diversion. *American Journal of Clinical Nutrition* **60**, 320–326.

Thiebaud, D., Schutz, Y., Acheson, K., Jacot, E., Defronzo, R.A., Felber, J.P. and Jecquier, E. (1983a) Energy cost of glucose storage in human subjects during glucose–insulin infusions. *American Journal of Physiology* **244**, E216–E221.

Thiebaud, D., Acheson, K., Schutz, Y., Felber, J.P., Golay, A., Defronzo, R.A. and Jecquier, E. (1983b) Stimulation of thermogenesis in men after combined glucose, long-chain triglyceride infusion. *American Journal of Clinical Nutrition* **37**, 603–611.

159

Vaz, M., Tunet, A., Kingwell, B., Chin, J., Koff, E., Cox, H., Jennings, G. and Esler, M. (1995) Postprandial sympathoadrenal activity: its relation to metabolic and cardiovascular events and to changes in meal frequency. *Clinical Science* **89**, 349–357.

Wade, A.J., Marbut, M.M. and Round, J.M. (1990) Muscle fibre type and aetiology of obesity. *Lancet* **335**, 805–808.

Webber, J. and Macdonald, I.A. (1993) Metabolic actions of catecholamines in man. *Baillière's Clinical Endocrinology and Metabolism* **7**, 393–413.

Welle, S., Forbes, G.B., Start, M., Barnard, R.R. and Amatruda, J.M. (1992) Energy expenditure under free-living conditions in normal weight and overweight women. *American Journal of Clinical Nutrition* **55**, 14–21.

Young, J.B. and Macdonald, I.A. (1992) Sympathoadrenal activity in human obesity: heterogeneity of findings since 1980. *International Journal of Obesity* **16**, 959–967.

Zurlo, F., Ferraro, R., Fontvieile, A.M., Rising, R., Bogardus, C. and Ravussin, E. (1992) Spontaneous physical activity and obesity: cross-sectional and longitudinal studies in Pima Indians. *American Journal of Physiology* **263**, E296–E300.

Obesity and disease

12 Obesity and dyslipidaemia: importance of body fat distribution

André Tchernof and Jean-Pierre Després

Overview of lipid and lipoprotein metabolism, 163

Dyslipidaemic states and the risk of coronary heart disease, 163

Obesity and dyslipidaemia: importance of visceral adipose tissue, 165

Measurement of visceral adipose tissue: age and gender differences, 165

Visceral obesity and related complications: the metabolic syndrome, 166

The insulin-resistant, dyslipidaemic, proinflammatory and prothrombotic state of abdominal obesity: an important cause of coronary heart disease, 170

Visceral adipose tissue and the insulin resistant–dyslipidaemic syndrome: physiopathology and causal relationships, 172

Genetic susceptibility to metabolic complications of visceral obesity, 174

Therapeutic implications, 175

Conclusions, 176

References, 177

Overview of lipid and lipoprotein metabolism

Cholesterol and triglycerides are hydrophobic compounds that are transported in the blood by lipoproteins. On the basis of their density and composition, four major subclasses of lipoproteins have been identified: chylomicrons, very low-density lipoproteins (VLDLs), low-density lipoproteins (LDLs) and high-density lipoproteins (HDLs) (Fig. 12.1).

Chylomicrons are the largest, most buoyant lipoproteins and contain mostly triglycerides. The protein constituents of these particles are apolipoprotein (Apo) E and C (II and III), as well as small intestine-synthesized Apo B48, which are responsible for lipoprotein catabolism and structural integrity. Chylomicrons are synthesized in the intestine shortly after a meal and represent the form by which most of the dietary fatty acids are transported in the plasma. Endothelial lipoprotein lipase (LPL) is responsible for the hydrolysis of triglycerides contained within chylomicrons. The resulting chylomicron remnants are taken up by remnant receptors in the liver. VLDLs are synthesized by the liver and contain Apo B100, E and C. VLDL synthesis rates rely mainly on the availability of neutral lipids from *de novo* lipogenesis, hepatocyte cytoplasmic triglyceride stores, fatty acids derived from lipoproteins taken up by the liver (mainly chylomicron remnants) or plasma free fatty acids.

The relative contribution of each of these sources varies upon nutritional, hormonal and metabolic status of the patient (Lewis, 1997). In the fasting state, most triglycerides are contained within VLDL particles. Intermediate-density lipoproteins (IDLs) and LDLs are the catabolic products of VLDLs, resulting from the hydrolysis of the triglyceride content of VLDL particles by both LPL and hepatic lipase (Shepherd and Packard, 1989). LDL particles are the main carriers of cholesterol in the blood. Apo B100 synthesized in the liver is their main protein constituent, and only one molecule of Apo B is found per LDL particle. IDL and LDL are taken up by the liver through binding to the hepatic Apo B/E receptor (LDL receptor). The formation of HDL particles results from the hydrolysis of VLDL to LDL, a process during which excess surface components aggregate to form nascent HDL particles (Fig. 12.1). The major apolipoproteins of HDL particles are Apo A-I and Apo A-II. According to the concept of reverse cholesterol transport (Reichl and Miller, 1989), HDL particles promote the net movement of cholesterol from extrahepatic tissues back to the liver (Lamarche *et al.*, 1999a).

Dyslipidaemic states and the risk of coronary heart disease

Coronary heart disease (CHD) is recognized as a major cause of mortality and morbidity in affluent societies. In this regard, the scientific evidence supporting the notion that high plasma cholesterol and LDL-cholesterol concentrations are associated

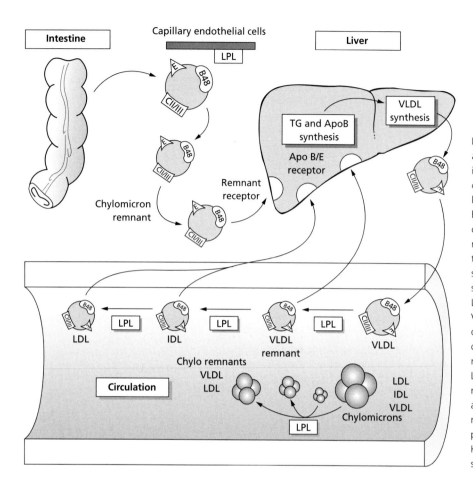

Fig 12.1 Overview of lipoprotein metabolism and lipid transport. Dietary fatty acids are incorporated in the form of triglycerides into chylomicrons in the intestine. Endothelial lipoprotein lipase (LPL) is responsible for the hydrolysis of the triglyceride content of chylomicrons. The resulting chylomicron remnants are taken up by the remnant receptor in the liver. Apo B100-containing VLDL particles are synthesized by the liver. These particles are submitted to the catabolic activity of endothelial LPL in the circulation, leading to the formation of VLDL remnants, IDL and LDL particles, which are depleted in triglycerides and enriched in cholesterol. VLDL remnants are taken up by the remnant receptor in the liver, whereas IDL and LDL bind to the hepatic Apo B/E receptor (LDL receptor). HDL particles are generated by aggregation of excess surface components resulting from the hydrolysis of Apo B-containing particles by LPL. The cholesterol ester content of HDL is also increased during this process (HDL$_2$ subfraction).

with an increased risk of CHD is unequivocal (Gotto *et al.*, 1990; Adult Treatment Panel III, 2002; Kwiterovich, 2002). Epidemiological studies have established that each 1% increase in LDL-cholesterol leads to a 1–2% increase in coronary artery disease mortality rate (Kwiterovich, 1998). Accordingly, interventions aimed at plasma LDL-cholesterol reduction have been shown to decrease significantly coronary artery disease events (Kwiterovich, 1998; 2002).

However, measuring LDL-cholesterol levels, along with traditional CHD risk factors such as cigarette smoking, hypertension, diabetes and family history of cardiovascular disease, enables the identification of only approximately 50% of the population that will eventually develop the disease (Wilson *et al.*, 1987). For instance, a study from Genest and colleagues (1991) has shown that there is considerable overlap in plasma cholesterol concentrations among subjects with and without CHD, as almost 50% of patients with the disease had rather 'normal' plasma cholesterol levels (Genest *et al.*, 1991). Accordingly, Sniderman and Silberberg (1990) have suggested that, although mean plasma cholesterol levels may be higher in patients with CHD than in healthy subjects, the overlap of cholesterol values in these two groups of individuals is such

that the ability of cholesterol alone to discriminate subjects at risk for CHD is relatively weak (Sniderman *et al.*, 1980; Sniderman and Silberberg 1990). With respect to cholesterol lowering, although the relative reduction in coronary heart disease event rate has been shown to reach about 25–30% in clinical trials, a relatively small percentage reduction in absolute CHD event rate has been observed, with a very significant number of treated patients developing either a first or a recurrent event (Kwiterovich, 2002). Consequently, beyond traditional risk factors and LDL-cholesterol levels, a collection of non-traditional risk factors has recently emerged including homocysteine levels, prothrombotic factors and proinflammatory markers, as well as measures reflecting lipoprotein heterogeneity, such as Apo B levels, triglyceride concentrations and small, dense LDL particles.

The study of apolipoprotein concentrations certainly provides some additional information on the risk of coronary heart disease, as these variables could be indicative of the concentrations of lipoproteins that promote or protect against premature atherosclerosis. Studies have shown that approximately one-half of patients with coronary artery disease have elevated LDL-Apo B levels (Sniderman *et al.*, 1980). Patients with elevated LDL-Apo B, but with LDL-cholesterol values within the normal range, are generally characterized by an elevated number of small, dense LDL particles, which have been shown in several studies to be associated with an increased risk of cardiovascular disease (Lamarche *et al.*, 1999b). The presence of these atherogenic LDL particles most likely arises from an increased flow of triglycerides from triglyceride-rich lipoproteins to LDLs, through the action of the cholesteryl ester transfer protein (CETP). Such transfer, which contributes to deplete LDL particles in cholesterol ester and increases their triglyceride content, is amplified in hypertriglyceridaemic states (Lamarche *et al.*, 1999b). LDL heterogeneity reflecting differences in LDL particle composition and density is now recognized as an important factor that contributes to the link between dyslipidaemic states and the risk of coronary heart disease.

Epidemiological studies have also clearly established that a low plasma HDL-cholesterol concentration is a very potent and independent risk factor for coronary heart disease (Gordon and Rifkind 1989; Després *et al.*, 2000). The levels of Apo A-I, the main protein component of HDL, are also reduced in patients with coronary heart disease (Rader *et al.*, 1994). Despite the fact that HDL-cholesterol has long been recognized as an independent risk factor, HDL particles are also heterogeneous in size and composition (Lamarche *et al.*, 1999a; Rader 2002). As for LDL, the presence of hypertriglyceridaemia also appears to be a major factor modulating HDL metabolism (Lamarche *et al.*, 1999a). There is a well-established negative relationship between plasma HDL-cholesterol level and triglyceride concentrations (Gordon *et al.*, 1977; Albrink *et al.*, 1980; Davis *et al.*, 1980; Petersson *et al.*, 1984), and patients characterized by high plasma triglyceride levels frequently have low HDL-cholesterol. Among mechanisms explaining this association, small HDL particles, which are the product of intravascular lipolysis of triglyceride-enriched HDL, could be cleared more rapidly, are less stable or are more prone to shed Apo A-I than large HDL particles (Lamarche *et al.*, 1999a). Thus, although the contribution of plasma triglyceride level itself as a risk factor for CHD remains equivocal—several studies have shown that high plasma triglyceride levels were no longer a risk factor for CHD after statistical adjustment for HDL-C concentration (Austin, 1991)—it appears that triglyceride enrichment of HDL particles plays a significant role in modulating HDL metabolism. The clinical importance of HDL particle composition and size remains to be established. Nevertheless, knowledge about lipid and lipoprotein metabolism has evolved considerably in recent years, and future studies are likely to further refine cardiovascular disease risk prediction through the measurement of additional lipid lipoprotein-related variables. It is increasingly clear that clinicians now need to go beyond simple plasma cholesterol level measurements in CHD risk assessment.

Obesity and dyslipidaemia: importance of visceral adipose tissue

Obesity is commonly associated with chronic diseases such as hypertension, type 2 diabetes and cardiovascular disease (Sims and Berchtold, 1982; Bray 1985; NIH Consensus Conference, 1985; Garrison *et al.*, 1987; Kissebah *et al.*, 1989). Excess body fatness has also been frequently associated with dyslipidaemic states and with alterations in other cardiovascular disease risk factors (Kissebah *et al.*, 1989; Després 1991; 1994a; Ford 1999). Some prospective studies have found that obesity was a significant predictor of cardiovascular disease-related mortality, although this association appears to be of lower magnitude than the relationships of cardiovascular disease mortality to well-known risk factors such as smoking, hypertension and dyslipidaemia (Bray *et al.* 1972; Barrett-Connor 1985; Kissebah *et al.* 1989; Manson *et al.* 1995). This section describes how the morphologic heterogeneity of obesity, more specifically regional body fat distribution, accounts for the most important part of the association between obesity and the related metabolic complications.

In 1947, Jean Vague (Vague, 1947) was the first to describe the sex-related difference in body fat distribution and to foresee its correlation with the complications of obesity. He defined the accumulation of upper body fat mostly found in men as android obesity, this type of obesity being more frequently associated with diabetes, hypertension and cardiovascular disease. He also referred to gynoid obesity to describe a condition in which body fat was preferentially accumulated in the gluteal–femoral region. He suggested that this pattern of fat distribution, mostly found in women, was not associated with the expected complications of obesity (Vague, 1947) (Fig. 12.2). Several prospective studies that have used the ratio of waist and hip circumferences (the widely used waist–hip ratio, WHR) have now confirmed that the android type of obesity, now referred to as abdominal obesity, is more closely associated with a cluster of metabolic complications such as dyslipidaemias, hyperinsulinaemia and a higher risk of diabetes and cardiovascular diseases than an excess of total body fatness per se (Kissebah *et al.*, 1982; Björntorp, 1984; Lapidus *et al.*, 1984; Larsson *et al.*, 1984; Ohlson *et al.*, 1985; Ducimetière *et al.*, 1986; Donahue *et al.*, 1987).

Measurement of visceral adipose tissue: age and gender differences

As mentioned above, the most widely used measurement of body fat distribution has been the WHR. The rationale for using this index is that the higher is the accumulation of abdominal fat, the higher is the ratio of waist–hip circumferences. However, this measurement does distinguish the

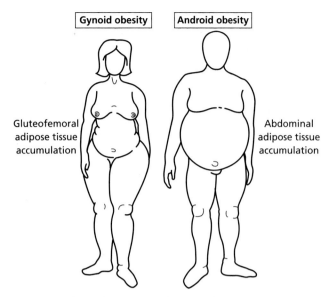

Fig 12.2 Android and gynoid types of obesity as first defined by Vague (1947), with preferential accumulation of adipose tissue in the abdominal and gluteofemoral region respectively. The android pattern of adipose tissue distribution is more closely associated with the metabolic complications of obesity.

amount of adipose tissue located in the abdominal cavity (the intra-abdominal or visceral adipose tissue) from the subcutaneous abdominal adipose tissue. With the development of imaging techniques such as computerized tomography and magnetic resonance, it has become possible to accurately quantify the amount of fat located in the various body compartments, including the abdominal cavity (Sjöström et al., 1986; Ferland et al., 1989; Després et al., 1991). On the basis of differences in the density of tissues, adipose tissue can be distinguished from bone and muscle, and the size of the visceral and subcutaneous adipose tissue compartments can be reliably estimated by measuring areas of the corresponding tissues on a single scan at the abdominal level, usually at the L4–L5 vertebrae (Sjöström et al., 1986; Ferland et al., 1989; Després et al., 1991) (Fig. 12.3).

Starting in the late 1980s, studies were published creating an increasingly large body of knowledge regarding correlates of abdominal visceral obesity in various populations and physiological conditions. These studies have indicated that age and gender are important correlates of visceral adipose tissue accumulation. Using computerized tomography methodology, Lemieux and colleagues (1993) have noted that for any given body fat mass value, men have at least twice the amount of visceral adipose tissue than that found in premenopausal women (Fig. 12.4). Whether such a gender difference in visceral adipose tissue accumulation could account for the well-known difference in cardiovascular risk factors between men and women has also been examined (Lemieux *et al.*, 1994). In a cross-sectional comparison of subgroups of men and women, matching for the level of visceral adipose tissue largely elimi-

nated most of the differences in plasma lipoprotein levels, with the exception of plasma HDL-C concentrations, which remained higher in women than in men (Lemieux *et al.*, 1994). Additional studies have been performed on the importance of visceral fat accumulation on sex differences in LDL particle size, which is generally lower in men than women (Lemieux *et al.*, 2002). When comparing subgroups of men and women with similar increases in triglyceride concentrations (> 2 mmol/L) and similarly elevated visceral adipose tissue areas (> 100 cm²), LDL particle size was significantly lower in men vs. women, suggesting that the gender differences in plasma triglyceride levels and visceral adipose tissue area could not entirely explain this sex difference (Lemieux *et al.*, 2002).

The prevalence of obesity increases with age (Reeder *et al.*, 1992), and total body fat mass as well as visceral adipose tissue accumulations are significant positive correlates of age (Enzi *et al.*, 1986; Seidell *et al.*, 1988; Schwartz *et al.*, 1990; Kotani *et al.*, 1994). Globally, the cardiovascular disease risk profile also deteriorates with age, and it has been shown that the concomitant increase in visceral adipose tissue was one of the important factors associated with the development of a more atherogenic metabolic profile (Lemieux *et al.*, 1995; DeNino *et al.*, 2001). However, it also appears that other age-related processes that are independent of the variation in total adiposity and visceral adipose tissue deposition contribute to the alterations in plasma lipid and lipoprotein concentrations as well as insulin sensitivity (Lemieux *et al.*, 1995; DeNino *et al.*, 2001). Thus, a substantial proportion of age and gender differences in the metabolic risk profile predictive of the risk of type 2 diabetes and cardiovascular disease could be attributed to concomitant variations in visceral adipose tissue accumulation.

Visceral obesity and related complications: the metabolic syndrome

It is now well established that visceral obesity is a critical correlate of several metabolic complications found in obesity (Kissebah *et al.*, 1989; Kissebah and Krakower, 1994). In order to sort out the relative contribution of total body fatness vs. visceral adipose tissue accumulation as correlates of metabolic alterations, we have used a simple approach in which we compared two subgroups of obese men matched for total body fat, but with either low or high levels of visceral adipose tissue measured by computerized tomography. These two groups were then compared to lean control subjects (Fig. 12.5). As shown in Fig. 12.5, only men with high levels of visceral adipose tissue displayed significantly higher plasma triglyceride levels and lower HDL-C concentrations as well as a reduced HDL$_2$-C/HDL$_3$-C ratio compared with the two other subgroups. Comparable results were obtained when similar analyses were conducted in women (not shown).

It is important to point out that plasma LDL-cholesterol levels are often within the normal range in subjects with visceral

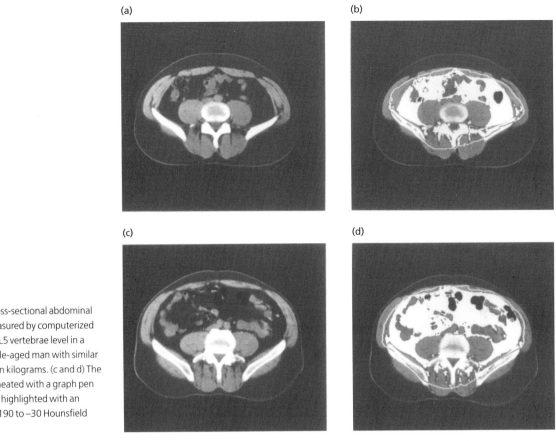

Fig 12.3 (a and b) Cross-sectional abdominal adipose tissue area measured by computerized tomography at the L4–L5 vertebrae level in a young man and a middle-aged man with similar levels of total body fat in kilograms. (c and d) The visceral cavity was delineated with a graph pen and adipose tissue was highlighted with an attenuation range of −190 to −30 Hounsfield units.

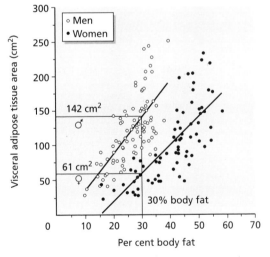

Fig 12.4 Relationships between visceral adipose tissue area and percentage body fat in men (○) and women (●) ($r = 0.71$, $P < 0.0001$ in men and $r = 0.76$, $P < 0.0001$) in women. At 30% body fat, regression equations predict a 142 cm^2 vs. 61 cm^2 visceral fat accumulation in men and women respectively. (Adapted from Lemieux *et al.*, 1993.)

obesity. However, we have reported that viscerally obese subjects were characterized by significant increases in Apo B as well as in LDL-Apo B concentrations (Fig. 12.6) (Pouliot *et al.*, 1992). Thus, visceral obesity is associated with an increased LDL-Apo B/LDL-C ratio, which is suggestive of alterations in the composition of LDL particles. Studies from our group (Tchernof *et al.*, 1996), in which a 2–16% polyacrylamide gradient gel electrophoretic procedure was used to assess the proportion of small, dense LDL particles as well as LDL particle size, have revealed that visceral obesity is also associated with the predominance of small, dense LDL particles in the plasma (Tchernof *et al.*, 1996; Lemieux *et al.*, 2002).

Visceral obesity is, therefore, associated with a dyslipidaemic state that includes hypertriglyceridaemia, hypoalphalipoproteinaemia, a reduced HDL$_2$-C/HDL$_3$-C ratio, elevated Apo B concentration, a greater proportion of small, dense LDL particles and an increased C/HDL-C ratio. How this dyslipidaemic phenotype substantially increases the risk of coronary heart disease will be discussed in a subsequent section of this chapter.

Using the approach described above to compare obese subjects with either low or high levels of visceral adipose tissue to lean control subjects, we have observed that obese men and women with high levels of visceral adipose tissue were also characterized by significantly higher fasting plasma insulin

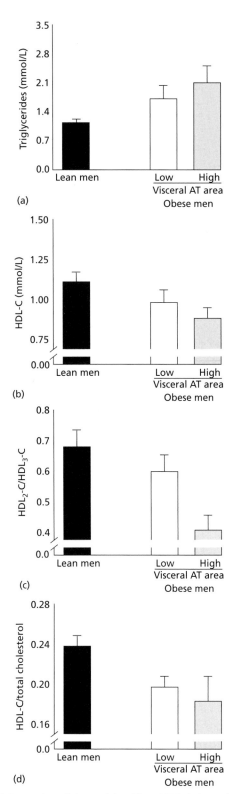

Fig 12.5 Comparison of plasma triglyceride and HDL-cholesterol concentrations as well as HDL_2-C/HDL_3-C and HDL/total cholesterol ratios among a subgroup of lean men and two subgroups of obese men with the same amount of total fat, but with either low or high levels of visceral adipose tissue (AT). 1, significantly different from lean control subjects. (Adapted from Pouliot *et al.*, 1992.)

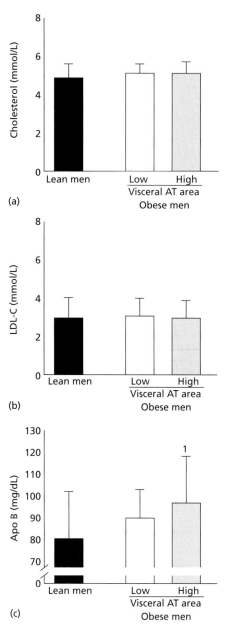

Fig 12.6 Comparison of plasma cholesterol, LDL-cholesterol and Apo B levels among a subgroup of lean men vs. two subgroups of obese men with the same amount of total fat, but with either low or high levels of visceral adipose tissue (AT). 1, significantly different from lean control subjects. (Adapted from Lemieux and Després, 1994.)

concentrations and by higher insulinaemic and glycaemic responses to a standard oral glucose load, suggesting a link between visceral fat accumulation and insulin resistance (Després *et al.*, 1989a; Pouliot *et al.*, 1992) (Fig. 12.7). In a recent study, Brochu and colleagues (2001) examined a subgroup of women who were obese but had a normal metabolic profile. Specifically, women who, despite being obese, were metabolically normal (normal insulin sensitivity) were compared with equally obese women who were insulin resistant and had

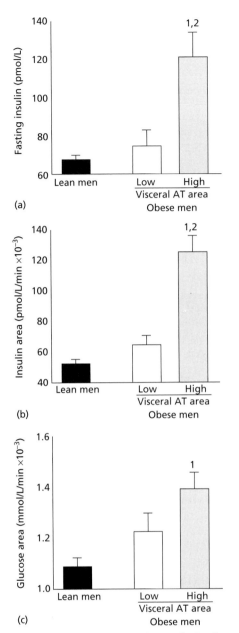

Fig 12.7 Comparison of fasting plasma insulin as well as insulinaemic and glycaemic responses to a 75-g oral glucose load (areas under the curves) among a subgroup of lean men and two subgroups of obese men with the same amount of total fat, but with either low or high levels of visceral adipose tissue (AT). 1, significantly different from lean control subjects; 2, significantly different from obese men with low levels of visceral adipose tissue, $P < 0.05$. (Adapted from Pouliot *et al.*, 1992.)

similar levels of obesity. It was found that the major feature of 'metabolically abnormal' (insulin-resistant) women was an increased visceral fat accumulation measured by computerized tomography (Brochu *et al.*, 2001). Other studies have now emphasized the importance of visceral fat accumulation in the association between obesity and risk factors for type 2 diabetes. Specifically, in both men and women, visceral adipose tissue

accumulation has been positively associated with fasting insulin and C-peptide levels, as well as with the insulin response to an oral glucose challenge (Després *et al.*, 1989a; Pouliot *et al.*, 1992). These associations appeared to be independent from concomitant variations in total body fat mass (Lemieux and Després, 1994; Wajchenberg, 2000). The negative correlations between CT-measured visceral fat accumulation and glucose disposal assessed with the hyperinsulinaemic–euglycaemic clamp technique is also a well-established phenomenon (Wilson *et al.*, 1987; Bonora *et al.*, 1992; Goodpaster *et al.*, 1997; Dvorak *et al.*, 1999; Brochu *et al.*, 2000; Sites *et al.*, 2000; DeNino *et al.*, 2001; Rendell *et al.*, 2001). In addition, prospective studies have shown that visceral obesity is associated with an increased risk of developing type 2 diabetes (Bergstrom *et al.*, 1990; Boyko *et al.*, 2000). Thus, individuals with visceral obesity are frequently characterized by both hyperinsulinaemia and insulin resistance.

Reaven was the first in 1988 (Reaven, 1988) to suggest the term 'insulin resistance syndrome' (or syndrome X) to describe a cluster of metabolic abnormalities including hypoalphalipoproteinaemia, hypertriglyceridaemia, hyperinsulinaemia and increased blood pressure. Through its strong relation with most components of the syndrome, visceral adipose tissue accumulation is now a recognized and perhaps central element of the cluster (Després 1993; 1994b; Lemieux and Després, 1994). In a recent report, experts from the American National Education Program (Adult Treatment Panel III, 2002) issued a new definition for the syndrome, now called 'metabolic syndrome', which included abdominal obesity, atherogenic dyslipidaemia, raised blood pressure, insulin resistance with or without glucose intolerance, and a prothrombotic/proinflammatory state. To screen for the presence of the metabolic syndrome, the ATPIII panel recommended the simultaneous occurrence of three or more of the following components: (a) abdominal obesity (as defined by a waist circumference greater than 102 cm in men and 88 cm in women); (b) elevated plasma triglyceride levels (greater than or equal to 1.69 mmol/L); (c) low HDL-cholesterol (below 1.04 mmol/L in men and below 1.29 mmol/L in women); (d) high blood pressure (greater than or equal to 130/85 mm Hg); and (e) elevated fasting plasma glucose (greater than or equal to 6.1 mmol/L) (Adult Treatment Panel III, 2002). Other components of the metabolic syndrome, such as insulin resistance, the proinflammatory state and the prothrombotic state, were not included in the clinical variables to identify individuals affected by the metabolic syndrome, as they cannot be used in routine clinical evaluation at the present time (Adult Treatment Panel III, 2002).

New additional components of the metabolic syndrome, such as the proinflammatory/prothrombotic states, are also closely correlated with the presence of excess body fatness and abdominal obesity. The acute phase reactant C-reactive protein (CRP) is a sensitive marker of inflammation (Gabay and Kushner, 1999). Circulating levels of this protein are generally low in patients without acute illness, but, using high-sensitivity assays, it has been possible to investigate the relationship between previously considered normal plasma CRP levels and cardiovascular disease (Ross, 1999). Several studies have now demonstrated that elevated high-sensitivity CRP levels are independently associated with an increased risk of cardiovascular disease mortality and morbidity, as well as with acute coronary events in both men and women (Ridker *et al.*, 1997; 1998; 2000; Koenig *et al.*, 1999; Thompson *et al.*, 2000). Elevated CRP levels are also correlated with body weight and body mass index (BMI) as well as insulin resistance (Ford, 1999; Hak *et al.*, 1999; Visser *et al.*, 1999; Yudkin *et al.*, 1999).

In a recent study, Lemieux and colleagues examined a sample of 159 men and found that, among subjects with a high body fat mass, those with high visceral adipose tissue areas had the highest CRP levels (Lemieux *et al.*, 2001). The nature of the relationship between CRP and adiposity has not been clearly established. However, it has been proposed that other adipose tissue-secreted proinflammatory cytokines such as interleukin 6 (IL-6), IL-1β or tumour necrosis factor alpha (TNF-α) may be involved in CRP level increases in obesity (Visser *et al.*, 1999; Yudkin *et al.* 1999; 2000). Accordingly, plasma levels of TNF-α) and IL-6 are increased in obese subjects (Bastard *et al.*, 2000; Hotamisligil, 2000). The haemostatic and fibrinolytic systems may also be affected in obese patients as these patients tend to have higher fibrinogen, factor VII, factor VIII, von Willebrand factor and plasminogen activator inhibitor levels than non-obese individuals. A close association has generally been observed between abdominal obesity and disturbances in plasminogen activator inhibitor, fibrinogen, factor VIII and von Willebrand factor, whereas less consistent results have been found for factor VII (Vague *et al.*, 1989; Juhan-Vague *et al.*, 1991; Mertens and Van Gaal, 2002). Adipose cells are responsible for plasminogen activator inhibitor-1 production, which possibly explains elevated levels found in abdominal obesity (Juhan-Vague *et al.*, 1991; Mertens and Van Gaal, 2002).

Thus, abdominal, visceral obesity appears to be closely associated with a cluster of metabolic abnormalities, including dyslipidaemia and insulin resistance, as well as a prothrombotic/proinflammatory state, which are also features of the metabolic syndrome. We suggest that excess visceral adipose tissue accumulation represents an important and perhaps central component of this constellation of high-risk metabolic features (Després 1993; 1994b; Lemieux and Després, 1994).

The insulin-resistant, dyslipidaemic, proinflammatory and prothrombotic state of abdominal obesity: an important cause of coronary heart disease

Although at present there is no prospective study having identified visceral obesity as an independent risk factor for cardiovascular disease and related mortality, several studies have suggested that a substantial increase in the risk of cardiovascular disease results from the cluster of metabolic abnormalities found in visceral obesity, namely hyperinsulinaemia, insulin resistance, hypertriglyceridaemia, hypoalphalipoproteinaemia, hyperapolipoprotein B and the dense LDL phenotype, as well as an altered proinflammatory cytokine production and a prothrombotic profile. The prevalence of the metabolic syndrome has recently been examined in a large US cohort (NHANES), and it was found that approximately 25% of the overall population was characterized by the metabolic syndrome. This proportion increased dramatically with age, as 43% of the population above 60 years of age were characterized by the metabolic syndrome (Ford *et al.*, 2002). The metabolic syndrome and its associated risk factors have now emerged as factors contributing to the same extent as cigarette smoking to premature CHD. This phenomenon will cause major prejudice to the trend for a reduction in CHD events, which has been observed over the past three decades and was largely explained by the management of hypertension and elevated LDL-cholesterol levels in the US population (Adult Treatment Panel III, 2002).

Few studies have examined the contribution of the various components of the clustering metabolic abnormalities found in visceral obesity to coronary heart disease risk. The Québec Cardiovascular Study examined this issue in a prospective design. In 1985, the cardiovascular disease risk profile of a random sample of 2443 middle-aged men living in the metropolitan area of Québec City was evaluated (Dagenais *et al.*, 1990). This evaluation included the measurement of fasting plasma lipid and lipoprotein levels. After exclusion of men who showed clinical signs of ischaemic heart disease (IHD) (exertional angina, coronary insufficiency, non-fatal myocardial infarction and coronary death) and of men with triglyceride concentrations above 4.5 mmol/L, the incidence of IHD over 5 years was studied in a sample of 2103 men initially free of IHD. Over the 5-year follow-up, 114 men developed clinical signs of IHD.

When comparing the risk profiles of these 114 men to the 1989 men who remained healthy over the 5 years, it was found that men who eventually developed IHD had an elevated systolic blood pressure and a much higher prevalence of diabetes (Lamarche *et al.*, 1995). Body fatness, at least as crudely assessed by the BMI, was not significantly different among these groups. Significant differences were found in the plasma lipoprotein and lipid profile between men with IHD and men who remained healthy. Plasma total cholesterol and triglyceride levels were significantly higher in men who developed IHD than in those who remained event free. The mean Apo B concentration was also 12% higher in men who developed IHD. In concordance with previous prospective data, plasma HDL-C concentrations were lower and the cholesterol/HDL-C ratio was substantially higher (by 16%) in men who developed IHD than in men who remained healthy over the 5-year follow-up (Lamarche *et al.*, 1995).

By classifying subjects according to various dyslipidaemic phenotypes, Lamarche and colleagues (1995) found that, whereas 51% of the 1989 men who remained healthy over the follow-up were normolipidaemic, less than one-third of men who developed IHD were initially characterized by a normal lipoprotein–lipid profile, emphasizing the importance of alterations in plasma lipoprotein–lipid levels as risk factors for the development of IHD (Lamarche *et al.*, 1995). An elevated Apo B concentration was also found in 42% of men who developed IHD (Lamarche *et al.*, 1996). Quantification of the relative risk of IHD associated with each dyslipidaemic phenotype indicated that, in accordance with previous studies, elevated LDL-cholesterol levels were associated with an increased risk of IHD. However, men with hypertriglyceridaemia, but with normal Apo B levels, were not characterized by a higher risk of IHD, whereas men with hyperapo B with or without high triglyceride concentrations had a 2.5- to 3.0-fold increase in IHD risk (Lamarche *et al.*, 1996). Multiple regression analyses revealed that after including Apo B level in a model to predict IHD risk, this variable was found to be the best metabolic predictor of IHD (Lamarche *et al.*, 1996). These results emphasize that an elevated plasma Apo B concentration, a frequent consequence of visceral obesity, is predictive of an increased IHD risk, even in the absence of marked elevation in total cholesterol or LDL-cholesterol levels.

As hyperinsulinaemia is commonly accompanied by insulin resistance, the fasting insulin concentration is often used as a crude index of *in vivo* insulin resistance. This assumption is especially valid in non-diabetic subjects with no impairment in glucose tolerance (Laakso, 1997). Some prospective studies have reported a significant association between fasting hyperinsulinaemia and mortality from coronary heart disease, although this relationship did not appear to be independent from other factors (Pyörälä 1979; Welborn and Wearne 1979; Eschwège *et al.*, 1985; Yarnell *et al.*, 1994). In the Québec Cardiovascular Study, fasting insulin levels were measured in the plasma of men who then developed ischaemic heart disease and in matched control subjects of the 1985 cohort. Diabetic patients were excluded from the analyses and IHD subjects were matched with control subjects for smoking habits, BMI, alcohol consumption and age. Fasting plasma insulin levels were 18% higher in men who then developed IHD than in men who remained asymptomatic. Furthermore, fasting plasma insulin concentration was found to be an independent predictor of IHD risk, even after control for other risk variables, including plasma lipid and lipoprotein concentrations (Després *et al.*, 1996). By performing stratified analyses, it was also found that the combination of both hyperinsulinaemia (upper tertile of fasting insulin values distribution) and elevated Apo B levels (above the 50th percentile of Apo B distribution) was associated with more than a 10-fold increase in IHD risk (Fig. 12.8) (Després *et al.*, 1996). It is also important to emphasize that this high-risk combination of hyperinsulinaemia and hyperapo B is frequently found in visceral obese

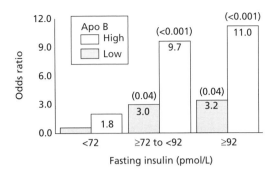

Fig 12.8 Odds ratios for ischaemic heart disease (IHD) according to plasma insulin and Apo B levels in the case–control prospective design of the Québec Cardiovascular Study. The cut-off point for low or high Apo B was the 50th percentile of Apo B distribution (119 mg/dL). *P*-values are given in parentheses. (Reproduced with permission from Després *et al.*, 1996.)

patients, even in the absence of glucose intolerance or type 2 diabetes.

As mentioned, the predominance of small, dense LDL particles in the plasma is another condition that has also been associated with an increase in the risk of IHD. Small, dense LDL particles have been reported to be more prevalent in coronary heart disease patients than in healthy control subjects (Fisher, 1983; Crouse *et al.*, 1985; Austin *et al.*, 1988; Griffin *et al.*, 1990; 1994; Tornvall *et al.*, 1991; Campos *et al.*, 1992; Coresh *et al.*, 1993; Jaakkola *et al.*, 1993), and there is evidence suggesting that these particles have atherogenic properties, which could be mediated by an increased filtration rate in the subendothelial space of the artery wall (Packard 1994; Rajman *et al.*, 1994), an increased susceptibility to oxidation (Chait *et al.*, 1993; Dejager *et al.*, 1993; de Graaf *et al.*, 1993), a reduced affinity for the LDL receptor (longer residence time in the plasma) (Silliman *et al.*, 1994) and an increased capacity to bind to intimal proteoglycans (La Belle and Krauss, 1990). Recent results from the Québec Cardiovascular Study have also shown that dense LDL particles are indeed predictive of a significant increase in the risk of IHD over 5 years (Lamarche *et al.*, 1997).

Furthermore, the simultaneous combination of small, dense LDL particles with elevated Apo B concentrations has been found to be associated with a sixfold increase in the risk of IHD (Lamarche *et al.*, 1997). The hypothesis that small, dense LDL particles may be associated with an increased risk of IHD was recently confirmed within the large-scale, population-based, prospective design of the Québec Cardiovascular Study (Lamarche *et al.*, 2001). Additional work by St Pierre and colleagues (2001) investigated further various electrophoretic characteristics of LDL particles and their relationship to the risk of IHD. In addition to having smaller and denser LDL particles, IHD cases also had a smaller number of LDL subclasses, and the higher LDL-cholesterol levels found in cases was mainly attributable to a 40% elevation of small LDL particle cholesterol content. Taking into account the amount of cholesterol located in the small, dense LDL fraction was found to markedly improve the ability to predict disease risk in the

Québec Cardiovascular Study (St Pierre *et al.*, 2001). As the predominance of small, dense LDL particles is closely associated with the hypertriglyceridaemic low HDL-cholesterol dyslipidaemic state of visceral obesity (Campos *et al.*, 1991; Katzel *et al.*, 1994; Tchernof *et al.*,1996), these recent results provide further support to the notion that small, dense LDL particles represent another component of the dyslipidaemic profile of visceral obesity that increases the risk of IHD.

The contribution of the inflammation marker CRP to the 5-year risk of developing IHD was also recently examined within the Québec Cardiovascular Study design (Pirro *et al.*, 2001; St Pierre *et al.*, 2003a). As mentioned, accumulating evidence indicates that inflammation may be involved in the aetiology of acute coronary syndromes and that plasma CRP is a significant predictor of future IHD events (Ridker *et al.*, 1997; 1998; 2000; Koenig *et al.*, 1999; Thompson *et al.*, 2000). However, only a few population-based studies had been published, and it was still unclear whether the age of the population and time of follow-up could modify the association of CRP to IHD. Recent results by Pirro *et al.* (2001) indicated that CRP level predicted the short-term risk for IHD (< 2 years), but not the long–term risk. Moreover, the risk associated with high CRP levels was independent of other known risk factors only in younger men (" 55 years). These results suggest that disease prediction by elevated CRP may be especially relevant for younger middle-aged men and in the case of events occurring early after the evaluation (Pirro *et al.*, 2001).

Finally, we found that the use of a particular combination of non-traditional risk factors, namely elevated insulin and Apo B levels and dense LDL particles, predicted a more than 20-fold increase in IHD risk than in those not showing this triad of metabolic abnormalities (Lamarche *et al.*, 1998). The strength of the relationship between non-traditional risk factors and IHD risk was not found to be affected by adjustment for traditional risk factors. Once again, these results emphasize the ability of features of the insulin resistant–dyslipidaemic state of visceral obesity to identify individuals at risk for cardiovascular disease (Lamarche *et al.*, 1998).

Visceral adipose tissue and the insulin resistant–dyslipidaemic syndrome: physiopathology and causal relationships

The physiological mechanisms underlying the relationship between abdominal obesity and clustering features of the metabolic syndrome have been extensively studied over recent years. Although several hypotheses have been put forward, some aspects of this relationship remain unclear at the present time. Hepatic VLDL synthesis is as a central factor in the dyslipidaemic state of abdominal obesity (Lewis 1997; Lewis *et al.*, 2002). In fact, the hypertriglyceridaemic state of this condition is primarily due to VLDL overproduction, whereas the concomitant low HDL-cholesterol levels and pre-

dominance of small, dense LDL particles appear to be consequences of high triglyceride levels (Lewis 1997; Lamarche *et al.*, 1999a; Lewis *et al.*, 2002). Availability of fatty acids in the liver is recognized as the primary determinant of reduced Apo B degradation and VLDL overproduction (Lewis, 1997), which has led to the hypothesis that an increased fatty acid flux from adipose tissue located within the abdominal cavity through the portal vein to the liver could potentially explain abdominal obesity-related hypertriglyceridaemia (Björntorp, 1990). Visceral adipose cells have a high lipolytic activity, which is poorly inhibited by insulin (Kissebah *et al.*, 1989; Kissebah and Peiris, 1989 Björntorp, 1990). This hypothesis is now known as the 'portal vein theory'.

The activity of the enzyme LPL is responsible for the catabolism of triglyceride-rich lipoproteins such as chylomicrons and VLDL. Its activity measured in post-heparin plasma has been reported to be lower in viscerally obese patients (Després *et al.*, 1989b), which contributes to the reduction in the catabolism of triglyceride-rich particles and to elevated plasma triglyceride concentrations. The high concentrations of triglyceride-rich lipoproteins found in visceral obesity also favour an increased lipid transfer by the cholesterol ester transfer protein (CETP) between VLDL particles and LDL as well as HDL particles. HDL particles then become relatively depleted in cholesterol esters and enriched in triglycerides. Triglycerides can also be transferred to LDL by CETP and this phenomenon also reduces the cholesterol to triglyceride ratio in LDL particles. As hepatic triglyceride lipase (HL) activity has been reported to be increased in visceral obesity (Després *et al.* 1989b; Després and Marette, 1994), triglyceride-rich HDL and LDL particles are then submitted to hydrolysis by this enzyme, generating small, dense LDL and HDL particles and, as a consequence, reduced HDL-cholesterol levels, especially in the HDL_2 subfraction (resulting in a reduced HDL_2-C/HDL_3-C ratio) (Fig. 12.9).

In recent years, some studies have suggested that the abdominal subcutaneous adipose tissue area was a better correlate of insulin resistance than visceral adipose tissue area (Abate *et al.*, 1995; Goodpaster *et al.*, 1997; Marcus *et al.*, 1999). In addition, morphological examination of subcutaneous fat has led to the identification of two distinct compartments within the subcutaneous anatomical region: a superficial layer of adipose tissue, evenly distributed under the abdominal skin layer, and a deeper subcutaneous adipose tissue compartment, located under the superficial adipose tissue layer (Markman and Barton, 1987), and reports by Misra *et al.* (1997) and Kelley and colleagues (2000) investigated whether estimating the area of the deep subcutaneous fat compartment could bring further insight into the relationship between abdominal obesity and metabolic risk factors. These investigators found that measures of the deep subcutaneous fat compartment were better predictors of insulin resistance than visceral adipose tissue area (Misra *et al.*,1997; Kelley *et al.*, 2000). These results were supported by some (Smith *et al.*, 2001;

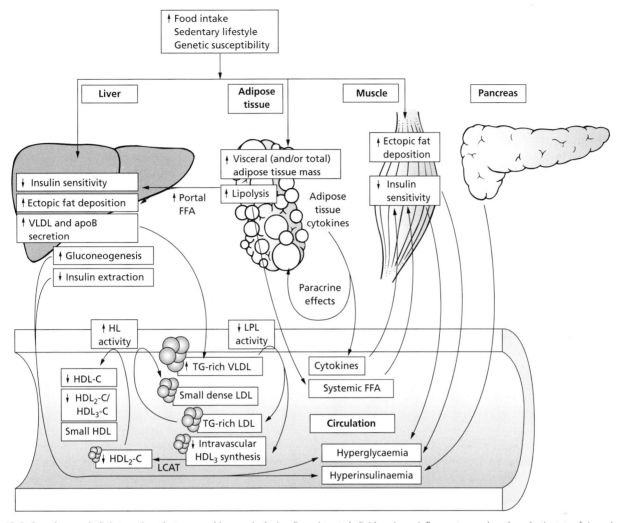

Fig 12.9 Complex metabolic interactions that presumably occur in the insulin-resistant, dyslipidaemic, proinflammatory and prothrombotic state of visceral obesity. Increased food intake and a sedentary lifestyle lead to excess accumulation of fat in the visceral compartments as well as ectopic fat deposition. As a result, the liver is exposed to high concentrations of free fatty acids (FFAs) generated by the highly lipolytic activity of the enlarged visceral adipose tissue mass and poor inhibition of lipolysis by insulin. This phenomenon stimulates VLDL synthesis and secretion as well as gluconeogenesis in the liver and inhibits hepatic extraction of insulin. The activity of lipoprotein lipase (LPL) is low, which leads to increased plasma concentrations of triglycerides (TG). The increased hepatic lipase (HL) activity contributes to the formation of small, dense LDL particles from TG-enriched LDL particles. It also leads to decreased HDL-cholesterol concentrations, HDL$_2$-C/HDL$_3$-C and HDL size. Adipose tissue releases cytokines that may modulate adipose tissue metabolism via paracrine effects, exert direct effects on the vascular endothelium and atherogenic plaque, or interfere with insulin signalling in the muscle, thereby contributing to peripheral insulin resistance.

Toth *et al.*, 2001), but not all, studies on this topic (Lovejoy *et al.*, 2001; Ross *et al.*, 2002), which contributed further to the controversy. However, a recent study by Jensen *et al.* (2003) examined the correlation between fat content of the two abdominal compartments and whole-body glucose disappearance during high- and low-dose insulin infusions. The study indicated that the correlation between deep subcutaneous abdominal adipose tissue and glucose disappearance, which was significant only at high insulin doses, was accounted for by the correlation between visceral fat and deep abdominal subcutaneous fat (Jensen *et al.*, 2003). Accordingly, Deschenes and colleagues (2003) found a relatively strong correlation between visceral

adipose tissue area and deep subcutaneous fat area, which could partly explain discrepancies among studies. They also found that visceral adipose tissue area was the best predictor of plasma lipid and lipoprotein levels, particularly with measures of hepatic lipoprotein synthesis. This relationship was independent of concomitant variation in other adiposity measures such as deep abdominal subcutaneous area or total body fat mass, which provides indirect support to the portal vein theory (Deschenes *et al.*, 2003).

On the other hand, whether such a theory is a plausible physiological mechanism to explain visceral obesity-related insulin resistance has been a matter of intense debate recently.

The excess free fatty acid release through the portal system to the liver may be associated with a reduced hepatic insulin extraction (Hennes *et al.*, 1990; Svedberg *et al.*, 1990), which could partly contribute to the hyperinsulinaemic state of this condition (Björntorp, 1990; Després, 1991). It may also be associated with an increased hepatic gluconeogenesis, leading to an elevated hepatic glucose production. This phenomenon could contribute to the deterioration in glucose tolerance frequently found in viscerally obese patients (Björntorp, 1992; Després and Marette, 1994) (Fig. 12.9). At present, the literature suggests that excess systemic free fatty acid release is involved in skeletal muscle insulin resistance through inhibition of insulin signalling and glucose transport, as well as inhibition of glycogen synthase, pyruvate dehydrogenase and hexokinase (Kelley *et al.*, 1993; Boden *et al.*, 1994; Griffin *et al.*, 1999; Thompson and Cooney, 2000). One would suggest that the highly lipolytic properties of visceral fat could account for an important part of these effects.

However, studies by Jensen and colleagues (Basu *et al.*, 2001) examined the relative contribution of splanchnic and non-splanchnic tissues to systemic free fatty acid (FFA) release and found that approximately 75% of fatty acids released originated from non-splanchnic tissues. Thus, further studies are required to elucidate the nature of the association between visceral adipose tissue accumulation, high FFA levels and peripheral insulin resistance. In this regard, recent results on lipodystrophic mice and ectopic fat accumulation have led to the suggestion that the appearance of insulin resistance in a high dietary fat intake context may be due to an increased lipid burden on skeletal muscle and liver resulting from a reduced capacity for excess fat storage when facing caloric excess (Reitman *et al.*, 1999; Nadler and Attie, 2001). Several papers have now emphasized that an increased muscle lipid content is closely associated with insulin resistance (Goodpaster *et al.*, 1997; Goodpaster and Kelley 2002). Moreover, a very elegant study by Kim and colleagues (2001), performed in mice overexpressing either liver or skeletal muscle LPL, showed insulin resistance specific to the tissue overexpressing LPL, suggesting a direct and causative relationship between the accumulation of intracellular fatty acids and insulin resistance (Kim *et al.*, 2001). Of note, these effects were independent from those of circulating adipocyte-derived hormones (see below). According to this hypothesis, insulin resistance could be due not only to lipids released from fat, but also to a reduced capacity for excess lipid storage (Nadler *et al.*, 2000; Kim *et al.*, 2001).

More recently, the increasingly recognized endocrine and paracrine nature of the adipose organ has emerged as a new line of investigation to elucidate the link between fat accumulation and the related metabolic complications. Adipose tissue-secreted cytokines (adipocytokines) have been proposed as potential links between the adipocyte, insulin resistance and atherosclerosis. For example, studies have shown that the secretion of TNF-α is increased in adipose tissue of obese rodents and humans, and that elevated levels of this cytokine may interfere with insulin signalling (Hotamisligil, 2000), or lead to insulin resistance in muscle by increasing nitric oxide production in this tissue through activation of inducible nitric oxide synthase (Perreault and Marette, 2001). A recent study by Weyer and colleagues (2000) provided additional support to the notion that the adipocyte plays a central role in the aetiology of insulin resistance. This study demonstrated that an enlarged subcutaneous adipocyte size was predictive of the risk of type 2 diabetes, independent from insulin resistance. The authors suggested that these findings may be attributable to the fact that enlarged adipocytes secrete increased amounts of TNF-α (Weyer *et al.*, 2000). Studies in humans and rodents also recently suggested that additional adipocytokines such as resistin, adiponectin and IL-6 may contribute to obesity-related insulin resistance (Fried *et al.*, 1998; Steppan *et al.*, 2001; Spranger *et al.*, 2003). Proinflammatory cytokines originating from adipose tissue have also been involved in the process of atherogenesis and linked to the previously discussed elevated plasma CRP found in patients with an increased risk for cardiovascular disease (Blake and Ridker, 2002).

Taken together, available data support the notion that several factors related to body fat accumulation and distribution may contribute to the cluster of metabolic abnormalities observed in the metabolic syndrome, and the related risk of type 2 diabetes and cardiovascular disease. Adipose tissue fatty acid release and storage capacity, as well as secreted cytokines, may be involved in the aetiology of the syndrome. The anatomical location of visceral adipocytes close to the liver, combined with possible depot-specific alterations in various adipocyte or adipose tissue features probably play important roles in this process. This highly complex aetiology is concordant with the rather heterogeneous clinical manifestations of the metabolic syndrome, and suggests the possibility of interindividual variability in the extent to which each pathophysiological mechanism is involved.

Genetic susceptibility to metabolic complications of visceral obesity

Some abdominally obese individuals may be especially prone to develop the clinical features of the metabolic syndrome, whereas others may appear to be relatively protected. As illustrated above, the cluster of metabolic abnormalities related to visceral obesity represents an extremely complex phenotype with a multifactorial aetiology. Although environmental factors obviously contribute to the development of obesity, genetic factors clearly modulate the susceptibility to this condition (Bouchard, 1991). In a similar manner, the magnitude of the metabolic complications found in a given viscerally obese patient partly depends upon his/her genetic predisposition. In this regard, several candidate genes could be responsible for the variability observed in the dyslipidaemic phenotype of visceral obesity. For example, genes coding for apolipoproteins, lipoprotein receptors, enzymes responsible for lipoprotein metabolism or genes that are expressed in adipose tissue could be involved in the development of the metabolic syndrome (Després *et al.*, 1992). In recent years, several publications from investigators in our group have identified genetic polymorphisms that are associated with the magnitude of the 'dysmetabolic' state found in visceral obesity (Pouliot *et al.*, 1990; 1994a; Després *et al.*, 1993; Vohl *et al.*, 1995; 1996; 1997; Berthier *et al.*, 2001; 2003; Engert *et al.*, 2002; St Pierre *et al.*, 2002; 2003b; Couillard *et al.*, 2003; Robitaille *et al.*, 2003; Tremblay *et al.*, 2003). The following section lists a few examples.

Apolipoprotein genes have proven to be interesting candidates. By studying isoforms of Apo E, it was found that excess visceral adipose tissue accumulation and hyperinsulinaemia were associated with hypertriglyceridaemia only in carriers of the Apo E_2 allele or among Apo E_3 homozygotes (Pouliot *et al.*, 1990; Després *et al.*, 1993), whereas Apo E_4 carriers did not show these associations. Thus, the Apo E polymorphism altered the expected relationship of visceral obesity and hyperinsulinaemia to hypertriglyceridaemia. We have also examined the potential contribution of an Apo B-100 gene *Eco*RI polymorphism in men (Pouliot *et al.*, 1994a). Our results indicated that among subjects who were heterozygous for the absence of the *Eco*RI restriction site, visceral obesity was associated with elevated Apo B concentrations. However, this relationship could not be found among homozygotes for the presence of this *Eco*RI restriction site. We have also shown that viscerally obese men heterozygous for the absence of this polymorphism were more likely to develop the dense LDL phenotype (Vohl *et al.*, 1996). The *Msp*I polymorphism of the Apo A-II gene has also been found to be a modulator of the dyslipidaemic state of visceral obesity, as carriers of the fairly frequent M1 allele with high levels of visceral fat were characterized by a lower HDL_2–cholesterol/HDL_3–cholesterol ratio than viscerally obese patients with other Apo A-II genotypes (Vohl *et al.*, 1997). More recently, a study of Apo CIII gene polymorphisms led to the identification of a *Sst*I polymorphism also modulating the association between visceral adipose tissue accumulation and plasma triglyceride levels in viscerally obese men. This polymorphism has also been associated with the presence of small, dense LDL particles (Couillard *et al.*, 2003).

Genes coding for enzymes involved in lipoprotein metabolism have also been studied, namely hepatic lipase, lipoprotein lipase and microsomal transfer protein (Vohl *et al.* 1995; St Pierre *et al.*, 2002; 2003b). Homozygous carriers of the *Hind*III polymorphism in the LPL gene characterized by visceral obesity were found to be more susceptible to hypertriglyceridaemia than heterozygous viscerally obese patients (Vohl *et al.*, 1995). The hepatic lipase −514C→T polymorphism, which is normally associated with increased HDL-C concentrations, was found to have no impact on HDL-C levels in the presence of visceral obesity (St Pierre *et al.*, 2003b). In a study on the microsomal transfer protein −493G→T polymorphism, it was found that the presence of visceral obesity modulated the impact of the mutation on total cholesterol and LDL-Apo B levels as well as on LDL particle size (St Pierre *et al.*, 2002). These results emphasize once again that the expression of a given atherogenic phenotype results from the complex interaction between genetic and environmental factors.

Important adipose tissue-expressed genes are also being investigated at present (Engert *et al.*, 2002; Berthier *et al.*, 2003; Robitaille *et al.*, 2003; Tremblay *et al.*, 2003). For example, the −174G→C polymorphism of IL-6 was significantly associated with indices of adiposity and parameters of glucose and insulin homeostasis (Berthier *et al.*, 2003). A number of polymorphisms have been identified in the resistin gene, and some of the 5'-flanking variants showed significant associations with BMI (Engert *et al.*, 2002). The IVS2–*Bcl*I polymorphism of the glucocorticoid receptor was associated with longitudinal changes in fatness through adolescence in women (Tremblay *et al.*, 2003). Finally, using a new paradigm in the study of gene and environment interactions, Robitaille and colleagues (2003) examined the interaction between a PPAR-gamma polymorphism and dietary fat intake. This study demonstrated that high dietary fat intake was associated with the presence of several metabolic abnormalities in patients with the P12/P12 genotype, whereas none of these associations was found in the A12 allele carriers, which suggested that the PPAR-gamma polymorphism could modulate the association between dietary fat intake and features of the metabolic syndrome (Robitaille *et al.*, 2003).

It should be pointed out that although not all of these polymorphisms have been associated with altered protein levels or enzyme activities, the associations found could be resulting from a linkage disequilibrium between these polymorphisms and other unknown genes significantly modulating genetic susceptibility to the dyslipidaemic state of visceral obesity. Future studies using new high-throughput methodologies, such as DNA microarrays and real-time PCR, are likely to accelerate research on the genetic susceptibility to the metabolic syndrome in abdominal obesity. Moreover, the combination of several gene variants (gene–gene interactions) or of genetic variants and variables of the environment, such as gene–diet interactions, may eventually lead to a better understanding of the variability in clinical manifestations of the metabolic syndrome. The challenge in clinical practice will be to integrate all of this genetic information in the evaluation of the risk associated with visceral obesity.

Therapeutic implications

As revised in this chapter, visceral obesity is associated with a cluster of metabolic abnormalities contributing to increase the risk of type 2 diabetes and IHD. The proper identification of patients with visceral obesity has important public health implications. The use of computerized tomography represents a precise and reliable procedure to identify viscerally obese patients. However, this expensive methodology is not readily available to most clinicians. Several studies have used the waist–hip ratio as a measurement of abdominal obesity and until recently, this variable had been considered as a relevant tool in the assessment of abdominal fat accumulation (Kissebah and Peiris, 1989). We and others have now demonstrated that the waist circumference by itself is a better correlate of visceral adipose tissue accumulation than the WHR or other anthropometric measures (Pouliot et al., 1994b; Rankinen et al., 1999; Chan et al., 2003).

As mentioned earlier, the combined use of a particular triad of non-traditional risk factors (elevated insulin, Apo B and small, dense LDL particles) has contributed to a better identification of patients at markedly elevated risk of developing IHD in the Québec Cardiovascular Study. Given that visceral fat accumulation generally predicts Apo B and fasting insulin levels and that there is a close correlation between fasting plasma triglyceride concentrations and the presence of the small, dense LDL phenotype, Lemieux and colleagues (2000) have attempted to predict the presence of this high-risk metabolic triad using waist circumference and triglyceride levels. These analyses were performed in a sample of healthy white middle-aged men. It was found that men with a low waist circumference (below 90 cm) and low triglyceride levels (below 2 mmol/L) had a low probability (approximately 10%) of being characterized by the atherogenic metabolic triad. On the other hand, using the same cut-off values, the probability of being characterized by the metabolic triad increased to 80% in men characterized by both an elevated waist circumference and increased triglyceride levels (Lemieux et al., 2000). This simple clinical phenotype termed 'hypertriglyceridaemic waist' will probably prove very useful in the identification of high-risk patients following further validation in other populations and longitudinal designs.

As discussed, excess visceral adipose tissue accumulation plays a significant role in the pathophysiology of a number of clustering abnormalities. Accordingly, weight loss therapy leading to a reduction in the visceral adipose tissue mass has been suggested to be associated with improvements in several aspects of the metabolic risk profile (Després and Lamarche, 1993; Heilbronn et al., 2001; Tchernof et al., 2002; Brochu et al., 2003; Kreisberg and Oberman, 2003). In this regard, a critical review of weight loss studies suggested that the visceral adipose tissue compartment may be preferentially mobilized in response to a negative energy balance (Smith and Zachwieja, 1999). Thus, it appears that interventions producing a significant mobilization of visceral adipose tissue may contribute to alleviate some of the abnormalities leading to type 2 diabetes and cardiovascular disease.

When considering weight reduction, however, the clinician is confronted with crucial questions: which mode of intervention should be chosen, how much weight loss would be enough to obtain significant health benefits, and how the high rate of relapse usually observed in the post-weight loss state should be approached. Definitive answers to these questions have not yet been provided. However, important studies on lifestyle intervention recently demonstrated that counselling patients with the aim of reducing weight, total intake of fat and saturated fat, while increasing fibre intake and physical activity, led to a significant reduction in the longitudinal risk of developing type 2 diabetes (Tuomilehto et al., 2001). Most interestingly, changes in the diabetes incidences were directly proportional to the extent to which patients were compliant to clinical recommendations. This highly effective intervention was even more effective than metformin therapy alone (Knowler et al., 2002). These results clearly emphasize that behavioural modifications have a high potential for health improvements. Although the aforementioned studies were not designed to evaluate the respective contributions of exercise, caloric restriction and weight loss on health outcomes, the inclusion of an exercise prescription probably played a significant role in the results achieved and long-term maintenance of a reduced body weight. In this regard, physical activity may represent an interesting adjunct to weight reduction interventions as it has been shown to have beneficial effects on carbohydrate and lipid metabolism, irrespective of the weight loss achieved (Lamarche et al., 1992).

Regarding the amount of weight loss required to obtain health-related benefits, studies tend to demonstrate that body weight normalization is not necessary to achieve substantial metabolic benefits (Poirier and Després, 2003). In a recent weight loss protocol in post-menopausal women, Brochu and colleagues (2003) examined whether it was necessary to reach a low value of visceral adipose tissue (below 110 cm^2 in that study) to induce favourable metabolic changes. Interestingly, results did not favour the necessity of reaching any given threshold of visceral adipose tissue to improve the risk profile. Moreover, moderate visceral fat losses yielded similar metabolic improvement compared with large losses (Brochu et al., 2003). These results suggest that moderate weight loss, specifically in the abdominal region, may represent an effective strategy for risk management in abdominal obesity. Keeping realistic expectations and objectives as far as weight loss is concerned, and adding a significant amount of exercise, may help in reducing the risk of relapse.

Conclusions

Excess visceral adipose tissue accumulation appears to represent a central component of the clustering metabolic abnormalities leading to an increased risk of type 2 diabetes and cardiovascular disease. When present, this condition is associated, in both men and women, with insulin resistance, compensatory hyperinsulinaemia, glucose intolerance, a dyslipidaemic state including high plasma triglycerides, low HDL-C, an increased cholesterol/HDL-C ratio, hyper-apolipoprotein B and an increased proportion of small, dense LDL particles, as well as with a prothrombotic and proinflammatory profile. Evidence from prospective studies including recent observations from the Québec Cardiovascular Study cohort have indicated that this cluster of metabolic abnormalities clearly increases the risk of IHD in men. It is therefore clinically relevant to identify and treat these high-risk patients. On the basis of its high prevalence in affluent societies, it is proposed that visceral obesity and the concomitant development of the metabolic syndrome will probably represent the most prevalent cause of type 2 diabetes and CHD in the coming years. Concerted efforts to prevent and treat this condition are needed.

References

Abate, N., Garg, A., Peshock, R.M., Stray-Gundersen, J. and Grundy, S.M. (1995) Relationships of generalized and regional adiposity to insulin sensitivity in men. *Journal of Clinical Investigation* **96**, 88–98.

Adult Treatment Panel III (2002) Third Report of the National Cholesterol Education Program (NCEP) Expert Panel on Detection, Evaluation, and Treatment of High Blood Cholesterol in Adults (Adult Treatment Panel III) final report. *Circulation* **106**, 3143–3421.

Albrink, M.J., Krauss, R.M., Lindgren, F.T., Von der Groeben, V.D. and Wood, P.D. (1980) Intercorrelation among high density lipoprotein, obesity, and triglycerides in a normal population. *Lipids* **15**, 668–678.

Austin, M.A. (1991) Plasma triglyceride and coronary heart disease. *Arteriosclerosis and Thrombosis* **11**, 2–14.

Austin, M.A., Breslow, J.L., Hennekens, C.H., Buring, J.E., Willet, W.C. and Krauss, R.M. (1988) Low-density lipoprotein subclass patterns and risk of myocardial infarction. *Journal of the American Medical Association* **260**, 1917–1921.

Barrett-Connor, E. (1985) Obesity, atherosclerosis, and coronary artery disease. *Annals of Internal Medicine* **103**, 1010–1019.

Bastard, J.P., Jardel, C., Bruckert, E., Blondy, P., Capeau, J., Laville, M. and Vidal, H. (2000) Elevated levels of interleukin 6 are reduced in serum and subcutaneous adipose tissue of obese women after weight loss. *Journal of Clinical Endocrinology and Metabolism* **85**, 3338–3342.

Basu, A., Basu, R., Shah, P., Vella, A., Rizza, R.A. and Jensen, M.D. (2001) Systemic and regional free fatty acid metabolism in type 2 diabetes. *American Journal of Physiology Endocrinology and Metabolism* **280**, E1000–E1006.

Bergstrom, R. W., Newell-Morris, L.L., Leonetti, D.L., Shuman, W.P., Wahl, P. W. and Fujimoto, W.Y. (1990) Association of elevated fasting C-peptide level and increased intra-abdominal fat distribution with development of NIDDM in Japanese-American men. *Diabetes* **39**, 104–111.

Berthier, M.T., Couillard, C., Prud'homme, D., Nadeau, A., Bergeron, J., Tremblay, A., Després, J.P. and Vohl, M.C. (2001) Effects of the FABP2 A54T mutation on triglyceride metabolism of viscerally obese men. *Obesity Research* **9**, 668–675.

Berthier, M.T., Paradis, A.M., Tchernof, A., Bergeron, J., Prud'homme, D., Després, J.P. and Vohl, M.C. (2003) The interleukin 6 -174G/C polymorphism is associated with indices of obesity in men. *Journal of Human Genetics* **48**, 14–19.

Björntorp, P. (1984) Hazards in subgroups of human obesity. *European Journal of Clinical Investigation* **14**, 239–241.

Björntorp, P. (1990) 'Portal' adipose tissue as a generator of risk factors for cardiovascular disease and diabetes. *Arteriosclerosis* **10**, 493–496.

Björntorp, P. (1992) Metabolic abnormalities in visceral obesity. *Annals of Medicine* **24**, 3–5.

Blake, G.J. and Ridker, P.M. (2002) Inflammatory bio-markers and cardiovascular risk prediction. *Journal of Internal Medicine* **252**, 283–294.

Boden, G., Chen, X., Ruiz, J., White, J.V. and Rossetti, L. (1994) Mechanisms of fatty acid-induced inhibition of glucose uptake. *Journal of Clinical Investigation* **93**, 2438–2446.

Bonora, E., Del Prato, S., Bonadonna, R.C., Gulli, G., Solini, A., Shank, M.L., Guitas, A.A., Lancaster, J.L., Kilcoyne, R.F., Alyassin, A.M. and DeFronzo, R. A. (1992) Total body fat content and fat topography are associated differently with *in vivo* glucose metabolism in nonobese and obese nondiabetic women. *Diabetes* **41**, 1151–1159.

Bouchard, C. (1991) Current understanding of the etiology of obesity: genetic and nongenetic factors. *American Journal of Clinical Nutrition* **53**, 1561S–1565S.

Boyko, E.J., Fujimoto, W.Y., Leonetti, D.L. and Newell-Morris, L. (2000) Visceral adiposity and risk of type 2 diabetes: a prospective study among Japanese Americans. *Diabetes Care* **23**, 465–471.

Bray, G.A. (1985) Complications of obesity. *Annals of Internal Medicine* **103**, 1052–1062.

Bray, G.A., Davidson, M.B. and Drenick, E.J. (1972) Obesity: A serious symptom. *Annals of Internal Medicine* **77**, 797–805.

Brochu, M., Starling, R.D., Tchernof, A., Matthews, D.E. and Poehlman, E.T. (2000) Visceral adipose tissue as an independent correlate of glucose disposal in older postmenopausal women. *Journal of Clinical Endocrinology and Metabolism* **85**, 2378–2384.

Brochu, M., Tchernof, A., Sites, C.K., Eltabbakh, G.H., Sims, E.A.H. and Poehlman, E.T. (2001) What are the physical characteristics associated with a normal metabolic profile despite a high level of obesity in postmenopausal women? *Journal of Clinical Endocrinology and Metabolism* **86**, 1020–1025.

Brochu, M., Tchernof, A., Turner, A.N., Ades, P. A. and Poehlman, E.T. (2003) Is there a threshold of visceral fat loss that improves the metabolic profile in obese postmenopausal women? *Metabolism* **52**, 599–604.

Campos, H., Bailey, S.M., Gussak, L.S., Siles, X., Ordovas, J.M. and Schaefer, E.J. (1991) Relations of body habitus, fitness level, and cardiovascular risk factors including lipoproteins in a rural and urban Costa Rican population. *Arteriosclerosis and Thrombosis* **11**, 1077–1088.

Campos, H., Genest, J.J., Blijlevens, E., McNamara, J.R., Jenner, J.L., Ordovas, J. M., Wilson, P.W. F. and Schaefer, E.J. (1992) Low density lipoprotein particle size and coronary artery disease. *Arteriosclerosis and Thrombosis* **12**, 187–195.

Chait, A., Brazg, R.L., Tribble, D.L. and Krauss, R.M. (1993) Susceptibility of small, dense, low-density lipoproteins to oxidative modification in subjects with the atherogenic lipoprotein phenotype, pattern B. *American Journal of Medicine* **94**, 350–356.

Chan, D.C., Watts, G.F., Barrett, P.H. and Burke, V. (2003) Waist circumference, waist-to-hip ratio and body mass index as predictors of adipose tissue compartments in men. *Quarterly Journal of Medicine* **96**, 441–447.

Coresh, J., Kwiterovich, Jr, P.O., Smith, H.H. and Bachorik, P.S. (1993) Association of plasma triglyceride concentration and LDL particle diameter, density, and chemical composition with premature coronary artery disease in men and women. *Journal of Lipid Research* **34**, 1687–1697.

Couillard, C., Vohl, M.C., Engert, J.C., Lemieux, I., Houde, A., Alméras, N., Prud'homme, D., Nadeau, A., Després, J.P. and Bergeron, J. (2003) Effect of apoC-III gene polymorphisms on the lipoprotein-lipid profile of viscerally obese men. *Journal of Lipid Research* **44**, 986–993.

Crouse, J.R., Parks, J.S. and Schey, H.M. (1985) Studies of low density lipoprotein molecular weight in human beings with coronary artery disease. *Journal of Lipid Research* **26**, 566–574.

Dagenais, G.R., Robitaille, N.M., Lupien, P.J., Christen, A., Gingras, S., Moorjani, S., Meyer, F. and Rochon, J. (1990) First coronary heart disease event rates in relation to major risk factors: Québec Cardiovascular Study. *Canadian Journal of Cardiology* **6**, 274–280.

Davis, C.E., Gordon, D., LaRosa, J.C., Wood, P.D. and Halperin, M. (1980) Correlation of plasma high density lipoprotein cholesterol levels with other plasma lipid and lipoprotein concentrations. *Circulation* **62** (Suppl. IV), 24–30.

Dejager, S., Bruckert, E. and Chapman, M.J. (1993) Dense low density lipoprotein subspecies with diminished oxidative resistance predominate in combined hyperlipidemia. *Journal of Lipid Research* **34**, 295–308.

DeNino, W.F., Tchernof, A., Dionne, I.J., Toth, M.J., Ades, P.A., Sites, C.K. and Poehlman, E.T. (2001) Contribution of abdominal adiposity to age-related differences in insulin sensitivity and plasma lipids in healthy nonobese women. *Diabetes Care* **24**, 925–932.

Deschenes, D., Couture, P., Dupont, P. and Tchernof, A. (2003) Subdivision of the subcutaneous adipose tissue compartment and lipid-lipoprotein levels in women. *Obesity Research* **11**, 469–476.

Després, J.P. (1991) Obesity and lipid metabolism: relevance of body fat distribution. *Current Opinion in Lipidology* **2**, 5–15.

Després, J.P. (1993) Abdominal obesity as important component of insulin- resistance syndrome. *Nutrition* **9**, 452–459.

Després, J.P. (1994a) Dyslipidaemia and obesity. *Baillières Clinical Endocrinology and Metabolism* **8**, 629–660.

Després, J.P. (1994b) Visceral obesity: a component of the insulin resistance- dyslipidemic syndrome. *Canadian Journal of Cardiology* **10** (Suppl.), 17B–22B.

Després, J.P. and Lamarche, B. (1993) Effects of diet and physical activity on adiposity and body fat distribution: implications for the prevention of cardiovascular disease. *Nutrition Research Reviews* **6**, 137–159.

Després, J.P. and Marette, A. (1994) Relation of components of insulin resistance syndrome to coronary disease risk. *Current Opinion in Lipidology* **5**, 274–289.

Després, J.P., Nadeau, A., Tremblay, A., Ferland, M., Moorjani, S., Lupien, P. J., Thériault, G., Pinault, S. and Bouchard, C. (1989a) Role of deep abdominal fat in the association between regional adipose tissue distribution and glucose tolerance in obese women. *Diabetes* **38**, 304–309.

Després, J.P., Ferland, M., Moorjani, S., Nadeau, A., Tremblay, A.,

Lupien, P. J., Thériault, G. and Bouchard, C. (1989b) Role of hepatic-triglyceride lipase activity in the association between intra-abdominal fat and plasma HDL-cholesterol in obese women. *Arteriosclerosis* **9**, 485–492.

Després, J.P., Prud'homme, D., Pouliot, M.C., Tremblay, A. and Bouchard, C. (1991) Estimation of deep abdominal adipose-tissue accumulation from simple anthropometric measurements in men. *American Journal of Clinical Nutrition*, **54**, 471–477.

Després, J.P., Moorjani, S., Lupien, P.J., Tremblay, A., Nadeau, A. and Bouchard, C. (1992) Genetic aspects of susceptibility to obesity and related dyslipidemias. *Molecular and Cellular Biochemistry* **113**, 151–169.

Després, J.P., Verdon, M.F., Moorjani, S., Pouliot, M.C., Nadeau, A., Bouchard, C., Tremblay, A. and Lupien, P.J. (1993) Apolipoprotein E polymorphism modifies relation of hyperinsulinemia to hypertriglyceridemia. *Diabetes* **42**, 1474–1481.

Després, J.P., Lamarche, B., Mauriège, P., Cantin, B., Dagenais, G.R., Moorjani, S. and Lupien, P.J. (1996) Hyperinsulinemia as an independent risk factor for ischemic heart disease. *New England Journal of Medicine* **334**, 952–957.

Després, J.P., Lemieux, I., Dagenais, G.R., Cantin, B. and Lamarche, B. (2000) HDL-cholesterol as a marker of coronary heart disease risk: the Quebec cardiovascular study. *Atherosclerosis* **153**, 263–272.

Donahue, R.P., Abbot, R.D., Bloom, E., Reed, D.M. and Yano, K. (1987) Central obesity and coronary heart disease in men. *Lancet* **1**, 821–824.

Ducimetière, P., Richard, J. and Cambien, F. (1986) The pattern of subcutaneous fat distribution in middle-aged men and the risk of coronary heart disease: the Paris prospective study. *International Journal of Obesity* **10**, 229–240.

Dvorak, R., DeNino, W.F., Ades, P.A. and Poehlman, E.T. (1999) Phenotypic characteristics associated with insulin resistance in metabolically obese but normal-weight young women. *Diabetes* **48**, 2210–2214.

Engert, J.C., Vohl, M.C., Williams, S.M., Lepage, P., Loredo-Osti, J.C., Faith, J., Doré, C., Renaud, Y., Burtt, N.P., Villeneuve, A., Hirschhorn, J.N., Altshuler, D., Groop, L.C., Després, J. P., Gaudet, D. and Hudson, T.J. (2002) 5′ flanking variants of resistin are associated with obesity. *Diabetes* **51**, 1629–1634.

Enzi, G., Gasparo, M., Biondetti, P.R., Fiore, D., Semisa, M. and Zurlo, F. (1986) Subcutaneous and visceral fat distribution according to sex, age and overweight, evaluated by computed tomography. *American Journal of Clinical Nutrition* **44**, 739–746.

Eschwège, E., Richard, J.L., Thibult, N., Ducimetière, P., Warnet, J.M. and Rosselin, G. (1985) Coronary heart disease mortality in relation with diabetes, blood glucose and plasma insulin levels: The Paris Prospective study, ten years later. *Hormone and Metabolic Research* **15** (Suppl.), 41–46.

Ferland, M., Després, J. P., Tremblay, A., Pinault, S., Nadeau, A., Moorjani, S., Lupien, P.J., Thériault, G. and Bouchard, C. (1989) Assessment of adipose tissue distribution by computed axial tomography in obese women: association with body density and anthropometric measurements. *British Journal of Nutrition* **61**, 139–148.

Fisher, W. R. (1983) Heterogeneity of plasma low density lipoproteins manifestations of the physiologic phenomenon in man. *Metabolism* **32**, 283–291.

Ford, E.S. (1999) Body mass index, diabetes, and C-reactive protein among US adults. *Diabetes Care* **22**, 1971–1977.

Ford, E.S., Giles, W.H. and Dietz, W.H. (2002) Prevalence of the metabolic syndrome among US adults. Findings from the third National Health and Nutrition Examination Survey. *Journal of the American Medical Association* **287**, 356–359.

Fried, S.K., Bunkin, D.A. and Greenberg, A.S. (1998) Omental and subcutaneous adipose tissues of obese subjects release interleukin-6: Depot difference and regulation by glucocorticoid. *Journal of Clinical Endocrinology and Metabolism* **83**, 847–850.

Gabay, C. and Kushner, I. (1999) Acute-phase proteins and other systemic responses to inflammation. *New England Journal of Medicine* **340**, 448–454.

Garrison, R.J., Kannel, W.B., Stokes, III, J. and Castelli, W.P. (1987) Incidence and precursors of hypertension in young adults: The Framingham offspring study. *Preventive Medicine* **16**, 235–251.

Genest, J.J., McNamara, J.R., Salem, D.N. and Schaefer, E.J. (1991) Prevalence of risk factors in men with premature coronary heart disease. *American Journal of Cardiology* **67**, 1185–1189.

Goodpaster, B.H. and Kelley, D.E. (2002) Skeletal muscle triglyceride: marker or mediator of obesity-induced insulin resistance in type 2 diabetes mellitus? *Current Diabetes Report* **2**, 216–222.

Goodpaster, B.H., Thaete, F.L., Simoneau, J.A. and Kelley, D.E. (1997) Subcutaneous abdominal fat and thigh muscle composition predict insulin sensitivity independently of visceral fat. *Diabetes* **46**, 1579–1585.

Gordon, D.J. and Rifkind, B.M. (1989) High-density lipoprotein: the clinical implications of recent studies. *New England Journal of Medicine* **321**, 1311–1316.

Gordon, T., Castelli, W.P., Hjortland, M.C., Kannel, W.B. and Dawber, T.R. (1977) High density lipoprotein as a protective factor against coronary heart disease: The Framingham Study. *American Journal of Medicine* **62**, 707–714.

Gotto, A.M., LaRosa, J.C., Hunninghake, D., Grundy, S.M., Wilson, P.R., Clarkson, T.B., Hay, J.W. and Goodman, D.S. (1990) The cholesterol facts: A summary of the evidence relating dietary fats, serum cholesterol and coronary heart disease. *Circulation* **81**, 1721–1733.

de Graaf, J., Hendriks, J.C.M., Demacker, P.N.M. and Stalenhoef, A.F. (1993) Identification of multiple dense LDL subfractions with enhanced susceptibility to *in vitro* oxidation among hypertriglyceridemic subjects. Normalization after clofibrate treatment. *Arteriosclerosis and Thrombosis* **13**, 712–719.

Griffin, B.A., Caslake, M.J., Yip, B., Tait, G.W., Packard, C.J. and Shepherd, J. (1990) Rapid isolation of low density lipoprotein (LDL) subfractions from plasma by density gradient ultracentrifugation. *Atherosclerosis* **83**, 59–67.

Griffin, B.A., Freeman, D.J., Tait, G.W., Thomson J, Caslake, M.J., Packard, C.J. and Shepherd, J. (1994) Role of plasma triglyceride in the regulation of plasma low density lipoprotein (LDL) subfractions: relative contribution of small dense LDL to coronary heart disease risk. *Atherosclerosis* **106**, 241–253.

Griffin, M.E., Marcucci, M.J., Cline, G.W., Bell, K., Barucci, N., Lee, D., Goodyear, L.J., Kraegen, E.W., White, M.F. and Shulman, G.I. (1999) Free fatty acid-induced insulin resistance is associated with activation of protein kinase C theta and alterations in the insulin signaling cascade. *Diabetes* **48**, 1270–1274.

Hak, A.E., Stehouwer, C.D.A., Bots, M.L., Polderman, K.H., Schalkijk, C.G., Westendorp, I.C.D., Hofman, A. and Witteman, J.C.M. (1999) Associations of C-reactive protein with measures of obesity, insulin resistance, and subclinical atherosclerosis in healthy, middle-aged women. *Arteriosclerosis, Thrombosis and Vascular Biology* **19**, 1986–1991.

Heilbronn, L.K., Noakes, M. and Clifton, P.M. (2001) Energy restriction and weight loss on very-low-fat diets reduce C-reactive protein concentrations in obese, healthy women. *Arteriosclerosis, Thrombosis and Vascular Biology* **21**, 968–970.

Hennes, M., Shrago, E. and Kissebah, A.H. (1990) Receptor and postreceptor effects of FFA on hepatocyte insulin dynamics. *International Journal of Obesity* **14**, 831–841.

Hotamisligil, G.S. (2000) Molecular mechanisms of insulin resistance and the role of the adipocyte. *International Journal of Obesity* **24** (Suppl.), S23–S27.

Jaakkola, O., Solakivi, T., Tertov, V.V., Orekhov, A.N., Miettinen, T.A. and Nikkari, T. (1993) Characteristics of low-density lipoprotein subfractions from patients with coronary artery disease. *Coronary Artery Disease* **4**, 379–385.

Jensen, M.D., Cardin, S., Edgerton, D. and Cherrington, A. (2003) Splanchnic free fatty acid kinetics. *American Journal of Physiology, Endocrinology and Metabolism* **284**, E1140–E1148.

Juhan-Vague, I., Alessi, M.C. and Vague, P. (1991) Increased plasma plasminogen activator inhibitor 1 levels. A possible link between insulin resistance and atherothrombosis. *Diabetologia* **34**, 457–462.

Katzel, L.I., Krauss, R.M. and Goldberg, A.P. (1994) Relations of plasma TG and HDL-C concentrations to body composition and plasma insulin levels are altered in men with small LDL particles. *Arteriosclerosis and Thrombosis* **14**, 1121–1128.

Kelley, D.E., Mokan, M., Simoneau, J.A. and Mandarino, L.J. (1993) Interaction between glucose and free fatty acid metabolism in human skeletal muscle. *Journal of Clinical Investigation* **92**, 91–98.

Kelley, D.E., Thaete, F.L., Troost, F., Huwe, T. and Goodpaster, B.H. (2000) Subdivisions of subcutaneous abdominal adipose tissue and insulin resistance. *American Journal of Physiology* **278**, E941–E948.

Kim, J.K., Fillmore, J.J., Chen, Y., Yu, C., Moore, I.K., Pypaert, M., Lutz, E.P., Kako, Y., Velez-Carrasco, W., Goldberg, I.J., Breslow, J.L. and Shulman, G.I. (2001) Tissue-specific overexpression of lipoprotein lipase causes tissue-specific insulin resistance. *Proceedings of the National Academy of Science of the USA* **98**, 7522–7527.

Kissebah, A.H. and Peiris, A.N. (1989) Biology of regional body fat distribution. Relationship to non-insulin-dependent diabetes mellitus. *Diabetes and Metabolic Reviews* **5**, 83–109.

Kissebah, A.H. and Krakower, G.R. (1994) Regional adiposity and morbidity. *Physiological Reviews* **74**, 761–811.

Kissebah, A.H., Vydelingum, N., Murray, R., Evans, D.J., Hartz, A.J., Kalkhoff, R.K. and Adams, P.W. (1982) Relation of body fat distribution to metabolic complications of obesity. *Journal of Clinical Endocrinology and Metabolism* **54**, 254–260.

Kissebah, A.H., Freedman, D.S. and Peiris, A.N. (1989) Health risks of obesity. *Medical Clinics of North America* **73**, 111–138.

Knowler, W.C., Barrett-Connor, E., Fowler, S.E., Hamman, R.F., Lachin, J.M., Walker, E.A. and Nathan, D.M. (2002) Reduction in the incidence of type 2 diabetes with lifestyle intervention or metformin. *New England Journal of Medicine* **346**, 393–403.

Koenig, W., Sund, M., Fröhlich, M., Fischer, H.G., Löwel, H., Döring, A., Hutchinson, W.L. and Pepys, M.B. (1999) C-reactive, a sensitive marker of inflammation, predicts future risk of coronary heart disease in initially healthy middle-aged men. Results from the MONICA (Monitoring Trends and Determinants in Cardiovascular Disease) Augsburg Cohort Study, 1984 to 1992. *Circulation* **99**, 237–242.

Kotani, K., Tokunaga, K., Fujioka, S., Kobatake, T., Keno, Y., Yoshida, S., Shimomura, I., Tarui, S. and Matsuzawa, Y. (1994) Sexual dimorphism of age-related changes in whole-body fat distribution in the obese. *International Journal of Obesity* **18**, 207–212.

Kreisberg, R.A. and Oberman, A. (2003) Medical management of hyperlipidemia/dyslipidemia. *Journal of Clinical Endocrinology and Metabolism* **88**, 2445–2461.

Kwiterovich, Jr, P.O.(1998) State-of-the-art update and review: clinical trials of lipid-lowering agents. *American Journal of Cardiology*, **82**, (12A), 3U–17U.

Kwiterovich, Jr, P.O. (2002) Clinical relevance of the biochemical, metabolic, and genetic factors that influence low-density lipoprotein heterogeneity. *American Journal of Cardiology* **90**, 30i–47i.

Laakso, M. (1997) How good a marker is insulin level for insulin resistance? *American Journal of Epidemiology* **137**, 959–965.

La Belle, M. and Krauss, R.M. (1990) Differences in carbohydrate content of low density lipoproteins associated with low density lipoprotein subclass patterns. *Journal of Lipid Research* **31**, 1577–1588.

Lamarche, B., Després, J. P., Pouliot, M.C., Moorjani, S., Lupien, P.J., Theriault, G., Tremblay, A., Nadeau, A. and Bouchard, C. (1992) Is body fat loss a determinant factor in the improvement of carbohydrate and lipid metabolism following aerobic exercise training in obese women? *Metabolism* **41**, 1249–1256.

Lamarche, B., Després, J.P., Moorjani, S., Cantin, B., Dagenais, G. R. and Lupien, P.J. (1995) Prevalence of dyslipidemic phenotypes in ischemic heart disease: prospective results form the Quebec Cardiovascular Study. *American Journal of Cardiology* **75**, 1189–1195.

Lamarche, B., Moorjani, S., Lupien, P.J., Cantin, B., Dagenais, G.R. and Després, J.P. (1996) Apolipoprotein A-I and B levels and the risk of ischemic heart disease during a five-year follow-up of men in the Québec Cardiovascular Study. *Circulation* **94**, 273–278.

Lamarche, B., Tchernof, A., Moorjani, S., Cantin, B., Dagenais, G.R., Lupien, P. J. and Després, J.P. (1997) Small, dense low-density lipoprotein particles as a predictor of the risk of ischemic heart disease in men. Prospective results from the Québec Cardiovascular Study. *Circulation* **95**, 69–75.

Lamarche, B., Tchernof, A., Mauriège, P., Cantin, B., Dagenais, G.R., Lupien, P. J. and Després, J.P. (1998) Fasting insulin and apolipoprotein B levels and low-density lipoprotein particle size as risk factors for ischemic heart disease. *Journal of the American Medical Association* **279**, 1955–1961.

Lamarche, B., Rashid, S. and Lewis, G.F. (1999a) HDL metabolism in hypertriglyceridemic states: an overview. *Clinica et Chimica Acta* **286**, 145–161.

Lamarche, B., Lemieux, I. and Després, J.P. (1999b) The small, dense LDL phenotype and the risk of coronary heart disease: epidemiology, patho-physiology and therapeutic aspects. *Diabetes Metabolism* **25**, 199–211.

Lamarche, B., St Pierre, A.C., Ruel, I.L., Cantin, B., Dagenais, G.R. and Després, J. P. (2001) A prospective, population-based study of low density lipoprotein particle size as a risk factor for ischemic heart disease in men. *Canadian Journal of Cardiology* **17**, 859–865.

Lapidus, L., Bengtsson, C., Larsson, B., Pennert, K., Rybo, E. and Sjöström, L. (1984) Distribution of adipose tissue and risk of cardiovascular disease and death: a 12-year follow up of participants in the population study of women in Gothenburg, Sweden. *British Medical Journal* **289**, 1261–1263.

Larsson, B., Svardsudd, K., Welin, L., Wilhemsen, L., Björntorp, P. and Tibblin, G. (1984) Abdominal adipose tissue distribution, obesity and risk of cardiovascular disease and death: 13-year follow-up of participants in the study of men born in 1913. *British Medical Journal* **288**, 1401–1404.

Lemieux, S. and Després, J.P. (1994) Metabolic complications of visceral obesity: contribution to the aetiology of type 2 diabetes and implications for prevention and treatment. *Diabète et Métabolisme* **20**, 375–393.

Lemieux, S., Prud'homme, D., Bouchard, C., Tremblay, A. and Després, J.P. (1993) Sex differences in the relation of visceral adipose tissue accumulation to total body fatness. *American Journal of Clinical Nutrition* **58**, 463–467.

Lemieux, S., Després, J.P., Moorjani, S., Nadeau, A., Theriault, G., Prud'homme, D., Tremblay, A., Bouchard, C. and Lupien, P.J. (1994) Are gender differences in cardiovascular disease risk factors explained by the level of visceral adipose tissue? *Diabetologia* **37**, 757–764.

Lemieux, S., Prud'homme, D., Moorjani, S., Tremblay, A., Bouchard, C., Lupien, P.J. and Després, J.P. (1995) Do elevated levels of abdominal visceral adipose tissue contribute to age-related differences in plasma lipoprotein concentrations in men? *Atherosclerosis* **118**, 155–164.

Lemieux, I., Pascot, A., Couillard, C., Lamarche, B., Tchernof, A., Alméras, N., Bergeron, J., Gaudet, D., Tremblay, G., Prud'homme, D., Nadeau, A. and Després, J.P. (2000) Hypertriglyceridemic waist. A marker of the atherogenic metabolic triad (hyperinsulinemia; hyperapolipoprotein B; small, dense LDL) in men? *Circulation* **102**, 179–184.

Lemieux, I., Pascot.A., Prud'homme, D., Alméras, N., Bogaty, P., Nadeau, A., Bergeron, J. and Després, J.P. (2001) Elevated C-reactive protein: another component of the atherothrombotic profile of abdominal obesity. *Circulation* **21**, 961–967.

Lemieux, I., Pascot, A., Lamarche, B., Prud'homme, D., Nadeau, A., Bergeron, J. and Després, J.P. (2002) Is the gender difference in LDL size explained by the metabolic complications of visceral obesity? *European Journal of Clinical Investigation* **32**, 909–917.

Lewis, G.F. (1997) Fatty acid regulation of very low density lipoprotein production. *Current Opinion in Lipidology* **8**, 146–153.

Lewis, G.F., Carpentier, A., Adeli, K. and Giacca, A. (2002) Disordered fat storage and mobilization in the pathogenesis of insulin resistance and type 2 diabetes. *Endocrine Reviews* **23**, 201–229.

Lovejoy, J.C., Smith, S.R. and Rood, J.C. (2001) Comparison of regional fat distribution and health risk factors in middle-aged white and African American women: The Healthy Transitions Study. *Obesity Research* **9**, 10–16.

Manson, J.E., Willet, W.C., Stampfer, M.J., Colditz, G.A., Hunter, D.J., Hankinson, S.E., Hennekens, C.H. and Speizer, F.E. (1995) Body weight and mortality among women. *New England Journal of Medicine* **333**, 677–685.

Marcus, M.A., Murphy, L., Pi-Sunyer, F.X. and Albu, J.B. (1999) Insulin sensitivity and serum triglyceride level in obese white and black women: relationship to visceral and truncal subcutaneous fat. *Metabolism* **48**, 194–199.

Markman, B. and Barton, Jr, F.E. (1987) Anatomy of the subcutaneous tissue of the trunk and lower extremity. *Plastic and Reconstructive Surgery* **80**, 248–254.

Mertens, I. and Van Gaal, L.F. (2002) Obesity, haemostasis and the fibrinolytic system. *Obesity Review* **3**, 85–101.

Misra, A., Garg, A., Abate, N., Peshock, R.M., Stray-Gundersen, J. and Grundy, S.M. (1997) Relationship of anterior and posterior subcutaneous abdominal fat to insulin sensitivity in nondiabetic men. *Obesity Research* **5**, 93–99.

Nadler, S.T. and Attie, A.D. (2001) Please pass the chips: genomic insights into obesity and diabetes. *Journal of Nutrition* **131**, 2078–2081.

Nadler, S.T., Stoehr, J.P., Chueler, K.L., Tanimoto, G., Yandell, B.S. and Attie, A. D. (2000)The expression of adipogenic genes is decreased in obesity and diabetes mellitus. *Proceedings of the National Academy of Science USA* **97**, 11371–11376.

NIH Consensus Conference (1985) Lowering blood cholesterol to prevent heart disease. *Journal of the American Medical Association* **253**, 2080–2086.

Ohlson, L.O., Larsson, B., Svardsudd, K., Welin, L., Eriksson, H., Wilhemsen, L., Björntorp, P. and Tibblin, G. (1985) The influence of body fat distribution on the incidence of diabetes mellitus 13.5 years of follow-up of the participants in the study of men born in 1913. *Diabetes* **34**, 1055–1058.

Packard, C.J. (1994) Plasma triglycerides, LDL heterogeneity and atherogenesis. *Therapies Experimentalles* **85**, 1–6.

Perreault, M. and Marette, A. (2001) Targeted disruption of inducible nitric oxide synthase protects against obesity-linked insulin resistance in muscle. *Nature Medicine* **7**, 1138–1143.

Petersson, B., Trell, E. and Hood, B. (1984) Premature death and associated risk factors in urban middle-aged men. *American Journal of Medicine* **77**, 418–426.

Pirro, M., Bergeron, J., Dagenais, G.R., Bernard, P.M., Cantin, B., Després, J.P. and Lamarche, B. (2001) Age and duration of follow-up as modulators of the risk for ischemic heart disease associated with high plasma C-reactive protein levels in men. *Archives of Internal Medicine* **161**, 2474–2480.

Poirier, P. and Després, J.P. (2003) Waist circumference, visceral obesity, and cardiovascular risk. *Journal of Cardiopulmonary Rehabilitation* **23**, 161–169.

Pouliot, M.C., Després, J.P., Moorjani, S., Lupien, P.J., Tremblay, A. and Bouchard, C. (1990) Apolipoprotein E polymorphism alters the association between body fatness and plasma lipoprotein in women. *Journal of Lipid Research* **31**, 1023–1029.

Pouliot, M.C., Després, J.P., Nadeau, A., Moorjani, S., Prud'homme, D., Lupien, P.J., Tremblay, A. and Bouchard, C. (1992) Visceral obesity in men: associations with glucose tolerance, plasma insulin, and lipoprotein levels. *Diabetes* **41**, 826–834.

Pouliot, M.C., Després, J.P., Dionne, F.T., Vohl, M.C., Moorjani, S., Prud'homme, D., Bouchard, C. and Lupien, P.J. (1994a) Apolipoprotein B-100 gene *Eco*RI polymorphism: relations to the plasma lipoprotein changes associated with abdominal visceral obesity. *Arteriosclerosis and Thrombosis* **14**, 527–533.

Pouliot, M.C., Després, J.P., Lemieux, S., Moorjani, S., Bouchard, C., Tremblay, A., Nadeau, A. and Lupien, P.J. (1994b) Waist circumference and abdominal sagittal diameter: best simple anthropometric indexes of abdominal visceral adipose tissue accumulation and related cardiovascular risk in men and women. *American Journal of Cardiology* **73**, 460–468.

Pyörälä, K. (1979) Relationship of glucose tolerance and plasma insulin to the incidence of coronary heart disease: Results from the two population studies in Finland. *Diabetes Care* **2**, 131–141.

Rader, D. J. (2002) High-density lipoproteins and atherosclerosis. *American Journal of Cardiology* **90**, 62i–70i.

Rader, D.J., Hoeg, J.M. and Brewer, H.M. (1994) Quantification of plasma apolipoproteins in the primary and secondary prevention of coronary artery disease. *Annals of Internal Medicine* **120**, 1012–1025.

Rajman, I., Maxwell, S., Cramb, R. and Kendall, M. (1994) Particle size: the key to the atherogenic lipoprotein? *Quarterly Journal of Medicine* **87**, 709–720.

Rankinen, T., Kim, S.Y., Pérusse, L., Després, J.P. and Bouchard, C. (1999) The prediction of abdominal visceral fat level from body composition and anthropometry: ROC analysis. *International Journal of Obesity* **23**, 801–809.

Reaven, G.M. (1988) Role of insulin resistance in human disease. *Diabetes* **37**, 1595–1607.

Reeder, B.A., Angel, A., Ledoux, M., Rabkin, S.W., Young, T.K. and Sweet, L.E. (1992) Obesity and its relation to cardiovascular disease risk factors in Canadian adults. Canadian Heart Health Surveys Research Group. *Canadian Medical Association Journal* **146**, 2009–2019.

Reichl, D. and Miller, N.E. (1989) Pathophysiology of reverse cholesterol transport. Insights from inherited disorders of lipoprotein metabolism. *Arteriosclerosis* **9**, 785–797.

Reitman, M.L., Mason, M.M., Moitra, J., Gavrilova, O., Markus-Samuels, B., Eckhaus, M. and Vinson, C. (1999) Transgenic mice lacking white fat: models for understanding human lipoatrophic diabetes. *Annals of the New York Academy of Sciences* **892**, 289–296.

Rendell, M., Hulthen, U.L., Tornquist, C., Groop, L. and Mattiasson, I. (2001) Relationship between abdominal fat compartments and glucose and lipid metabolism in early postmenopausal women. *Journal of Clinical Endocrinology and Metabolism* **86**, 744–749.

Ridker, P.M., Cushman, M., Stampfer, M.J., Tracy, R.P. and Hennekens, C.H. (1997) Inflammation, aspirin, and the risk of cardiovascular disease in apparently healthy men. *New England Journal of Medicine* **336**, 973–979.

Ridker, P.M., Glynn, R.J. and Hennekens, C.H. (1998) C-reactive protein adds to the predictive value of total and HDL cholesterol in determining risk of first myocardial infarction. *Circulation* **97**, 2007–2011.

Ridker, P.M., Hennekens, C.H., Buring, J.E. and Rifai, N. (2000) C-reactive protein and other markers of inflammation in the prediction of cardiovascular disease in women. *New England Journal of Medicine* **342**, 836–843.

Robitaille, J., Després, J.P., Pérusse, L. and Vohl, M.C. (2003) The PPAR-gamma P12A polymorphism modulates the relationship between dietary fat intake and components of the metabolic syndrome: results from the Quebec Family Study. *Clinical Genetics* **63**, 109–116.

Ross, R. (1999) Atherosclerosis – an inflammatory disease. *New England Journal of Medicine* **340**, 115–126.

Ross, R., Aru, J., Freeman, J., Hudson, R. and Janssen, I. (2002) Abdominal adiposity and insulin resistance in obese men. *American Journal of Physiology* **282**, E657–E663.

Schwartz, R.S., Shuman, W.P., Bradbury, V.L., Cain, K.C., Fellingham, G.W., Beard, J.C., Kahn, S.E., Stratton, J.R., Cerqueira, M.D. and Abrass, I.B. (1990) Body fat distribution in healthy young and older men. *Journal of Gerontology* **45**, M181–M185.

Seidell, J.C., Oosterlee, A., Deurenberg, P., Hautvast, J.G.A. and Ruijs, J.H.J. (1988) Abdominal fat depots measured with computed tomography: Effects of degree of obesity, sex, and age. *European Journal of Clinical Nutrition* **42**, 805–815.

Shepherd, J. and Packard, C.J. (1989) Lipoprotein metabolism. In: Fruchart, J.C., Shepherd, J., eds. *Human Plasma Lipoproteins*. Berlin: De Gruyter, 55–78.

Silliman, K., Shore, V. and Forte, T.M. (1994) Hypertriglyceridemia during late pregnancy is associated with the formation of small dense low-density lipoproteins and the presence of large buoyant high-density lipoproteins. *Metabolism* **43**, 1035–1041.

Sims, E.A.H. and Berchtold, P. (1982) Obesity and hypertension: mechanisms and implications for management. *Journal of the American Medical Association* **247**, 49–52.

Sites, C.K., Calles-Escandon, J., Brochu, M., Butterfield, M., Ashikaga, T. and Poehlman, E.T. (2000) Relation of regional fat distribution to insulin sensitivity in postmenopausal women. *Fertility and Sterility* **73**, 61–65.

Sjöström, L., Kvist, H., Cederblad, A. and Tylen, U. (1986) Determination of total adipose tissue and body fat in women by computed tomography, 40K, and tritium. *American Journal of Physiology* **250**, E736–E745.

Smith, S.R. and Zachwieja, J.J. (1999) Visceral adipose tissue: a critical review of intervention strategies. *International Journal of Obesity* **23**, 329–335.

Smith, S.R., Lovejoy, J.C., Greenway, F., Ryand, D., deJonge, L., de la Bretonne, J., Volafova, J. and Bray, G.A. (2001) Contributions of total body fat, abdominal subcutaneous adipose tissue compartments, and visceral adipose tissue to the metabolic complications of obesity. *Metabolism* **50**, 425–435.

Sniderman, A.D. and Silberberg, J. (1990) Is it time to measure apolipoprotein B? *Arteriosclerosis* **10**, 665–667.

Sniderman, A., Shapiro, S., Marpole, D., Skinner, B., Teng, B. and Kwiterovich, Jr, P.O. (1980) Association of coronary atherosclerosis with hyperapobetalipoproteinemia [increased protein but normal cholesterol levels in human plasma low density (β) lipoproteins]. *Proceedings of the National Academy of Science of the USA* **77**, 604–608.

Spranger, J., Kroke, A., Mohlig, M., Bergmann, M.M., Ristow, M., Boeing, H. and Pfeiffer, A.F. (2003) Adiponectin and protection against type 2 diabetes mellitus. *Lancet* **361**, 226–228.

St Pierre, A.C., Ruel, I.L., Cantin, B., Dagenais, G.R., Bernard, P.M., Després, J. P. and Lamarche, B. (2001) Comparison of various electrophoretic characteristics of LDL particles and their relationship to the risk of ischemic heart disease. *Circulation* **104**, 2295–2299.

St Pierre, J., Lemieux, I., Miller-Félix, I., Prud'homme, D., Bergeron, J., Gaudet, D., Nadeau, A., Després, J.P. and Vohl, M.C. (2002) Visceral obesity and hyperinsulinemia modulate the impact of the microsomal triglyceride transfer protein -493G/T polymorphism on plasma lipoprotein levels in men. *Atherosclerosis* **160**, 317–324.

St Pierre, A.C., Bergeron, J., Pirro, M., Cantin, B., Dagenais, G.R., Després, J.P. and Lamarche, B. (2003a) Effect of plasma C-reactive protein levels in modulating the risk of coronary heart disease associated with small, dense, low-density lipoproteins in men (The Quebec Cardiovascular Study). *American Journal of Cardiology* **91**, 555–558.

St Pierre, J., Miller-Félix, I., Paradis, M.E., Bergeron, J., Lamarche, B., Després, J.P., Gaudet, D. and Vohl, M.C. (2003b) Visceral obesity attenuates the effect of the hepatic lipase -514C>T polymorphism on plasma HDL-cholesterol levels in French-Canadian men. *Molecular Genetics and Metabolism* **78**, 31–36.

Steppan, C.M., Bailey, S.T., Bhat, S., Brown, E.J., Banerjee, R.R.,

Wright, C.M., Patel, H.R., Ahima, R.S. and Lazar, M.A. (2001) The hormone resistin links obesity to diabetes. *Nature* **409**, 307–312.

Svedberg, J., Björntorp, P., Smith, V. and Lonnroth, P. (1990) FFA inhibition of insulin binding, degradation, and action in isolated hepatocytes. *Diabetes* **39**, 570–574.

Tchernof, A., Lamarche, B., Prud'homme, D., Nadeau, A., Moorjani, S., Labrie, F., Lupien, P.J. and Després, J.P. (1996) The dense LDL phenotype: Association with plasma lipoprotein levels, visceral obesity, and hyperinsulinemia in men. *Diabetes Care* **19**, 629–637.

Tchernof, A., Nolan, A., Sites, C.K., Ades, P.A. and Poehlman, E.T. (2002) Weight loss reduces C-reactive protein levels in obese postmenopausal women. *Circulation* **105**, 564–569.

Thompson, A.L. and Cooney, G.J. (2000) Acyl-CoA inhibition of hexokinase in rat and human skeletal muscle is a potential mechanism of lipid-induced insulin resistance. *Diabetes* **49**, 1761–1765.

Thompson, S.G., Kienast, J., Pyke, S.D.M., Haverkate, F. and van de Loo, J.C.W. (2000) Hemostatic factors and the risk of myocardial infarction or sudden death in patients with angina pectoris. *New England Journal of Medicine* **332**, 635–641.

Tornvall, P., Karpe, F., Carlson, L.A. and Hamsten, A. (1991) Relationships of low density lipoprotein subfractions to angiographically defined coronary artery disease in young survivors of myocardial infarction. *Atherosclerosis* **90**, 67–80.

Toth, M.J., Sites, C.K., Cefalu, W.T., Matthews, D.E. and Poehlman, E.T. (2001) Determinants of insulin-stimulated glucose disposal in middle-aged, premenopausal women. *American Journal of Physiology* **281**, E113–E121.

Tremblay, A., Bouchard, L., Bouchard, C., Després, J.P., Drapeau, V. and Pérusse, L. (2003) Long-term adiposity changes are related to a glucocorticoid receptor polymorphism in young females. *Journal of Clinical Endocrinology and Metabolism* **88**, 3141–3145.

Tuomilehto, J., Lindstrom, J., Eriksson, J.G., Valle, T.T., Hamalainen, H., Ilanne-Parikka, P., Keinanen-Kiukaanniemi, S., Laakso, M., Louheranta, A., Rastas, M., Salminen, V. and Uusitupa, M. (2001) Prevention of type 2 diabetes mellitus by changes in lifestyle among subjects with impaired glucose tolerance. *New England Journal of Medicine* **344**, 1343–1350.

Vague, J. (1947) La différenciation sexuelle, facteur déterminant des formes de l'obésité. *La Presse Médicale* **30**, 339–340.

Vague, P., Juhan-Vague, I., Chabert, V., Alessi, M.C. and Atlan, C. (1989) Fat distribution and plasminogen activator inhibitor activity in nondiabetic obese women. *Metabolism* **38**, 913–915.

Visser, M., Bouter, L.M., McQuillan, G.M., Wener, M.H. and Harris, T.B. (1999) Elevated C-reactive protein levels in overweight and obese adults. *Journal of the American Medical Association* **282**, 2131–2135.

Vohl, M.C., Lamarche, B., Moorjani, S., Prud'homme, D., Nadeau, A., Bouchard, C., Lupien, P.J. and Després, J.P. (1995) The lipoprotein lipase *HindIII* polymorphism modulates plasma triglyceride levels in visceral obesity. *Arteriosclerosis, Thrombosis and Vascular Biology* **15**, 714–720.

Vohl, M.C., Tchernof, A., Dionne, F.T., Moorjani, S., Prud'homme, D., Bouchard, C., Nadeau, A., Lupien, P.J. and Després, J.P. (1996) The ApoB-100 gene *EcoRI* polymorphism influences the relationship between features of the insulin resistance syndrome and the hyper-ApoB and dense LDL phenotype in men. *Diabetes* **45**, 1405–1411.

Vohl, M.C., Lamarche, B., Bergeron, J., Moorjani, S., Prud'homme, D.,

Nadeau, A., Tremblay, A., Lupien, P.J., Bouchard, C. and Després, J.P. (1997) The MspI polymorphism of the apolipoprotein A-II gene as a modulator of the dyslipidemic state found in visceral obesity. *Atherosclerosis* **128**, 183–190.

Wajchenberg, B.L. (2000) Subcutaneous and visceral adipose tissue: their relation to the metabolic syndrome, *Endocrine Reviews* **21**, 697–738.

Welborn, T.A. and Wearne, K. (1979) Coronary heart disease incidence and cardiovascular mortality in Busselton with reference to glucose and insulin concentrations. *Diabetes Care* **2**, 154–160.

Weyer, C., Foley, J.E., Bogardus, C., Tataranni, P.A. and Pratley, R.E. (2000) Enlarged subcutaneous abdominal adipocyte size, but not obesity itself, predicts type II diabetes independent of insulin resistance. *Diabetologia* **43**, 1498–1506.

Wilson, P.W., Castelli, W.P. and Kannel, W.B. (1987) Coronary risk prediction in adults (the Framingham Heart Study). *American Journal of Cardiology* **59**, 91G–94G.

Yarnell, J.W.G., Sweetnam, P.M., Marks, V., Teale, J.D. and Bolton, C.H. (1994) Insulin in ischemic heart disease: Are associations explained by triglyceride concentrations? The Carphilly Prospective Study. *British Heart Journal* **71**, 293–296.

Yudkin, J.S., Stehouwer, C.D.A., Emeis, J.J. and Coppack, S.W. (1999) C-reactive protein in healthy subjects: associations with obesity, insulin resistance, and endothelial dysfunction. A potential role for cytokines originating from adipose tissue? *Arteriosclerosis, Thrombosis and Vascular Biology* **19**, 972–978.

Yudkin, J.S., Kumari, M., Humphries, S.E. and Mohamed-Ali, V. (2000) Inflammation, obesity, stress and coronary heart disease: is interleukin-6 the link? *Atherosclerosis* **148**, 209–214.

13 Obesity and disease: insulin resistance, diabetes, metabolic syndrome and polycystic ovary syndrome

Joseph Proietto

Introduction, 184

Obesity and insulin resistance, 184
  What causes insulin resistance in
  obese subjects?, 184
  Tumour necrosis factor alpha, 186
  Resistin, 186
  Adiponectin, 186

Interleukin 6, 187
Leptin, 187

Obesity and diabetes, 188

Obesity and the metabolic
syndrome, 189
  What is the link between obesity
  and the metabolic syndrome?, 189

Obesity and polycystic ovary
syndrome, 190

Conclusion, 191

References, 191

Introduction

Obesity has been recognized by the World Health Organization as one of the world's major health problems. The prevalence of obesity [defined as a body mass index (BMI) $>30 \, kg/m^2$] is rising in many regions of the world, with rates of around 20% in many Western countries (Gutierrez-Fisac et al., 2000; Torrance et al., 2002). Prevalence levels are higher in some selected populations, such as Polynesians (McAnulty and Scragg, 1996; Leonard et al., 2002), Australian Aborigines (McDermott et al., 2000), Pima Indians (Krosnick, 2000) and other groups. The causes of this epidemic are multifactorial and discussed elsewhere in this book (Chapters 1, 7 and 9) but involve the interaction of an increasingly 'obesogenic' environment with genetic predisposition.

This rising tide of obesity is of great concern because of its multiple health consequences, including insulin resistance, type 2 diabetes, hypertension, dyslipidaemia, sleep apnoea and polycystic ovary syndrome (Pi-Sunyer, 2002). It can aggravate the symptoms of arthritis and has been associated with increased risk of breast cancer and of other cancers. This chapter will discuss some of the known mechanisms by which obesity causes its many metabolic consequences.

Obesity and insulin resistance

The relationship between obesity and insulin resistance has been known for many years (Rabinowitz and Zierler, 1962).

More recently, Ferrannini and colleagues (1997) reported on behalf of the European Group for the study of insulin resistance that insulin sensitivity declines linearly with BMI at an age-adjusted rate of 1.2 mol/min/kg of fat-free mass. This study used the 'gold standard' measurement of insulin action, the euglycaemic hyperinsulinaemic clamp, to measure insulin sensitivity in a large group of normotensive Caucasian men and women aged 18–85 years with BMIs ranging from 15 to $55 \, kg/m^2$.

What causes insulin resistance in obese subjects?

A surprising large number of different causes for obesity-induced insulin resistance have been described including excess availability of free fatty acids (FFAs), overproduction of some cytokines and reduced production of others.

Free fatty acids

Lipolysis from an enlarged fat mass leads to an increase in circulating FFA levels in obesity (Gorden, 1960; Groop et al. 1991; Baldeweg et al., 2000). Several well-designed studies have shown that elevation of FFAs can cause insulin resistance rapidly (Thiebaud et al., 1982; Boden et al., 1994; Roden et al., 1996). When FFAs are elevated acutely to 1.9 mM, insulin action declines and glycogen synthesis diminishes after a delay of 3 h. Preceding this is a decrease in glucose oxidation and a reduction in glucose-6-phosphate concentration, suggesting that the reduced rate of glycogen synthesis is due to an impairment of glucose transport into the muscle cell rather than a

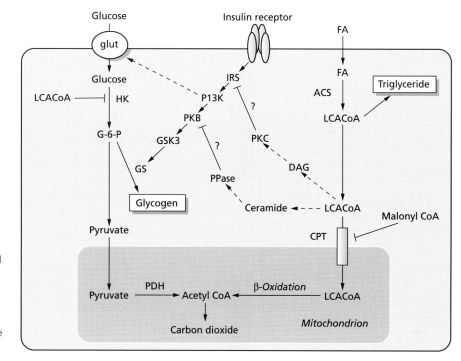

Fig 13.1 Some of the interactions whereby lipid metabolism may inhibit insulin action on glucose metabolism in muscle. LCACoA, long-chain fatty acyl CoAs; DAG, diacylglycerol; PKC, protein kinase C; IRS, insulin receptor substrate; PKB, protein kinase B; GSK3, glycogen synthase kinase 3. (From Cooney *et al.*, 2002, with permission.)

defect in the activity of glycogen synthase (Roden *et al.*, 1996) as had been proposed previously (Boden *et al.*, 1994). In the converse situation, lowering of elevated FFA levels in obese subjects by 60–70% using the anti-lipolytic drug acipimox improved oral glucose tolerance and insulin action as measured by the hyperinsulinaemic clamp (Santomauro *et al.*, 1999).

The specific mechanisms by which excess FFA supply to muscle tissue leads to insulin resistance are multiple (Fig. 13.1). Possibly central to these is the overproduction of long-chain acyl CoA (LCACoA) secondary to oversupply of FFA. These metabolically active lipids have been proposed to lead to activation of protein kinase C_θ (Griffin *et al.*, 1999), which in turn impairs the action of the insulin signalling cascade possibly by serine phosphorylation of insulin receptor substrate (IRS) proteins. Excess accumulation of LCACoAs may also lead to increased production of ceramide (Schmitz-Peiffer *et al.*, 1999), a derivative of palmitate. It has been shown that ceramide can inhibit protein kinase B (PKB) (or Akt) (Zhou *et al.*, 1998), which, among other signalling functions, is an important intermediary in the transduction of the insulin signal (Summers *et al.*, 1998). LCACoAs have also been shown to inhibit hexokinase, the enzyme responsible for the first step in glucose metabolism in muscle (Thompson and Cooney, 2000) providing another mechanism for fat-induced muscle insulin resistance.

FFAs also stimulate gluconeogenesis (Chen *et al.*, 1999). In a process termed *autoregulation*, an acute elevation in gluconeogenesis does not lead to an increase in endogenous glucose production (Clore *et al.*, 1991; Roden *et al.*, 2000). Hepatic au-

toregulation has been proposed to be due to either (or both) extrahepatic or intrahepatic mechanisms. The extrahepatic mechanism is an elevation in insulin levels, possibly stimulated by FFA (Boden and Jadali, 1991), whereas the intrahepatic mechanism has been proposed to be secondary to activation of glycogen synthase and inactivation of glycogen phosphorylase by increased concentrations of glucose-6-phosphate secondary to increased gluconeogenesis (Youn and Bergman, 1990). However, chronic exposure to FFA such as in obesity or after consumption of a high-fat diet does result in both increased gluconeogenesis and endogenous glucose production (Fig. 13.2) (Andrikopoulos and Proietto, 1995: Song *et al.*, 2001; Lam *et al.*, 2002). Multiple mechanisms have been proposed (Lam *et al.*, 2003) including elevation of acetyl-CoA, citrate, NADH or ATP (Lam *et al.*, 2002; 2003), accumulation of PKCδ (Lam *et al.*, 2002) and increased protein levels of the gluconeogenic enzyme fructose-1,6-bisphosphatase (Song *et al.*, 2001) among others.

Irrespective of the mechanism by which excess fat stimulates gluconeogenesis, the consequences are greater than just an increase in endogenous glucose production. Chronic stimulation of gluconeogenesis in the kidney, induced in transgenic rats by the overexpression of phosphoenol pyruvate carboxykinase (PEPCK), has been shown to result in marked peripheral insulin resistance, especially in brown and white adipose tissue (Lamont *et al.*, 2003) as well as some features of the metabolic syndrome (Thorburn *et al.*, 1999).

Thus, in summary an important way that obesity causes insulin resistance is by the excessive circulation of FFAs, which cause peripheral insulin resistance directly and which also

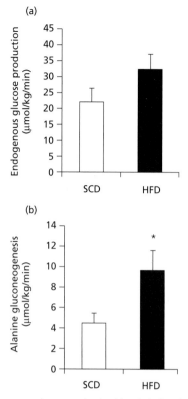

Fig 13.2 Endogenous glucose production (a) and alanine gluconeogenesis (b) in rats ($n = 8$) that were fed a standard chow (SCD, open bars) or high-fat (HFD, closed bars) diet for 14 days. EGP was assessed using [6-^{3}H]-glucose, and alanine gluconeogenesis was determined using [U-^{14}C]-alanine. *$P < 0.05$. (Modified from Song et al., 2001, with permission.)

stimulate gluconeogenesis. Secondarily, such enhanced gluconeogenesis can cause a further increase in the severity of peripheral insulin resistance. However, excess circulating FFAs are not the only way by which obesity causes insulin resistance.

Adipokines

One of the most interesting and surprising developments in the understanding of the link between obesity and insulin resistance was the discovery that adipocytes make and secrete a series of cytokines and other hormones that impact either positively or negatively on insulin sensitivity, and that the expression of these cytokines is altered by weight gain or weight loss. These molecules include tumour necrosis factor alpha (TNF-α), resistin, adiponectin, interleukin 6 (IL-6) and leptin (Bastard et al., 2000; Bruun et al., 2003).

Tumour necrosis factor alpha

In the early 1990s, it was shown that TNF-α could modulate glucose transport in cultured cells (Stephens and Pekala, 1991) and that chronic infusion of human recombinant TNF into rats induced both hepatic and muscle insulin resistance (Lang

et al., 1992). Hotamisligil and colleagues (1993) then reported overexpression of TNF-α in adipose tissue from four different rodent models of obesity and insulin resistance. Mechanisms of TNF-α-induced insulin resistance include reduction in GLUT4 expression (Stephens and Pekala, 1991) and reduced tyrosine phosphorylation of the insulin receptor, in particular of its first downstream substrate IRS-1 (Hotamisligil et al., 1994a,b) and upregulation of suppressor of cytokine signalling (SOCS-3) proteins (Emanuelli et al., 2001).

The role of TNF-α-induced insulin resistance in human obesity and type 2 diabetes has been more controversial, with some studies finding elevated expression in obesity (Kern et al., 1995; Dandona et al., 1998; Kopp et al., 2003) and type 2 diabetes (Miyazaki et al., 2003), whereas others have reported no reliable relationship between elevated TNF-α levels and obesity (Koistinen et al., 2000) or a failure of removal of TNF-α using a specific antibody to improve insulin sensitivity in subjects with type 2 diabetes (Ofei et al., 1996).

Resistin

Resistin is a member of a novel family of secreted proteins that includes resistin-like molecule alpha (RELMα, known also as FIZZ1), RELMβ (FIZZ2) and resistin (FIZZ3). In rodents, resistin has been shown to be secreted by adipocytes, and to impair glucose tolerance and insulin action when infused into mice (Steppan et al., 2001). Studies on L6 rat skeletal muscle cells have demonstrated that resistin impairs glucose transport without altering insulin signalling, suggesting that the reduction in glucose transport is due to a decrease in the intrinsic activity of cell surface glucose transporters (Moon et al., 2003). In in vivo studies, however, Rajala and colleagues (2003) report that resistin and RELMβ infusion powerfully stimulates endogenous glucose production without impairing peripheral (mainly muscle) glucose clearance. One study has also reported increased resistin expression in human abdominal tissue (McTernan et al., 2002). In contrast with these findings, several studies have reported reduced resistin expression in human (Nagaev and Smith, 2001; Savage et al., 2001; Way et al. 2001; Janke et al., 2002) and rat (Milan et al., 2002) obesity. Insulin (Haugen et al., 2001), free fatty acids (Juan et al. 2001) and TNF-α (Fasshauer et al., 2001) have all been shown to inhibit resistin expression, providing a mechanism for the reduced resistin levels, as all of these factors are elevated in obesity. Thus, even if resistin does induce insulin resistance in some tissues, the fact that it is downregulated in obesity makes it unlikely that resistin plays a major role in the insulin resistance of obesity.

Adiponectin

Adiponectin (Acrp30), first reported in 1995, is a 30-kDa secretory protein made exclusively in adipocytes. It is structurally similar to complement factor C1q and forms large homooligomers (Scherer *et al.*, 1995). Secretion of adiponectin is stimulated by PPARγ agonists (Maeda *et al.*, 2001; Yang *et al.*, 2002) and decreased by androgens (Nishizawa *et al.*, 2002), corticosteroids (Fasshauer *et al.*, 2002) and TNF-α (Maeda *et al.*, 2001). Adiponectin has been shown to be reduced in patients with obesity (Arita *et al.*, 1999; Weyer *et al.*, 2001) or type 2 diabetes (Hotta *et al.*, 2000) and in relatives of patients with type 2 diabetes (Lihn *et al.*, 2003), and to increase with weight reduction (Yang *et al.*, 2001). A study conducted on obese, diabetic monkeys showed that, like humans, these animals have reduced adiponectin levels and demonstrate a positive relationship between adiponectin levels and insulin sensitivity measured with a hyperinsulinaemic, euglycaemic clamp (Hotta *et al.*, 2001), a relationship later confirmed in humans (Tschritter *et al.*, 2003). Knockout of the adiponectin gene in mice causes moderate insulin resistance (Kubota *et al.*, 2002), whereas in the converse situation, administration of adiponectin has been shown to reverse insulin resistance in mice (Yamauchi *et al.*, 2001), possibly by enhancing the effect of insulin to suppress endogenous glucose production (Berg *et al.*, 2001; Combs *et al.*, 2001), and by stimulating AMP kinase in skeletal muscle and liver (Yamauchi *et al.*, 2002). Two receptors have been cloned: AdipoR1 is expressed in skeletal muscle, whereas AdipoR2 is found in liver (Yamauchi *et al.*, 2003a). Two recent studies have reported a possible protective effect of adiponectin on the development of type 2 diabetes (Daimon *et al.*, 2003; Spranger *et al.*, 2003). This is consistent with a study showing that overexpression of the globular domain of adiponectin protects *ob/ob* mice from becoming diabetic (Yamauchi *et al.*, 2003b).

In addition to its effects of improving insulin sensitivity, adiponectin has effects on the vasculature to reduce the risk of atherosclerosis. Thus, in atherosclerosis-prone apolipoprotein E-deficient mice, overexpression of adiponectin reduced lesion formation in the aortic sinus by 30% compared with control mice, and the lipid droplets became smaller (Okamoto *et al.*, 2002). Using another model of atherosclerosis induced by mechanically damaging the neointimal vascular lining, it was shown that adiponectin deficiency led to a marked neointimal thickening and increased proliferation of vascular smooth muscle cells, which was attenuated by adenoviral expression of adiponectin (Matsuda *et al.*, 2002). Adiponectin inhibits DNA synthesis in cultured smooth muscle cells induced by a variety of growth factors (Matsuda *et al.*, 2002).

Interleukin 6

Type 2 diabetes is associated with features of the acute-phase response. One of the mediators of the acute-phase response is interleukin 6 (IL-6) (Baumann and Gauldie, 1994). Elevated circulating levels of IL-6 were found in patients with features of the metabolic syndrome (compared with age and sex-matched control subjects) (Pickup *et al.*, 1997). IL-6 is secreted by adipocytes (Mohamed-Ali *et al.*, 2001) and is elevated in

obesity (Vgontzas *et al.*, 1997). Subsequently, there have been several reports of a positive relationship between IL-6 levels and insulin resistance (Fernandez-Real *et al.*, 2001; Kern *et al.*, 2001; Vozarova *et al.*, 2001), suggesting that overproduction of IL-6 in obese subjects was one cause of insulin resistance in obesity. This conclusion was reinforced by the findings that IL-6 levels fall after weight loss (Bastard *et al.*, 2000; Bruun *et al.*, 2003) and that IL-6 induces defects in insulin signalling in hepatocytes (Senn *et al.*, 2002).

This view of the insulin resistance-inducing role of IL-6 has been challenged by studies showing that IL-6 is secreted by muscle tissue (Ostrowski *et al.*, 1998), that its secretion is dependent on the glycogen content of muscle (Steensberg *et al.*, 2001) and that IL-6 inhibits the secretion of TNF-α (Starkie *et al.*, 2003). Indeed it has been shown that IL-6-deficient mice develop obesity and glucose intolerance. This effect of IL-6 was shown to be centrally acting, as intracerebroventricular, but not intraperitoneal, administration of IL-6 partly reversed the defect by increasing energy expenditure (Wallenius *et al.*, 2002). The recent demonstration that insulin dramatically stimulates IL-6 mRNA production in insulin-resistant but not control muscle tissue (Carey *et al.*, 2003) may offer an explanation for the reported relationship between insulin resistance and IL-6 levels. Thus, contrary to IL-6 being a cause of insulin resistance, it has now been proposed that IL-6 may be used as a therapy for the treatment of metabolic disorders (Febbraio and Pedersen, 2002).

Leptin

Leptin was discovered in 1994 as the mutated gene causing severe obesity in the *ob/ob* mouse (Zhang *et al.*, 1994). It is a 16-kDa peptide, cytokine-like hormone produced in fat cells and secreted into the bloodstream. It is transported into the brain through the choroid plexus, using a saturable mechanism, and it reduces food intake and stimulates energy expenditure. Leptin functions as a long-term regulator of energy balance rather than a short-term satiety signal. Complete deficiency of leptin leads to severe obesity in both humans (Montague *et al.*, 1997) and mice (Zhang *et al.*, 1994). Leptin has many other actions apart from its anorectic activity. These include effects on bone turnover (Blain *et al.*, 2002), regulation of puberty and fertility (Moschos *et al.*, 2002), and modulation of the acute-phase response by its capacity to modulate cytokine production (Faggioni *et al.*, 1999).

The effects of leptin on glucose metabolism and insulin sensitivity have been thoroughly studied but the results have been confusing and at times contradictory (for a review, see Ceddia *et al.*, 2002). Thus, in some studies, leptin has been shown to profoundly impair the action of insulin to stimulate glucose transport (Fig. 13.3), glycogen synthase, lipogenesis and protein synthesis in isolated adipocytes (Muller *et al.*, 1997), and exposure of human liver cells to leptin impairs insulin action (Cohen *et al.*, 1996). These *in vitro* investigations

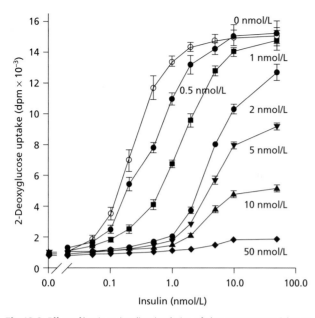

Fig 13.3 Effect of leptin on insulin stimulation of glucose transport. Primary cultures of rat adipocytes were incubated for 16.5 h in the absence or presence of the indicated concentrations of leptin. Subsequently, the cells were washed and assayed for glucose transport activation by various concentrations of insulin. Glucose transport activity is given as 2-[^{3}H]-deoxyglucose specifically associated with the cells. Each point represents the mean value; each error bar represents the half-range of two independent adipocyte cultures, with glucose transport determinations performed in quadruplicate. (From Muller *et al.*, 1997, with permission.)

are consistent with studies showing a relationship between insulin resistance and leptin levels independent of body fat mass (Segal *et al.*, 1996; Fischer *et al.*, 2002). Although this relationship has been attributed to the action of insulin to increase leptin levels (Mohamed-Ali *et al.*, 1997; Fischer *et al.*, 2002), other studies have failed to find a stimulatory effect of insulin on leptin production (Pratley *et al.*, 1996; Segal *et al.*, 1996).

Although data from some studies suggest that leptin causes insulin resistance, other studies have shown the opposite. When leptin-deficient *ob/ob* mice were treated with leptin, there was a dramatic lowering of glucose and insulin. This could not be reproduced in pair-fed animals, leading the authors to suggest that the hypoglycaemic affect of leptin is partly independent of its weight-reducing effect in these animals (Schwartz *et al.*, 1996). Similarly, intravenous and intraventricular administration of leptin to wild-type mice (Kamohara *et al.*, 1997) and subcutaneous administration of leptin in rats (Sivitz *et al.*, 1997) increased glucose turnover, glucose uptake and insulin sensitivity. In other studies, leptin has been reported to enhance the suppression of endogenous glucose production by insulin but to have no effect on glucose transport (Rossetti *et al.*, 1997).

Thus, many mechanisms have been described that may explain the relationship between obesity and insulin resistance. The view of the adipocyte as a simple repository for fat has

been dramatically changed by the discovery that fat cells can manufacture and secrete powerful molecules, many related to the cytokine system, which can modulate insulin action and glucose metabolism. In addition, these compounds can have powerful effects on nutrient intake and vascular health.

Obesity and diabetes

Although obesity almost always causes insulin resistance, only a subset of obese, insulin-resistant subjects develop diabetes. These often have a family history, suggesting the need for a genetically determined tendency to develop the disorder. It is now clear that diabetes can only occur if there is a defect in insulin secretion (Groop, 2000; Boitard, 2002). Therefore, it appears that a genetic tendency to develop beta cell failure is necessary for the development of diabetes, but the triggers for this failure are environmental. Excess fat is a powerful factor in triggering beta cell failure in genetically susceptible individuals.

There is evidence that FFA excess can contribute to beta cell failure. In the diabetes-prone zucker diabetic fatty (ZDF) rats, an elevation of FFAs precedes the development of hyperglycaemia by 2 weeks (Lee *et al.*, 1994). The excess FFAs accumulate in the beta cell to 10 times that measured in control islets, and are associated with impaired glucose-mediated insulin secretion (Lee *et al.*, 1994). Normalization of FFA levels by dietary energy restriction in these hyperphagic animals reduced circulating FFA levels, normalized beta cell abnormalities and prevented the development of hyperglycaemia (Lee *et al.*, 1994).

Several different mechanisms have been proposed by which excessive fat accumulation in islets leads to impaired insulin secretion. These include increased production of ceramide leading to apoptosis (Maedler *et al.*, 2001) by a variety of mechanisms, including increased nitric oxide formation (Shimabukuro *et al.*, 1998a), inhibition of mitochondrial respiratory chain complex 3 (Gudz *et al.*, 1997), or by inhibition of Akt kinase activity (Kulik *et al.*, 1997; Zhou *et al.*, 1998). In addition, there may be direct apoptotic effects of free fatty acyl moieties via lipid peroxidation (Das, 1999) and by reducing Bcl2 expression (Shimabukuro *et al.*, 1998b). Figure 13.4 shows one hypothetical mechanism by which excess non-esterified fatty acids lead to apoptosis via the production of ceramide and the activation of NFκB, resulting in the increased expression of inducible nitric oxide synthase (iNOS) and overproduction of nitric oxide, leading to apoptosis (Unger and Orci, 2002). Figure 13.4 also shows evidence that *fa/fa* rats that are severely obese because of a mutation of the leptin receptor have upregulation of the initial enzyme in this pathway, serine-palmitoyl transferase (Fig. 13.4b) and evidence that this is associated with an increased production of ceramide (Fig. 13.4c).

Interestingly, on day 2 of an 8-day FFA incubation, an inverse relationship has been found between intracellular

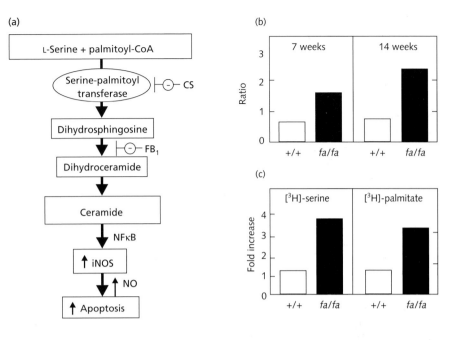

Fig 13.4 (a) Putative pathway of lipoapoptosis. Condensation of unoxidized palmitoyl-CoA and L-serine catalysed by serine-palmitoyl transferase generates ceramide. Ceramide upregulates the expression of inducible nitric oxide synthase (iNOS) by activating NFκB. Alternatively, it may reduce Akt phosphorylation, thereby reducing its antiapoptotic effects. Apoptosis can be prevented by inhibiting ceramide synthesis with cycloserine (CS) or fumonisin-B1 (FB1). (b) mRNA of serine-palmitoyl transferase, the enzyme that catalyses condensation of L-serine and palmitoyl CoA, in 7- and 14-week-old normal (+/+) and obese (*fa/fa*) ZDF rats. *fa/fa* rats become diabetic at the age of 14 weeks as a consequence of apoptotic depletion of their cells. (c) Comparison of [³H]-ceramide formation for [³H]-serine or [³H]-palmitate. (From Unger and Orci, 2002, with permission.)

triglyceride content and the percentage of dead beta cells, suggesting that the ability to store triglyceride is protective and that it is non-esterified FFAs that are harmful (Cnop *et al.*, 2001; Listenberger *et al.*, 2003). Thus, prolonged exposure of FFAs may be more toxic if the ability to esterify fatty acids is limiting. This was confirmed recently by the overexpression of hormone-sensitive lipase in beta cells. This led to beta cell damage in high-fat fed mice. Interestingly, the higher expression of hormone-sensitive LPL resulted in more mobilization of FFAs and lower triglycerides in the islets of transgenic mice, suggesting that it is the FFAs that are harmful and not stored triglyceride (Winzell *et al.*, 2003).

In conclusion, excess fat availability predisposes to diabetes by inducing insulin resistance and by causing beta cell failure in some genetically susceptible individuals.

Obesity and the metabolic syndrome

The metabolic syndrome refers to a cluster of disorders often occurring together in the one individual, which include central obesity, impaired glucose tolerance or insulin resistance, hypertension, dyslipidaemia, hyperuricaemia and elevation of plasminogen activator inhibitor-1 (PAI-1) (Ford and Giles, 2003). The metabolic syndrome is thus a major risk factor for cardiovascular disease. The syndrome is highly prevalent. In the USA, a survey conducted between 1988 and 1994 of 8814 men and women aged over 20 years looked in each individual for the presence of at least three of the following: elevated waist circumference (> 102 cm men and > 88 cm in women), low HDL (< 1.04mmol/L), hypertension (BP > 130/85) or elevated fasting glucose (> 6.1 mmol/L), and found a prevalence

of 21.8%, rising from 6.7% in subjects 20–29 years of age to 42% in those aged 60–69 years (Ford *et al.*, 2002). The association of the metabolic syndrome with obesity was clearly demonstrated in the same dataset, in which only 4% of lean adolescents had the metabolic syndrome compared with 30% in overweight adolescents (Cook *et al.*, 2003). Furthermore, a prospective population-based cohort study on 937 individuals aged 40–65 years concluded that BMI was the central feature of the syndrome in both sexes (Maison *et al.*, 2001).

What is the link between obesity and the metabolic syndrome?

A clue to the relationship between obesity and the metabolic syndrome is provided by the fact that the strongest relationship is between the metabolic syndrome and visceral adipose tissue (for a review, see Wajchenberg, 2000; von Eyben *et al.*, 2003). Visceral adiposity has been linked to insulin resistance (Fujioka *et al.*, 1987; Pouliot *et al.*, 1992), and primary insulin resistance generated by production of transgenic animals has been shown to result in features of the metabolic syndrome (Bruning *et al.*, 1998; Thorburn *et al.*, 1999). This suggests that one way in which obesity can cause the metabolic syndrome is by causing insulin resistance. In addition, another feature of the metabolic syndrome, elevated circulating PAI-1 levels may be caused by excessive production of PAI-1 in visceral fat. In rats, PAI-1 mRNA has been found to be increased only in visceral fat during the development of obesity (Shimomura *et al.*, 1996).

There is a surprising emerging association between obesity, insulin resistance, features of a low-grade inflammatory state and the metabolic syndrome. There is a relationship between elevated C-reactive protein and obesity (Visser *et al.*, 1999) and a significant positive correlation has been found between C-reactive protein and several features of the metabolic syndrome, including total cholesterol, triglyceride, glucose and uric acid levels, with a negative correlation with HDL-cholesterol levels (Frohlich *et al.*, 2000). This study also confirmed the relationship between C-reactive protein and BMI (Frohlich *et al.*, 2000). These relationships have also recently been demonstrated in a different population (Tamakoshi *et al.*, 2003). The relationship of obesity with this mild inflammatory state may be via the production of insulin resistance, as it has been shown that the elevated levels of PAI-1, another characteristic of the metabolic syndrome, are related to insulin resistance independent of obesity (Nakamura *et al.*, 2003; Solano *et al.*, 2003). However, associations do not provide information as to what is cause and what is effect. A clue to the direction of this relationship is given by studies showing that the administration of croton oil to rabbits to initiate an acute-phase response resulted in a sixfold increase in triglycerides and a decrease in HDL-cholesterol (Cabana *et al.*, 1989), suggesting that an increase in acute-phase proteins causes some features of the metabolic syndrome.

How could acute-phase proteins induce features of the metabolic syndrome? One potential mechanism is the overexpression of 11β-hydroxysteroid dehydrogenase type-1 (11β-HSD-1), an enzyme that locally converts the inactive cortisone to the active cortisol (Stewart, 2003). Inflammatory stimuli increase the expression of 11β-HSD-1 in a variety of tissues, including aortic smooth muscle cells (Cai *et al.*, 2001), osteoblasts (Cooper *et al.*, 2001) and cultured human amnion fibroblasts (Sun and Myatt, 2003). Transgenic mice overexpressing 11β-HSD-1 in adipose tissue to the same extent as that found in obese humans developed visceral obesity, insulin resistance, diabetes, hyperlipidaemia, hyperphagia (Masuzaki *et al.*, 2001) and hypertension (Masuzaki *et al.*, 2003). Recently, elevated 11β-HSD-1 activity and mRNA levels have been reported to correlate with adiposity, fasting glucose, insulin and insulin resistance in human subjects, showing that the level of 11β-HSD-1 expression is associated with the metabolic syndrome in human subjects (Lindsay *et al.*, 2003).

Thus, a testable hypothesis for the relationship between obesity and the metabolic syndrome can be presented as in Fig. 13.5. Much remains to be discovered, including how insulin resistance causes the mild inflammatory state, how inflammatory markers upregulate 11β-HSD-1 and how excess local production of corticosteroid causes the features of the metabolic syndrome.

Obesity and polycystic ovary syndrome

Polycystic ovary syndrome (PCOS) is a common condition affecting women of reproductive age that causes anovulation, menstrual irregularities, infertility, hirsutism and acne (Hull,

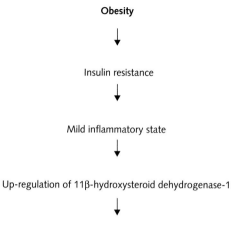

Obesity

↓

Insulin resistance

↓

Mild inflammatory state

↓

Up-regulation of 11β-hydroxysteroid dehydrogenase-1

↓

Metabolic syndrome

Fig 13.5 Hypothesized mechanism for the development of the metabolic syndrome in obesity.

1987; Polson *et al.*, 1988). Approximately 50% of women with PCOS are overweight or obese, and these women are more likely to have more hirsutism and menstrual irregularities (Franks *et al.*, 1991; Gambineri *et al.*, 2002). Obesity is a risk factor for POCS because obesity is a cause of insulin resistance.

The association of insulin resistance with hirsutism and menstrual irregularities has long been known (called 'la diabète des femme à barbe'—the diabetes of bearded women) (Achard and Thiers, 1921). The presence of hyperinsulinaemia in hyperandrogenic women with PCOS was reported in 1980 (Burghen *et al.*, 1980). Insulin has been shown to stimulate androgen production from both ovarian stroma and thecal tissue (Barbieri *et al.*, 1984; Willis *et al.*, 1996; Nestler *et al.*, 1998) (Fig. 13.6). Hyperinsulinaemic clamps performed on small groups of intact or oophorectomized women confirmed that the androgenic effect of hyperinsulinaemia was due to the action of insulin on the ovary rather than on the adrenal gland (Stuart and Nagamani, 1990).

In obese women, insulin resistance is likely to be secondary to the excess adipose tissue by mechanisms discussed above. Consistent with this is the fact that weight loss (Huber-Buchholz *et al.*, 1999; Crosignani *et al.*, 2003) and insulin-sensitizing agents such as metformin (Velazquez *et al.*, 1994) and thiazolidenediones (Dunaif *et al.*, 1996) all lower insulin levels and have been shown to reverse features of the PCOS and lead to ovulation in a substantial proportion of women.

It has also been shown that insulin resistance is a feature of non-obese women with PCOS. It has been postulated that in these women, the action of insulin is disrupted by excessive serine phosphorylation of the insulin receptor, presumably secondary to an overactive serine/threonine kinase. As P450c17, an important regulatory enzyme of androgen biosynthesis, is modulated by serine phosphorylation, it has been proposed that in these women a single defect could

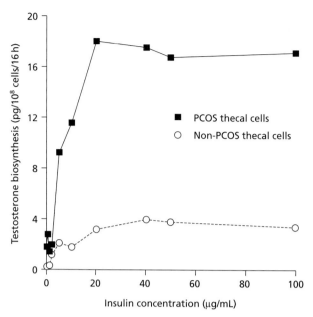

Fig 13.6 Dose–response study of insulin's stimulation of testosterone biosynthesis in PCOS and non-PCOS thecal cells. Thecal cells were isolated from one woman with PCOS (PCOS) and one healthy woman (non-PCOS) and cultured in the absence or presence of various concentrations of insulin. After 16 h, cells were quickly frozen and thawed, and the testosterone content of cells and media was assayed by radioimmunoassay (RIA). Net steroid synthesis was calculated by subtracting the steroid content of cells and media at time zero. (From Nestler *et al.*, 1998, with permission.)

explain both insulin resistance and hyperandrogenism (Dunaif, 1997).

Conclusion

Obesity can cause many serious metabolic complications including many key features of the metabolic syndrome such as insulin resistance, type 2 diabetes and dyslipidaemia and polycystic ovary syndrome. Recent work is unravelling the many and complex mechanisms responsible for this relationship. The facts that the adipocyte manufactures and secretes many compounds that can modify insulin action and that obesity is associated with a mild inflammatory state are two of the most surprising outcomes of recent research in this area.

References

Achard, C. and Thiers, J. (1921) Le virilisme pilaire et son association a l'insuffisance glycolytique (diabete des femmes a bard). *Bulletin of the National Academy Medicine* **86**, 51–64.

Andrikopoulos, S. and Proietto, J. (1995) The biochemical basis of increased hepatic glucose production in a mouse model of type 2 (non-insulin-dependent) diabetes mellitus. *Diabetologia* **38**, 1389–1396.

Arita, Y., Kihara, S., Ouchi, N., Takahashi, M., Maeda, K., Miyagawa, J., Hotta, K., Shimomura, I., Nakamura, T., Miyaoka, K., Kuriyama, H., Nishida, M., Yamashita, S., Okubo, K., Matsubara, K., Muraguchi, M., Ohmoto, Y., Funahashi, T. and Matsuzawa, Y. (1999) Paradoxical decrease of an adipose-specific protein, adiponectin, in obesity. *Biochemical and Biophysical Research Communications* **257**, 79–83.

Baldeweg, S.E., Golay, A., Natali, A., Balkau, B., Del Prato, S. and Coppack, S.W. (2000) Insulin resistance, lipid and fatty acid concentrations in 867 healthy Europeans. European Group for the Study of Insulin Resistance (EGIR). *European Journal of Clinical Investigation* **30**, 45–52.

Barbieri, R.L., Makris, A. and Ryan, K.J. (1984) Insulin stimulates androgen accumulation in incubations of human ovarian stroma and theca. *Obstetrics and Gynecology* **64**, 73S–80S.

Bastard, J.P., Jardel, C., Bruckert, E., Blondy, P., Capeau, J., Laville, M., Vidal, H. and Hainque, B. (2000) Elevated levels of interleukin 6 are reduced in serum and subcutaneous adipose tissue of obese women after weight loss. *Journal of Clinical Endocrinology and Metabolism* **85**, 3338–3342.

Baumann, H. and Gauldie, J. (1994) The acute phase response. *Immunology Today* **15**, 74–80.

Berg, A.H., Combs, T.P., Du, X., Brownlee, M. and Scherer, P.E. (2001) The adipocyte-secreted protein Acrp30 enhances hepatic insulin action. *Nature Medicine* **7**, 947–953.

Blain, H., Vuillemin, A., Guillemin, F., Durant, R., Hanesse, B., de Talance, N., Doucet, B. and Jeandel, C. (2002) Serum leptin level is a predictor of bone mineral density in postmenopausal women. *Journal of Clinical Endocrinology and Metabolism* **87**, 1030–1035.

Boden, G. and Jadali, F. (1991) Effects of lipid on basal carbohydrate metabolism in normal men. *Diabetes* **40**, 686–692.

Boden, G., Chen, X., Ruiz, J., White, J. V. and Rossetti, L. (1994) Mechanisms of fatty acid-induced inhibition of glucose uptake. *Journal of Clinical Investigation* **93**, 2438–2446.

Boitard, C. (2002) Insulin secretion in type 2 diabetes: clinical aspects. *Diabetes and Metabolism* **28**, 4S33–4S38.

Bruning, J.C., Michael, M.D., Winnay, J.N., Hayashi, T., Horsch, D., Accili, D., Goodyear, L.J. and Kahn, C. R. (1998) A muscle-specific insulin receptor knockout exhibits features of the metabolic syndrome of NIDDM without altering glucose tolerance. *Molecular Cell* **2**, 559–569.

Bruun, J.M., Verdich, C., Toubro, S., Astrup, A. and Richelsen, B. (2003) Association between measures of insulin sensitivity and circulating levels of interleukin-8, interleukin-6 and tumor necrosis factor-alpha. Effect of weight loss in obese men. *European Journal of Endocrinology* **148**, 535–542.

Burghen, G.A., Givens, J.R. and Kitabchi, A.E. (1980) Correlation of hyperandrogenism with hyperinsulinism in polycystic ovarian disease. *Journal of Clinical Endocrinology and Metabolism* **50**, 113–116.

Cabana, V.G., Siegel, J.N. and Sabesin, S.M. (1989) Effects of the acute phase response on the concentration and density distribution of plasma lipids and apoliporoteins. *Journal of Lipid Research* **30**, 39–49.

Cai, T.Q., Wong, B., Mundt, S.S., Thieringer, R., Wright, S.D. and Hermanowski-Vosatka, A. (2001) Induction of 11 beta-hydroxysteroid dehydrogenase type 1 but not -2 in human aortic smooth muscle cells by inflammatory stimuli. *Journal of Steroid Biochemistry and Molecular Biology* **77**, 117–122.

Carey, A.L., Lamont, B., Andrikopoulos, S., Koukoulas, I., Proietto, J. and Febbraio, M.A. (2003) Interleukin-6 gene expression is increased in insulin-resistant rat skeletal muscle following insulin stimulation. *Biochemical and Biophysical Research Communications* **302**, 837–840.

Ceddia, R.B., Koistinen, H.A., Zierath, J. R. and Sweeney, G. (2002) Analysis of paradoxical observations on the association between leptin and insulin resistance. *FASEB J* **16**, 1163–1176.

Chen, X., Iqbal, N. and Boden, G. (1999) The effects of free fatty acids on gluconeogenesis and glycogenolysis in normal subjects. *Journal of Clinical Investigation* **103**, 365–372.

Clore, J.N., Glickman, P.S., Nestler, J.E. and Blackard, W.G. (1991) In vivo evidence for hepatic autoregulation during FFA-stimulated gluconeogenesis in normal humans. *American Journal of Physiology* **261**, E425–E429.

Cnop, M., Hannaert, J. C., Hoorens, A., Eizirik, D. L. and Pipeleers, D. G. (2001) Inverse relationship between cytotoxicity of free fatty acids in pancreatic islet cells and cellular triglyceride accumulation. *Diabetes* **50**, 1771–1777.

Cohen, B., Novick, D. and Rubinstein, M. (1996) Modulation of insulin activities by leptin. *Science* **274**, 1185–1188.

Combs, T.P., Berg, A.H., Obici, S., Scherer, P.E. and Rossetti, L. (2001) Endogenous glucose production is inhibited by the adipose-derived protein Acrp30. *Journal of Clinical Investigation* **108**, 1875–1881.

Cook, S., Weitzman, M., Auinger, P., Nguyen, M. and Dietz, W.H. (2003) Prevalence of a metabolic syndrome phenotype in adolescents: findings from the third National Health and Nutrition Examination Survey, 1988–1994. *Archives of Pediatric and Adolescent Medicine* **157**, 821–827.

Cooney, G.J., Thompson, A.L., Furler, S.M., Ye, J. and Kraegen, E.W. (2002) Muscle long-chain acyl CoA esters and insulin resistance. *Annals of the New York Academy of Science* **967**, 196–207.

Cooper, M.S., Bujalska, I., Rabbitt, E., Walker, E.A., Bland, R., Sheppard, M.C., Hewison, M. and Stewart, P.M. (2001) Modulation of 11 beta-hydroxysteroid dehydrogenase isozymes by proinflammatory cytokines in osteoblasts: an autocrine switch from glucocorticoid inactivation to activation. *Journal of Bone and Mineral Research* **16**, 1037–1044.

Crosignani, P.G., Colombo, M., Vegetti, W., Somigliana, E., Gessati, A. and Ragni, G. (2003) Overweight and obese anovulatory patients with polycystic ovaries: parallel improvements in anthropometric indices, ovarian physiology and fertility rate induced by diet. *Human Reproduction* **18**, 1928–1932.

Daimon, M., Oizumi, T., Saitoh, T., Kameda, W., Hirata, A., Yamaguchi, H., Ohnuma, H., Igarashi, M., Tominaga, M. and Kato, T. (2003) Decreased serum levels of adiponectin are a risk factor for the progression to Type 2 diabetes in the Japanese population: The Funagata study. *Diabetes Care* **26**, 2015–2020.

Dandona, P., Weinstock, R., Thusu, K., Abdel-Rahman, E., Aljada, A. and Wadden, T. (1998) Tumor necrosis factor-alpha in sera of obese patients: fall with weight loss. *Journal of Clinical Endocrinology and Metabolism* **83**, 2907–2910.

Das, U.N. (1999) Essential fatty acids, lipid peroxidation and apoptosis. *Prostaglandins, Leukotrienes and Essential Fatty Acids* **61**, 157–163.

Dunaif, A. (1997) The insulin-sensitizing agent troglitazone improves metabolic and reproductive abnormalities in the polycystic ovary syndrome. *Endocrine Reviews* **18**, 774–800.

Dunaif, A., Scott, D., Finegood, D., Quintana, B. and Whitcomb, R. (1996) Insulin resistance and the polycystic ovary syndrome:

mechanism and implications for pathogenesis. *Journal of Clinical Endocrinology and Metabolism* **81**, 3299–3306.

Emanuelli, B., Peraldi, P., Filloux, C., Chavey, C., Freidinger, K., Hilton, D.J., Hotamisligil, G.S. and Van Obberghen, E. (2001) SOCS-3 inhibits insulin signaling and is up-regulated in response to tumor necrosis factor-alpha in the adipose tissue of obese mice. *Journal of Biological Chemistry* **276**, 47944–47949.

von Eyben, F.E., Mouritsen, E., Holm, J., Montvilas, P., Dimcevski, G., Suciu, G., Helleberg, I., Kristensen, L. and von Eyben, R. (2003) Intra-abdominal obesity and metabolic risk factors: a study of young adults. *International Journal of Obesity and Related Metabolic Disorders* **27**, 941–949.

Faggioni, R., Fantuzzi, G., Gabay, C., Moser, A., Dinarello, C.A., Feingold, K.R. and Grunfeld, C. (1999) Leptin deficiency enhances sensitivity to endotoxin-induced lethality. *American Journal of Physiology* **276**, R136–R142.

Fasshauer, M., Klein, J., Neumann, S., Eszlinger, M. and Paschke, R. (2001) Tumor necrosis factor alpha is a negative regulator of resistin gene expression and secretion in 3T3-L1 adipocytes. *Biochemical and Biophysical Research Communications* **288**, 1027–1031.

Fasshauer, M., Klein, J., Neumann, S., Eszlinger, M. and Paschke, R. (2002) Hormonal regulation of adiponectin gene expression in 3T3-L1 adipocytes. *Biochemical and Biophysical Research Communications* **290**, 1084–1089.

Febbraio, M.A. and Pedersen, B.K. (2002) Muscle-derived interleukin-6: mechanisms for activation and possible biological roles. *FASEB J* **16**, 1335–1347.

Fernandez-Real, J.M., Vayreda, M., Richart, C., Gutierrez, C., Broch, M., Vendrell, J. and Ricart, W. (2001) Circulating interleukin 6 levels, blood pressure, and insulin sensitivity in apparently healthy men and women. *Journal of Clinical Endocrinology and Metabolism* **86**, 1154–1159.

Ferrannini, E., Natali, A., Bell, P., Cavallo-Perin, P., Lalic, N. and Mingrone, G. (1997) Insulin resistance and hypersecretion in obesity. European Group for the Study of Insulin Resistance (EGIR). *Journal of Clinical Investigation* **100**, 1166–1173.

Fischer, S., Hanefeld, M., Haffner, S. M., Fusch, C., Schwanebeck, U., Kohler, C., Fucker, K. and Julius, U. (2002) Insulin-resistant patients with type 2 diabetes mellitus have higher serum leptin levels independently of body fat mass. *Acta Diabetologica* **39**, 105–110.

Ford, E.S. and Giles, W.H. (2003) A comparison of the prevalence of the metabolic syndrome using two proposed definitions. *Diabetes Care* **26**, 575–581.

Ford, E.S., Giles, W.H. and Dietz, W. H. (2002) Prevalence of the metabolic syndrome among US adults: findings from the third National Health and Nutrition Examination Survey. *Journal of the American Medical Association* **287**, 356–359.

Franks, S., Kiddy, D., Sharp, P., Singh, A., Reed, M., Seppala, M., Koistinen, R. and Hamilton-Fairley, D. (1991) Obesity and polycystic ovary syndrome. *Annals of the New York Academy of Science* **626**, 201–206.

Frohlich, M., Imhof, A., Berg, G., Hutchinson, W.L., Pepys, M.B., Boeing, H., Muche, R., Brenner, H. and Koenig, W. (2000) Association between C-reactive protein and features of the metabolic syndrome: a population-based study. *Diabetes Care* **23**, 1835–1839.

Fujioka, S., Matsuzawa, Y., Tokunaga, K. and Tarui, S. (1987) Contribution of intra-abdominal fat accumulation to the impairment of glucose and lipid metabolism in human obesity. *Metabolism* **36**, 54–59.

Gambineri, A., Pelusi, C., Vicennati, V., Pagotto, U. and Pasquali, R. (2002) Obesity and the polycystic ovary syndrome. *International Journal of Obesity and Related Metabolic Disorders* **26**, 883–896.

Gorden, E.S. (1960) Non-esterified fatty acids in blood of obese and lean subjects. *American Journal of Clinical Nutrition* **8**, 740–747.

Griffin, M.E., Marcucci, M.J., Cline, G.W., Bell, K., Barucci, N., Lee, D., Goodyear, L.J., Kraegen, E.W., White, M.F. and Shulman, G.I. (1999) Free fatty acid-induced insulin resistance is associated with activation of protein kinase C theta and alterations in the insulin signaling cascade. *Diabetes* **48**, 1270–1274.

Groop, L. (2000) Role of free fatty acids and insulin in determining free fatty acid and lipid oxidation in man. *International Journal of Clinical Practice* **113** (Suppl.), 3–13.

Groop, L., Bonadonna, R., Shank, M., Petrides, A. and De Fronzo, R. (1991) Pathogenesis of type 2 diabetes: the relative contribution of insulin resistance and impaired insulin secretion. *Journal of Clinical Investigation* **87**, 83–89.

Gudz, T.I., Tserng, K.Y. and Hoppel, C.L. (1997) Direct inhibition of mitochondrial respiratory chain complex III by cell-permeable ceramide. *Journal of Biological Chemistry* **272**, 24154–24158.

Gutierrez-Fisac, J.L., Banegas Banegas, J.R., Artalejo, F.R. and Regidor, E. (2000) Increasing prevalence of overweight and obesity among Spanish adults, 1987–1997. *International Journal of Obesity and Related Metabolic Disorders* **24**, 1677–1682.

Haugen, F., Jorgensen, A., Drevon, C.A. and Trayhurn, P. (2001) Inhibition by insulin of resistin gene expression in 3T3-L1 adipocytes. *FEBS Letters* **507**, 105–108.

Hotamisligil, G.S., Shargill, N.S. and Spiegelman, B.M. (1993) Adipose expression of tumor necrosis factor-alpha: direct role in obesity-linked insulin resistance. *Science* **259**, 87–91.

Hotamisligil, G.S., Budavari, A., Murray, D. and Spiegelman, B.M. (1994a) Reduced tyrosine kinase activity of the insulin receptor in obesity-diabetes. Central role of tumor necrosis factor-alpha. *Journal of Clinical Investigation* **94**, 1543–1549.

Hotamisligil, G.S., Murray, D.L., Choy, L.N. and Spiegelman, B.M. (1994b) Tumor necrosis factor alpha inhibits signaling from the insulin receptor. *Proceedings of the National Academy of Science of the USA* **91**, 4854–4858.

Hotta, K., Funahashi, T., Arita, Y., Takahashi, M., Matsuda, M., Okamoto, Y., Iwahashi, H., Kuriyama, H., Ouchi, N., Maeda, K., Nishida, M., Kihara, S., Sakai, N., Nakajima, T., Hasegawa, K., Muraguchi, M., Ohmoto, Y., Nakamura, T., Yamashita, S., Hanafusa, T. and Matsuzawa, Y. (2000) Plasma concentrations of a novel, adipose-specific protein, adiponectin, in type 2 diabetic patients. *Arteriosclerosis Thrombosis and Vascular Biology* **20**, 1595–1599.

Hotta, K., Funahashi, T., Bodkin, N.L., Ortmeyer, H.K., Arita, Y., Hansen, B.C. and Matsuzawa, Y. (2001) Circulating concentrations of the adipocyte protein adiponectin are decreased in parallel with reduced insulin sensitivity during the progression to type 2 diabetes in rhesus monkeys. *Diabetes* **50**, 1126–1133.

Huber-Buchholz, M.M., Carey, D.G. and Norman, R.J. (1999) Restoration of reproductive potential by lifestyle modification in obese polycystic ovary syndrome: role of insulin sensitivity and luteinizing hormone. *Journal of Clinical Endocrinology and Metabolism* **84**, 1470–1474.

Hull, M. G. (1987) Epidemiology of infertility and polycystic ovarian

disease: endocrinological and demographic studies. *Gynecology and Endocrinology* **1**, 235–245.

Janke, J., Englei, S., Gorzelniak, K., Luft, F.C. and Sharma, A.M. (2002) Resistin gene expression in human adipocytes is not related to insulin resistance. *Obesity Research* **10**, 1–5.

Juan, C.C., Au, L.C., Fang, V.S., Kang, S.F., Ko, Y.H., Kuo, S.F., Hsu, Y.P., Kwok, C.F. and Ho, L.T. (2001) Suppressed gene expression of adipocyte resistin in an insulin-resistant rat model probably by elevated free fatty acids. *Biochemical and Biophysical Research Communications* **289**, 1328–1333.

Kamohara, S., Burcelin, R., Halaas, J.L., Friedman, J. M. and Charron, M.J. (1997) Acute stimulation of glucose metabolism in mice by leptin treatment. *Nature* **389**, 374–377.

Kern, P.A., Saghizadeh, M., Ong, J.M., Bosch, R.J., Deem, R. and Simsolo, R.B. (1995) The expression of tumor necrosis factor in human adipose tissue. Regulation by obesity, weight loss, and relationship to lipoprotein lipase. *Journal of Clinical Investigation* **95**, 2111–2119.

Kern, P.A., Ranganathan, S., Li, C., Wood, L. and Ranganathan, G. (2001) Adipose tissue tumor necrosis factor and interleukin-6 expression in human obesity and insulin resistance. *American Journal of Physiology, Endocrinology and Metabolism* **280**, E745–E751.

Koistinen, H.A., Bastard, J.P., Dusserre, E., Ebeling, P., Zegari, N., Andreelli, F., Jardel, C., Donner, M., Meyer, L., Moulin, P., Hainque, B., Riou, J.P., Laville, M., Koivisto, V.A. and Vidal, H. (2000) Subcutaneous adipose tissue expression of tumour necrosis factor-alpha is not associated with whole body insulin resistance in obese nondiabetic or in type-2 diabetic subjects. *European Journal of Clinical Investigation* **30**, 302–10.

Kopp, H.P., Kopp, C.W., Festa, A., Krzyzanowska, K., Kriwanek, S., Minar, E., Roka, R. and Schernthaner, G. (2003) Impact of weight loss on inflammatory proteins and their association with the insulin resistance syndrome in morbidly obese patients. *Arteriosclerosis, Thrombosis and Vascular Biology* **23**, 1042–1047.

Krosnick, A. (2000) The diabetes and obesity epidemic among the Pima Indians. *New England Journal of Medicine* **97**, 31–37.

Kubota, N., Terauchi, Y., Yamauchi, T., Kubota, T., Moroi, M., Matsui, J., Eto, K., Yamashita, T., Kamon, J., Satoh, H., Yano, W., Froguel, P., Nagai, R., Kimura, S., Kadowaki, T. and Noda, T. (2002) Disruption of adiponectin causes insulin resistance and neointimal formation. *Journal of Biological Chemistry* **277**, 25863–25866.

Kulik, G., Klippel, A. and Weber, M.J. (1997) Antiapoptotic signalling by the insulin-like growth factor I receptor, phosphatidylinositol 3-kinase, and Akt. *Molecular Cell Biology* **17**, 1595–1606.

Lam, T.K., Yoshii, H., Haber, C.A., Bogdanovic, E., Lam, L., Fantus, I.G. and Giacca, A. (2002) Free fatty acid-induced hepatic insulin resistance: a potential role for protein kinase C-delta. *American Journal of Physiology Endocrinology and Metabolism* **283**, E682–E691.

Lam, T.K., Carpentier, A., Lewis, G.F., van de Werve, G., Fantus, I.G. and Giacca, A. (2003) Mechanisms of the free fatty acid-induced increase in hepatic glucose production. *American Journal of Physiology, Endocrinology and Metabolism* **284**, E863–E873.

Lamont, B.J., Andrikopoulos, S., Funkat, A., Favaloro, J., Ye, J.M., Kraegen, E.W., Howlett, K.F., Zajac, J. D. and Proietto, J. (2003) Peripheral insulin resistance develops in transgenic rats overexpressing phosphoenolpyruvate carboxykinase in the kidney. *Diabetologia* **46**, 1338–1347.

Lang, C.H., Dobrescu, C. and Bagby, G.J. (1992) Tumor necrosis factor

193

impairs insulin action on peripheral glucose disposal and hepatic glucose output. *Endocrinology* **130**, 43–52.

Lee, Y., Hirose, H., Ohneda, M., Johnson, McGarry, J. and Unger, R. (1994) β-cell lipotoxicity in the pathogenesis of non-insulin dependent diabetes mellitus of obese rats: impairment in adipocyte-β-cell relationships. *Proceedings of the National Academy of Science* **91**, 10878–10882.

Leonard, D., McDermott, R., Odea, K., Rowley, K. G., Pensio, P., Sambo, E., Twist, A., Toolis, R., Lowson, S. and Best, J.D. (2002) Obesity, diabetes and associated cardiovascular risk factors among Torres Strait Islander people. *Australia and New Zealand Journal of Public Health* **26**, 144–149.

Lihn, A.S., Ostergard, T., Nyholm, B., Pedersen, S.B., Richelsen, B. and Schmitz, O. (2003) Adiponectin expression in adipose tissue is reduced in first-degree relatives of type 2 diabetic patients. *American Journal of Physiology, Endocrinology and Metabolism* **284**, E443–E448.

Lindsay, R.S., Wake, D.J., Nair, S., Bunt, J., Livingstone, D.E., Permana, P. A., Tatarranni, P. A. and Walker, B.R. (2003) Subcutaneous adipose 11 beta-hydroxysteroid dehydrogenase type 1 activity and messenger ribonucleic acid levels are associated with adiposity and insulinemia in Pima Indians and Caucasians. *Journal of Clinical Endocrinology and Metabolism* **88**, 2738–2744.

Listenberger, L.L., Han, X., Lewis, S.E., Cases, S., Farese, Jr, R.V., Ory, D. S. and Schaffer, J.E. (2003) Triglyceride accumulation protects against fatty acid-induced lipotoxicity. *Proceedings of the National Academy of Science of the USA* **100**, 3077–3082.

McAnulty, J. and Scragg, R. (1996) Body mass index and cardiovascular risk factors in Pacific Island Polynesians and Europeans in New Zealand. *Ethnic Health* **1**, 187–195.

McDermott, R., Rowley, K.G., Lee, A.J., Knight, S. and O'Dea, K. (2000) Increase in prevalence of obesity and diabetes and decrease in plasma cholesterol in a central Australian aboriginal community. *Medical Journal of Australia* **172**, 480–484.

McTernan, P.G., McTernan, C.L., Chetty, R., Jenner, K., Fisher, F.M., Lauer, M.N., Crocker, J., Barnett, A.H. and Kumar, S. (2002) Increased resistin gene and protein expression in human abdominal adipose tissue. *Journal of Clinical Endocrinology and Metabolism* **87**, 2407.

Maeda, N., Takahashi, M., Funahashi, T., Kihara, S., Nishizawa, H., Kishida, K., Nagaretani, H., Matsuda, M., Komuro, R., Ouchi, N., Kuriyama, H., Hotta, K., Nakamura, T., Shimomura, I. and Matsuzawa, Y. (2001) PPARgamma ligands increase expression and plasma concentrations of adiponectin, an adipose-derived protein. *Diabetes* **50**, 2094–2099.

Maedler, K., Spinas, G.A., Lehmann, R., Sergeev, P., Weber, M., Fontana, A., Kaiser, N. and Donath, M.Y. (2001) Glucose induces beta-cell apoptosis via upregulation of the Fas receptor in human islets. *Diabetes* **50**, 1683–1690.

Maison, P., Byrne, C.D., Hales, C.N., Day, N.E. and Wareham, N.J. (2001) Do different dimensions of the metabolic syndrome change together over time? Evidence supporting obesity as the central feature. *Diabetes Care* **24**, 1758–1763.

Masuzaki, H., Paterson, J., Shinyama, H., Morton, N.M., Mullins, J.J., Seckl, J.R. and Flier, J.S. (2001) A transgenic model of visceral obesity and the metabolic syndrome. *Science* **294**, 2166–2170.

Masuzaki, H., Yamamoto, H., Kenyon, C.J., Elmquist, J.K., Morton, N. M., Paterson, J.M., Shinyama, H., Sharp, M.G., Fleming, S., Mullins, J. J., Seckl, J.R. and Flier, J.S. (2003) Transgenic amplification of glucocorticoid action in adipose tissue causes high blood pressure in mice. *Journal of Clinical Investigation* **112**, 83–90.

Matsuda, M., Shimomura, I., Sata, M., Arita, Y., Nishida, M., Maeda, N., Kumada, M., Okamoto, Y., Nagaretani, H., Nishizawa, H., Kishida, K., Komuro, R., Ouchi, N., Kihara, S., Nagai, R., Funahashi, T. and Matsuzawa, Y. (2002) Role of adiponectin in preventing vascular stenosis. The missing link of adipo-vascular axis. *Journal of Biological Chemistry* **277**, 37487–37491.

Milan, G., Granzotto, M., Scarda, A., Calcagno, A., Pagano, C., Federspil, G. and Vettor, R. (2002) Resistin and adiponectin expression in visceral fat of obese rats: effect of weight loss. *Obesity Research* **10**, 1095–1103.

Miyazaki, Y., Pipek, R., Mandarino, L.J. and DeFronzo, R.A. (2003) Tumor necrosis factor alpha and insulin resistance in obese type 2 diabetic patients. *International Journal of Obesity and Related Metabolic Disorders* **27**, 88–94.

Mohamed-Ali, V., Pinkney, J. H., Panahloo, A., Goodrick, S., Coppack, S. W. and Yudkin, J. S. (1997) Relationships between plasma leptin and insulin concentrations, but not insulin resistance, in non-insulin-dependent (type 2) diabetes mellitus. *Diabetic Medicine* **14**, 376–380.

Mohamed-Ali, V., Flower, L., Sethi, J., Hotamisligil, G., Gray, R., Humphries, S.E., York, D.A. and Pinkney, J. (2001) Adrenergic regulation of IL-6 release from adipose tissue: in vivo and in vitro studies. *Journal of Clinical Endocrinology and Metabolism* **86**, 5864–5869.

Montague, C.T., Farooqi, I.S., Whitewhead, J.P., Soos, M. A., Rau, H., Wareham, N.J., Sewter, C.P., Digby, J.E., Mohammed, S.N., Hurst, J. A., Cheetham, C.H., Earley, A.R., Barnett, A.H., Prins, J.B. and O'Rahilly, S. (1997) Congenital leptin deficiency is associated with severe early-onset obesity in humans. *Nature* **387**, 903–908.

Moon, B., Kwan, J.J., Duddy, N., Sweeney, G. and Begum, N. (2003) Resistin inhibits glucose uptake in L6 cells independently of changes in insulin signaling and GLUT4 translocation. *American Journal of Physiology, Endocrinology and Metabolism* **285**, E106–E115.

Moschos, S., Chan, J.L. and Mantzoros, C.S. (2002) Leptin and reproduction: a review. *Fertility and Sterility* **77**, 433–444.

Muller, G., Ertl, J., Gerl, M. and Preibisch, G. (1997) Leptin impairs metabolic actions of insulin in isolated rat adipocytes. *Journal of Biological Chemistry* **272**, 10585–10593.

Nagaev, I. and Smith, U. (2001) Insulin resistance and type 2 diabetes are not related to resistin expression in human fat cells or skeletal muscle. *Biochemical and Biophysical Research Communications* **285**, 561–564.

Nakamura, T., Adachi, H., Hirai, Y., Satoh, A., Ohuchida, M. and Imaizumi, T. (2003) Association of plasminogen activator inhibitor-1 with insulin resistance in Japan where obesity is rare. *Metabolism* **52**, 226–229.

Nestler, J.E., Jakubowicz, D.J., de Vargas, A.F., Brik, C., Quintero, N. and Medina, F. (1998) Insulin stimulates testosterone biosynthesis by human thecal cells from women with polycystic ovary syndrome by activating its own receptor and using inositolglycan mediators as the signal transduction system. *Journal of Clinical Endocrinology and Metabolism* **83**, 2001–2005.

Nishizawa, H., Shimomura, I., Kishida, K., Maeda, N., Kuriyama, H., Nagaretani, H., Matsuda, M., Kondo, H., Furuyama, N., Kihara, S., Nakamura, T., Tochino, Y., Funahashi, T. and Matsuzawa, Y. (2002) Androgens decrease plasma adiponectin, an insulin-sensitizing adipocyte-derived protein. *Diabetes* **51**, 2734–2741.

Ofei, F., Hurel, S., Newkirk, J., Sopwith, M. and Taylor, R. (1996) Effects of an engineered human anti-TNF-alpha antibody (CDP571) on insulin sensitivity and glycemic control in patients with NIDDM. *Diabetes* **45**, 881–885.

Okamoto, Y., Kihara, S., Ouchi, N., Nishida, M., Arita, Y., Kumada, M., Ohashi, K., Sakai, N., Shimomura, I., Kobayashi, H., Terasaka, N., Inaba, T., Funahashi, T. and Matsuzawa, Y. (2002) Adiponectin reduces atherosclerosis in apolipoprotein E-deficient mice. *Circulation* **106**, 2767–2770.

Ostrowski, K., Rohde, T., Zacho, M., Asp, S. and Pedersen, B.K. (1998) Evidence that interleukin-6 is produced in human skeletal muscle during prolonged running. *Journal of Physiology* **508**, 949–953.

Pickup, J.C., Mattock, M.B., Chusney, G. and Burt, D. (1997) NIDDM as a disease of the innate immune system: association of acute-phase reactants and interelukin-6 with metabolic syndrome X. *Diabetologia* **40**, 1286–1292.

Pi-Sunyer, F.X. (2002) The medical risk of obesity. *Obesity and Surgery* **12**, 6S–11S.

Polson, D.W., Adams, J., Wadsworth, J. and Franks, S. (1988) Polycystic ovaries – a common finding in normal women. *Lancet* **1**, 870–872.

Pouliot, M.-C., Despres, J.-P., Nadeau, A., Moorjani, S., Prud'homme, D., Lupien, P., Tremblay, A. and Bouchard, C. (1992) Visceral obesity in men. Associations with glucose tolerance, plasma insulin and lipoprotein levels. *Diabetes* **41**, 826–834.

Pratley, R.E., Nicolson, M., Bogardus, C. and Ravussin, E. (1996) Effects of acute hyperinsulinemia on plasma leptin concentrations in insulin-sensitive and insulin-resistant Pima Indians. *Journal of Clinical Endocrinology and Metabolism* **81**, 4418–4421.

Rabinowtiz, D. and Zierler, K.L. (1962) Forearm metabolism in obesity and its response to intra-arterial insulin. Characterization of insulin resistance and evidence for adaptive hyperinsulinism. *Journal of Clinical Investigation* **12**, 2173–2181.

Rajala, M. W., Obici, S., Scherer, P.E. and Rossetti, L. (2003) Adipose-derived resistin and gut-derived resistin-like molecule-beta selectively impair insulin action on glucose production. *Journal of Clinical Investigation* **111**, 225–230.

Roden, M., Price, T.B., Perseghin, G., Petersen, K.F., Rothman, D.L., Cline, G.W. and Shulman, G.I. (1996) Mechanism of free fatty acid-induced insulin resistance in humans. *Journal of Clinical Investigation* **97**, 2859–2865.

Roden, M., Stingl, H., Chandramouli, V., Schumann, W. C., Hofer, A., Landau, B.R., Nowotny, P., Waldhausl, W. and Shulman, G.I. (2000) Effects of free fatty acid elevation on postabsorptive endogenous glucose production and gluconeogenesis in humans. *Diabetes* **49**, 701–7.

Rossetti, L., Massillon, D., Barzilai, N., Vuguin, P., Chen, W., Hawkins, M., Wu, J. and Wang, J. (1997) Short term effects of leptin on hepatic gluconeogenesis and in vivo insulin action. *Journal of Biological Chemistry* **272**, 27758–27763.

Santomauro, A.T., Boden, G., Silva, M.E., Rocha, D.M., Santos, R.F., Ursich, M.J., Strassmann, P.G. and Wajchenberg, B.L. (1999) Overnight lowering of free fatty acids with Acipimox improves insulin resistance and glucose tolerance in obese diabetic and nondiabetic subjects. *Diabetes* **48**, 1836–41.

Savage, D.B., Sewter, C.P., Klenk, E.S., Segal, D.G., Vidal-Puig, A., Considine, R.V. and O'Rahilly, S. (2001) Resistin / Fizz3 expression in relation to obesity and peroxisome proliferator-activated receptor-gamma action in humans. *Diabetes* **50**, 2199–202.

Scherer, P.E., Williams, S., Fogliano, M., Baldini, G. and Lodish, H.F. (1995) A novel serum protein similar to C1q, produced exclusively in adipocytes. *Journal of Biological Chemistry* **270**, 26746–26749.

Schmitz-Peiffer, C., Craig, D.L. and Biden, T.J. (1999) Ceramide generation is sufficient to account for the inhibition of the insulin-stimulated PKB pathway in C2C12 skeletal muscle cells pretreated with palmitate. *Journal of Biological Chemistry* **274**, 24202–24210.

Schwartz, M.W., Seeley, R.J., Campfield, L.A., Burn, P. and Baskin, D.G. (1996) Identification of targets of leptin action in rat hypothalamus. *Journal of Clinical Investigation* **98**, 1101–1106.

Segal, K.R., Landt, M. and Klein, S. (1996) Relationship between insulin sensitivity and plasma leptin concentration in lean and obese men. *Diabetes* **45**, 988–991.

Senn, J.J., Klover, P.J., Nowak, I.A. and Mooney, R.A. (2002) Interleukin-6 induces cellular insulin resistance in hepatocytes. *Diabetes* **51**, 3391–3399.

Shimabukuro, M., Zhou, Y.T., Levi, M. and Unger, R.H. (1998a) Protection against lipoapoptosis of beta cells through leptin-dependent maintenance of Bcl-2 expression. *Proceedings of the National Academy of Science of the USA* **95**, 2498–2502.

Shimabukuro, M., Wang, M.Y., Zhou, Y.T., Newgard, C.B. and Unger, R. H. (1998b) Fatty acid-induced beta cell apoptosis: a link between obesity and diabetes. *Proceedings of the National Academy of Science of the USA* **95**, 9558–9561.

Shimomura, I., Funahashi, T., Takahashi, M., Maeda, K., Kotani, K., Nakamura, T., Yamashita, S., Miura, M., Fukuda, Y., Takemura, K., Tokunaga, K. and Matsuzawa, Y. (1996) Enhanced expression of PAI-1 in visceral fat: possible contributor to vascular disease in obesity. *Nature Medicine* **2**, 800–803.

Sivitz, W.I., Walsh, S.A., Morgan, D.A., Thomas, M.J. and Haynes, W.G. (1997) Effects of leptin on insulin sensitivity in normal rats. *Endocrinology* **138**, 3395–3401.

Solano, M.P., Perry, A.C., Wang, X., Ross, R. and Goldberg, R.B. (2003) Insulin resistance but not visceral adipose tissue is associated with plasminogen activator inhibitor type 1 levels in overweight and obese premenopausal African-American women. *International Journal of Obesity and Related Metabolic Disorders* **27**, 82–87.

Song, S., Andrikopoulos, S., Filippis, C., Thorburn, A.W., Khan, D. and Proietto, J. (2001) Mechanism of fat-induced hepatic gluconeogenesis: effect of metformin. *American Journal of Physiology, Endocrinology and Metabolism* **281**, E275–E282.

Spranger, J., Kroke, A., Mohlig, M., Bergmann, M.M., Ristow, M., Boeing, H. and Pfeiffer, A.F. (2003) Adiponectin and protection against type 2 diabetes mellitus. *Lancet* **361**, 226–228.

Starkie, R., Ostrowski, S.R., Jauffred, S., Febbraio, M. and Pedersen, B.K. (2003) Exercise and IL-6 infusion inhibit endotoxin-induced TNF-alpha production in humans. *FASEB Journal* **17**, 884–886.

Steensberg, A., Febbraio, M.A., Osada, T., Schjerling, P., van Hall, G., Saltin, B. and Pedersen, B.K. (2001) Interleukin-6 production in contracting human skeletal muscle is influenced by pre-exercise muscle glycogen content. *Journal of Physiology* **537**, 633–639.

Stephens, J.M. and Pekala, P.H. (1991) Transcriptional repression of the GLUT4 and C/EBP genes in 3T3-L1 adipocytes by tumor necrosis factor-alpha. *Journal of Biological Chemistry* **266**, 21839–21845.

Steppan, C.M., Bailey, S.T., Bhat, S., Brown, E.J., Banerjee, R.R., Wright, C.M., Patel, H.R., Ahima, R.S. and Lazar, M.A. (2001) The hormone resistin links obesity to diabetes. *Nature* **409**, 307–312.

Stewart, P.M. (2003) Tissue-specific Cushing's syndrome, 11beta-hydroxysteroid dehydrogenases and the redefinition of corticosteroid hormone action. *European Journal of Endocrinology* **149**, 163–168.

Stuart, C. A. and Nagamani, M. (1990) Insulin infusion acutely augments ovarian androgen production in normal women. *Fertility and Sterility* **54**, 788–792.

Summers, S.A., Garza, L.A., Zhou, H. and Birnbaum, M.J. (1998) Regulation of insulin-stimulated glucose transporter GLUT4 translocation and Akt kinase activity by ceramide. *Molecular and Cellular Biology* **18**, 5457–5464.

Sun, K. and Myatt, L. (2003) Enhancement of glucocorticoid-induced 11-hydroxysteroid dehydrogenase type 1 expression by pro-inflammatory cytokines in cultured human amnion fibroblasts. *Endocrinology* **144**, 5568–5577.

Tamakoshi, K., Yatsuya, H., Kondo, T., Hori, Y., Ishikawa, M., Zhang, H., Murata, C., Otsuka, R., Zhu, S. and Toyoshima, H. (2003) The metabolic syndrome is associated with elevated circulating C-reactive protein in healthy reference range, a systemic low-grade inflammatory state. *International Journal of Obesity and Related Metabolic Disorders* **27**, 443–449.

Thiebaud, D., DeFronzo, R. A., Jacot, E., Golay, A., Acheson, K., Maeder, E., Jequier, E. and Felber, J.P. (1982) Effect of long chain triglyceride infusion on glucose metabolism in man. *Metabolism* **31**, 1128–1136.

Thompson, A.L. and Cooney, G.J. (2000) Acyl-CoA inhibition of hexokinase in rat and human skeletal muscle is a potential mechanism of lipid-induced insulin resistance. *Diabetes* **49**, 1761–1765.

Thorburn, A.W., Baldwin, M.E., Rosella, G., Zajac, J.D., Fabris, S., Song, S. and Proietto, J. (1999) Features of syndrome X develop in transgenic rats expressing a non-insulin responsive phosphoenolpyruvate carboxykinase gene. *Diabetologia* **42**, 419–426.

Torrance, G.M., Hooper, M.D. and Reeder, B.A. (2002) Trends in overweight and obesity among adults in Canada (1970–1992): evidence from national surveys using measured height and weight. *International Journal of Obesity and Related Metabolic Disorders* **26**, 797–804.

Tschritter, O., Fritsche, A., Thamer, C., Haap, M., Shirkavand, F., Rahe, S., Staiger, H., Maerker, E., Haring, H. and Stumvoll, M. (2003) Plasma adiponectin concentrations predict insulin sensitivity of both glucose and lipid metabolism. *Diabetes* **52**, 239–243.

Unger, R.H. and Orci, L. (2002) Lipoapoptosis: its mechanism and its disease. *Biochimica et Biophysica Acta* **1585**, 202–212.

Velazquez, E.M., Mendoza, S., Hamer, T., Sosa, F. and Glueck, C.J. (1994) Metformin therapy in polycystic ovary syndrome reduces hyperinsulinemia, insulin resistance, hyperandrogenemia, and systolic blood pressure, while facilitating normal menses and pregnancy. *Metabolism* **43**, 647–654.

Vgontzas, A.N., Papanicolaou, D.A., Bixler, E.O., Kales, A., Tyson, K. and Chrousos, G.P. (1997) Elevation of plasma cytokines in disorders of excessive daytime sleepiness: role of sleep disturbance and obesity. *Journal of Clinical Endocrinology and Metabolism* **82**, 1313–1316.

Visser, M., Bouter, L.M., McQuillan, G.M., Wener, M.H. and Harris, T.B. (1999) Elevated C-reactive protein levels in overweight and obese adults. *Journal of the American Medical Association* **282**, 2131–2135.

Vozarova, B., Weyer, C., Hanson, K., Tataranni, P.A., Bogardus, C. and Pratley, R.E. (2001) Circulating interleukin-6 in relation to adiposity, insulin action, and insulin secretion. *Obesity Research* **9**, 414–417.

Wajchenberg, B.L. (2000) Subcutaneous and visceral adipose tissue: their relation to the metabolic syndrome. *Endocrinology Review* **21**, 697–738.

Wallenius, V., Wallenius, K., Ahren, B., Rudling, M., Carlsten, H., Dickson, S.L., Ohlsson, C. and Jansson, J.O. (2002) Interleukin-6-deficinet mice develop mature-onset obesity. *Nature Medicine* **8**, 75–79.

Way, J.M., Gorgun, C.Z., Tong, Q., Uysal, K.T., Brown, K.K., Harrington, W.W., Oliver, Jr, W.R., Willson, T.M., Kliewer, S.A. and Hotamisligil, G.S. (2001) Adipose tissue resistin expression is severely suppressed in obesity and stimulated by peroxisome proliferator-activated receptor gamma agonists. *Journal of Biological Chemistry* **276**, 25651–25653.

Weyer, C., Funahashi, T., Tanaka, S., Hotta, K., Matsuzawa, Y., Pratley, R.E. and Tataranni, P.A. (2001) Hypoadiponectinemia in obesity and type 2 diabetes: close association with insulin resistance and hyperinsulinemia. *Journal of Clinical Endocrinology and Metabolism* **86**, 1930–1935.

Willis, D., Mason, H., Gilling-Smith, C. and Franks, S. (1996) Modulation by insulin of follicle-stimulating hormone and luteinizing hormone actions in human granulose cells of normal and polycystic ovaries. *Journal of Clinical Endocrinology and Metabolism* **81**, 302–309.

Winzell, M.S., Svensson, H., Enerback, S., Ravnskjaer, K., Mandrup, S., Esser, V., Arner, P., Alves-Guerra, M.C., Miroux, B., Sundler, F., Ahren, B. and Holm, C. (2003) Pancreatic beta-cell lipotoxicity induced by overexpression of hormone-sensitive lipase. *Diabetes* **52**, 2057–2065.

Yamauchi, T., Kamon, J., Waki, H., Terauchi, Y., Kubota, N., Hara, K., Mori, Y., Ide, T., Murakami, K., Tsuboyama-Kasaoka, N., Ezaki, O., Akanuma, Y., Gavrilova, O., Vinson, C., Reitman, M. L., Kagechika, H., Shudo, K., Yoda, M., Nakano, Y., Tobe, K., Nagai, R., Kimura, S., Tomita, M., Froguel, P. and Kadowaki, T. (2001) The fat-derived hormone adiponectin reverses insulin resistance associated with both lipoatrophy and obesity. *Nature Medicine* **7**, 941–946.

Yamauchi, T., Kamon, J., Minokoshi, Y., Ito, Y., Waki, H., Uchida, S., Yamashita, S., Noda, M., Kita, S., Ueki, K., Eto, K., Akanuma, Y., Froguel, P., Foufelle, F., Ferre, P., Carling, D., Kimura, S., Nagai, R., Kahn, B. B. and Kadowaki, T. (2002) Adiponectin stimulates glucose utilization and fatty-acid oxidation by activating AMP-activated protein kinase. *Nature Medicine* **8**, 1288–1295.

Yamauchi, T., Kamon, J., Ito, Y., Tsuchida, A., Yokomizo, T., Kita, S., Sugiyama, T., Miyagishi, M., Hara, K., Tsunoda, M., Murakami, K., Ohteki, T., Uchida, S., Takekawa, S., Waki, H., Tsuno, N. H., Shibata, Y., Terauchi, Y., Froguel, P., Tobe, K., Koyasu, S., Taira, K., Kitamura, T., Shimizu, T., Nagai, R. and Kadowaki, T. (2003a) Cloning of adiponectin receptors that mediate antidiabetic metabolic effects. *Nature* **423**, 762–769.

Yamauchi, T., Kamon, J., Waki, H., Imai, Y., Shimozawa, N., Hioki, K., Uchida, S., Ito, Y., Takakuwa, K., Matsui, J., Takata, M., Eto, K., Terauchi, Y., Komeda, K., Tsunoda, M., Murakami, K., Ohnishi, Y., Naitoh, T., Yamamura, K., Ueyama, Y., Froguel, P., Kimura, S., Nagai, R. and Kadowaki, T. (2003b) Globular adiponectin protected ob/ob mice from diabetes and ApoE-deficient mice from atherosclerosis. *Journal of Biological Chemistry* **278**, 2461–2468.

Yang, W.S., Lee, W.J., Funahashi, T., Tanaka, S., Matsuzawa, Y., Chao, C. L., Chen, C.L., Tai, T.Y. and Chuang, L.M. (2001) Weight reduction increases plasma levels of an adipose-derived anti-inflammatory protein, adiponectin. *Journal of Clinical Endocrinology and Metabolism* **86**, 3815–3819.

Yang, W.S., Jeng, C.Y., Wu, T.J., Tanaka, S., Funahashi, T., Matsuzawa, Y., Wang, J.P., Chen, C.L., Tai, T.Y. and Chuang, L.M. (2002) Synthetic peroxisome proliferator-activated receptor-gamma agonist, rosiglitazone, increases plasma levels of adiponectin in type 2 diabetic patients. *Diabetes Care* **25**, 376–380.

Youn, J. and Bergman, R. (1990) Enhancement of hepatic glycogen by gluconeogenic precursors: substrate flux or metabolic control? *American Journal of Physiology* **258**, E899–E906.

Zhang, Y., Proenca, R., Maffei, M., Barone, M., Leopold, L. and Friedman, J. M. (1994) Positional cloning of the mouse obese gene and its human homologue. *Nature* **372**, 425–432.

Zhou, H., Summers, S.A., Birnbaum, M.J. and Pittman, R.N. (1998) Inhibition of Akt kinase by cell-permeable ceramide and its implications for ceramide-induced apoptosis. *Journal of Biological Chemistry* **273**, 16568–16575.

14 Obesity and disease: hormones and obesity

Jonathan Pinkney

Introduction, 198

Primary endocrine disease and
obesity, 198

Endocrine consequences of
obesity, 200
    Pituitary–adrenal axis, 200
    Growth hormone–insulin-like
    growth factor-1 axis, 201
    Pituitary–gonadal axis, 202

Pituitary–thyroid axis, 204
Endocrine functions of adipose
tissue, 205

Endocrine testing in obese patients, 206
    Interpreting endocrine tests in
    obese patients, 207
    Endocrine testing in the obese
    child, 208

References, 209

Introduction

A question often asked by patients is whether a hormonal abnormality has caused their obesity. Although endocrine disorders are often associated with characteristic changes in body composition and body weight, these disorders—and so far as we know, abnormalities of the major neuroendocrine circuits in the brain controlling energy balance—play little role in the pathogenesis of common obesity, which is overwhelmingly the consequence of environmental and behavioural factors. This is a point of clinical significance because classical endocrine disorders are now being diagnosed with increasing frequency in overweight and obese subjects, simply because the prevalence of obesity in the population is rising. In this situation, both patient and doctor may consider a relationship between the two, whereas there is usually very little or none. The great majority of the endocrine abnormalities that are observed in patients with obesity are caused by the obesity. These endocrine abnormalities are mostly maladaptive and are responsible for many of the metabolic complications of obesity.

This chapter first considers the rare endocrine disorders that can play primary aetiological roles in the development of obesity. The main focus of the chapter—endocrine changes that are brought about as direct consequences of common obesity—are then considered in detail, and points of clinical relevance are highlighted. The important effects of obesity on insulin secretion and action, and its role in the pathogenesis of the metabolic syndrome and diabetes, are dealt with elsewhere in this book and will not be considered here. Finally, the question concerning which biochemical and other clinical investigations are worthwhile in obese patients will be examined, together with the everyday clinical problem of interpreting endocrine test results in obese patients.

Primary endocrine disease and obesity

In the weight reduction clinic, routine investigation for classical endocrine diseases seldom yields a diagnosis that explains a patient's obesity. At first sight this can seem surprising, as adipose tissue differentiation, and uptake and storage of fatty acids are controlled by sophisticated endocrine mechanisms involving the brain, the foregut and the autonomic nervous system (Fig. 14.1). Although it is not unusual for morbidly obese subjects to be screened biochemically for hypothyroidism and hypogonadism, and if there is clinical suspicion to investigate for Cushing's syndrome, these diagnoses are very rarely made. Rather, the clinical history usually identifies longstanding lifestyle-related factors as the principal cause of weight gain. Weight gain is a common presenting symptom of primary hypothyroidism, but it is usually modest, seldom more than a few kilograms, unless the diagnosis remains overlooked for a long period, by which time other symptoms are obvious. Similarly, although hypogonadism can be associated with weight gain, it is not usually a major factor in obesity, rather redistribution of body fat. Obesity also clouds the biochemical diagnosis of hypogonadism, particularly in men in whom obesity suppresses levels of sex hormone-binding globulin (SHBG), and total and free testosterone.

Panhypopituitarism has more potential for weight gain, although secondary hypoadrenalism may offset this. However, in the absence of delayed diagnosis, panhypopituitarism is a very rare cause of obesity, and in the absence of hypothalamic

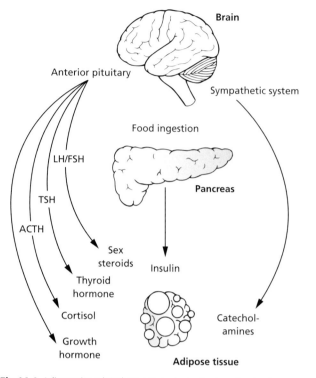

Fig 14.1 Adipose tissue has three principal sets of external endocrine regulatory mechanisms, coming from the central nervous system via the anterior pituitary and the sympathetic nervous system, and from the foregut. Short-term metabolic responses are dominated by insulin and noradrenaline, whereas longer term adaptations are also influenced by the anterior pituitary endocrine pathways.

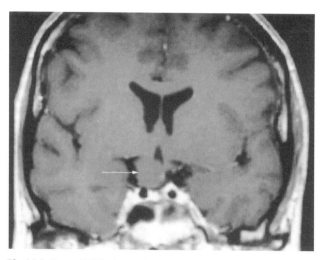

Fig 14.2 Coronal MRI brain scan in a patient with a glioma compressing the basal hypothalamus. The tumour (arrowed) has disrupted the medial basal hypothalamus, breached the floor of the third ventricle and disturbed the normal configuration of the ventricle. Hypothalamic lesions are extremely rare causes of obesity.

Table 14.1 Primary endocrine causes of obesity in humans.

Structural diseases of the hypothalamus
Craniopharyngioma
Pituitary macroadenomas with suprasellar extension
Other primary tumours, infiltrations, inflammatory diseases of the
  hypothalamus
Trauma, surgery and radiotherapy to hypothalamus

Other endocrine factors that can contribute to weight gain
Hypothyroidism
Hypogonadism
Growth hormone deficiency
Panhypopituitarism

Genetic forms of obesity associated with hypothalamic dysfunction
Prader–Willi syndrome
Leptin mutation
Leptin receptor mutation
Proopiomelanocortin mutation
Prohormone convertase mutation
MC4 receptor mutation

---

damage can not be considered a sufficient cause of morbid obesity.

Cushing's syndrome is also a rare diagnosis in patients referred for morbid obesity alone, as it is more usually associated with fat redistribution and muscle wasting. In Liverpool, a diagnosis of pituitary Cushing's disease was made only once from 400 patients referred for assessment of morbid obesity. Except for research purposes, there is little merit in routine biochemical screening of obese patients for hypothyroidism, hypogonadism, growth hormone (GH) deficiency or Cushing's syndrome. The presence of other typical clinical features will suggest the need for biochemical investigation, just as in non-obese patients.

The hypothalamus plays a critical role in the regulation of food intake, energy expenditure and in regulating the internal metabolic milieu via the autonomic nervous system and the anterior pituitary gland. Not surprisingly, hypothalamic dysfunction, caused by acquired insults or by genetic defects, principally affecting the mediobasal hypothalamus in the region of the arcuate, ventromedial, dorsomedial and paraventricular nuclei can cause major disturbances of energy regulation, culminating in obesity (Pinkney *et al.*, 2002). The magnetic resonance imaging (MRI) scan of a patient with a

glioma compressing the hypothalamus is shown in Fig. 14.2. Table 14.1 summarizes the principal endocrine disorders known to lead to significant weight gain and obesity, including structural lesions of the hypothalamus. The majority of patients with acquired structural hypothalamic damage will gain weight, and weight gain correlates with more extensive endocrine dysfunction, including the presence of diabetes insipidus and growth hormone deficiency, and perhaps the radiological extent of the lesions (de Vile *et al.*, 1996; Lustig *et al.*,

Table 14.2 Principal characteristics of the pituitary–adrenal axis in obesity.

Normal 24-h urinary cortisol excretion
Flat diurnal plasma cortisol profile
Reduced morning plasma cortisol peak
Increased stress-induced ACTH secretion
Resistance of ACTH to cortisol feedback
Impaired low-dose dexamethasone suppression
Decreased cortisol-binding globulin
Increased cortisol clearance
Increased adrenal androgen production

2003; Daousi *et al.*, 2005). Such is the rarity of structural hypothalamic disease, however, that in the absence of suggestive clinical features, brain imaging does not have a routine role in the investigation of morbid obesity.

Prader–Willi syndrome is one of the commoner genetic causes of obesity that is associated with hypothalamic dysfunction. This diagnosis is usually suggested by characteristic phenotypic features, including a history of hyperphagia, and is confirmed by genetic testing. All the other genetic forms are rare, with the possible exception of mutations in the melanocortin 4 receptor (Farooqi *et al.*, 2003). Although the number of recognized monogenic forms of obesity is likely to increase further, this group of diseases makes only a very small contribution to the overall prevalence of morbid obesity in the population.

Endocrine consequences of obesity

The endocrine consequences of obesity can be viewed broadly as physiological adaptations to positive energy balance. However, obesity is far from a transient physiological state, and many of these adaptations are ultimately maladaptive, either opposing attempts at weight loss or contributing in various ways to the metabolic complications of obesity.

Pituitary–adrenal axis

Glucocorticoids profoundly influence fat distribution and are therefore of interest to clinicians and researchers. Obesity is associated with complex changes in the pituitary–adrenal (PA) axis (Table 14.2). Although obese subjects usually have normal basal plasma and urinary cortisol levels, a variety of more subtle changes in the axis have been reported in obese subjects, including accelerated cortisol production and degradation (Migeon *et al.*, 1963; Galvao-Tales *et al.*, 1976), reduced daytime variation with diminished morning peaks (Strain *et al.*, 1980; Marin *et al.*, 1992; Ljung *et al.*, 1996) and modest elevation of plasma adrenocorticotropic hormone (ACTH) levels (Slavnov and Epstein, 1977). The PA axis is often described as being 'hyper-reactive' in obesity. For example, the ACTH response

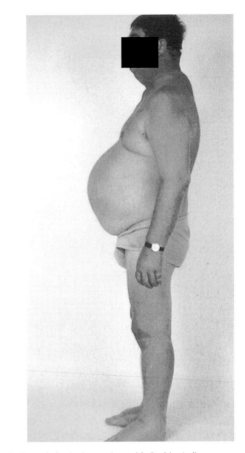

Fig 14.3 Central obesity in a patient with Cushing's disease caused by an ACTH-secreting adenoma of the pituitary gland. Redistribution of body fat to the abdomen and the back of the neck ('buffalo hump'), with loss of peripheral fat and muscle are evident. Recently, the patient had also developed diabetes and hypertension.

to insulin-induced hypoglycaemia has been found to correlate positively with body weight (Weaver *et al.*, 1993). Meal-induced activation is also greater in women with central obesity (Korbonits *et al.*, 1996), and hyper-responsiveness of the PA axis has been observed in obese subjects in response to stimulation by neuropeptides and stress (Pasquali *et al.*, 1993; 1998). Elevations in salivary cortisol profiles have also been associated with stress and central obesity in men (Rosmond *et al.*, 1998), in support of the concept that stress may contribute to central obesity through activation of the PA axis. The distinction between cause and effect in the relationship between obesity and defects in the PA axis is problematic, however, and although the hypothesis that stress-induced PA defects play a primary role, particularly in the development of central obesity, is plausible, it awaits convincing proof.

There are many similarities between central obesity and Cushing's syndrome, and it is important not to miss a diagnosis of Cushing's syndrome in centrally obese patients. Cushing's syndrome, which is typically associated with marked central obesity (Fig. 14.3), is characterized also by insulin resistance, hyperinsulinaemia, impaired glucose tolerance, hypertension and dyslipidaemia (Rebuffe-Scrive *et al.*, 1988). This similarity has led to the suggestion that central obesity might be a localized form of Cushing's syndrome affecting central adipose tissue (Bujalska *et al.*, 1997).

There are several additional lines of evidence that support an association of increased PA activity and central obesity. Cushing's syndrome has been associated with diminished lipolysis, and this may lead to a decreased capacity of abdominal adipocytes to mobilize fat, contributing to the development of central obesity. Other abnormalities described in Cushing's syndrome include decreased plasma SHBG and raised free testosterone levels, and this also clearly has the potential to influence fat distribution. Furthermore, the action of sex steroids is also regulated at tissue level. Glucocorticoids are dependent not only on pituitary drive and adrenal secretion, but also upon receptor binding and local metabolism. Thus, the enzyme 11-β-hydroxysteroid dehydrogenase converts cortisol to cortisone, and regulates tissue steroid availability. Evidence to support the hypothesis that such a mechanism could determine visceral fat accumulation comes from transgenic studies in mice that overexpress 11-β-hydroxysteroid dehydrogenase in fat. These animals developed central obesity and the metabolic syndrome (Masuzaki *et al.*, 2001). The significance of this mechanism in human central obesity remains uncertain.

Changes in skeletal muscle in central obesity and Cushing's syndrome also show intriguing similarities. A relative decrease in type 1 muscle fibres was seen in central obesity and Cushing's syndrome (Rebuffe-Scrive *et al.*, 1988). Type 1 fibres have greater insulin sensitivity and bind insulin more efficiently. Insulin sensitivity correlates positively with the proportion of type 1 fibres and inversely with that of type 2b fibres. Thus, muscle fibre composition in Cushing's syndrome resembles that seen in central obesity, again implying that increased tissue exposure to glucocorticoids occurs in centrally obese subjects, perhaps from increased PA axis activation.

Differences in the secretion and action of sex steroids are thought to be primarily responsible for the gender difference in fat distribution, and the adrenal cortex contributes significantly to androgen production in women. The principal adrenal androgens, dehydroepiandrosterone (DHEA) and androstenedione can be converted to testosterone in adipose tissue stromal cells, acting directly on neighbouring adipocytes. The obesity-related changes in PA function also include increased adrenal androgen production and urinary 17-ketosteroid excretion (Simkin 1961; Kurtz *et al.*, 1987). In premenopausal women, serum levels of the adrenal androgen DHEA correlate positively with truncal fat accumulation, but these effects are not seen in men (Usiskin *et al.*, 1990; Williams *et al.*, 1993). In women, in whom adrenal androgen production is proportionately more important than gonadal androgen production, a shift towards central obesity may be an effect of increased adrenal androgen output. Thus, in healthy postmenopausal women, androgen levels have also been found to

predict the subsequent development of central obesity (Khaw and Barret-Connor, 1991). The stimulation of DHEA and DHEA/17-hydroxyprogesterone ratio after administration of ACTH has also been correlated with body weight (Brody *et al.*, 1987). Androgens impair insulin sensitivity, and the resulting hyperinsulinaemia leads to suppression of levels of SHBG, resulting, in turn, in increased free testosterone levels and further visceral fat accumulation. Thus, adrenal androgens are likely to play a significant role in the development of central obesity in women.

In summary, complex dysregulation of the PA axis is apparent in subjects with central obesity, and could play a primary role, either alone or in combination with additional endocrine mechanisms described below, in the pathogenesis of central obesity. Cause and effect are difficult to distinguish. The two principal changes in this axis are increased central activation with resistance to glucocorticoid feedback, and increased adrenal and tissue responsiveness.

Growth hormone–insulin-like growth factor-1 axis

Multiple changes in the GH–IGF axis—especially reduced GH secretion—are present in obese individuals (Table 14.3). As with the pituitary–adrenal axis, these changes are consequences of common obesity, rather than factors with any primary causal role. However, deficient GH secretion is certainly relevant to increasing body fatness. Subcutaneous fat is markedly increased in GH-deficient subjects (Tanner and Whitehouse, 1967) and central rather than peripheral adiposity is closely associated with GH hyposecretion (Vahl *et al.*, 1997). In one study of GH-deficient subjects, visceral fat was decreased by 30% after 6 months of treatment with GH (Bengtsson *et al.*, 1994). GH deficiency is associated with impairments of lipolysis in fat and protein synthesis in muscle—an unfavourable combination in the context of obesity. Several mechanisms contribute to reduced GH levels in obesity including inhibition of secretion by nutrient and neuro-endocrine signals, increased binding and clearance. GH secretion is reduced in response to both pharmacological and physiological stimuli (Maccario *et al.*, 2000). The reduction in GH secretion is due mainly to a reduction in pulse amplitude rather than frequency (Veldhuis *et al.*, 1995). The clearance of both exogenous GH and endogenous GH is also increased in

Table 14.3 Principal abnormalities of the GH–IGF axis in obesity.

Decreased pituitary GH secretion
Increased GHBP production
Decreased IGFBP-1
Decreased IGFBP-3
Low/normal total serum IGF-1
Increased levels of free IGF-1
Decreased gastric ghrelin secretion

obesity (Veldhuis *et al.*, 1991, Langendonk *et al.*, 1999), and the consequences of reduced GH secretion are further amplified by increased levels of GH-binding protein (GHBP) (Postel-Vinay *et al.*, 1995), particularly in central obesity (Fisker *et al.*, 1997).

Circulating fatty acid (FA) levels are typically increased in obesity, and also contribute to the downregulation of GH secretion. A direct inhibitory effect of FA on pituitary GH secretion could explain this phenomenon (Alvarez *et al.*, 1991). Chronic carbohydrate overfeeding also impairs GH responses without any increase in body weight (Merimee and Fineberg, 1973). At present, it is unclear whether this results from direct nutrient effects or neuroendocrine mechanisms. Insulin also suppresses GH secretion *in vitro* (Yamashita and Melmed, 1986), and so hyperinsulinaemia may contribute to GH hyposecretion in obesity. Other factors involved in the downregulation of GH secretion are insulin-like growth factor (IGF)-1 and its binding proteins. IGF-binding proteins 1 and 3 (IGFBP-1, IGFBP-3) are reduced in obesity, with serum IGFBP-1 inversely related to fasting insulin levels and central fat distribution (Weaver *et al.*, 1990; Bang *et al.*, 1994). Insulin stimulates synthesis of IGF-1 and suppresses that of IGFBP-1. Thus, the hyperinsulinaemia of obesity, in conjunction with increased IGF-1 output from an expanded adipose tissue mass, may explain the elevated levels of free IGF-1 observed in obesity (Frystyk *et al.*, 1995). Free IGF-1 exerts negative feedback on GH secretion in pituitary cells. Confirming this mechanism, the GH response to GHRH in obese humans is suppressed by exogenous IGF-1 (Maccario *et al.*, 2001). A final mechanism for GH hyposecretion is suggested by the recent finding in obesity of reduced plasma levels of the gut hormone ghrelin (see below).

Evidence that GH hyposecretion contributes to the maintenance, and perhaps the pathophysiology of the obese state is provided by clinical trials of GH in obese subjects. In a 9-month duration study of GH in men with central obesity, total body and visceral fat declined by 9.2% and 18.1%, with improved glucose tolerance, lipid profile and blood pressure (Johansson *et al.*, 1997). The mechanisms responsible for the beneficial effect on fat mass are probably multiple, including increased lipolysis, increased lean body mass and resting metabolic rate. There is evidence that GH may augment plasma leptin levels in GH-deficient humans (Bianda *et al.*, 1997), which could promote negative energy balance. Furthermore, in preadipocytes, IGF-1 promotes and GH suppresses adipocyte differentiation (Smith *et al.*, 1988; Richelsen, 1997), raising the interesting possibility that the high IGF-1/low GH environment of obesity favours adipocyte differentiation. Finally, the observation that weight loss reverses the defects in GH and IGF-1 secretion and reduces GHBP levels (Rasmussen *et al.*, 1995; 1996) confirms that these abnormalities are indeed secondary to obesity.

In addition to GHRH and somatostatin, ghrelin has emerged recently as a third major regulator of GH secretion. Ghrelin is a 28-amino-acid peptide expressed in neuroen-docrine cells of the gut—mainly in the gastric fundus—but it is also expressed in the arcuate nucleus of the hypothalamus (Kojima *et al.*, 1999). Ghrelin is the endogenous ligand for the growth-hormone-secretagogue receptor. Whether administered to pituicytes *in vitro*, ICV to animals or by peripheral injection to animals and humans, ghrelin provokes growth hormone secretion. Unexpectedly, both ICV and peripheral injection of ghrelin in animals and humans also elicited feeding responses, and weight gain was observed in animals. Gastric ghrelin expression and secretion increase with fasting and decline in the postprandial state. In the stomach, ghrelin has a prokinetic effect, whereas circulating ghrelin appears to stimulate feeding and induce weight gain and gastric acid secretion through central effects. The effect on weight is mediated through central antagonism of leptin and other anorectic cytokines through signals delivered via vagal afferents, rather than a direct blood-borne effect on the hypothalamus (Shintani *et al.*, 2001). This action appears to be mediated through increased expression of hypothalamic neuropeptide-Y and Agouti-related protein (AGRP) (Kamegai *et al.*, 2000). Ghrelin may also stimulate feeding through the orexin system of the lateral hypothalamus (Toshinai *et al.*, 2003). In human obesity, reduced plasma ghrelin concentrations have been reported (Tschöp *et al.*, 2001). This apparently appropriate adaptation may be caused in part by the hyperinsulinaemia of obesity (Flanagan *et al.*, 2003).

While the role of ghrelin in energy homeostasis remains to be fully clarified, it appears that ghrelin links feeding and GH secretion. Although increased ghrelin secretion may elicit hunger, and ghrelin downregulation in the stomach may be an appropriate adaptation to the fed state, long-term suppression of ghrelin in the obese state clearly does not prevent continued food consumption and may be maladaptive. Low ghrelin secretion might also contribute to the reduction of growth hormone secretion observed in the obese state. An interesting recent observation has been the finding of increased plasma ghrelin levels in Prader–Willi syndrome (Cummings *et al.*, 2003). This finding could explain the marked hyperphagia characteristic of this syndrome.

Pituitary–gonadal axis

Sex steroids are important regulators of adipose tissue metabolism and play a significant role in some of the endocrine consequences of obesity, especially in women. The production of 17β-oestradiol and its precursors, including androstenedione and testosterone, decreases in women with normal ageing and the menopause. However, obesity in women is associated with subtle and complex changes in the pituitary–ovarian axis and ovarian function (Aziz, 1989). These will be considered in detail.

Androstenedione and testosterone concentrations are often elevated, and the plasma ratio of oestrone to oestradiol is increased. In postmenopausal obese women, serum oestrone and oestradiol also correlate with fat mass (Meldrum *et al.*, 1981). Levels of free oestrogen are increased, in conjunction with reduced SHBG—a pattern similar to the one observed in women with polycystic ovary syndrome (see below). In both women and men, altered production of SHBG in the obese state leads to major changes in sex steroid dynamics. Levels of SHBG are inversely related to fat mass and waist–hip ratio (Evans *et al.*, 1983), and so obesity results in increased free steroid levels and clearance. Body weight and waist–hip ratio correlate inversely with SHBG levels and directly with free testosterone. The clearance of testosterone increases as the availability of SHBG decreases, the consequence of an increased fraction of unbound testosterone available for hepatic extraction and clearance (Vermulen and Ando, 1979). Obesity probably influences SHBG production by several mechanisms. Insulin directly inhibits SHBG synthesis (Plymate *et al.*, 1988), and hyperinsulinaemia is probably the main mechanism responsible for the characteristic reduction of SHBG production in obesity. Hyperinsulinaemia, in conjunction with increased tissue free IGF-1 at ovarian level, further increases thecal androgen secretion (Barbieri *et al.*, 1986; Barbieri and Hornstein, 1988). Central obesity in women is characterized by higher total testosterone, increased oestradiol and reduced SHBG rather than lower body obesity (Kirschner *et al.*, 1990). In men, obesity is also associated with reductions in circulating concentrations of SHBG, but androgen levels (total and free testosterone) are also reduced (Zumoff *et al.*, 1990; Haffner *et al.*, 1993). In this situation, gonadotrophin levels and stimulated androgen secretion are usually normal. Obese men with lower free testosterone have lower lipolytic responses to catecholamines and higher LPL activity in adipose tissue. These metabolic adaptations may contribute to lower triglyceride turnover and further fat accumulation in obese subjects.

Adipose tissue is also able to sequester steroids, including androgens, because of their high lipid solubility, and most sex steroids are preferentially concentrated within adipocytes rather than plasma (Wahrenberg *et al.*, 1989). As a result, the steroid pool is significantly greater in obese than in lean subjects—the fat volume in obese subjects is much larger than the intravascular space and tissue steroid levels are many times higher than plasma (Feher and Brodrogi, 1982). However, adipose tissue serves not only as a reservoir but also as an important site for steroid metabolism—androgens are irreversibly aromatized to oestrogens or reversibly converted to other androgens (Longcope *et al.*, 1969; Schinder *et al.*, 1972). Aromatization increases with age and is two to four times higher in postmenopausal women. Androstenedione is the major substrate for oestrogen formation. The interconversion of oestrone to oestradiol is greater in omental than subcutaneous fat (Deslypere *et al.*, 1987). Furthermore, adipose tissue 17-hydroxysteroid dehydrogenase activity, determined by the conversion of oestrone to oestradiol, is higher in premenopausal than postmenopausal women, and women have higher activity than men. Oestrogens are not passive by-products of obesity because they positively promote preadipocyte proliferation, preservation and further expansion of adipose tissue.

There are two potential explanations for the increase in androgen production rate in female obesity. One is increased pituitary–gonadal and/or pituitary–adrenal drive. Alternatively, the increase in ovarian and adrenal production is stimulated by peripheral factors such as insulin, and with falling SHBG production, increased bioactivity and clearance of free steroid. Increased androgen levels may favour central fat deposition with an additional increase in steroid clearance through adipose tissue sequestration and metabolism. Unlike most hormone receptors, the number of androgen receptors in fat cells increases with exposure to testosterone. Interestingly, hypogonadism in men is associated with a significant decrease in the lipolytic response to catecholamines, whereas treatment with testosterone normalizes this response and increases triglyceride turnover. The lipolytic effect of testosterone is mediated by an increase in beta-adrenoceptor numbers and the activity of adenylate cyclase, protein kinase A and hormone-sensitive lipase. The density of abdominal subcutaneous adipose tissue alpha-adrenoceptors is higher in men than women and, although the main effect of androgens is lipolytic, these hormones also increase the number of anti-lipolytic α_2-adrenoceptors. Long-term treatment with testosterone of hypogonadal men leads to a marked decrease in both LPL activity and FA uptake in abdominal but not femoral subcutaneous fat. Thus, androgen deficiency in men and androgen excess in women both have significant impacts on fat distribution. Such results are in keeping with studies that show an increased density of androgen receptors in visceral compared to subcutaneous fat (Sjögren *et al.*, 1995).

The obesity-related abnormalities of the pituitary–gonadal axis are of major clinical importance in women. This subject is discussed in more detail in Chapters 13 and 20, and so only the principal endocrine issues will be summarized here. Hyperandrogenism, ovulatory and menstrual disturbances are common consequences of obesity, and can be viewed as additional aspects of the metabolic syndrome with which they are closely associated. Female hirsutism is one of the most common causes of referral to an endocrinologist, and menstrual disturbance, obesity, diabetes and cardiovascular risk factors are identified frequently in this group. In women, obesity is also associated with an increased risk of hormone-sensitive carcinomas. Menarche frequently occurs at a young age in obese girls and oligomenorrhoea and amenorrhoea are common in adulthood. Weight loss has a salutary effect on ovulatory function with the return of menses in previously amenorrhoeic obese women. Polycystic ovary syndrome (PCOS) is the most common endocrine disorder of reproduction, and is discussed further in Chapter 13. Moderate degrees of excess body weight are frequently observed in the syndrome, fuelling speculation that obesity is a causal factor. The multiple endocrine and

Table 14.4 Principal endocrine and metabolic abnormalities associated with PCOS.

Increased adrenal androgen secretion
Increased ovarian testosterone secretion
Increased aromatization of androstenedione
Increased oestrone/oestradiol ratio
Increased LH/FSH ratio
Decreased SHBG
Increased free steroid concentrations
Decreased IGFBP-1
Insulin resistance
Hyperinsulinaemia
Type 2 diabetes
Dyslipidaemia

---

metabolic defects associated with PCOS are summarized in Table 14.4.

In PCOS, the ovaries show thickened cortices, thecal hyperplasia, immature granulosa cells and increased numbers of atretic follicles. In contrast with obesity, the ovaries are the major source of androgens in PCOS, with LH-dependent testosterone production. Also in contrast with obesity, many subjects with PCOS exhibit increased LH secretion. PCOS is characterized also by increased plasma androstenedione and testosterone, and a reversed oestradiol–oestrone ratio. SHBG levels are also reduced in PCOS as in obesity. Testosterone is formed in peripheral tissues by conversion from androstenedione and DHEA, whereas oestrone is both secreted by the ovaries and derived from extragonadal aromatization. In both PCOS and obesity, aromatization rates of androstenedione to oestrone by adipose tissue rise with increasing body weight.

The aetiology of PCOS is controversial. Much evidence supports a role for insulin resistance, and this may explain the association of PCOS with central obesity. Insulin increases free testosterone levels in PCOS by increasing production of testosterone and suppressing that of SHBG (Nestler *et al.*, 1991). Women with PCOS are insulin resistant and hyperinsulinaemic, and often develop impaired glucose tolerance and type 2 diabetes (Oberfield, 2001). Although the degree of hyperinsulinaemia is proportional to body weight, lean women with PCOS are also insulin resistant. However, obese women with PCOS are significantly more hyperinsulinaemic than non-obese women with PCOS (Franks *et al.*, 1991). Suppression of gonadal steroidogenesis with a long-acting gonadotrophin-releasing hormone (GnRH) analogue does not affect plasma insulin levels or insulin sensitivity (Geffner *et al.*, 1986), which argues against hyperandrogenism as a cause of insulin resistance. Hyperinsulinaemia is thought to promote ovarian steroidogenesis. Consistent with this mechanism, Nestler and colleagues (1989) observed a fall in plasma insulin and testosterone levels in obese women with PCOS given diazoxide, with no effect on gonadotrophin release.

Subsequent studies with insulin-sensitizing agents, metformin and thiazolidinediones (Velasquez *et al.*, 1994; Dunaif *et al.*, 1996; Iunro and Nestler, 2001) confirm these results. Metformin has also been shown to have a favourable effect on hirsutism in PCOS (Kelly and Gordon, 2003). An additional mechanism by which insulin influences androgen secretion involves IGFBP-1. Lean women with PCOS show a positive correlation between plasma insulin and IGF-1 concentrations and a negative one with IGFBP-1, a pattern identical to that in obesity (Conway *et al.*, 1990). IGF-1 is a potent amplifier of LH-induced androgen synthesis (Erickson *et al.*, 2001), and as IGFBP-1 acts as an inhibitor of IGF-1 action, its suppression by insulin favours increased androgen production by increasing ovarian levels of free IGF-1.

In conclusion, obesity and insulin resistance play important roles in the pathogenesis of female hyperandrogenism and infertility. The observation that weight loss improves menstrual function in obese women with PCOS supports a causal role for obesity in the reproductive disturbance.

Pituitary–thyroid axis

Although hypothyroidism can present with modest weight gain, primary disorders of the pituitary–thyroid (PT) axis do not play any significant role in the aetiology of common obesity. Thyroid hormone is an important physiological regulator of energy balance (Zhang and Lazar, 2000), and during fasting, overfeeding and in obesity, adaptations occur at all levels of the PT axis. The availability of free hormone measurements and more sensitive thyroid-stimulating hormone (TSH) assays over the last two decades has aided research in this area. A study of lean and obese children has reported that the median TSH and thyroid hormone levels were elevated in obese subjects, although still within the conventional laboratory reference range (Stichel *et al.*, 2000).

Increased TSH and decreased prolactin responses to TRH are also seen in obesity (Scaglione *et al.*, 1991), suggesting central upregulation. Levels of TSH also correlated with body fat and plasma leptin in obese subjects (Pinkney *et al.*, 1998) consistent with central upregulation. Experimental data in humans confirm that the PT axis is under nutritional control. Overfeeding increases total levels of thyroid hormone and reduces levels of reverse-T_3 (Davidson and Chopra, 1979), whereas fasting reduces free T_3 and free T_4 levels in obese subjects (Kvetny, 1995). Although 5′-deiodinase activity is under nutritional control, and regulates T_4–T_3 conversion, the fasting-induced fall in T_3 is mainly due to reduced thyroid secretion (Kinlaw *et al.*, 1985).

Therefore, the main nutritional and obesity-related changes in the PT axis occur centrally. The mechanism for this involves the action of leptin in the arcuate nucleus on proopiomelanocortin (POMC) and NPY-containing neurons (Legradi *et al.*, 1998; Fekete *et al.*, 2000). Thus, the PT axis makes appropriate adaptations to fasting, defending body weight and muscle mass. As with other endocrine mechanisms, the PT axis has little capacity for the opposite adaptation in obesity. Although thyroid hormones have attracted interest in obesity treatment, their primary effect is to reduce lean rather than fat mass. This and other side-effects, particularly cardiac arrhythmias, mean that therapeutic hyperthyroidism is neither an effective nor safe treatment for obesity.

Endocrine functions of adipose tissue

The discovery of leptin by Friedman (Zhang *et al.*, 1994) confirmed the previous predictions of Coleman (1973), that adipose tissue had an endocrine role in the control of energy balance. Table 14.5 summarizes some of the principal hormones and other substances known to be expressed in, or released from, adipocytes. Some of these factors have local autocrine and paracrine roles within adipose tissue, whereas others are released from adipose tissue into the general circulation, where they exert a variety of remote effects, many of which are endocrine in nature. Some of the main relationships are summarized in Fig. 14.4. The clinical relevance of many of these mediators is not yet established, but given their potential clinical importance they will be discussed briefly.

Although the adipose tissue–brain axis is clearly of major physiological importance in the control of energy balance and reproduction, it is far less clear whether many of the other endocrine effects for which there is evidence are of primary physiological significance in the lean state, as opposed to representing maladaptive 'spillover effects' in the obese state. These mediators have attracted great interest because some of

them may contribute directly to the pathophysiology of obesity. Apart from leptin, the other adipose tissue peptides that best fit the classical definition of hormones are adiponectin, IL-6 and resistin. TNF-α, several other cytokines and angiotensinogen may also be released from adipose tissue and possibly also fit this definition.

Leptin is the best characterized endocrine product of the adipocyte, the main function of which is to act as a blood-borne

Table 14.5 Classical and local hormones released by adipose tissue.

Hormones
Leptin
Adiponectin
IL-6
IGF-1
Resistin
Angiotensinogen
Paracrine/autocrine mediators
TNF-α
IL-1β
IL1ra
IL-8
Prostanoids
Products of local steroid metabolism
Oestrogens
Glucocorticoids
Other molecules with distant metabolic effects
Fatty acids

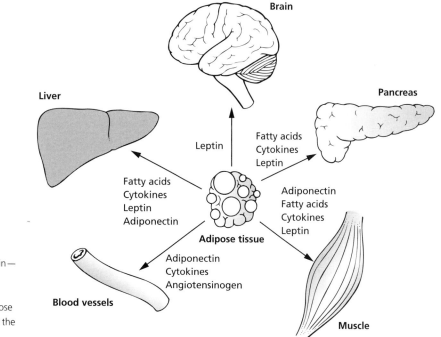

Fig 14.4 Endocrine targets of adipose tissue. The principal physiological endocrine target is that of leptin — the brain. Fatty acids also affect insulin secretion and action, thereby influencing carbohydrate and lipid oxidation. Increased or decreased production by adipose tissue of other mediators probably also contributes to the metabolic and vascular complications of obesity.

signal to the brain to indicate the level of fat storage, and enable the organism to adapt its behaviour and metabolism accordingly. Thus, leptin, acting principally through the arcuate nucleus of the hypothalamus, suppresses feeding and increases energy expenditure. Short-term fasting or overfeeding are sufficient to down- or upregulate leptin production in advance of major weight change. The two main pathways mediating these effects are the NPY–AGRP pathway and the MSH–CART pathway (Schwartz et al., 2000). Whether the hyperleptinaemia of obesity is of any clinical consequence is controversial, although it is obvious that hyperleptinaemia alone is unable to offset weight gain. This may be because of leptin resistance at receptor level, induced either by diet or supranormal leptin concentrations. Soon after its discovery, leptin was found to promote glucose uptake in vivo (Kamohara et al., 1997). Since then, many other groups have examined the effects of leptin on insulin action with varying results. However, in leptin-deficient subjects with lipodystrophy the administration of recombinant leptin clearly improved glycaemic control and lipid profiles (Oral et al., 2002), in keeping with an important effect of leptin on insulin sensitivity. Thus, in contrast with hyperleptinaemia, leptin deficiency has a clear deleterious effect on glucose homeostasis and lipid metabolism.

Leptin is also an important link between fuel storage and reproductive function, playing a pivotal role in initiating the onset of puberty in humans by stimulating pulsatile gonadotrophin secretion (Farooqi, 2002). Thus, mutations in leptin and its receptor are associated with hypogonadotrophic hypogonadism as well as severe obesity. It is plausible also that hyperleptinaemia contributes to the earlier onset of menarche seen in females with common obesity. Although it is not known whether leptin contributes directly to the ovarian dysfunction that is common in obesity, both leptin and its receptor are expressed in ovarian tissue. At present, the principal significance of leptin in the clinic is that severe early-onset obesity and hypogonadotrophic hypogonadism should prompt consideration of one of the rare genetic forms of obesity.

Adipose tissue expresses a variety of cytokines and other molecules (Mohamed-Ali et al., 1998), and these are still being discovered. IL-6 has been shown to be released into the circulation in humans (Mohamed–Ali et al., 1997) and therefore clearly could play an endocrine role. Both IL-6 and TNF-α are important mediators of inflammation and could contribute to insulin resistance and the increased risks of cardiovascular disease that accompany obesity. Adiponectin (formerly also known as acrp30, GBP28 and AdipoQ) is a 28-kDa peptide expressed principally by adipocytes (Scherer et al., 1995) and has attracted great interest. This peptide hormone is secreted by adipocytes and circulates in plasma. Its physiological role remains uncertain. Adiponectin levels are reduced in obesity (Arita et al., 1999) and in a variety of groups of subjects with type 2 diabetes or coronary heart disease. The regulation of adiponectin remains to be fully characterized, but weight loss increases adiponectin production (Yang et al., 2001). The function of adiponectin remains controversial, but it has been shown to enhance insulin sensitivity in several situations (Berg et al., 2001; Yamauchi et al., 2001) and to have antiatherogenic effects (Yamauchi et al., 2003). Therefore, a reduced output of adiponectin from adipose tissue in obesity may be yet another maladaptive effect of obesity, and predispose to the metabolic syndrome and vascular dysfunction. At present there are no clinical applications for adiponectin.

Resistin was first characterized as an adipocyte product that was suppressed by treatment with the thiazolidinedione drug rosiglitazone (Steppan et al., 2001), and is therefore a good candidate as another hormone linking obesity to insulin resistance. Although a modulator of insulin action in animals (Steppan et al. 2001; Moon et al. 2003), the role of this hormone in humans remains undecided.

Adipose tissue also expresses components of the renin–angiotensin system. Angiotensinogen is expressed and secreted by adipocytes, and angiotensin II promotes adipocyte differentiation (Ailhaud et al., 2000). Obese subjects have increased adipose tissue expression of several components of the renin–angiotensin system and it has been suggested that this may contribute to the pathogenesis of hypertension in obese subjects (Gorzelniak et al., 2002). If so, this would be another maladaptive endocrine consequence of obesity.

Apart from increased fuel storage, obesity clearly leads to a wide variety of changes in adipose tissue. In addition to obesity-associated changes in insulin secretion and action, the up- and downregulation of a range of adipocyte hormones and other mediators is also likely to have deleterious metabolic consequences, and probably contributes towards much of the pathophysiology of obesity (Fig. 14.5). Before leaving the endocrinology of adipose tissue, the question remains—why is central obesity more harmful than excess subcutaneous fat accumulation? There appear to be two reasons for this. Although difficult to study non-invasively in humans, visceral adipose tissue (VAT) possesses a different set of regulatory and secretory characteristics from subcutaneous adipose tissue, including increased adrenergic sensitivity (Lonnqvist et al., 1995) and reduced expression of leptin (Montague et al., 1997). Secondly, VAT is better placed anatomically to influence hepatocellular function. This led Bjorntorp to formulate the portal hypothesis of insulin resistance (Bjorntorp, 1990). Thus, the 'first pass effect' of fatty acids, cytokines and other VAT-derived mediators is more likely to impair hepatic insulin sensitivity, in turn leading to disorders like diabetes and the metabolic syndrome discussed in Chapters 12, 13 and 18.

Endocrine testing in obese patients

There are two common clinical situations in which it may be necessary to undertake and interpret basal or dynamic

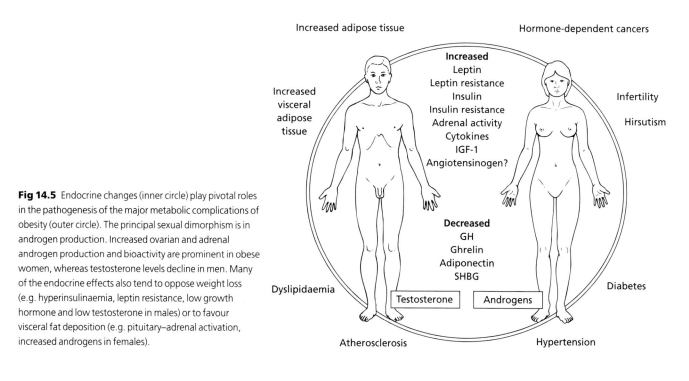

Fig 14.5 Endocrine changes (inner circle) play pivotal roles in the pathogenesis of the major metabolic complications of obesity (outer circle). The principal sexual dimorphism is in androgen production. Increased ovarian and adrenal androgen production and bioactivity are prominent in obese women, whereas testosterone levels decline in men. Many of the endocrine effects also tend to oppose weight loss (e.g. hyperinsulinaemia, leptin resistance, low growth hormone and low testosterone in males) or to favour visceral fat deposition (e.g. pituitary–adrenal activation, increased androgens in females).

Table 14.6 Abnormalities of common endocrine tests in obese subjects.

Unstimulated tests
Low testosterone (males)
Low SHBG (males and females)
Raised adrenal androgens and testosterone (females)
Low growth hormone
Raised/normal ACTH

Dynamic tests
Reduced growth hormone response to insulin or glucagon
Increased cortisol response to ACTH
Increased cortisol response to CRF
Reduced suppression of cortisol with low-dose dexamethasone

endocrine tests on patients with obesity (Table 14.6). The first is the patient with an endocrine problem who also happens to be obese, in which case the interpretation of many common endocrine tests will be confounded. As obesity is becoming more and more common, this situation is frequently encountered in the endocrine clinic, and the problem is most acute in the morbidly obese. The second situation in which the question of endocrine testing may arise is in the assessment of a new patient referred with obesity. Patients themselves often ask if there is a hormonal cause for their weight gain, and it is not unusual for referring doctors to ask if the patient could have Cushing's syndrome. In this case, before the patient steps aboard the investigational conveyer belt, the clinician should bear in mind that the great majority of the endocrine abnormalities that will be identified in an obese patient are only consequences of the obesity, without any primary aetiological significance, and

with no therapeutic implications at present. Careful history and examination by an endocrinologist should exclude endocrine disease in most cases.

Interpreting endocrine tests in obese patients

Low total testosterone levels, mainly secondary to suppression of SHBG, are the rule in obese males. In morbidly obese males, levels as low as 5 nmol/L, and sometimes lower, are not uncommon, and as there is no 'cut-off' value in obesity this may cause diagnostic uncertainty. Free testosterone levels are also suppressed, and so this assay is probably not a satisfactory substitute for total testosterone measurements. It is always important to measure testosterone in the morning as levels decline throughout the day. However, the suppression of testosterone in obesity is insufficient to cause clinical hypogonadism, and usually this will be ruled out by the concurrent demonstration of normal concentrations of gonadotrophins. Therefore, the appropriate test, if required, is measurement of both testosterone (free or total) and gonadotrophins. Routine measurement of SHBG in obese males adds little to clinical decision-making. There is no good reason routinely to measure testosterone in obese males unless there is a reason to suspect hypogonadism, for example failure to develop/loss of secondary sexual characteristics, small testes, gynaecomastia, female body habitus, loss of libido or erectile dysfunction. This is not to say that the low-testosterone state in obese males may not have a deleterious long-term effect on health, or perpetuate the obese state by impairing lipolysis. There is no rationale at present for testosterone administration in obese males with suppressed testosterone levels, although there is much more to be learned about pituitary–gonadal interactions in male obesity.

A measurement of TSH is always worthwhile because hypothyroidism is common, and with increasing obesity in the population, both hypothyroidism and hyperthyroidism are now presenting in more obese patients. In morbidly obese subjects it is appropriate also to measure free T_3 or free T_4 so that rare instances of secondary hypothyroidism are not overlooked. Given an obese population, patients with previous hypothyroidism may ask if this endocrine abnormality is relevant to the development of obesity. The answer to this is usually no, although significant weight gain (not enough to cause obesity on its own) is not unusual after the treatment of hyperthyroidism. Whether this is because previous hyperthyroidism has prevented weight gain that otherwise would have occurred, or because a rapid decline in thyroid hormone feedback resets energy balance around a new level, is not clear. In the occasional obese patient, subclinical hypothyroidism may contribute a small amount to weight gain, but is most unlikely to be a sufficient explanation for obesity, and certainly not for morbid obesity. In obesity, the PTA can be upregulated, and this may give rise to a small increase in concentrations of TSH, although the total level rarely exceeds 5 iu/L. Although it is not known whether obese hypothyroid patients might require supranormal thyroxine replacement, thyroxine is an ineffective treatment for obesity. Furthermore, given the effects of thyroid hormone on lean body mass, and its potential for cardiac arrhythmias, supraphysiological thyroid supplementation has no place in the treatment of obesity.

Cushing's syndrome causes central obesity, but on its own it is not a sufficient explanation for morbid obesity. Nevertheless, Cushing's syndrome clearly can occur in individuals who happen also to be obese. Cushing's syndrome can be extremely subtle, and its investigation is not necessarily straightforward, even in lean subjects. Unless there is other clinical evidence of Cushing's syndrome there is a very low yield from investigating morbidly obese patients routinely for this diagnosis. Moreover, given the high prevalence of pituitary and adrenal 'incidentalomas', such investigations can be misleading. Diagnostic doubt most commonly arises in females with central obesity and hyperandrogenism who are often hirsute and hypertensive, and may have cutaneous striae. Appropriate endocrine screening tests include serial urinary free cortisol (UFC) excretion, diurnal cortisol studies, low-dose dexamethasone suppression testing, and plasma or urinary androgen profiles. However, the major caveats are that obesity may result in borderline UFC excretion and impaired low-dose dexamethasone suppression testing, requiring repeat tests or additional diagnostic procedures. Simple observation may be the best course of action when endocrine screening tests for Cushing's syndrome are inconclusive.

If pituitary function testing is required in obese individuals, there are several important caveats, principally the probability of false-positive diagnosis of GH or testosterone deficiency.

This is a problem in obese patients with suprasellar structural lesions or Prader–Willi syndrome, who are often GH- and/or testosterone-deficient. Growth hormone secretion is suppressed in obesity and fails to increase normally in response to the usual provocative stimuli (Maccario *et al.*, 2000). Ghrelin appears to be the only stimulus that overcomes this, although its clinical use has yet to be assessed in detail. Reliable ranges for IGF-1 in obesity are lacking, and the interpretation of GH and IGF-1 levels in obesity is not straightforward. Most IGF-1 assays measure total serum IGF-1, and this does not reflect the bioactive free fraction.

In view of the high prevalence of diabetes in obese subjects, it is mandatory to screen for diabetes using fasting blood glucose or a glucose tolerance test. We also routinely measure the fasting lipid profile, with measurement of LDL and HDL-cholesterol and triglyceride, because of the high risk of cardiovascular disease associated with obesity.

Endocrine testing in the obese child

In children, the classical causes of morbid obesity include diagnoses such as Prader–Willi syndrome and craniopharyngioma, and the other causes listed in Table 14.1. However, in the absence of suggestive clinical features, such as growth failure, visual field defects or a characteristic phenotype, there is little point in routine endocrine screening for every obese child, given the relative rarity of these diagnoses. Failure of linear growth or pubertal progression clearly are important features that may be indicative of hypothalamic disease. Although dependent upon age and severity of the obesity, the overwhelming majority of children referred at present for evaluation of severe obesity appear to have 'lifestyle-related' obesity, inherited from their parents and the home environment.

As in adults, TSH is a worthwhile test in children. Sex steroid and gonadotrophin levels have to be interpreted with caution, recognizing the stage of pubertal development. As for adults, children need to be screened for complications of obesity. Type 2 diabetes, caused by obesity, is becoming increasingly common in children, and so screening for diabetes is also essential in obese children. Likewise, dyslipidaemia and hypertension have their origins in childhood, and should be measured.

Various features that should prompt consideration of one of the rare monogenic obesity syndromes include severe early-onset obesity, a family history of severe obesity—especially in the presence of consanguinity, and hypogonadotrophic hypogonadism. At present, genetic testing in obesity is a research tool. If advances in understanding the genetic influences on common obesity, such as melanocortin-4 receptor mutations (Farooqi *et al.*, 2003), eventually lead to the development of specific therapeutic interventions, as has been the case already with mutations in the leptin gene (Farooqi *et al.*, 1999), it is possible that an increased role for genetic testing might come into play in assessing children with severe early onset obesity.

References

Ailhaud, G., Fukamizu, A., Massiera, F., Negrel, F., Saint-Marc, P. and Teboul, M. (2000) Angiotensinogen, angiotensin II and adipose tissue development. *International Journal of Obesity* **24**, S33–S35.

Alvarez, C.V., Mallo, F., Burguera, B., Caciedo, L., Dieguez, C. and Casanueva, F.F. (1991) Evidence for a direct pituitary inhibition by free fatty acids of *in vivo* growth hormone responses to growth hormone-releasing hormone in the rat. *Neuroendocrinology* **53**, 185–189.

Arita, Y., Kihara, S., Ouchi, N., Takahashi, M., Maeda, K., Miyagawa, J., Hotta, K., Shimomura, I., Nakamura, T., Miyaoka, K., Kuriyama, H., Nishida, M., Yamashita, S., Okubo, K., Matsubara, K., Muraguchi, M., Ohmoto, Y., Funahashi, T. and Matsuzawa, Y. (1999) Paradoxical decrease of an adipose-specific protein, adiponectin. *Biochemical and Biophysical Research Communications* **257**, 79–83.

Aziz, R. (1989) Reproductive endocrinologic alterations in female asymptomatic obesity. *Fertility and Sterility* **52**, 703–725.

Bang, P., Brismar, K., Rosenfeld, R.G. and Hall, K. (1994) Fasting affects serum insulin-like growth factors (IGFs) and IGF-binding proteins in patients with non-insulin dependent diabetes versus healthy nonobese and obese subjects. *Journal of Clinical Endocrinology and Metabolism* **78**, 960–967.

Barbieri, R.L. and Hornstein, M.D. (1988) Hyperinsulinaemia and ovarian hyperandrogenism: cause and effect. *Endocrinology and Metabolism Clinics of North America* **17**, 685–703.

Barbieri, R.R., Makris, A., Randall, R.W, Daniels, G., Kistner, R.W. and Ryan, K.J. (1986) Insulin stimulates androgen accumulation in incubations of ovarian stroma obtained from women with hyperandrogenism. *Journal of Clinical Endocrinology and Metabolism* **62**, 904–910.

Bengtsson, B.A., Eden, S., Lonn, L., Kvist, H., Stokland, A., Lindstedt, G., Boseaus, I., Tolli, J., Sjostrom, L. and Isaksson, O.G. (1994) Treatment of adults with growth hormone deficiency with recombinant human GH. *Journal of Clinical Endocrinology and Metabolism* **78**, 960–967.

Berg, A.H., Combs, T.P., Du, X., Brownlee, M. and Scherer, P. (2001) The adipocyte-secreted protein Acrp30 enhances hepatic insulin action. *Natural Medicine* **7**, 947–953.

Bianda, T.L., Glatz, Y., Boeni-Schnetzler, M., Froesch, E.R. and Schmid, C. (1997) Effects of growth hormone (GH) and insulin like growth factor-1 on serum leptin in GH-deficient adults. *Diabetologia* **40**, 363–364.

Bjorntorp, P. (1990) 'Portal' adipose tissue as a generator of risk factors for cardiovascular disease and diabetes. *Arteriosclerosis* **10**, 493–496.

Brody, S., Carlstrom, K., Lagrelius, K., Lunell, N.O. and Mollerstrom, G. (1987) Adrenal steroid in postmenopausal women: relation to obesity and bone mineral content. *Maturitas* **9**, 25–32.

Bujalska, I.J., Kumar, S. and Stewart, P.M. (1997) Does central obesity reflect Cushing's disease of the omentum? *Lancet* **349**, 1210–1213.

Coleman, D.L. (1973) Effects of parabiosis of obese with diabetic and normal mice. *Diabetologia* **9**, 294–298.

Conway, G.S., Jacobs, H.S., Holly, J.M.P. and Wass, J.A.H. (1990) Effects of luteining hormone, insulin insulin-like growth factor small binding protein-1 in the polycystic ovary syndrome. *Clinical Endocrinology* **33**, 593–603.

Cummings, D.E., Clement, K., Purnell, J.Q., Vaisse, C., Foster, K.E., Frayo, R.S., Schwartz, M., Basdevant, A. and Weigle, D.S. (2003) Elevated plasma ghrelin levels in Prader Willi syndrome. *Natural Medicine* **8**, 643–644.

Daousi, C., Dunn, A.J., Foy, P.M., MacFarlane, I.A. and Pinkney, J.H. (2005) Endocrine and neuroanatomic features associated with weight gain and obesity in adult patients with hypothalamic damage. *American Journal of Medicine* (in press).

Davidson, M.B. and Chopra, I.J. (1979) Effect of carbohydrate and non-carbohydrate sources of calories on plasma 3,5,3-triiodothyronine concentrations in man. *Journal of Clinical Endocrinology and Metabolism* **48**, 577–581.

Deslypere, J.P., Verdonek, L. and Vermulen, A. (1987) Fat tissue: a steroid reservoir and site of steroid metabolism. *Journal of Clinical Endocrinology and Metabolism* **61**, 564–570.

Dunaif, A., Scott, D., Finegood, D., Quintana, B. and Whitcomb, R. (1996) The insulin-sensitizing agent troglitazone improves metabolic and reproductive abnormalities in polycystic ovary syndrome. *Journal of Clinical Endocrinology and Metabolism* **81**, 3299–3306.

Erickson, G.F., Magoffin, D.A., Dyer, C.A. and Hofeditz, C. (2001) The ovarian androgen producing cells: a review of structure/function relationships. *Endocrine Reviews* **6**, 371–399.

Evans, D.J., Hoffman, R.G., Kalkhoff, R. and Kissebah, A.H. (1983) Relationship of androgenic activity of body fat topography, fat cell morphology and metabolic aberrations in postmenopausal women. *Journal of Clinical Endocrinology and Metabolism* **57**, 304–310.

Farooqi, I.S. (2002) Leptin and the onset of puberty: insights from rodent and human genetics. *Seminar in Reproductive Medicine* **20**, 139–144.

Farooqi, I.S., Jebb, S.A., Langmack, G., Lawrence, E., Cheetham, C.H., Prentice, A.M., Highes, I.A., McCamish, M.A. and O'Rahilly, S. (1999) Effects of recombinant leptin therapy in a child with congenital leptin deficiency. *New England Journal of Medicine* **341**, 879–884.

Farooqi, I.S., Keogh, J.M., Yeo, G.S., Lank, E.J., Cheetham, T. and O'Rahilly, S. (2003) Clinical spectrum of obesity and mutations in the melanocortin 4 receptor gene. *New England Journal of Medicine* **348**, 1085–1095.

Feher, T. and Brodrogi, L. (1982) A comparative study of steroid concentrations in human adipose tissue and peripheral circulation. *Clinica Chimica Acta* **126**, 135–141.

Fekete, C., Legradi, G., Mihaly, E., Huang, Q.H., Tatro, J.B., Rand, W.M., Emerson, C.H. and Lechan, R.M. (2000) Alpha-melanocyte-stimulating hormone is contained in nerve terminals in the hypothalamic paraventricular nucleus and prevents fasting-induced suppression of prothyrotropin-releasing hormone gene expression. *Journal of Neuroscience* **20**, 1550–1558.

Fisker, S., Vahl, N., Jorgense, J.O., Christiansen, J.S. and Orskov, H. (1997) Abdominal fat determines growth hormone-binding protein levels in healthy non-obese adults. *Journal of Clinical Endocrinology and Metabolism* **82**, 123–128.

Flanagan, D.E., Evans, M.L., Monsod, T.P., Rife, F., Heptulla, R.A., Tamborlane, W.V. and Sherwin, R.S. (2003) The influence of insulin on circulating ghrelin. *American Journal of Physiology* **284**, E313–E316.

Franks, S., Kiddy, D., Sharp, P., Singh, A., Reed, M., Seppala, M., Koistinen, R. and Hamilton-Fairley, D. (1991) Obesity and polycystic ovary syndrome. *Annals of the New York Academy of Science* **626**, 201–206.

Frystyk, J., Skjaerbaek, E., Mogensen, C.E. and Orskov, H. (1995) Free insulin-like growth factor in human obesity. *Metabolism* **44**, 37–44.

Galvao-Tales, A., Graves, L. and Burke, C., Fotherby, K. and Fraser, R. (1976) Free cortisol in obesity: effect of fasting. *Acta Endocrinologica* **81**, 321–329.

Geffner, M.E., Kaplan, S.A., Bersch, N., Golde, D.W., Landaw, E.M. and Chang, R.J. (1986) Persistence of insulin resistance in polycystic ovary disease after inhibition of ovarian steroid secretion. *Fertility and Sterility* **45**, 327–333.

Gorzelniak, K., Englei, S., Janke, J., Luft, F.C. and Sharma, A.M. (2002) Hormonal regulation of the human adipose-tissue renin-angiotensin system: relationship to obesity and hypertension. *Journal of Hypertension* **20**, 839–841.

Haffner, S.M., Valdez, R.A., Stern, M.P. and Katz, M.S. (1993) Obesity, body fat distribution and sex hormones in men. *International Journal of Obesity* **17**, 643–649.

Iuonro, M.J. and Nestler, J.E. (2001) Insulin-lowering drugs in polycystic ovary syndrome. *Obstetrics and Gynecology Clinics of North America* **28**, 153–164.

Johansson, G., Marin, P., Lonn, L., Ottosson, M., Stenlof, K., Bjorntorp, P., Sjostrom, L. and Bengtsson, B.A. (1997) Growth hormone treatment of abdominally obese men reduces abdominal fat mas, improves glucose and lipoprotein metabolism, and reduces diastolic blood pressure. *Journal of Clinical Endocrinology and Metabolism* **82**, 727–734.

Kamegai, J., Tamura, H., Shimizu, T., Ishii, S., Sugihara, H. and Wakabayashi, I. (2000) Central effects of ghrelin, an endogenous growth hormone secretagogue, on hypothalamic peptide gene expreison. *Endocrinology* **141**, 4797–4800.

Kamohara, S., Burcelin, R., Halaas, J.L., Friedman, J.M. and Charrron. M.J. (1997) Acute stimulation of glucose metabolism in mice by leptin. *Nature* **389**, 374–377.

Kelly, C.J. and Gordon, D. (2003) The effect of metformin on hirsutism in polycystic ovary syndrome. *European Journal of Endocrinology* **147**, 217–221.

Khaw, K.-T. and Barret-Connor, E. (1991) Fasting plasma glucose levels and endogenous androgens in non-diabetic postmenopausal women. *Clinical Science* **80**, 199–203.

Kinlaw, W.B., Schwartz, H.L. and Oppenheimer, J.H. (1985) Decreased serum triiodothyronine in starving rats is due primarily to diminished thyroidal secretion of thyroxine. *Journal of Clinical Investigation* **75**, 1238–1241.

Kirschner, M.A., Samojlik, M., Drejka, M., Szmal, E., Schneider, G. and Ertel, N. (1990) Androgen-oestrogen metabolism in women with upper body obesity versus lower body obesity. *Journal of Clinical Endocrinology and Metabolism* **70**, 479.

Kojima, M., Hosoda, H., Date, Y., Nakazato, M., Matsuo, H. and Kangawa, K. (1999) Ghrelin is a growth-hormone-releasing acylated peptide from stomach. *Nature* **402**, 656–660.

Korbonits, M., Trainer, P.J., Nelson, M.I., Howse, I., Kopelman, P.G., Besser, G.M., Grossman, A.B. and Svec, F. (1996) Differential stimulation of cortisol and dehydroepiandrosterone levels by food

in obese and normal subjects: relation to body fat distribution. *Clinical Endocrinology* **45**, 699–706.

Kurtz, B.R., Givens, J.R., Kominder, S., Stevens, M.D., Karas, J.G., Bittle, J.B., Judge, D. and Kitabchi, A.E. (1987) Maintenance of normal circulating levels of Δ-androstenedione and dehydroepiandrosterone in simple obesity despite increased metabolic clearance rates: evidence for a servo-controlled mechanism. *Journal of Clinical Endocrinology and Metabolism* **64**, 1261–1267.

Kvetny, J. (1995) Nuclear tyroxine receptors and cellular metabolism of thyroxine in obese subjects before and after fasting. *Hormone Research* **21**, 60–65.

Langendonk, J.G., Meinders, A.E., Burggraaf, J., Frolich, M., Roelen, C.A.M., Schoemaker, R.C., Cohen, A.F. and Pijl, H. (1999) Influence of obesity and body fat distribution on growth hormone kinetics in humans. *American Journal of Physiology* **277**, E824–E829.

Legradi, G., Emerson, C.M., Ahima, R.S., Rand, W.M., Flier, J.S. and Lechan, R.M. (1998) Arcuate nucleus ablation prevents fasting-induced suppression of proTRH in the hypothalamic paraventricular nucleus. *Neuroendocrinology* **68**, 89–97.

Ljung, T., Andersson, B., Bengtsson, B.-A., Bjorntorp, P. and Marin, P. (1996) Inhibition of cortisol secretion by dexamethasone in relation to body fat distribution: a dose response study. *Obesity Research* **4**, 277–282.

Longcope, C., Kato, T. and Orton, R. (1969) Conversion of blood androgens to estrogens in normal adult men and women. *Journal of Clinical Investigation* **48**, 2191–2201.

Lonnqvist, F., Thorne, A., Nilsell, K., Hoffstedt, J. and Arner, P. (1995) A pathogenic role of visceral adipose fat β₃-adrenoceptors in obesity. *Journal of Clinical Investigation* **95**, 1109–1116.

Lustig, R.H., Post, S.R., Srivannaboon, K., Rose, S.R., Danish, R.K., Burghen, G.A., Xiong, X., Wu, S. and Merchant, T.E. (2003) Risk factors for the development of obesity in children surviving brain tumours. *Journal of Clinical Endocrinology and Metabolism* **88**, 611–616.

Maccario, M., Grotolli, S., Procopio, M., Oleandri, S.E., Rossetto, R., Gauna, C., Arvat, E. and Ghigo, E. (2000) The GH/IGF-1 axis in obesity: influence of neuroendocrine and metabolic factors. *International Journal of Obesity* **24**, S96–S99.

Maccario, M., Tassone, F., Gianotti, L., Lanfranco, F., Grottoli, S., Arvat, E., Muller, E.E. and Ghigo, E. (2001) Effects of recombinant human insulin-like growth factor 1 administration on the growth hormone (gh) response to GH-releasing hormone in obesity. *Journal of Clinical Endocrinology and Metabolism* **86**, 167–171.

Marin, P., Darin, N., Amemiya, T., Andersson, B., Jern, S. and Bjorntorp, P. (1992) Cortisol secretion in relation to body fat distribution in obese premenopausal women. *Metabolism* **41**, 882–886.

Masuzaki, H., Paterson, J., Shinyama, H., Mullins, J.J., Seckl, J.R. and Flier, J.S. (2001) A transgenic model of visceral obesity and the metabolic syndrome. *Science* **294**, 2166–2170.

Meldrum, D.R., Davidson, B.J., Tatryn, I.V. and Judd, H.L. (1981) Changes in circulating steroids with ageing in post-menopausal women. *Obstetrics and Gynecology* **57**, 404–408.

Merimee, T.J. and Fineberg, S.E. (1973) Dietary regulation of human growth hormone secretion. *Metabolism* **22**, 1491–1497.

Migeon, C.J., Green, O.C. and Eckert, J.P. (1963) Study of adrenocortical function in obesity. *Metabolism* **12**, 718–730.

Mohamed-Ali, V., Goodrick, S., Rawesh, A., Katz, D.R., Miles, J.M., Yudkin, J.S., Klein, S. and Coppack, S.W. (1997) Subcutaneous adipose tissue releases interleukin-6, but not tumor necrosis factor-α, *in vivo*. *Journal of Clinical Endocrinology and Metabolism* **82**, 4196–4200.

Mohamed-Ali, V., Pinkney, J.H. and Coppack, S.W. (1998) Adipose tissue as an endocrine and paracrine organ. *International Journal of Obesity* **22**, 1145–1158.

Montague, C.T., Prins, J.B., Sanders, L., Digby, J.E. and O'Rahilly, S. (1997) Depot and sex specific differences in human leptin mRNA expression: implications for the control of regional fat distribution. *Diabetes* **46**, 342–347.

Moon, B., Kwan, J.J., Duddy, N., Sweeney G. and Begum, N. (2003) Resistin inhibits glucose uptake in L6 skeletal muscle cells independent of changes in insulin signalling components and Glut 4 translocation. *American Journal of Physiology* (in press).

Nestler, J.E., Barlascini, C.O., Matt, D.W., Steingold, K.A., Plymate, S.R., Clore, J.N. and Blackard, W.G. (1989) Suppression of serum insulin by diazoxide reduces serum testosterone levels in obese women with PCOS. *Journal of Clinical Endocrinology and Metabolism* **68**, 1027–1032.

Nestler, J.E., Powers, L.P., Matt, D.W., Steingold, K.A., Plymate, S.R., Rittmaster, R.S., Clore, J.N. and Blackard, W.G. (1991) A direct effect of hyperinsulinemia on serum sex hormone binding globulin levels in obese women with polycystic ovary syndrome. *Journal of Clinical Endocrinology and Metabolism* **72**, 83–89.

Oberfield, S.E. (2001) Metabolic lessons from the study of young adolescents with polycystic overy syndrome—Is insulin, indeed, the culprit? *Journal of Clinical Endocrinology and Metabolism* **85**, 3520–3525.

Oral, E.A., Simha, V., Ruiz, E., Andewelt, A., Premkumar, A., Snell, P., Wagner, A.J., DePaoli, A.M., Reitman, M.L., Taylor, S.I., Gorden, P. and Garg, A. (2002) Leptin-replacement for lipodystrophy. *New England Journal of Medicine* **346**, 570–578.

Pasquali, R., Cantobelli, S., Casimirri, S. Capieeli, M., Bortoluzzi, L., Flamia, R., Labate, A. and Barbara, L. (1993) The hypothalamic-pituitary-adrenal axis in obese women with different patterns of body fat distribution. *Journal of Clinical Endocrinology and Metabolism* **77**, 341–346.

Pasquali, R., Biscotti, M., Spinucci, G., Vicennati, V., Genazzani. A.D., Sgarbi, L. and Casimirri, F. (1998) Pulsatile rhythm of ACTH and cortisol in premenopausal women: effect of obesity and body fat distribution. *Clinical Endocrinology* **48**, 603–612.

Pinkney, J.H., Goodrick, S.J., Katz, J.R., Johnson, A., Lightman, S.L., Coppack, S.C. and Mohamed-Ali, V. (1998) Leptin and the pituitary-thyroid axis: A comparative study in lean, obese, hypothyroid and hyperthyroid subjects. *Clinical Endocinology* **49**, 583–589.

Pinkney, J.H., Wilding, J.P.H., Williams, G. and MacFarlane, I. (2002) Hypothalamic obesity: What do we know and what can be done? *Obesity Reviews* **3**, 27–34.

Plymate, S.R., Matej, L.A., Jones, R.A. and Friedl, K.E. (1988) Inhibition of sex hormone binding globulin production in human hepatoma (HepG2) cell line by insulin and prolactin. *Journal of Clinical Endocrinology and Metabolism* **67**, 460–464.

Postel-Vinay, M.C., Saab, C. and Gourmelen, M. (1995) Nutritional status and growth hormone binding protein. *Hormone Research* **44**, 177–181.

Rasmussen, M.H., Hvidberg, A.J.A., Main, K.M., Gotfredsen, A.,

Skakkebaek, N.E. and Hilsted, J. (1995) Massive weight loss restores 24-hour growth hormone release profiles and serum insulin-like-growth factor-1 levels in obese subjects. *Journal of Clinical Endocrinology and Metabolism* **80**, 1407–1415.

Rasmussen, M.H., Ho, K.K., Kjems, L. and Hilsted, J. (1996) Serum growth hormone-binding protein in obesity: effect of short term, very low calorie diet and diet-induced weight loss. *Journal of Clinical Endocrinology and Metabolism* **81**, 1519–1524.

Rebuffe-Scrive, M., Krotkiewski, M., Elfverson, J. and Bjorntorp, P. (1988) Muscle and adipose tissue morphology and metabolism in Cushing's syndrome. *Journal of Clinical Endocrinology and Metabolism* **67**, 1122–1128.

Richelsen, B. (1997) Action of growth hormone in adipose tissue. *Hormone Research* **48**, 105–110.

Rosmond, R., Dallman, M.F. and Bjorntorp, P. (1998) Stress-related cortisol secretion in men: relationships with abdominal obesity and endocrine, metabolic and hemodynamic abnormalities. *Journal of Clinical Endocrinology and Metabolism* **83**, 1853–1859.

Scaglione, R., Averna, M.R., Dichiara, M.A.,Barbagallo, C.M., Mazzola, G., Montalto, G., Licata, G. and Notarbartolo. A. (1991) Thyroid function and release of thyroid-stimulating hormone and prolactin from the pituitary in human obesity. *Journal of International Medicine Research* **19**, 389–394.

Scherer, P.E., Williams, S., Fogliano, M., Baldini. G. and Lodish, H.F. (1995) A novel serum protein similar to C1q, produced exclusively in adipocytes. *Journal of Biological Chemistry* **270**, 26746–26749.

Schinder, A.E., Ebert, A. and Friedrich, E. (1972) Conversion of androstenedione to oestrone by human fat tissue. *Journal of Clinical Endocrinology and Metabolism* **35**, 627–630.

Schwartz, M.W., Woods, S.C., Porte, D., Seeley, R.J. and Baskin, D.G. (2000) Central nervous system control of food intake. *Nature* **404**, 661–671.

Shintani, M., Ogawa, Y., Ebihara, K., Aizawa-Abe, M., Miyanaga, F., Takaya, K., Hayashi, T., Inoue, G., Hosoda, K., Kojima, M., Kangawa, K. and Nakao, K. (2001) Ghrelin, an endogenous growth hormone secretagogue, is a novel orexigenic peptide that antagonizes leptin action through the activation of hypothalamic neuropeptide Y/Y1 receptor pathways. *Diabetes* **50**, 227–232.

Simkin, V. (1961) 17-ketosteroid and 17-ketogenic steroid excretion in obese patients. *New England Journal of Medicine* **264**, 974–977.

Sjögren, J., Min, L. and Bjorntorp, P. (1995) Androgen hormone binding to adipose tissue in rats. *Biochimica et Biophysica Acta* **1244**, 117–120.

Slavnov, V.N. and Epstein, E.V. (1977) Somatotrophic, thyrotrophic and adenotrophic functions of the anterior pituitary in obesity. *Endocrinologie* **15**, 213–218.

Smith, P.J., Wise, L.S., Berkowitz, R., Wan, C. and Rubin, C.S. (1988) Insulin-like growth factor-1 is an essential regulator of the differentiation of 3T3-L1 adipocytes. *Journal of Biological Chemistry* **263**, 9402–9408.

Steppan, C.M., Bailey, S.T., Bhat, S., Brown, E.J., Banerjee, R.R., Wright, C.M., Patel, H.R., Ahima, R.S. and Lazar, M.A. (2001) The hormone resistin links obesity to diabetes. *Nature* **409**, 307–312.

Stichel, H., l'Allemand, D. and Gruters, A. (2000) Thyroid function and obesity in children and adolescents. *Hormone Research* **54**, 14–19.

Strain, G.W., Zumoff, B., Strain, J.J., Levin, J. and Fukushima, D.K. (1980) Cortisol production in obesity. *Metabolism* **29**, 980–985.

Tanner, J.M. and Whitehouse, R.H. (1967) The effect of human growth hormone on subcutaneous fat thickness in hyposomatrophic and hypopituitary dwarfs. *Journal of Endocrinology* **39**, 263–275.

Toshinai, K., Date, Y., Murakami, N., Shimada, M., Mondal, M.S., Shimbara, T., Guan, J.L., Wang, Q.P., Funahashi, H., Sakurai, T., Shioda, S., Matsukura, S., Kangawa, K. and Nakazato, M. (2003) Ghrelin-induced food intake is mediated via the orexin pathway. *Endocrinology* **144**, 1506–1512.

Tschöp, M., Weyer, C., Tataranni, P.A., Devanarayan, V., Ravussin, E. and Heiman, M.L. (2001) Circulating ghrelin levels are decreased in human obesity. *Diabetes* **50**, 707–709.

Usiskin, K.S., Butterworth, S., Clore, J.N., Arad, Y., Ginsberg, H.N., Blackard, W.G. and Nestler, J.E. (1990) Lack of effect of dehydroepiandrosterone sulphate in obese men. *International Journal of Obesity* **14**, 457–463.

Vahl, N., Jorgensen, J.O.L., Skjaerbaek, C., Veldhuis, J.D., Orskov, H. and Christiansen, J.S. (1997) Abdominal adiposity rather than age and sex predicts mass and regularity of GH secretion in healthy adults. *American Journal of Physiology* **272**, E1108–E1116.

Velasquez, E.M., Mendoza, S. and Hamer, T. (1994) Metformin therapy in polycystic ovary syndrome reduces hyperinsulinemia, hyperandrogenemia and systolic blood pressure while facilitating menses and pregnancy. *Metabolism* **43**, 647–654.

Veldhuis, J.D., Iranmanesh, A., Ho, K.K., Waters, M.J., Johnson, M.L. and Lizarralde, G. (1991) Dual defects in pulsatile growth hormone secretion and clearance subserve the hyposomatotropism of obesity in man. *Journal of Clinical Endocrinology and Metabolism* **72**, 51–59.

Veldhuis, J., Liem, A., South, S., Weltman, A., Weltman, J., Clemmons, D.A., Abbott, R., Mulligan, T., Johnson, M.L. and Pincus, S. (1995) Differential impact of age, sex steroid hormones, and obesity on basal vs. pulsatile growth hormone secretion in men as assessed in an ultrasensitive chemiluminescence assay. *Journal of Clinical Endocrinology and Metabolism* **80**, 3209–3222.

Vermulen, A. and Ando, S. (1979) Metabolic clearance rate and interconversion of androgens and the influence of free androgen fractions. *Journal of Clinical Endocrinology and Metabolism* **48**, 320–326.

de Vile, C.J., Grant, D.B., Hayward, R.D., Kendall, B.E., Neville, B.G. and Stanhope, R. (1996) Obesity in childhood craniopharyngioma: relation to post-operative hypothalamic damage shown by magnetic resonance imaging. *Journal of Clinical Endocrinology and Metabolism* **81**, 2734–2737.

Wahrenberg, H., Lonnqvist, F. and Arner, P. (1989) Mechanisms underlying regional differences in lipolysis in human adipose tissue. *Journal of Clinical Investigation* **84**, 458–467.

Weaver, J.U., Kopelman, P.G., Holly, J.M.P., Noonan, K., Giadom, C.G., White, N., Virdee, S. and Wass, J.A. (1990) Decreased sex hormone binding globulin (SHBG) and insulin-like growth factor-1 (IGFBP-1) in extreme obesity. *Clinical Endocrinology* **32**, 641–646.

Weaver, J.U., Kopelman, P.G., McLoughlin, L., Forsling, M.L. and Grossman, A. (1993) Hyperactivity of the hypothalamo-pituitary-adrenal axis in obesity: a study of ACTH, AVP, β-lipotropin and cortisol responses to insulin-induced hypoglycaemia. *Clinical Endocrinology* **39**, 345–350.

Williams, D.P., Boyden, T.W., Pamenter, R.W., Lohman, T.G. and Going, S.B. (1993) Relationship of body fat percentage and fat distribution with dehydroepiandrosterone sulphate in premenopausal females. *Journal of Clinical Endocrinology and Metabolism* **77**, 80–85.

Yamashita, S. and Melmed, S. (1986) Effect of insulin on rat anterior pituitary cells. *Diabetes* **35**, 440–447.

Yamauchi, T., Kamon, J., Waki, H., Terauchi, Y., Kubota, N., Hara, K., Mori, Y., Ide, T., Murakami, K., Tsuboyama-Kasaoka, N., Ezaki, O., Akanuma, Y., Gavrilova, O., Vinson, C., Reitman, M.L., Kagechika, H., Shudo, K., Yoda, M., Nakano, Y., Tobe, K., Nagai, R., Kimura, S., Tomota, M., Froguel, P. and Kadowaki, T. (2001) The fat-derived hormone adiponectin reverses insulin resistance associated with both lipoatrophy and obesity. *Natural Medicine* **7**, 941–946.

Yamauchi, T., Kamon, J., Waki, H., Imai, Y., Shimozawa, N., Hioki, K., Uchida, S., Ito, Y., Takakuwa, K., Matsui, J., Takata, M., Eto, K., Terauchi, Y., Komeda, K., Tsunoda, M., Murakami, K., Ohnishi, Y., Naitoh, T., Yamamura, K., Ueyama, Y., Froguel, P., Kimura, S., Nagai, R. and Kadowaki, T. (2003) Globular adiponectin protected o/ob mice from diabetes and ApoE-deficient mice from atherosclerosis. *Journal of Biological Chemistry* **278**, 2461–2468.

Yang, W.S., Lee, W.J., Funahashi, T., Tanaka, S., Matsuzawa, Y., Chao, C.L., Chen, C.L., Tai, T.Y. and Chuang, L.M. (2001) Weight reduction increases plasma levels of an adipose-derived anti-inflammatory protein, adiponectin. *Journal of Clinical Endocrinology and Metabolism* **86**, 3815–3819.

Zhang, J. and Lazar, M.A. (2000) The mechanism of action of thyroid hormones. *Annual Review of Physiology* **62**, 439–466.

Zhang, Y., Proenca, R., Maffei, M., Barone, M., Leopold, L. and Friedman, J.M. (1994) Positional cloning of the mouse obese gene and its human homologue. *Nature* **372**, 425–432.

Zumoff, B., Strain, G.W., Miller, L.K., Rosner, W., Senie, R., Seres, D.S. and Rosenfeld, R.S. (1990) Plasma free and non-sex hormone binding globulin bound testosterone are decreased in obese men in proportion to their degree of obesity. *Journal of Clinical Endocrinology and Metabolism* **71**, 929–931.

Childhood obesity

15

Childhood obesity: definition, classification and assessment

Aviva Must and Sarah E. Anderson

Definition and classification, 215
  Measures of body fatness, 216
  Child and adolescent obesity:
  definition and classification, 217
  Choosing a cut-off point, 221
  Sensitivity and specificity, 222

Assessment, 223
  BMI-for-age assessment, 223
  Other anthropometric assessment
  measures, 224

Regional adiposity, 224
Medical assessment, 225
Lifestyle assessments, 226
Family readiness, 226
Clinician deportment and choice
of terms, 227
Future directions, 227

References, 227

Definition and classification

At its simplest level, obesity in children, as in adults, arises when there is an excess of body fat. Setting a definition of obesity for children that will have utility in a clinical setting presents a formidable task; it is far more complicated than in adults for several reasons. Ideally, a definition of obesity for children should accurately reflect body fatness, and have cut-off points that are predictive of adverse health. Each of these requirements is difficult to meet in the paediatric population.

Because children are growing, all body compartments are increasing in size, although at variable rates. Thus, any measure of excess weight is a moving target and needs to be tied to age. A further complexity arises because biological age and chronological age, although closely correlated, are not interchangeable—a problem that is particularly apparent around the time of puberty, when body composition changes are dramatic.

In adults, the universally recognized body mass index (BMI) cut-off points to define overweight and obesity are based on research evidence that links BMI levels to health risks, and are also convenient whole numbers. A BMI of 25–29 defines overweight and a BMI of 30 or above defines obesity (NHLBI Obesity Education Initiative Expert Panel, 1998). In adults, mortality risk increases with increasing BMI (Calle *et al.*, 1999), and a BMI above 25 is associated with elevated risk for cardiovascular disease (Seidell *et al.*, 1996) and diabetes (Colditz *et al.*, 1995). In children, although there are substantial immediate and remote health consequences to obesity, data are not adequate to set cut-off points based on health effects.

As will be discussed in detail in later sections, BMI-for-age has been adopted as the basic measure for clinical assessment of obesity in children and adolescents. BMI-for-age is well correlated with adiposity (Pietrobelli *et al.*, 1998) and has been linked to morbidity (Freedman *et al.*, 1999). BMI-for-age percentile charts for boys and girls are available for a number of reference populations (Rolland-Cachera *et al.*, 1991; Cole *et al.*, 1995; Kuczmarski *et al.*, 2000). Monitoring of childhood growth with percentile charts is a familiar activity for health practitioners who have used height and weight percentile charts for several decades. BMI-for-age growth charts are structured like the weight-for-age and stature-for-age charts. This should make adoption of monitoring this aspect of a child's growth relatively straightforward.

Standard practice tends to resist change, however. In 2001, an estimated 19% of US paediatricians reported using BMI to monitor obesity and 12.5% reported using BMI-for-age percentiles (Barlow *et al.*, 2002). The explosion of articles on childhood obesity and its alarming increase may lead to more rapid adoption of BMI-for-age monitoring. Like any screening tool, BMI-for-age represents a trade-off between precision and accuracy on the one hand, and ease of use on the other. The American Academy of Paediatrics recommends annual monitoring of BMI in youth (Committee on Nutrition, 2003). The use of BMI-for-age is justified by its comparison to criterion measures of fatness. These measures are discussed in the following section.

Table 15.1 Strengths and limitations of laboratory methods for assessing body fatness in children and adolescents.

Method	Strengths	Limitations	Type
Underwater weighing (hydrodensitometry)	Measures body density Highly reproducible Accurate	Requires high subject compliance Unsuitable for use in young children Relies on assumption of composition of fat-free mass, which is unsystematically influenced by age, sex and ethnicity	Whole body
Air-displacement plethysmography	Measures body density Quick Non-invasive Minimal subject compliance needed	High cost Accuracy in children has not been established Instrument designed for adults Relies on assumption of composition of fat-free mass, which is unsystematically influenced by age, sex and ethnicity	Whole body
Dual energy X-ray absorptiometry (DXA)	Highly reproducible Accurate Quick Minimal subject compliance needed	High cost Slight radiation exposure	Whole body and regional
Total body water – isotope dilution (^{2}H, ^{18}O)	Direct measure of body water Provides estimates of fat-free mass, fat mass and percentage body fat	High cost Difficult analysis (mass spectrometer needed) Relies on assumption of composition of fat-free mass, which is unsystematically influenced by age, sex and ethnicity	Whole body
^{40}K counting	Measure of body cell mass	Shielded room Scary for children	Whole body
Computerized tomography (CT)	Accurate Regional/visceral adiposity can be measured	Exposure to radiation High cost Requires high subject compliance	Regional
Magnetic resonance imaging (MRI)	Accurate Regional/visceral adiposity can be measured No exposure to radiation	High cost Requires high subject compliance	Regional

Measures of body fatness

In a laboratory setting, in contrast with a clinical or field setting, direct measures of body fatness are possible. Such methods conceptualize the human body as having two or more compartments: a fat compartment, and at least one compartment for fat-free mass. Although these body composition analysis methods are more precise than the anthropometric measures discussed in the following section, they are not without their own limitations (Table 15.1). Whole-body methods of fatness include underwater weighing (hydrodensitometry), isotopic dilution and dual energy X-ray absorptiometry (DXA). Regional and visceral adiposity can be assessed with computerized tomography (CT), magnetic resonance imaging (MRI) or DXA. Table 15.1 describes these methods and lists some of their advantages and disadvantages for measurement in children. Although these methods, when applied by trained technicians, provide more accurate measures

of body fatness than do non-laboratory methods, none is broadly applicable to clinical use owing to the interrelated issues of cost, technical requirements and time, as well as limitations due to their invasiveness, necessity of subject cooperation and, for some (such as the CT scan), the associated health risks (Goran, 1998; Ellis, 2000). Furthermore, because such methods are not widely used, population-based reference data are not available.

Non-laboratory methods are those applicable to field and clinical studies. These methods are validated against the laboratory methods summarized above. Bioelectric impedance analysis is a non-laboratory method that has gained widespread use because it is non-invasive (surface electrodes on hand and foot) and rapid. Impedance analysis is based on electrical resistance, which is directly related to total body water. Several equations to relate impedance measures to percentage body fat have been published for use in children and adolescents (Houtkooper *et al.*, 1989; Deurenberg *et al.*, 1989; 1990;

1991; Kushner *et al.*, 1992). Experience to date suggests that caution is warranted when applying equations that have been developed in one study population to other groups (Pietrobelli *et al.*, 1998; Phillips *et al.*, 2003).

Anthropometric measures, such as height, weight, circumferences and skinfolds, represent low-cost, minimally invasive measures of nutritional status in general, and of obesity in particular. For children, these measures are moving targets; all will increase with age, and will do so at variable rates.

Weight-for-height indices do not measure fatness directly but are correlated with direct measures of body fatness (Cole, 1991). Many indices, derived from combinations of height and weight, have been proposed for use in adults dating back to the nineteenth century (Cole, 1991). These include weight/height, weight/height^2 (Quetelet's index or BMI), weight/height^3 (Rohrer or Khosla–Lowe index), weight$^{1/3}$/height (ponderal index) and height/weight$^{1/3}$ (Sheldon's index) (Smalley *et al.*, 1990). Weight/height^P (Benn index) establishes the power to which height is raised, based on a population-specific analysis, which minimizes the residual correlation of the index with height. These various indices based on height and weight have been proposed to meet two non-interchangeable goals: to be maximally correlated with a criterion measure of body fatness or to be minimally correlated with height (Cole and Rolland-Cachera, 2003). In adults, there is a general consensus for use of the body mass index to assess relative weight. BMI meets both goals: it is correlated with adiposity and largely uncorrelated with height.

In children, changing relationships between height and weight with age complicate the situation. Whereas in adults adjusting weight by height raised to the power of 2 best reduces correlation with height, in children the 'best' power changes with age, such that for young children it is of the order of 2, and in puberty it is closer to 3 (Rolland-Cachera *et al.*, 1982). It would be possible to use Rohrer's index (weight/height^3) for early adolescents and BMI (weight/height^2) for children, or to have a continually changing exponent across childhood and adolescence. However, for consistency with adult definitions, and because BMI is more strongly correlated with adiposity in adolescence than is Rohrer's index, BMI is used for children and adolescents as it is for adults.

Child and adolescent obesity: definition and classification

In children, the choice of BMI-for-age to assess obesity offers continuity for the measure of obesity across the lifespan. Weight and height can be measured accurately with relative ease. BMI can be calculated as weight in kilograms divided by squared height in metres, or weight in pounds divided by squared height in inches, with the quotient multiplied by 703 (see formulas below). Because weight and height are highly correlated (about 0.7 in childhood), a measure of relative weight needs to account for the increases in weight that increased height brings, which are independent of fatness.

$$BMI = weight\ (kg) / height\ (m)^2$$
$$BMI = [weight\ (lb) / height\ (in)^2] \times 703$$

Another method for determining relative weight in children that adjusts weight for height is *weight-for-stature*, but it is not recommended for clinical assessment of obesity. BMI-for-age compares children of the same age but not necessarily of the same height. Weight-for-stature compares children of the same height but not necessarily of the same age. In the widely adopted United States 1977 National Centre for Health Statistics growth charts, weight-for-stature percentiles were available for boys up to 58 in tall and girls up to 54 in tall (Hamill *et al.*, 1979). With the 2000 growth chart revision and the introduction of the BMI-for-age growth charts for boys and girls ages 2–20 years (Ogden *et al.*, 2002), weight-for-stature charts were retained for children of 30–48 in in height, due to the widespread programmatic use of weight-for-stature in nutritional assessment of US pre-school children. In the US, approximately 5% of 5-year-old children are taller than 48 in (Flegal *et al.*, 2002).

It is important to recognize that the BMI-for-age and weight-for-stature charts are *not* equivalent for the centile of relative weight into which an individual child will fall. Differences between weight-for-stature centiles and BMI-for-age centiles have been compared in US children aged 2–5 years. Weight-for-stature percentiles tend to be lower than BMI-for-age percentiles, with larger differences between the two measures at 4 and 5 years of age; between 2 and 3 years of age the difference between percentile measures is highly dependent upon the child's height (Flegal *et al.*, 2002). BMI-for-age charts are recommended for classification of overweight in US children and adolescents.

BMI rises rapidly from birth to about the age of 2, and then declines gradually until about the age of 6—the adiposity rebound—when it then begins to increase again throughout childhood and adolescence (Fig. 15.1). In adults, there is general consensus that a BMI above 25 indicates overweight and a BMI above 30 indicates obesity. In children and adolescents, it is not possible to identify a single BMI cut-off point as a threshold for defining obesity because BMI is changing with age across development. Instead, centile charts, based on a large set of reference data, are constructed.

Plotting height and weight on growth charts is a familiar practice in paediatrics. To determine a child's centile for height, the intersection of the child's age and height is plotted on a growth chart and the corresponding centile is read off. Thus, using the United States Centres for Disease Control (CDC) 2000 growth charts (Kuczmarski *et al.*, 2000), a 10-year-old boy who is 1.43 m tall would be at approximately the 75th percentile of height for his age, and a boy of the same age who is 1.25 m tall would be below the 3rd percentile of height for his age. To construct centile charts, a representative sample of

(a)

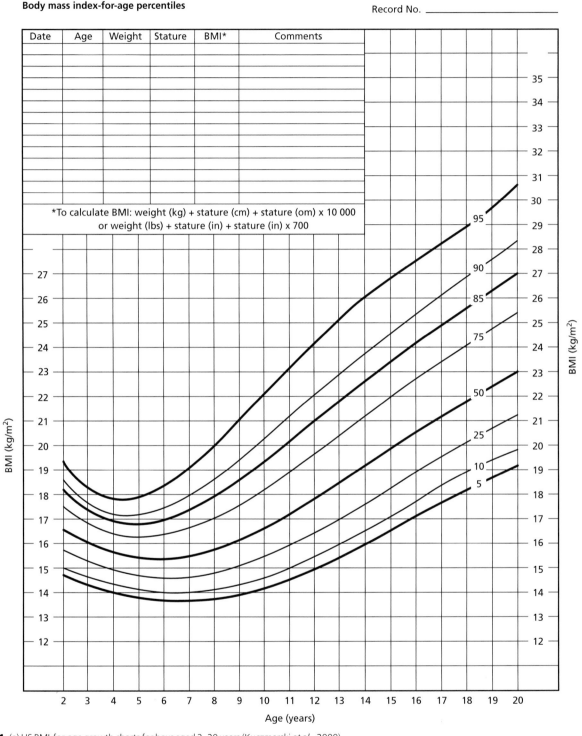

2 to 20 years: Boys
Body mass index-for-age percentiles

Name _____

Record No. _____

*To calculate BMI: weight (kg) + stature (cm) + stature (om) x 10 000
or weight (lbs) + stature (in) + stature (in) x 700

Age (years)

BMI (kg/m²)

Fig 15.1 (a) US BMI-for-age growth charts for boys aged 2–20 years (Kuczmarski *et al.*, 2000).

(b)

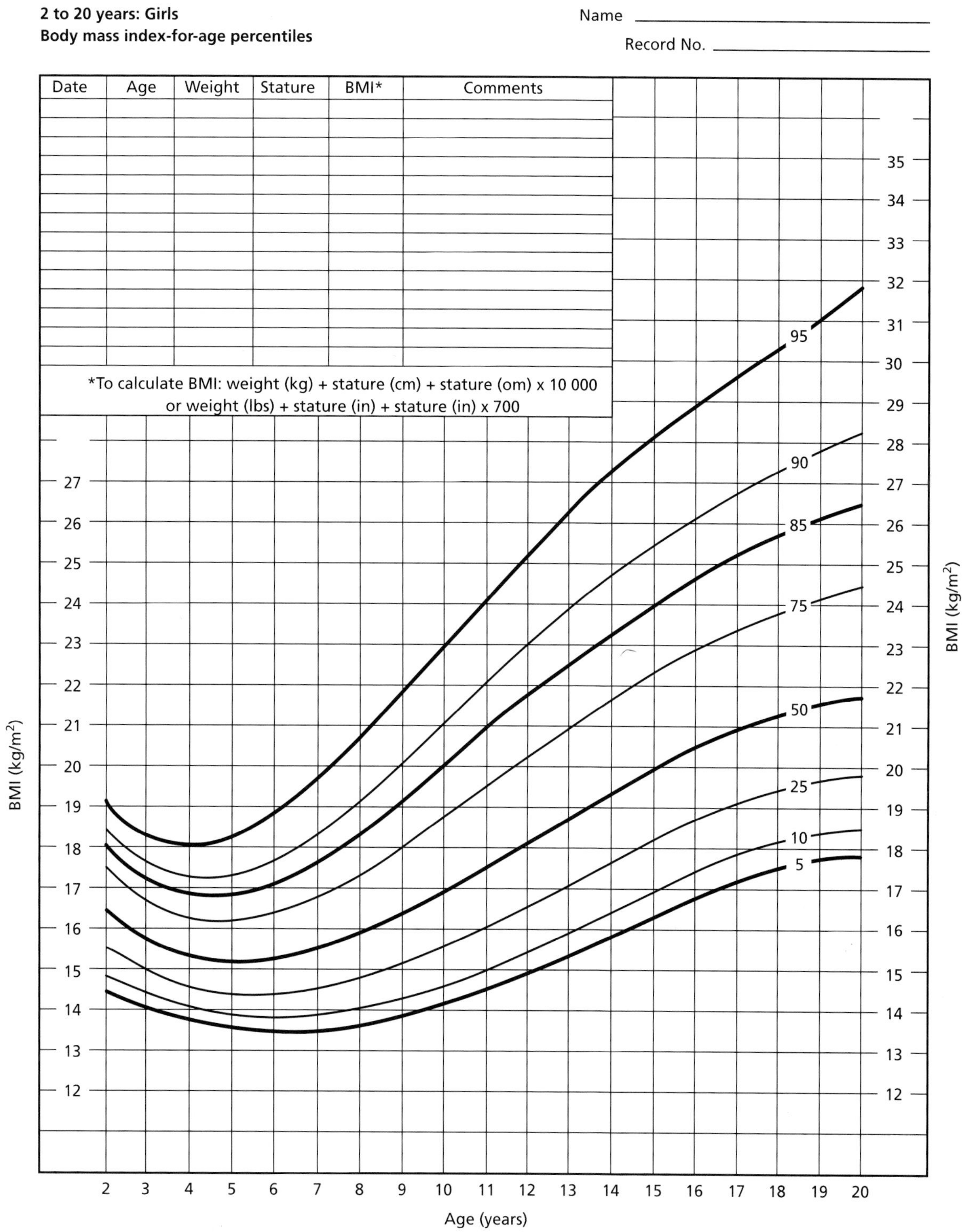
2 to 20 years: Girls
Body mass index-for-age percentiles
Name
Record No.
Date
Age
Weight
Stature
BMI*
Comments
*To calculate BMI: weight (kg) + stature (cm) + stature (om) x 10 000
or weight (lbs) + stature (in) + stature (in) x 700
95
90
85
75
50
25
10
5
BMI (kg/m²)
Age (years)
2 3 4 5 6 7 8 9 10 11 12 13 14 15 16 17 18 19 20
12 13 14 15 16 17 18 19 20 21 22 23 24 25 26 27 28 29 30 31 32 33 34 35

Fig 15.1 (b) US BMI-for-age growth charts for girls aged 2–20 years (Kuczmarski *et al.*, 2000).

children in the population for which charts are being developed is measured. Then, using the LMS method (Cole, 1990), smoothed curves can be constructed for any centile. The LMS method requires construction of curves describing the median (M), the coefficient of variation (S) and the degree of skewness or power (L) of the distribution. Given these three curves (Fig. 15.2 provides LMS curves for US BMI), an anthropometric measurement can be converted to a z-score (also called standard deviation score, SDS) with the following formula, where z is z-score, A is the anthropometric measure (e.g. BMI), M is the median, L is the power and S is the coefficient of variation read from the curves appropriate to the child's age and sex:

$$z = [(A/M)^L - 1]/L \times S$$

z-scores can then be converted to centiles by referring to a table of probabilities of the standard normal distribution: a z-score of 0 corresponds to the 50th percentile, −0.67 to the 25th percentile, −1.28 to the 10th percentile, 1.04 to the 85th percentile and 1.65 to the 95th percentile. In clinical practice, percentiles can be read directly off the growth charts.

Until the release of the CDC 2000 growth charts (Kuczmarski et al., 2000), reference curves for BMI were not available for clinical use in the USA; however, they have been available longer in the UK and France. US growth charts and corresponding LMS values and percentiles are available online (http://www.cdc.gov/growthcharts), as are the charts for the UK (http://www.health-for-all-children.co.uk).

Rather than calculating and plotting BMI, some clinicians determine whether a large difference exists between a child's weight and height centiles (Hulse and Schilg, 1996; Mulligan and Voss, 1999). Although there is intuitive appeal to directly comparing weight-for-age centiles with height-for-age centiles to assess obesity, this approach is not recommended. The notion is that for a child whose weight-for-age percentile exceeds the height-for-age percentile, excess weight or adiposity is likely. Although this approach of subtracting weight-for-age centile from height-for-age centile (W–H index) and then looking at the magnitude of the difference does not require the calculation of BMI, the W–H index has the undesirable properties of being only weakly correlated with weight and negatively correlated with height (Cole, 2002). Cole has constructed charts linking weight and height centiles to BMI centile for UK and US reference data (Fig. 15.3). These charts can be used to estimate BMI centile from weight centile and height centile, and should be used if BMI is not directly calculated. The point at which a child's height and weight centiles intersect on the chart can be plotted and then BMI centile read off, following the slanted lines up to the right. Using these charts, BMI centiles based on height and weight centiles can be calculated accurately enough for clinical purposes (Cole, 2002).

The dashed line in Fig. 15.3a is the line of identity, indicating where weight and height centiles are equal (W–H index of 0).

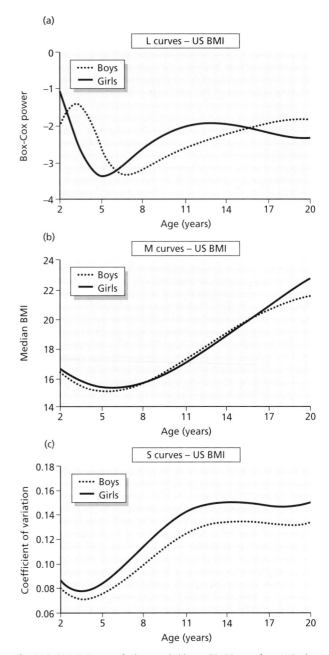

Fig 15.2 BMI LMS curves for boys and girls aged 2–20 years from United States 2000 CDC BMI growth reference (Kuczmarski et al., 2000). (a) Box-Cox power; (b) median BMI; (c) coefficient of variation.

The four points shown on the UK chart (Fig. 15.3a) indicate where a short lean, short heavy, tall heavy and tall lean child would fall on the chart. It is clear that the line of identity is closer to the tall heavy child than to the short heavy child, even though both have the same BMI centile. This means that using the W–H index, the tall heavy child would be less likely to be characterized as overweight than the short heavy child, even though they both have a BMI above the 99th percentile for age. Therefore, BMI centiles rather than the W–H index should be used to define obesity in children and adolescents.

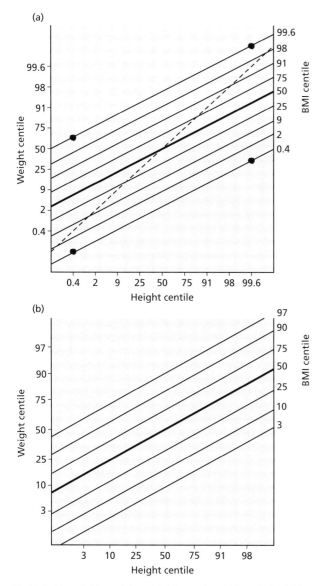

Fig 15.3 Charts linking weight and height centile to BMI centile for children and adolescents for UK (a) and USA (b) reference data (Cole, 2002). Dashed line in (a) indicates line of identity where weight centile equals height centile. Points described in the text. (Figures reprinted with permission.)

Choosing a cut-off point

BMI centiles or *z*-scores are useful to compare relative weights among children or to monitor a child's growth across time, but to use BMI centiles or *z*-scores to define obesity, a cut-off point must be determined. Although an ideal cut-off point to define obesity in children and adolescents would be related to risk for present or future morbidity, this is not possible at this time for three reasons:

1 Children and adolescents experience less obesity-related morbidity than do adults.

2 Long-term health risks of childhood obesity are mediated through adult obesity, and therefore separating the effect of obesity in childhood from the effect of obesity in adulthood on adult morbidity is difficult.

3 Health risk increases linearly with increasing adiposity, and there does not exist a clear threshold above which level adiposity has deleterious health effects.

Thus, it is not possible at present to provide a cut-off point for defining obesity in children and adolescents that is linked to risk; the choice of a cut-off point is essentially arbitrary.

Although BMI is a measure of relative weight and not adiposity, it is correlated with adiposity as measured by skinfold thickness, percentage body fat from DXA and bioelectrical impedance analysis (BIA), and total fat mass from DXA. Correlations between BMI-for-age and average triceps and subscapular skinfold thicknesses range from 0.68 in 2- to 5-year-old boys to 0.85 in 6- to 19-year-old girls (Mei *et al.*, 2002). The correlation of BMI-for-age with percentage body fat by DXA is about 0.81 in boys aged 6–19 years and about 0.86 in girls aged 6–19 years, with slightly lower correlations in children aged 3–5 years; similar results were found for total fat mass measured by DXA (Mei *et al.*, 2002). In a research setting, the 95th percentile BMI cut-off point of the US growth reference has been shown to increase the risk of obesity persistence into adulthood (Guo *et al.*, 2002), and is linked with elevated cardiovascular risk factor levels, such as blood pressure, cholesterol and blood glucose (Freedman *et al.*, 1999). It should be noted that although the adequacy of BMI to assess adiposity has been well evaluated in black and white youth, there has been limited research on the use of BMI in other racial-ethnic groups (Dietz and Robinson, 1998).

Using reference curves for BMI, a specific centile (e.g. the 95th percentile) is chosen as the threshold to indicate overweight or obesity. Obviously, which centile is chosen as the cut-off point affects the proportion of children and adolescents who are declared overweight. It is also important to keep in mind that a centile-based definition sets the prevalence of obesity for boys and girls at all ages to the proportion above the cut-off centile (e.g. 5% if 95th percentile). This statistical definition requires the same proportion of boys and girls at all ages to be declared as above the cut-off point at the time the reference is constructed. The 'true' prevalence of excess adiposity is unlikely to be independent of sex and age (Cole and Rolland-Cachera, 2003). Choice of the reference population will also affect obesity rates. BMI reference curves for childhood and adolescence are available for the US (Kuczmarski *et al.*, 2000), France (Rolland-Cachera *et al.*, 1991) and the UK (Cole *et al.*, 1995). An international BMI reference (Cole *et al.*, 2000) has also been developed and will be discussed in the next section. Although all these reference curves are of similar shape, the location of a particular centile for a given age and sex will correspond to different BMI values. A 10-year-old girl at the 95th percentile of BMI on the US charts would have a BMI of 23, a 10-year-old girl at the 95th percentile of BMI on the UK

Table 15.2 Comparison of BMI centiles that have been used as cut-off points to define obesity from the USA (Kuczmarski *et al.*, 2000), UK (Cole *et al.*, 1995), France (Rolland-Cachera *et al.*, 1991) and the International Obesity Task Force (Cole *et al.*, 2000) for boys and girls aged 9 and 15 years.

	Centile	Age 9		Age 15		Centile	Age 9		Age 15	
	Overweight	Boys	Girls	Boys	Girls	Obesity	Boys	Girls	Boys	Girls
US	85th	18.6	19.1	23.5	24.1	95th	21.1	21.8	26.8	28.1
UK	91st	19.0	19.8	23.1	24.1	98th	21.0	22.0	26.0	27.0
French	90th	18.0	17.4	22.4	22.5	97th	19.7	19.5	23.8	25.2
IOTF	BMI = 25 at age 18	19.1	19.1	23.3	23.9	BMI = 30 at age 18	22.8	22.8	28.3	29.1

charts would have a BMI of ~22, and on the French curve the corresponding BMI would be less than 19.

In order to facilitate global comparisons of trends in childhood and adolescent obesity rates (Prentice, 1998; Guillaume, 1999), the International Obesity Task Force (IOTF) developed BMI centile curves based on pooled data for children and adolescents aged 2–18 years from nationally representative surveys conducted in Brazil, Great Britain, Hong Kong, the Netherlands, Singapore and the USA (Cole *et al.*, 2000). The IOTF BMI curves were drawn using the LMS method individually for the six national samples, which were then averaged; centiles corresponding to a BMI of 25 and a BMI of 30 at age 18 were fit to the data. That is, these centiles were chosen as extrapolations into childhood of the well-accepted adult BMI cut-off points of 25 and 30 to define overweight and obesity respectively. Unlike other child references, the IOTF curves have continuity from childhood into adulthood. These international standards are useful for allowing obesity rates in different countries to be meaningfully compared, but there is controversy about whether they should be used clinically to classify children and adolescents as overweight or obese (Jebb and Prentice, 2001; Reilly, 2002; Rona and Chinn, 2002). There are strong arguments in favour of using national, rather than international, standards to define childhood and adolescent obesity clinically (Reilly, 2002; Reilly *et al.*, 2002). The international BMI reference curves have not been sufficiently evaluated to determine their validity for obesity classification in children and adolescents, whereas national BMI reference standards in the US and the UK have been well-evaluated (Freedman *et al.*, 1999; Reilly, 2002; Wright *et al.*, 2002).

Although few studies have directly compared national and international reference curves, it appears that the sensitivity of the international standard is lower than national standards, and that sensitivity and specificity differ by sex (Reilly *et al.*, 2000). Variability within the individual country curves that make up the international BMI reference requires caution when applying this international definition to clinical classification of obesity in children and adolescents, particularly during early adolescence when population differences in the timing of puberty may limit applicability (Reilly, 2002).

Various cut-off points have been used to define overweight and obesity depending upon the reference population used. Table 15.2 provides a comparison of BMI values for 9- and 15-year-old boys and girls using the US (Kuczmarski *et al.*, 2000), UK (Cole *et al.*, 1995), French (Rolland-Cachera *et al.*, 1991) and IOTF (Cole *et al.*, 2000) reference curves at cut-off points that have been used to classify children and adolescents as overweight or obese. The US 85th percentile, UK 91st percentile, and IOTF centile corresponding to a BMI of 25 at age 18 are broadly equivalent; the French 90th percentile runs at a lower level of BMI. At the higher obesity definition of the US 95th percentile, UK 98th percentile, French 97th percentile and IOTF centile corresponding to a BMI of 30 at age 18, the French cut-off point has the lowest BMI values and the IOTF has the highest—the US and UK references are intermediate.

It should be noted that centile curves for BMI provide a growth reference rather than a growth standard. Whereas a growth standard would delineate 'optimal' growth, a growth reference describes the population for which it is constructed without any implication that it would be 'best' for individuals to follow the pattern of growth depicted. It has been recommended that national BMI references be 'frozen' at their present-day levels (Wright *et al.*, 2002) to facilitate comparisons within a population across time.

Sensitivity and specificity

A screening test for obesity in children and adolescents should have high specificity (low false-positive rate) in order to minimize the number of children and adolescents who are incorrectly labelled as overweight or obese (Himes and Dietz, 1994). The potential negative psychological effects of labelling youth as overweight or obese argue for maximizing specificity instead of sensitivity. Although maximization of specificity over sensitivity means that this screen will miss a large number of truly overweight children, the assumption is that with annual rescreening, these children will be identified.

The sensitivity and specificity of 'BMI-based' definitions of overweight and obesity have been evaluated against 'gold standard' definitions of adiposity. Using a gold standard definition of obesity as greater than the age- and sex-specific 85th percentile of total body fat as measured by DXA, the false-positive rates of using the 85th and 95th percentiles of BMI from NHANES I were calculated as about 5% for the 85th percentile and less than 1% for the 95th percentile (Lazarus *et al.*, 1996).

Sensitivities and specificities of the 85th percentile from the CDC 2000 BMI reference have been calculated using the 85th percentile of NHANES III triceps and subscapular skinfold thickness measurements, and the 85th percentile of percentage body fat from DXA (Mei *et al.*, 2002). Using sum of skinfolds as the gold standard, sensitivities were 78.3%, 92.7% and 84.7% for BMI-for-age in 2- to 5-year-olds, 6- to 11-year-olds and 12- to 19-year-olds respectively; corresponding specificities were 88.3%, 91.5% and 90.5% (Mei *et al.*, 2002). Using percentage body fat from DXA as the gold standard, sensitivities were 88.5%, 98.6% and 100%, with specificities of 79.4%, 67.7% and 72.2% in children aged 2–5 years, 6–11 years and 12–19 years respectively (Mei *et al.*, 2002). This illustrates that the 85th percentile BMI is more specific and will decrease the proportion of individuals incorrectly classified as overweight as compared to DXA.

Use of the 95th percentile of the US BMI reference will minimize the number of children and adolescents who are classified as overweight when they do not have excess adiposity. Children and adolescents whose BMI falls at a lower percentile may have excess adiposity, and US screening guidelines at present recommend further evaluation if a youth's BMI is between the 85th and 95th percentile and secondary risk characteristics are present (Barlow and Dietz, 1998). The assessment section that follows describes how these cut-off points are integrated into a comprehensive obesity assessment.

Assessment

In addition to measurement of height and weight to calculate BMI, comprehensive assessment requires a more detailed medical evaluation, including a medical history. Further, before any treatment plan is considered, a family history and 'lifestyle' assessments should be undertaken. Finally, readiness for change, on the part of the child, and of the child's parents should be evaluated. This comprehensive assessment should be repeated annually.

BMI-for-age assessment

Accurate measurement of weight and height are needed for calculation of BMI. Both height and weight should be obtained with the child in light clothing and without shoes. Large hair arrangements can present a challenge for the measurement of height.

The CDC website (http://www.cdc.gov/growthcharts) contains tables in multiple formats and other supporting materials for calculating BMI percentiles in children using the US growth reference. The clinical charts are also available in Spanish and French. There are several on-line BMI-for-age percentile calculators as well. Clinicians are encouraged to calculate BMI at all well-child visits and plot the value on a sex-specific BMI-for-age chart (Fig. 15.1). As discussed above, despite its intuitive appeal, the discrepancy between weight-for-age and height-for-age percentile is not directly equivalent to BMI-for-age and should not be used to identify overweight. Cole (2002) has developed an equation and nomogram that approximates BMI-for-age based on the weight-for-age and height-for-age percentiles (Fig. 15.3).

Although there is general agreement about the use of BMI-for-age to identify excess weight in children, the terminology differs. In the US, the terms *at-risk-for-overweight* and *overweight* are used to designate the 85th and 95th percentile cut-off points. In the UK, the terminology is overweight and obesity, similar to the adult terminology, and the terms *overweight* and *obese* generally signify the 91st and 98th percentiles of the UK90 reference (Gibson *et al.*, 2002). Scottish guidelines proposed in 2003 (Scottish Intercollegiate Guidelines Network, 2003) have not been adopted throughout the United Kingdom (to date) (Table 15.3).

A set of recommendations for the evaluation and treatment of paediatric obesity were developed by an expert panel under the auspices of the United States Department of Health and Human Services (Barlow and Dietz, 1998) (Fig. 15.4). These practical recommendations start with assessment of age- and sex-specific BMI percentile. The 85th and 95th percentiles are recommended to designate *at-risk-for-overweight* (85th percentile) and *overweight* (95th percentile). These cut-offs are statistical definitions, based on an external reference population. In the US, the CDC 2000 growth reference, which was developed with pooled data from several nationally representative surveys conducted between 1964 and 1980, is used (Kuczmarski *et al.*, 2000). The 95th percentile BMI cut-off point was selected to screen for overweight. As can be seen in the top of Fig. 15.4, children and adolescents whose BMI exceeds the 95th percentile should undergo an in-depth medical assessment.

Children who screen between the 85th and 95th percentile BMI are considered 'at risk of overweight'. For these children,

Table 15.3 Initial screening clinical recommendations for assessment of obesity in children and adolescents (US).

1 Measure child's weight and height
2 Calculate BMI [BMI = weight (kg)/height (m)²]
3 Plot BMI-for-age on BMI growth chart appropriate for child's sex and determine BMI centile
4 Determine if child's BMI is above the 95th percentile (overweight), between the 85th and 95th percentiles (at risk for overweight) or below the 85th percentile (not at risk of overweight).

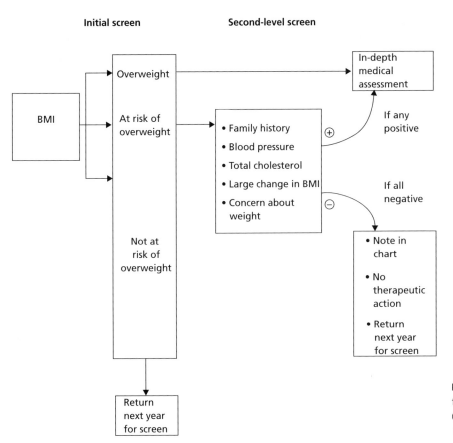

Initial screen   **Second-level screen**

Fig 15.4 Recommended overweight screening for children and adolescents—US guidelines. (Reprinted with permission from Himes and Dietz, 1994.)

a second level of screening is appropriate. Additional parameters should be considered: family history of obesity, elevated blood pressure levels, elevated total serum cholesterol, concern about weight or large incremental increases in BMI. When BMI-for-age is monitored, a large change in BMI (in excess of 3 or 4 BMI units over 1 year) suggests excess fat accretion. Concern about weight by the child or the child's parent is considered a positive second-level screening attribute. A child with a BMI between the 85th and 95th percentile who presents with any of these second-level screening attributes should be referred for in-depth medical assessment.

All children, regardless of their weight status, should be reevaluated every year (Committee on Nutrition, 2003). The BMI and BMI percentile should be recorded in the patient's chart. BMI can be monitored longitudinally by plotting BMI on the BMI-for-age charts. The National Obesity Forum (UK) (Gibson *et al.*, 2002) and Scottish Intercollegiate Guidelines Network (SIGN) (2003) have also promulgated assessment guidelines based on BMI-for-age. The SIGN guidelines for management of paediatric obesity are evidence based, and the quality of evidence for each recommendation is graded. At present, the evidence base for the recommendations is acknowledged to be poor, as it was derived from observational studies, non-analytic studies (e.g. case reports and case series) and expert opinion.

Other anthropometric assessment measures

Because BMI is a measure of weight adjusted for height rather than adiposity, under some circumstances it may be useful to assess fatness using skinfold thickness. Skinfolds measure the subcutaneous fat depot, which correlates with overall percentage body fat. For children or adolescents with large amounts of muscle mass, an elevated BMI will be misleading. When a child with BMI-for-age in excess of the 95th percentile is clearly not overfat, no further assessment will be needed. For the rare circumstance when a muscular child is suspected of excess adiposity, assessment of skinfold thickness may be helpful in confirming excess fatness. Taking skinfolds properly requires training to minimize measurement error. Nationally representative reference data for skinfolds at selected sites are available (Must *et al.*, 1991, National Center for Health Statistics, 1982). These measurements are not part of routine obesity assessment.

Regional adiposity

Regional adiposity, or fat distribution, may also be of importance in obesity assessment. As is seen consistently in studies of adults, a central pattern of fat distribution, or abdominal adiposity, is associated with adverse levels of classic cardiovascular risk factors, independent of total fatness or weight status. Elevations in LDL and total cholesterol, triglycerides and insulin as well as lower levels of HDL are associated with more centralized fat patterning (Freedman *et al.*, 1999). Central adiposity is also associated with higher diastolic and systolic blood pressure (Morrison *et al.*, 1999a). Some researchers have suggested that indirect measures of abdominal fatness, such as skinfold ratios, waist–hip ratio or waist circumference, could be as useful as BMI in early identification of children who would benefit from lifestyle interventions (McCarthy *et al.*, 2001). The criterion measures used to assess abdominal adiposity are MRI, CT scan and regional DXA (Table 15.1). Anthropometric measures that correlate with abdominal adiposity include waist circumference, waist–hip ratio and a number of skinfold ratios, including subscapular/triceps and (subscapular + suprailiac)/triceps. Of the various anthropometric measures of abdominal adiposity, waist circumference appears to be the best based on its strong correlation with regional DXA and its weak correlation with sex, race and overall fatness (Daniels *et al.*, 2000). Although some reference data for waist circumference in children are available from several countries (Zannolli and Morgese, 1996; Moreno *et al.*, 1999; McCarthy *et al.*, 2001; Pietrobelli *et al.*, 2002), waist circumference assessment is not recommended at present as part of routine screening.

Medical assessment

Obesity in the vast majority of children will be of the simple or primary sort, not associated with another disease state. Although the line of demarcation is not always clear, obesity that presents with psychological problems or accompanies Down's syndrome or non-specific mental retardation is considered simple. Obesity due to other pathology is far less common, but these exogenous causes must be ruled out as an early step in assessment. As part of differential diagnosis, the conditions to be ruled out fall into two main categories: genetic syndromes and endocrinological abnormalities.

Of the genetic syndromes, Prader–Willi (or Prader–Labhart–Willi) is the most common specific syndrome, with prevalence estimated at one per 10 000 to one per 15 000 (Burd *et al.*, 1990). Two chromosomal abnormalities seem to account for the syndrome, which presents with a range of symptoms in addition to obesity, including neonatal hypotonia, orthopaedic abnormalities, excessive appetite and hyperphagia, temper tantrums and self-abusive behaviours (Cassidy, 1997). Other genetic syndromes occur with far lower frequency and include Bardet–Biedl, Cohen (or Pepper), Alstrom, Biemond, Laurence–Moon, Börjeson–Forssman–Lehmann and Carpenter. These syndromes all present with other symptoms, such as abnormalities of facial appearance, polydactyly, hypogenitalism or neurological deficits (Chiumello and Poskitt, 2003).

Endocrine disorders that present with obesity in childhood include Cushing's syndrome, hypothyroidism or growth hormone deficiency. These rare conditions may be suspected when weight gain is normal but linear growth is poor. These characteristics contrast with simple obesity; before puberty, obese children tend to be taller than their peers. Also exceedingly rare are abnormalities associated with the hormone leptin. Leptin deficiency will be evident as low serum leptin accompanied by severe early-onset obesity and hyperinsulinaemia. Leptin receptor abnormalities are often accompanied by central hypothyroidism and hypercortisolism, as well as delayed sexual maturation (Yanovski, 2001). Finally, certain hypothalamic tumours may be associated with obesity. It is important to stress that these conditions are exceedingly rare. In the absence of other clinical signs, a search for genetic, neurological or endocrine abnormalities is not part of standard diagnostic assessment.

A medical assessment, including a medical history, is an important aspect of comprehensive obesity assessment for several reasons. First, it is necessary to identify patients with rare medical conditions that predispose the child to obesity. Second, where obesity is present, health may already be adversely affected. The presence of either exogenous causes or of significant obesity-related comorbidities will influence to whom the child is referred and how aggressively the condition is treated.

Adverse health effects of obesity, affecting many organ systems of the body, may already be present at the time of assessment. Chapter 16 details the health consequences of obesity in childhood, and therefore these are considered only very briefly here. Immediate health consequences, which may be present at the time of obesity assessment, include certain lower extremity orthopaedic conditions, sleep disordered breathing and sleep apnoea, and non-alcoholic steatohepatitis (Must and Strauss, 1999). Also seen are adverse levels of classic cardiovascular risk factors, including systolic and diastolic blood pressure, total cholesterol and subfractions, triglycerides and blood glucose (Smoak *et al.*, 1987; Morrison *et al.*, 1999a,b). Impaired glucose tolerance and frank type 2 diabetes are increasingly seen in obese children, and may be present at diagnosis, especially where there is a family history of type 2 diabetes with onset before age 40 (Mitchell *et al.*, 1994). Certain psychological disorders may be associated with obesity and should be routinely assessed as part of the medical history. Bulimic eating disorders, including binge eating, may be associated with adolescent obesity, particularly in girls (Friedman *et al.*, 1995). When discontent about weight is internalized, poor self-esteem may result. Depression scores can also be elevated in overweight children (Erickson *et al.*, 2000).

In addition to the full medical history that is part of standard clinical assessment, additional items of relevance for obesity evaluation should be included. Height and weight or obesity status of the biological and non-biological mother and father should be obtained, if possible. Parental obesity has been linked to childhood overweight, as it reflects both heritability of the condition and the influence of shared environment.

Parental obesity is strongly associated with child overweight in younger children; its influence appears to dissipate as the child ages (Whitaker *et al.*, 1997). Information on the age at obesity onset in the child should be obtained, by review of the growth chart if available, or by parent report. In addition to parental obesity, family history of other chronic conditions, such as type 2 diabetes, hyperlipidaemia, heart disease, stroke, hypertension and thyroid disease should be obtained. When these conditions are present, the risk for the overweight child is further elevated. Overweight onset before the age of 8 has been linked to its likelihood of persistence into adulthood (Freedman *et al.*, 2001). When BMI has been monitored and plotted, examination of the growth chart provides an objective tool for looking at relative weight status over time. In addition, the medical history may provide important information regarding family history of obesity-related comorbidities, such as type 2 diabetes, as well as disordered eating and depression.

Lifestyle assessments

Weight management, whether weight maintenance or weight loss is indicated, relies on sustained changes in diet and activity. For this reason, assessment of present-day diet, eating behaviours, physical activity and sedentary behaviours is a key aspect of evaluation for treatment. Efforts at standard assessment guides for diet and activity for use in paediatric practice are under way (International Life Sciences Institute Center for Health Promotion, 2002).

At the time of writing, we do not know which aspects of diet are the most useful for assessment, so a global assessment of diet and eating patterns is recommended. For younger children, the information should be obtained from the parent or primary caregiver. Assessment of frequency with which fruits, vegetables, sweets, salty snacks, fried foods, low-fat milk, whole milk and soda are consumed will provide an overall picture of food choices, and the likelihood of excess caloric intake. Beverage choice may be an important source of excess calories (Mrdjenovic and Levitsky, 2003). The frequency of breakfast consumption, meals eaten away from home and meals eaten 'as a family' should be assessed (Siega-Riz *et al.*, 1998; Neumark-Sztainer *et al.*, 2003). Food eaten or prepared outside of the home is more likely to be higher in calories, due to menu offerings, lack of parental control and large portion sizes (French *et al.*, 2001; Young and Nestle, 2003). The information obtained from this assessment may offer useful entry points for discussion and more constructive counselling.

Activity assessment should include both physical activity and sedentary behaviour. Information on structured activity, such as physical education at school, team sports, lessons or hobbies, should be complemented by information about unstructured time. This includes activities of daily living, such as household chores, walking to school or yard work. Time spent in sedentary behaviour, particularly television viewing, should be assessed, given its direct association with overweight (Gortmaker *et al.*, 1990). The child and parent should be asked about the frequency with which meals are eaten in front of the television (Coon *et al.*, 2001). Similarly, time spent playing computer or video games should be assessed. The presence of a television and/or computer in the child's bedroom is also of interest given its relation to time spent viewing (Dennison *et al.*, 2002). Knowledge of household structure, neighbourhood safety and who, if anyone, is at home after school will help the clinician provide realistic observations and should make any counselling on these issues more relevant to the child and the family.

Family readiness

Assessment of family readiness for change could be seen as the final step of obesity assessment or as the first step of obesity therapy. Behaviour change theory suggests that change will not occur until the individual is ready. Attempts at weight management counselling or referral to a weight management programme may alienate families who are not ready, and/or may contribute to the child's negative self-concept. As such, these attempts may compromise weight management efforts in the future. Assessment of readiness to make change should be included as part of comprehensive obesity assessment (Barlow and Dietz, 1998; Dietz, 1999). In the context of childhood obesity, motivation to address a child's weight problem requires that both the child and the child's family are ready to address the issue with concrete changes.

Motivational interviewing, borrowed from the treatment of addictive behaviours, grew out of the conviction that advice-giving is undermined by the nature of the clinician–patient encounter. By encouraging the patient to actively engage in problem analysis and goal-setting, behaviour change is more likely to occur (Emmons and Rollnick, 2001). In the area of obesity, motivational interviewing has the potential to increase readiness for change among individuals and their families. Training programmes that teach motivational interviewing skills are available throughout the US and Europe.

As with any clinical encounter, the clinician's skill at engaging the patient and the patient's parents is central to getting valid information and setting an environment that will promote effective counselling. Provider questions should be open ended and non-judgmental. The parents should be asked if they deem the child's weight to be a problem. If they do, they should be asked what changes in the family would be needed to help the child address his or her weight problem. If the parents do not see the child's weight as a problem, the clinician should enquire as to what might occur to make them see it as something to be addressed. Depending on the child's age, a similar exchange should be initiated directly with the child.

Clinician deportment and choice of terms

Obesity in childhood was dubbed 'the dismal condition' by Dwyer and Mayer 30 years ago (1973). Despite the rising prevalence of childhood overweight, discrimination is widespread: the overweight child is often socially isolated (Strauss and Pollack, 2003), the target of teasing and bullying by peers (Neumark-Sztainer *et al.*, 1998) and is assumed to be 'lazy and dishonest' by children (Staffieri, 1967; Latner and Stunkard, 2003) and even by adults (Neumark-Sztainer *et al.*, 1999). Health-care professionals are not immune to 'anti-fat' bias (Harvey and Hill, 2001; Teachman and Brownell, 2001). It seems likely that the overweight child and perhaps the child's parents have internalized this negative societal reaction.

The clinician who discusses weight with paediatric patients and their family members should appreciate the importance of an accepting, non-judgmental tone. Recognizing that the weight problem may be a highly sensitive and emotionally charged issue, the clinician should handle the assessment carefully. In particular, because obesity runs in families, many parents will be obese themselves and will have experienced their own frustrations and negative societal reaction. For adolescents who are trying to separate from their parents, navigating the role of family involvement in weight management is challenging (Frelut and Flodmark, 2003). The advice for health-care professionals recommended by the National Task Force on the Prevention and Treatment of Obesity for adults (2002) is broadly applicable to those who treat children. Some adaptations of the physical office space such as large-size examination gowns, and large blood pressure cuffs, are relevant to those who treat children and adolescents (National Task Force on the Prevention and Treatment of Obesity, 2002). Weight should be assessed in a private setting and recorded without comment. Every opportunity for enhancing self-esteem and self-acceptance during the medical encounter should be exploited.

The words to describe or talk about the child's weight should also be chosen carefully. Most of the terms used to describe excess weight appear to be offensive to obese adults, as shown by Wadden and Didie (2003); to date no similar study has been conducted with children or adolescents. Particularly undesirable for the obese individuals surveyed were the terms *fatness*, *excess fat*, *obesity* and *large size*. The term *weight* was most preferred. If weight and lifestyle assessment is to be a positive, or at least a neutral, experience, clinicians are encouraged to avoid potentially offensive terminology.

Future directions

Increasing rates of child and adolescent obesity in many countries make the need for screening and assessment protocols all the more urgent. At present there is reasonably good consensus about the use of BMI-for-age and percentile cut-off points for defining obesity in children. The availability of nationally representative data for the US and several European countries represents an encouraging beginning. Application of reference curves developed in one population to assessment of a different population can present difficulties due to variability in growth by race and differences in maturational timing. The global nature of the present epidemic makes for a pressing need for nationally relevant reference curves.

It is unlikely that all countries will have the resources to create their own growth curves. With continued usage by the obesity research community, we may better understand the strengths and limitations of the International Obesity Task Force growth standards and the implications of their utilization for clinical assessment. Incorporating what has been learned from the initial international standards, a second international reference could be undertaken with more countries and with better representation from around the world.

Reference data for waist circumference may prove useful as a second-level screen for central adiposity, and to identify children at particular risk for obesity-related comorbidities. As the reference data available at present for waist circumference (Zannolli and Morgese, 1996; Moreno *et al.*, 1999; McCarthy *et al.*, 2001; Pietrobelli *et al.*, 2002) are used by researchers and clinicians, the utility of this information should become apparent.

As suggested by James (2003), the possibility of an improved height–weight index that exploits the ease of computation that computers provide is real. With improvements in technology, it may also be possible to develop a clinically useful, direct measure of body fat. It seems certain that a measure that directly reflects adipose tissue, rather than weight, will be more strongly linked to disease outcomes.

Finally, whatever measures and definitions of obesity are developed in the future, the present explosion of childhood obesity is likely to provide the evidence base needed to tie cut-off points to physical and psychosocial health risk. Ironically, a 'benefit' of high rates of childhood obesity worldwide may be to improve screening and diagnosis of the condition.

References

Barlow, S.E. and Dietz, W.H. (1998) Obesity evaluation and treatment: expert committee recommendations. *Pediatrics* **102**, 1–11.

Barlow, S.E., Dietz, W.H., Klish, W.J. and Trowbridge, F.L. (2002) Medical evaluation of overweight children and adolescents: reports from pediatricians, pediatric nurse practitioners, and registered dietitians. *Pediatrics* **110**, 222–228.

Burd, L., Vesely, B., Martsolf, J. and Kerbeshian, J. (1990) Prevalence study of Prader-Willi syndrome in North Dakota. *American Journal of Medical Genetics* **37**, 97–99.

Calle, E.E., Thun, M.J., Petrelli, J.M., Rodriguez, C. and Heath, C.W. (1999) Body-mass index and mortality in a prospective cohort of US adults. *New England Journal of Medicine* **341**, 1097–1105.

Cassidy, S.B. (1997) Prader-Willi syndrome. *Journal of Medical Genetics* **34**, 917–923.

Chiumello, G. and Poskitt, E.M.E. (2003) Prader-Willi and other syndromes. In: Burniat, W., Cole, T.J., Lissau, I., Poskitt, E.M.E., eds. *Child and Adolescent Obesity*. Cambridge: Cambridge University Press, 171–188.

Colditz, G.A., Willett, W.C., Rotnitzky, A. and Manson, J.E. (1995) Weight gain as a risk factor for clinical diabetes mellitus in women. *Annals of Internal Medicine* **122**, 481–486.

Cole, T.J. (1990) The LMS method for constructing normalized growth standards. *European Journal of Clinical Nutrition* **44**, 45–60.

Cole, T.J. (1991) Weight-stature indices to measure underweight, overweight, and obesity. In: Himes, J.H. ed. *Anthropometric Assessment of Nutritional Status*. New York: Wiley-Liss, 83–111.

Cole, T.J. (2002) A chart to link child centiles of body mass index, weight and height. *European Journal of Clinical Nutrition* **56**, 1194–1199.

Cole, T.J. and Rolland-Cachera, M.F. (2003) Measurement and definition. In: Burniat, W., Cole, T.J., Lissau, I., Poskitt, E.M.E., eds. *Child and Adolescent Obesity*. Cambridge: Cambridge University Press, 3–27.

Cole, T.J., Freeman, J.V. and Preece, M.A. (1995) Body mass index reference curves for the UK, 1990. *Archives of Disease in Childhood* **73**, 25–29.

Cole, T.J., Bellizzi, M.C., Flegal, K.M. and Dietz, W.H. (2000) Establishing a standard definition for child overweight and obesity worldwide: international survey. *British Medical Journal* **320**, 1240–1243.

Committee on Nutrition (2003) Prevention of pediatric overweight and obesity: policy statement. *Pediatrics* **112**, 424–430.

Coon, K.A., Goldberg, J., Rogers, B.L. and Tucker, K.L. (2001) Relationships between use of television during meals and children's food consumption patterns. *Pediatrics* **107**, e7.

Daniels, S.R., Khoury, P.R. and Morrison, J.A. (2000) Utility of different measures of body fat distribution in children and adolescents. *American Journal of Epidemiology* **152**, 1179–1184.

Dennison, B.A., Erb, T.A. and Jenkins, P.L. (2002) Television viewing and television in bedroom associated with overweight risk among low-income preschool children. *Pediatrics* **109**, 1028–1035.

Deurenberg, P., Smit, H.E. and Kusters, C. (1989) Is the bioelectrical impedance method suitable for epidemiological field studies? *European Journal of Clinical Nutrition* **43**, 647–654.

Deurenberg, P., Kusters, C. and Smit, H.E. (1990) Assessment of body composition by bioelectrical impedance in children and young adults is strongly age-dependent. *European Journal of Clinical Nutrition* **44**, 261–268.

Deurenberg, P., van der Kooy, K., Leenen, R., Westrrate, J.A. and Seidell, J.C. (1991) Sex and age specific prediction formulas for estimating body composition from bioelectrical impedance: a cross-validation study. *International Journal of Obesity* **15**, 17–25.

Dietz, W. (1999) How to tackle the problem early? The role of education in the prevention of obesity. *International Journal of Obesity* **23**, S7–9.

Dietz, W.H. and Robinson, T.N. (1998) Use of the body mass index (BMI) as a measure of overweight in children and adolescents. *Journal of Pediatrics* **132**, 191–193.

Dwyer, J. and Mayer, J. (1973) The dismal condition: problems faced by obese adolescent girls in American society. In: Bray, G.A. ed. *Obesity in Perspective*. Washington, DC: DHEW Publication.

Ellis, K.J. (2000) Human body composition: *in vivo* methods. *Physiological Reviews* **80**, 649–680.

Emmons, K.M. and Rollnick, S. (2001) Motivational interviewing in health care settings: opportunities and limitations. *American Journal of Preventive Medicine* **20**, 68–74.

Erickson, S.J., Robinson, T.N., Haydel, K.F. and Killen, J.D. (2000) Are overweight children unhappy? Body mass index, depressive symptoms, and overweight concerns in elementary school children. *Archives of Pediatrics and Adolescent Medicine* **154**, 931–935.

Flegal, K.M., Wei, R. and Ogden, C.L. (2002) Weight-for-stature compared with body mass index-for-age growth charts for the United States from the Centers for Disease Control and Prevention. *American Journal of Clinical Nutrition* **75**, 761–766.

Freedman, D.S., Dietz, W.H., Srinivasan, S.R. and Berenson, G.S. (1999) The relation of overweight to cardiovascular risk factors among children and adolescents: the Bogalusa Heart Study. *Pediatrics* **103**, 1175–1182.

Freedman, D.S., Khan, L.K., Dietz, W.H., Srinivasan, S.R. and Berenson, G. S. (2001) Relationship of childhood obesity to coronary heart disease risk factors in adulthood: the Bogalusa Heart Study. *Pediatrics* **108**, 712–718.

Frelut, M.-L. and Flodmark, C.-E. (2003) The obese adolescent. In: Burniat, W., Cole, T.J., Lissau, I., Poskitt, E.M.E., eds. *Child and Adolescent Obesity*. Cambridge: Cambridge University Press, 154–170.

French, S.A., Story, M. and Jeffery, R.W. (2001) Environmental influences on eating and physical activity. *Annual Review of Public Health* **22**, 309–335.

Friedman, M.A., Wilfley, D.E., Pike, K.M., Striegel-Moore, R.H. and Rodin, J. (1995) The relationship between weight and psychological functioning among adolescent girls. *Obesity Research* **3**, 57–62.

Gibson, P., Edmunds, L., Haslam, D.W. and Poskitt, E. (2002) An approach to weight management in children and adolescents (2–18 years) in primary care. *Journal of Family Health Care* **12**, 108–109.

Goran, M.I. (1998) Measurement issues related to studies of childhood obesity: assessment of body composition, body fat distribution, physical activity, and food intake. *Pediatrics* **101**, 505–518.

Gortmaker, S., Must, A., Cheung, L., Peterson, K., Colditz, G. and Dietz, W. (1990) *Increasing Childhood Obesity and TV Viewing in the United States, 1990*. Boston: Harvard School of Public Health.

Guillaume, M. (1999) Defining obesity in childhood: current practice. *American Journal of Clinical Nutrition* **70**, 126S–130S.

Guo, S., Wu, W., Chumlea, W.C. and Roche, A.F. (2002) Predicting overweight and obesity in adulthood from body mass index values in childhood and adolescence. *American Journal of Clinical Nutrition* **76**, 653–658.

Hamill, P.V., Drizd, T.A., Johnson, C.L., Reed, R.B., Roche, A.F. and Moore, W.M. (1979) Physical growth: National Center for Health Statistics percentiles. *American Journal of Clinical Nutrition* **32**, 607–629.

Harvey, E.L. and Hill, A.J. (2001) Health professionals' views of overweight people and smokers. *International Journal of Obesity* **25**, 1253–1261.

Himes, J.H. and Dietz, W.H. (1994) Guidelines for overweight in adolescent preventive services: recommendations from an expert committee. *American Journal of Clinical Nutrition* **59**, 307–316.

Houtkooper, L.B., Lohman, T.G., Going, S.B. and Hall, M.C. (1989) Validity of bioelectric impedance for body composition assessment in children. *Journal of Applied Physiology* **66**, 814–821.

Hulse, J.A. and Schilg, S. (1996) Relation between height and weight centiles may be more useful. *British Medical Journal* **312**, 122.

International Life Sciences Institute Center for Health Promotion (2002) *Assessment and Counseling Guide.*

James, W.P.T. (2003) The future. In: Burniat, W., Cole, T.J., Lissau, I., Poskitt, E.M.E., eds. *Child and Adolescent Obesity.* Cambridge: Cambridge University Press, 389–402.

Jebb, S.A. and Prentice, A.M. (2001) Single definition of overweight and obesity should be used. *British Medical Journal* **323**, 999.

Kuczmarski, R.J., Ogden, C.L., Grummer-Strawn, L.M., Flegal, K.M., Guo, S.S., Wei, R., Mei, Z., Curtin, L.R., Roche, A.F. and Johnson, C.L. (2000) CDC Growth Charts: United States. In: *Advance Data from Vital and Health Statistics*, Vol. 314. Hyattsville, MD; National Center for Health Statistics.

Kushner, R., Schoeller, D., Fjeld, C. and Danford, L. (1992) Is the impedance index (ht2/R) significant in predicting total body water? *American Journal of Clinical Nutrition* **56**, 835–839.

Latner, J. and Stunkard, A. (2003) Getting worse: the stigmatization of obese children. *Obesity Research* **11**, 452–456.

Lazarus, R., Baur, L., Webb, K. and Blyth, F. (1996) Body mass index in screening for adiposity in children and adolescents: systematic evaluation using receiver operating characteristic curves. *American Journal of Clinical Nutrition* **63**, 500–506.

McCarthy, H.D., Jarrett, K.V. and Crawley, H.F. (2001) The development of waist circumference percentiles in British children aged 5.0–16.9 years. *European Journal of Clinical Nutrition* **55**, 902–907.

Mei, Z., Grummer-Strawn, L.M., Pietrobelli, A., Goulding, A., Goran, M.I. and Dietz, W.H. (2002) Validity of body mass index compared with other body-composition screening indexes for the assessment of body fatness in children and adolescents. *American Journal of Clinical Nutrition* **75**, 978–985.

Mitchell, B.D., Kammerer, C.M., Reinhart, L.J. and Stern, M.P. (1994) NIDDM in Mexican-American families. Heterogeneity by age of onset. *Diabetes Care* **17**, 567–573.

Moreno, L.A., Fleta, J., Mur, L., Rodriquez, G., Sarria, A. and Bueno, M. (1999) Waist circumference values in Spanish children—gender related differences. *European Journal of Clinical Nutrition* **53**, 429–433.

Morrison, J.A., Barton, B.A., Biro, F.M., Daniels, S.R. and Sprecher, D.L. (1999a) Overweight, fat patterning, and cardiovascular disease risk factors in black and white boys. *Journal of Pediatrics* **135**, 451–457.

Morrison, J.A., Sprecher, D.L., Barton, B.A., Waclawiw, M.A. and Daniels, S.R. (1999b) Overweight, fat patterning, and cardiovascular disease risk factors in black and white girls: The National Heart, Lung, and Blood Institute Growth and Health Study. *Journal of Pediatrics* **135**, 458–464.

Mrdjenovic, G. and Levitsky, D. (2003) Nutritional and energetic consequences of sweetened drink consumption in 6- to 13-year-old children. *Journal of Pediatrics* **142**, 604–610.

Mulligan, J. and Voss, L.D. (1999) Identifying very fat and very thin children: test of criterion standards for screening test. *British Medical Journal* **319**, 1103–1104.

Must, A. and Strauss, R.S. (1999) Risks and consequences of childhood and adolescent obesity. *International Journal of Obesity* **23**, S2-S11.

Must, A., Dallal, G.E. and Dietz, W. (1991) Reference data for obesity: 85th and 95th percentiles of body mass index (wt/ht²) and triceps skinfold thickness. *American Journal of Clinical Nutrition* **53**, 839–846.

National Center for Health Statistics (1982) Plan and operation of the Second Health and Nutrition Examination Survey, United States, 1976–1980. *Vital and Health Statistics 1.*

National Task Force on the Prevention and Treatment of Obesity (2002) Medical care for obese patients: advice for health care professionals. *American Family Physician* **65**, 81–88.

Neumark-Sztainer, D., Story, M. and Faibisch, L. (1998) Perceived stigmatization among overweight African-American and Caucasian adolescent girls. *Journal of Adolescent Health* **23**, 264–270.

Neumark-Sztainer, D., Story, M. and Harris, T. (1999) Beliefs and attitudes about obesity among teachers and school health care providers working with adolescents. *Journal of Nutrition Education* **31**, 3–9.

Neumark-Sztainer, D., Hannan, P.J., Story, M., Croll, J. and Perry, C. (2003) Family meal patterns: associations with sociodemographic characteristics and improved dietary intake among adolescents. *Journal of the American Dietetic Association* **103**, 317–322.

NHLBI Obesity Education Initiative Expert Panel (1998) Clinical guidelines on the identification, evaluation, and treatment of overweight and obesity in adults: the evidence report. *Obesity Research* **6**, 51S–209S.

Ogden, C.L., Kuczmarski, R.J., Flegal, K.M., Mei, Z., Guo, S., Wei, R., Grummer-Strawn, L.M., Curtin, L.R., Roche, A.F. and Johnson, C.L. (2002) Centers for Disease Control and Prevention 2000 growth charts for the United States: improvements to the 1977 National Center for Health Statistics version. *Pediatrics* **109**, 45–60.

Phillips, S.M., Bandini, L.G., Compton, D.V., Naumova, E.N. and Must, A. (2003) A longitudinal comparison of body composition by total body water and bioelectrical impedance in adolescent girls. *Journal of Nutrition* **133**, 1419–1425.

Pietrobelli, A., Faith, M.S., Allison, D.B., Gallagher, D., Chiumello, G. and Heymsfield, S.B. (1998) Body mass index as a measure of adiposity among children and adolescents: a validation study. *Journal of Pediatrics* **132**, 204–210.

Pietrobelli, A., Fernández, J.R., Redden, J.T. and Allison, D.B. (2002) Waist circumference percentiles in nationally representative samples of black, white, and Hispanic children. *International Journal of Obesity and Related Metabolic Disorders* **26**, S93.

Prentice, A.M. (1998) Body mass index standards for children: are useful for clinicians but not yet for epidemiologists. *BMI* **317**, 1401–1402.

Reilly, J.J. (2002) Assessment of childhood obesity: national reference data or international approach? *Obesity Research* **10**, 838–840.

Reilly, J.J., Dorosty, A.R., Emmett, P.M. and ALSPAC Study Team (2000) Identification of the obese child: adequacy of the body mass index for clinical practice and epidemiology. *International Journal of Obesity* **24**, 1623–1627.

Reilly, J.J., Wilson, M.L., Summerbell, C.D. and Wilson, D.C. (2002) Obesity: diagnosis, prevention, and treatment; evidence-based answers to common questions. *Archives of Disease in Childhood* **86**, 392–395.

Rolland-Cachera, M.F., Sempe, M., Guilloud-Batalle, M., Patois, E., Pequignot-Guggenbuhi, F. and Faurad, V. (1982) Adiposity indices in children. *American Journal of Clinical Nutrition* **36**, 178–184.

Rolland-Cachera, M.F., Cole, T.J., Sempe, M., Tichet, J., Rossignol, C. and Charraud, A. (1991) Body mass index variations: centiles from birth to 87 years. *European Journal of Clinical Nutrition* **45**, 13–21.

Rona, R.J. and Chinn, S. (2002) One cheer for the international definitions of overweight and obestiy. *Archives of Disease in Childhood* **87**, 390–391.

Scottish Intercollegiate Guidelines Network (2003) *Management of Obesity in Children and Young People*. Edinburgh: Royal College of Physicians, 1–23.

Seidell, J.C., Verschuren, W.M.M., van Leer, E.M. and Kromhout, D. (1996) Overweight, underweight, and mortality: a prospective study of 48 287 men and women. *Archives of Internal Medicine* **156**, 958–960.

Siega-Riz, A.M., Popkin, B.M. and Carson, T. (1998) Trends in breakfast consumption for children in the United States from 1965–1991. *American Journal of Clinical Nutrition* **67**, 748S–756S.

Smalley, K.J., Knerr, A.N., Kendrick, Z.V., Colliver, J.A. and Owen, O.E. (1990) Reassessment of body mass indices. *American Journal of Clinical Nutrition* **52**, 405–408.

Smoak, C.G., Burke, G.L., Webber, L.S., Harsha, D.W., Srinivasan, S.R. and Berenson, G.S. (1987) Relation of obesity to clustering of cardiovascular disease risk factors in children and young adults. *American Journal of Epidemiology* **125**, 364–372.

Staffieri, J.R. (1967) A study of social stereotype of body image in children. *Journal of Personality and Social Psychology* **7**, 101–104.

Strauss, R.S. and Pollack, H. (2003) Social marginalization of overweight adolescents. *Archives of Pediatrics and Adolescent Medicine* **157**, 746–752.

Teachman, B.A. and Brownell, K.D. (2001) Implicit anti-fat bias among health professionals: is anyone immune? *International Journal of Obesity* **25**, 1525–1531.

Wadden, T.A. and Didie, M.A. (2003) What's in a name? Patient's preferred terms for describing obesity. *Obesity Research* **11**, 1140–1146.

Whitaker, R.C., Wright, J.A., Pepe, M.S., Seidel, K.D. and Dietz, W.H. (1997) Predicting obesity in young adulthood from childhood and parental obesity. *New England Journal of Medicine* **337**, 869–873.

Wright, C.M., Booth, I.W., Buckler, J.M.H., Cameron, N., Cole, T.J., Healy, M.J.R., Hulse, J.A., Preece, M.A., Reilly, J.J. and Williams, A.F. (2002) Growth reference charts for use in the United Kingdom. *Archives of Disease in Childhood* **86**, 11–14.

Yanovski, J.A. (2001) Pediatric obesity. *Reviews in Endocrine and Metabolic Disorders* **2**, 371–383.

Young, L.R. and Nestle, M. (2003) Expanding portion sizes in the US marketplace: Implications for nutrition counseling. *Journal of the American Dietetic Association* **103**, 231–234.

Zannolli, R. and Morgese, G. (1996) Waist percentiles: a simple test for atherogenic disease? *Acta Paediatrica* **85**, 1368–1369.

16 Childhood obesity: consequences and physical and psychosocial complications

Kate Steinbeck

Consequences of childhood
obesity, 231
   Adult obesity, 231
   Belonging to an obese family, 232
   Puberty is a risk time for further
   weight gain, 232
   Fat distribution matters, 232
   Increased adult morbidity and
   mortality, 233
   Disadvantaged in health-care
   provision, 234
   Adverse adult psychological
   outcomes, 235

Complications of childhood
obesity, 235

Physical complications of
childhood obesity, 235
   Morbidities of significant medical
   importance, 236
   Specific genetic defects, 241
   The effect of weight
   management on obesity-related
   comorbidities, 241

Psychosocial complications of
childhood obesity, 242
   Stigmatization and
   stereotypes, 242
   How do the responses by others
   and their own responses affect the
   obese child?, 243

What do obese children and
adolescents think about their
obesity?, 243
Are there any formal
psychiatric disorders that are more
prevalent in obese children and
adolescents?, 244
Does treatment of obesity make a
difference?, 244
Childhood and adolescent obesity
and disordered eating, 245

Summary and conclusions, 245

References, 245

Obese children and adolescents have ongoing existing medical and psychosocial morbidity and the risks for adult ill health are increased. The increasing prevalence of obesity in childhood and adolescence has heightened the awareness of conditions that are known to be associated with childhood and adolescent obesity. Of considerable concern is the emergence of conditions that were previously considered relevant only to adult obesity.

The true prevalence of obesity-related morbidities remains largely unknown. Most data come from clinical studies representing highly selected patient groups. As the prevalence of childhood and adolescent obesity increases and as the percentage of children and adolescents in the heavier weight categories also increases, true prevalence data can be obtained as a result of population-based methods.

This chapter will examine both the physical and the psychosocial consequences and complications of childhood obesity, with an emphasis on recognition and diagnosis.

Consequences of childhood obesity

The consequences of childhood and adolescent obesity are detailed below (for a summary, see Table 16.1).

Adult obesity

The first consequence of childhood and adolescent obesity is adult obesity. Tracking studies have used variable definitions of obesity, different length of follow-up and many of the large cohort studies commenced well before the worldwide increase in obesity began. There have been variable predictions of adult obesity tracking through from childhood obesity, but no study has demonstrated the absence of a relationship between childhood and adult weight.

Earlier studies found that less than one-third of obese adults were obese in childhood. More recent studies show that over 75% of obese children remain obese as adults and that they are more obese than adults who had adult onset obesity (Freedman *et al.*, 2001). Up to 50% of obese adolescents remain obese in adulthood, and the later in adolescence that overweight persists and the greater the degree of overweight, the more likely it is that an individual will be an obese adult (Power *et al.*, 1997; Guo *et al.*, 2000).

Tracking studies are unable to distinguish between the influences of genes, environment and social behaviours on the tracking of body weight. It is likely that other lifestyle habits that impact on obesity, including physical activity, track into

Table 16.1 The consequences of childhood and adolescent obesity.

Adult obesity
Belonging to an obese family
Puberty is a risk time for further weight gain
Fat distribution already matters
Increased adult morbidity and mortality
Disadvantaged in health-care provision
Adverse adult psychological outcomes

adulthood. Childhood may be a more flexible time to permanently alter tracking trajectories.

Clinical highlight
Tracking data support intervention in and prevention of childhood and adolescent obesity.

Belonging to an obese family

The second consequence of childhood and adolescent obesity is that the child or adolescent is likely to be part of an obese family.

There is strong evidence for a significant genetic component to obesity in children and adolescents, from family, twin and adoptee studies (Stunkard *et al.*, 1990). The offspring of two obese parents have an 80% chance of becoming obese (Garn and Clark, 1976). This compares with a less than 10% chance for the offspring of two lean parents and an intermediary risk for the offspring of one lean and one obese parent. By the age of 17 years, the children of two obese parents are three times as obese as the children of two lean parents. Genes may not be expressed fully until adulthood but when obesity has been present from childhood it tends to be more severe.

In longitudinal studies in children, for which parental weights are available and used for their predictive value, parental obesity more than doubles the risk of adult obesity among both obese and non-obese children under 10 years of age (Whitaker *et al.*, 1997; Margarey *et al.*, 2003). This is a lifetime, rather than an immediate risk. Obese children under 3 years of age without obese parents appear at lower risk of obesity in adulthood, but among older children obesity is an increasingly important predictor of adult obesity.

The predictive power of parental morbidity is also seen in cardiovascular risk (Bao *et al.*, 1997). Children of parents with documented coronary artery disease have significantly higher body weight and body mass index (BMI) from childhood. They also have higher mean blood pressure, total cholesterol, LDL-cholesterol, glucose and insulin, but these differences may not become clinically significant until late adolescence.

Clinical highlight
In the management of childhood and adolescent obesity, take a family weight history and a family metabolic risk history.

Puberty is a risk time for further weight gain

The third consequence of childhood obesity is that the onset of adolescence is not associated with more favourable body composition. Body fatness changes throughout childhood and adolescence, with gender differences (Dugdale and Payne, 1976). There is a predominance of fat deposition in the first 12 months of life: it is normal for a baby to look chubby. From 12 months until approximately 4–6 years of age the percentage of body fat reduces, with lean tissue deposition more marked, and then from about 6 to 10 years fat deposition predominates. Adiposity rebound describes the point of reversion from a tendency to increasing leanness to one of increasing fatness around 4–6 years (Rolland-Cachera *et al.*, 1990). An earlier age at adiposity rebound is associated with greater adiposity in later adolescence. The adiposity rebound may simply be the description of an epiphenomenon; children who are genetically predisposed to obesity, who mature early as a result of higher body weight and who are exposed to certain environmental risks go on to become fatter earlier.

Girls show an increase in fat-free mass that slows over adolescence. Boys, in contrast, have a continuing increase in fat-free mass into young adulthood. Total body fat increases with age in adolescent girls and produces the long-observed adult gender dimorphism in body composition (Guo *et al.*, 1998). Gender dimorphism begins before puberty, with girls as young as 4 years having a higher body fat than boys, when matched for age, height, weight and BMI (Byrnes *et al.*, 1999).

Adipose tissue studies parallel clinical observation. The adipocyte size peaks first around 12 months of age, followed by a fall and then a second rise starting from peri-puberty. Up to about 10 years of age most of the increase in fat depot in lean subjects is from increased cell size. The next major increase in fat cell number is at puberty. In obese subjects the number of fat cells increases throughout childhood and adolescence, and by the end of puberty they have over twice as many fat cells as lean subjects (Knittle *et al.*, 1979). This proliferation can be modified by lifestyle intervention.

Clinical highlight
'Puppy fat' is a myth and adolescence is a high-risk time for excessive fat deposition. Upward crossing of BMI centiles in a child or adolescent is a time for action.

Fat distribution matters

The fourth consequence of childhood and adolescent obesity is that it matters where the fat is distributed. Obese children and adolescents show a variation in fat distribution, which is present prior to adolescence, and there is a genetic influence on this distribution of body fat. Deep visceral fat depots in children, whatever their degree of obesity, are much less than those seen in adults, so that subcutaneous fat is predominant in both the obese and the non-obese children when compared with intra-abdominal fat. The waist–hip ratio is lower in females aged 6–17 years than in males and the ratio falls with age, levelling out at mid-adolescence (Gillum, 1987). Waist circumference measures in childhood track into adulthood. Waist circumference in mid-childhood is predictive of overweight at early puberty indicating tracking of abdominal distribution of fat. Subscapular–triceps skinfold ratio is also a good discriminator of centralized fat distribution. The use of skinfold callipers, however, requires practice and callipers may not be wide enough in obese children and adolescents.

Anthropometric markers of central fat distribution correlate with markers of the metabolic syndrome, including blood pressure and HDL-cholesterol (Freedman *et al.*, 1999). Central obesity in children is also associated with adverse haemostatic factors, as measured by fibrinogen and plasminogen activator inhibitor-1. The waist circumference appears the most significant predictor for all cardiovascular risk factors, with BMI having a much lower predictive value (Savva *et al.*, 2000). There are no accepted cut-off points for waist circumference in children and adolescents because the relationship between waist measure and metabolic complications in children and adolescents remains undefined. It has been suggested that children with 33% or more body fat and a waist circumference of 71 cm or more are likely to have an adverse cardiovascular risk profile (Higgins *et al.*, 2001).

Clinical highlight
Waist circumference may indicate cardiovascular risk in obese children and adolescents and certainly can be used for longitudinal assessment in weight management.

Increased adult morbidity and mortality

The fifth consequence of obesity in childhood and adolescence is an increased risk of morbidity and mortality in adulthood, with origins in childhood. These long-term consequences of childhood and adolescent obesity are difficult to study, because of the time delay between origins of disease and disease appearance. In a 40-year follow-up of overweight children born in Europe in the first half of last century there were two clear findings. There was an increased mortality in adult life in children whose standard deviation weight score was > +3 in puberty and a significant increase in chronic disease in adulthood, as well as an earlier appearance of that chronic disease (Mosberg, 1989).

A review of the subjects from the third American Harvard Growth Study (1922–1935) also provides an example of the long-term risks associated with overweight in adolescence (Must *et al.*, 1992). For men, but not for women, there was an increased risk for all cause mortality and colorectal cancer. For both men and women there was an increased risk of morbidity from coronary artery disease and vascular disease, and for women an increased risk of arthritis.

A retrospective study, based on over 13 000 individuals measured as children or adolescents between 1933 and 1945 in Maryland, USA, also had similar findings (Nieto, 1992). There was a linear increase in adult mortality with increasing relative weight before puberty for both genders, and for relative weight in adolescent females only.

Clinical highlight
Obesity in childhood and adolescence confers a disease risk in adulthood, irrespective of adult weight status.

Not all future disease risk for obese children and adolescents is cardiovascular and not all cardiovascular risk in children and adolescents is associated with obesity. Cardiovascular risk factors are influenced by obesity and fat distribution, and they place the child and/or adolescent into an overall worse lifetime risk category.

The most consistent evidence comes from the Bogalusa Heart Study, Louisiana, a cross-sectional plus longitudinal epidemiological survey of the early natural history of atherosclerosis. Autopsy findings from young subjects in the Bogalusa study, who died predominantly from trauma, demonstrated the presence of fatty streaks and fibrous plaques in the coronary arteries, which increased with age, with detectable abnormalities in the 2–15 years age group (Berenson *et al.*, 1998). There were strongly significant correlations between the presence of cardiovascular risk factors and this atherosclerotic change. Subjects with zero, one, two and three or four risk factors had 19.1%, 30.3%, 37.9% and 30.5%, respectively, of the intimal surface of the aorta covered in fatty streaks. In the Muscatine study from Iowa, coronary calcification was more prevalent in young adults, who, as children, had elevated cardiovascular risk factors (Mahoney *et al.*, 1996).

Increasing body fatness in children is associated with an increase in cardiovascular risk factors (Fig. 16.1). Risk factor

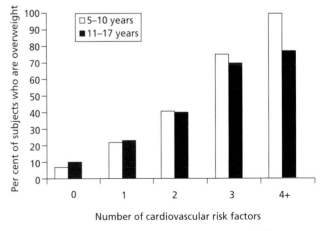

Fig 16.1 Overweight (BMI > 95th percentile) in children and adolescents and the number of cardiovascular risk factors (elevated blood pressure, LDL-cholesterol, triglycerides and insulin and low HDL-cholesterol). (Adapted from Freedman *et al.*, 1999a.)

prevalence increases with a BMI above the 85th percentile, but children with a BMI above the 95th percentile are 2.4 times more likely to have elevated cholesterol than children with a BMI less than the 85th percentile, with even higher estimated risks for systolic blood pressure, LDL-cholesterol, diastolic blood pressure and fasting insulin (Freedman *et al.*, 1999a,b; 2001). The cardiovascular risk associations do not always vary linearly with age: associations for blood pressure and triglyceride tend to be stronger in the younger children, whereas LDL-cholesterol and insulin are stronger in older groups. An increase in adiposity is the second most significant predictive variable for serum lipids and lipoprotein levels, after the initial lipid and lipoprotein values. The strength of the relationship increases from adolescence into young adulthood and the relationship appears stronger among males. Cardiovascular risk factors in parents further predict the presence of such risk factors in their offspring.

Clustering and tracking of cardiovascular risk factors in children and adolescents and associations with obesity have been described in other populations. The Muscatine study showed that adolescent obesity, especially in males, is associated with higher levels of total and LDL-cholesterol in adulthood. Hypertensive children who continue to have high blood pressure in adulthood are more likely to have higher body weight, BMI and waist circumferences. In the Netherlands, the Amsterdam Growth and Health Study demonstrated strong tracking of lipoproteins and body fatness (Twisk *et al.*, 1997).

Clinical highlight
A fasting lipid profile should be considered in obese children and adolescents, particularly those who have a family history of cardiovascular risk factors. The levels of lipids are unlikely to be at the levels at which pharmacotherapy is indicated but these levels can be used both as an indicator of risk and a monitor of successful intervention.

Insulin is an independent risk factor for cardiovascular disease in adults, and insulin resistance also predicts the future risk of type 2 diabetes in adults. Hyperinsulinaemia in childhood has been found in several populations known to be at high risk for type 2 diabetes (McCance *et al.*, 1994). Hyperinsulinaemia is a common finding in childhood and adolescent obesity (Fig. 16.2) and may be the initial signal of the metabolic syndrome. Hyperinsulinaemia in children and adolescents is associated with adverse lipid and lipoprotein levels, and this association is independent of obesity, age or glucose level (Jiang *et al.*, 1995). In the context of obesity, the development of the metabolic syndrome in adults is associated with childhood BMI and childhood insulin levels, but the relationship with insulin disappears after adjustment for childhood BMI (Srinivasan *et al.*, 2002). The relationship between BMI and insulin levels appears non-linear, with a sharp increase at about the 95th BMI centile. Whether hyperinsulinaemia with insulin resistance increases efficiency of fat storage or decreases risk for further weight gain is unclear.

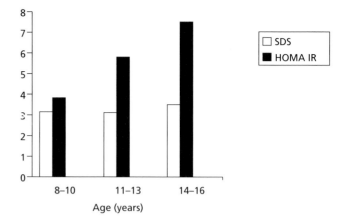

Fig 16.2 BMI SD score and insulin resistance score as measured by homeostasis model assessment (HOMA) in non-diabetic children and adolescents attending a teaching hospital weight management service (unpublished data from K. Steinbeck, 2003).

Clinical highlight
A fasting insulin should be considered in obese children and adolescents, particularly those who have a family history of type 2 diabetes or cardiovascular disease.

Disadvantaged in health-care provision

The sixth consequence of child and adolescent obesity is the difficulties in providing health care, particularly in the hospital setting. The main difficulties relate to anaesthesia, equipment and accommodation, and drug dosage. The anaesthetic care of the obese adult has been well considered, but obese children and adolescents are likely to experience similar risks and difficulties. These include pre-existing abnormal lung function, difficulties in ventilation (especially when supine), difficulties with intubation and with venous access. Standard paediatric equipment may be too small to use in obese children and adolescents. Hospital furniture may not accommodate body size and in extreme circumstances may require premature admission to adult facilities, often a very inappropriate placement. Paediatric dosing is carried out on a weight basis. As the proportion of lean to fat mass in obese children and adolescents is altered, the dosage assumptions may be incorrect. Thus, a chance for both therapeutic overdosing and underdosing exists. In situations in which protein intake is adequate it should be assumed that about 30% of excess weight is lean body mass. As the rest is increased fat mass there is the chance of an increased volume of distribution, particularly for more lipophilic drugs.

Clinical highlight
Manage the obese child and adolescent both age and weight appropriately.

Adverse adult psychological outcomes

The seventh consequence of childhood and adolescent obesity is adverse psychosocial outcomes in adult life. Just as the medical consequences of childhood obesity extend into adulthood, so do the psychosocial impacts. A study of American women who were obese as adolescents found that they achieved a lower final educational level, had lower incomes and greater rates of poverty and were less likely to marry when compared with peers of lower body weight (Gortmaker *et al.*, 1993). Similar findings have been described in European studies. Although outside the scope of this chapter, discriminatory practices against obese youths and young adults have been described in health facilities, teaching, employment, rental applications and admission to tertiary education. Obesity is not associated with lower intellectual function, as an explanation for poorer personal achievement. These findings represent a high personal cost of obesity with significant societal implications. These costs are even more difficult to define than those related to physical morbidity and mortality.

Complications of childhood obesity

An important part of the management of childhood and adolescent obesity is the diagnosis and management of existing obesity-related comorbidity. Complications of obesity are physical and non-physical. The greater the degree of obesity, the greater the likelihood of obesity-related comorbidity and the greater the chance of multiple comorbidities. Symptoms need to be actively sought. Children may not perceive symptoms as abnormal. Adolescents may be reticent to discuss symptomatology owing to concerns that it may represent something serious or that they may be ridiculed. The symptoms of some obesity-related comorbidities may be different in children and adolescents from those in adults. Physical complications may be of minor medical significance but of major importance to the individual (Table 16.2).

Physical complications of childhood obesity

The following complications are morbidities of minor medical significance but of major importance to management. Little research has been directed to these complications and there are no data related to prevalence. These complications will be familiar to those clinicians who manage child and adolescent obesity.

Heat intolerance

Adipose tissue acts as insulation, and inhibits the natural dissipation of body heat. Any increase in physical activity and muscle use increases superficial skin perfusion and sweating, in order to lose body heat (Haymes *et al.*, 1975). In child and

Table 16.2 Complications of minor medical significance.

Heat intolerance*
Heat rash and intertrigo*
Breathlessness on minimal exertion*
Tiredness*
Musculoskeletal discomfort*
Pseudogynaecomastia
Male genitalia of small appearance
Cutaneous striae

*May impact on activity management in obesity.

adolescent obesity, heat intolerance is seen at rest and further exacerbated by physical activity. Sweating and perceptions of hotness, together with excessive facial flushing are common. These symptoms and signs may be the reason that physical activity is avoided or terminated early.

Heat rash and other skin lesions

Overheating and sweating combined with deeper skinfolds increase the likelihood of intertrigo and heat rash in obese children and adolescents. Fungal infections are common in the groin and axilla and under breast tissue in both sexes. Obese children and adolescents have a greater body surface area than their leaner peers and lose more fluid by perspiration and insensible fluid loss. In clinical practice, obese children and adolescents are frequently described as always thirsty and drinking copious volumes of liquid. Obese children and adolescents often wear cover-up clothing to hide their body size and shape, which further exacerbates heat-related symptoms. This makes physical examination harder. Tact and sensitivity are required to ensure that an adequate examination is performed.

Breathlessness

In the absence of lung pathology, shortness of breath on exertion is a common morbidity in obese adults. There are no published data to confirm this in children, although it is often observed in clinical practice. Increased respiratory effort will be required at rest because of chest wall mechanics and visceral fat. The situation is worsened by physical activity—another reason why obese children and adolescents avoid physical activity.

Tiredness

Tiredness is a prevalent general symptom in obese children and adolescents. The presence of obstructive sleep apnoea should be considered. Tiredness may also be secondary to the increased physical effort of daily lifestyle activity and is exacerbated by low levels of physical fitness and exercise tolerance in obese children and adolescents.

Musculoskeletal discomfort

Obese children and adolescents on questioning will regularly admit to general musculoskeletal discomfort in feet, ankles and calves, which is exacerbated by physical activity. Back, knee and hip discomfort are uncommon, even in high grades of obesity, unless there is associated trauma or orthopaedic abnormality. This non-specific discomfort is likely due to soft-tissue strain and distortion, as a result of the physical forces of excess weight, altered centre of gravity (with pronounced lumbar lordosis) and gait abnormalities. These factors increase the risk of falls and soft-tissue injury and contribute towards the perception of clumsiness in obese children and adolescents. Musculoskeletal discomfort is another deterrent to physical activity, the body is more comfortable at rest and when supported.

Staging of puberty

Published data suggest that older children and adolescents are competent at self-grading against line drawings of the Tanner stages of pubertal development. It is often difficult clinically to assess breast stage in obese children and adolescents. Assessment of secondary sexual hair (adrenarche) may be discordant with gonadarche, and a bone age and biochemical assessment of gonadal function may be required, particularly if precocious puberty is a concern. Obese girls overestimate breast development by self-assessment in about 40% of cases, much higher than for non-obese girls of similar age.

Pseudogynaecomastia in males

A general increase in subcutaneous truncal fat can simulate gynaecomastia. Pseudogynaecomastia is differentiated from true gynaecomastia initially by palpation. Ultrasound of the chest wall will define fat and glandular tissue if palpation is equivocal. The sequelae of pseudogynaecomastia are psychosocial rather than medical, and the psychological impact may determine surgical intervention. Weight loss may improve the appearance.

Small genitalia in males

Obese prepubertal males may have the appearance of an abnormally small penis. The vast majority of obese boys will have a normal size penis for age, buried in a large pubic fat pad. Appearances will improve with the pubertal increase in penile size. Applying downwards pressure towards the pubic symphysis will allow better determination of penile size. Some boys will experience difficulties in micturition when standing. Obesity and true micropenis may co-exist—either as two unrelated conditions or as part of a hypogonadal state such as Klinefelter's or Bardet–Biedl syndrome.

Cutaneous striae

Cutaneous striae, or stretch marks, occur as a result of dermal collagen disruption (Sheu *et al.*, 1991). These are a response to rapid deposition of fat. In obesity these are most likely seen over the abdomen and hips. Striae occur in pathological states such as Cushing's syndrome with obesity. In this situation, striae have a different distribution, being in the axillae and groin as well as on the abdomen, and are combined with other dermal abnormalities (such as skin fragility and bruising) that are not generally present in obesity. Striae will fade with weight loss and/or stabilization but will not disappear completely.

Clinical highlight
There is a higher level of chronic physical discomfort in the obese child and adolescent, which has the potential to greatly affect the lifestyle of obese children and adolescents. These discomforts will counteract attempts to increase physical activity as part of a management programme and are likely to further impair self-esteem.

Morbidities of significant medical importance

Obesity in children and adolescents is associated with major medical comorbidity. Comorbidities are more likely to be present in the higher grades of obesity and in the older child or adolescent. There is not an obesity threshold below which a child or adolescent can be assumed to be free of morbidity. Table 16.3 shows the major medical complication groupings.

Cardiovascular

Hypertension
In parallel with the increasing prevalence of childhood and adolescent obesity is the change in the epidemiology of hypertension in these age groups. Most hypertension is now essential or primary, rather than secondary to renal disease, and generally clustering with other cardiovascular risk factors (Rosner *et al.*, 2000; Sorof and Daniels, 2002). Obese children and adolescents have higher blood pressures and higher prevalence rates for hypertension than children of leaner body weight. About one-third of obese children and half of obese adolescents are hypertensive. There is a doubling of prevalence between the 75th and 95th BMI percentiles. Initially, hypertension in childhood obesity is predominantly systolic. Isolated systolic hypertension is an independent risk factor for cardiovascular disease in adults, and in children it may well contribute to their total cardiovascular burden as adults.

Hypertension is probably underdiagnosed in obese children and adolescents. Blood pressure rises with age and height, and age-related percentile charts are required. The

Table 16.3 Significant medical complications present in childhood and adolescent obesity.

Cardiovascular
Hypertension
Cardiac muscle abnormalities
Abnormal blood vessel structure and function
Increased heart rate variability

Respiratory
Sleep-disordered breathing
Pickwickian syndrome
Asthma

Endocrine
Type 2 diabetes (and acanthosis nigricans)
Changed onset of puberty
Polycystic ovaries

Orthopaedic
Foot pronation
Tibia vara (Blount's disease)
Slipped capital epiphysis

Gastrointestinal
Hepatic steatosis
Gastro-oesophageal reflux
Cholelithiasis

Neurological
Benign intracranial hypertension

---

arbitrary cut-off points are >90th for high normal blood pressure and >95th for hypertension.

The accurate measurement of blood pressure in obese children and adolescents requires the correct blood pressure cuff (both width and length). If it is too large, the blood pressure reading will be falsely low; if it is too narrow then the reading will be falsely elevated. The width of the cuff bladder should be 40% of the circumference of the mid upper arm. Blood pressure seems more variable in obese children than in their leaner peers, and standardization of measuring conditions is also important.

Cardiac abnormalities

The effects of obesity on the adult heart are well documented, including left ventricular hypertrophy, right ventricular hypertrophy and cardiac failure. Controlled echocardiography studies in obese children and adolescents show that mean left ventricular mass, ventricular septal and posterior wall thickness and the internal dimension of the left ventricle in diastole are all greater in severely obese children than in their lean counterparts (Alpert, 2001). These studies have small subject numbers and it is not possible to generalize these findings. Echocardiography should be considered in children and adolescents with severe obesity, particularly if they are hypertensive and have additional symptoms such as palpitations,

shortness of breath and syncope. A referral for specialist assessment would also be appropriate under these circumstances.

Blood vessel structure and function

Increased intimal–medial thickness and reduced vascular compliance are present in children with diabetes and familial hypercholesterolaemia—both are known risk factors for early-onset adult cardiovascular morbidity. Obese adolescents have decreased maximum forearm blood flow and increased forearm vascular resistance (Rocchini *et al.*, 1992). Increased vascular stiffness and endothelial dysfunction are best correlated with abdominal fat and insulin levels (Tounian *et al.*, 2001).

Heart rate variability

There is an increased heart rate variability in obese children and adolescents when compared with leaner peers (Martini *et al.*, 2001). On formal testing there are abnormalities of sympathetic and parasympathetic function. The significance of these findings is unknown and variations in heart rate are not associated with consistent clinical symptoms. Physical training in obese children alters these autonomic findings by decreasing the ratio of sympathetic to parasympathetic activity.

Respiratory

Obesity increases the work or effort required to breathe. Mechanical forces such as the weight of the chest wall and the narrowing of airways are coupled with diffusion abnormalities. Lung function is altered in obese children (Inselma *et al.*, 1993). Airway narrowing, reduced diffusion capacity and ventilatory tiring are common.

Sleep-disordered breathing

Sleep-associated breathing disorders are frequently found in child and adolescent obesity in clinical practice. These disorders include increased air flow resistance in the upper airways, reduction in air flow, regular heavy snoring and multiple and brief cessations of breathing during sleep (apnoeas) with compensatory arousals.

Although obesity is considered a risk factor for sleep-associated breathing disorders in children and adolescents, the prevalence of these disorders is less clear. In one case–control study of children and adolescents recruited from families with and without sleep apnoea, obesity is a risk with an odds ratio of over 4.5 (Redline *et al.*, 1999). If the study population is selected for obesity, the prevalence of an abnormal sleep study in such children is between 30% and 50% (Marcus *et al.*, 1996). There is also a correlation between the degree of obesity and the severity of the documented sleep disturbance, with 5–10% having severe obstructive sleep apnoea, and 50% of severely obese children having a degree of central hypoventilation. Daytime somnolence and tiredness are not commonly reported in children with established obstructive sleep apnoea.

Neurocognitive deficits (memory and learning performance) may be present in morbidly obese children with obstructive sleep apnoea (Rhodes *et al.*, 1995). Sleeping in the upright position and adenotonsillar hypertrophy increase the chances of obstructive sleep apnoea. Truncal obesity, a short broad neck and a crowded oropharynx are other clinical clues to the presence of sleep apnoea, and the degree of fasting hyperinsulinaemia may predict severity.

If sleep-disordered breathing is suspected, referral to a paediatric sleep unit is necessary, as diagnosis will require an overnight sleep study. Tonsillectomy and adenoidectomy will reduce the symptoms of obstructive sleep apnoea in obese children, even in the absence of weight reduction. In fact, tonsillectomy and/or adenoidectomy may be associated with a further increase in BMI (Soultan *et al.*, 1999).

Pickwickian syndrome

The Pickwickian syndrome is present when ventilation capacity cannot be increased to overcome chronic hypoxia and to normalize blood carbon dioxide. It is characterized by severe obesity, hypersomnolence, pulmonary hypertension and right-sided heart failure, polycythaemia, daytime hypoxaemia and hypercapnia. The syndrome is associated with pulmonary embolism and sudden death in children. It is uncommon and is most likely to be diagnosed in secondary obesity, including hypothalamic hyperphagia syndromes and Prader–Willi syndrome.

Asthma

It has been suggested that a causal relationship exists between asthma and obesity in children, although not all studies are supportive of this. Both conditions are increasing in prevalence. There may be complicated causality in that those children who have asthma may be less physically active because of their respiratory condition, thus increasing their risk of obesity. Additionally, drugs used to treat asthma, glucocorticoids in particular, may also increase a child's risk of obesity. There may be other common lifestyle markers or links that are not readily apparent, especially as the link between the two conditions is a recent one.

Using doctor-diagnosed asthma as the criterion, American data in over 12 000 children and adolescents aged between two months and 16 years found that the highest risk for asthma was a family history, but a BMI > 85th percentile almost doubled the risk (Rodriguea *et al.*, 2002). This study identified some ethnic differences in risk and presentation. Others have identified female gender as a risk for obesity-associated asthma. In a study of 600 children, girls who were obese at 11 years were more likely to have asthma between the ages of 11 and 13 years, and more so if they entered puberty early (Castro-Rodriguez *et al.*, 2001). In a cross-sectional study on over 9000 German boys and girls at school entry, the female gender risk for asthma was also identified (von Kries *et al.*, 2001). Obesity in girls did not increase the risk of other atopic phenomena and this suggests that the aetiology of obesity-related asthma may be related to fat mass and possibly its distribution.

Exercise induces a greater frequency and degree of bronchospasm in obese children who are not known to have asthma (Gokbal and Atas, 1999). Obese children who experience shortness of breath and chest discomfort, with physical activity in particular, should be considered for assessment and management of exercise-induced bronchospasm, with a particular emphasis on its prevention.

Weight reduction improves lung function in obese adults, so it is likely that weight management in children and adolescents will reduce the impact of asthma.

Endocrine

Type 2 diabetes

In 1996, Pinhas-Hamiel and colleagues published a paper describing an increase in the incidence of type 2 diabetes in adolescents over the previous decade. The proportion of newly diagnosed patients with type 2 diabetes rose from 4% to 16%, but if the age group of 10–19 years was selected, the figure was 33%. Both obesity and a family history of type 2 diabetes are strongly associated with type 2 diabetes in children and adolescents. Type 2 diabetes is associated with excess body weight in 95% of cases, whereas type 1 diabetes is associated with excess body weight in only 20% of cases.

Ethnicity is also a strong risk factor. Indigenous populations are at greater risk of developing type 2 diabetes in young age groups (Harris *et al.*, 1996). British case report studies have identified South Asian and Middle Eastern ethnicity as a major risk group (Ehtisham *et al.*, 2000). An increase in the incidence of type 2 diabetes in children has occurred in Japan with Westernization of the diet (Kitigawa *et al.*, 1998). Additional risk factors for the development of type 2 diabetes in children and adolescents are female gender, puberty and acanthosis nigricans as the external expression of insulin resistance.

Puberty is a state of transient physiological insulin resistance, primarily due to the increased production of growth hormone and insulin-like growth factor-1 (IGF-1). This phenomenon is more marked in females than in males. When insulin resistance is extreme prior to puberty, the onset of pubertal insulin resistance may be enough to induce type 2 diabetes. Diabetes does not resolve following puberty and cessation of growth.

Acanthosis nigricans is a dermatological abnormality that, in children and adolescents, has to date almost exclusively been described in insulin-resistant states. *Acanthosis nigricans* has a darkened, velvety, raised appearance and is most easily seen in darker skinned individuals; in lighter skinned individuals, the ridges of dermal overgrowth may be more easily palpated than visualized. Acanthosis nigricans may be associated with truncal skin tags in the adolescent. In obesity, it is commonly found around the neck, and in the flexures including the groin and axillae. Scrubbing in an attempt to reduce it will exacerbate the condition. In severe cases cracking and fissuring of the skin may appear and expert dermatological input may be required. The pathophysiology of acanthosis nigricans is not completely understood. It has been suggested that the elevated insulin levels act through the IGF-1 receptor to cause dermal overgrowth, but this does not explain the predilection for certain areas or the racial predilection. The management is weight loss and the reduction of insulin resistance. Metformin can be used as adjunctive therapy.

It is not practicable to perform a standard oral glucose tolerance test in all obese children and adolescents. A fasting blood glucose should be performed in obese children and adolescents from minority groups, in those with acanthosis nigricans and in those with a family history of diabetes.

Prevalence data for type 2 diabetes in children and adolescents are likely to be underestimated because of the insidious onset of type 2 diabetes, making diagnosis difficult unless it is entertained. The majority of cases are asymptomatic or present with fungal or other skin infections, rather than with the classic symptoms of hyperglycaemia—polydipsia, polyuria and weight loss.

In a representative sample of 2867 US adolescents from the National Health and Nutrition Examination Survey III (1988–1994) the estimated prevalence of type 2 diabetes was 0.41% and similar prevalence figures are being reported elsewhere (Fagot-Campagna, 2001). Rates as high as 5% have been found among adolescents in native American populations. In an obesity clinic population of 167 obese American children and adolescents, 25% of younger obese children and 21% of obese adolescents had impaired glucose tolerance diagnosed by 2-h glucose tolerance test (Sinha *et al.*, 2002). Undiagnosed diabetes was present in 4% of the adolescents. Similar findings have been described in older studies.

Lifestyle intervention is the cornerstone of management in type 2 diabetes. Adherence to such regimens, particularly when there may be no perceived clinical benefit is difficult in adolescence. Adolescence is a period of change in lifestyle behaviours with increasing independence from family and reduction in physical activity, particularly in females. The standard drug therapies in adult type 2 diabetes have never been evaluated for safety or efficacy in children and adolescents. Relatively higher doses of pharmacotherapy are required during puberty. Adolescent females require counselling about pregnancy—the risk of fetal abnormalities and overgrowth syndrome with poor control of diabetes, and the requirement for insulin therapy prior to conception.

The early onset of a progressive, chronic disease will increase the number of younger adults presenting with both the macrovascular and microvascular complications of diabetes, and the ensuing coronary and cerebrovascular events, visual impairment, limb amputations and chronic renal failure.

Puberty and reproduction

Puberty in females

It is well recognized in adults that body weight at both extremes influences menstrual function and fertility. There is also evidence that weight status influences menarche. Over the last 10–15 years, there has been a decrease in the mean age of menarche. It is likely that this lowering of menarchal age is associated with the rise in the prevalence of obesity over the same time. Best evidence for this comes from the analysis of data from the United States NHANES (Adair and Gordon-Larsen, 2001; Wang, 2002). The effect of body weight on early maturation is evident at BMI > 85th percentile. One-third of overweight girls could be expected to reach menarche before the age of 11 years and in those who reach menarche before the age of 10 years the prevalence of overweight is even higher.

These are population trends and menarche is still falling within the normal age range (9–16 years). True precocious puberty with sexual maturation apparent before the age of 8 years should be referred for specialist assessment whatever the BMI percentile of the child.

Early menarche is associated with earlier onset of sexual activity and its attendant risks. Adolescents who experience earlier menarche are more likely to have depression and substance abuse and eating disorders. Endometriosis, increased severity of dysmenorrhoea and menstrual cramping and increased risk of spontaneous abortion are more common in young adulthood. Early menarche is a well-established risk factor for breast cancer and has been linked to other cancers, including those of the ovary and thyroid.

Puberty in males

Although early maturation is twice as likely to occur in overweight females, the reverse is true in boys. Overweight boys are less likely to have early maturation than their leaner peers. The physiological explanation for this observation is unclear but does parallel the gender differences in pubertal body composition. Girls increase fat mass during puberty and higher, earlier fat mass may signal readiness for sexual maturation. Conversely, for males lean body mass increases with sexual maturity and boys with a relatively higher lean body mass are the earlier maturers. Increased adipose tissue aromatase activity and conversion of androgen to oestrogen could theoretically impact on sexual maturation in males at a hypothalamic level.

Reproductive

Polycystic ovary syndrome

The polycystic ovary syndrome (PCOS) comprises late menarche, oligomenorrhoea or amenorrhoea, with hirsutism, acne, abdominal obesity, acanthosis nigricans and insulin resistance (Arslanian and Witchel, 2002). Hyperinsulinaemia increases ovarian thecal androgen production and induces the characteristic endocrine pattern of elevated free androgen and increased luteinizing hormone (LH)/follicle-stimulating hormone (FSH) ratio. This pattern is increasingly being described in younger obese adolescents. The true prevalence of PCOS in adolescents is unknown. It is probably underdiagnosed because adolescents are less likely have to the characteristic ultrasound changes (Rosenfield *et al.*, 2000). Elevated free testosterone levels are the most consistent finding. Oligomenorrhoea or delayed menstruation may be dismissed as normal for adolescents, and it may be difficult to distinguish clinically between adolescent anovulation and PCOS. Insulin resistance can be significant in this situation, with a 50% reduction in peripheral tissue insulin sensitivity and hepatic insulin resistance (Lewy *et al.*, 2001) and is further manifested in a reduced sex hormone-binding globulin (SHBG), which magnifies androgen effects. Fasting insulin and other measures of insulin resistance remain significantly higher in adolescent females with hyperandrogenism than in age-matched control subjects, even when corrected for BMI. There is an association between premature adrenarche and subsequent ovarian hyperandrogenism (Ibanez *et al.*, 1998), although body weight is not a strong discriminator in this group.

The efficacy of weight reduction alone in obese adolescents with PCOS has not been demonstrated. The most commonly used medication is the oral contraceptive to suppress ovarian androgen production, with or without an anti-androgen. The oral contraceptive in some adolescents can cause weight gain, as can the anti-androgen, cyproterone acetate. Metformin therapy has been reported to induce ovulation and improve the endocrine profile in obese adolescents with PCOS. There has also been recent interest in thiazoledinediones. Pharmacotherapy must be prescribed with lifestyle change, given the longer term risks of type 2 diabetes and heart disease.

Orthopaedic

Obese children also have a characteristic walking pattern, with longer cycle duration, lower cadence, lower velocity and a longer stance period than normal-weight subjects and they often display forms of gait asymmetry (Hills and Parker, 1992).

Foot pronation

Foot pronation, or flat feet, is more common in obese children and adolescents, often associated with genu valgus and lax ligaments (Napolitano *et al.*, 2000). The longitudinal arch of the foot is low or absent in the 'flat foot'. There is significant eversion of the subtalar complex during weight-bearing, with a dorsiflexed and abducted navicular bone. A decreased footprint angle and an increased surface area of the foot in contact with the ground are characteristic, as are increased static and dynamic plantar pressures (Dowling *et al.*, 2001). This functional deformity produces non-specific joint and ligamentous discomfort and pain. Management involves attention to risk factors, the use of orthotics and stretching exercises. Suppor-

tive, enclosed footwear will also counteract a tendency to pronation and improve comfort during physical activity. Obese children and adolescents tend to have a broad foot, which further limits their choice of footwear.

The primary orthopaedic morbidities associated with overweight and obesity in children and adolescents are Blount's disease (Thompson and Carter, 1990) and slipped capital femoral epiphysis (Loder *et al.*, 1993).

Blount's disease

Blount's disease, or idiopathic tibia vara, is a pathological bowing of the tibia. The condition is classified according to the age of onset. Infantile (3 years or younger), juvenile (between 4 and 10 years) and adolescent (11 years and older). All affected older patients are obese, and there is a 2:1 male preponderance.

Tibial bowing is initiated by suppression of epiphyseal growth as a result of abnormal pressures causing repetitive trauma to the growth plate. There is then failure to adequately ossify the endochondrium, exacerbated by the adolescent growth spurt. The presentation is knee pain, with slowly progressive clinical deformity. Radiological examination will show wedging of the epiphysis. Histological changes include abnormal cellular islands of hyaline cartilage, foci of necrotic cartilage, prominent intertrabecular vascularity and premature closure of the medial aspects of the epiphysis. The treatment is surgical and if obesity persists there is a high degree of recurrence, particularly in younger males.

Slipped capital femoral epiphysis (Fig. 16.3)

The presentation for slipped capital femoral epiphysis is hip pain (or referred knee pain) and limitation of movement. The histological and radiological appearances are similar to those described for Blount's disease. The condition is also associated with endocrine disorders, including hypothyroidism and growth hormone therapy for short stature. Hypothyroidal slippage is usually bilateral and is associated with obesity, short stature and skeletal immaturity. Obese children present earlier, at a mean age of 12 years (13 years for non-obese children) and are more likely to have bilateral slippage (in >40% of cases). The clinical threshold for radiological assessment should be low and the films reviewed by a radiologist with paediatric expertise. If the diagnosis is missed, the hip joint will develop early degenerative change with further impairment of function. The treatment is surgical. It is important to minimize the period of immobility post surgery in the obese child or adolescent in order not to aggravate weight gain.

Gastrointestinal

Gastrointestinal morbidity is almost certainly underdiagnosed in child and adolescent obesity. Gastro-oesophageal reflux is the most common clinical condition, and hepatic steatosis is the greatest long-term risk.

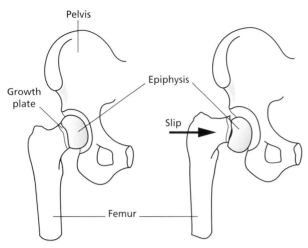

Fig 16.3 Slipped femoral capital epiphysis.

Hepatic steatosis (fatty liver)

Hepatic steatosis has been described in children and adolescents as an important obesity comorbidity (Guzzaloni *et al.*, 2000; Rashid and Roberts, 2000). The prevalence of fatty liver as diagnosed by ultrasound is 33% in obese prepubertal children and rises to nearly 50% in late puberty. BMI and the level of elevation of hepatic transaminases both correlate with the degree of fatty liver across all age groups. The liver is palpable in only a minority of cases. There is limited liver biopsy information in children and adolescents and no formal criteria for when this should be performed. In one small biopsy study of obese children, inflammatory changes were present in 88% of cases and fibrosis in 75%. One 10-year-old had established cirrhosis. These findings suggest that fatty accumulation in the young liver may be particularly damaging.

Little is known of the impact of intervention in hepatic steatosis in children and adolescents, but weight loss of approximately 10% of body weight has been shown to reduce both hepatic size and transaminase levels. There is unlikely to be spontaneous resolution.

Gastro-oesophageal reflux

There are no studies of the prevalence or health sequelae of gastro-oesophageal reflux in obese children and adolescents, although it is well recognized clinically. Children and adolescents will not spontaneously offer symptoms of reflux but readily identify when questioned discomfort or burning with meals, certain foods or with postural change. Weight management, the avoidance of overeating episodes and antacids are the first-line therapy. Ranitidine is commonly used in paediatric practice and should be prescribed if symptoms persist to avoid ulceration. Endoscopy should only be considered if symptoms persist. There is a case report of a Nissen fundoplication procedure in an obese 10-year-old boy who had pain and apnoea that were secondary to reflux and not responsive to medical therapy (Lobe and Schropp, 1993).

Cholelithiasis

In children and adolescents, gall bladder disease is more commonly found in girls, but the overall prevalence rate is low (0.13%) (Palasciano *et al.*, 1989). Obesity is associated with higher gall bladder volumes in children and adolescents. In established cholelithiasis, obesity and hypertriglyceridaemia are the most common predisposing factors. Over 10% of subjects who have gallstones will develop pancreatitis. Laparoscopic cholecystectomy is considered the surgical intervention of choice for children and adolescents. Older adolescents who are treated with very low-energy diets may have an exacerbation of underlying gall bladder pathology. An ultrasound should be performed if abdominal pain occurs during this therapy.

Neurological complications

Benign intracranial hypertension

Benign intracranial hypertension is more common in women and more so in obese women. There are limited data on the occurrence of benign intracranial hypertension in children and adolescents (Lessell, 1992), but the condition should be considered in obese adolescent females presenting with either persistent headache (in over 90% of cases), visual disturbance and/or papilloedema. Associated hypothyroidism will increase the risk of benign intracranial hypertension. It is not a benign condition, despite its name, and formal assessment of visual fields and visual acuity are mandatory.

Specific genetic defects

It is beyond the scope of this chapter to consider specific obesity syndromes in detail. Intellectual disability and short stature with unusual physical stigmata should arouse a high level of clinical suspicion. These syndromes include Prader–Willi, Bardet–Biedl, Alstrom and Cohen syndromes. The single gene defects that cause severe, early-onset obesity with unrelenting weight gain include leptin deficiency, leptin resistance, proopiomelanocortin mutations (subjects have bright red hair), proconvertase-1 defect and peroxisome proliferative-activated receptor-gamma 2 defect. These are all extremely rare. The most common single gene defect is the incidence of mutations involving the melanocortin-4 receptor. The phenotype includes increased linear growth, increased fat-free mass, severe hyperinsulinaemia and increased bone mineral density.

The effect of weight management on obesity-related comorbidities

There is evidence that cardiovascular risk factors—blood pressure, total and HDL-cholesterol, triglycerides and insulin in children and adolescents can be favourably altered by weight management (Epstein *et al.*, 1989; Knip and Nuutinen 1993). The percentage loss of body fat or body weight required to improve metabolic risk is generally modest, about 5–10%. The metabolic improvement in obese children and adolescents is more likely to be significant if there is an exercise component to management. Children seem to be able to maintain this metabolic improvement for some years, following intervention. The fall in insulin levels correlates with the decrease in relative overweight, although levels do not return to normal control values. The effects of such metabolic changes with respect to the long-term macrovascular morbidity are not known.

Psychosocial complications of childhood obesity

It is easier to document the physical comorbidities of childhood obesity than it is to describe the psychological and social consequences of childhood obesity. Research into the psychological complications of obesity in children and adolescents has usually considered stigmatization, self-esteem and friendship rather than formal diagnostic criteria for psychiatric pathology.

It is clear in clinical practice that obese children and adolescents suffer distress. The type and degree of that distress is harder to quantify. Less clear too are the psychological consequences of child and adolescent obesity. Physical comorbidity persists into adulthood but there is much less information on long-term psychological sequelae of childhood obesity.

It is likely that the earliest complications or consequences of childhood and adolescent obesity are in the psychological and social arenas (Fig. 16.4). Studies that assessed the psychosocial impact of obesity were often performed when obesity was less prevalent. It is not known how the increasing prevalence of obesity in children and adolescents might impact on societal responses to obesity.

Stigmatization and stereotypes

This is what others think about obese children and adolescents. Stigmatization by the peers of obese children and adolescents is well recognized and documented. Obesity in children is more stigmatized than clear, single physical disabilities (Goodman *et al.*, 1963). Children aged 10–11 years show a remarkably consistent ranking of drawings of disability, which is independent of age, gender, ethnicity and socioeconomic status. Obesity is ranked lowest when compared with amputation, crutches, physical abnormality and severe scarring. When children assign descriptions to three silhouettes—thin, muscular and fat—the fat silhouette is most likely to receive the epithets of 'gets teased' and least likely to be described as a 'best friend' (Staffieri, 1967). Cheating, lazy, lying, naughty, mean or stupid were other descriptors.

Older children are more likely to display negative views about obesity (Lawson, 1980). However, this stereotyping has some abstract qualities about it, as children do not necessarily

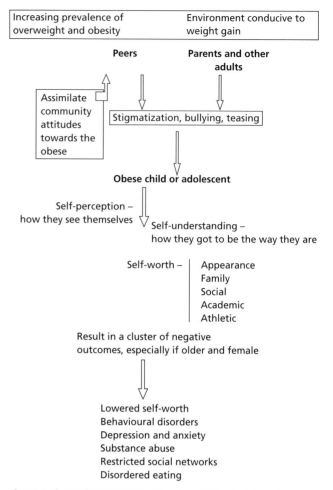

Fig 16.4 The psychosocial world of the obese child and adolescent.

apply it to classmates. Despite an overweight silhouette being associated with negative stereotypes, stereotyping is relatively independent of the rater's own body weight (Hill and Silver, 1995). Children at an early age have assimilated both health messages and societal messages related to fatness and thinness. Less is known about how the obese child or adolescent feels about themselves, because this question is not directly asked in studies. Providing children with medical explanations for obesity does not reduce stereotyping and does not influence their aversion for sharing activities with an obese peer.

The obese child and adolescent also have to cope with negative perceptions from adults—parents, health providers and others. Clinically, it is often observed that one child or adolescent is presented for management despite siblings of similar obesity who are not. This discrepancy is probably due to parental perception of obesity and is more likely to be directed at girls. Boys are more likely to be described as strong and solid. There are often significant parenting and control issues with the presenting child, which may both initiate referral and interfere with management. Between 50% and 75% of parents do not identify an overweight child as overweight and this finding is more prevalent in the lower socioeconomic classes (Baughcum *et al.*, 2000), despite parents being able to weight classify themselves accurately. Reasons for this inaccurate perception of their child's weight status are likely to be complex. These include denial (too hard to deal with), a belief (unfounded) that their child will grow out of their obesity, a belief that a big child is a healthy and loved child, and failure to perceive obesity as a high future physical health risk. Those parents who do perceive their children as obese are more likely to report poorer health and well-being for their child, particularly boys (Wake *et al.*, 2002). The level of concern in parents who report their child as obese is higher for more obese children. Health providers are likely to hold stereotypic views about childhood and adolescent obesity, as reflected in some referral letters and, until recently, obesity has not occupied much of the content in medical education.

In clinical practice this antipathy is not usually spontaneously described by the child or adolescent, and parents may be unaware of the extent of their child's distress. Not only is the obese child receiving messages of unacceptability about their physical appearance, but also they are most unhappy to share that experience.

How do the responses by others and their own responses affect the obese child?

The prejudice and discrimination directed towards the obese are well established by the time children have reached primary school age. Research into childhood obesity has generally not examined the specific problems related to being an obese child in our society (Friedman and Brownell, 1995). Forty years ago, obese adolescents were described as having personality traits that were similar to those seen in persecuted minorities (Monello and Mayer, 1963).

The term *self-esteem* is frequently used in discussion about childhood obesity, but it may be used with limited understanding. How self-esteem is measured varies from study to study. It may be a global measure of self-esteem or self-worth, or may concentrate on specific areas such as academic performance, body appearance, sporting prowess or social competence (French *et al.*, 1995).

There is little evidence to support the notion that self-esteem is significantly affected in obese pre-school children (Klesges *et al.*, 1992). In children of primary school age the relationship between self-esteem and body weight is generally inverse, but not strong. Many obese children have measures within the accepted ranges, but a positive relationship between relative weight and self-esteem has never been shown. If a distinction is made between general self-esteem and body self-esteem, relationships between body self-esteem and weight are much clearer. Generally, no gender differences are identified in this age group, but there is a trend towards girls exhibiting higher body dissatisfaction (Hill *et al.*, 1994). Although obese primary school children have lower self-esteem in relation to physical

appearance and athletic competence, they do seem to differ from their leaner peers in popularity, but they are judged as less 'pretty' (Phillips and Hill, 1998).

The inverse relationship between self-esteem and body weight becomes much stronger and clearer in adolescents, as social acceptance, athletic competence and physical appearance become more significant to the individual. A sense of social well-being and a sense of psychological wholeness are major tasks of adolescence. This fall in self-esteem at the start of the second decade is more pronounced in females, is present in males to a lesser degree and with some variation by race (Kimm *et al.*, 1997; Strauss, 2000). Obese adolescents who exhibit decreasing levels of self-esteem are more likely to smoke and drink alcohol than those who maintain self-esteem during adolescence, which may further compromise weight management. High-level physical activity in children and adolescents is an important determinant of self-esteem and obesity makes such activity difficult, despite its multifactorial benefits (Strauss *et al.*, 2001). Intuitively stereotyping and discrimination might lead to fewer friends or less satisfactory peer relationships for obese children and adolescents. Although not found in younger children, obese adolescents have less robust social networks, which may predispose to the social isolation characteristic of many obese adults.

What do obese children and adolescents think about their obesity?

This aspect is much harder to assess. Dissatisfaction with body size and a desire to lose weight have been found even in young children, particularly in girls. Young boys often express a desire to be heavier, but equate this with muscularity, not fatness. A wish to change body size or shape is found in all weight groups, not just obese children. There is no evidence that overweight children or adolescents have a distorted body image. Overweight children are more accurate at estimating their real body shape than lean children (Probst *et al.*, 1995). Overweight children do, however, express greater dissatisfaction with their body size (Probst *et al.*, 1995; van der Wal and Thelen, 2000).

There is little information as to what children or adolescents might believe is the cause of their obesity, how their obesity might be reduced and what future effects their obesity may have. To understand beliefs, a knowledge of cognitive development is important. Younger children may have simplistic and concrete views about aetiology and may well believe that obesity is somehow their fault. If their parents are obese they may well incorporate parental views into their belief system. Their world is very immediate and the concept of long-term behaviours and the impacts of these on weight will be poorly perceived. Children who internalize their obesity—believe that they are responsible for it—score lower on self-esteem measures (Pierce and Wardle, 1997). Older adolescents may have a better understanding of aetiology and future

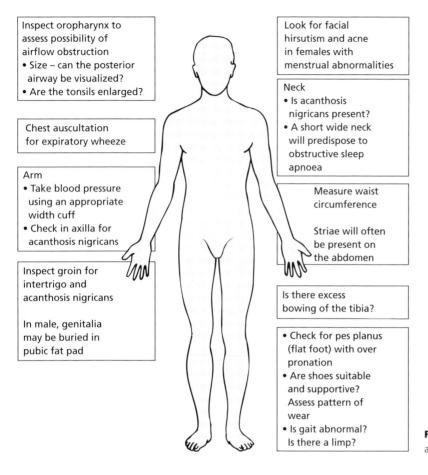

Fig 16.5 Clinical examination of the obese child and adolescent.

Labels in figure:

Inspect oropharynx to assess possibility of airflow obstruction
• Size – can the posterior airway be visualized?
• Are the tonsils enlarged?

Chest auscultation for expiratory wheeze

Arm
• Take blood pressure using an appropriate width cuff
• Check in axilla for acanthosis nigricans

Inspect groin for intertrigo and acanthosis nigricans

In male, genitalia may be buried in pubic fat pad

Look for facial hirsutism and acne in females with menstrual abnormalities

Neck
• Is acanthosis nigricans present?
• A short wide neck will predispose to obstructive sleep apnoea

Measure waist circumference

Striae will often be present on the abdomen

Is there excess bowing of the tibia?

• Check for pes planus (flat foot) with over pronation
• Are shoes suitable and supportive? Assess pattern of wear
• Is gait abnormal? Is there a limp?

---

implications, but this does not generally translate into behaviours necessary for weight control. Many day-to-day behaviour traits seen in obese children and adolescents are a result of the behaviour of others towards them. These traits include not eating in public and including at school, dressing in loose, cover-up clothing even when the weather is hot, avoiding situations when they may have to undress in front of others and avoidance of situations in which their lack of physical skills will be noted.

Are there any formal psychiatric disorders that are more prevalent in obese children and adolescents?

Behavioural problems diagnosed by parental report seem to be more common in obese children, with oppositional conduct disorder more frequent (Braet and Van Strien, 1997; Mustillo et al., 2003). It is not clear whether this behaviour stems from parental attempts at weight regulation. Depression and anxiety might be expected in obese children and adolescents and there is evidence that BMI is positively correlated with depression in older children and adolescents. Depression in these age groups may present differently to adults. Depression is also more common in obese children and adolescents presenting for weight management than in BMI-matched children and adolescents in the community. The relationship is clearer in females. Causality is hard to define as overeating and reduced physical activity may be part of a depressive complex, rather than the other way around.

Does treatment of obesity make a difference?

Improving self-efficacy and self-competency are accepted general approaches when working with children in whom behaviour change is desired (Harter, 1982). Such an approach requires that effort is rewarded with some form of success. There is a lack of evidence available on the impact of weight management interventions on child and adolescent well-being and body image, or for that matter on parenting capacity, confidence and satisfaction. It is not possible to say whether weight management will improve or worsen a child's or adolescent's psychosocial well-being, as there is evidence for both outcomes (Mellin et al., 1987; O'Brien et al., 1990; Cameron, 1999). To avoid further compromise of a sense of well-being, strategies that focus on a variety of outcomes besides weight change should be employed.

Childhood and adolescent obesity and disordered eating

Restrained eating and dieting behaviours are already present in pre-adolescent children (Hill and Oliver, 1992; Braet and Wydhooge, 2000). Age, female gender and increasing weight have all been associated with a greater frequency of weight control behaviours and concerns. By adolescence, dieting behaviours are well entrenched, sometimes with purging behaviours (Field *et al.*, 1999). There are differences between eating styles in obese and normal-weight children and adolescents (Braet and Van Strien, 1997). Obese children and adolescents have more emotional and external cued eating. Clinically, these behaviours include sneaky eating, stealing of food and constant complaints about hunger. It is important to encourage parents to understand non-hunger eating, even in small children. Obese adolescent females exhibit psychological features that predate the development of eating disorders, including concerns about self-esteem based on physical appearance. Obesity in adolescence is a risk factor for eating disorders in adulthood (Burrows and Cooper, 2002).

Eating is not driven by hunger alone but is also controlled by restraint (self-imposed eating controls) and by disinhibition (loss of control of intake in the presence of certain cues). Parental eating behaviours influence those of their offspring, with the mother/daughter combination being the strongest (Cutting *et al.*, 1999; Hood *et al.*, 2000). Disinhibition in the parent predicts both obesity and excess weight gain in offspring. High restraint and low disinhibition in parents is protective against excess weight gain in their offspring. High levels of parental restriction and disinhibition—the classical combination for binge eating—increases the likelihood of excessive weight gain in their offspring. It is not possible to say whether parental influence is by modelling of parental behaviours or whether genetic factors around eating control also come into play.

Summary and conclusions

Obesity in childhood and adolescence is not a healthy state and the degree of obesity is related to the presence of comorbidity. Comorbidities in childhood obesity are likely to be underdiagnosed. This is a complex result of failure to perceive the seriousness of the condition (education), prejudice and stigmatization by health professionals. Obese children and adolescents often do not voice their symptoms as they are unaware of their significance. Change in associated morbidities is one outcome indicator for successful weight management. Children do not grow out of obesity, and obesity in adolescence is a dangerous situation, as it will persist into adulthood.

References

Adair, L.S. and Gordon-Larsen, P. (2001) Maturational timing and overweight prevalence in US adolescent girls. *American Journal of Public Health* **91**, 642–644.

Alpert, M.A. (2001) Obesity cardiomyopathy: pathophysiology and evolution of the clinical syndrome. *American Journal of Medical Science* **321**, 225–236.

Arslanian SA and Witchel SF. (2002) Polycystic ovary syndrome in adolescents: Is there an epidemic? *Current Opinions in Endocrinology and Diabetes* **9**, 33–42.

Bao, W., Srinivasan, S.R., Valdez, R., Greenlund, K.J., Wattigney, M.S. and Berenson, G.S. (1997) Longitudinal changes in cardiovascular risk from childhood to young adulthood in offspring of parents with coronary artery disease. *Journal of the American Medical Association* **278**, 1749–1754.

Baughcum, A.E., Chamberlin, L.A., Deeks, C.M., Powers, S.W. and Whitaker, R.C. (2000) Maternal perceptions of overweight preschoolers. *Pediatrics* **106**, 1380–1386.

Berenson, G.S., Srinivasan, S.R., Bao, W.H., Newman, W.P., Tracey, R.E. and Wattigney, W.A. (1998) Association between multiple cardiovascular risk factors and atherosclerosis in children and young. *New England Journal of Medicine* **338**, 1650–1656.

Braet, C. and Van Strien, T. (1997) Assessment of emotional, externally induced and restrained eating behaviour in nine to twelve-year-old obese and non-obese children. *Behavioural Research and Therapy* **35**, 863–873.

Braet, C. and Wydhooge, K. (2000) Dietary restraint in normal weight and overweight children: A cross-sectional study. *International Journal of Obesity* **24**, 314–318.

Burrows, A. and Cooper, M. (2002) Possible risk factors in the development of eating disorders in overweight pre-adolescent girls. *International Journal of Obesity and Related Metabolic Disorders* **26**, 1268–1273.

Byrnes, S.E., Baur, L.A., Bermingham, M., Brock, K. and Steinbeck, K. (1999) Leptin and total cholesterol are predictors of weight gain in pre-pubertal children. *International Journal of Obesity* **23**, 146–150.

Cameron, J.W. (1999) Self-esteem changes in children enrolled in weight management programs. *Issues in Comparative Pediatric Nursing* **22**, 75–85.

Castro-Rodriguez, J.A., Holberg, C.J., Morgan, W.J., Wright, A.L. and Martinez, F.D. (2001) Increased incidence of asthma like symptoms in girls who become overweight or obese during the school years. *American Journal of Respiratory and Critical Care Medicine* **163**, 1344–1349.

Cutting, T.M., Fisher, J.O., Grimm-Thomas, K. and Birch, L.L. (1999) Like mother, like daughter: familial patterns of overweight are mediated by mothers' dietary disinhibition. *American Journal of Clinical Nutrition* **69**, 608–613.

Dowling, A.M., Steele, J.R. and Baur, L.A. (2001) Does obesity influence foot structure and plantar pressure patterns in pre-pubescent children? *International Journal of Obesity* **25**, 845–852.

Dugdale, A.E. and Payne, P.R. (1976) Pattern of fat and lean deposition in children. *Nature* **256**, 725–727.

Ehtisham, S., Barrett, T.G. and Shaw, N.J. (2000) Type 2 diabetes mellitus in UK children—an emerging problem. *Diabetic Medicine* **17**, 867–871.

Epstein LH, Kuller LH, Wing RR, Valoski A, McCurley J (1989) The effect of weight control on lipid changes in obese children. *American Journal of Diseases in Childhood* **143**, 454–457.

Fagot-Campagna, A., Narayan, K.M.V. and Imperatore, G. (2001) Type 2 diabetes in children. *British Medical Journal* **322**, 377–378.

Field, A.E., Camargo, C.A., Taylor, C.B., Berkey, C.S., Frazier, A.L., Gillman, M.W. and Colditz, G.A. (1999) Overweight, weight concerns and bulimic behaviours among girls and boys. *Journal of the American Academy of Child and Adolescent Psychiatry* **38**, 754–760.

Freedman, D.S., Dietz, W.H., Srinivasan, S.R. and Berenson, G.S. (1999a) The relation of overweight to cardiovascular risk factors among children and adolescents: the Bogalusa Heart Study. *Pediatrics* **103**, 1175–1182.

Freedman, D.S., Serdula, M.K., Srinivasan, S.R. and Berenson, G.S. (1999b) Relation of circumferences and skinfold thicknesses to lipid and insulin concentrations in children and adolescents: the Bogalusa Heart Study. *American Journal of Clinical Nutrition* **69**, 308–317.

Freedman, D.S., Khan, L.K., Dietz, W.H., Srinivasan, S.R. and Berenson, G.S. (2001) Relationship of childhood obesity to coronary heart disease risk factors in adulthood: The Bogalusa Heart Study. *Pediatrics* **108**, 712–718.

French, S.A., Story, M. and Perry, C. (1995) Self-esteem and obesity in children and adolescents: A literature review. *Obesity Research* **3**, 479–490.

Friedman, M.A. and Brownell, K.D. (1995) Psychological correlates of obesity: moving to the next research generation. *Psychological Bulletin* **117**, 3–20.

Garn, S.M. and Clark, D.C. (1976) Trends in fatness and origins of obesity. *Pediatrics* **57**, 443–456.

Gillum, R.F. (1987) The association of the ratio of waist to hip girth with blood pressure, serum cholesterol and serum uric acid in children and youths aged 6–17 years. *Journal of Chronic Diseases* **40**, 413–420.

Gokbal, H. and Atas, S. (1999) Exercise-induced bronchospasm in nonasthmatic obese and non-obese boys. *Journal of Sports Medicine and Physical Fitness* 1999; **39**, 361–364.

Goodman, N., Richardson, S.A., Dornbusch, S.M. and Hastorf, A.H. (1963) Variant reactions to physical disabilities. *American Sociological Review* **28**, 429–435.

Gortmaker, S.L., Must, A., Perrin, J.M., Sobol, A.M. and Dietz, W.H. (1993) Social and economic consequences of overweight in adolescence and young adulthood. *New England Journal of Medicine* **329**, 1008–1012.

Guo, S.S., Chumlea, W.C., Roche, A.F. and Siervogel, R.M. (1998) Age and maturity related changes in body composition during adolescence into adulthood. The Fels Longitudinal Study. *Applied Radiation Isotopes* **49**, 581–585.

Guo, S.S., Huang, C., Maynard, L.M., Demerath, E., Towne, B., Chumlea, W.C. and Siervogel, R.M. (2000) Body mass index during childhood, adolescence and young adulthood in relation to adult overweight and adiposity: the Fels Longitudinal Study. *International Journal of Obesity and Related Metabolic Disorders* **24**, 1628–1635.

Guzzaloni, G., Grugni, G., Minocci, A., Moro, D. and Morabitio, F. (2000) Liver steatosis in juvenile obesity: correlations with lipid profile, hepatic biochemical parameters and glycemic and insulinemic responses to an oral glucose tolerance test. *International Journal of Obesity and Related Metabolic Disorders* **24**, 772–776.

Harris, S.B., Perkins, B.A. and Whalen-Brough, E. (1996) Non-insulin dependent diabetes mellitus among First Nations children: new entity among First Nations people of north-western Ontario. *Canadian Family Physician;* **42**, 869–876.

Harter, S. (1982) Developmental perspectives on the self-esteem. In: Karoly, P., Kanfer, F.H. eds. *Self-management and Behaviour Change: from Theory to Practice.* New York: Pergamon, 165–204.

Haymes, E.M., McCormick, R.J. Buskirk. (1975) Heat tolerance of exercising lean and obese prepubertal boys. *Journal of Applied Physiology* **39**, 457–461.

Higgins, P.B., Gower, B.A., Hunter, G.R. and Goran, M.I. (2001) Defining health-related obesity in children. *Obesity Research* **94**, 233–240.

Hill, A.J. and Oliver, S. (1992) Eating in the adult world: The rise of dieting in childhood and adolescence. *British Journal of Clinical Psychology* **31**, 95–105.

Hill, A.J. and Silver, E.K. (1995) Fat, friendless and unhealthy: 9 year old children's perception of body shape stereotypes. *International Journal of Obesity* **19**, 423–430.

Hill, A.J., Draper, E. and Stack, J. (1994) A weight on children's minds: body shape dissatisfactions at 9 years old. *International Journal of Obesity* **18**, 383–389.

Hills, A.P. and Parker, A.W. (1992) Locomotor characteristics of obese children. *Child Care, Health and Development* **18**, 29–34.

Hood, M.Y., Moore, L.L., Sundarajan-Ramamurti, A., Singer, M., Cupples, L.A. and Ellison, R.C. (2000) Parental eating attitudes and the development of obesity in children: The Framingham Children's Study. *International Journal of Obesity* **24**, 1319–1325.

Ibanez, L., de Zegher, F. and Potau, N. (1998) Premature pubarche, ovarian hyperandrogenism, hyperinsulinism and the polycystic ovary syndrome: from a complex constellation to a simple sequence of prenatal onset. *Journal of Endocrinological Investigation* **21**, 558–566.

Inselma, L.S., Milanese, A. and Deurloo, A. (1993) Effect of obesity on pulmonary function in childhood. *Pediatric Pulmonology* **16**, 130–137.

Jiang, X., Srinivasan, S.R., Webber, L.S., Wattigney, W.A. and Berenson, G.S. (1995) Association of fasting insulin level with serum lipid and lipoprotein levels in children, adolescents and young adults. *Archives of Internal Medicine* **155**, 190–196.

Kimm, S.Y., Barton, B.A., Berhane, K., Ross, J.W., Payne, G.H. and Schreiber, G.B. (1997) Self-esteem and adiposity in black and white girls: the NHLBI Growth and Health Study. *Annals of Epidemiology* **7**, 550–560.

Kitigawa, T., Owada, M., Urakami, T. and Yamauchi K. (1998) Increased incidence of non-insulin-dependent diabetes mellitus among Japanese school children correlates with an increased intake of animal protein and fat. *Clinical Pediatrics* **37**, 111–115.

Klesges, R.C., Haddock, C.K., Stein, R.J., Klesges, L.M., Eck, L.H. and Hanson, C.L. (1992) Relationship between psychosocial functioning and body fat in preschool children: a longitudinal investigation. *Journal of Consulting Clinical Psychology* **60**, 793–796.

Knip, M. and Nuutinen, O. (1993) Long-term effects of weight reduction on serum lipids and plasma insulin in obese children. *American Journal of Clinical Nutrition* **57**, 490–493.

Knittle, J.L., Timmers, K., Ginsberg-Fellner, F., Brown, R.E. and Katz, D.P. (1979) The growth of adipose tissue in children and adolescents: Cross-sectional and longitudinal studies of adipose cell number and size. *Journal of Clinical Investigation* **63**, 239–246.

von Kries, R., Hermann, M., Grunert, V.P. and von Mutius, E. (2001) Is obesity a risk factor for childhood asthma? *Allergy* **56**, 318–322.

Lawson, M.C. (1980) Development of body build stereotypes, peer rating and self esteem in Australian children. *Journal of Psychology* **104**, 111–118.

Lessell, S. (1992) Pediatric pseudotumor cerebri (idiopathic intracranial hypertension). *Survey of Ophthalmology* **37**, 155–166.

Lewy. V.D., Danadian, K., Witchel, S.F. and Arslanian, S. (2001) Early metabolic abnormalities in adolescent girls with polycystic ovarian syndrome. *Journal of Pediatrics* **138**, 38–44.

Lobe, T.E. and Schropp, K.P. (1993) Laparoscopic Nissen fundoplication in childhood. *Journal of Pediatric Surgery* **28**, 358–360.

Loder, R.T., Aronson, D.D. and Greenfield, M.L. (1993) The epidemiology of bilateral slipped capital epiphyses. A study of children in Michigan. *Journal of Bone and Joint Surgery of America* **75**, 1141–1147.

McCance, D.R., Pettit, D.J., Hanson, R.L., Jacobsson, L.T.H., Bennett, P.H. and Knowler, W.C. (1994) Glucose, insulin concentrations and obesity in childhood and adolescence as predictors of NIDDM. *Diabetologia* **37**, 617–623.

Magarey, A.M., Daniles, L.A., Boulton, T.J. and Cockington, R.A. (2003) Predicting obesity in early adulthood from childhood and parental obesity. *International Journal of Obesity* **27**, 505–513.

Mahoney, L.T., Burns, T.L. and Stanford, W. (1996) Coronary risk factors in childhood and young adult life are associated with coronary artery calcification in young adults : the Muscatine Study. *Journal of the American College of Cardiology* **27**, 277–284.

Marcus, C.L., Curtis, S., Koerner, C.B., Joffe, A., Serwint, J.R. and Loughlin, G.M. (1996) Evaluation of pulmonary function and polysomnography in obese children and adolescents. *Pediatric Pulmonology* **21**, 176–183.

Martini, G., Riva, P., Rabbia, F., Molini, V., Ferrero, G.B., Cerutti, F., Carra, R. and Veglio, F. (2001) Heart rate variability in childhood obesity. *Clinical Autonomy Research* **11**, 87–91.

Mellin, L.M., Slinkard, L.A. and Irwin, C.E. (1987) Adolescent obesity intervention: validation of the SHAPEDOWN program. *Journal of the American Dietetics Association* **87**, 333–338.

Monello, L.F. and Mayer, J. (1963) Obese adolescent girls. An unrecognised 'minority' group? *American Journal of Clinical Nutrition* **13**, 35–39.

Mosberg, H.-O. (1989) 40 year follow up of overweight children. *Lancet* **ii**: 491–493.

Must, A., Jacques, P.F., Dallal, G.E., Bajema, C.J. and Dietz, W.H. (1992) Long term morbidity and mortality of overweight adolescents. A follow up of the Harvard Growth Study. *New England Journal of Medicine* **327**, 1350–1355.

Mustillo, S., Worthman, C., Erkanli, A., Keeler, G., Angold, A. and Costello, E.J. (2003) Obesity and psychiatric disorder: developmental trajectories. *Pediatrics* **111**, 851–859.

Napolitano, C., Walsh, S., Mahoney, L. and McCrea, J. (2000) Risk factors that may adversely modify the natural history of the pediatric pronated foot. *Clinical Podiatric Medicine and Surgery* **17**, 397–417.

Nieto, F.J., Szklo, M. and Comstock, G.W. (1992) Childhood weight and growth rate as predictors of adult mortality. *American Journal of Epidemiology* **136**, 201–213.

O'Brien, R.W., Smith, S.A., Bush, P.J. and Peleg, E. (1990) Obesity, self-esteem and health locus of control in black youths during transition to adolescence. *American Journal of Health Promotion* **5**, 133–139.

Palasciano, G., Portincasa, P., Vinciguerra, V., Velardi, A., Tardi, S., Baldassarre, G. and Albano, O .(1989) Gallstone prevalence and gall bladder volume in children and adolescents: an epidemiological ultrasonographic survey and relationship to body mass index. *American Journal of Gastroenterology* **84**, 1378–1382.

Phillips, R.G. and Hill, A.J. (1998) Fat, plain, but not friendless: self-esteem and peer acceptance of pre-adolescent girls. *International Journal of Obesity and Related Disorders* **22**, 287–293.

Pierce, J.W. and Wardle, J. (1997) Cause and effect beliefs and self-esteem of overweight children. *Journal of Child Psychology and Psychiatry* **38**, 645–650.

Pinhas-Hamiel, O., Dolan, L.M., Daniles, S.R., Standiford, D., Khoury, P.R. and Zeitler, P. (1996) Increased incidence of non-insulin dependent diabetes mellitus among adolescents. *Journal of Pediatrics* **128**, 608–615.

Power, C., Lake, J.K. and Cole, T.J. (1997) Body mass index and height from childhood to adulthood in the 1958 British birth cohort. *American Journal of Clinical Nutrition* **66**, 1094–1101.

Probst, M., Braet, C., Vandereycken, W., De Vos, P., Van Coppenolle, H. and Verhofstadt-Deneve, L. (1995) Body size estimation in obese children: a controlled study with video distortion method. *International Journal of Obesity and Related Metabolic Disorders* **19**, 820–824.

Rashid, M. and Roberts, EA. (2000) Non-alcoholic steatohepatitis in children. *Journal of Pediatric Gastroenterology* **30**, 48–53.

Redline, S., Tishler, P.V., Schluchter, M., Aylor, J., Clark, K. and Graham, G. (1999) Risk factors for sleep-disordered breathing in children. Associations with obesity, race and respiratory problems. *American Journal of Respiratory and Critical Care Medicine* **159**, 1527–1532.

Rhodes, S.K., Shimoda, K.C., Waid, L.R., O'Neil, P.M., Oxeman, M.J., Collop, N.A. and Willi, S.M. (1995) Neurocognitive deficits in morbidly obese children with obstructive sleep apnea. *Journal of Pediatrics* **127**, 741–744.

Rocchini, A.P., Moorehead, C., Katch, V., Key, J. and Finta, K.M. (1992) Forearm resistance vessel abnormalities and insulin resistance in obese adolescents. *Hypertension* **19**, 615–620.

Rodriguez, M.A., Winkleby, M.A., Ahn, D., Sundquist, J. and Kraemer, H.C. (2002) Identification of population subgroups of children and adolescents with high asthma prevalence: findings from the Third National Health and Nutrition Examination Survey. *Archives of Pediatric and Adolescent Medicine* **156**, 269–275.

Rolland-Cachera, M.-F., Bellisle, F., Deheeger, M. Pequignot-Guggenbuhi, F. and Sempe, M. (1990) Influence of body fat distribution during childhood on body fat distribution in adulthood: a two decade follow up study. *International Journal of Obesity* **14**, 473–481.

Rosenfield, R.L., Ghai, K., Ehrmann, D.A. and Barnes, R.B. (2000) Diagnosis of the polycystic ovarian syndrome in adolescence: comparison of adolescent and adult hyperandrogenism. *Journal of Pediatric Endocrinology* **13** (Suppl. 5), 1285–1289.

Rosner, B., Prineas, R., Daniels, S.R. and Loggie, J. (2000) Blood pressure differences between blacks and whites in relation to body size among US children and adolescents. *American Journal of Epidemiology* **151**, 1007–1019.

Savva, S.C., Tornitis, M., Savva, M.E., Kourides, Y., Panagi, A., Silikiotou, N., Georgiou, C. and Kafatos, A. (2000) Waist circumference and waist to height ratio are better predictors of cardiovascular disease risk factors in children than body mass. *International Journal of Obesity* **24**, 1453–1458.

Sheu, H.M., Yu, H.S. and Chang, C.H. (1991) Mast cell degranulation and elastolysis in the early stage of striae distensae. *Journal of Cutaneous Pathology* **18**, 410–416.

Sinha, R., Fisch, G., Teague, B., Tamborlane, W.V., Banyas, B., Allen, K., Savoye, M., Rieger, V., Taksali, S., Barbetta, G., Sherwin, R.S. and Caprio, S. (2002) Impaired glucose tolerance among children and adolescents with marked obesity. *New England Journal of Medicine* **346**, 802–810.

Sorof, J. and Daniels, S. (2002) Obesity hypertension in children: a problem of epidemic proportions. *Hypertension* **40**, 441–447.

Soultan, Z., Wadowski, S., Rao, M., Kravath, R.E. (1999) Effect of treating obstructive sleep apnea by tonsillectomy and/or adenoidectomy in children. *Archives of Pediatric and Adolescent Medicine* **153**, 33–37.

Srinivasan, S.R., Myers, L. and Berenson, G.S. (2002) Predictability of childhood adiposity and insulin for developing insulin resistance syndrome (syndrome X) in young adulthood: the Bogalusa Heart Study. *Diabetes* **51**, 204–209.

Staffieri, J.R. (1967) A study of social stereotype of body image in children. *Journal of Personal and Social Psychology* **7**, 101–4.

Strauss, R.S. (2000) Childhood obesity and self esteem. *Pediatrics* **105**, e111.

Strauss, R.S., Rodzilsky, D., Burack, G. and Colin, M. (2001) Psychosocial correlates of physical activity in healthy children. *Archives of Pediatric and Adolescent Medicine* **155**, 897–902.

Stunkard, A.J., Harris, J.R., Pedersen, N.L. and McClearn, G.E. (1990) The body mass index of twins who have been reared apart. *New England Journal of Medicine* **322**, 1483–1487.

Thompson, G.H. and Carter, J.R. (1990) Late-onset tibia vara (Blount's disease). Current concepts. *Clinical Orthopaedics* **255**, 24–35.

Tounian, P., Aggoun, Y., Dubern, B., Varille, V., Guy-Grand, B., Sidi, D., Girardet, J.P. and Bonnet, D. (2001) Presence of increased stiffness in the common carotid artery and endothelial dysfunction in severely obese children: a prospective study *Lancet* **358**, 1400–1404.

Twisk, J.W.R., Kemper, H.C.G., van Mechelen, W. and Post, G.B. (1997) Which lifestyle parameters discriminate high- from low risk participants for coronary heart disease risk factors. Longitudinal analysis covering adolescence and young adulthood. *Journal of Cardiovascular Risk* **4**, 393–400.

van der Wal, J.S. and Thelen, M.H. (2000) Eating and body image concerns among obese and average-weight children. *Addictive Behaviour* **25**, 775–778.

Wake, M., Salmon, L., Waters, E., Wright, M. and Hesketh, K.I. (2002) Parent-reported health status of overweight and obese Australian primary school children: a cross-sectional population survey. *International Journal of Obesity* **26**, 717–724.

Wang, Y. (2002) Is obesity associated with early sexual maturation? A comparison of the association in American boys versus girls. *Pediatrics* **110**, 903–910.

Whitaker, R.C., Wright, J.A., Pepe, M.S., Seidel, K.D. and Dietz, W.H. (1997) Predicting obesity in young adulthood from childhood and parental obesity. *New England Journal of Medicine* **337**, 869–873.

Adult obesity

17 Adult obesity: metabolic syndrome, diabetes and non-alcoholic steatohepatitis

Shivani Dewan and John Wilding

Introduction, 251

Epidemiological associations, 252
Obesity, 252
Type 2 diabetes, 252
The importance of fat
distribution, 253
Metabolic syndrome, 253

Pathophysiological links between
obesity, type 2 diabetes and the
metabolic syndrome, 254
Insulin synthesis and secretion, 254
Metabolic effects of insulin, 255
Normal glucose homeostasis, 255

Pathogenesis of type 2 diabetes, 255

Insulin resistance, 256
Insulin resistance and metabolic
syndrome, 256
Insulin resistance and lipid
metabolism, 256
Insulin resistance and
hypertension, 257

Insulin resistance and
prothrombotic state, 257

How does obesity lead to insulin
resistance?, 257
Free fatty acids and the Randle
cycle, 257
Adipokines, 257
Systemic hormones and
neurotransmitters, 258

Does obesity lead to β-cell
dysfunction?, 258
Lipotoxicity, 259
Islet amyloid polypeptide, 259
Fetal malnutrition, 259

Drugs as a cause of weight gain
and type 2 diabetes, 259

Management of obesity in patients
with diabetes, 260

Benefits of weight loss, 260
Glycaemic control, 260

Blood pressure, 260
Lipids, 260

Treatment of obesity in diabetes, 261
Lifestyle modification, 261
Very low-calorie diets, 261
Physical activity and exercise, 261
Pharmacotherapy in the obese
diabetic patient, 261
Use of anti-obesity drugs in
diabetes, 262
Who should be offered
pharmacotherapy for weight loss
in diabetes?, 262
Other agents and the future, 263
Surgical treatment in morbidly
obese patients with type 2
diabetes, 263

Weight loss and diabetes
prevention, 263

Non-alcoholic fatty liver disease, 263

References, 264

Introduction

Associations have been recognized for centuries between obesity and diabetes — indeed, Hindu physicians of 1500 years ago described a syndrome affecting older overweight patients who passed large volumes of sweet-tasting urine. Type 2 diabetes may be the most important medical consequence of obesity because it is common, can adversely affect health in many ways and is expensive to manage.

Most of this chapter focuses on type 2 diabetes; however, it has become increasingly recognized that type 2 diabetes is often part of a more complex syndrome of insulin resistance, dyslipidaemia, hypertension and vascular dysfunction, together termed the *metabolic syndrome*. We shall first review the evidence that obesity leads to type 2 diabetes and then discuss in detail how an increased fat mass leads to an increased risk of diabetes and other features of the metabolic syndrome. Other mechanisms, including the effects of diabetogenic drugs, will also be discussed. Management of both type 1 and type 2 diabetes can be complicated by co-existing obesity, and present-day and future approaches, including the role of diet, physical activity, anti-obesity drugs and obesity surgery, will be described with specific reference to diabetes. The importance of weight loss in diabetes prevention has recently been highlighted following publication of the results from diabetes prevention trials, which will be discussed.

Finally, the syndrome of non-alcoholic fatty liver disease (NAFLD), which may lead to non-alcoholic steatohepatitis (NASH) and eventually cirrhosis, is becoming increasingly recognized. This syndrome shares many clinical features with obesity, insulin resistance and the metabolic syndrome, so it has been included in this chapter and its management is discussed.

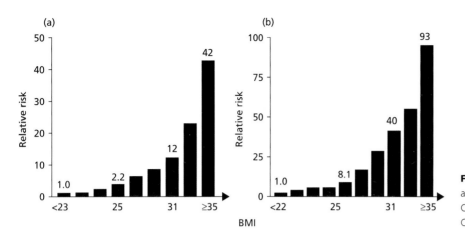

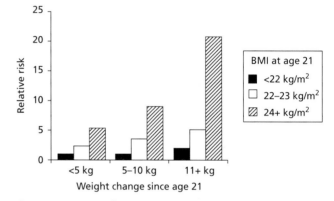

Fig 17.1 Relative risk of developing diabetes according to body mass BMI. (a) Data for men from Colditz *et al.* (1995). (b) Data for women from Chan *et al.* (1994).

Epidemiological associations

This section looks at the epidemiological associations of obesity, type 2 diabetes and the metabolic syndrome.

Obesity

Obesity has reached epidemic proportions globally, and all evidence suggests that the situation is likely to deteriorate (WHO, 1998). In the USA alone, more than 97 million adults are obese, and more than one-half of the population is overweight. Data from the third National Health and Nutrition Examination Survey (NHANES III: 1988–1994) showed that 20% of US men and 25% of US women are obese (Kuczmarski *et al.*, 1994). In England and Wales, the prevalence of obesity has increased in adults from 6% in men and 8% in women in 1980 to 21% of men and 23.5% of women in 2001. The Health Survey for England (2003) from 1993 to 2001 also reported an increase in the prevalence of obesity in older people. In 2001, 24.5% of men aged 65–74 years had a body mass index (BMI) >30 kg/m^2 compared with 15.2% in 1993. Likewise, in women the rise was seen from 21.5% in 1993 to 30.2% in 2001. It is this rise in obesity that appears to be the driving force behind the epidemic of type 2 diabetes at present.

Type 2 diabetes

Type 2 diabetes comprises about 70–90% of all cases of diabetes, approximately one-half of which are undiagnosed (Jervell, 1997). Coincident with the high rates of obesity, the prevalence of type 2 diabetes is also escalating and this increase is expected to continue, so that that by the year 2010 it is predicted that a total of 216 million people worldwide will have type 2 diabetes (Amos *et al.*, 1997). There is enormous variation in type 2 diabetes prevalence between populations, and especially populations who have changed from a traditional to a modern 'Westernized' lifestyle, for example

Fig 17.2 Importance of weight gain in adult life as a predictor of diabetes risk. (Data from Chan *et al.*, 1994.)

American Pima Indians, Micronesians, migrant Asian Indians, Mexican Americans and other Pacific Islanders (King and Rewers, 1993). The prevalence of type 2 diabetes ranges from zero in rural Melanesia (the highland population of Papua New Guinea) to 40% in Micronesians (Nauru) and more than 50% in the population of Pima Indians of the USA (King and Rewers, 1993). This variation in prevalence results from a combination of differences in genetic susceptibility, changes in diet, obesity, physical inactivity and, in certain situations, factors relating to intrauterine development.

Obesity and overweight have been closely associated with the development of type 2 diabetes in epidemiological surveys. For example both the nurses' health study and the physicians' health study in the USA showed an exponential relationship between BMI and the relative risk of developing type 2 diabetes (Chan *et al.*, 1994; Colditz *et al.*, 1995). The risk is increased two- to eightfold at a BMI of 25 (compared with a relative risk of 1 at BMI 22 kg/m^2), rising dramatically to 40- to 90-fold at a BMI above 35 kg/m^2 (Fig. 17.1). Weight gain in adult life appears to be a particularly important predictive factor, perhaps of greater importance than BMI itself (Fig. 17.2).

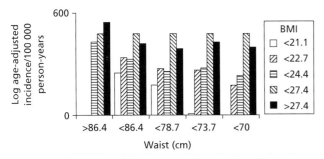

Fig 17.3 Role of abdominal obesity assessed by waist circumference in determining the risk for developing diabetes. (Data from Calle *et al.*, 1999.)

Table 17.1 Diagnostic criteria for the metabolic syndrome*.

Abdominal obesity [waist circumference > 102 cm (40 in) in men, > 88 cm (35 in) in women]
Hypertriglyceridaemia ≥ 1.7 mmol/L (150 mg/dL)
Low HDL-cholesterol [< 1.04 mmol/L (40 mg/dL) in men, < 1.3 mmol/L (50 mg/dL) in women]
High blood pressure (≥ 130/85 mmHg)
High fasting glucose [IGT – blood sugar ≥ 6.1 mmol/L (110 mg/dL)]

*The presence of three or more of these factors defines a subject as having metabolic syndrome.

The increased prevalence of type 2 diabetes in obese and overweight subjects is also dependent upon ethnicity. For example, the prevalence of diabetes associated with an increase in desirable body weight from 100% to > 140% is higher among Mexican Americans than amon African Americans and European Americans in the USA (Fujimoto, 1996). The risk for Asian populations is also greater at a lower BMI, to the extent that cut-off levels for obesity have recently been redefined in these populations, largely as a result of the strong associations with diabetes and the metabolic syndrome (WHO, 2000).

The importance of fat distribution

Although obesity is traditionally defined by the presence of excessive total body fat, the pattern of body fat distribution seems to be particularly important in terms of diabetes risk. Vague (1956) first described the association with diabetes of 'android' (upper body or truncal) obesity characterized by distribution of subcutaneous and visceral fat around the abdomen. Central adiposity is an important clue to the presence of insulin resistance and hyperinsulinaemia. By contrast, 'gynoid' obesity in the gluteofemoral region is only weakly associated with insulin resistance. Although most epidemiological surveys have only used BMI as a predictor of diabetes risk, there is also good evidence that subjects with central adiposity, as assessed by measurements of waist circumference or waist–hip ratio (WHR), are at greater risk of type 2 diabetes, cardiovascular disease (CVD) and stroke, independently of the risk associated with a raised BMI (Fig. 17.3) (Lapidus *et al.*, 1984; Larsson *et al.*, 1984; Ohlson *et al.*, 1985; Calle *et al.*, 1999). A waist circumference above 104 cm (40 in) for men and above 88 cm (35 in) for women indicates abdominal obesity/visceral obesity. A healthy WHR is considered to be < 0.95 for men and < 0.80 for women (National Institute of Health, 1998; Despres *et al.*, 2001).

Metabolic syndrome

The metabolic syndrome (syndrome X, insulin resistance syndrome) describes a cluster of metabolic alterations associated with excess body weight. The typical abnormalities include impaired glucose tolerance, upper body obesity, dyslipidaemia, insulin resistance, hypertension, coagulation abnormalities, hyperuricaemia and polycystic ovary syndrome in women. The Third Report of the National Cholesterol Education Program Expert Panel on Detection, Evaluation and Treatment of High Blood Cholesterol in Adults (Adult Treatment Panel III [ATP III]) has defined individuals with the metabolic syndrome as having three or more of the criteria listed in Table 17.1 (ATP III, 2001).

Insulin resistance has been proposed to be the underlying feature that links all the manifestations of metabolic syndrome. Much research in the last 10 years or so has focused on the features and complications of the syndrome (Reaven, 1988; Zavaroni *et al.*, 1999).

The hallmarks of the metabolic syndrome include increased body weight and waist circumference (abdominal obesity), raised fasting or postprandial blood glucose concentrations (glucose intolerance), an adverse lipid profile, including high blood triglyceride levels and low concentrations of HDL-cholesterol, and increased blood pressure (hypertension). The common underlying element linking these adverse risk factors for progression of atherosclerosis appears to be insulin resistance (Reaven, 2001).

The prevalence of metabolic syndrome is increasing. Approximately 47 million Americans (including 10–15 million individuals with type 2 diabetes), or about 1 : 4 adults, have the metabolic syndrome (Ford *et al.*, 2002). As the US population ages and becomes more obese, the prevalence of metabolic syndrome is likely to increase steadily. As with diabetes, ethnicity is also an important factor when considering the risk of developing the metabolic syndrome. African-American women have an approximately 57% higher prevalence than men, and Hispanic women have a 26% higher prevalence than men (Ford *et al.*, 2002). High rates are also seen in some Asian populations (Das, 2002).

Of the 23% of men and women in the USA with metabolic syndrome, approximately 50% showed evidence of insulin resistance (Ford *et al.*, 2002). Therefore being overweight and obese is associated with insulin resistance and a cluster of

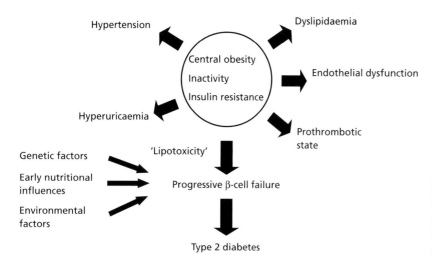

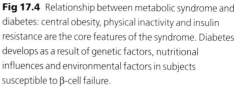

Fig 17.4 Relationship between metabolic syndrome and diabetes: central obesity, physical inactivity and insulin resistance are the core features of the syndrome. Diabetes develops as a result of genetic factors, nutritional influences and environmental factors in subjects susceptible to β-cell failure.

metabolic disorders, including type 2 diabetes (Fig. 17.4). This is important in terms of disease risk, particularly as the metabolic syndrome is associated with a greater risk of developing complications of atherosclerosis, such as myocardial infarction, peripheral vascular disease and stroke.

Overall, these data indicate that obesity, (especially truncal) is associated with an increased risk of type 2 diabetes and the metabolic syndrome. However, it is important to remember that this does not prove a causative link. Many obese subjects will not develop type 2 diabetes or complications of the metabolic syndrome: other factors, both inherited (such as β-cell reserve) and acquired (such as physical activity levels), determine whether or not an individual will develop these conditions.

Pathophysiological links between obesity, type 2 diabetes and the metabolic syndrome

This section will first review normal glucose metabolism, with reference to the key role of insulin, and then focus on abnormalities found in type 2 diabetes and the metabolic syndrome, reviewing some of the key research that supports a pathophysiological link between obesity, type 2 diabetes and risk of vascular disease.

Insulin synthesis and secretion

Insulin is synthesized and secreted by the β-cells of the islets of Langerhans. The precursor of insulin in the β-cells is the single chain preproinsulin. During insulin synthesis, a 24-amino-acid signal sequence is first cleaved from preproinsulin by a peptidase yielding proinsulin. Proinsulin splits releasing equimolar amounts of insulin and C-peptide. Basal insulin secretion in healthy subjects is pulsatile in nature, with a cycle

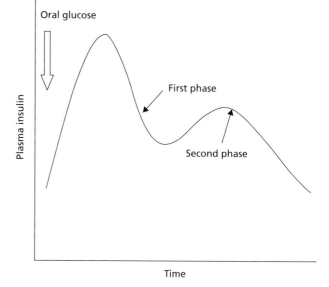

Fig 17.5 Insulin secretion.

of 8–9 min. During a meal, insulin is released from the pancreatic β-cell in response to increased concentrations of glucose and amino acids. Already before glucose is absorbed, various signals lead to insulin release. These include vagal nerve activation during swallowing, and release of glucagon-like peptide 1 (7–36) amide (GLP-1) and gastric inhibitory polypeptide (GIP) upon contact of the duodenum with food (Creutzfeldt and Nauck, 1992). An identical amount of glucose given by mouth elicits about twice as much insulin release as when given intravenously, which underlines the physiological importance of these mechanisms. Insulin release after a meal is biphasic, with an initial peak followed by a trough, and a second, later peak (Fig. 17.5).

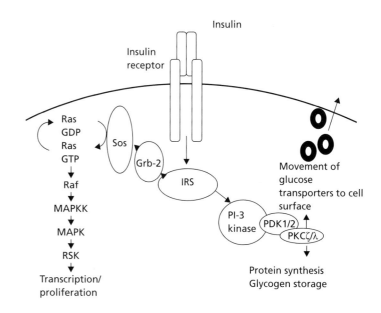

Fig 17.6 The effects of insulin on intracellular biochemical pathways that mediate insulin signalling.

Metabolic effects of insulin

Insulin acts on three main target tissues—the liver, muscle and adipose tissue. As the first step in its action insulin binds to a four-subunit protein membrane receptor. The β-subunit of the receptor contains a transmembrane protein with an adenosine triphosphate (ATP) binding site and has latent tyrosine kinase activity. Binding of insulin to the receptor activates tyrosine kinase that can phosphorylate other proteins such as the insulin receptor substrate (IRS-1). IRS-1 generates a cascade of signals within the target cell, which affect glucose transport, glycogen synthesis and many other key metabolic processes in lipid and protein metabolism (Fig. 17.6).

Normal glucose homeostasis

The plasma glucose concentration reflects the balance between intake (glucose absorption from the gut), tissue utilization (glycolysis, pentose phosphate pathway, TCA cycle, glycogen synthesis) and endogenous production (glycogenolysis and gluconeogenesis). Glucose homeostasis entails an intricate interplay of various mechanisms, which can be divided into glucose-elevating and glucose-lowering mechanisms, for which the liver plays a central role (Gerich, 1993). The liver normally contains a large amount of carbohydrate in the form of glycogen, and is capable of converting glucose into glycogen and of converting glycogen back into glucose. Moreover, the liver is equipped with the machinery of gluconeogenesis.

Insulin will rapidly diminish hepatic gluconeogenesis and glycogen breakdown, even at low plasma insulin levels. After an overnight fast, plasma insulin levels are sufficient to keep hepatic glucose production at about one-third of its maximum capacity (DeFronzo, 1988). In the liver, insulin stimulates glycogen synthesis and also promotes the synthesis of long chain fatty acids. The lipids are then packaged into very low-density lipoproteins (VLDL), which are secreted into the blood. In adipose tissue, insulin induces lipoprotein lipase, an enzyme that 'offloads' triglycerides by hydrolysing them into glycerol and fatty acids in adipose tissue. At the higher plasma insulin levels seen after a meal, insulin will also stimulate muscle and adipocyte glucose uptake, by activating glucose transporter-4 (GLUT-4) (Kahn, 1992). In muscle, insulin increases glucose transport, glucose metabolism and glycogen synthesis. Insulin also increases cellular uptake of amino acids and stimulates protein synthesis in many tissues (Fig. 17.7).

Pathogenesis of type 2 diabetes

Hyperglycaemia in type 2 diabetes results from a malfunction of the inter-relationship between insulin secretion and insulin action; it is characterized by both β-cell dysfunction and insulin resistance (Bergman, 1989; Kahn and Porte, 1996). The β-cells of the islets of Langerhans act as glucose sensors to maintain a balance between hepatic glucose production and the rate of insulin-dependent utilization of glucose by muscle and adipose tissue. When islet β-cell function is impaired, insulin secretion is inadequate. Consequently, hepatic glucose production increases and this increase correlates directly with the degree of fasting hyperglycaemia.

There has been much debate as to whether insulin resistance is the primary defect that precedes β-cell failure in the evolution of hyperglycaemia in type 2 diabetes or vice versa. The initial idea that insulin resistance could be the primary defect (Himsworth and Kerr, 1939), whereas β-cell dysfunction was a late phenomenon due to exhaustion after years of compensatory hypersecretion (DeFronzo, 1988; Reaven, 1995) has been challenged by accumulating evidence from cross-sectional

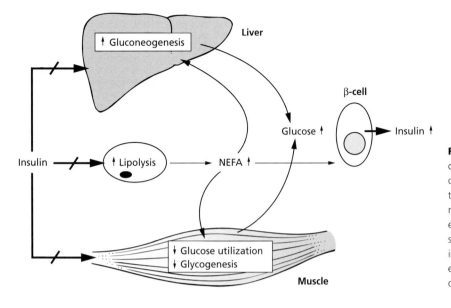

Fig 17.7 Effects of insulin resistance on lipid and carbohydrate metabolism. Insulin resistance leads to decreased glucose uptake into skeletal muscle and thus to hyperglycaemia. Lipolysis is disinhibited, resulting in increased NEFA levels, which may further exacerbate insulin resistance. Insulin secretion is stimulated by hyperglycaemia and increased NEFAs; initially insulin resistance can be overcome, but eventually β-cell failure supervenes, leading to diabetes.

and longitudinal studies examining β-cell function and insulin sensitivity, suggesting that impaired β-cell function is necessary for the development of type 2 diabetes (Gerich, 1998; Kahn, 2001; Pratley and Weyer, 2001).

The UKPDS (UK Prospective Diabetes Study Group, 1995) evaluation of β-cell function using the homeostasis model assessment (HOMA) indicated that β-cell function was already reduced by 50% at diagnosis, and there was subsequent further deterioration regardless of therapy. Commonly found defects in β-cell function include reduced or absent first-phase insulin responses to intravenous glucose, delayed responses to ingestion of mixed meals, decreased pulsatile and oscillatory insulin release, increased release of proinsulin-like molecules and impaired ability to compensate for superimposed tissue insulin resistance (Brunzell *et al.*, 1976; Polonsky *et al.*, 1996). Second-phase insulin release may also be reduced.

Normally there is a curvilinear hyperbolic relationship between β-cell function and insulin sensitivity, so that as insulin sensitivity decreases, β-cell function increases in a compensatory fashion to maintain normal glucose (Bergman *et al.*, 1981). People who develop impaired glucose tolerance (IGT) and progress to type 2 diabetes fall off this curve owing to an inability of β-cells to compensate for insulin resistance.

Insulin resistance

Insulin resistance can be defined as the inability of the insulin to produce its usual biological actions at circulating concentrations that are effective in normal subjects. Insulin resistance in the context of glucose metabolism is characterized by an inability of insulin to lower plasma glucose levels through suppression of hepatic glucose production and stimulation of glucose utilization in skeletal muscle and adipose tissue. Both

inherited and acquired influences contribute to the development of insulin resistance. Mutations in insulin receptors, glucose transporters and signalling proteins have been identified but these are relatively rare. The acquired causes of insulin resistance include obesity, reduced physical activity, hyperglycaemia, ageing, increased levels of free fatty acids (FFA), glucocorticoids and other drugs, pregnancy and smoking.

Insulin resistance and metabolic syndrome

Insulin resistance is viewed as a common denominator for the various components of the metabolic syndrome. A clustering of risk factors, including elevated triglycerides, decreased HDL-cholesterol, hypertension and hyperinsulinaemia, is often observed in patients who are found to be insulin resistant. However, although obese patients with metabolic syndrome are frequently insulin resistant, not all individuals with obesity and insulin resistance develop the metabolic syndrome.

Insulin resistance and lipid metabolism

There is growing evidence that hypertriglyceridaemia is a marker for increased risk of coronary artery disease (Austin, 1991). This is particularly the case if it is associated with visceral obesity (Despres *et al.*, 2001). The lipid triad consists of elevated serum triglycerides, small LDL particles and low HDL-cholesterol. These abnormalities appear to be caused by the insulin-resistant state itself rather than by elevated insulin concentrations or obesity. Insulin resistance impairs lipoprotein lipase. Increased FFA flux induces accumulation of triglycerides and VLDL particles in the liver. Thus, reduced lipoprotein lipase activity and excessive liver output of triglycerides results in elevated plasma triglyceride concentrations. Cholesterol ester transfer proteins (CETPs) mediate exchange of triglycerides for cholesterol esters with LDL and HDL, resulting in accumulation of triglycerides and loss of cholesterol esters content in LDL and HDL, thus explaining the lowering of HDL-cholesterol levels and small dense LDL particles (see Chapter 12).

Insulin resistance and hypertension

Elevated blood pressure is commonly associated with other risk factors of the metabolic syndrome (Reaven *et al.*, 1996). However, there is some dispute whether hypertension is the product of the insulin resistance state. Several possible mechanisms have been proposed. Insulin resistance has been shown to enhance sympathetic adrenergic activity (Reaven *et al.*, 1996), and to upregulate angiotensin II receptors by a post-translational mechanism (Nickenig *et al.*, 1998). Recent studies have shown that stress activates the hypothalamic–pituitary–adrenal axis (HPA) and sympathetic nervous system. Thus, it is suggested that metabolic syndrome results from HPA activation, and that hypertension develops as a consequence of sympathetic nervous system activation, which is amplified by insulin and leptin (Chrousos and Gold, 1992; Ljung *et al.*, 2000). An alternative (but not mutually exclusive) hypothesis is that sodium retention associated with impaired vasodilatation also predisposes to blood pressure elevation in insulin resistance.

Insulin resistance and prothrombotic state

A prothrombotic state predisposes to atherosclerotic plaque formation and cardiovascular events. The link between a pro-thrombotic state and other metabolic risk factors is not clearly understood. Possibly, overloading of the liver with lipids in patients with insulin resistance may stimulate the synthesis of various coagulation factors. The observation that increased plasma plasminogen activator inhibitor 1 (PAI-1) levels were associated with insulin resistance and atherothrombosis added for the first time a pathological basis for an association of the insulin resistance syndrome not only with metabolic, atherosclerotic risk but also with atherothrombotic risk (Shimomura *et al.*, 1996).

How does obesity lead to insulin resistance?

The mechanisms whereby increased adipose tissue mass results in a reduction in insulin action in adipose tissue and at other sites, especially skeletal muscle and liver are becoming better understood. It is now clear that multiple factors are involved, including metabolic factors, principally free fatty acids, local production of adipocyte hormones, collectively known as adipokines, and effects mediated by altered secretions and action of systemic hormones and neurotransmitters, such as cortisol and noradrenaline. This section will describe how these factors are altered in obesity and how these changes result in insulin resistance.

Free fatty acids and the Randle cycle

A rise in adipose tissue mass is associated with an increase in circulating free fatty acids; the large adipocytes typical of obesity secrete greater quantities of free fatty acids (Weyer *et al.*, 2000). High concentrations of free fatty acids have been shown to inhibit glucose metabolism in muscle *in vitro* and *in vivo*, but the precise mechanisms have not been fully elucidated. The concept of substrate competition between FFA and glucose metabolism to explain this effect was proposed by Randle *et al.* (1963), but the original description has now been refined, and it appears that there are many points at which this could occur (reviewed in Boden and Shulman, 2002). One possibility is that reduced sensitivity to insulin's effects on skeletal muscle is due to inhibition of glucose transport or its phosphorylation by hexokinase, thus reducing the amount of glucose being metabolized by the glycolytic pathway, and also reducing glycogen synthesis. Most experimental evidence now points towards the defect being in glucose transport, rather than hexokinase activity (Cline *et al.*, 1999; Dresner *et al.*, 1999). An alternative explanation is that FFA directly interfere with insulin signalling, perhaps via PKCθ, resulting in reduced IRS-1 tyrosine phosphorylation (Griffin *et al.*, 1999). The net result is that muscle selectively uses more FFA to generate ATP and reduces the ability of insulin to promote glucose uptake. In liver, the effect of raised FFA is to promote both gluconeogenesis and glycogenolysis, resulting in an increase in hepatic glucose production for a given concentration of insulin. In uncomplicated obesity, this insulin resistance is compensated for by increased insulin secretion, so circulating glucose concentrations remain normal, but hyperglycaemia develops if there is a co-existing defect in insulin secretion (Fig. 17.8).

Adipokines

Recent years have seen rapid advances in our understanding of the adipocyte as an endocrine organ; many of these hormonal products have been found to influence insulin sensitivity in experimental animal models, and there is increasing evidence that some may also be important in humans. Tumour necrosis factor alpha (TNF-α) was one of the first adipokines to be identified that also caused insulin resistance. TNF-α may act in part by interfering with phosphorylation of the insulin receptor, thus reducing insulin action directly (Hotamisligil *et al.*, 1993). Its production is increased in animal models of obesity and insulin resistance, such as the Zucker fatty rat, and treatment of these animals with antibodies to TNF-α improves insulin resistance (Hotamisligil and Spiegelman, 1994).

Plasma concentrations are also increased in humans with obesity and type 2 diabetes (Miyazaki *et al.*, 2003). Resistin was

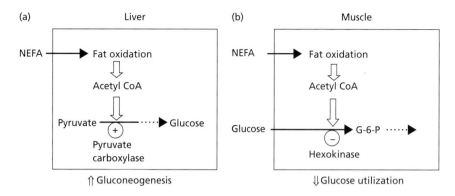

Fig 17.8 The Randle cycle in liver (a) and muscle (b). CoA, coenzyme A; NEFA, non-esterified fatty acids.

recently identified as an adipocyte product—initial reports based on work in rodents suggested that it might be an important mediator of insulin resistance, as resistin expression is related to fat mass, and administration of resistin impaired insulin action in mice (Steppan *et al.*, 2001). However, circulating resistin concentrations are low in humans, casting some doubt on its pathophysiological role in insulin resistance (Ukkola, 2002).

Adiponectin has also attracted recent interest; this peptide is inversely related to insulin resistance—concentrations fall as fat mass increases, and it has also been found to improve insulin action experimentally. It is also of note that polymorphisms of the adiponectin gene have been associated with insulin resistance and type 2 diabetes in some human populations (Weyer *et al.*, 2001; Hara *et al.*, 2002). Adiponectin may also protect against the vascular dysfunction that is frequently present in association with insulin resistance, as it has been found to inhibit cell adhesion and other pro-inflammatory processes in vessel walls (Okamoto *et al.*, 2000).

Leptin may also play a role, as leptin has been shown to directly stimulate fat oxidation in skeletal muscle, probably through stimulation of α-AMP kinase, which reduces the activity of acetyl CoA carboxylase, leading to preferential use of lipid as a metabolic fuel (Minokoshi and Kahn, 2003). Other adipocyte products such as interleukins 1 and 6 may also have indirect effects on insulin action, but at present the evidence that they are major players in the process is less convincing.

Systemic hormones and neurotransmitters

Increased circulating levels of cortisol, due to activation of the hypothalamic–pituitary–adrenal (HPA) axis have long been recognized to be present in obesity, and the association of hypercortisolaemia with insulin resistance and diabetes is well known (Bjorntorp, 1995). It is less clear whether the subtle abnormalities play a significant role in causing insulin resistance in obese subjects, but recent work demonstrating increased activity of 11β-hydroxysteroid dehydrogenase in omental adipocytes, thus enhancing steroid action in this

tissue is of some interest (Bujalska *et al.*, 1997). Despite insulin resistance in peripheral tissues, other sites, notably the central nervous system, appear to remain insulin sensitive in obesity.

The hyperinsulinaemia of insulin resistance may thus result in an exaggerated response to insulin at these protected sites. One of the effects of this is an increase in sympathetic nervous system activity, which is thought to be one mechanism that explains the increase in blood pressure seen in obesity (Anderson *et al.*, 1991; Reaven *et al.*, 1996). It is less widely appreciated, however, that this might also contribute to insulin resistance in skeletal muscle, and an increase in hepatic glucose production, thus tending to increase circulating glucose and stimulate further insulin secretion (Koopmans *et al.*, 1998). Hyperleptinaemia may also contribute to increased sympathetic nervous system (SNS) activity in these circumstances.

Does obesity lead to β-cell dysfunction?

As long as insulin resistance is compensated for by increased insulin secretion then obese subjects will remain euglycaemic. It is only when β-cell failure supervenes that glucose tolerance becomes impaired, eventually leading to diabetes. This raises the important question as to whether obesity itself is a factor in the development of β-cell failure, or whether the processes of insulin resistance and β-cell dysfunction develop as a result of different pathological processes. As with the pathophysiology of insulin resistance, the processes described here are not mutually exclusive, and it is likely that a combination of factors is involved.

One of the earliest abnormalities of insulin secretion seen in obesity is a loss of the first phase of insulin secretion; this is also associated with loss of the usual pulsatility of insulin secretion and an increase in the release of split pro-insulin products. This suggests disruption of the usually tightly regulated patterns of insulin secretion, which heralds a progressive decline in all β-cell functions. Evidence from the UKPDS study suggests that β-cell reserve is already reduced to 50% of normal at the time of diagnosis of diabetes (Holman, 1998).

Table 17.2 Drugs associated with weight gain.

Class	Examples
Anticonvulsants	Sodium valproate, phenytoin, gabapentin
Antidepressants	Citalopram, mirtazepine
Antipsychotics	Chlorpromazine, risperidone*, olanzepine*
Beta-blockers	Atenolol
Corticosteroids	Prednisolone*, dexamethasone*
Insulin	All formulations
Sex steroids	Medroxyprogesterone acetate, progesterone, combined oral contraceptives
Oral hypoglycaemic drugs	Glibenclamide, gliclazide, repaglinide, rosiglitazone, pioglitazone
Antiretroviral drugs	Indinavir*, ritonavir*, didanosine*

Those marked with an asterisk have also been associated with increased diabetes risk.

Lipotoxicity

Evidence from animal models of type 2 diabetes, particularly those due to deficiency or resistance to the fat-derived hormone, leptin, such as the *db/db* mouse and OLETF rat, shows that triglyceride becomes deposited within the islets, particularly in β-cells (Man *et al.*, 1997). It is suggested that this can result in metabolic changes that reduce glucose responsiveness, and that high concentrations of oxidized lipid may promote an inflammatory response involving nitric oxide and free radical production, ultimately leading to β-cell apoptosis. This is supported by experimental data showing that when lipotoxicity is reduced using a thiazolidinedione drug, nitric oxide production and apoptotic rates fall (Pickavance *et al.*, 2003). In humans, the response to an acute lipid infusion is an initial increase in insulin secretion, but this response is lost with prolonged elevation of non-esterified fatty acid (NEFA), giving additional weight to the possibility that raised NEFA contributes to loss of β-cell function (Carpentier *et al.*, 1999).

Islet amyloid polypeptide

Islet amyloid polypeptide (IAPP), also known as amylin, was identified as the principal component of islet amyloid, a frequent finding in islets of subjects with type 2 diabetes. IAPP is a peptide product of the β-cell that is co-secreted with insulin. Although IAPP has been reported to have a number of effects as a circulating hormone, including effects on gastric emptying, its main role appears to be as an autocrine regulator of insulin secretion. Accumulation of IAPP as amyloid fibrils appears to occur as a consequence of increased insulin secretion, and might contribute to the progressive development of β-cell dysfunction that is characteristic of type 2 diabetes (Marzban *et al.*, 2003).

Fetal malnutrition

The observation that infants of low birth weight have a greater risk of developing diabetes in later life has led to the suggestion that early influences may affect β-cell reserve and other metabolic factors that might predipose to insulin resistance and diabetes (Hales and Barker, 1992). This remains a controversial area, and evidence at present makes it difficult to precisely define the magnitude of this effect (see Chapter 7).

Drugs as a cause of weight gain and type 2 diabetes

When considering the causes of obesity and type 2 diabetes, it is important that iatrogenic causes are not forgotten. A large number of drugs (Table 17.2) have been shown to cause weight gain, and some of these have also been found to contribute to insulin resistance and other metabolic abnormalities that might predispose to the metabolic syndrome and type 2 diabetes. The potential role of glucocorticoids has already been discussed above, as the doses necessary to treat inflammatory and other disease are often diabetogenic. Another group of drugs that deserves special mention are drugs used to treat psychiatric disease, particularly the so-called 'atypical' antipsychotic drugs, such as olanzapine and risperidone. A number of case reports have highlighted the fact that use of these agents may precipitate uncontrolled diabetes, sometimes with ketoacidosis, both in subjects with known diabetes and in previously undiagnosed patients (Wirshing *et al.*, 1998). These have been supported by surveys showing a higher than expected prevalence of diabetes in patients taking such agents (Kornegay *et al.*, 2002). The mechanisms underlying this association seem complex. They may include an effect to increase food intake and thus weight gain, exacerbating insulin resistance, but may also include inhibitory effects on β-cell function (Baptista *et al.*, 2002).

Protease inhibitors and nucleoside reverse transcriptase inhibitors used to treat HIV infection have been associated with alterations in fat distribution, notably an increase in central adiposity and loss of subcutaneous fat from the face, arms and legs. This lipodystrophy has also been associated with an increase in insulin resistance, dyslipidaemia and a greater risk of diabetes (Galli *et al.*, 2001). With prolonged survival now becoming commonplace in HIV infection, the problem of long-term adverse metabolic effects of this drug-induced lipodystrophy is becoming increasingly recognized; such patients should be assessed for cardiovascular and diabetes risk, and counselled and treated appropriately (Justman *et al.*, 2003).

In general it is important to avoid using potentially diabetogenic drugs in obese patients, or drugs that might cause weight gain in patients with diabetes, particularly if they are already obese. Alternatives are frequently available, and health professionals should be aware of this issue, and be prepared to adapt their usual prescribing when appropriate.

Management of obesity in patients with diabetes

Most patients with type 2 diabetes are significantly overweight; around 80–90% are obese (National Diabetes Data Group, 1985). Promoting weight loss in people with type 2 diabetes is proposed as the cornerstone of therapy, yet is one of the most difficult goals to accomplish in patient management. Weight loss of as little as 5–10% will improve glucose control, reduce blood pressure and improve lipid profiles, thereby being of particular benefit to people with diabetes. There is also the likelihood that improvement or elimination of other obesity-related comorbid conditions such as cardiovascular disease, stroke, sleep apnoea and certain types of cancer (such as colon, rectum, breast and gall bladder) can be achieved if sustained weight loss can be achieved (National Institute of Health, 1998; Lean *et al.*, 1999).

This section focuses on different therapeutic strategies in the management of obesity in patients with diabetes. Lifestyle modifications using a hypocaloric diet and exercise are considered the primary objective. This may need to be followed by use of antiobesity drugs or drugs that reduce insulin resistance, treating commonly associated risk factors such as hypertension and dyslipidaemia. In case of morbid obesity, bariatric surgery plays a major role.

Benefits of weight loss

The benefits of weight loss are detailed below.

Glycaemic control

Several studies have demonstrated that many patients with type 2 diabetes who achieve substantial weight loss can discontinue oral hypoglycaemic medication or insulin therapy (Pi-Sunyer, 1993a). A behavioural study conducted by Wing

and colleagues (1987a) using intensified dietetic and lifestyle measures showed that a 10% initial weight loss could improve glycaemic control (Dattilo and Kris-Etherton, 1992). In the same study patients who achieved more than 14 kg of weight loss had near normalization of HBA_c levels with reduction in blood pressure and improvement in insulin sensitivity and dyslipidaemia. However, it should be noted that the proportion of patients who achieve these goals is low, and there are few data on long-term effects beyond about 12 months.

A 32-week study also undertaken by Wing and colleagues (1994) has shown that improvement in measures of glycaemic control associated with weight loss can be enhanced when weight loss is achieved through extreme calorie restriction (400 cal per day). In an effort to determine how much weight loss is required to achieve fasting plasma glucose of <6.0 mmol/L, the UKPDS (UK Prospective Diabetes Study Group, 1990) showed that a 10-kg weight loss (16% of ideal body weight) was necessary if individuals had initial fasting plasma glucose of 6–8 mmol/L compared with a weight loss of 26 kg (41%) if initial blood glucose was more than 14 mmol/L.

Blood pressure

Patients with type 2 diabetes are frequently also hypertensive, and lowering of blood pressure to < 140/80 mmHg is an important treatment target. Most of the studies on the benefits of weight loss on blood pressure have been conducted in people without diabetes. A meta-analysis by MacMohan *et al.* (1987) showed the benefits of dietary intervention on blood pressure. Weight loss of 9.2 kg in hypertensive patients resulted in a reduction of 6.3 mmHg systolic and 3.1 mmHg diastolic blood pressure compared with control subjects (MacMohan *et al.*, 1987). This reduction in blood pressure was demonstrated regardless of sodium intake (Maxwell *et al.*, 1984). In the Dietary Intervention Study in Hypertension (DISH) and Hypertension Control Program (HCP), overweight patients with controlled hypertension were withdrawn from antihypertensive drug treatment. Subsequent modest weight loss by diet therapy resulted in a significant reduction in redevelopment of hypertension after 1 year (Langford *et al.*, 1985; Stamler *et al.*, 1987). For non-hypertensive obese subjects, weight loss is a very effective way to prevent hypertension (Cutler, 1991); according to this study, each kilogram of weight loss results in an approximately 0.45 mmHg reduction in diastolic blood pressure. It is disappointing that there is remarkably little published information on the effects of dietary-induced weight loss on blood pressure in people with diabetes.

Lipids

Modest weight loss induced by either dieting or exercise is associated with an increase in HDL-cholesterol and reduction in LDL-cholesterol. Serum triglycerides are also reduced (Pi-Sunyer, 1993b; National Institute of Health, 1998). A meta-analysis by Dattilo and Kris-Etherton (1992) showed that weight reduction was associated with significant decrease in LDL and VLDL-cholesterol and increase in HDL by 0.0007 mmol/L for every kilogram of weight loss. Early data from the UKPDS clearly demonstrated the beneficial effects of dietary change and weight loss on plasma lipids in the short term (Manley *et al.*, 2000).

Treatment of obesity in diabetes

The following approaches are considered in the treatment of diabetes.

Lifestyle modification

Weight loss is a key therapeutic objective. Even modest weight reductions in the range of 5–10% of initial body weight are associated with significant clinical improvements in a wide range of comorbid conditions (Wing *et al.*, 1987a; Goldstein, 1992). Successful weight loss requires that more energy be expended than is consumed over a period of time. Patients need to modify their dietary intake to achieve a decrease in energy intake while maintaining a nutritionally adequate diet. The target of a weight loss programme should initially be to decrease body weight by 10% (National Institute of Health, 1998; WHO, 1998). However, even a 5% weight reduction improves risk factors and risk of comorbidities. Several factors should be taken into consideration, for example the patient's risk factors, degree of obesity, previous attempts at weight loss and personal and social capacity to undertake lifestyle changes. Changes in lifestyle may be encouraged by using communications and counselling skills to promote behavioural change; it should be remembered that some patients may not be motivated to lose weight—it is therefore important to assess 'readiness to change' before giving detailed advice about lifestyle changes.

The first step in dietary therapy is an estimate of patient's actual energy requirements and to recommend a diet with a defined energy deficit. This can be estimated from self-reported 3- to 7-day food diaries, but under-reporting is quite common; energy expenditure can be accurately estimated using formulas based on body weight, height, age, sex and physical activity levels (Lean and James, 1986) (see Chapter 9). A deficit of 300–500 kcal/day will produce a weight loss of 300–500 g/week, and a deficit of 500–1000 kcal/day will produce a weight loss of 500–1000 g/week (National Institute of Health, 1998). It is important to encourage patients to move away from a 'Western' diet to a diet centred on fruits, vegetables, whole grains, fish and poultry. Limiting dietary fat equal to or less than 30% of total calories can help patients reduce energy intake and achieve weight loss. There has been recent controversy as to whether this degree of fat restriction is necessary, and it may be possible to

achieve significant improvements in risk factors and weight loss by substituting saturated fats with mono- and polyunsaturated fats, particularly those containing fish oils (omega-3 polyunsaturated fatty acids, PUFAs), provided that the total energy intake is also reduced (Reaven, 2003). Increasing the proportion of low glycaemic index foods may also help metabolic control, but is unlikely to influence weight loss (Brand-Miller and Foster-Powell, 1999).

Very low-calorie diets

Very low-calorie diets (VLCDs) are defined as diets of 400–800 kcal/day. They can be helpful in achieving weight loss goals in obese persons with type 2 diabetes and improving glycaemic control independent of weight loss (Wing, 1995). VLCDs are usually recommended for persons who are 30% or more above their ideal body weight (National Task Force on the Prevention and Treatment of Obesity, 1993). They can induce rapid weight loss over a 2- to 3-month period but they do not seem to facilitate weight maintenance.

VLCDs are mainly used to replace one or two meals per day. Their use is contraindicated in renal disease, cerebrovascular disease and type 1 diabetes because of the potential risk of ketosis and hypoglycaemia. However, when used with carefully selected persons and appropriate medical monitoring VLCDs appear to be relatively safe (Wadden *et al.*, 1983). Therefore they are mainly reserved for the induction of a medically indicated rapid weight loss in patients with BMI > 40 kg/m^2, for example prior to surgery or for the rapid improvement of comorbidities and glycaemic control.

Physical activity and exercise

Regular exercise improves body weight, plasma lipids, blood pressure, insulin sensitivity and glucose tolerance. It also maintains general fitness, balance, mobility and sense of well-being. WHO guidelines state that moderate exercise such as brisk walking for 30–60 min three or four times per week is beneficial and easier to maintain. The general consensus at the International Association for the Study of Obesity, May 2002, was that 30 min of moderate exercise intensity activity daily, preferably all days of the week, is of importance for limiting health risks for coronary heart disease and diabetes. However, prevention of weight gain in formerly obese individuals requires 60–90 min of moderate intensity activity (Saris *et al.*, 2003).

Pharmacotherapy in the obese diabetic patient

When treating patients with type 2 diabetes it is important to consider whether the drugs prescribed, particularly those used to treat hyperglycaemia and hypertension, may predispose to weight gain and thus compromise attempts to improve glycaemic control and other risk factors. This is one reason why metformin is considered the first-line pharmacological treatment for hyperglycaemia in overweight and obese patients with type 2 diabetes, and is supported by positive benefits on complication rates, including macrovascular disease seen in UKPDS (1998). α-Glucosidase inhibitors such as acarbose are also weight neutral, and are worthy of consideration, although gastrointestinal tolerability can be a significant problem (Holman *et al.*, 1999). When prescribing agents that might predispose to weight gain, such as sulphonylureas, thiazolidinediones and insulin, it is important to discuss this with patients, and consider specific additional dietary input at that time.

Combination therapy is often now used in patients who require insulin; combining metformin and insulin has the particular advantage that weight gain is significantly attenuated and glycaemic control improved. Thiazolidinediones are worthy of a particular mention, because although they cause weight gain, with an increase in adipose tissue mass, the amount of visceral adipose tissue is decreased, which may partly explain how they improve insulin sensitivity (Kelly *et al.*, 1999). When treating hypertension, the use of beta-blockers may also cause modest weight gain, although it is important to note that atenolol showed similar efficacy in terms of reduction in complications in the UKPDS study (1999).

Use of anti-obesity drugs in diabetes

The evidence base for using pharmacotherapy specifically targeted to produce weight loss as an adjunct to diet and physical activity for patients with type 2 diabetes is steadily growing. The two drugs that are licensed at present for long-term use (up to 2 years) are *orlistat* and *sibutramine*. The pharmacology of these and other drugs that produce weight loss is described in detail in Chapter 25.

Orlistat is an inhibitor of intestinal lipases, which produces weight loss via fat malabsorption. The main side-effects are GI related, and due to an increase in fat in the stool. Orlistat has been evaluated in combination with sulphonylureas, metformin and insulin in studies of up to 12 months' duration. In general, weight loss is greater with orlistat than with placebo, although the degree of weight loss is less than that seen in studies of non-diabetic patients, consistent with the observation that subjects with type 2 diabetes find it more difficult to lose weight than people without the condition (Wing *et al.*, 1987b). Despite a modest placebo-subtracted weight loss of about 2–3 kg in these studies, about twice as many patients (50% of the total) achieved a weight loss of 5% or greater, and this was associated with significant improvements in glycaemic control (HbA_{1c} falls of about 0.5%), blood pressure and improved lipid profiles (Hollander *et al.*, 1998; Miles *et al.*, 2001) (Fig. 17.9).

Sibutramine is a centrally acting serotonin and noradrenaline reuptake inhibitor; it is thought to cause weight loss by increasing satiety after meals, and by increasing thermogenesis.

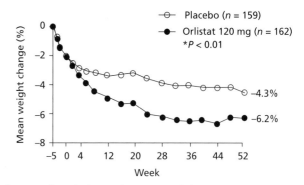

Fig 17.9 Effect of orlistat in the treatment of obese patients with type 2 diabetes on sulphonylurea medication. After 1 year of treatment, the orlistat group lost 6.2% of initial body weight vs. 4.3% in the placebo group.

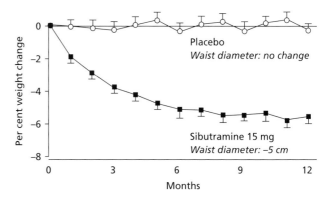

Fig 17.10 Sibutramine in the management of obese patients with type 2 diabetes treated with metformin. Sibutramine induced significant weight loss with 15 mg/day (6% of initial body weight at 12 months), whereas placebo did not.

It can cause dry mouth, constipation, difficulty sleeping, and also results in a modest rise in pulse and in some patients, blood pressure. It has been evaluated in patients with type 2 diabetes treated with diet alone, sulphonylureas or metformin in studies of 6–12 months' duration. The placebo-subtracted weight loss in these studies was in the range of 4–5 kg, with 2.5–3 times as many patients than placebo losing 5% of body weight (Serrano-Rios *et al.*, 2002; McNulty *et al.*, 2003) (Fig. 17.10). This was associated with improvements in HbA_{1c} of 0.5%, with greater falls in those who lost 10% of body weight or more. Lipid profiles were improved; notably triglycerides fell by up to 20% and HDL-cholesterol increased by about 10%. These benefits were partly offset by small increases in blood pressure, and the contraindication in subjects with established cardiovascular disease and uncontrolled hypertension may limit its use in the diabetic population.

Who should be offered pharmacotherapy for weight loss in diabetes?

Pharmacotherapy available at present, as described above, is likely to benefit a significant proportion of obese patients with type 2 diabetes, but translating these trial results into clinical practice is difficult. Furthermore, the lack of long-term outcome data is a barrier to widespread adoption given the costs of such treatment. Pharmacotherapy should be considered in those patients who are motivated to enter a weight loss programme, where such facilities exist, and only used within the terms of the product licence. Drugs should not be continued long term in patients who obtain no weight loss benefit, although it may be reasonable to allow diabetic patients longer than 3 months to achieve a 5% weight loss, given the difficulty these patients have in losing weight.

Other agents and the future

Other drugs for obesity, such as phentermine, are only licensed for short-term use, and there is no evidence of their effectiveness in patients with diabetes, so it is not possible to recommend their use. Many other drugs, including cannabinoid receptor antagonists, cholecystokinin, GLP-1 analogues and the anticonvulsants zonisamide and topiramate are undergoing clinical trials, and may yet expand the range of drugs available to treat the obese diabetic patient.

Surgical treatment in morbidly obese patients with type 2 diabetes

A recent survey in a diabetic clinic in Liverpool, UK, indicated that 8% of patients with type 2 diabetes had morbid obesity (BMI > 40 kg/m^2), compared with only 1–2% expected in the population; such patients are rarely included in clinical trials of pharmacotherapy, so it is worth considering what is the best treatment for such individuals. Surgical approaches to obesity management are becoming increasingly sophisticated and are now much safer than previously (see Chapter 26), with many procedures carried out laparoscopically. Furthermore, there is now increasing evidence that they may be a very effective treatment for morbidly obese patients with type 2 diabetes. For example, in a retrospective series of nearly 800 patients treated with a Roux-en-Y gastric bypass, one-quarter of whom had type 2 diabetes, over two-thirds of the diabetic patients were normoglycaemic and off treatment after up to 14 years of follow-up (Pories *et al.*, 1995). Unfortunately there are no prospective data on surgical treatment of morbidly obese patients with diabetes, or comparisons with medical treatment, but this option should certainly be seriously considered for such patients.

Weight loss and diabetes prevention

There is overwhelming evidence from dietary, pharmacological and surgical studies of weight loss that the onset of type 2 diabetes can be substantially delayed, and sometimes prevented by weight loss in susceptible subjects with impaired glucose tolerance. Two studies of dietary, exercise and behavioural intervention, the Finnish and the American diabetes prevention studies both demonstrated that a weight loss of about 7%, maintained for 4–6 years, reduced the incidence of new diabetes by 58% in subjects with IGT (Tuomilheto *et al.*, 2001; Diabetes Prevention Program Research Group, 2002). Interestingly, the lifestyle programmes were more effective than metformin, which only reduced diabetes by 30%. A 4-year study with orlistat, the XENDOS study, included over 3000 patients, 21% of whom had IGT, and showed an additional 37% reduction over and above that of lifestyle intervention (Anon, 2002). In the Swedish Obese Subjects study of surgery for morbid obesity, after 2 years the incidence of new-onset diabetes was 6.5% in the control group, compared with less than 0.5% in the intervention group, a 16-fold relative risk reduction (Sjöstrom *et al.*, 1999). These findings appear to persist for up to 10 years following surgery. The challenge is how to put these important findings into practice. Large-scale screening for glucose intolerance has been considered, but given that it is likely to affect 20–30% of the population screened, this is unlikely to be adopted. More targeted screening and intervention might be appropriate, but the ideal strategy is yet to be devised. It is also unlikely that the resources will be available to deliver the intensity of intervention used in the DPP study, so more general, population-based approaches seem more likely to be used. Specific interventions, such as drug treatment and surgery, might be used in those individuals deemed to be at greatest risk.

Non-alcoholic fatty liver disease

Non-alcoholic fatty liver disease (NAFLD) is a generic term used to describe a spectrum of pathological changes that may occur in the liver in association with obesity and insulin resistance. It is recognized that a spectrum of changes may be present, ranging in severity from a simple 'fatty liver', through to a hepatitic-type picture, or non-alcoholic steatohepatitis (Fig. 17.11), to a more complex picture with fibrosis and, ultimately, cirrhosis (reviewed by Day, 2002). At present there is nothing to distinguish the changes seen in the liver in association with NAFLD from those seen with alcohol excess; it is therefore important to exclude an alcoholic aetiology and other causes of chronic liver disease (such as viral hepatitis or haemochromatosis) when assessing such patients. Patients may present with isolated increases in hepatic enzymes, often as an incidental finding (particularly a raised AST) or with more severe forms of the disease, such as cirrhosis. The evidence linking obesity to the presence of NAFLD is now becoming stronger: most patients are obese, and the incidence appears to be rising together with that of obesity; one survey in patients undergoing surgery for morbid obesity suggested that 25% of such patients have NASH (Dixon *et al.*, 2001). Patients are nearly always insulin resistant, and some go on to

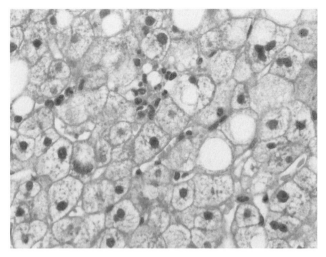

Fig 17.11 Macrovesicular steatosis with foci of hepatitis where the hepatocytes are surrounded by neutrophills. The appearances are consistent with non alcoholic steatohepatitis (NASH). Haematoxylin and eosin stain, magnification X350. Image courtesy of Dr Mustafa Haqqani, University Hospital Aintree, Liverpool.

develop type 2 diabetes (Comert *et al.*, 2001). It is presently unclear what leads up to 25% of subjects to progress to fibrosis and cirrhosis, whereas the majority follow a relatively benign course; increases in adipose tissue and gut-derived cytokines, notably TNF-α have been implicated in precipitating fibrosis and progression of disease, possibly by activating pathways of oxidative stress; genetically determined responses, including polymorphisms in liver enzymes, may determine the ultimate response to these stressors but, given a strong enough stimulus (such as that seen following jejuno-ileal bypass), most subjects will develop NASH (de Knegt, 2001).

Obese patients with clinically significant persistent elevations in liver enzymes (greater than two times the upper limit of normal) therefore warrant investigation to exclude other forms of liver disease, and possibly a liver biopsy to determine prognosis and help decide whether treatment is indicated. Most treatments at present have been tried on an empirical basis, and there is only limited evidence to support their use. Metformin has been used in a number of small trials with good effect (Nair *et al.*, 2002; Urso and Visco-Comandini, 2002); early reports also suggest that thiazolidinediones, such as rosiglitazone and pioglitazone, may also be of benefit (Neuschwander-Tetri *et al.*, 2003). Probucol, a lipid lowering agent with antioxidant properties, has been shown to lower ALT in one study (Merat *et al.*, 2003). Most authorities support modest, gradual weight loss (Sasaki *et al.*, 2003); diets high in fat, such as the Atkins diet, and approaches that result in rapid weight loss, such as the use of VLCDs or bariatric surgery, should probably be avoided. One small study has suggested that orlistat is effective; this has the theoretical advantage of reducing lipid supply to the liver (Assy *et al.*, 2001). Other suggestions, not yet subjected to randomized trials, might be use of anti-bodies to TNF-α, or use of antioxidants, to delay or prevent the progression to fibrosis.

References

Amos, A.F., McCarty, D.J. and Zimmet, P. (1997) The rising global burden of diabetes and its complications: estimates and projections to the year 2010. *Diabetic Medicine* **14**, (Suppl.), S1–85.

Anderson, E.A., Hoffman, R.F., Balon, T.W., Sinkey, C.A. and Mark, A.L. (1991) Hyperinsulinaemia produces both sympathetic neural activation and vasodilation in normal humans. *Journal of Clinical Investigation* **87**, 2246–2252.

Anon. (2002) Xendos study: Orlistat plus diet prevents, delays diabetes onset in obese patients. *Formulary* **37**, 504.

Assy, N., Svalb, S. and Hussein, O. (2001) Orlistat (Xenical) reverse fatty liver disease and improve hepatic fibrosis in obese patients with NASH. *Hepatology* **34**, 1146.

ATP III (2001) Adult Treatment Panel III. Executive Summary of the Third Report of the National Cholesterol Education Program (NCEP) Expert Panel on Detection, Evaluation, and Treatment of High Blood Cholesterol in Adults. *Journal of the American Medical Association* **285**, 2486–2497.

Austin, M.A. (1991) Plasma triglyceride and coronary heart disease. *Arteriosclerosis and Thrombosis* **11**, 2–14.

Baptista, T., Kin, N.M.K.N., Beaulieu, S. and de Baptista, E.A. (2002) Obesity and related metabolic abnormalities during antipsychotic drug administration: Mechanisms, management and research perspectives. *Pharmacopsychiatry* **35**, 205–219.

Bergman, R.N. (1989) Lilly lecture 1989. Toward physiological understanding of glucose tolerance. Minimal-model approach. *Diabetes* **38**, 1512–1527.

Bergman, R.N., Phillips, L.S. and Cobelli, C. (1981) Physiologic evaluation of factors controlling glucose tolerance in man: measurement of insulin sensitivity and beta-cell glucose sensitivity from the response to intravenous glucose. *Journal of Clinical Investigation* **68**, 1456–1467.

Bjorntorp, P. (1995) Endocrine abnormalities of obesity. *Metabolism* **44**, 21–23.

Boden, G. and Shulman, G.I. (2002) Free fatty acids in obesity and type 2 diabetes: defining their role in the development of insulin resistance and beta-cell dysfunction. *European Journal of Clinical Investigation* **32**, 14–23.

Brand-Miller, J.C. and Foster-Powell, K. (1999) Diets with a low glycaemic index: from theory to practice. *Nutrition Today* **34**, 64–72.

Brunzell, J.D., Robertson, R.P., Lerner, R.L., Hazzard, W.R., Ensinck, J.W., Bierman, E.L. and Porte, Jr, D. (1976) Relationships between fasting plasma glucose levels and insulin secretion during intravenous glucose tolerance tests. *Journal of Clinical Endocrinology and Metabolism* **42**, 222–229.

Bujalska, I.J., Kumar, S. and Stewart, P.M. (1997) Does central obesity reflect 'Cushing's disease of the omentum'? *Lancet* **349**, 1210–1213.

Calle, E.E., Thun, M.J. and Petrelli, J.M. (1999) Body mass index and mortality in a prospective cohort of obese adults. *New England Journal of Medicine* **341**, 1097–1105.

Carpentier, A., Mittelman, S.D., Lamarche, B., Bergman, R.N., Giacca,

A. and Lewis, G.F. (1999) Acute enhancement of insulin secretion by FFA in humans is lost with prolonged FFA elevation. *American Journal of Physiology, Endocrinology and Metabolism* **276**, E1055–E1066.

Chan, J.M., Stampfer, M.J., Ribb, E.B., Willett, W.C. and Colditz, G.A. (1994) Obesity, fat distribution and weight gain as risk factors for clinical diabetes in man. *Diabetes Care* **17**, 961–969.

Chrousos, G.P. and Gold, P.W. (1992) The concepts of stress and stress system disorders. Overview of physical and behavioral homeostasis. *Journal of the American Medical Association* **267**, 1244–1252.

Cline, G.W., Petersen, K.F., Krssak, M., Shen, J., Hundal, R.S., Trajanoski, Z., Inzucchi, S., Dresner, A., Rothman, D.L. and Shulman, G.I. (1999) Impaired glucose transport as a cause of decreased insulin- stimulated muscle glycogen synthesis in type 2 diabetes. *New England Journal of Medicine* **341**, 240–246.

Colditz, G.A., Willett, W.C., Rotnitzky, A. and Manson, J.E. (1995) Weight-gain as a risk factor for clinical diabetes-mellitus in women. *Annals of Internal Medicine* **122**, 481–486.

Comert, B., Mas, M.R., Erdem, H., Dinc, A., Saglamkaya, U., Cigerim, M., Kuzhan, O., Unal, T. and Kocabalkan, F. (2001) Insulin resistance in non-alcoholic steatohepatitis. *Digestive and Liver Disease* **33**, 353–358.

Creutzfeldt, W. and Nauck, M. (1992) Gut hormones and diabetes mellitus. *Diabetes Metabolic Review* **8**, 149–177.

Cutler, J. (1991) Randomised clinical trials of weight reduction in non hypertensive persons. *Annals of Epidemiology* **1**, 363–370.

Das, U.N. (2002) Metabolic syndrome X is common in South Asians, but why and how? *Nutrition* **18**, 774–776.

Dattilo, A.M. and Kris-Etherton, P.M. (1992) Effects of weight reduction on blood lipids and lipoproteins: a meta-analysis. *American Journal of Clinical Nutrition* **56**, 320–328.

Day, C.P. (2002) Non-alcoholic steatohepatitis (NASH): where are we now and where are we going? *Gut* **50**, 585–588.

DeFronzo, R. (1988) The triumvirate: β cell, muscle, liver. A collusion responsible for NIDDM. *Diabetes* **37**, 667–687.

Despres, J.P., Lemieux, I. and Prud'homme, D. (2001) Treatment of obesity: need to focus on high risk abdominally obese patients. *British Medical Journal* **322**, 716–720.

Diabetes Prevention Program Research Group (2002) Reduction in the incidence of type 2 diabetes with lifestyle intervention or metformin. *New England Journal of Medicine* **346**, 393–403.

Dixon, J.B., Bhathal, P.S. and O'Brien, P.E. (2001) Non-alcoholic fatty liver disease: Predictors of non-alcoholic steatohepatitis and liver fibrosis in the severely obese. *Gastroenterology* **121**, 91–100.

Dresner, A., Laurent, D., Marcucci, M., Griffin, M.E., Dufour, S., Cline, G.W., Slezak, L.A., Andersen, D.K., Hundal, R.S., Rothman, D.L., Petersen, K.F. and Shulman, G.I. (1999) Effects of free fatty acids on glucose transport and IRS-1-associated phosphatidylinositol 3-kinase activity. *Journal of Clinical Investigation* **103**, 253–259.

Ford, E.S., Giles, W.H. and Dietz, W.H. (2002) Prevalence of the metabolic syndrome among US adults: findings from the third National Health and Nutrition Examination Survey. *Journal of the American Medical Association* **287**, 356–359.

Fujimoto, W.Y. (1996) Overview of non-insulin-dependent diabetes mellitus (NIDDM) in different populations. *Diabetic Medicine* **13**, (Suppl.) S7–S10.

Galli, M., Ridolfo, A.L. and Gervasoni, C. (2001) Cardiovascular disease risk factors in HIV-infected patients in the HAART era.

HIV-Associated Cardiovascular Disease: Clinical and Biological Insights **946**, 200–213.

Gerich, J. (1993) Control of glycaemia. *Baillière's Clinical Endocrinology and Metabolism* **7**, 551–556.

Gerich, J. (1998) The genetic basis of type 2 diabetes mellitus: impaired insulin secretion versus impaired insulin sensitivity. *Endocrinology Review* **19**, 491–503.

Goldstein, D.J. (1992) Beneficial health effects of modest weight loss. *International Journal of Obesity and Related Metabolic Disorders* **16**, 397–415.

Griffin, M.E., Marcucci, M.J., Cline, G.W., Bell, K., Barucci, N., Lee, D., Goodyear, L.J., Kraegen, E.W., White, M.F. and Shulman, G.I. (1999) Free fatty acid-induced insulin resistance is associated with activation of protein kinase C theta and alterations in the insulin signaling cascade. *Diabetes* **48**, 1270–1274.

Hales, C.N. and Barker, D.J.P. (1992) Type 2 (non-insulin dependent) diabetes mellitus: the thrifty phenotype hypothesis. *Diabetologia* **35**, 595–601.

Hara, K., Boutin, P., Mori, Y., Tobe, K., Dina, C., Yasuda, K., Yamauchi, T., Otabe, S., Okada, T., Eto, K., Kadowaki, H., Hagura, R., Akanuma, Y., Yazaki, Y., Nagai, R., Taniyama, M., Matsubara, K., Yoda, M., Nakano, Y., Kimura, S., Tomita, M., Kimura, S., Ito, C., Froguel, P. and Kadowaki, T. (2002) Genetic variation in the gene encoding adiponectin is associated with an increased risk of type 2 diabetes in the Japanese population. *Diabetes* **51**, 536–540.

Himsworth, H. and Kerr, R. (1939) Insulin-sensitive and insulin-insensitive types of diabetes mellitus. *Clinical Science* **4**, 119–152.

Hollander, P.A., Elbein, S.C., Hirsch, I.B., Kelley, D., McGill, J., Taylor, T., Weiss, S.R., Crockett, S.E., Kaplan, R.A., Comstock, J., Lucas, C.P., Lodewick, P.A., Canovatchel, W., Chung, J. and Hauptman, J. (1998) Role of orlistat in the treatment of obese patients with type 2 diabetes: A 1-year randomized double-blind study. *Diabetes Care* **21**, 1288–1294.

Holman, R.R. (1998) Assessing the potential for alpha-glucosidase inhibitors in prediabetic states. *Diabetes Research and Clinical Practice* **40**, S21–S25.

Holman, R.R., Cull, C.A. and Turner, R.C. (1999) A randomized double-blind trial of acarbose in type 2 diabetes shows improved glycemic control over 3 years (UK Prospective Diabetes Study 44). *Diabetes Care* **22**, 960–964.

Hotamisligil, G.S. and Spiegelman, B.M. (1994) Tumor-necrosis-factor alpha — a key component of the obesity–diabetes link. *Diabetes* **43**, 1271–1278.

Hotamisligil, G.S., Shargill, N.S. and Spiegelman, B.M. (1993) Adipose expression of tumor-necrosis-factor alpha — direct role in obesity-linked insulin resistance. *Science* **259**, 87–91.

Jervell, J. (1997) Type 2 diabetes (NIDDM) can be prevented. *IDF Bulletin* **42**, 1–3.

Justman, J.E., Benning, L., Danoff, A., Minkoff, H., Levine, A., Greenblatt, R.M., Weber, K., Piessens, E., Robison, E. and Anastos, K. (2003) Protease inhibitor use and the incidence of diabetes mellitus in a large cohort of HIV-infected women. *Journal of Acquired Immune Deficiency Syndromes* **32**, 298–302.

Kahn, B. (1992) Facilitative glucose transporters: regulatory mechanisms and dysregulation in diabetes. *Journal of Clinical Investigation* **89**, 1367–1374.

Kahn, S. (2001) The importance of β-cell failure in the development and progression of type 2 diabetes. *Journal of Clinical Endocrinology and Metabolism* **86**, 4047–4058.

Kahn, S.E. and Porte, Jr, D. (1996) The pathophysiology of type II (non insulin-dependent diabetes mellitus): implications for treatment. In: Porte, Jr, D. and Sherwin, R.S. eds. *Diabetes Mellitus*. New York: Elsevier, 487–512.

Kelly, I.E., Han, T.S., Walsh, K. and Lean, M.E.J. (1999) Effects of a thiazolidinedione compound on body fat and fat distribution of patients with type 2 diabetes. *Diabetes Care* **22**, 288–293.

King, H. and Rewers, M. (1993) Diabetes in adults is now a Third World problem. World Health Organization Ad Hoc Diabetes Reporting Group. *Ethnic Disease* **3** (Suppl.), S67–S74.

de Knegt, R.J. (2001) Non-alcoholic steatohepatitis: Clinical significance and pathogenesis. *Scandinavian Journal of Gastroenterology* **36**, 88–92.

Koopmans, S.J., Leighton, B. and DeFronzo, R.A. (1998) Neonatal de-afferentation of capsaicin-sensitive sensory nerves increases insulin sensitivity in conscious adult rats. *Diabetologia* **41**, 813–820.

Kornegay, C.J., Vasilakis-Scaramozza, C. and Jick, H. (2002) Incident diabetes associated with antipsychotic use in the United Kingdom General Practice Research Database. *Journal of Clinical Psychiatry* **63**, 758–762.

Kuczmarski, R.J., Flegal, K.M., Campbell, S.M. and Johnson, C.L. (1994) Increasing prevalence of overweight among US adults. The National Health and Nutrition Examination Surveys (1960 to 1991). *Journal of the American Medical Association* **272**, 205–211.

Langford, M.G., Blaufox, M.D., Oberman, A., Hawkins, C.M., Curb, J.D., Cutter, G.R., Wassertheilsmoller, S., Pressel, S., Babcock, C., Abernethy, J.D., Hotchkiss, J. and Tyler, M. (1985) Dietary therapy slows the return of hypertension after stopping prolonged medication. *Journal of the American Medical Association* **253**, 657–664.

Lapidus, L., Bengtsson, C., Larsson, B., Rybo, E. and Sjöström, L. (1984) Distribution of adipose tissue and risk of cardiovascular disease and death: a 12 year follow up of participants in the population study of women in Gothenberg, Sweden. *British Medical Journal* **289**, 1257–1261.

Larsson, B., Svardsudd, K., Welin, L., Wilhelmsen, L., Bjorntorp, P. and Tibblin, G. (1984) Abdominal adipose tissue distribution, obesity, and risk of cardiovascular disease and death: 13 year follow up of participants in the study of men born in 1913. *British Medical Journal* **288**, 1401–1404.

Lean, M.E.J. and James, W.P.T. (1986) Presription of diabetic diets in the 1980s. *Lancet* **1**, 723–725.

Lean, M.E., Han, T.S. and Seidell, J.C. (1999) Impairment of health and quality of life using new US federal guidelines for the identification of obesity. *Archives of Internal Medicine* **159**, 837–843.

Ljung, T., Holm, G., Friberg, P., Andersson, B., Bengtsson, B.A., Svensson, J., Dallman, M., McEwen, B. and Bjorntorp, P. (2000) The activity of the hypothalamic-pituitary-adrenal axis and the sympathetic nervous system in relation to waist/hip circumference ratio in men. *Obesity Research* **8**, 487–495.

MacMohan, S., Cutler, J., Brittain, E. and Higgin, M. (1987) Obesity and hypertension: epidemiological and clinical issues. *European Heart Journal* **8** (Suppl. B), 57S–70S.

McNulty, S.J., Ur, E. and Williams, G. (2003) A randomized trial of sibutramine in the management of obese type 2 diabetic patients treated with metformin. *Diabetes Care* **26**, 125–131.

Man, Z.W., Zhu, M., Noma, Y., Toide, K., Sato, T., Asahi, Y., Hirashima, T., Mori, S., Kawano, K., Mizuno, A., Sano, T. and Shima, K. (1997) Impaired beta-cell function and deposition of fat droplets in the pancreas as a consequence of hypertriglyceridemia in OLETF rat, a model of spontaneous NIDDM. *Diabetes* **46**, 1718–1724.

Manley, S.E., Stratton, I.M., Cull, C.A., Frighi, V., Eeley, E.A., Matthews, D.R., Holman, R.R., Turner, R.C. and Neil, H.A. (2000) Effects of three months' diet after diagnosis of Type 2 diabetes on plasma lipids and lipoproteins (UKPDS 45). UK Prospective Diabetes Study Group. *Diabetic Medicine* **17**, 518–523.

Marzban, L., Park, K. and Verchere, C.B. (2003) Islet amyloid polypeptide and type 2 diabetes. *Experimental Gerontology* **38**, 347–351.

Maxwell, H., Kushiro, T., Dornfield, L.P., Tuck, M.L. and Waks, A.U. (1984) Blood pressure changes in obese hypertensive subjects during rapid weight loss; comparison of restricted versus unchanged salt intake. *Archives of Internal Medicine* **144**, 1581–1584.

Merat, S., Malekzadeh, R., Sohrabi, M.R., Sotoudeh, M., Rakhshani, N., Sohrabpour, A.A. and Naserimoghadam, S. (2003) Probucol in the treatment of non-alcoholic steatohepatitis: a double-blind randomized controlled study. *Journal of Hepatology* **38**, 414–418.

Miles, J.M., Aronne, L.J., Hollander, P. and Klein, S. (2001) Effect of orlistat in overweight and obese type 2 diabetes patients treated with metformin. *Diabetes* **50**, A442–A443.

Minokoshi, Y. and Kahn, B.B. (2003) Role of AMP-activated protein kinase in leptin-induced fatty acid oxidation in muscle. *Biochemical Society Transactions* **31**, 196–201.

Miyazaki, Y., Pipek, R., Mandarino, L.J. and DeFronzo, R.A. (2003) Tumor necrosis factor alpha and insulin resistance in obese type 2 diabetic patients. *International Journal of Obesity* **27**, 88–94.

Nair, S., Diehl, A.M. and Perrillo, R. (2002) Metformin in non alcoholic steatohepatitis (NASH): Efficacy and safety: A preliminary report. *Gastroenterology* **122**, 4.

National Diabetes Data Group. (1985) *Diabetes in America*. Bethesda, MD: US Department of Health and Human Services.

National Institute of Health. (1998) Clinical guidelines on the identification, evaluation, and treatment of overweight and obesity in adults: the evidence report. *Obesity Research* **6** (Suppl.), 51S–209S.

National Task Force on the Prevention and Treatment of Obesity. (1993) Very low-calorie diets. *Journal of the American Medical Association* **270**, 967–974.

Neuschwander-Tetri, B.A., Brunt, E.M., Wehmeier, K.R., Sponseller, C.A., Hampton, K. and Bacon, B.R. (2003) Interim results of a pilot study demonstrating the early effects of the PPAR-gamma ligand rosiglitazone on insulin sensitivity, aminotransferases, hepatic steatosis and body weight in patients with non-alcoholic steatohepatitis. *Journal of Hepatology* **38**, 434–440.

Nickenig, G., Roling, J., Strehlow, K., Schnabel, P. and Bohm, M. (1998) Insulin induces upregulation of vascular AT1 receptor gene expression by posttranscriptional mechanisms. *Circulation* **98**, 2453–2460.

Ohlson, L.O., Larsson, B., Svardsudd, K., Welin, L., Eriksson, H., Wilhelmsen, L., Bjorntorp, P. and Tibblin, G. (1985) The influence of body fat distribution on the incidence of diabetes mellitus. 13.5 years of follow-up of the participants in the study of men born in 1913. *Diabetes* **34**, 1055–1058.

Okamoto, Y., Arita, Y., Nishida, M., Muraguchi, M., Ouchi, N., Takahashi, M., Igura, T., Inui, Y., Kihara, S., Nakamura, T., Yamashita, S., Miyagawa, J., Funahashi, T. and Matsuzawa, Y. (2000) An adipocyte-derived plasma protein, adiponectin, adheres to injured vascular walls. *Hormone and Metabolism Research* **32**, 47–50.

Pi-Sunyer, F.X. (1993a) Medical hazards of obesity. *Annals of Internal Medicine* **119**, 655–660.

Pi-Sunyer, F.X. (1993b) Short-term medical benefits and adverse effects of weight loss. *Annals of Internal Medicine* **119**, 722–726.

Pickavance, L.C., Widdowson, P.S., Foster, J.R., Williams, G. and Wilding, J. P.H. (2003) Chronic treatment with the thiazolidinedione, MCC-555, is associated with reductions in nitric oxide synthase activity and beta-cell apoptosis in the pancreas of the Zucker Diabetic Fatty rat. *International Journal of Experimental Pathology* **84**, 83–89.

Polonsky, K.S., Sturis, J. and Bell, G.I. (1996) Seminars in Medicine of the Beth Israel Hospital, Boston. Non-insulin- dependent diabetes mellitus—a genetically programmed failure of the beta cell to compensate for insulin resistance. *New England Journal of Medicine* **334**, 777–783.

Pories, W.J., Swanson, M.S., MacDonald, K.G., Long, S.B., Morris, P.G., Brown, B.M., Barakat, H.A., Deramon, R.A., Israel, G., Dolezal, J.M. and Dohm, L. (1995) Who would have thought it—an operation proves to be the most effective therapy for adult-onset diabetes-mellitus. *Annals of Surgery* **222**, 339–352.

Pratley, R.E. and Weyer, C. (2001) The role of impaired early insulin secretion in the pathogenesis of type II diabetes mellitus. *Diabetologia* **44**, 929–945.

Randle, P.J., Garland, P.B., Hales, C.N. and Newsholme, C.A. (1963) The glucose fatty-acid cycle. Its role in insulin sensitivity and the metabolic disturbances of diabetes mellitus. *Lancet* **1**, 785–789.

Reaven, G.M. (1988) Banting lecture 1988. Role of insulin resistance in human disease. *Diabetes* **37**, 1595–1607.

Reaven, G. (1995) Physiology of insulin resistance in human disease. *Physiology Review* **75**, 473–486.

Reaven, G.M. (2001) Insulin resistance, compensatory hyperinsulinaemia, and coronary heart disease: syndrome X revisited. In: Jefferson, L.S., Cherrington, A.D. eds. *Handbook of Physiology*. Oxford: Oxford University Press, 1169–1197.

Reaven, G.M. (2003) Effect of variations in the amount and kind of dietary fat and carbohydrate in the dietary management of type 2 diabetes. In: Frost, G., Dornhorst, A., Moses, R. eds. *Nutritional Management of Diabetes Mellitus*, 1st edn. Chichester: John Wiley, 189–200.

Reaven, G.M., Lithell, H. and Landsberg, L. (1996) Hypertension and associated metabolic abnormalities: the role of insulin resistance and the sympathoadrenal system. *New England Journal of Medicine* **334**, 374–381.

Saris, W.H.M., Blair, S.N., van Baak, M.A., Eaton, S.B., Davies, P.S.W., Di Pietro, L., Fogelholm, M., Rissanen, A., Schoeller, D., Swinburn, B., Tremblay, A., Westerterp, K.R. and Wyatt, H. (2003) How much physical activity is enough to prevent unhealthy weight gain? Outcome of the IASO 1st Stock Conference and consensus statement. *Obesity Reviews* **4**, 101–114.

Sasaki, N., Ueno, T., Morita, Y., Yoshiok, S., Nagata, E. and Sata, M. (2003) Therapeutic effects of restricted diet and exercise is of benefit to patients with non-alcoholic steatohepatitis (NASH). *Journal of Hepatology* **38**, 696.

Serrano-Rios, M., Meichionda, N. and Moreno-Carretero, E. (2002) Role of sibutramine in the treatment of obese type 2 diabetic patients receiving sulphonylurea therapy. *Diabetic Medicine* **19**, 119–124.

Shimomura, I., Funahashi, T., Takahashi, M., Maeda, K., Kotani, K., Nakamura, T., Yamashita, S., Miura, M., Fukuda, Y., Takemura, K., Tokunaga, K. and Matsuzawa, Y. (1996) Enhanced expression of PAI-1 in visceral fat: possible contributor to vascular disease in obesity. *Nature Medicine* **2**, 800–803.

Sjöstrom, C.D., Lissner, L., Wedel, H. and Sjöstrom, L. (1999) Reduction in incidence of diabetes, hypertension and lipid disturbances after intentional weight loss induced by bariatric surgery: The SOS Intervention Study. *Obesity Research* **7**, 477–484.

Stamler, R., Stamler, J., Grimm, R., Gosch, F.C., Elmer, P., Dyer, A., Berman, R., Fishman, J., Van Heel, N. and Civinelli, J. (1987) Nutritional therapy for high blood pressure. Final report of a four- year randomized controlled trial: the Hypertension Control Program. *Journal of the American Medical Association* **257**, 1484–1491.

Steppan, C.M., Bailey, S.T., Bhat, S., Brown, E.J., Banerjee, R.R., Wright, C.M., Patel, H.R., Ahima, R.S. and Lazar, M.A. (2001) The hormone resistin links obesity to diabetes. *Nature* **409**, 307–312.

Tuomilheto, J., Lindstrom, J., Erickson, J.G., Valle, T.T., Hamalainen, H., Ilanne-Perikha, P., Keinanen-Kiukaanniemi, S., Laakso, M., Louheranta, A., Rastas, M., Salminen, V., Uusitupa, M. for the Finnish Diabetes Prevention Study Group (2001) Prevention of type 2 diabetes mellitus by changes in lifestyle amongst subjects with impaired glucose tolerance. *New England Journal of Medicine* **344**, 1343–1350.

UK Prospective Diabetes Study Group (1990) UK Prospective Diabetes Study 7. Response of fasting plasma glucose to diet therapy in newly presenting type II diabetic patients. *Metabolism* **39**, 905–912.

UK Prospective Diabetes Study Group (1995) UK Prospective Diabetes Study 16. Overview of 6 years therapy of type II diabetes: a progressive disease. *Diabetes* **44**, 1249–1258.

UK Prospective Diabetes Study Group (1998) Effect of intensive blood-glucose control with metformin on complications in overweight patients with type 2 diabetes (UKPDS 34). *Lancet* **352**, 854–865.

UK Prospective Diabetes Study Group (1999) Tight blood pressure control and risk of macrovascular and microvascular complications in type 2 diabetes: UKPDS 38, vol. 317, p. 703, 1998. *British Medical Journal* **318**, 29.

Ukkola, O. (2002) Resistin—a mediator of obesity-associated insulin resistance or an innocent bystander? *European Journal of Endocrinology* **147**, 571–574.

Urso, R. and Visco-Comandini, U. (2002) Metformin in non-alcoholic steatohepatitis. *Lancet* **359**, 355–356.

Vague, J. (1956) The degree of masculine differentiation of obesities, a factor determining predisposition to diabetes, athersclerosis, gout and uric calculous disease. *American Journal of Clinical Nutrition* **4**, 20–34.

Wadden, T.A., Stunkard, A.J. and Brownell, K.D. (1983) Very low calorie diets: their efficacy, safety, and future. *Annals of Internal Medicine* **99**, 675–684.

Weyer, C., Foley, J.E., Bogardus, C., Tataranni, P.A. and Pratley, R.E. (2000) Enlarged subcutaneous abdominal adipocyte size, but not obesity itself, predicts type II diabetes independent of insulin resistance. *Diabetologia* **43**, 1498–1506.

Weyer, C., Funahashi, T., Tanaka, S., Hotta, K., Matsuzawa, Y., Pratley, R.E. and Tataranni, P.A. (2001) Hypoadiponectinemia in obesity and type 2 diabetes: close association with insulin resistance and hyperinsulinemia. *Journal of Clinical Endocrinology and Metabolism* **86**, 1930–1935.

WHO (1998) *Obesity: Preventing and Managing the Global Epidemic*. Report of a World Health Organization consultation on obesity. Geneva: WHO.

WHO (2000) *The Asia-Pacific Perspective: Redefining Obesity and its Treatment*. Australia: Health Communications Australia Pty.

Wing, R.R. (1995) Use of very low calorie diets in the treatment of obese persons with non-insulin dependent diabetes mellitus. *Journal of the American Dietetics Association* **95**, 569–572.

Wing, R.R., Koeske, R., Epstein, L.H., Nowalk, M.P., Gooding, W. and Becker, D. (1987a) Long-term effects of modest weight loss in type II diabetic patients. *Archives of Internal Medicine* **147**, 1749–1753.

Wing, R.R., Marcus, M.D., Epstein, L.H. and Salata, R. (1987b) Type-II diabetic subjects lose less weight than their overweight nondiabetic spouses. *Diabetes Care*, **10**, 563–566.

Wing, R.R., Blair, E.H., Bononi, P., Marcus, M.D., Watanabe, R. and Bergman, R.N. (1994) Caloric restriction per se is a significant factor in improvements in glycemic control and insulin sensitivity during weight loss in obese NIDDM patients. *Diabetes Care* **17**, 30–36.

Wirshing, D.A., Spellberg, B.J., Erhart, S.M., Marder, S.R. and Wirshing, W.C. (1998) Novel antipsychotics and new onset diabetes. *Biological Psychiatry* **44**, 778–783.

Zavaroni, I., Bonini, L., Gasparini, P., Barilli, A.L., Zuccarelli, A., Dall'Aglio, E., Delsignore, R. and Reaven, G.M. (1999) Hyperinsulinemia in a normal population as a predictor of non-insulin-dependent diabetes mellitus, hypertension, and coronary heart disease: the Barilla factory revisited. *Metabolism* **48**, 989–994.

18 Cardiovascular consequences of obesity

Ian Wilcox

Introduction, 269

Physical fitness and obesity as predictors of mortality risk in obesity, 269

Obesity and sudden death, 269

Obesity and vascular disease, 271

Obesity and hypertension, 272

Obesity, hypertension and patterns of cardiac hypertrophy, 274

Obesity and stroke, 275

Obesity and congestive heart failure, 275

Effects of obesity on intra-abdominal pressure, 276

Effects of obesity on lung function, 277

Obesity, sleep-disordered breathing and cardiorespiratory disease, 278

Sleep apnoea and pulmonary hypertension, 278

Summary, 279

References, 279

Introduction

Obesity is a well-recognized cardiovascular risk factor that exerts effects on the heart and circulation both directly and also by its association with other known risk factors such as hypertension or diabetes (Eckel *et al.*, 2002). Impaired cardiovascular fitness is also common in obese subjects and is an adverse factor that appears to predict increased mortality from cardiovascular disease independently of the degree of obesity, and thus both 'fatness' and 'fitness' are important independent and modifiable risk factors for heart disease (Stevens *et al.*, 2002). This is clearly of major importance to both obese individuals and to the health of the community as a whole.

In the past, the effects of obesity on respiratory function have been considered separately from the cardiovascular effects of obesity; however, in this chapter we will explore the interaction between obesity, heart and lung disease in an attempt to better understand the cardiorespiratory consequences of obesity. Obesity, especially upper body obesity, is linked with snoring, sleep-disordered breathing (SDB) and cardiovascular disease, and thus has important influences on cardiorespiratory function, both while awake and asleep (Wilcox *et al.*, 1998a).

Physical fitness and obesity as predictors of mortality risk in obesity

A sedentary lifestyle and consequent lack of physical fitness is believed to be a predictor of increased mortality. A series of reports from a longitudinal study of a population that consisted of predominantly white US male college graduates (Aerobics Centre Longitudinal Study) showed that performance on a maximal treadmill test indicated that those individuals in the lowest quartile of fitness had an increased mortality risk independent of their degree of obesity. These findings were confirmed and extended subsequently in a report from the Lipid Research Study (Stevens *et al.*, 2002), which used data from 7589 subjects (2506 women, 2860 men) aged between 30 and 75 years, examined in eight US centres between 1972 and 1976 and followed until 1988. The subjects had a mean age of 46 years and body mass indices (BMIs) of 27.4 for men and 24.9 for women, perhaps reflecting a clinical trial bias in favour of healthier subjects; 12% of subjects were obese (BMI ≥ 30), whereas 33% of women and 50% of men were overweight (BMI = 25–29.9 kg/m²). The adjusted mortality hazard ratio for 'fit–fat' women was 1.3 compared with 1.30 for 'unfit–not fat' women and 1.57 for 'unfit–fat' women. The values for men were 1.44, 1.25 and 1.49, respectively, with no significant interaction between fitness or fatness in men or women.

Physical fitness does not completely ameliorate the health hazard of obesity (Eckel *et al.*, 2002; Stevens *et al.*, 2002). Therefore, it appears that both fatness and fitness are potentially modifiable risk factors for mortality.

Obesity and sudden death

Obesity increases the risk of sudden death (Messerli *et al.*, 1987). A variety of mechanisms have been suggested which include increased sympathetic nerve activity, prolongation of the QT interval and structural heart disease such as coronary artery disease and cardiomyopathy. Snoring and obstructive sleep apnoea (OSA) are common in obese subjects and have been linked to an increased risk of sudden death, and therefore the association of obesity with OSA is likely to be another factor contributing to the risk of sudden death in obesity (Seppala *et al.*, 1991).

The US Nurses Health study is a prospective study of a cohort of 121701 nurses aged 30–55 years who completed a questionnaire about their medical history, coronary heart disease (CHD) risk factors, lifestyle and menopausal status at entry in 1976 and have been followed up at 2-year intervals by mail. In this cohort, the risk of sudden death increased with age and was associated with at least one known CHD risk factor in most instances, of which smoking, hypertension and diabetes conferred a 2.5- to fourfold increase in risk of sudden death. Obesity and a family history of myocardial infarction before the age of 60 years each conferred a moderate (1.6-fold) increase in risk. These data showed that, as in men, the risk of sudden death was associated with risk factors for CHD, including obesity, and, as expected, most deaths (88%) were classified as arrhythmic (Alpert, 2001; Albert *et al.*, 2003). Given that other vascular risk factors are common in obese people, the total risk of sudden death in obese women is likely to be substantially increased. Although coronary heart disease is the underlying heart disease responsible for sudden death in most instances, other diseases such as cardiomyopathy are also common in obese people.

Increased sympathetic nerve activity promotes cardiac arrhythmias and has been shown to be increased in obesity in normotensive (Grassi *et al.*, 1995) and hypertensive subjects, whereas weight reduction tends to normalize these changes. The degree of sympathetic nerve overactivity during sleep and while awake is further increased by coexistent OSA that occurs in a significant proportion of obese people (Grunstein *et al.*, 1993).

The long QT syndrome is a genetically diverse inherited disorder of cardiac myocyte ion channels which leads to prolonged ventricular repolarization, and predisposes individuals with it to a characteristic type of ventricular tachycardia (torsades de pointes) and sudden death (Schwartz *et al.*, 2000). In susceptible individuals, changes in autonomic nerve activity (sympathetic overactivity) and electrolyte disturbances can prolong the duration of ventricular repolarization to a critical degree, causing serious and potentially fatal cardiac arrhythmias.

The use of diuretics and laxatives is well known to cause electrolyte changes, particularly hypokalaemia and hypomagnesaemia, which prolong ventricular repolarization, lengthen the QT interval on the surface electrocardiogram (ECG) and increase the risk of ventricular tachycardia/fibrillation, especially in those with the long QT syndrome (Schwartz *et al.*, 2000). Treatment of obesity with ultra low-energy diets has been reported in some, but not many, studies to be associated with a risk of sudden death, and changes in electrolytes caused by these types of diets may be the mechanism responsible for this risk of death, especially in susceptible subjects.

In a study of both obese and non-obese women with a normal QT interval corrected for heart rate (QTc) at rest, Corbi and colleagues compared free fatty acid (FFA) and catecholamine levels in women, separated by the presence and pattern of obesity, and examined the effects of weight loss (approximately 12 kg over 12 months) in obese people. Obese women were subdivided into either peripheral (waist–hip ratio, WHR, ″ 0.85) or central (WHR > 0.85) fat distributions, and it was demonstrated that there was a close positive relationship between obesity and FFA levels and the QTc (Corbi *et al.*, 2002). There was a similar relationship with plasma catecholamines, including both adrenaline (mainly originating in the adrenal glands) and noradrenaline (which spills over from sympathetic nerves). The authors showed that with weight reduction of the same magnitude over 12 months in both groups of obese women, reduced QTc, FFAs and both noradrenaline and adrenaline levels were significantly more in women with central obesity. These findings suggest that weight reduction may reduce the risk of sudden death in obese people by modifying increased sympathetic nerve activity and its effects on ventricular repolarization.

It is likely that the changes in sympathetic nerve activity and QTc in obese subjects, particularly those with abdominal obesity, are most important in the subgroup with an inherited ion channel disorder. Although patients in this study had a normal QT interval at rest, this group can be assumed to contain subjects with inherited ion channel abnormalities, in whom these changes are potentially very important.

Dietary fat and fatty acid content have been linked to risk of CHD and sudden death in the population in general, and may also be important in obese people. Although the traditional view of the 'diet–heart hypothesis' focused on the importance of unsaturated fat intake, there have been a number of recent studies that have demonstrated that dietary intake of *n*-3 polyunsaturated fatty acids (PUFAs) may be an important factor in sudden death in those with or without known CHD. Of special interest have been the long-chain *n*-3 PUFAs (mainly derived from seafood) and intermediate chain *n*-3 PUFAs (derived from canola oil and walnuts in Western diets). None of these is synthesized by humans and they are therefore essential fatty acids. Recently, Leaf and colleagues (2003) proposed a cellular mechanism to explain the link between dietary intake of fat and risk of sudden death based on observations from a number of animal and human studies that suggest that *n*-3 PUFAs reduce the risk of ventricular fibrillation and therefore sudden death by stabilizing myocyte ion channels.

Taken together, these findings suggest that the diet of obese subjects is likely to affect their health in a number of ways. Given that obesity is associated with an increased risk of sudden death, consideration should be given to measures such as improving physical fitness and increasing the dietary intake of intermediate and long-chain essential PUFAs, which may reduce the risk of sudden death without necessarily leading to loss of adipose tissue. Finally, the health benefits of weight reduction using caloric restriction may also be adversely affected by the composition of the diet used to achieve it.

Obesity and vascular disease

For many years, obesity has been suspected to confer an increased risk of morbidity and mortality due to coronary artery and peripheral vascular diseases. However, because of differences in the way obesity was defined and measured, and of specific methodological problems, proving the validity of this apparent relationship has been difficult. As has been discussed earlier, obesity often occurs in a cluster with established metabolic vascular risk factors and lack of physical fitness, making it more difficult to establish whether the presence and pattern of obesity is an *independent* vascular risk factor.

A number of studies have reported that predominantly abdominal fat distribution may be at least as important as BMI as a determinant of cardiac risk. The Gothenburg study reported by Larsson and co-workers (1984) was an early epidemiological study of men, which demonstrated that abdominal fat distribution was a risk factor for CHD, but, once the data had been adjusted for smoking, blood pressure and total cholesterol levels, this was not statistically significant.

In a prospective study of a cohort of middle-aged Finnish men who were followed for 11 years, two indices of abdominal obesity (waist measurement and waist–hip ratio) were used, and coronary events that were defined using MONICA criteria (Lakka *et al.*, 2002) were reported. The study showed that the risk of coronary events in men with a waist–hip ratio of 0.91 was increased almost threefold and that the waist–hip ratio was more powerful and consistent than BMI in predicting the risk of future CHD events. In this study, smoking and poor fitness were not only more common in obese people but, as in other studies, were independent risk factors for CHD, augmenting the risk of CHD and increasing the potential benefits of identifying and modifying all of these risk factors in obese people.

The effects of obesity in general, and its distribution in particular, on CHD risk have also been shown to occur in women. In an 8-year follow-up of the US Nurses Health Study, Rexrode and co-workers (1998) reported that among women the waist circumference and waist–hip ratio were strongly and independently associated with an increased age-adjusted risk of CHD. The adverse effects of abdominal fat distribution were also seen in relatively lean women (BMI < 25 kg/m²). For example, after adjusting for BMI and other cardiac risk factors, women with a waist–hip ratio of 0.88 or higher had a relative risk of CHD of 3.25 compared with those with a ratio of below 0.72 (Fig. 18.1).

Detection of coronary artery calcification using X-rays has been used as a marker of atherosclerotic coronary artery disease in the past but, although highly specific, this method lacked sensitivity. The advent of modern CT scanners, particu-

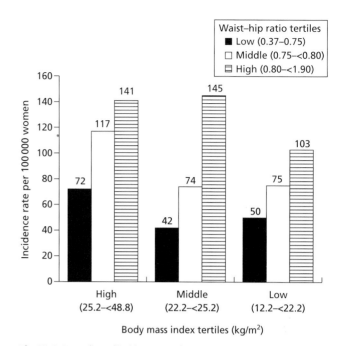

Fig 18.1 Age-adjusted incidence rates for CHD according to BMI and WHR tertiles. Numbers at the top of each bar indicate incidence. (From Rexrode *et al.*, 1998.) At each level of obesity, risk of CHD was significantly increased by an abdominal fat distribution.

larly those using electron beam technology, has increased the sensitivity of this non-invasive method to detect CHD without apparent loss in specificity. In a study of 1160 asymptomatic men, Arad and co-workers (2001) compared anthropomorphic, metabolic and insulin resistance measurements with coronary calcium scores derived from electron beam CT examinations, and showed that coronary calcium scores were positively and independently correlated with visceral obesity, glucose levels and insulin resistance. The relationship between visceral obesity and coronary calcification as a measure of CHD was present whether subjects had elevated glucose levels or not.

A critical question in those at risk of vascular disease is the mode of presentation. Calcification is a marker of relatively stable plaques and therefore although it identifies those with risk factors who have actually developed vascular disease, these individuals are not necessarily those at highest risk and are therefore most likely to benefit from interventions to reduce risk. The development of acute coronary syndromes in patients with vascular disease identifies a group of patients with a markedly increased temporal risk of adverse outcomes. The spectrum of presentations of acute coronary syndromes includes sudden death and acute myocardial infarction with either ST elevation or depression and unstable angina. Acute rupture of an atherosclerotic plaque is well known to be responsible for the clinical manifestations of acute coronary syndromes in most patients; although this is usually a single lesion, multiple unstable plaques can occur in some patients. It

Table 18.1 Components of a proposed 'syndrome Z'.

Obstructive sleep apnoea
Hypertension
Increased sympathetic nerve activity
Central (visceral) obesity
Insulin resistance
Dyslipidaemia

From Wilcox *et al.* (1998a).

is also clear that subclinical plaque rupture can occur. Identifying the factors responsible for the development of acute phases in the course of otherwise stable disease has been the subject of intensive investigation.

Inflammation is increasingly understood to be an important factor in the pathophysiology of atherosclerosis and in the development of acute vascular syndromes (Eckel *et al.*, 2002). Elevated inflammatory markers such as C-reactive protein and cytokines have been shown to occur not only in acute vascular syndromes but also in people at future risk of developing acute vascular events.

Interleukin (IL) 6 is a cytokine that is produced in response to several factors, including infection, IL-1, interferon-γ and tumour necrosis factor alpha (TNF-α), and it has pleiotropic effects on cellular and humoral immunity in response to infection, inflammation and tissue injury. IL-6 is a central mediator of the acute-phase response and a primary determinant of production of C-reactive protein by the liver.

The Physicians' Health Study was a randomized, double-blind, placebo-controlled trial of the effectiveness of aspirin and β-carotene in the primary prevention of cardiovascular disease and cancer in 22 071 US male physicians, aged 40 to 84 years, with no prior history of myocardial infarction, stroke, transient ischaemic attack or cancer. As part of this study a prospective, nested, case–control study of IL-6 as a potential marker for future myocardial infarction among participants was performed and this showed that IL-6 levels at baseline appeared to identify men at future risk of acute myocardial infarction (Ridker *et al.*, 2000).

Adipose tissue is now well recognized to be a source of inflammatory mediators with production of TNF-α and IL-6. Increased production and release of these mediators may play a significant role in promoting the development of atherosclerosis and its complications (Loskutoff and Samad, 1998).

The effect of obesity on the risk of developing atherosclerosis and its acute and chronic complications is compounded by the apparent prothrombotic effects of obesity, meaning that the consequences of plaque rupture are likely to be more adverse than in lean subjects. The identification of adipose tissue as a source of inflammatory mediators with production of pro-inflammatory cytokines, such as TNF-α, interleukins (including IL-6) and also C-reactive protein, provides a conceptual framework linking obesity, insulin resistance and atherosclerosis (Rader, 2000).

Cholesterol lowering has been shown to reduce the risk of future vascular events and in obese subjects, relatively modest weight loss achieved by diet, drugs (Marks *et al.*, 1998), or a combination of the two, is associated with significant changes in lipid levels, which, if sustained, would have major beneficial effects on future risk of vascular events.

Drugs such as statins (HMG CoA reductase inhibitors) appear to have pleiotropic effects, which include stabilization or 'passivization' of potentially vulnerable atherosclerotic plaques. Inflammatory markers such as C-reactive protein have been shown to be reduced during statin treatment and may be a marker of risk reduction.

OSA appears to confound the relationship between obesity, inflammation and cardiovascular risk (Lattimore *et al.*, 2003). In a Japanese study of 30 men with OSA and 14 obese control subjects (mean BMI = 27.7 kg/m^2), levels of C-reactive protein and IL-6 produced from peripheral blood monocytes were significantly higher in obese subjects with OSA than in control subjects, and the levels fell after a month's treatment of OSA using nasal continuous positive airway pressure (Yokoe *et al.*, 2003), an effect independent of the effects of obesity.

Our understanding of the relationship between obesity and risk of CHD has advanced substantially in recent years. Evidence that obesity, especially abdominal obesity, is related to increased risk of atherosclerotic vascular disease has become increasingly convincing and accepted. Advances in our understanding of the key role inflammation plays in the development and course of atherosclerosis have allowed us to examine the potential mechanisms by which obesity may contribute to this process, and perhaps provide clinicians with better measures to assess the risk reduction conferred by modification of obesity and other factors, such as smoking and physical inactivity, which commonly cluster with it.

Obesity and hypertension

Obesity is associated with increased blood pressure levels in both normotensive and hypertensive children and adults in a large number of studies. Although the mechanisms by which obesity leads to higher blood pressure levels are not completely understood, studies of weight reduction have shown that it can lower blood pressure and some of its effects on the heart and circulation.

In the US, obesity in childhood has increased dramatically since the 1960s and similar trends have been noted in other countries. In children, obesity increases the risk of hypertension approximately threefold across all levels of BMI with no threshold of effect, and interventional studies have shown that blood pressure reduction can be achieved (Sorof and Daniels, 2002), as has been reported more extensively in adults. Whereas hypertension in paediatric practice was formerly considered more likely in children with genetic hypertension and those with renal disease, this pattern has changed and obesity-related hypertension has assumed much more importance.

The diagnosis of hypertension in adults is relatively straightforward but in children, blood pressure values have to be adjusted for age, gender and height, making accurate diagnosis of hypertension more difficult than in adults, and the significance of borderline elevated blood pressure in children is potentially more important as it appears to be a precursor of hypertension in adulthood. Unlike in adults, it has been reported that the early pattern of hypertension in childhood has been that of systolic rather than diastolic hypertension. The use of an appropriate blood pressure cuff size is relatively more important than in adult practice; blood pressure will tend to be overestimated if the cuff is too small, seen commonly in adults, but, more importantly, it can be underestimated if the cuff is too large. The recommended cuff size is one with a bladder width that is approximately 40% of the arm circumference midway between the olecranon and the acromion process (Sorof and Daniels, 2002).

The pathophysiology of hypertension in obesity hypertension in children and adults remains to be fully elucidated. Characteristically, such patients have increased sympathetic nerve activity, increased insulin levels and increased activity of the renin–angiotensin–aldosterone system. Obesity hypertension is one of the salt-sensitive variants of essential hypertension. Although there is clearly a strong association between obesity hypertension, sodium sensitivity and insulin resistance, there is no simple relationship that integrates these observations into an explanation of why blood pressure is increased in these patients.

Activation of the sympathetic nervous system occurs early in the course of obesity and is involved in many of its chronic manifestations, including the cardiovascular complications of hypertension, left ventricular hypertrophy, congestive heart failure and arrhythmias. Recent research interest has focused on the role of leptin, produced in adipocytes, in the regulation of the sympathetic nervous system in obesity.

Leptin is a 16-kDa peptide produced mainly in adipose tissue and has been conceived to play a regulatory role ('adipostat') (see Chapter 6) in determining fat mass by reducing appetite and thus inhibiting food intake—probably in the hypothalamus—and by increasing thermogenesis via increased sympathetic nerve activity. However, many of the results of studies in animal and human subjects have been contradictory.

In a recent study by Eikelis and co-workers (2003), adrenaline secretion and leptin levels were measured in a range of healthy obese subjects who had a wide variety of leptin levels, normal-weight healthy subjects and patients with heart failure (high noradrenaline levels), essential hypertension (high noradrenaline levels), pure autonomic failure (low noradrenaline levels) and healthy elderly subjects (reduced adrenaline levels). Leptin levels were not low in the two models of high

sympathetic tone (heart failure and hypertension). In fact, elevated leptin levels found in heart failure were due to reduced renal clearance. Plasma leptin levels were normal in autonomic failure and in the elderly. Thus, the concept that leptin directly stimulates sympathetic efferent activity appears to be overly simplistic. Clearly, further studies are needed to clarify the relationship, in obesity, of total fat mass, fat distribution and the autonomic nervous system.

A series of studies in obese adults have shown that short-term weight loss reduces blood pressure substantially (Dahl *et al.*, 1958; Tuck *et al.*, 1981; MacMahon *et al.*, 1986; Rocchini *et al.*, 1989; Kotchen *et al.*, 1993). Typically, there is a fall in both weight and blood pressure that is associated with a natriuresis, which is most marked in the acute phase and increases gradually thereafter.

In a study of 26 Japanese obese women, mean age of 50 years with BMI of 34 kg/m^2 (Kanai), an average weight loss of 9 kg reduced mean blood pressure by 11 mmHg. In this study, the fall in blood pressure did not correlate with weight or BMI but did correlate with reduction in intra-abdominal obesity measured by CT scan. These results do not exclude the possibility that weight and adiposity expressed as BMI are important, but do suggest that fat distribution is a more important factor than obesity alone in affecting blood pressure in obese people.

End-stage renal disease and congestive heart failure are major consequences of chronic essential hypertension. When hypertension and diabetes are both present, as they commonly are in obesity, the risk of end-stage renal disease is substantially increased. Obesity has a number of effects on renal function which promote an increase in blood pressure, including increasing renal tubular sodium reabsorption, impairing pressure natriuresis and intravascular volume expansion due to activation of the sympathetic nervous system and renin–angiotensin system and by physical compression of the kidneys, particularly when visceral obesity is present (Hall *et al.*, 2003). Early functional changes of microalbuminuria and expression of growth- and/or fibrosis-promoting factors precede major histological changes in the kidney (Eckel *et al.*, 2002). It is believed that chronic obesity promotes gradual loss of nephron numbers and function.

In animal studies, a relationship can be shown between caloric intake and renal disease. Excess intake promotes and energy restriction protects against glomerular injury. Long-term studies of the effects of caloric restriction or weight reduction in human subjects are lacking (Eckel *et al.*, 2002; Hall *et al.*, 2003).

Prevention of end-stage renal disease is a major objective of treatment in hypertension. In obese people, treatment goals in hypertension should include not only weight reduction and good blood pressure control, but also correction of the associated metabolic abnormalities to try to prevent further renal injury and consequent irreversible nephron loss (Hall *et al.*, 2003).

Obesity, hypertension and patterns of cardiac hypertrophy

Obesity when predominantly central in distribution is characteristically associated with a number of cardiac structural changes, which include right and left ventricular dilatation and hypertrophy, left atrial dilatation and fatty infiltration of the conducting system. Peripheral (lower body) obesity appears not to be associated with hypertension or structural changes in the heart and circulation.

The effect of obesity on blood pressure begins early in the course of this disorder. Hypertension occurs commonly in obese children and adults of all ages but daytime hypertension is not a prerequisite for the presence of left ventricular hypertrophy in obese subjects, and this observation, along with an apparent increase in cardiomyopathy and heart failure in obese subjects led to the notion of the 'cardiomyopathy of obesity' (Alpert, 2001). An additional factor contributing adversely to the severity of left ventricular hypertrophy and systolic dysfunction in obese patients is coexistent OSA (Wilcox *et al.*, 1998b).

Remodelling of the heart occurs in response to *chronic* changes in distending pressure in systole, diastole or both. This is distinct from the changes in cardiac function which occur in response to an *acute* load. At a cellular level, this process is due to hypertrophy of cardiac myocytes in a configuration that depends on the type of load to which the heart is responding (Figs 18.2 and 18.3).

Isolated pressure overload of the left ventricle, such as that which occurs in hypertension in the absence of obesity, produces a pattern of hypertrophy in which the left ventricle remodels with a symmetrical increase in wall thickness, without an increase in diastolic diameter, but a reduction in end-systolic diameter or concentric hypertrophy. At a cellular level, this pattern of hypertrophy results from addition of new myofibrils in a parallel pattern. This change in geometry has the effect of reducing left ventricular systolic wall stress and therefore is an adaptation that reduces the left ventricular work in response to this pressure overload (Fig. 18.2).

Volume overload of the left ventricle occurs typically in mitral or aortic regurgitation, when the ventricle has to generate a greater stroke volume because of valvular regurgitation in order to maintain net forward stroke volume and cardiac output. Therefore the overload of the ventricle occurs in diastole, causing increased diastolic wall stress. The heart responds to this stress by adding new sarcomeres in series. Dilatation of the ventricle in response to this chronic volume overload increases diastolic wall stress, but typically end-systolic diameter and volume are unchanged. Left ventricular wall mass increases to a greater degree despite apparently more modest increases in wall thickness (Fig. 18.3).

Obesity has been associated with eccentric ventricular hypertrophy in which both the diameter and wall thickness of

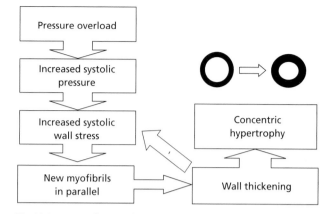

Fig 18.2 Pattern of ventricular remodelling: response to pressure overload. In this setting, the pressure overload occurs in systole, leading to increased systolic wall stress. (Adapted from Grossman *et al.*, 1993.)

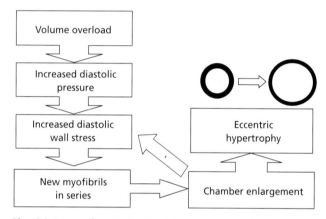

Fig 18.3 Pattern of ventricular remodelling: response to volume. In this setting, the pressure overload occurs in diastole, resulting in increased diastolic wall stress to which the heart responds by 'eccentric' hypertrophy. (Adapted from Grossman *et al.*, 1993.)

the left ventricle are increased at all levels of blood pressure. The apparently different effects of obesity and hypertension on left ventricular geometry led to the concept of the 'dimorphic' effects of obesity and hypertension on left ventricular hypertrophy and systolic function. Thus, lean hypertensive individuals are expected to have concentric hypertrophy, centrally obese but normotensive individuals have eccentric hypertrophy, and the combination of obesity and hypertension produces an unfavourable situation of both volume and pressure overload (or systolic and diastolic pressure overload), resulting in dilatation and dysfunction and potentially earlier heart failure in the course of their disease. However, the relationship between central obesity and left ventricular hypertrophy is not as simple as first thought and many obese subjects have concentric hypertrophy even if they are normotensive.

The importance of left ventricular hypertrophy lies in its value as an adverse prognostic factor in hypertension. In hypertensive subjects, echocardiographically measured left ventricular mass is a more powerful prognostic factor than systolic or diastolic blood pressure (Levy *et al.*, 1991). Antihypertensive drugs vary in their effects on regression of ventricular hypertrophy, and regression of cardiac and vascular hypertrophy is considered to be an important goal in treating hypertension (Levy *et al.*, 1994).

Studies of the effect of weight reduction have provided evidence supporting the notion that obesity causes both hypertension and left ventricular hypertrophy. The effects of weight reduction (average of 8 kg) on left ventricular hypertrophy were examined by MacMahon and co-workers (MacMahon *et al.*, 1986) in a population of young obese, predominantly male, subjects (mean age 42 years and BMI of 33 kg/m^2). Obesity, expressed as BMI, was independently associated with systolic, diastolic blood pressure and left ventricular mass. Following weight reduction, blood pressure fell by an average of 13/14 mmHg (systolic/diastolic) and echocardiographic left ventricular mass by 20%. The effects of weight reduction on left ventricular mass were reported to be statistically independent of effects on blood pressure.

In clinical practice, interventions to reduce weight typically involve a combination of increased exercise, and potentially fitness, as well as weight loss, with variable effects on fat mass and distribution in individual subjects. Although assessing the relative impacts of these different factors on blood pressure and cardiac structure may be a relevant research question, in practice they are usually combined and therefore the total benefit that this approach can achieve is more clinically relevant. Exercise itself has effects on cardiac structure, which vary with the type and intensity of the exercise programme undertaken.

Hinderliter and colleagues (2002) studied the effect of either improved fitness through regular aerobic exercise or exercise plus a behavioural weight reduction programme with waitlisted control subjects in a randomized controlled study of 82 overweight or obese men and women (mean BMI = 31 kg/m^2) who were sedentary and included normotensive and hypertensive subjects. Patients with hypertension had no drug treatment for at least 6 weeks. Over 6 months, blood pressure fell (6/7 mmHg in the weight management group and 3/4 mmHg in the aerobic exercise group) and both groups had significant reductions in left ventricular septal and posterior wall thickness, but not indexed left ventricular mass, compared with the control subjects. Although previous studies have shown that weight reduction promotes ventricular remodelling in obese people, this study showed that regular aerobic exercise had beneficial effects on ventricular remodelling whether or not weight loss occurred.

There is increasing evidence that factors other than blood pressure itself lead to left ventricular hypertrophy. Only approximately 50% of hypertensive subjects have left ventricular hypertrophy, suggesting there may be genetic and other factors that determine the hypertrophic response to a given blood pressure load in an individual. The results of a number of studies in animals and human subjects have suggested that increased sympathetic nerve activity leads to left ventricular

hypertrophy, and a recent study that separately examined the role of cardiac sympathetic nerve activity showed that the degree to which this was increased was a major determinant of left ventricular hypertrophy (Schlaich *et al.*, 2003).

Thus, obese subjects who appear to have increased sympathetic nerve activity independently of the presence of hypertension would be more likely to have increased left ventricular mass, regardless of geometric changes, provided that this involved cardiac as well as peripheral sympathetic nerve activity. Such a situation has usually been measured using microneurographic techniques.

Obesity and stroke

Obesity is well recognized to be a risk factor for coronary artery disease as described earlier; however, the relationship between obesity and stroke has been less clear-cut. Established stroke risk factors, such as hypertension, left ventricular hypertrophy, diabetes and hypercholesterolaemia, are common in obese people and these associated stroke risk factors have been considered to explain the increased risk of stroke in obese subjects. As in other vascular consequences of obesity, OSA is a potential confounder of this association given that it is common in obese people and in patients with stroke or transient ischaemic attacks (Harbison and Gibson, 2000).

In a prospective study from the Physicians Health Study, Kurth and co-workers (2002) examined the relationship between increasing adiposity, measured as BMI, and self-reported stroke over a period of 12.5 years in the 21 414 participating US physicians. The study population was relatively healthy and although 38% were overweight, only 6% of the subjects were obese. There was little change in BMI during the course of the study. For each 1-unit increase in BMI, total, ischaemic and haemorrhagic stroke risk increased by 6%, and after adjusting for hypertension this reduced to 4%. This was unaffected by diabetes, alcohol consumption and smoking status for total and ischaemic stroke, but the risk of haemorrhagic stroke remained increased by 6%. There is no equivalent study in women; those studies that have been published have shown variable and inconclusive results.

The mechanism by which obesity might mediate an increased risk of stroke independent of associated hypertension or diabetes remains to be established, but elevated inflammatory markers, cytokines and pro-thrombotic factors observed in obese subjects are all possibilities that might be involved in increasing the risk of acute vascular disease, including ischaemic stroke in obese people.

Obesity and congestive heart failure

Congestive heart failure is a major cause of morbidity and mortality, whether manifested as predominantly systolic or diastolic heart failure. Given the ominous prognosis of this condition, prevention of this disorder is now considered to be a major medical health issue. The cardiac response to obesity is characterized by left ventricular dilatation and hypertrophy, which are known precursors to later congestive heart failure. The progression from risk factor to heart failure has been shown clearly in systemic hypertension (Levy *et al.*, 1996; Lloyd-Jones, 2002), in which pressure overload leads to concentric hypertrophy with early diastolic dysfunction and late systolic dysfunction.

As in other disease processes linked with obesity, heart failure is complicated by coexistent other risk factors, which include not only hypertension and diabetes, but also sleep apnoea. Patients with severe congestive heart failure are often cachectic and this has the potential to complicate our understanding of a possible link between increasing adiposity and congestive heart failure. Therefore, it is important to distinguish between obesity as a possible factor leading to heart failure and the effects of established heart failure on metabolism and body composition.

Obesity has been identified as a risk factor for heart failure in extremely obese patients and more recently this relationship has been shown to hold for patients with less severe obesity (a recently published report from the Framingham study by Kenchaiah and co-workers (2002) in which 5881 subjects were followed for a mean of 14 years). Criteria used to define overweight and obesity as well as those to define heart failure have varied in previous studies. The authors excluded underweight subjects (BMI < 18.5 kg/m^2) and used BMI to define overweight (BMI = 25–29.9 kg/m^2) and obesity (BMI ≥ 30 kg/m^2). Presentation with an initial episode of heart failure was classified by a panel of three experienced cardiologists, using criteria previously used as part of the Framingham Heart Study. Peripheral oedema, common in obese subjects without heart failure, is only a minor criterion in this definition in which this is only included if not attributable to another cause.

Only 16% of the subjects in this study were obese; one-half of the men and one-third of the women were overweight and extreme obesity (BMI ≥ 40) was rare (only eight men). After adjustment for known heart failure risk factors (mainly hypertension and diabetes, both of which increased with increasing BMI) there was an incremental increase in risk of developing heart failure of approximately 5% for women and 7% for men for each increase of BMI by 1 kg/m^2. Compared with normal-weight women, overweight women had a 50% increase in congestive heart failure risk and obese women had a doubling of risk. In men, overweight analysed as a categorical variable was associated with a 20% increase, and obesity a 90% increase in risk of congestive heart failure. Analysed as a continuous variable, there did not appear to be a threshold of effect of obesity on the risk of developing congestive heart failure in men or women.

From this study, based on an accepted normal study population, obesity could be attributed as the cause of congestive heart failure in approximately 11% of men and 14% of women. The prospective nature of the study, demonstration of a progressive, stepwise increase in risk with increasing BMI and the temporal relationship between documentation of obesity and the subsequent development of heart failure are clearly strengths of this study.

The 'obesity paradox' in congestive heart failure lies in the observation that although obesity is a risk factor for the development of heart failure among patients with heart failure, those with a higher BMI have a better prognosis. Another factor that complicates our understanding of the relationship between adiposity and heart failure is OSA. As previously discussed, snoring and sleep apnoea occur commonly in obese subjects and when such patients have a dilated cardiomyopathy or left ventricular systolic dysfunction due to another factor such as coronary heart disease, the combination is an adverse one (Malone *et al.*, 1991; Wilcox *et al.*, 1998b; Kaneko *et al.*, 2003).

As a consequence of the development of congestive heart failure, some patients develop periodic breathing and central apnoeas (Cheyne–Stokes respiration) during sleep, and such patients are typically normal or underweight, have worse systolic function, typically quite severe (left ventricular ejection fraction < 20%) and have a worse prognosis than those with or without OSA.

Exercise capacity or 'fitness' is a prognostic factor in patients with heart failure and is independent of left ventricular systolic function. Patients with a lower maximal exercise capacity (often measured as maximal oxygen uptake or $\dot{V}_{O_2 \, max}$) have a worse prognosis. Although cachexia is a recognized adverse prognostic factor in patients with heart failure, this relationship persists even among patients who are not cachectic (Davos *et al.*, 2003).

Therefore, even in patients with established systolic heart failure, fitness and fatness remain important prognostic factors, as they are present in obese people who have apparently normal cardiac function. However, in heart failure, fitness and fatness have discordant effects on prognosis, with fatness being not only a predictor of risk of developing heart failure, but also a marker of lower risk once heart failure develops. Given the major burden imposed by congestive heart failure on patients, their families and the community in general, physicians increasingly understand the importance of intervening to prevent the development of heart failure and obesity needs to be understood in this context.

Effects of obesity on intra-abdominal pressure

Abdominal pressure can be measured in various ways and intravesical and rectal pressures correlate well with directly measured intra-abdominal pressure. Increasing abdominal obesity not only increases intra-abdominal pressure significantly, but also intrathoracic pressure and central venous, pulmonary arterial and pulmonary venous pressure.

The effects of obesity on intra-abdominal pressure may be an important factor contributing to cardiac, respiratory and other consequences of obesity. Raised intra-abdominal pressure is likely to be another factor causing breathlessness in obese people and, for example, it partly explains why obese subjects commonly develop marked increases in dyspnoea with postural changes such as stooping or bending or lying down in the prone or supine position.

Studies in dogs have shown that increasing intra-abdominal pressure using an implanted balloon that was progressively inflated to a pressure of 25 mmHg resulted in elevated systolic and diastolic blood pressure in the systemic circulation, which returned to baseline values 2 weeks after balloon deflation (Bloomfield *et al.*, 2000). These changes in blood pressure occurred without changes in renin, aldosterone, natriuretic peptides or catecholamines, suggesting that intra-abdominal pressure affects blood pressure by other means and may be an independent factor contributing to elevated blood pressures that are common in many, but not all, obese subjects.

Elevated abdominal and thoracic pressure results in increased cerebral venous pressure, and therefore increased intracranial pressure, and at least partly explains the association of obesity with increased intracranial pressure in pseudo-tumour cerebri (Sugerman *et al.*, 1997).

Effects of obesity on lung function

Symptoms of breathlessness are a common complaint in overweight and obese subjects, and these may be cardiac or respiratory in origin or a combination of the two. General deconditioning is not unusual in obese people and therefore fitness, or rather lack of it, rather than 'fatness', may be an important factor in some patients with obesity and complaints of effort intolerance.

Obesity has a number of effects on respiratory function, which can interact with the effects of obesity on the heart and circulation to cause breathlessness (Fig. 18.4). The distribution of body fat in obese subjects has specific effects on heart and lung function (Unterborn, 2001). Obesity influences upper airway reflexes, lung function and lung mechanics, and may affect the central control of breathing primarily. Body posture is an important modulating factor in obese people, which can be critically important in sedated or sleeping obese subjects.

The effects of obesity on lung function include a reduction in forced expiratory volume at 1 sec (FEV_1) and forced vital capacity (FVC), with a normal spirometric ratio (FEV_1/FVC), an increased residual volume and a normal diffusing capacity for carbon monoxide (DLCO). Measurement of the DLCO can be useful in distinguishing those obese patients who have

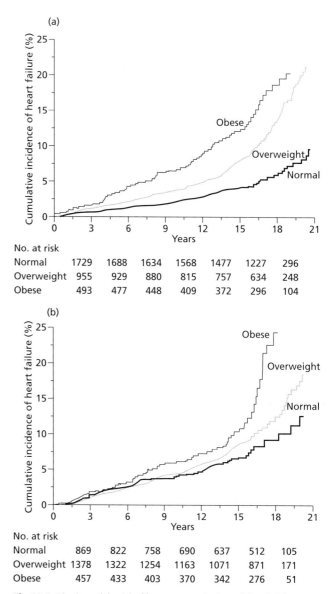

No. at risk

Normal	1729	1688	1634	1568	1477	1227	296
Overweight	955	929	880	815	757	634	248
Obese	493	477	448	409	372	296	104

No. at risk

Normal	869	822	758	690	637	512	105
Overweight	1378	1322	1254	1163	1071	871	171
Obese	457	433	403	370	342	276	51

Fig 18.4 Obesity and the risk of future congestive heart failure in (a) women and (b) men. (From Kenchaiah *et al.*, 2002.) Obesity was associated with an increased risk of heart failure in both men and women, without evidence of a threshold effect.

parenchymal lung disease. Complaints of wheezing and the use of bronchodilator drugs are common in obese people, but whether or not obesity is associated with airway hyper-responsiveness has been controversial. A series of recent studies tends to support the view that although complaints of asthma and the use of treatments for it are common in obese people, objectively measured airway hyper-responsiveness is not (Schachter *et al.*, 2001; Sin *et al.*, 2002).

The major effect on lung mechanics is a decrease in overall compliance, mainly due to the effects of obesity on the chest and abdominal wall rather than on the lungs as such. There are also effects of obesity on upper airway tone and hence resis-

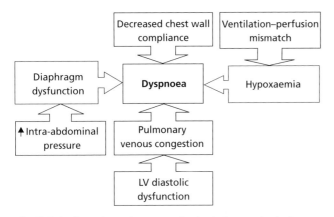

Fig 18.5 Cardiorespiratory factors contributing to dyspnoea in obesity. LV, left ventricular.

tance, which add a mechanical load that increases the work of breathing. Thus, healthy obese but eucapneic subjects can be demonstrated to have increased work of breathing at rest. Maximum voluntary ventilation can also be shown to be reduced.

Obesity leads to mismatch of blood flow and air flow in the lungs, resulting in an increased alveolar–arterial oxygen (A-aO$_2$) difference; this ventilation–perfusion mismatch, although present in the upright position, is worsened significantly when supine (Unterborn, 2001).

A proportion of obese people will progress to develop the obesity–hypoventilation or 'Pickwickian' syndrome. The factors responsible for development of hypercapnic respiratory failure in obese people are not entirely understood, but in the past the importance of OSA in combination with morbid obesity with or without parenchymal lung disease has been greatly underestimated (Piper and Sullivan, 1994).

Obesity, sleep-disordered breathing and cardiorespiratory disease

Obesity is known to be associated with cardiovascular disease, including systemic hypertension, pulmonary hypertension, atherosclerosis and congestive heart failure. Understanding the pathophysiological basis of this relationship is potentially compounded by emerging knowledge of the importance of the link between obesity, particularly central or upper body obesity, and SDB, including sleep apnoea and hypercapnic respiratory failure.

Obesity is strongly linked with OSA as defined by obstructed breathing efforts typically associated with snoring, and either partial (50% reduction in breathing amplitude — hypopnoea) or complete apnoea for 10 s or more (Grunstein et al., 1993). An apnoea–hypopnoea index of > 5/h has been used to define 'sleep apnoea', and when associated with symptoms of tiredness or sleepiness this is known as the 'sleep apnoea

syndrome'. Only a minority of patients with sleep apnoea have symptoms of sleepiness and not all patients who are obese and who may snore have sleep apnoea.

The definition of sleep apnoea, based on these respiratory parameters, has been empirical and almost certainly overly simplistic. In making comparisons between the cardiovascular and respiratory consequences of SDB, it becomes clear that the cardiovascular consequences of OSA are much more serious than the respiratory consequences, mainly hypercapnic respiratory failure with/without associated lung disease ('overlap syndrome').

The prevalence of OSA increases with age and obesity. Epidemiological studies have shown that OSA (apnoea–hypopnoea index ≥ 5/h) affects up to 24% of men and 12% of women between the ages of 30 and 65 years; the 'OSA syndrome' affects 4% of men and 2% of women in this age range. Among morbidly obese people, the proportion who present with OSA rises to approximately 50%. It is important to note that obesity is less clearly related to OSA in older patients. Data from the Sleep Heart Health Study (Young et al., 2002) showed that OSA in older people (age > 60 years) was poorly predicted by higher BMI, neck circumference, waist–hip ratio and self-reported breathing pauses. The reason for the differences in the SDB risk factors by age was not clear. However, it is clear that OSA is a significant factor that interacts with obesity and its cardiorespiratory consequences.

OSA is now established as a risk factor for systemic hypertension during the day, as well as cyclical blood pressure and heart rate fluctuations at night. This understanding is based on animal and human studies that include cross-sectional and prospective epidemiological studies and treatment trials using nasal continuous positive airway pressure (nCPAP) treatment. Human studies have shown that nCPAP eliminates the nocturnal blood pressure changes and lowers daytime blood pressure independently of other factors such as obesity itself and antihypertensive drugs. The mechanism by which OSA causes hypertension is not known, but increased peripheral sympathetic nerve activity has been shown to be present night and day and to be reduced by nCPAP treatment (Hedner et al., 1995; Narkiewicz et al., 1998). In rats, sympathetic blockade or adrenalectomy prevents the blood pressure increase in response to repetitive hypoxia during sleep. There is also evidence that beta-blockers are more effective antihypertensive drugs in OSA (Kraiczi et al., 2000), providing additional support for the notion that the sympathetic nervous system is critically important for the development of systemic hypertension in OSA.

Sleep apnoea and pulmonary hypertension

Pulmonary hypertension is associated with OSA, occurring in 20–40% of patients; although this is typically mild to moderate in severity, it can be severe. The prevalence of pulmonary hypertension in OSA is increased by increasing obesity and by the presence of parenchymal lung disease such as chronic obstructive pulmonary disease.

Evidence in favour of a causal relationship includes observation of pulmonary hypertension in animals exposed to repetitive hypoxia, regression of pulmonary hypertension in children with OSA due to enlarged tonsils and adenoids, and some studies of the effect of treatment of OSA with nCPAP in human subjects.

Given what is known about the relationship between increasing obesity and OSA, approximately 50% of morbidly obese subjects would be expected to have OSA, and approximately 25% of these subjects would have pulmonary hypertension, or at least 1 in 10 morbidly obese subjects overall unselected for a history of snoring or sleep apnoea.

Summary

Obesity has a plethora of effects on the heart, circulation, respiratory function and sleep, which combine to reduce quality and length of life for the obese individuals who form an ever-increasing proportion of the population, particularly in more industrially developed nations. In considering the cardiovascular effects of obesity, it is clearly important to understand the respiratory effects of obesity, given the physiological importance of these heart–lung interactions. In addition, increasing recognition of snoring and sleep apnoea among obese subjects (especially those with abdominal or visceral fat distributions) presents an opportunity to advance our understanding of the circadian health consequences of obesity and offers new opportunities to intervene to improve it. The fact that many different cardiovascular risk factors 'cluster' together in obese subjects enables these to be identified more readily and, more importantly, modified.

References

Albert, C.M., Chae, C.U. *et al.* (2003) Prospective study of sudden cardiac death among women in the United States. *Circulation* **107**, 2096–2101.

Alpert, M.A. (2001) Obesity cardiomyopathy: pathophysiology and evolution of the clinical syndrome. *American Journal of Medical Sciences* **321**, 225–236.

Arad, Y., Newstein, D. *et al.* (2001) Association of multiple risk factors and insulin resistance with increased prevalence of asymptomatic coronary artery disease by an electron-beam computed tomographic study. *Arteriosclerosis, Thrombosis and Vascular Biology* **21**, 2051–2058.

Bloomfield, G., Sugerman, H. *et al.* (2000) Chronically increased intra-abdominal pressure produces systemic hypertension in dogs. *International Journal of Obesity and Related Metabolic Disorders* **24**, 819–824.

Corbi, G.M., Carbone, S. *et al.* (2002) FFAs and QT intervals in obese women with visceral adiposity, effects of sustained weight loss over 1 year. *Journal of Clinical Endocrinology and Metabolism* **87**, 2080–2083.

Dahl, L.K., Silver, L. *et al.* (1958) The role of salt in the fall of blood pressure accompanying reduction in obesity. *New England Journal of Medicine* **258**, 1186–1192.

Davos, C.H., Doehner, W. *et al.* (2003) Body mass and survival in patients with chronic heart failure without cachexia: the importance of obesity. *Journal of Cardiac Failure* **9**(1), 29–35.

Eckel, R.H., Barouch, W.W. *et al.* (2002) Report of the National Heart, Lung, and Blood Institute–National Institute of Diabetes and Digestive and Kidney Diseases Working Group on the pathophysiology of obesity-associated cardiovascular disease. *Circulation* **105**, 2923–2928.

Eikelis, N., Schlaich, M. *et al.* (2003) Interactions between leptin and the human sympathetic nervous system. *Hypertension* **41**, 1072–1079.

Grassi, G., Seravalle, G. *et al.* (1995) Sympathetic activation in obese normotensive subjects. *Hypertension* **25**, 560–563.

Grossman, W., Carabello, B.A. *et al.* (1993) *Ventricular Wall Stress and the Development of Cardiac Hypertrophy and Failure.* New York: Raven Press.

Grunstein, R., Wilcox, I. *et al.* (1993) Snoring and sleep apnea in men: interaction with central obesity and hypertension. *International Journal of Obesity* **17**, 503–540.

Hall, J.E., Jones, D.W. *et al.* (2003) Impact of the obesity epidemic on hypertension and renal disease. *Current Hypertension Reports* **5**, 386–392.

Harbison, J.A. and Gibson, G.J. (2000) Snoring, sleep apnoea and stroke: chicken or scrambled egg? *Quarterly Journal of Medicine* **93**, 647–654.

Hedner, J.A., Darpo, B. *et al.* (1995) Reduction in sympathetic activity after long-term CPAP treatment in sleep apnoea: cardiovascular implications. *European Respiratory Journal* **8**, 222–229.

Hinderliter, A., Sherwood, A. *et al.* (2002) Reduction of left ventricular hypertrophy after exercise and weight loss in overweight patients with mild hypertension. *Archives of Internal Medicine* **162**, 1333–1339.

Kaneko, Y., Floras, J.S. *et al.* (2003) Cardiovascular effects of continuous positive airway pressure in patients with heart failure and obstructive sleep apnea. *New England Journal of Medicine* **348**, 1233–1241.

Kenchaiah, S., Evans, J.C. *et al.* (2002) Obesity and the risk of heart failure. *New England Journal of Medicine* **347**, 305–313.

Kotchen, J.M., Cox-Ganser, J. *et al.* (1993) Gender differences in obesity-related cardiovascular disease risk factors among participants in a weight loss programme. *International Journal of Obesity and Related Metabolic Disorders* **17**, 145–151.

Kraiczi, H., Hedner, J. *et al.* (2000) Comparison of atenolol, amlodipine, enalapril, hydrochlorothiazide, and losartan for antihypertensive treatment in patients with obstructive sleep apnea. *American Journal of Respiratory and Critical Care Medicine* **161**, 1423–1428.

Kurth, T., Gaziano, J.M. *et al.* (2002) Body mass index and the risk of stroke in men. *Archives of Internal Medicine* **162**, 2557–2562.

Lakka, H.-M., Lakka, T.A. *et al.* (2002) Abdominal obesity is associated with increased risk of acute coronary events in men. *European Heart Journal* **23**, 706–713.

Larsson, B., Svardsudd, K. *et al.* (1984) Abdominal adipose tissue distribution, obesity, and risk of cardiovascular disease and death:

13 year follow up of participants in the study of men born in 1913. *British Medical Journal* **289**, 1257–1261.

Lattimore, J.-D., Celermajer, D.S. *et al.* (2003) Obstructive sleep apnea and cardiovascular disease. *Journal of the American College of Cardiology* **41**, 1429–1437.

Leaf, A., Kang, J.X. *et al.* (2003) Clinical prevention of sudden cardiac death by n-3 polyunsaturated fatty acids and mechanism of prevention of arrhythmias by n-3 fish oils. *Circulation* **107**, 2646–2652.

Levy, D., Anderson, K. *et al.* (1991) Prognostic implications of echocardiographically determined left ventricular mass in the Framingham Heart Study. *New England Journal of Medicine* **322**, 1561–1566.

Levy, D., Salomon, M. *et al.* (1994) Prognostic implications of baseline echocardiographic features and their serial changes in subjects with left ventricular hypertrophy. *Circulation* **90**, 1786–1793.

Levy, D., Larson, M.G. *et al.* (1996) The progression from hypertension to congestive heart failure. *Journal of the American Medical Association* **275**, 1557–1562.

Lloyd-Jones, D.M., Larson, M.G. *et al.* (2002) Lifetime risk for developing congestive heart failure: The Framingham Heart Study. *Circulation* **106**, 3068–3072.

Loskutoff, D.J. and Samad, F. (1998) The adipocyte and hemostatic balance in obesity: studies of PAI-1. *Arteriosclerosis, Thrombosis and Vascular Biology* **18**, 1–6.

MacMahon, S.W., Wilcken, D.E.L. *et al.* (1986) The effect of weight reduction on left ventricular mass. *New England Journal of Medicine* **314**, 334–343.

Malone, S., Liu, P.P. *et al.* (1991) Obstructive sleep apnoea in patients with dilated cardiomyopathy: effects of continuous positive airway pressure. *Lancet* **338**, 1480–1484.

Marks, S.J., Chin, S. *et al.* (1998) The metabolic effects of preferential reduction of visceral adipose tissue in abdominally obese men. *International Journal of Obesity and Related Metabolic Disorders* **22**, 893–898.

Messerli, F.H., Nunez, B.D. *et al.* (1987) Overweight and sudden death: increased ventricular ectopy in cardiomyopathy of obesity. *Archives of Internal Medicine* **147**, 1725–1728.

Narkiewicz, K., van de Borne, P.J.H. *et al.* (1998) Sympathetic activity in obese subjects with and without obstructive sleep apnea. *Circulation* **98**, 772–776.

Piper, A.J. and Sullivan,C.E. (1994) Effects of short-term NIPPV in the treatment of patients with severe obstructive sleep apnea and hypercapnia. *Chest* **105**, 434–440.

Rader, D.J. (2000) Inflammatory markers of coronary risk. *New England Journal of Medicine* **343**, 1179–1182.

Rexrode, K.M., Carey, V.J. *et al.* (1998) Abdominal adiposity and coronary heart disease in women. *Journal of the American Medical Association* **280**, 1843–1848.

Ridker, P.M., Rifai, N. *et al.* (2000) Plasma concentration of interleukin-6 and the risk of future myocardial infarction among apparently healthy men. *Circulation* **101**, 1767–1772.

Rocchini, A., Key, J. *et al.* (1989) The effect of weight loss on the sensitivity of blood pressure to sodium in obese adolescents. *New England Journal of Medicine* **321**, 580–585.

Schachter, L.M., Salome, C.M. *et al.* (2001) Obesity is a risk for asthma and wheeze but not airway hyperresponsiveness. *Thorax* **56**, 4–8.

Schlaich, M.P., Kaye, D.M. *et al.* (2003) Relation between cardiac sympathetic activity and hypertensive left ventricular hypertrophy. *Circulation* **108**, 560–565.

Schwartz, P.J., Priori, S.G. *et al.* (2000) The long QT syndrome. In: Zipes, D.P., Jalife, J. eds. *Cardiac Electrophysiology: from Cell to Bedside*. Philadelphia: WB Saunders, 597–615.

Seppala, T., Partinen, M. *et al.* (1991) Sudden death and sleeping history among Finnish men. *Journal of Internal Medicine* **229**(1), 23–28.

Sin, D.D., Jones, R.L. *et al.* (2002) Obesity is a risk factor for dyspnoea but not airflow obstruction. *Archives of Internal Medicine* **162**, 1477–1481.

Sorof, J. and Daniels, S. (2002) Obesity hypertension in children, a problem of epidemic proportions. *Hypertension* **40**, 441–447.

Stevens, J., Cai, J. *et al.* (2002) Fitness and fatness as predictors of mortality from all causes and from cardiovascular disease in men and women in the lipid research clinics study. *American Journal of Epidemiology* **156**, 832–841.

Sugerman, H., DeMaria, E. *et al.* (1997) Increased intra-abdominal pressure and cardiac filling pressure in obesity-associated pseudotumor cerebri. *Neurology* **49**, 507–511.

Tuck, M.L., Sowers, J. *et al.* (1981) The effect of weight reduction on blood pressure, plasma renin activity, and plasma aldosterone levels in obese patients. *New England Journal of Medicine* **304**, 930–933.

Unterborn, J. (2001) Pulmonary function testing in obesity, pregnancy, and extremes of body habitus. *Clinics in Chest Medicine* **22**, 759–767.

Wilcox, I., McNamara, S.G. *et al.* (1998a) Syndrome Z, the interaction of sleep apnoea, vascular risk factors and heart disease. *Thorax* **53**, 25S–28S.

Wilcox, I., McNamara, S.G. *et al.* (1998b) Prognosis and sleep disordered breathing in heart failure. *Thorax* **53**, 33S–36S.

Yokoe, T., Minoguchi, K. *et al.* (2003) Elevated levels of C-reactive protein and interleukin 6 in patients with obstructive sleep apnea syndrome are decreased by nasal continuous positive airway pressure. *Circulation* **107**, 1129–1134.

Young, T., Shahar, E. *et al.* (2002) Predictors of sleep-disordered breathing in community-dwelling adults: The Sleep Heart Health Study. *Archives of Internal Medicine* **162**, 893–900.

Adult obesity: fertility

Stephen Robinson, Stephen Franks and Jasmine Leonce

Introduction, 281

Obesity and fertility, 281
  Nutrition and ovarian
  function, 281
  Hyperinsulinaemia and
  obese polycystic ovary
  syndrome, 282
  Metformin and obesity, 282
  Leptin and ovulation, 282
  Energy expenditure in
  obese polycystic ovary
  syndrome, 282

Pregnancy, 283
  Maternal body composition, 283
  Metabolism during normal and
  obese pregnancy, 284
  Fetal growth, 285
  The effects of obesity, 286

Maternal complications, 286
  Gestational diabetes and
  pregestational diabetes, 286
  Hypertensive disorders of
  pregnancy, 286
  Infections, 287
  Anaemia, 288
  Thromboembolic disease, 288
  Mode of delivery and postpartum
  complications, 288
  Breast-feeding, 288
  Weight gain of pregnancy, 288
  Long-term effect of pregnancy on
  maternal obesity, 289
  Pregnancy after adjustable
  gastric banding and weight
  control, 289

Effect of obesity on the fetus, 289
  Fetal macrosomia, 289

Congenital abnormalities, 290
  Perinatal morbidity and
  mortality, 290

Long-term consequences of maternal
obesity for the fetus, 290

Cost of maternal obesity, 290

Contraception in the obese
woman, 291
  Combined oral contraceptive
  pills, 291
  Progesterone-only contraceptive
  pills, 291
  Injectables, 291
  Intrauterine devices, 291

Summary, 292

References, 292

Introduction

England and Scotland together have one of the fastest growing obesity rates in the world. Women of the reproductive age group are also susceptible to the epidemic of obesity as the rates of childhood obesity increase. Furthermore, women are having children when they are older when they are more likely to be obese. Of 287 213 singleton pregnancies in the North West Thames (London) area, 27.5% of the women had a body mass index (BMI) of 25–29.9 and 10.9% had a BMI > 30. Obesity carries significant health consequences for fertility and pregnancy outcome with increased perinatal morbidity and mortality, as well as increased costs for the health service.

Obesity and fertility

The effects of obesity on fertility are detailed below.

Nutrition and ovarian function

Nutritional status has a considerable influence on female reproduction. In most mammals this is a means of ensuring that the pregnant mother and her newborn have access to enough food to maximize the chances of survival. Not only is being underweight associated with amenorrhoea as with anorexia nervosa through hypothalamic mechanisms, but also obesity is associated with anovulation. In obesity, the mechanisms of anovulation are complex, involving both peripheral and central pathways.

Body fat and body fat as a percentage of total weight are important to ovulation; however, polycystic ovaries have an effect additional to that of obesity. The term *polycystic ovaries* refers to the typical ovarian morphology—enlarged ovaries with increased stroma and increased follicle number. Polycystic ovary syndrome (PCOS) is conventionally defined as the combination of hyperandrogenism (hirsutism and acne) and anovulation (oligomenorrhoea, infertility and dysfunctional uterine bleeding) with polycystic ovaries on ultrasound scanning (Franks, 1989). The aetiology of polycystic ovary and PCOS appears to be genetic, with environmental precipitants.

Obesity is a common feature, occurring in 35–40% of cases of PCOS (Franks, 1989). It is not clear whether obesity acts to amplify the effects of PCOS or whether the mechanisms of obesity and the aetiology of PCOS are linked. Obese women presenting with PCOS are more likely to have menstrual disturbance and more likely to be hirsute than lean PCOS women. Total testosterone and luteinizing hormone are similar in the two groups (Kiddy *et al.*, 1990). But sex hormone-binding globulin concentrations (SHBG) are lower in obese women. SHBG levels were inversely correlated with BMI in PCOS women and control subjects, the values being lower in PCOS women. Insulin may be the factor that links the SHBG and obesity, and hyperinsulinaemia may be related to the anovulation in these women. Indeed, hyperinsulinaemia and insulin resistance may be the final common pathway by which anovulation occurs in women with obesity or in women with PCOS.

Hyperinsulinaemia and obese polycystic ovary syndrome

Hyperinsulinaemia and insulin insensitivity are well-recognized features of uncomplicated obesity (see Chapter 8), although the primary abnormality is unknown.

Women with polycystic ovaries are hyperinsulinaemic (Dunaif *et al.*, 1987; Mahabeer *et al.*, 1989) but, unlike type 2 diabetes, this is associated with a normal proportion of split proinsulin and concentrations of specific insulin are significantly elevated (Conway *et al.*, 1993; Robinson *et al.*, 1993a). Women with polycystic ovaries are more insulin resistant than weight-matched control women, the obese PCOS women having a degree of insulin insensitivity similar to that found in type 2 diabetes (Dunaif *et al.*, 1989). The hyperinsulinaemia is associated with insulin resistance in terms of glucose and lipid metabolism (Robinson *et al.*, 1996). Oligomenorrhoeic PCOS women, but not PCOS women with regular menstrual cycles, are more insulin resistant than weight-matched control women (Robinson *et al.*, 1993b). Menstrual dysfunction does not appear to affect insulin sensitivity. Amenorrhoea due to suppression of the pituitary–ovarian axis does not alter insulin levels or action (Geffner *et al.*, 1986). It seems more likely that hyperinsulinaemia and/or insulin resistance contributes to menstrual disturbance.

Weight loss following calorie restriction in obese PCOS subjects is associated with improvement in ovulatory function and a reduction in insulin concentrations (Kiddy *et al.*, 1990). The reduced hyperinsulinaemia precedes improved ovulatory function (Kiddy *et al.*, 1992). The common occurrence of insulin resistance in PCOS and the link between hyperinsulinaemia and PCOS provide the rationale for the use of insulin-sensitizing agents in the treatment of PCOS. The clinical relationship of insulin and ovarian action would seem to be in accord with *in vitro* experiments demonstrating that insulin augments luteinizing hormone-driven oestrogen secretion from granulosa cells (Willis *et al.*, 1996). The interaction of gonadotrophin and insulin action on the ovaries is summarized by Franks and colleagues (2000). Insulin resistance is usually measured in terms of glucose effect. The possibility exists therefore that insulin action on ovarian function is not influenced by insulin insensitivity in other tissues.

Metformin and obesity

Metformin has been used in several studies in PCOS women (summarized in Table 19.1). Although some biochemical parameters improve in women who use metformin, there has not been a clear benefit in terms of ovulation or hirsutism. A trial of metformin may well be used on an individual basis. Diarrhoea and gastrointestinal upset were reported in 10–40% of PCO subjects (Moghetti *et al.*, 2000; Pasquali *et al.*, 2000). Metformin has been shown to improve insulin secretion in obese PCOS women (Nestler and Jakubowicz, 1997). A recent meta-analysis has shown metformin treatment to be associated with improved ovulation rates. However, the authors also concluded that better ovulation rates could be achieved by weight loss.

Leptin and ovulation

Increased leptin concentrations are found in obesity. Leptin is secreted by white adipocytes acting on the hypothalamus to influence energy intake and energy expenditure (see Chapter 3). Reduced leptin during undernutrition is associated with decreased satiety and decreased energy expenditure. Decreased leptin concentrations are associated with anovulation, a mechanism of reducing the chance of pregnancy when calorie stores are low. The physiological role of the high level of leptin found in obesity is probably limited. PCOS subjects, especially obese women, have increased leptin concentrations (Muhittin *et al.*, 2002).

Energy expenditure in obese polycystic ovary syndrome

Total energy expenditure can be considered to have three main contributors: resting energy expenditure (REE), exercise and thermogenic activities such as postprandial thermogenesis (PPT) (see Chapter 6). PPT is believed to have an obligate and facultative component and the latter may be reduced in obese and pre-obese subjects, although there is considerable debate about this point. PPT and REE have been measured in women with PCOS and compared with weight-matched control subjects (Robinson *et al.*, 1992). The REE was similar in PCOS subjects and control subjects, but PPT was reduced in women with PCOS. PPT correlated negatively with insulin sensitivity in the women with PCOS but not in the control group. The association between glucose-induced thermogenesis and insulin resistance has been demonstrated in a large group of subjects (Camastra *et al.*, 1999). Reduced PPT may predispose to obesity although the obese woman clearly has an increased energy intake compared with the lean woman by virtue of increased lean body mass. Reduced PPT may be a marker for an associated reduction of satiety acting at a hypothalamic level.

Table 19.1 Summary of studies of metformin use in PCOS. NA, not applicable; TDS, three times daily.

Authors	Design	Patient no treatment: controls	Metformin, dose, duration	Insulin resistance	BMI	Testosterone	Ovulation rate	Menstrual loss
Chou *et al.* (2003)	Randomized double-blind placebo	32 (15:17)	500 mg, TDS, 3 months	No change	No change	Decrease	NA	No change
Vandermolen *et al.* (2001)	Randomized double-blind placebo	28	500 mg, TDS, 7 weeks	No change	No change	No change	Increase	NA
Kolodziejczyk *et al.* (2000)	Observational	39	500 mg, TDS, 3 months	Decrease	Decrease	NA	NA	Increased cycle length
Moghetti *et al.* (2000)	Randomized double-blind placebo	23	500 mg, TDS, 6 months	Decrease	No change	NA	NA	No change
Pasquali *et al.* (2000)	Double-blind	40 (20:20)	850 mg, BD, 6 months	Decrease	Decrease	NA	NA	Increased frequency
Unluhizarci *et al.* (1999)	Observational	17	500 mg, TDS, 4–5 weeks	Decrease	No change	Decrease	NA	NA
Morin-Papunen *et al.* (1998)	Observational	20	500 mg, TDS, 4–6 months	Decrease	No change	Decrease	NA	Increased cycles
Nestler *et al.* (1998)	Randomized placebo	61	500 mg, TDS, 4–5 weeks	Decrease	No change	No change	NA	NA
Ehrman *et al.* (1997)	Observational	20	850 mg, TDS, 3 months	No change	No change	No change	NA	NA

Pregnancy

The effects of obesity on pregnancy are discussed below.

Maternal body composition

The weight gain of the maternofetal unit is a function of the accumulated energy stores and the energy required to maintain these stores (Hytten and Leitch, 1971). Protein and fat are accumulated through pregnancy, whereas the increased lean body mass demands an increase in resting energy expenditure. There is also an increase in PPT associated with the increased energy intake. In order to measure the fat stores and to facilitate assessment of basal metabolic rate per unit lean body mass, body composition has been measured. The measurement of body composition should allow for the increase in water content of lean tissue during pregnancy, from 72.5% at 10 weeks to 75% at 40 weeks' gestation (van Raaij *et al.*, 1988). Two whole-body methods combined give the best estimate of fat gained during pregnancy (Prentice *et al.*, 1996), with an average total fat gain of 3.0 kg by late pregnancy and a gain in maternal fat stores of 2.6 kg.

The total energy needs of pregnancy amount to 360 MJ or about 1.2 MJ/day (Hytten and Chamberlain, 1980). This was later modified (Hytten, 1991) and gives values of a 2.7-kg increase in fat stores for a pregnancy in which the weight gain was 12.4 kg with a baby delivered of 3.3 kg. The extra requirements of energy through pregnancy are not equal to the increased energy intake of normal pregnancy and there is a large field of work on why this should be the case.

Basal metabolic rate (BMR) or resting metabolic rate (RMR) has been measured in several longitudinal studies. There were differences in the developed compared with the developing world; this review will concentrate on the 'developed' world. In a serial study using 24-h calorimetry, it was concluded that there were highly characteristic changes with each subject and large intersubject differences (Prentice *et al.*, 1989). Lean women tended to have a decrease in BMR early in pregnancy before the rise beyond 20 weeks' gestation, whereas women with an increased BMI and increased fat mass showed an increased basal metabolic rate from the beginning of gestation. The energy maintenance costs of pregnancy were strongly correlated with the degree of fat mass of the women before they became pregnant ($r = 0.72$) and the weight gained during pregnancy ($r = 0.79$) (Prentice *et al.*, 1996).

Diet-induced thermogenesis (DIT) and PPT have been studied in pregnancy. This is the increment in energy expenditure after consumption of a meal. Two studies have demonstrated no change in DIT during pregnancy (Nagy and King, 1984; Spaaij *et al.*, 1994). Two other studies have demonstrated decreased PPT during pregnancy (Illingworth *et al.*, 1987; Robinson *et al.*, 1993a). The latter study also demonstrated the reduction in PPT to correlate with the degree of insulin insensitivity during normal pregnancy. There has been no specific study of obesity and PPT in pregnancy, but obese women are more insulin resistant, consistent with reduced PPT found in other settings (Camastra *et al.*, 1999).

The thermogenic response to weight-bearing or non-weight-bearing exercise appears to change little during pregnancy. Energy intake is difficult to establish, although there is little evidence for increased error in longitudinal studies through pregnancy. Prentice and colleagues (1996) conclude that an energy intake increment of between 0.3 and 0.5 MJ/day is needed, representing 84–140 MJ through pregnancy. The increased intake does not meet the increased energy needs.

Metabolism during normal and obese pregnancy

Normal pregnancy is characterized by significant changes to intermediary metabolism wherein insulin resistance appears to play a central role. Fasting blood glucose levels are decreased in normal pregnancy, reaching a nadir at 12 weeks' gestation and remaining at this level until term. The mechanism for this is uncertain. It does not appear to be related to fetal demand (the fetus weighs 16 g at 12 weeks) or to changes in insulin concentration. Plasma glucose excursions around the fasting level are not great after food until the third trimester and cumulative glucose concentrations over 24 h have been reported to be slightly increased (Cousins *et al.*, 1980) or decreased (Gillmer *et al.*, 1975) compared with non-pregnant levels.

After a glucose load, peripheral glucose uptake is enhanced in insulin-sensitive tissues (largely skeletal muscle), whereas hepatic glucose production is suppressed. During pregnancy, compared with the same postpartum women, the peak glucose concentration was increased by approximately 0.5 mmol/L and delayed, from 30 to 60 min (Lind, 1975). No data are available for obese pregnant women. In the non-pregnant state, however, obesity is associated with similar post-glucose load plasma glucose concentrations to lean subjects, but insulin concentrations are increased.

Fasting plasma insulin levels increase through pregnancy but these changes do not occur at the same stage of pregnancy as the decrease in glucose concentrations. This would seem to preclude any cause and effect relationship between the two unless insulin sensitivity is also changing and the pancreatic β-cell glucostat is set at a different level (Lind *et al.*, 1973; Kuhl and Holst, 1976). For a given glucose challenge, the pregnant woman is stimulated to produce more insulin so that plasma insulin concentrations may be double those observed in the non-pregnant (Lind, 1975; Freinkel, 1980). A cohort of obese women [>150% ideal body weight (IBW), roughly equivalent to BMI of 33 kg/m^2] have been studied through pregnancy (Kalkhoff *et al.*, 1988). The same pattern of changes in plasma glucose and hyperinsulinaemia was seen compared with a non-obese control group.

Obese premenopausal women are insulin resistant compared with non-obese control women (Ludvik *et al.*, 1995). Uncomplicated pregnancy is an insulin-resistant state, demonstrated by the euglycaemic clamp (Ryan *et al.*, 1985) intravenous glucose tolerance test with minimal modelling (Buchanan *et al.*, 1990) and the short insulin tolerance test (Robinson *et al.*, 1993a). The insulin resistance of pregnancy is associated with a lower apparent volume of distribution for insulin and decreased insulin clearance (Jolly *et al.*, 2003). The importance of this for insulin resistance in pregnancy is not clear. The insulin resistance is more marked in obese women before and during otherwise uncomplicated pregnancy, but the effects of the increased insulin resistance are unknown.

Glucose turnover in pregnant women has been assessed with non-radioactive stable isotopes (Kalhan *et al.*, 1979). The isotopic enrichment of a glucose tracer primed infusion method allows the calculation of systemic glucose production or hepatic glucose output. Although one would expect hepatic glucose output to be similar in obese and lean pregnant women, there are no data regarding this. Hepatic glucose output is not elevated in subjects with type 2 diabetes until the fasting plasma glucose is greater than 8 mmol/L (DeFronzo, 1988).

Non-esterified fatty acid (NEFA) concentrations are variable in non-pregnant normal subjects and the length of fasting has a major influence. There is no agreement in the literature as to whether post-absorptive NEFA concentrations are altered in normal pregnancy. NEFA levels rise more quickly in pregnant women fasting from 12 to 18 h compared with non-pregnant control women (Metzger *et al.*, 1982).

Triglyceride levels fall in early pregnancy and then rise to term; by the third trimester of pregnancy, there is a two- to threefold increase in plasma triglyceride (Herrera *et al.*, 1987). There are lesser increases in cholesterol concentrations. Very low-density lipoprotein (VLDL), low-density lipoprotein (LDL) and high-density lipoprotein (HDL) all show increased concentrations in normal pregnancy. VLDL and IDL levels are increased but compositionally unchanged (Warth *et al.*, 1975). Triglyceride rises more than cholesterol and phospholipid in LDL and HDL. Cholesterol levels rise through pregnancy mainly as LDL-cholesterol. HDL-cholesterol levels peak in mid-pregnancy then fall towards term. The hypertriglyceridaemia probably is a result of three factors. Increased adipose tissue lipolysis, related to insulin insensitivity, enhances NEFA delivery to the liver and contributes to the increased VLDL (Kissebah *et al.*, 1982).

Maternal hyperphagia and unmodified lipid absorption from the gut lead to increased chylomicron concentrations.

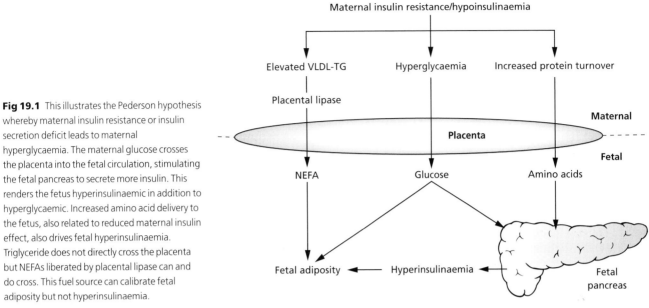

Fig 19.1 This illustrates the Pederson hypothesis whereby maternal insulin resistance or insulin secretion deficit leads to maternal hyperglycaemia. The maternal glucose crosses the placenta into the fetal circulation, stimulating the fetal pancreas to secrete more insulin. This renders the fetus hyperinsulinaemic in addition to hyperglycaemic. Increased amino acid delivery to the fetus, also related to reduced maternal insulin effect, also drives fetal hyperinsulinaemia. Triglyceride does not directly cross the placenta but NEFAs liberated by placental lipase can and do cross. This fuel source can calibrate fetal adiposity but not hyperinsulinaemia.

Reduced lipoprotein lipase activity, especially in adipose tissue, means there is reduced capacity for triglyceride removal (Herrera *et al.*, 1987). Maternal hypertriglyceridaemia is present in the second and third trimesters of normal pregnancy, and is associated with the degree of maternal insulin resistance (Robinson *et al.*, 1993a). Maternal BMI correlates with triglyceride concentrations ($r = 0.58$, $P < 0.01$) in the second trimester but this association is lost in the third trimester.

Obese pregnant women had increased concentrations of branched-chain amino acids compared with lean pregnant control women (Felig *et al.*, 1969). During normal pregnancy, total plasma amino acid concentrations decrease compared with non-pregnant women (Kalkhoff *et al.*, 1988). During the second trimester of non-diabetic pregnancy, total amino acid concentrations were reduced in obese women compared with the lean group. There was no significant difference in total amino acid concentrations during the third trimester, but histidine concentrations were increased in the obese women. Although there are several studies of protein turnover in normal pregnancy using stable non-radioactive tracers (Thompson and Halliday, 1992), there are no specific studies of the effects of obesity. One would predict that the insulin resistance of normal pregnancy would be associated with increased amino acid turnover and this would be further elevated in insulin-resistant obese women.

Fetal growth

Glucose has been believed to be the main fuel for fetal growth (Fig. 19.1) (Ginsberg and Cramp, 1977). Although other fuels are now believed to be important, the relative caloric load to the fetus from glucose, fat and protein is unknown (Sheath *et al.*, 1972; Kalkhoff *et al.*, 1988; Knopp *et al.*, 1992). Increased

serum triglyceride concentrations in the mother were thought to be an indicator of the increased importance of maternal lipid oxidation, sparing carbohydrate and protein for fetal use (Warth *et al.*, 1975). Furthermore, the propensity for ketosis is more rapid and profound in the post-absorptive state than in non-pregnant women and the term 'accelerated starvation' was coined to describe these changes (Metzger and Freinkel, 1987). It was suggested that the increased ketone body and free fatty acid concentrations in the post-absorptive state represent increased oxidation by the mother of these metabolites, and that this more rapid adjustment to fat catabolism allows glucose to be spared for transplacental transfer. The other side of this process was said to be 'facilitated anabolism'. The increased postprandial rise in glucose and other fetal fuels was hypothesized to be a mechanism for promoting fetal growth.

Maternal regional adiposity is also associated with fetal growth. The influence of regional distribution of fat on newborn size was investigated in a sample of 702 women whose preconceptual nutritional characteristics were recorded. Each 0.1 unit increase in pregravid waist–hip ratio predicted a 120-g greater birth weight, a 0.51-cm greater length and a 0.3-cm greater head circumference (Brown *et al.*, 1996).

In the placenta of the guinea pig, which is haemochorial and therefore similar to the human, hydrolysis of maternal triglyceride in very low-density lipoprotein (VLDL) liberates NEFA in the placental bed and is potentially a major fetal fuel (Thomas, 1987). In support of this hypothesis is the observation that maternal triglyceride concentrations measured in the second trimester correlate better with fetal birth weight than does maternal glucose (Knopp *et al.*, 1992; Nolan *et al.*, 1995).

Fetal macrosomia will be discussed under the effects of obesity on pregnancy.

The effects of obesity

The adverse consequences of obesity in pregnancy can be divided broadly into maternal complications and fetal complications. The complications of maternal obesity are shown in Table 19.2.

Maternal complications

The following complications may arise.

Gestational diabetes and pregestational diabetes

Gestational diabetes has an incidence of 14–25% in pregnancies complicated by obesity (Table 19.2). Maternal diabetes is associated with an increased incidence of fetal macrosomia, polycythaemia, intrauterine death, birth trauma and neonatal hypoglycaemia. In the medium term, the infant may have developmental delay (Rizzo et al., 1991). In the long term there may be metabolic complications for the offspring of the diabetic mother as adults in terms of obesity or early diabetes (Pettitt et al., 1983; 1988). The mothers have an increased risk of birth trauma due to the macrosomic infant and have an increased chance of developing type 2 diabetes in later life.

Gestational diabetes mellitus (GDM) can be defined as diabetes first discovered during pregnancy; it usually remits after pregnancy but this is not required to make the diagnosis. The increased incidence of GDM in obese pregnant women has been ascribed to increased insulin resistance combined with an insulin secretory deficit. Increasing BMI is associated with insulin insensitivity in normal pregnancy (Robinson et al., 1993a). As there is considerable evidence that GDM precedes type 2 diabetes (O'Sullivan, 1984; Dornhorst et al., 1990) these women probably represent a subset of insulin-resistant women who have inadequate insulin secretion in the face of insulin resistance. That being the case, the increased prevalence of obesity in women with GDM may represent a combined predisposition to both obesity and type 2 diabetes rather than obesity increasing the risk of type 2 diabetes per se.

The prevalence of diabetes in pregnancy, mostly gestational diabetes, with maternal obesity was found to be 10.6% compared with 2.8% in lean women (Edwards et al., 1978). When obesity is defined as 135% or more of IBW the relative risk for GDM is 6.57 (Abrams and Parker, 1988).

The logical treatments of obesity and gestational diabetes are not clear as there are no randomized studies of diet treatment in obese subjects with or without GDM. Maternal obesity and excessive weight gain in pregnancy are associated with fetal macrosomia and treatment should be directed to avoid this (Boyd et al., 1983), although the long-term outcome of such treatment is unknown. The US Institute of Sciences has made recommendations for weight gain during pregnancy, including obese women (BMI > 26–29) of 7.0–11.5 kg. This is not the practice of the authors: many UK units observe good outcome with mothers gaining less than 6.8 kg (Pimblett, 1996).

Total energy intake is crucial in pregnancy complicated by diabetes or obesity. Women with gestational diabetes are often treated with energy restriction. In a trial of hypocaloric diets for women with gestational diabetes, women gained a mean of 2 kg from 28 weeks' gestation (Dornhorst et al., 1991). The incidence of macrosomia was reduced to that of the general population when no infant was small for gestational age. Maternal ketosis should be avoided as this may be detrimental to the fetus (Rizzo et al., 1991). When the maternal energy intake was restricted to 5.02 MJ/day, improved glycaemic control was accompanied by increased maternal ketonaemia (Magee et al., 1990). However, when energy was restricted to 6.92 MJ/day, there was an improvement in glycaemic control with reduced triglyceride levels, which was not accompanied by increased maternal ketonaemia (Knopp et al., 1991). Women with pre-existing type 1 or type 2 diabetes (most of whom will need insulin before and during the pregnancy) will have dietary prescriptions on the basis of their weight. Hypoglycaemia can be a problem, especially in the first trimester, and the dietary prescription should take this into account. Insulin treatment of gestational diabetes is required more often in obese women than in lean women (Comtois et al., 1993). Exercise is a useful adjunct to dietary management of gestational diabetes and has been shown to improve glycaemic control (Jovanovic-Peterson and Peterson, 1991).

Most would recommend a diet high in complex carbohydrate, around 50% of the total energy intake. This should also be combined with an effort to reduce refined carbohydrate although moderate amounts of sucrose are not harmful. Soluble fibre reduces glucose and triglycerides but this has not been specifically tested in the obese woman with diabetes. Most women in the UK consume more than the recommended 51 g of protein per day prior to pregnancy. There is a theoretical concern that excessive protein restriction could lead to fetal insulin resistance/insulin secretion programming for that infant as an adult and increase the likelihood of adult diabetes (Hales and Barker, 1992). Protein restriction should therefore be avoided.

Hypertensive disorders of pregnancy

The relationship between essential hypertension and obesity in non-pregnant subjects is well recognized (Kannel et al., 1967). Hypertension during pregnancy may be pre-existing or pregnancy associated; the two conditions are not entirely separate and the studies do not always differentiate them. Pre-eclampsia has an incidence of 6–14% (Bianco et al., 1998; Beaten et al., 2001; Kumari, 2001).

The prevalence of hypertension in severely obese pregnant women varies between 5% and 66% (Edwards et al., 1978; Gross et al., 1980; Garbaciak et al., 1985; Abrams and Parker, 1988). The relative risk of hypertension (compared to a lean control group) is 4.49 when obesity is defined as a BMI

Table 19.2 Various pregnancy complications of maternal obesity are illustrated, categorized according to BMI 20–25, 25–30 and >30. For each BMI, the proportion of women having a particular complication is shown. The odds ratio is given numerically and graphically, with BMI 20–25 defined as OR = 1.

	BMI	Proportion	OR (99% CI)	Graphical representation of previous column
Antenatal complications				
Gestational diabetes	20–25	0.75		
	25–30	1.70	1.68 (1.53–1.84)	
	>30	3.50	3.6 (3.25–3.98)	
Pre-eclampsia	20–25	0.70		
	25–30	0.97	1.44 (1.28–1.62)	
	>30	1.43	2.14 (1.85–2.47)	
Maternal complications				
Wound infection	20–25	0.39		
	25–30	0.59	1.27 (1.09–1.48)	
	>30	1.34	2.24 (1.91–2.64)	
Urinary tract infection	20–25	0.69		
	25–30	0.84	1.17 (1.04–1.33)	
	>30	1.10	1.39 (1.18–1.63)	
Pulmonary embolism	20–25	0.04		
	25–30	0.07	1.41 (0.91–2.19)	
	>30	0.08	1.48 (0.82–2.69)	
Delivery complications				
Induction of labour	20–25	15–26		
	25–30	19–24	1.27 (1.23–1.30)	
	>30	24.65	1.70 (1.64–1.76)	
Emergency caesarean section	20–25	7.83		
	25–30	10.25	1.30 (1.25–1.34)	
	>30	13.40	1.83 (1.74–1.93)	
Postpartum haemorrhage	20–25	10.38		
	25–30	13.19	1.16 (1.12–1.21)	
	>30	17.07	1.39 (1.32–1.46)	
Neonatal complications				
Birth weight >90th centile	20–25	9.03		
	25–30	13.41	1.57 (1.50–1.64)	
	>30	17.46	2.36 (2.23–2.50)	
Admission to SCBU >24 h	20–25	5.14		
	25–30	5.52	1.22 (1.16–1.28)	
	>30	6.48	1.34 (1.25–1.44)	
Breast-feeding	20–25	65.5		
	25–30	60.3	0.86 (0.84–0.88)	
	>30	50.1	0.58 (0.56–0.60)	
				0.5 1.0 1.5 2 3 4

>33 kg/m^2 (Abrams and Parker, 1988) and 8.70 (Garbaciak *et al.*, 1985) and 2.42 (Edwards *et al.*, 1978) when obesity is defined as a BMI >37 kg/m^2.

In a Swedish population, hypertensive disease among nulliparous women was 2.8% in lean women compared with 10.2% in obese women (Cnattingius *et al.*, 2001). In a multiethnic UK population, the relative risk of pre-eclampsia was 1.44 in an overweight group and increased to 2.14 in an obese group (Sebire *et al.*, 2001).

Infections

Women with a BMI of 30 or more have two to three times more postoperative infections than thinner women (Myles *et al.*, 2002). Urinary tract infections (UTIs) include urethritis, cystitis and pyelonephritis. The relative risk of UTI in mild obesity is 1.42 (Abrams and Parker, 1988). Some (Garbaciak *et al.*, 1985; Abrams and Parker, 1988; Sebire *et al.*, 2001), but not all (Edwards *et al.*, 1978) workers have found a further increase in the incidence of UTI in severely obese women during pregnancy. Wound infections are also more common in obese women (Sebire *et al.*, 2001).

Anaemia

Anaemia is less common in obese non-pregnant women than in lean women (Rimm *et al.*, 1975); this may be related to oligomenorrhoea and therefore reduced menstrual blood loss prior to conception. Obese pregnant women also have a reduced prevalence of anaemia. It is not clear whether this relates to obese women starting pregnancy with more iron stores than lean women (Edwards *et al.*, 1978; Garbaciak *et al.*, 1985; Abrams and Parker, 1988). The relative risk for anaemia in severely obese pregnant women is between 0.56 and 0.72.

Thromboembolic disease

Thromboembolic disease is rare in pregnancy, therefore large studies are required to have the power necessary to demonstrate any increase in prevalence. In a study of the North West Thames area of London, the prevalence of thromboembolism was 0.05% in a normal-weight population compared with 0.06% in moderately obese women, but 0.12% in the very obese group [odds ratio (OR) 1.60, 1.01–2.56, $P < 0.001$], with smoking being included in the regression model (Sebire *et al.*, 2001). Thromboembolism in pregnancy is most likely to occur post partum and obesity is a major risk factor. In the most recent Confidential Enquiry into Maternal Deaths in the United Kingdom (1997–1999), there were 35 deaths from thromboembolism; risk factors were present in 25 out of the 35 and 13 women were overweight. Obese women undergoing caesarean section should receive thromboembolic prophylaxis in the form of early mobilization, compression stockings and prophylactic heparin where necessary.

Mode of delivery and postpartum complications

An increased rate of induction of labour has been reported in obese women compared with normal-weight women (Gross *et al.*, 1980; Sebire *et al.*, 2001), whereas the duration of labour and percentage of instrumental deliveries are the same. The caesarean section rates are increased in obese women and include both emergency and elective caesarean sections with a 1.15- to 3-fold increase over the rates in lean women (Bianco *et al.*, 1998; Sebire *et al.*, 2001). In three US studies, the non-obese caesarean section rate was between 8.6% and 13.3% (Edwards *et al.*, 1978; Garbaciak *et al.*, 1985; Abrams and Parker, 1988). In moderately obese women, the caesarean section rate was 12.4–16.9%, rising to 11.0–21.5% in the very obese group. Reasons for increased caesarean section rates in the obese women included macrosomia-associated cephalopelvic disproportion, fetal distress and slow progress of induced labour (Galtier-Dereure *et al.*, 1995). For morbidly obese women (mean BMI 57.2 ± 9.2) who are attempting a successful vaginal delivery after a previous caesarean section, vaginal delivery is 13%, which is significantly lower than the quoted success rate of 70–80% in a leaner population (Chauhan *et al.*, 2001). Endometritis is also more common in obese women post caesarean sections but tends to follow the emergency operations. Prophylactic antibiotics is routine practice for women undergoing surgical delivery in many obstetric units.

Breast-feeding

Maternal obesity appears to be associated with a reduction in breast-feeding (Donath and Amir, 2000; Sebire *et al.*, 2001; Li *et al.*, 2003). Matched records from the Paediatric Nutrition Surveillance System and the Pregnancy Nutrition Surveillance System from seven US states were obtained over the period 1996–1998. Maternal characteristics were identified and women who were obese (BMI > 29) before pregnancy breast fed for ~2 weeks less than pre-pregnancy normal-weight subjects. Those women who failed to reach the recommended weight gain during pregnancy, and those who exceeded the recommended gestational weight gain, breast fed for 1 week less than those who gained the recommended weight (Li *et al.*, 2003). Other significant risk factors were identified for failure to initiate breast-feeding: these included low infant birth weight, smoking, late introduction of prenatal care and poverty. Although there may be an association between obesity and poor breast-feeding practices, the mechanisms are unclear. Poor milk production, mechanical difficulties of breast-feeding and psychological factors have been suggested but were not assessed in this study. Further studies are required to test the mechanisms of poor breast-feeding practices in obese women.

Weight gain of pregnancy

Normal pregnant women gain a mean weight of 10–12 kg during their pregnancy. Women with severe obesity (> 37 kg/m^2 pre-pregnancy weight) had a higher prevalence of low weight gain (5.5 kg) during pregnancy (31.2%) than to a non-obese control group (4.3%) (Edwards *et al.*, 1978). Women weighing over 90 kg were more likely to have low weight gain than those mothers weighing less than 90 kg (Gross *et al.*, 1980). However, it is not clear whether this low weight gain can be labelled inadequate, and the optimal weight gain in obese women is therefore controversial. The Institute of Medicine recommends a minimum of 6.8 kg, even for massively obese women to improve fetal outcome (Institute of Medicine, 1990). A randomized trial looking at low-fat eating in pregnancy, in an attempt to uphold these recommendations, also incorporated educational interventions and exercise programmes. Although the intervention seemed to have some benefit in normal-weight women there was no significant benefit in overweight women (Polley *et al.*, 2002).

Although many clinicians would treat maternal obesity and

gestational diabetes with energy restriction, formal randomized control trials of maternal calorie restriction on maternal and fetal outcome are required. Certainly, the meals should be spread through the day to avoid ketosis.

Long-term effect of pregnancy on maternal obesity

Many women attribute long-term weight gain to a previous pregnancy. In a study of 7000 women who had two pregnancies within 6 years, a weight gain of 9 kg in the first pregnancy had a significant effect on body weight prior to the second pregnancy. Therefore, weight gain in excess of 9 kg during pregnancy is more likely to be retained after pregnancy (Greene *et al.*, 1988). There is a strong association between weight gain in pregnancy and postpartum weight retention (Polley *et al.*, 2002). A weight gain of 10 kg is statistically associated with best fetal outcome, but those data are based on the whole population, lean and obese. The ideal weight gain for the mother may not be the same as the ideal weight gain for the fetus.

Pregnancy after adjustable gastric banding and weight control

Pregnancy has been investigated after laparoscopic banded gastroplasty (LBG). The aim of the operation is to produce early satiety and decrease food consumption. In a study of 265 fertile couples with an obese female who had had gastric banding performed between 1990 and 1998, there were 23 completed pregnancies. The average weight loss was 10–12 kg over 4 months to 4 years. Of the pregnancies that went to full term (18), none had complications related to obesity. Of the 18, there were 14 vaginal deliveries and four caesarean sections, with a mean birth weight of 3.6 kg (range 2381–3912 g). Two subjects who gained the most weight during pregnancy had no fluid in their bands and hence no restriction of food intake with weight gain of 31–39 kg. Of the women (12) who kept the diameter of their bands constant during the pregnancy, three subjects lost weight (1.8–7.6 kg) and nine gained weight (1.4–25 kg). Three women required removal of fluid because of nausea and vomiting (Martin *et al.*, 2000).

Effect of obesity on the fetus

Maternal obesity may cause fetal macrosomia, congenital abnormalities and perinatal morbidity and mortality.

Fetal macrosomia

Fetal macrosomia has been defined by a variety of methods; the relative importance of each may depend on the outcome of interest. For example, a fetal weight greater than 4 kg will have 'mechanical' implications for safe delivery and beyond. The centiles for gestational age, birth weight or a more sophisticated birth weight ratio based on gestation, maternal weight, maternal height, parity and ethnic group have more predictive power (Sanderson *et al.*, 1994). Macrosomia can also be defined in terms of relative fetal obesity (for example, skinfold thickness or magnetic resonance imaging-based abdominal fat) and one may hypothesize that the long-term outcome for the infant is more dependent on relative obesity.

The main risk factors for fetal macrosomia are maternal diabetes and maternal obesity (Fig. 19.1). The original Pederson hypothesis (Pederson *et al.*, 1954) suggested that the increased glucose concentrations in the diabetic mother led to fetal hyperglycaemia. The hypothesis suggested that the fetal pancreas is able to respond to hyperglycaemia from the 20th week of gestation, and this leads to fetal hyperinsulinaemia. The fetus then uses the glucose to increase fat stores. The hyperinsulinaemia is to an extent autonomous and this leads to neonatal hypoglycaemia. Maternal obesity may have a role in fetal macrosomia, but what are the mechanisms involved when the mother's glucose concentration is normal? Maternal obesity is more important to fetal macrosomia than GDM, when the glucose is only slightly elevated. GDM is associated with a greater risk of neonatal hypoglycaemia. Maternal obesity is associated with fetal hyperinsulinaemia, even in the absence of maternal diabetes (Hoegsburg *et al.*, 1993). Fetal macrosomia may involve glucose protein and lipid metabolism (Fig. 19.1). Maternal insulin resistance is associated with elevated VLDL triglyceride and increased energy delivery to the fetus. The insulin resistance may lead to increased protein turnover, which in turn could lead to fetal hyperinsulinaemia.

The association of maternal obesity and fetal macrosomia is independent of maternal diabetes mellitus, but the effects are additive. Fetal macrosomia is more common in the obese non-diabetic mother than in the lean mother with gestational diabetes (Maresh *et al.*, 1989). Indeed, the risk of fetal macrosomia is greater for the infant of the non-diabetic obese mother than for the infant of a lean mother with gestational diabetes. One study looking at morbidly obese women with a BMI > 40 at booking showed the incidence of fetal macrosomia to be 32% compared with 9.3% in the non-obese group (Kumari, 2001).

When macrosomia is defined in terms of birth weight greater than 4000 g, the prevalence is 1.3–1.7% and mothers are more likely to be obese. Mothers are also more likely to be older, have greater parity, have a greater prevalence of maternal diabetes and more likely to be post mature (>42 weeks' gestation) (Spellacy *et al.*, 1985).

There is a relationship between maternal weight gain and birth weight for mothers who are underweight, normal weight and mildly obese (Abrams and Laros, 1986). However, very obese mothers (greater than 33 kg/m² IBW) demonstrate no correlation between weight gain during pregnancy and fetal weight.

Clinical methods or special investigation poorly predict

fetal macrosomia. Recent studies indicate that fasting maternal triglyceride concentrations taken in the first or second trimester of pregnancy may be a better predictor of fetal macrosomia than maternal glucose concentrations (Knopp et al., 1992; Nolan et al., 1995; Kitajima et al., 2001). Ultrasound prediction of birth weight is particularly poor for macrosomic infants (Grandjean et al., 1980). Macrosomia is a major cause of obstructed labour (Boyd et al., 1983), and there is a higher rate of induction of labour and a higher rate of operative delivery. The induction of labour solely on the grounds of fetal macrosomia appears counterproductive. Expectant management is associated with fewer caesarean sections without compromising neonatal outcomes. Other delivery and post-natal complications in the macrosomic infant include shoulder dystocia, low Apgar scores at 1 and 5 min, birth asphyxia, fractured clavicle and brachial cord injuries.

One study that looked at the contributing factors to shoulder dystocia found that maternal obesity was not a significant independent risk factor for shoulder dystocia (OR 0.5), but that fetal macrosomia was the single most important predictor. The adjusted ORs were 39.5 for birth weight greater than 4500 g and 9 for birth weight between 4000 and 4499 g (Robinson et al., 2003).

Congenital abnormalities

There is still much debate as to whether obesity is an independent risk factor for non-chromosomal congenital abnormalities in the offspring. Case–control studies based on patient questionnaire and interview data have reported higher risks of neural tube defects (Shaw et al., 1996; 2000; Werler et al., 1996). In contrast, two studies involving several thousands of women failed to confirm this association (Feldman et al., 1999; Moore et al., 2000). The contribution of diabetes, or the predisposition to diabetes, to the positive association with neural tube defects is still uncertain and may have been an as yet unidentified confounding variable. Controlling for folate usage was included in the analysis.

Perinatal morbidity and mortality

Perinatal mortality is defined as the number of stillbirths and deaths within the first week of life per 1000 births. Although all studies that include a non-obese control group demonstrate an increased perinatal mortality rate, this is only significant in studies of larger numbers of women. The overall perinatal mortality is increased and related to the degree of obesity. The presence of other antenatal complications is additive to the perinatal mortality. In a retrospective cohort of 8000–16 000 women with a prenatal weight > 100 kg, the relative risk for neonatal death increased from 0.8 in 1980–1984 to 1.6 in the period 1995–1999, whereas that for fetal death remained the same (Lu et al., 2001). In this study, the proportion of women with a BMI > 29 increased from 16.3% in 1980–1984 to 36.4% in

the 4-year period of 1995–1999, which again reflects the increasing prevalence of obesity in pregnancy. One large study reported that only late fetal deaths are significantly higher in overweight women (OR 1.7) (Cnattingius et al., 1998).

There is some conflict with respect to rates of premature delivery before 32 weeks. One large study involving thousands of women by Sebire and colleagues showed that maternal obesity reduced the risk of preterm delivery (OR 0.81); Cnattingius also reported a decrease (OR 1.6). The latter found this association in nulliparous women but not in parous women (Cnattingius et al., 1998). In a study of survival in 771 infants delivered preterm, the number of deaths after 48 h to 18 months was increased in obese mothers. Maternal obesity and gestational age at delivery were associated with an increased death rate.

Most studies report a beneficial effect of maternal obesity on delivery of the small for gestational age (SGA) infant (Beaten et al., 2001; Sebire et al., 2001).

Long-term consequences of maternal obesity for the fetus

Infants of obese mothers are at higher risk of being overweight at 12 months of age than are infants of normal-weight mothers (Edwards et al., 1978). Both environmental and genetic factors are important in the development of obesity. The intrauterine environment may be an important non-genetic factor in the development of adult obesity. Low birth weight is associated with increased prevalence of several adult conditions, including diabetes, although the relative contribution of maternal energy intake and genetic factors to birth weight are not clear (Hales and Barker, 1992). Birth weight is a crude measure of the effect of the intrauterine environment on metabolic programming and the relative increase in fat mass with low lean body mass of the macrosomic infant may be as important.

Maternal diabetes during pregnancy is associated with increased fetal calorie delivery. The offspring are more likely to be obese as children, adolescents and as young adults (Pettitt et al., 1983). Diabetes during pregnancy in Pima Indian women results in a higher prevalence of type 2 diabetes (45%) in the offspring at age 20–24 years than in non-diabetic women (1.4%) or women who later became diabetic (prediabetic, 8.6%) (Pettitt et al., 1988). It is not possible to attribute the increased risk to maternal diabetes or the resulting fetal macrosomia.

Cost of maternal obesity

A House of Commons Public Accounts Committee in the UK has recently published a report which suggests that obesity costs society at least £2.5 billion per year. In a retrospective study, the cost of prenatal care in overweight women exceeded that in normal-weight control subjects by 5.4- to 16.2-fold and this was dependent on the degree of obesity (Galtier-Dereure *et al.*, 1995). In another prospective study conducted by the previous author, the average cost of hospital antenatal care was five times higher in mothers who were overweight before pregnancy than in normal-weight control women. The duration of hospital stay both day and night was also higher by 3.9- and 6.2-fold respectively (Galtier-Dereure *et al.*, 2000). Increased rates of caesarean sections and infectious morbidity may also contribute to prolonged hospital stay. Another potential contributor to the cost associated with maternal obesity is the increased number of neonatal admissions to special-care baby units.

Contraception in the obese woman

Pregnancy carries higher risks for the obese mother than the lean mother; it would therefore be prudent for a mother to conceive at a time when these risks can be minimized and if possible not conceive when overweight. In total, 10 women per 100 000 die from complications of pregnancy, whereas 1.3 non-smoking women per 100 000 may die of circulatory disease when taking combined oral contraception (Guillebaud, 1995). It should be emphasized that any risk to the women from side-effects of her contraceptive methods are small compared to her obesity, and her infant's risk from pregnancy.

Combined oral contraceptive pills

Combined (oestrogen and progestogen containing) oral contraceptives increase the blood pressure (within the normotensive range) and increase venous thromboembolic disease risk. These risks are greater in obesity. However, the same precautions regarding advice for contraceptive measures should be applied to obese women as non-obese women. Therefore, previous venous thromboembolic disease, present hypertension and present smoking should be taken into account when prescribing oestrogen-containing contraception (Vessey *et al.*, 1977). Although there are large epidemiological studies of the use of combined oral contraception and the relative effects of obesity, randomized studies for obese women are lacking. A woman without previous thromboembolic disease, hypertension or smoking may use standard combined oral contraception (containing ethinylestradiol, 30 or 35 μg). Desogestrel and gestodene are associated with around a twofold increase in risk of thromboembolic disease compared with those containing the other progestogens. It is advisable for obese women (BMI > 30 kg/m²) not to use combined oral contraception containing gestodene or desogestrel, but they may use levonorgestrel, norethisterone or ethynodiol. Using the last three, the excess risk of thromboembolic disease is about 5–10 cases per 100 000 women per annum. The risk of deep vein thrombosis is relatively high in obese subjects having surgery

or after leg immobilization. Contraception should be stopped prior to surgery and heparin prophylaxis considered.

Yasmin contains drosperinone and ethynylestradiol. Drosperinone has diuretic properties due to antimineralocorticoid activity and is also an antiandrogen. It is being used at present as an alternative to *Dianette* (lyproterone acetate and ethinylestradiol) in PCOS and is reported not to be associated with weight gain (Foidart, 2000). The suppression of ovulation by oral contraceptives is not affected by orlistat therapy (Hartman *et al.*, 1996).

Progesterone-only contraceptive pills

The progestogen-only pill (POP) has a higher failure rate than the combined oral contraceptive—3.1 compared with 0.38 user failure rates per 100 woman-years (Vessey *et al.*, 1982). A non-significant increase in failure rate was found in overweight users of the progestogen-only pill compared with non-obese users. Cerazette, containing desogestrel, is the first POP to be primarily anovulant. If no other form of contraception is suitable it is recommended that overweight (>70 kg) women take two progestagen-only pills per day, especially in the under 30-year-old group (Guillebaud, 1995). Both progestogen ring and norplant have increased failure rates in obese women compared with lean women. The effectiveness of progestagen-only contraception in obese women is therefore dependent on the method of delivery.

Injectables

Injectables include depoprovera (medroxyprogesteroneacetate) and implanon (etonogestrel). Depoprovera is administered every 12 weeks and is a very popular choice among obese women in whom the oral contraceptive pill is contraindicated. Depoprovera is equally effective in obese and non-obese women. The side-effect profile in overweight and obese women may be better with respect to uterine bleeding than in control women (Connor *et al.*, 2002).

Implanon, which is a single 40-mm by 20-mm subdermal rod releases etonorgestrel (the biologically active metabolite of desogestrel) over 3 years. The blood levels of etonorgestrel are certainly lower in women of very high BMI, and it has been suggested that those women with increased body mass (i.e. >100) may need to discuss changing their implanon early, at about 2 years instead of 3 years. However, if the woman is amenorrhoeic, which is highly suggestive of anovulation, it might be appropriate for her to continue to the third year, even if she weighs over 100 kg.

Intrauterine devices

These include the copper intrauterine devices (IUDs) and, more recently, the hormone-releasing intrauterine systems. The product licence for the levornorgestrel intrauterine system (Mirena) indicates effectiveness for 5 years, although efficacy for 7 years has been reported. The system has an additional benefit in improving menorrhagia with a reduction in blood loss of up to 90% (Rybo, 1995). An advantage of the system is that it releases progesterone locally into the uterine cavity, thereby reducing the systemic side-effects associated with oral contraceptive pills.

Summary

Obesity in pregnancy is a major public heath issue, both in terms of the number of obese women involved and the severity of the potential complications. Prevention of adult obesity may start as early as the intrauterine environment, and this poses a challenge to the medical profession with respect to intervention strategies. Other intervention endpoints include diet and exercise, beginning in childhood and adolescence. Despite these strategies, obesity will remain an antenatal high-risk factor which all obstetric personnel should be able to identify and monitor.

Any obese women planning pregnancy should be educated about the potential complications of obesity in pregnancy, and should embark on a weight-reducing programme prior to becoming pregnant. A reliable contraceptive method should be used in the interim. It is recommended that at least 6 months be allowed to achieve a 10% reduction in body weight. Dietary advice about energy restriction is required prepregnancy but weight reduction in pregnancy is not recommended. Dietary advice should be supported with an exercise programme. A multidisciplinary health-care team is required for the management of the obese pregnant woman.

Adequate screening programmes should be in place for the detection of pre-eclampsia and gestational diabetes, and the sequelae of these. Judicious decisions are required about the timing and mode of delivery, which bear in mind the possibility of fetal macrosomia and the increased infectious morbidity associated with caesarean section.

References

Abrams, B.F. and Laros, R.K. (1986) Prepregnancy weight, weight gain, and birth weight. *American Journal of Obstetrics and Gynecology* **154**, 503–509.

Abrams, B. and Parker, J. (1988) Overweight and pregnancy complications. *International Journal of Obesity* **12**, 293–303.

Beaten, J.M., Bukusi, E.A., Lambe, M. (2001) Pregnancy complications and outcomes among overweight and obese nulliparous women. *American Journal of Public Health* **91**, 436–444.

Bianco, A.T., Smilen, S.W., Davis, Y., Lopez, S., Lapinski, R. and Lockwood, J. (1998) Pregnancy outcome and weight gain recommendations for the morbidly obese woman. *Obstetrics and Gynecology* **91**, 97–102.

Boyd, M.E., Usher, R.H. and McLean, F.H. (1983) Fetal macrosomia: prediction, risks, proposed management. *Obstetrics and Gynecology* **61**, 715–722.

Brown, J.E., Potter, J.D., Jacobs, Jr, D.R., Kopher, R.A., Rourke, M.J., Barosso, G.M., Hannan, P.J. and Schmid, L.A. (1996) Maternal waist-to-hip ratio as a predictor of newborn size: results of the Diana project. *Epidemiology* **7**, 62–66.

Buchanan, T.A., Metzger, B.E., Frienkel, N. and Bergman, R.N. (1990) Insulin sensitivity and B-cell responsiveness to glucose during late pregnancy in lean and moderately obese women with normal glucose tolerance or mild gestational diabetes. *American Journal of Obstetrics and Gynecology* **162**, 1008–1014.

Camastra, S., Bonora, E., Del Prato, S., Weck, M. and Ferranni, E. (1999) Effect of obesity and insulin resistance and glucose induced thermogenesis in man, EGIR (European Group for the study of Insulin Resistance). *International Journal of Obesity* **23**, 1307–1313.

Chauhan, S.P., Magann, E.F., Caroll, C.S., Barilleaux, P.S., and Scardo, J.A. (2001) Mode of delivery for the morbidly obese with prior caesarean delivery; Vaginal versus repeat caesarean section. *American Journal of Obstetrics and Gynaecology* **185**, 349–354.

Chou, K.H., Eye Corleta, H., von Capp, E. and Spritzer, P.M. (2003) Clinical, metabolic and endocrine parameters in response to metformin in obese women with polycystic ovary syndrome: a randomized, double-blind and placebo-controlled trial. *Hormonal Metabolism Research* **35**, 86–91.

Cnattingius, S., Bergstrom, R., Lipworth, L. and Kramer, M. (1998) Prepregnancy weight and the risk of adverse pregnancy outcomes. *New England Journal of Medicine* **338**, 147–152.

Comtois, R., Seguin, M.C., Aris-Jilwan, N., Couturier M. and Beauregard, H. (1993) Comparison of obese and non-obese patients with gestational diabetes. *International Journal of Obesity* **17**, 605–608.

Connor, P., Tavernia, L.A., Thomas, S., Gates, D. and Lytton, S. (2002) Dertermining risk between Depo-Provera use and increased uterine bleeding in obese and overweight women. *Journal of the American Board of Family Practice* **15**, 7–10.

Conway, G.S., Clark, S. and Wong, D. (1993) Hyperinsulinaemia in the polycystic ovary syndrome confirmed with a specific immunoradiometric assay for insulin. *Clinical Endocrinology* **38**, 219–222.

Cousins, L., Rigg, L., Hollingsworth, D., Brink, G., Aurand, J. and Yen, S.S.C. (1980) The 24-hour excursion and diurnal rhythm of glucose, insulin, and C-peptide in normal pregnancy. *American Journal of Obstetrics and Gynecology* **136**, 483–488.

DeFronzo, R. (1988) The triumvirate, B cell, muscle and liver: A collusion responsible for NIDDM. *Diabetes* **37**, 667–687.

Donath, S.M. and Amir, L.H. (2000) How does maternal obesity adversely affect breastfeeding initiation and duration. *Journal of Paediatrics and Child Health* **36**, 482–486.

Dornhorst, A., Bailey, P.C., Anyaoku, V., Elkeles, R.S., Johnston, D.G. and Beard, R.W. (1990) Abnormalities of glucose tolerance following gestational diabetes. *Quarterly Journal of Medicine* **77**, 1219–1228.

Dornhorst, A., Nicholls, J.S., Probst, F., Paterson, C.M., Hollier, K.L., Elkeles, R.S. and Beard, R.W. (1991) Calorie restriction for treatment of gestational diabetes. *Diabetes* **40** (Suppl. 2), 161–164.

Dunaif, A., Graf, M., Mandeli, J., Laumas, V. and Dobrjansky, A. (1987) Characterisation of groups of hyperandrogenic women with acanthosis nigricans, impaired glucose tolerance, and/or hyperinsulinaemia. *Journal of Clinical Endocrinology and Metabolism* **65**, 449–507.

Dunaif, A., Segal, K.R., Futterweit, W. and Dobrjansky, A. (1989) Profound peripheral insulin resistance, independent of obesity, in polycystic ovary syndrome. *Diabetes* **38**, 1165–1174.

Edwards, L.E., Dickes, W.F., Alton, I.R. and Hakanson, E.Y. (1978) Pregnancy in the massively obese: Course, outcome and obesity prognosis of the infant. *American Journal of Obstetrics and Gynecology* **131**, 479–483.

Ehrmann, D.A., Cavaghan, M.K., Imperial, J., Sturis, J., Rosenfield, R.L. and Polonsky, K.S. (1997) Effects of metformin on insulin secretion, insulin action, and ovarian steroidogenesis in women with polycystic ovary syndrome. *Journal of Clinical Endocrinology and Metabolism* **82**, 524–530.

Feldman, B., Yaron, Y. and Critchfield, G. (1999) Distribution of neural defects as a function of maternal weight: no apparent correlation. *Fetal Diagnosis Therapy* **14**, 185–189.

Felig, P., Marliss, E. and Cahill, G.F. (1969) Plasma amino acid levels and insulin secretion in obesity. *New England Journal of Medicine* **281**, 811–816.

Foidart, J.M. (2000) The contraceptive profile of a new oral contraceptive with antimineralocorticoid and antiandrogenic effects. *European Journal of Contraception and Reproductive Heath Care* **3**, 25–33.

Franks, S. (1989) Polycystic ovary syndrome: a changing perspective. *Clinical Endocrinology* **31**, 87–120.

Franks, S., Mason, S. and Willis, D. (2000) Follicular dynamics in the polycystic ovary syndrome. *Molecular and Cellular Endocrinology* **163**, 49–52.

Freinkel, N. (1980) Of pregnancy and progeny. *Diabetes* **29**, 1023–1035.

Galtier-Dereure, F., Montpeyroux, F., Boulot, P., Bringer, J. and Jaffiol, C. (1995) Weight excess before pregnancy: complications and cost. *International Jounal of Obesity Related Metabolic Disorders* **19**, 443–448.

Galtier-Dereure, F., Boegner, C. and Bringer, J. (2000) Obesity and pregnancy: complications and cost. *American Journal of Clinical Nutrition* **71**, 1242S–1248S.

Garbaciak, J.A., Ritchter, M., Miller, S. and Barton, J.J. (1985) Maternal weight and pregnancy complications. *American Journal of Obstetrics and Gynecology* **152**, 238–245.

Geffner, M.E., Kaplan, S.A., Bersch, N., Golde, D.W., Landaw, E.M. and Chang, R.J. (1986) Persistence of insulin resistance in polycystic ovarian disease after inhibition of ovarian steroid secretion. *Fertility and Sterility* **45**, 327–333.

Gillmer, D.G., Beard, R.W., Brooke, F.M. and Oakley, N.W. (1975) Carbohydrate metabolism in pregnancy. Part 1-Diurnal plasma glucose profile in normal and diabetic women. *British Medical Journal* **3**, 399–404.

Ginsberg, J. and Cramp, D.G. (1977) Carbohydrate metabolism. In: Phillip, E.E., Barnes, J. and Newton, M. eds. *Scientific Foundations of Obstetrics and Gynaecology*. London: Heinemann, 467–479.

Grandjean, H., Sarramon, M.-F., de Mouzon, J., Reme, J.-M. and Pontonnier, G. (1980) Detection of gestational diabetes by means of ultrasonic diagnosis of excessive fetal growth. *American Journal of Obstetrics and Gynecology* **138**, 790–792.

Greene, G.W., Smiciklas-Wright, H., Scholl, T.O. and Karp, R.J. (1988) Postpartum weight change: How much of the weight gained in pregnancy will be lost after delivery? *Obstetrics and Gynecology* **71**, 701–707.

Gross, T., Sokol, R.J. and King, K.C. (1980) Obesity in pregnancy: risks and outcome. *Obstetrics and Gynecology* **56**, 446–450.

Guillebaud, J. (1995) *Contraception*. Edinburgh: Churchill Livingstone.

Hales, C.N. and Barker, D.J.P. (1992) Type 2 (non-insulin dependent) diabetes mellitus: the thrifty phenotype. *Diabetologia* **35**, 595–601.

Hartman, D., Güzelham, C., Zuiderwij, K. and Odink, J. (1996) Lack of interaction between or listat and oral contraceptives. *European Journal of Clinical Pharmacology* **50**, 421–424.

Herrera, E., Gomez-Coronado, D. and Lasuncion, M.A. (1987) Lipid metabolism in pregnancy. *Biology of the Neonate* **51**, 70–77.

Hoegsburg, B., Gruppuso, P.A. and Coustan, D.R. (1993) Hyperinsulinaemia in macrosomic infants of non-diabetic mothers. *Diabetes Care* **16** (1), 32–36.

Hytten, F.E. (1991), Weight gain in pregnancy. In: Hytten, F.E., Chamberlain, G. eds. *Clinical Physiology in Obstetrics*. Oxford: Blackwell Scientific Publications, 173–203.

Hytten, F.E. and Chamberlain, G. (1980) *Clinical Physiology in Obstetrics*. Oxford: Blackwell Scientific Publications.

Hytten, F.E. and Leitch, I. (1971) *The Physiology of Human Pregnancy*. Oxford: Blackwell Scientific Publications.

Illingworth, P.J., Jung, R.T., Howie, P.W. and Isles, T.E. (1987) Reduction in postprandial energy expenditure during pregnancy. *British Medical Journal* **294**, 1573–1576.

Institute of Medicine, Subcommittee on Nutritional Status and Weight Gain During Pregnancy (1990) *Nutrition During Pregnancy*. Washington, DC: National Academy Press.

Jolly, M., Hovorka, R., Godsland, I., Amin, R., Lawrence, N., Anyaoku, V., Johnston, D. and Robinson, S. (2003) *European Journal of Clinical Investigation* **8**, 698–703.

Jovanovic-Peterson, L. and Peterson, C.M. (1991) Is exercise safe or useful for gestational diabetic women? *Diabetes* **20**, 179–181.

Kalhan, S.C., D'Angelo, L.J., Savin, S.M. and Adam, P.A.J. (1979) Glucose production in pregnant women at term gestation. *Journal of Clinical Investigation* **63**, 388–394.

Kalkhoff, R.K., Kandaraki, E., Marrow, P.G., Mitchell, T.H., Kelber, S. and Borkowf, H. I. (1988) Relationship between neonatal birth weight and maternal plasma amino acid profiles in lean and obese nondiabetic women and in type 1 diabetic pregnant women. *Metabolism* **37**, 234–239.

Kannel, W.B., Brand, N., Skinner, J.J.J., Dawber, T.R. and McNamara, P.M. (1967) The relation of adiposity to blood pressure and development of hypertension. The Framingham Study. *Annals of Internal Medicine*, **67**, 48–59.

Kiddy, D., Hamilton-Fairley, D., Bush, A., Anyaoku, V., Short, F., Reed, M.J. and Franks, S. (1990) Improvement in menstrual function and fertility in obese women with polycystic ovary syndrome treated with a 1000 calorie diet. *Clinical Endocrinology* **124**, 253.

Kiddy, D.S., Hamilton-Fairley, D., Seppala, M., Koistinen, R., James, V.H.T. and Reed, M.J. (1992) Diet-induced changes in sex hormone-binding globulin and free testosterone in women with normal or polycystic ovaries: correlation with insulin and insulin-like growth factor 1. *Clinical Endocrinology* **1989**, 757–763.

Kissebah, A.H., Vydelingum, N., Murray, R., Evans, D.J., Hartz, A.J., Kalkhoff, R.K. and Adams, P.W. (1982) Relation of body fat distribution to metabolic complications of obesity. *Journal of Clinical Endocrinology and Metabolism* **54**, 254–260.

Kitajima, M., Oka, S., Yasuhi, I., Fukuda, M., Rii, Y. and Ishimaru, T. (2001) Maternal serum triglyceride at 24–32 weeks' gestation and newborn weight in nondiabetic women with positive screens. *Obstetrics and Gynecology* **97** (5 Pt 1), 776–780.

Knopp, R.H., Magee, M.S., Raisys, V., Benedetti, T. and Bonet, B. (1991) Hypocaloric diets and ketogenesis in the management of obese gestational diabetic women. *Journal of American College of Nutrition* **10**, 649–667.

Knopp, R.H., Magee, M.S., Walden, C.E., Bonet, B. and Benedetti, T.J. (1992) Prediction of infant birth weight by GDM screening tests. *Diabetes Care* **15**, 1605–1613.

Kolodziejczyk, B., Duleba, A.J., Spaczynski, R.Z. and Pawelczyk, L. (2000) Metformin therapy decreases hyperandrogenism and hyperinsulinemia in women with polycystic ovary syndrome. *Fetility and Sterility* **73**, 1149–1154.

Kuhl, C. and Holst, J.J. (1976) Plasma glucagon and the insulin–glucagon ratio in gestational diabetes. *Diabetes* **25**, 16–23.

Kumari, A.S. (2001) Pregnancy outcome in women with morbid obesity. *International Journal of Obesity* **73**, 101–107.

Li, R., Jewell, S. and Grummer-Strawn, L. (2003) Maternal obesity and breast-feeding practices. *American Journal of Clinical Nutrition* **77**, 931–936.

Lu, G.C., Rouse, D.J., Dubard, M., Cliver, S., Kimberlin, D. and Hauth, J.C. (2001) The effect of the increasing prevalence of maternal obesity on perinatal morbidity. *American Journal of Obstetrics and Gynecology* **185**, 845–849.

Lind, T. (1975) Changes in carbohydrate metabolism during pregnancy. *Clinical Obstetrics and Gynecology* **395**, 1023–1028.

Lind, T., Billewicz, W.Z. and Brown, G. (1973) A serial study of changes occuring in the oral glucose tolerance test in pregnancy. *Journal of Obstetrics and Gynaecology of the British Commonwealth* **80**, 1033–1039.

Ludvik, B., Nolan, J.J., Baloga, J., Sacks, D. and Olefsky, J. (1995) Effect of obesity on insulin resistance in normal subjects and patients with NIDDM. *Diabetes* **44**, 1121–1125.

Magee, M.S., Knopp, R.H. and Benedetti, T.J. (1990) Metabolic effects of 1200-kcal diet in obese pregnant women with gestational diabetes. *Diabetes* **39**, 234–240.

Mahabeer, S., Jialal, I., Norman, J., Naidoo, C., Reddi, K. and Joubert, S.M. (1989) Insulin and C-peptide secretion in non-obese patients with polycystic ovarian disease. *Hormone and Metabolic Research* **21**, 502–506.

Maresh, M., Beard, R.W., Bray, C.S., Elkeles, R.S. and Wadsworth, J. (1989) Factors predisposing to and outcome of gestational diabetes. *Obstetrics and Gynecology* **74**, 342–346.

Martin, L., Finnigan, K. and Nolan, T. (2000) Pregnancy after adjustable gastric banding. *Obstetrics and Gynecology* **95**, 927–930.

Metzger, B.E. and Frienkel, N. (1987) Accelerated starvation in pregnancy: Implications for dietary treatment of obesity and gestational diabetes mellitus. *Biology of the Neonate* **51**, 78–85.

Metzger, B.E., Ravinikar, V., Vileisis, R.A. and Freinkel, N. (1982) Accelerated starvation and the skipped breakfast in late normal pregnancy. *Lancet* **i**, 588–592.

Moghetti, P., Castello, R., Negri, C., Tosi, F., Perrone, F., Caputo, M., Zanol, and Muggeo, M. (2000) Metformin effects on clinical features, endocrine and metabolic profiles, and insulin sensitivity in polycystic ovary syndrome: A randomized, double-blind, placebo-controlled 6 month trial, followed by open, long-term

clinical evaluation. *Journal of Clinical Endocrinology and Metabolism* **85**, 139–146.

Moore, L.L., Singer, M.R., Bradlee, M.L., Rothman, K.J. and Milunsky, A. (2000) A prospective study of the risk of congenital defects associated with maternal obesity and diabetes mellitus. *Epidemiology* **11**, 669–694.

Morin-Panunen, L.C., Koivunen, R.M., Rvokonen, A. and Martikainen, H.K. (1998) Metformin therapy improves the menstrual pattern with minimal endocine and metabolic effects in women with polycystic ovary syndrome. *Fertility and Sterility* **69**, 691–696.

Muhittin, H., Telli, M.D., Mulazim Yildirim, M.D. and Volken Noyan, M.D. (2002) Serum leptin levels in patients with polycystic ovary syndrome. *Fertility and Sterility* **77**, 932–935.

Myles, T.D., Gooch, J. and Santolaya, J. (2002) Obesity as an independent risk factor for infectious morbidity in patients who undergo caesarean delivery. *Obstetrics and Gynecology* **100**, 959–964.

Nagy, L.E. and King, J.C. (1984) Postprandial energy expenditure and respiratory quotient during early and late pregnancy. *American Journal of Clinical Nutrition* **40**, 1258–1263.

Nestler, J.E. and Jakubowicz, D.J. (1997) Lean women with polycystic ovary syndrome respond to insulin reduction with decreases in ovarian P450c17 alpha activity and serum androgens. *Journal of Clinical Endocrinology and Metabolism* **82**, 4075–4079.

Nestler, J.E., Jakubowicz, D.J., Evans, W.S. and Pasquali, R. (1998) Effects of metformin on spontaneous and clomiphene-induced ovulation in the polycystic ovary syndrome. *New England Journal of Medicine* **338**, 1876–1880.

Nolan, C.J., Riley, S.F., Sheedy, M.T., Walstab, J.E. and Beischer, N.A. (1995) Maternal serum triglyceride, glucose tolerance, and neonatal birthweight ratio in pregnancy. *Diabetes Care* **18**, 1551–1556.

O'Sullivan, J.B. (1984), Subsequent morbidity among gestational diabetic women. In: Sutherland, H.W., Towers, J.M. eds. *Carbohydrate Metabolism in Pregnancy and the Newborn*. Edinburgh: Churchill Livingstone, 174–180.

Pasquali, R., Gambineri, D., Biscotti, V., Vicennati, L., Gagliardi, D., Colitta, Fiorini, S., Cognigni, G.E., Filicori, M. and Morselli-Labate, A.M. (2000) Effect of long term treatment with Metformin added to hypocaloric diet on body composition, fat distribution, and androgen and insulin levels in abdominally obese women with and without the polycystic ovary syndrome. *Journal of Clinical Endocrinology and Metabolism* **85**, 2767–2774.

Pederson, J., Bojsen-Moller, B. and Poulsen, H. (1954) Blood sugar in newborn infants of diabetic infants of diabetic mothers. *Acta Endocrinologica* **15**, 33–52.

Pettitt, D.J., Baird, H.R., Aleck, K.A., Bennett, P.H. and Knowler, W.C. (1983) Excessive obesity in offspring of Pima Indian women with diabetes during pregnancy. *New England Journal of Medicine* **308**, 242–245.

Pettitt, D.J., Aleck, K.A., Baird, R., Carraher, M.J., Bennett, P.H. and Knowler, W.C. (1988) Congenital susceptibility to NIDDM. Role of intrauterine environment. *Diabetes* **37**, 622–628.

Pimblett, C. (1996), The dietary management of diabetes and pregnancy. In: Dornhorst, A., Hadden, D.R. eds. *Diabetes and Pregnancy. An International Approach to Diagnosis and Management.* Chichester: John Wiley and Sons, 139–153.

Polley, B.A., Wing, R.R. and Sims, C.J. (2002) Randomised controlled trial to prevent excessive weight gain in pregnant women. *International Journal of Obesity* **26**, 1494–1502.

Prentice, A.M., Golberg, G.R., Davies, H.L., Murgatroyd, P.R. and Scott, W. (1989) Energy-sparing adaptations in human pregnancy assessed by whole body calorimetry. *British Journal of Nutrition* **62** (1), 5–22.

Prentice, A.M., Spaaij, C.J.K., Goldberg, G.R., Poppitt, S.D., van Raaij, J.M.A., Totton, M., Swann, D. and Black, A.E. (1996) Energy requirements of pregnant and lactating women. *European Journal of Clinical Nutrition* **50**, S82–S111.

van Raaij, J.M.A., Peek, M.E.M., Vermaat-Miedema, S.H., Schonk, C.M. and Hautvast, J.G.A.J. (1988) New equations for estimating body fat mass in pregnancy from body density or total body water. *American Journal of Clinical Nutrition* **48**, 24–29.

Rimm, A.A., Werner, Y.B.V. and Bernstein, R.A. (1975) Relationship of obesity and disease in 73 532 weight-conscious women. *Public Health of Reproduction* **90** (1), 44–54.

Rizzo, T., Metzger, B.E., Burns, W.J. and Burns, K. (1991) Correlation between antepartum maternal metabolism and intelligence of offspring. *New England Journal of Medicine* **325**, 911–916.

Robinson, S., Coldham, L., Gelding, S.V., Murphy, C., Halliday, D. and Johnston, D.G. (1992) Leucine flux is increased whilst glucose turnover is normal in pregnancy complicated by gestational diabetes. *Diabetologia* **35** (Suppl. 1), A683.

Robinson, S., Viira, J., Learner, J., Chan, S.-P., Anyaoku, V., Beard, R.W. and Johnston, D.G. (1993a) Insulin insensitivity is associated with a decrease in postprandial thermogenesis in normal pregnancy. *Diabetic Medicine* **10**, 139–145.

Robinson, S., Kiddy, D., Gelding, S.V., Willis, D., Niththyananthan, R., Bush, A., Johnston, D.G. and Franks, S. (1993b) The relationship of insulin sensitivity to menstrual pattern in women with hyperandrogenism and polycystic ovaries. *Clinical Endocrinology* **39**, 351–355.

Robinson, S., Henderson, A.D., Gelding, S.V., Kiddy, D., Niththyananthan, R., Bush, A., Richmond, W., Johnston, D.G. and Franks, S. (1996) Dyslipidaemia is associated with insulin resistance in women with polysystic ovaries. *Clinical Endocrinology* **44**, 277–284.

Robinson, H., Tkatch, S., Mayes, D.C., Bott, N. and Okun, N. (2003) Is maternal obesity a predictor of shoulder dystocia? *Obstetrics and Gynecology* **101**, 24–27.

Ryan, E.A., O'Sullivan, M.J. and Skyler, J.S. (1985) Insulin action during pregnancy. Studies with the euglycemic clamp technique. *Diabetes* **34**, 380–389.

Rybo, G. (1995) Treatment of menorrhagia in Chinese women: efficacy versus acceptability. *Contraception* **51**, 231–235.

Sanderson, D.A., Wilcox, M.A. and Johnson, I.R. (1994) Relative macrosomia identified by the individualised birthweight ratio (IBR). *Acta Obstetrica et Gynecologica Scandinavica* **73**, 246–249.

Sebire, N.J., Jolly, M., Harris, J.P., Wadsworth, J., Joffe, M., Beard, R.W., Regan, L. and Robinson, S. (2001) Maternal obesity and pregnancy outcome: a study of 287 213 pregnancies in London. *International Journal of Obesity* **25**, 1175–1182.

Shaw, G.M., Todoroff, K. and Schaffer, D. (1996) Risk of neural tube defect-affected pregnancies among obese women. *Journal of the American Medical Association* **275**, 1093–1096.

Shaw, G.M., Todoroff, K., Schaffer, D.M. and Selvin, S. (2000) Maternal height and prepregnancy body mass index as risk factors for selected congenital anomalies. *Paedatric and Perinatal Epidemiology* **14**, 234–239.

Sheath, J., Grimwade, J., Waldron, K., Bickley, M., Taft, P. and Wood, C. (1972) Arteriovenous nonesterified fatty acids and glycerol difference in the umbilical cord at term and their relationship to fetal metabolism. *American Journal of Obstetrics and Gynecology* **113**, 358–362.

Spaaij, C.J.K., van Raaij, J.M.A., van der Heijden, L.J.M., Schouten, F.J.M., Drijvers, J.J.M.M., de Groot, L.C.P.G.M., Boekholt, H.A. and Hautvast, J.G.A.J. (1994) No substantial reduction of the thermic effect of a meal during pregnancy in well-nourished Dutch women. *British Journal of Nutrition* **71**, 335–344.

Spellacy, W.N., Miller, S., Winegar, A. and Peterson, P.Q. (1985) Macrosomia—maternal characteristics and infant complications. *Obstetrics and Gynecology* **66**, 158–161.

Thomas, C.R. (1987) Placental transfer of non-esterified fatty acids in normal and diabetic pregnancy. *Biology of the Neonate* **51**, 94–101.

Thompson, G.N. and Halliday, D. (1992) Protein turnover in pregnancy. *European Journal of Clinical Nutrition* **46**, 411–417.

Unluhizarci, K., Keletimur, F., Bayram, F., Sahin, Y. and Tutus, A. (1999) The effects of metformin on insulin resistance and ovarian steroidogenesis in women with the polycystic ovary syndrome. *Clinical Endocrinology* **51**, 231–236.

Vandermolen, D.T., Ratts, V.S., Evans, W.S., Stovall, D.W., Kauma, S.W. and Nestler, J.E.N. (2001) Metformin increases the ovulatory rate and pregnancy rate from clomiphene citrate in patients with polycystic ovary syndrome who are resistant to clomiphene citrate alone. *Fertility and Sterility* **75**, 310–315.

Vessey, M.P., McPherson, K. and Johnson, B. (1977) Mortality in women participating in the Oxford/family planning association contraceptive study. *Lancet* **ii**, 731–733.

Vessey, M., Lawless, M. and Yeates, D. (1982) Efficacy of different contraceptive methods. *The Lancet* **1**, 841–842.

Warth, M.R., Arky, R.A. and Knopp, R.H. (1975) Lipid metabolism in pregnancy. III. Altered lipid composition in intermediate, very low, low and high-density lipoprotein fractions. *Journal of Clinical Endocrinology and Metabolism* **41**, 649–655.

Werler, M.M., Louik, C., Shapiro, S. and Mitchell, A.A. (1996) Prepregnant weight in relation to risk of neural tube defects. *Journal of the American Medical Association* **275**, 1089–1092.

Willis, D., Mason, H., Gilling-Smith, C. and Franks, S. (1996) Modulation by insulin of follicle stimulating hormone and luteinising hormone actions in human granulosa cells of normal and polycystic ovaries. *Journal of Clinical Endocrinology and Metabolism* **81**, 302–309.

20 Obstructive sleep apnoea

Brendon J. Yee and Ronald R. Grunstein

Sleep-disordered breathing:
pathogenesis, 296
  The physiology of sleep, 296
  Definitions in sleep-disordered
  breathing, 296
  Pathogenesis of obstructive sleep
  apnoea: general, 298
  Pathogenesis of obstructive
  sleep apnoea: the role of
  obesity, 298
  Obesity hypoventilation
  syndrome, 299

Sleep-disordered breathing:
epidemiology, 300
  Epidemiology in the general
  community, 300

Epidemiology in the obese
population, 300

Epidemiology: other risk factors for
obstructive sleep apnoea, 301

Sleep-disordered breathing: clinical
aspects, 302
  Symptoms and signs of sleep-
  disordered breathing, 302
  Diagnosis of sleep-disordered
  breathing, 302
  Consequences of sleep-disordered
  breathing, 303

Sleep-disordered breathing:
treatment, 306
  Weight loss, 306

Other general measures, 307
Continuous positive airway
pressure, 307
Mandibular advancement
devices, 308
Tracheostomy, 308
Uvulopalatopharyngoplasty and
other upper airway surgery, 309
Pharmacological treatment, 309
Management of obstructive sleep
apnoea with daytime respiratory
failure (including obesity
hypoventilation syndrome), 309

Conclusion, 310

References, 310

Sleep-disordered breathing: pathogenesis

The details of pathogenesis are outlined below.

The physiology of sleep

To sleep physiologists, humans exist in three states: wakefulness, non-rapid eye movement (NREM) sleep and rapid eye movement (REM or dreaming) sleep. There are marked differences between these three states in many aspects of physiology. Sleep has profound effects on breathing and these effects are usually greatest during REM sleep. Sleep can amplify the effects on breathing of drugs such as alcohol and opiates.

In normal subjects, sleep is associated with a fall in minute ventilation, primarily due to a drop in tidal volume. As a result, there is a small rise in arterial blood carbon dioxide tension ($P_a\text{co}_2$) and a small fall in arterial blood oxygen tension ($P_a\text{o}_2$). During NREM sleep, the hypoxic drive to breathe is reduced and the ventilatory response to hypercapnia is diminished. This depression of chemosensitivity is greatest during REM sleep.

Sleep is also associated with a reduction in tone of the upper airway dilator muscles, with a resulting increase in resistance to air flow. REM sleep is characterized by postural muscle atonia, with bursts of eye movements and associated peripheral muscle twitches (phasic REM). Phasic REM is associated with marked breathing irregularity. The loss of postural muscle tone during REM sleep leaves us largely reliant on the diaphragm (a non-postural muscle) for maintaining ventilation. An individual with abnormal diaphragm function, either due to neuromuscular disease or to mechanical disadvantage (kyphoscoliosis, lung disease or obesity) will have impaired breathing in sleep, particularly during REM sleep. A combination of these factors, such as an obese patient with lung disease, will be at even greater risk of developing sleep-related respiratory failure.

Definitions in sleep-disordered breathing

Sleep-disordered breathing is defined by the loss of a normal pattern of breathing during sleep and ranges from snoring through to profound nocturnal hypoventilation and respiratory failure during sleep. Intermittent snoring, with no associated sleep fragmentation (so called 'simple snoring') is common and generally not considered part of the spectrum of sleep-disordered breathing. On the other hand, heavy snoring can result in arousals from sleep with accompanying sleep disruption (Guilleminault *et al.*, 1992) and should be considered part of the disease state.

Obstructive sleep apnoea (OSA) is characterized by repetitive episodes of a complete cessation of air flow (apnoea) during sleep, due to collapse of the upper airway generally at the level of the pharynx (Remmers *et al.*, 1978). During an apnoea,

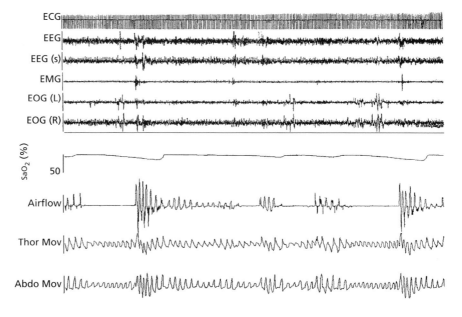

Fig 20.1 A 5-min tracing of a patient with typical severe OSA. The upper traces show the variables used for sleep staging (ECG, electrocardiogram; EEG, electroencephalogram; EMG, electromyogram; EOG, electro-oculogram) and indicate this patient is in REM sleep. The apnoeas are indicated by intermittent cessation of air flow (air flow: nasal air flow) and are obstructive in nature, as continued respiratory effort is seen when air flow is absent (Thor Mov, thoracic movement or effort; Abdo Mov, abdominal movement or effort). Repetitive falls in oxygen saturation (S_aO_2) are seen following each apnoea.

Table 20.1 Definitions in sleep-disordered breathing.

Apnoea
Complete cessation of air flow for at least 10 s

Hypopnoea
Reduction in air flow for at least 10 s, ending with an arousal or associated with oxygen desaturation of at least 3%

Obstructive event
Continued respiratory effort occurs despite reduced air flow as above

Central event
Respiratory effort is absent, with absent air flow

Periodic breathing (Cheyne–Stokes respiration)
Respiration that waxes and wanes, alternating between hyperventilation and central apnoea — seen in patients with heart failure or neurological disease

Hypoventilation
An abnormal rise in P_aCO_2 during sleep, usually associated with oxygen desaturation, with or without discrete respiratory events

Apnoea–hypopnoea index (AHI) (respiratory disturbance index, RDI)
Number of apnoeic and hypopnoeic episodes per hour of sleep; >5 is usually considered abnormal

continued respiratory efforts occur against the closed airway (Table 20.1), with resulting hypoxaemia, until the apnoea is terminated by arousal from sleep with restoration of upper airway patency. Typically, after a few deep breaths, this cycle is repeated, often hundreds of times through the night (Fig. 20.1). The recurrent arousals cause sleep fragmentation resulting in daytime sleepiness (McNamara *et al.*, 1993).

Significant upper airway obstruction can occur in the absence of complete collapse of the upper airway. Increased airway resistance can produce a measurable reduction in air flow (hypopnoea) with the same consequences (hypoxaemia and arousal) as an apnoea. Even very minor increases in airway resistance (without detectable reductions in air flow) can produce recurrent arousals and excessive daytime sleepiness; the *upper airway resistance syndrome* (Guilleminault *et al.*, 1992).

Patients with impaired daytime respiratory function, whatever the cause, will have abnormal breathing, and will often develop impaired gas exchange during sleep. These patients may have prolonged periods of hypoxaemia lasting minutes, usually due to reduced ventilation (hypoventilation), although worsening ventilation–perfusion mismatch may also contribute. Hypercapnia also develops during sleep owing to hypoventilation. These prolonged episodes of sleep-related hypercapnic hypoxia can lead to a *resetting* of chemoreceptors with subsequent blunted daytime chemosensitivity and the development or worsening of daytime hypercapnic respiratory failure. In addition, the prolonged exposure to hypoxaemia and hypercapnia may lead to pulmonary hypertension and right-sided heart failure, *cor pulmonale*. Patients with these severe forms of respiratory failure in sleep include patients with many types of chronic lung disease, respiratory muscle failure due to neuromuscular disorders and, importantly, the obesity hypoventilation syndrome (OHS) (see below).

Central apnoea refers to cessation of air flow with no detectable respiratory effort (in contrast with obstructive apnoeas in which breathing efforts are often vigorous). There is some confusion surrounding this term as it has been used to describe the patterns of breathing in patients where hypoventilation is the predominant pathology. This pattern of breathing, which tends to occur in patients with awake hypercapnia and reduced respiratory drive, should be differentiated from the 'true' central apnoeas that classically occur as part of the periodic breathing seen in patients with cardiac failure (Rubinstein *et al.*, 1989) (also called Cheyne–Stokes breathing). In this breathing pattern, ventilation waxes and wanes from hyperventilation to central apnoea. Periodic breathing can also occur in patients with neurological disease due to strokes or rarely as an idiopathic form. Sporadic central apnoeas may also occur in patients with severe OSA and usually disappear when the OSA is treated. The aetiology of central apnoea in the patient with cardiac failure is complex involving interplay between circulation time, brisk chemoreceptor drive and upper airway narrowing (Rubinstein *et al.*, 1989).

Pathogenesis of obstructive sleep apnoea: general

Upper airway collapse occurs when the negative (or suction) pressure applied to the upper airway during inspiration is greater than the dilating forces applied by the upper airway muscles, such as genioglossus (Remmers *et al.*, 1978; Sullivan *et al.*, 1990). Collapse of the upper airway usually occurs in the retropalatal or retroglossal areas, and most patients have more than one site of collapse. Less frequently, upper airway collapse can occur at the epiglottis or glottis (Rubinstein *et al.*, 1989). The determinants of the site of collapse in individual patients are unclear. Any factors that reduce airway size, decrease airway muscle tone, increase upper airway compliance or lead to the generation of a greater inspiratory pressure will predispose to the development of OSA (Sullivan *et al.*, 1990). Muscle tone and suction pressure are influenced by sleep stage and the relative respiratory drive to the diaphragm versus that to the upper airway dilator muscles.

Several studies have shown that the pharyngeal airway is smaller in patients with OSA than in normal subjects (Fleetham, 1992; Schwab *et al.*, 1993). When the airway size is reduced, a greater suction pressure is required during inspiration. In the awake state, patients with OSA have increased upper airway dilator muscle activity that normalizes air flow resistance despite the anatomically smaller airway (Horner *et al.*, 1991; Mezzanotte *et al.*, 1992). This compensatory increased upper airway muscle activity is lost during sleep, particularly in the genioglossus (Remmers *et al.*, 1978), resulting in airway closure. However, although the increased waking genioglossus activity is seen in some patients with OSA (Mezzanotte *et al.*, 1992), some patients have similar genioglossus muscle activity values to control subjects. Compensatory muscle activity may be increased in other muscle groups, or other mechanisms may be important in such patients.

Patients with OSA may also have defects in the sensory mechanisms that normally protect the upper airway from closure (Larsson *et al.*, 1992). However, it is difficult to determine whether identified defects in sensory control (based on both clinical and histopathological changes) in patients with OSA have a role in the genesis of OSA or are due to chronic airway vibration from snoring.

Pathogenesis of obstructive sleep apnoea: the role of obesity

Obesity is one of the strongest risk factors for OSA and there are a number of ways in which obesity can reduce upper airway size and therefore predispose the upper airway to collapse. External neck circumference is increased in patients with OSA and this measurement may explain some of the link between obesity and sleep apnoea (Davies *et al.*, 1990; Katz *et al.*, 1990). Neck circumference is an index of neck fat deposition, particularly in the lateral pharyngeal fat pads, and this fat deposition may lead to airway narrowing and OSA (Koenig and Thach, 1988). Imaging studies have shown that these fat pads are increased in size in obese patients with OSA (Brown *et al.*, 1986). However, excess fat deposition around the airway is not a universal finding in obese OSA patients (Ciscar *et al.*, 2001) and well-matched control subjects are often difficult to obtain. Other studies have shown that obese sleep apnoea patients have larger tongues (Do *et al.*, 2000) and smaller upper airway volumes (Fleetham, 1992) than non-obese patients. Obesity may predispose to OSA by increasing the size of upper airway soft-tissue structures, although the cause of this increased size is unknown. There may be soft-tissue oedema from the repeated vibration of snoring and apnoea. Human upper airway pathological studies have been described infrequently in sleep apnoea, although in one report more fat and muscle was observed in the uvula of sleep apnoea patients (Schwab *et al.*, 1995; Do *et al.*, 2000).

Recently, a case–control study examining the upper airway using a sophisticated volumetric analysis magnetic resonance imaging (MRI) scan found that OSA patients had a larger volume of soft tissue surrounding the upper airway than control subjects. Control subjects were matched in terms of sex, age, ethnicity and for craniofacial size and visceral neck fat. They concluded that OSA is associated with a significantly larger tongue, lateral pharyngeal walls and total amount of soft tissue. In a multivariable logistic regression, the volume of the tongue and lateral walls was shown to independently increase the risk of sleep apnoea (Schwab *et al.*, 2003).

Apart from upper airway narrowing, fat deposition in the chest and abdomen contribute to OSA. In morbidly obese patients, neck size is a better predictor of sleep apnoea than other body anthropomorphic measures (Grunstein *et al.*, 1995a). However, in a wide weight range of clinic patients with sleep apnoea, we observed that waist measurement provided similar or better statistical correlations with sleep apnoea (Grunstein *et al.*, 1993a). Abdominal obesity may reduce lung volumes, particularly in the supine posture, and so reduce upper airway size. Lung volume directly influences upper airway size during respiration. Thoracic inspiratory activity produces caudal traction on the trachea, increasing the pharyngeal cross-sectional area (Van de Graaff, 1988). This effect may be reduced in obese patients, as impaired respiratory muscle force has been noted in obese patients (Lopata and

Onal, 1982). Cephalad movement of the trachea, as would occur with a decrease in lung volume, decreases upper airway size and increases pharyngeal resistance (Series *et al.*, 1990). Passive inflation of the lung producing an increase in end-expiratory lung volume increases the size of the retropalatal airway (Begle *et al.*, 1990).

It is likely that obesity promotes sleep apnoea through a variety of mechanisms. In some patients, subcutaneous neck or peripharyngeal fat may be the critical load that tips the balance in favour of upper airway closure in sleep. In other patients, abdominal fat loading may be important. As yet there are no data on how weight loss relates to changes in the upper airway fat.

In addition, more speculatively, the central obesity–sleep apnoea link may be related to abnormal upper airway muscle function. Obesity is associated with changes in relative muscle fibre composition in skeletal muscle (Wade *et al.*, 1990). Some studies of sleep apnoea patients before and after weight loss have shown changes in upper airway function rather than structure (Begle *et al.*, 1990), supporting a hypothesis of abnormal upper airway muscle function in obese patients with sleep apnoea.

Obesity hypoventilation syndrome

The majority of patients with OSA have normal arterial carbon dioxide ($P_a\text{CO}_2$) tensions when awake. The term obesity hypoventilation syndrome (OHS) describes those patients with obesity and daytime hypercapnia (and usually hypoxaemia) in the absence of lung or muscle disease. This association between obesity, hypersomnolence and hypercapnia was recognized for many years, and was labelled *Pickwickian syndrome* (in honour of Joe, the fat boy, in Dickens' *Pickwick Papers*). However, the pathogenesis of the condition was poorly understood and the link with OSA not recognized. Early theories were that obesity produced a load to breathing, which, together with depressed chemosensitivity, produced OHS. The recognition that sleep apnoea was present in these patients and that relief of upper airway obstruction by tracheostomy effectively treated the respiratory failure altered our understanding of OHS. Upper airway obstruction is a crucial factor in the pathogenesis of OHS (Sullivan *et al.*, 1990).

However, most patients with OSA do not have hypercapnia when awake and so upper airway obstruction alone is not enough to produce OHS. In addition, the majority of patients with obesity and eucapnia have normal resting ventilation and occlusion pressures, and normal or increased responses to hypoxia and hypercapnia. The prevalence of OHS in the obese population is unknown but it is probably underdiagnosed. A recent study found that 31% of obese patients (BMI > 35 kg/m^2) admitted to medical wards had OHS (Nowbar *et al.*, 2000).

There are no longitudinal studies on the development of OHS but, almost certainly, OHS starts out as heavy snoring

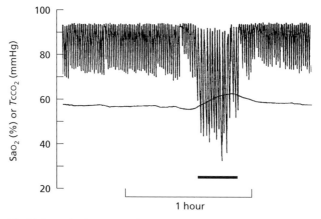

Fig 20.2 A 2-h oximetry recording, with transcutaneous (tc) CO_2 monitoring in a patient with severe OSA and OHS (obesity hypoventilation syndrome). The black bar indicates a period of REM sleep. There are repetitive arterial oxygen desaturations, with profound hypoxaemia in REM sleep, associated with a marked rise in $tcCO_2$, indicating hypoventilation.

and then OSA, and sleep-induced respiratory abnormalities occur before the development of daytime respiratory failure. During an apnoeic period, $P_a\text{CO}_2$ rises acutely and $P_a\text{O}_2$ falls (Fig. 20.2). When the apnoea is terminated by an arousal, ventilation increases and oxygen and carbon dioxide levels can return to normal. If arousal responses *or* ventilatory responses to hypoxia or hypercapnia are depressed, the apnoeic periods will be longer, the degree of blood gas derangement greater and the normalization of blood gases in the period following arousal compromised (Sullivan *et al.*, 1990). In those patients who are able to compensate for the loss of ventilation during apnoeic periods by increased ventilation between events, overall eucapnia will be maintained. In contrast, if the compensatory mechanisms are poor then overall ventilation will be reduced during sleep, with the development of persistent hypercapnia and hypoxia during sleep. This will result in resetting of the chemoreceptors (Berthon-Jones and Sullivan, 1987) and progression to daytime carbon dioxide retention. Sleep fragmentation as a result of repetitive arousals will also depress arousal responses. Arousal responses can be further impaired in patients who are prescribed sedatives/hypnotics to improve insomnia, opiate analgesics to ease musculoskeletal pain or by consumption of alcohol. The term *Pickwickian syndrome* should be replaced by OHS or OSA with awake respiratory failure, which better describes the syndrome within the spectrum of sleep-disordered breathing.

It is likely that the development of OHS is multifactorial, with the key elements being a combination of obesity (increased upper airway loading and reduced lung volumes), OSA, poor chemoreceptor function (particularly defective arousal responses to hypoxia) and possibly alcohol consumption (reducing upper airway tone and arousal responses to asphyxia) (Sullivan *et al.*, 1990). Assessment of chemoreceptor function in this patient group is made difficult as prolonged exposure to hypoxia and hypercapnia will alter ventilatory responses, but studies in other diseases have shown familial clustering in the level of chemosensitivity, suggesting a genetic component (Fleetham *et al.*, 1984) as well.

It is important to stress that awake hypercapnia can occur in obese patients in the absence of any smoking history or lung/muscle disease (Leech *et al.*, 1987). More recently, leptin has been implicated in sleep-disordered breathing in obese subjects. In obese, leptin-deficient mice with OHS, leptin replacement resulted in an increase in minute ventilation (awake and asleep) and increased chemosensitivity to carbon dioxide during sleep (Leech *et al.*, 1987). These changes were independent of food intake, weight and carbon dioxide production. Patients with OSA have higher leptin levels than subjects with similar obesity without OSA (O'Donnell *et al.*, 1999). Leptin levels fell significantly in a group of 22 patients with OSA after 4 days of treatment with continuous positive airway pressure (CPAP) (Phillips *et al.*, 2000) possibly due to reduced sympathetic activity. OSA may well be a confounder in some of the hormonal associations observed in central obesity and is possibly associated with resistance to the weight-reducing effects of leptin. In this context, hyperleptinaemia and accelerated weight gain appear closely associated with worsening of sleep apnoea (Chin *et al.*, 1999). Recently, we observed that higher circulatory leptin levels were associated with hypoventilation in obesity. In human obesity, leptin resistance is common and leptin may well act as a respiratory stimulant so that deficiency or resistance to the effects of leptin may promote OHS (Phipps *et al.*, 2002).

Sleep-disordered breathing: epidemiology

Epidemiology in the general community

Studies examining prevalence in the area of sleep-disordered breathing have largely concentrated on self-reported estimates of snoring and daytime sleepiness. These symptoms are commonly reported in the general community, including obese subjects, and sleepiness may have many causes (Table 20.2). In addition, snoring may be underestimated if history from a bed partner is unavailable. Therefore, questionnaire estimates of OSA are difficult to interpret and are of limited usefulness.

The Wisconsin Sleep Cohort Study (Young *et al.*, 1993) is the largest reported prevalence study in which sleep studies were performed. This group found an apnoea index of > 5 events per hour in 9% of female and 24% of male middle-aged public servants. The *OSA syndrome* (daytime sleepiness and an apnoea index of > 5 per hour) was found in 2% of women and 4% of men. An apnoea index of > 15 events was found in 4% of women and 9% of men. Our group has found a similar prevalence of OSA in an Australian rural community using home monitoring of breathing (Bearpark *et al.*, 1995).

Table 20.2 Sleepiness in the obese patient.

Inadequate amounts of sleep
Lifestyle (especially shift work and commercial drivers), insomnia

Drugs (causing sleepiness/disrupting sleep)
Hypnotics, alcohol, drug abuse

Disorders disrupting sleep
OSA, PLMS

Primary brain disorders
Narcolepsy, IHS

IHS, idiopathic hypersomnolence; OSA, obstructive sleep apnoea; PLMS, periodic leg movement disorder.

Even when sleep studies are performed, estimates of prevalence are made difficult by the varying definitions of OSA used. In the past, researchers have used an apnoea index of > 5 events per hour to define OSA. However, given that hypopnoeas and even increased upper airway resistance can produce the OSA syndrome, that definition is probably inadequate. Other measurements may be important, such as arousal index or changes in heart rate and blood pressure through the night. In addition, more recent work (see later) has suggested that an apnoea index as low as 1–5 events per hour may influence the development of hypertension (Peppard *et al.*, 2000b).

Epidemiology in the obese population

Multiple investigations have consistently shown that obesity, particularly central obesity, is strongly associated with sleep-disordered breathing in adults (Grunstein *et al.*, 1993a; 1995a. Measurements of central obesity such as waist or neck measurements are closely linked to OSA in sleep clinic populations, and this association remains tight in the general population, although not as strong as in sleep clinic cohorts. In the Busselton Sleep Survey there was a strong effect of body mass index (BMI) in increasing the risk of sleep-disordered breathing in the community (Bearpark *et al.*, 1995) (Fig. 20.3).

There are limited data on the prevalence of sleep apnoea in the obese population. The Swedish Obese Subjects study, which examined 3034 subjects with BMIs > 35, found that over 50% of obese men reported habitual loud snoring (Grunstein *et al.*, 1995b) compared with 15% in age-matched non-obese subjects. Similarly, 33% of men and 12% of women in this study reported a history of frequent witnessed apnoeas. Questionnaires tend to underestimate the prevalence of OSA. The exact prevalence of the spectrum of sleep-breathing disorders in obese individuals is unknown, but it is clear that OSA and related conditions occur in a very high proportion of obese subjects.

More recent longitudinal studies have demonstrated a strong association between weight gain and the development

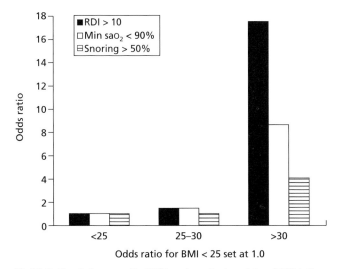

Fig 20.3 Obesity (measured by BMI) is an important predictor of OSA in the Busselton Sleep Survey. With the odds ratio for BMI < 25 set at 1.0, a BMI > 30 increased the odds ratio of either OSA (respiratory disturbance index, RDI, >10), desaturation during the night (minimum Sao_2 < 90%) or heavy snoring (snoring for more than 50% of the night) by 4–18 times, depending on the variable.

of sleep-disordered breathing. The Wisconsin group prospectively twice evaluated 690 randomly selected local residents at 4-year intervals for the presence of sleep-disordered breathing (Peppard *et al.*, 2000a). They found that weight gain of 10% predicted an approximate 32% increase in the apnoea–hypopnoea index (AHI), and similarly, weight loss of 10% predicted a 26% fall in the AHI. Therefore, even relatively small changes in baseline weight have a powerful impact on the degree of sleep-disordered breathing.

Epidemiology: other risk factors for obstructive sleep apnoea

Age

The prevalence of OSA increases with age. Some of this association may be due to increased central fat deposition with age, but other factors, such as changes in tissue elasticity and ventilatory control and cardiopulmonary and neurological comorbidity, may be important.

Gender

In the middle-aged population, the risk of OSA is three to four times greater in males than in females (Redline *et al.*, 1994). However, the prevalence of OSA increases in women after the menopause, suggesting a protective role for female hormones (hormone replacement therapy, HRT) or an OSA-promoting role for male hormones. These effects may be due to hormonal influences on ventilatory control and mechanical behaviour of

the upper airway (Brooks and Strohl, 1992) or on patterns of body fat deposition. The redistribution of fat from peripheral to central sites that occurs with menopause may lead to increased prevalence of sleep apnoea due to upper airway mass loading. Alternatively, the change in hormonal status may affect the arousal of ventilatory responses to blood gas changes during sleep. Finally, after menopause, the female airway may be more collapsible due to changes in upper airway mechanical properties from lowered female hormone levels.

Recently, a number of large epidemiological studies have indicated that female HRT in menopause may protect against OSA (Bixler *et al.*, 2001; Shahar *et al.*, 2003). However, clinical trials of oestrogen administration in menopausal OSA have been disappointing (Cistulli *et al.*, 1994).

Familial, genetic and maxillofacial factors

Familial clustering of OSA has been noted, independent of age and obesity. This association is probably due to similarities in facial structure affecting upper airway dynamics during sleep. Certain maxillofacial appearances such as class 2 malocclusion and retroposed mandible are strongly linked to OSA in non-obese subjects (Nelson and Hans, 1997). In obese patients, certain familial maxillofacial structures will further increase the likelihood of OSA.

Some congenital conditions are linked to OSA. The Pierre Robin sequence is strongly associated with OSA owing to mandibular shortening. Patients with Down's syndrome are predisposed to OSA due to oropharyngeal crowding and obesity. Nearly two-thirds of patients with Marfan's syndrome have OSA (Cistulli and Sullivan, 1995), despite a thin body habitus, due to abnormal compliance of upper airway tissue.

Any conditions causing narrowing of the upper airway, such as tonsillar and adenoidal hypertrophy, macroglossia and high-arched palates, will predispose to the development of OSA. Nasal obstruction is also a significant risk factor for OSA (Lofaso *et al.*, 2000). Again, the presence of these abnormalities will interact with obesity to produce a greater risk for OSA (Ferguson *et al.*, 1995).

Comorbid conditions

Many endocrine abnormalities are associated with an increased prevalence of OSA. Hypothyroidism reduces chemosensitivity and promotes airway narrowing by upper airway myopathy and myxoedematous infiltration (Grunstein and Sullivan, 1988). More than 50% of patients with acromegaly have OSA, and an increased prevalence of central sleep apnoea has been seen associated with increased disease activity (as assessed by biochemical markers) (Grunstein *et al.*, 1991). Cushing's disease is also associated with OSA (Rosenow *et al.*, 1998).

Cardiac failure (whatever the cause) is associated with a high incidence of sleep-disordered breathing. In a recent study of 450 patients with cardiac failure referred to a sleep laboratory (either with sleep symptoms or persistent dyspnoea), 72% had more than 10 apnoeas/hypopneas per hour (Sin *et al.*, 1999). Patients had OSA or central sleep apnoea (Cheynes–Stokes respiration), with OSA more common in those patients with BMI > 35 kg/m^2.

Cerebrovascular disease is associated with the presence of sleep-disordered breathing. A recent report examined patients in both the acute and convalescent stages of a first-ever stroke (haemorrhagic or ischaemic) (Parra *et al.*, 2000). In the acute phase, 71% of patients had an AHI greater than 10, with an AHI > 30 in 28%. Cheyne–Stokes breathing was seen in 26%. In the convalescent phase (3 months later), the overall AHI and the amount of Cheyne–Stokes breathing had fallen, but the obstructive apnoea index was unchanged. Some patients had persistent central apnoeas following their stroke.

Sleep-disordered breathing: clinical aspects

The clinical aspects are detailed below.

Symptoms and signs of sleep-disordered breathing

History and physical examination have fairly poor sensitivity and specificity for the detection of sleep-disordered breathing (Redline and Strohl, 1998). The typical symptoms associated with OSA are heavy snoring and excessive daytime sleepiness (EDS). The reporting of witnessed apnoeas is a relatively specific symptom but is also relatively insensitive. Other symptoms are listed in Table 20.3. Nocturnal symptoms include those related to the breathing disorder, such as choking and gasping, nocturia and nocturnal gastro-oesophageal reflux. Daytime symptoms are related to the effects of sleep fragmentation and include morning headaches, fatigue, poor memory and concentration, alteration in mood and impotence (McNamara *et al.*, 1993). Importantly, the arousal responses to

Table 20.3 Symptoms of sleep-disordered breathing.

Snoring
Daytime sleepiness
Disrupted sleep
Choking or gasping during sleep
Dry throat/mouth in morning
Morning headaches
Nocturia
Heartburn
Poor memory/concentration
Fatigue
Impotence
Altered mood/irritability

upper airway narrowing during sleep can be so brisk that some patients (particularly women) can present with insomnia, restless sleep or anxiety (Ambrogetti *et al.*, 1991).

These symptoms emphasize the importance of obtaining a confirmatory history from the spouse, bed partner and other family members. Few people are aware that they snore or stop breathing during sleep. The initial consultation is often precipitated by the bed partner's concerns about snoring and apnoea. Excessive sleepiness may be recognized by the patient, but may be under-reported if patients are unaware that their sleepiness is abnormal or are afraid of the potential consequences of excessive daytime sleepiness (EDS) (such as loss of driving licence or work).

Examination of the upper airway may be important. Obvious pharyngeal crowding and tonsillar enlargement suggest upper airway obstruction (Hoffstein and Szalai, 1993). The vibration of soft tissues due to heavy snoring can lead to a reddened and oedematous uvula and soft palate. Systemic hypertension is commonly associated with OSA. Detailed cephalometric measurements, as predictors for OSA, seem to be more useful in the non-obese populations (Redline and Strohl, 1998).

Diagnosis of sleep-disordered breathing

The *gold standard* approach for the investigation of sleep-disordered breathing is an overnight in-laboratory sleep study (polysomnography, PSG). Sleep stage, sleep architecture and arousals from sleep are monitored during a full sleep study by two electroencephalogram (EEG) channels, two electro-oculogram (EOG) channels and one electromyogram (EMG) channel. Breathing during sleep is usually monitored qualitatively with a measure of air flow at the nose/mouth, usually two measures of respiratory effort, such as diaphragm EMG and chest wall and abdominal movement, and oxygen saturation. Other variables measured include ECG, leg EMG, transcutaneous carbon dioxide, body position and snoring. A sleep study should be scored manually and, as a minimum, the report should include the total amount of sleep and proportions of different sleep stages, the number of respiratory events seen (apnoeas and hypopneas per hour both in REM and non-REM sleep), the degree of oxygen desaturation recorded, the number of EEG arousals and the presence or absence of periodic leg movements. Definitions of events are not standard across all sleep laboratories and different methods for measuring air flow and other respiratory variables have differing sensitivities.

In the area of sleep-disordered breathing, the definitions of normal and abnormal sleep are under constant revision. In general, an AHI of less than 5 events per hour would be considered normal, with an AHI of greater than 15 events per hour considered to represent at least moderate disease. An AHI of 5–15 events per hour would be considered mild disease, but there is significant individual variability in the symptoms re-

Table 20.4 Reasons for false-negative sleep studies.

Poor sleep efficiency (laboratory effect)
Little or no REM sleep seen
Usual sedatives or alcohol not taken
Patient not sleeping in usual position (especially supine)
Occurrence of *subcriterion events*
Night-to-night variability in the severity of OSA (significant in milder disease)

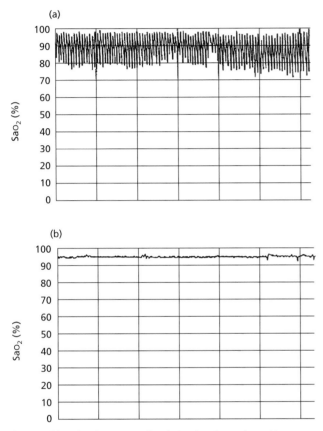

Fig 20.4 (a) A 1-h oximetry recording during sleep in a patient with severe OSA, showing typical repetitive arterial oxygen desaturations. (b) A 1-h oximetry recording during sleep in the same patient during treatment with nasal CPAP, with desaturations abolished and Sao_2 maintained above 90%.

lated to this mild degree of OSA. If a patient is symptomatic, then a trial of treatment is warranted. However, more recent studies have suggested that an AHI of between 1 and 5 may significantly increase the risk of developing hypertension, regardless of symptoms (Redline *et al.*, 1994).

Although polysomnography (PSG) is considered the best available test for the diagnosis of OSA, patients with OSA can have significant night-to-night variability in the severity of their disease, with the potential for a false-negative study (see Table 20.4). A negative PSG with high clinical suspicion warrants further review and often even a repeat sleep study.

The expense and inconvenience of polysomnography has

led to a search for alternative tools for the diagnosis of OSA. Overnight oximetry can detect repetitive oxygen desaturations seen in OSA (Fig. 20.4) and can be diagnostic in some patients (Gyulay *et al.*, 1993). However, not all apnoeic events produce significant desaturation and so a normal oximetry study does not exclude OSA. Similarly limited, portable or 'at-home' systems have had some success in the diagnosis of OSA but again do not necessarily exclude the diagnosis if negative. Currently, they are probably most useful in patients in whom the clinical suspicion is high or patients who cannot readily be studied in a laboratory, such as the immobile or medically unstable patient.

Consequences of sleep-disordered breathing

Psychosocial effects

Excessive daytime sleepiness is characteristic of sleep apnoea. However, sleepiness and fatigue are commonly reported symptoms in the general community, particularly in the obese population. The sleepiness seen in patients with OSA is predominantly related to repetitive arousal and sleep fragmentation, but a direct effect of hypoxaemia is possible (Montplaisir *et al.*, 1992). However, OSA is characterized by a range of EDS and there is a relatively poor correlation between markers of severity of OSA, such as AHI, and daytime sleepiness. It seems likely that people vary in their susceptibility to the effects of sleep fragmentation and sleep deprivation. There are no simple tests to accurately quantify daytime sleepiness. Sleepiness may lead to both impaired work performance and driving (Findley *et al.*, 1989). Patients with untreated OSA form an important risk group for motor vehicle accidents. Driving performance on various simulators is impaired in patients with OSA (Juniper *et al.*, 2000). Treatment with nasal CPAP dramatically improves daytime sleepiness and driving simulator performance (Findley *et al.*, 2000; Juniper *et al.*, 2000).

Many studies have found that OSA patients perform poorly on psychometric tests compared with control subjects. Sleep apnoea leads to defects in executive function and working memory in both adults and children (Beebe and Gozal 2002). There is a variable degree of improvement in cognitive function with nasal CPAP (Montplaisir *et al.*, 1992). The detrimental effects of OSA have other social implications, with data from the Swedish Obese Subjects study showing that, in equally obese men and women, OSA is associated with impaired work performance, increased sick leave and a higher divorce rate (Grunstein *et al.*, 1995a).

Cardiovascular effects

Acute effects

The acute cardiovascular effects seen during obstructive events have been well characterized, with marked changes in both systemic and pulmonary arterial blood pressure. As an

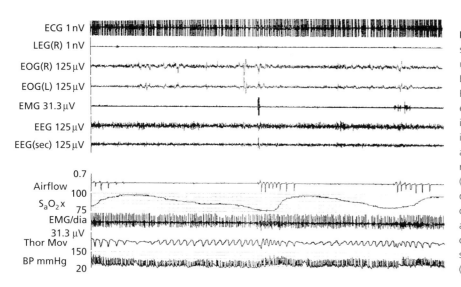

Fig 20.5 A 5-min tracing of a patient with typical severe OSA. The upper traces show the variables used for sleep staging (ECG, electrocardiogram; LEG, leg electromyogram; EOG, electro-oculogram; EMG, submental electromyogram; EEG, electroencephalogram) and indicate this patient is in REM sleep. The apnoeas are indicated by intermittent cessation of air flow (autoflow: nasal air flow) and are obstructive in nature, as continued respiratory effort is seen when air flow is absent (Thor Mov, thoracic movement or effort; EMG/dia, diaphragm electromyogram). Repetitive falls in oxygen saturation (S_aO_2) are seen following each apnoea. The lowest trace is a non-invasive recording of blood pressure (BP) showing an increase in both systolic (> 50 mmHg) and diastolic blood pressure (> 25 mmHg) at the end of an apnoea.

obstructive apnoea progresses, there are increasing swings in pleural pressure, worsening hypoxaemia, bradycardia (vagally mediated) and increased sympathetic nerve activity. As the apnoea is terminated by arousal, with increased ventilation, heart rate increases and both systolic and diastolic blood pressure increase markedly (Fig. 20.5), often by more than 100 mmHg. These profound haemodynamic fluctuations are largely due to surges in sympathetic nerve activity resulting from the combination of blood gas derangement, large swings in intrathoracic pressure and arousals. Patients with OSA have increased sympathetic activity through the night, with persistence of this increased activity into wakefulness (Carlson *et al.*, 1993). In addition, these patients have a potent pressor response to hypoxia compared with normal subjects (Hedner *et al.*, 1992), possibly due to repetitive nocturnal hypoxia. Studies using an elegant canine model of OSA have shown that sustained hypertension develops after 1–3 months of OSA (Brooks *et al.*, 1997). Studies in rats have found that intermittent hypoxia induces a persistent increase in diurnal blood pressure, mediated through renal sympathetic nerve activity and the renin–angiotensin system (Fletcher *et al.*, 1999).

Chronic effects
The chronic cardiovascular effects are detailed below.

Hypertension
Sleep apnoea is a common finding among patients in hypertension clinics and similarly, many patients with OSA have hypertension (Stradling and Crosby, 1991; Worsnop *et al.*, 1998). A cross-sectional study of 1400 patients who were referred for a sleep study showed that the degree of OSA was an independent predictor of morning blood pressure (Grunstein *et al.*, 1993a). Left-ventricular hypertrophy (as assessed by echocardiography), an important outcome of hypertension,

was shown to be increased in normotensive patients with OSA compared with matched control subjects without OSA (Hedner *et al.*, 1990). Studies of blood pressure as measured by intra-arterial monitoring, automated daytime blood pressure readings or 24-h ambulatory blood pressure have demonstrated a fall in blood pressure levels after CPAP treatment (Working Group on OSA and Hypertension, 1993). Despite these studies, a causal link between OSA and hypertension has been disputed due to the presence of important confounders such as obesity and age. However, more recently published data from two large epidemiological studies have provided stronger evidence that OSA is an independent risk factor for hypertension, regardless of obesity. Data from the Sleep Heart Health Study, a large cross-sectional community-based study with more than 6000 subjects, found that AHI and percentage of sleep time with an oxygen saturation below 90% were significantly associated with systemic hypertension, independent of anthropomorphic variables such as BMI, waist–hip ratio and neck circumference (Nieto *et al.*, 2000).

Similarly, prospective data from the Wisconsin Sleep Cohort Study (Bixler *et al.*, 2001), which followed more than 700 subjects over 4–8 years, have found a dose–response association between sleep-disordered breathing and hypertension, independent of measures of obesity. In this study, an AHI < 4.9 events per hour had an odds ratio for hypertension at follow-up of 1.42, with odds ratios of 2.03 and 2.89 for AHIs of 5.0–14.9 and >15 respectively. Therefore, it is likely that the acute nocturnal surges in blood pressure in response to chemoreflex-medicated hypoxic stimulation of sympathetic activity lead to chronic hypertension (Somers *et al.*, 1989). A number of mechanisms have been postulated for this process, including enhanced vasoconstriction and endothelial dysfunction (Kato *et al.*, 2000; Wolk *et al.*, 2003). Further support for an independent effect of OSA on blood pressure has been provided by recent studies showing that effective nasal CPAP reduces blood pressure compared with subtherapeutic CPAP (Pepperell *et al.*, 2002; Becker *et al.*, 2003).

Cardiovascular disease and mortality

As with hypertension, cause-and-effect relationships between OSA and other cardiovascular endpoints are difficult to establish. A number of groups have reported an increased risk of myocardial infarction and stroke in sleep apnoea (Hung *et al.*, 1990; Palomaki *et al.*, 1992). Potential mechanisms of atherosclerosis include endothelial dysfunction and a vascular inflammatory response from hypoxia. C-reactive protein level (CRP) (an index of the presence of systemic inflammation and probably atherogenesis) is elevated in OSA (Shamsuzzamam *et al.*, 2002). Effective CPAP therapy was associated with a reduction in CRP in a population with severe OSA (Yokoe *et al.*, 2003). A number of pro-atherogenic factors have been shown to be promoted by untreated OSA (Dyugovskaya *et al.*, 2002). Data from the Sleep Heart Health Study have demonstrated a relationship between AHI and prevalent cardiovascular disease (as defined by various manifestations of ischaemic heart disease, heart failure and stroke) (Shahar *et al.*, 2001). The odds ratios were fairly modest and surprisingly there did not appear to be a dose–response ratio above an AHI of 10. However, a criticism of this study is the mean age of the group (65 years). Prior work has suggested that the effects of OSA on cardiovascular disease, including mortality, are most marked in those patients under 50 years.

A prospective study of more than 1600 patients found that age, BMI, hypertension and apnoea index were independent predictors of death (Lavie *et al.*, 1995). He and colleagues (1988) observed an increased cumulative mortality in untreated patients with an apnoea index > 20 compared with AHI < 20, again most marked in patients under 50 years. Treatment with CPAP or tracheostomy reduced the mortality. Snoring is a strong risk factor for sleep-related strokes, whereas sleep apnoea symptoms (snoring plus reported apnoeas or EDS) increase the risk of cerebral infarction, with an odds ratio of 8.0. Mechanisms other than increased blood pressure and sympathetic activity may be involved. Tests of platelet aggregation increased overnight in a group of patients with OSA compared with decreasing overnight in control subjects (Sanner *et al.*, 2000). Treatment with CPAP decreased the night-time level of platelet aggregability and reversed the overnight rise seen pretreatment.

Other studies of vascular responsiveness have demonstrated impaired vasodilatation in patients with OSA, both with and without hypertension (Carlson *et al.*, 1996). These findings have implications in analysis of data linking obesity and cardiac disease. More recently, Peker and colleagues (2002) did a 7-year follow-up study of 182 middle-aged men. They concluded that the risk for cardiovascular disease is increased fivefold in middle-aged men with OSA, and that effective treatment decreases the risk to one-tenth of that in untreated men. More difficult still is the issue of treating patients with OSA who do not have significant sleepiness, with the aim of preventing the effects of sleep-disordered breathing on cardiovascular outcomes (Hedner, 2001).

Pulmonary hypertension and lung disease

Obstructive apnoeas can produce pulmonary hypertension acutely, largely due to hypoxic pulmonary vasoconstriction although hypercapnia may also play a role. A number of studies have found a relationship between OSA and the development of daytime pulmonary hypertension (PHT), with the prevalence of PHT ranging from 10% to 70% in patients presenting with OSA (Weitzenblum *et al.*, 1988; Sajkov *et al.*, 1994; 1999). Some of these studies have included patients with lung disease, particularly chronic obstructive pulmonary disease (COPD), as well as OSA, possibly confounding the results. However, there are several studies that carefully excluded patients with any lung disease and these studies have found PHT in 10–40% of patients with OSA (Bady *et al.*, 2000). It seems likely that individual variation in the response of the pulmonary vasculature to hypoxia accounts for the development of PHT in some patients with OSA. Sleep-disordered breathing should therefore be excluded in any patient who has PHT.

The *overlap syndrome* describes those patients with both OSA and lung disease, particularly COPD. The combination of these diseases results in a greater degree of pulmonary hypertension and blood gas abnormality than expected for each disease alone. In general, patients with COPD develop daytime hypercapnia only when their lung function falls below 30% of their predicted level. However, patients with only moderate COPD (lung function > 40% predicted) can develop significant awake hypercapnic hypoxic respiratory failure if they have coexistent OSA. The hypercapnia is due to hypoventilation secondary to changes in ventilatory control and can be partly or fully reversed with effective treatment of the sleep apnoea.

Endocrine abnormalities

Impaired growth hormone (GH) secretion in adults can lead to central obesity and reduced bone and muscle mass; patients with obesity have low levels of GH. Men with OSA have a defect in both GH and testosterone secretion (Grunstein *et al.*, 1989; 1993b) that can be reversed with CPAP treatment, independent of any weight change. The low GH levels in OSA patients may be additive to the already low levels of obesity, but it remains unknown whether the changes in GH and testosterone in OSA result in any measurable changes in body composition or body fat distribution.

In a group of patients with a high likelihood of OSA, based on questionnaire data, plasma insulin levels were found to be increased in both men and women, independent of obesity (Schwab *et al.*, 1995). Recently, Ip and colleagues (2002) studied 250 consecutive subjects from a sleep clinic who did not knowingly have diabetes mellitus. They essentially found that obesity and also sleep apnoea severity and minimum oxygen

Table 20.5 Effects of dietary weight change on severity of OSA.

Study	Participants	Follow-up (months)	Intervention	Weight change, kg (%)	AHI change, events/hour (%)
Smith *et al.* (1985)	15	5.3	Diet instruction	9.6 (9)	25.8 (47)
Pasquali *et al.* (1990)	23	?	VLCD	18.5 (61)	33.5 (49)
Schwartz *et al.* (1990)	13	16	DIET	7.3 (17)	50.8 (61)
Suratt *et al.* (1992)	8	24	VLCD	20.6 (13)	28 (30)
Kansanen *et al.* (1998)	15	3	Diet	9.2 (8)	12 (38.7)

VLCD, very low-calorie diet.

saturation were independent determinants of insulin resistance. In another study of 150 mildly obese subjects, sleep-disordered breathing was independently associated with glucose intolerance and insulin resistance (Punjabi *et al.*, 2002). A further study examined patients with type 2 diabetes mellitus and OSA, and found an improvement in insulin sensitivity after treatment with CPAP (Brooks *et al.*, 1994). This improvement again was independent of any changes in weight or other treatment. These data suggest that OSA has an effect on insulin resistance, possibly through increased sympathetic nerve activity. Some of the hormonal abnormalities in central obesity may be attributable to OSA.

Sleep-disordered breathing: treatment

The approach to any treatment should be tailored to suit the individual patient and in sleep-disordered breathing it will be determined primarily by the severity of symptoms and the severity of the OSA. A secondary consideration is the presence or absence of cardiovascular risk factors. The question as to whether patients should be treated for this latter reason alone, regardless of symptoms, remains unanswered and this area is made more difficult by the fact that compliance with the most successful form of treatment available (CPAP) is related to the relief of symptoms. However, patient denial, either conscious or not, may produce an *asymptomatic* patient and, if possible, family input should be sought when a patient with a highly positive study denies symptoms. Patient occupation may also influence the decision to treat, particularly given data regarding motor vehicle accidents and OSA, and the fact that sleep deprivation, which is common in commercial drivers, may act synergistically with even mild OSA to increase daytime sleepiness.

Weight loss

Weight loss is an important part of any treatment regime in which the disease is related to obesity. Weight loss, either by caloric restriction (Smith *et al.*, 1985; Pasquali *et al.*, 1990; Schwartz *et al.*, 1991; Suratt *et al.*, 1992; Kansanen *et al.*, 1998; Sampol *et al.*, 1998) (Table 20.5) or bariatric surgery (Harman *et al.*, 1982; Charuzi *et al.*, 1985; Sugerman *et al.*, 1992; Pillar *et al.*, 1994) (Table 20.6), significantly reduces the severity of OSA. Even moderate weight loss (10%) can decrease the AHI and improve daytime alertness. Recently published longitudinal data on 690 subjects, followed over 8 years with sleep studies, showed that a 10% weight gain predicted an increase in the AHI of around 32% and a 10% weight loss predicted a decrease of 26% in the AHI (Peppard *et al.*, 2000a; Shahar *et al.*, 2001).

Short-term effects of weight loss

Several small clinical studies have evaluated the short-term effects of varying degrees of weight loss in patients with OSA. The majority of these studies all demonstrated that weight loss was associated with an improvement in OSA. However, these studies are uncontrolled, as they have varying degrees of obesity at baseline. Smith and colleagues (1985) demonstrated not only a reduction in OSA with weight loss, but also a reduction in pharyngeal critical closing pressure, which indicated a reduction in upper airway collapsibility.

Several case series of significant weight loss following bariatric surgical procedures have been published. Although there was an improvement in OSA with dramatic weight loss, the amount of weight loss did not always correlate with the degree of improvement in OSA.

Long-terms effects of weight loss

Detailed long-term studies of weight loss are lacking. In a group of 313 patients with BMI > 35 kg/m² assessed by questionnaire 1 year after bariatric surgery, there were marked improvements in habitual snoring (82% preoperatively to 14% at follow-up), observed sleep apnoea (33% to 2%) and

Table 20.6 Effects of surgical weight change on severity of OSA.

Study	Baseline	Follow-up	Comment
Harman *et al.* (1982)	AHI: 78	AHI: 1.4	Jejuno-ileal bypass, mean weight loss 108 kg
Pillar *et al.* (1994)	AHI: 40 BMI: 45	AHI: 11 BMI: 33	Gastric bypass/gastroplasty (14 patients), initial results at 4/12
		AHI: 24 BMI: 35	Same group at follow-up at 7 years: note non-significant change in weight, but significantly worse OSA
Sugerman *et al.* (1992)	AHI: 64	AHI: 26	Gastric bypass/gastroplasty (40 patients), mean weight loss 57 kg
Charuzi *et al.* (1985)	AHI: 89	AHI: 8	Gastric bypass (13 patients), mean weight change 73%

daytime sleepiness (39% to 4%) (Dixon *et al.*, 2001). This group had lost an average of 48% of their excess weight. However, the effects of weight loss on OSA are variable, and many patients have significant residual disease that warrants further treatment. In addition, there have been reports of OSA recurring, despite maintenance of weight loss (Pillar *et al.*, 1994; Sampol *et al.*, 1998). For these reasons, patients should be re-assessed after weight loss and regularly during weight maintenance.

Other general measures

Alcohol and sedatives such as benzodiazepines should be avoided in patients with sleep-disordered breathing. These drugs can reduce pharyngeal muscle tone and depress arousal responses, resulting in more and longer apnoeas during sleep. Similarly sleep deprivation can impair upper airway muscle tone and increase arousal thresholds, increasing any tendency to OSA. Smoking cessation can reduce self-reported snoring possibly by effects of smoke on airway inflammation and should be encouraged (as always).

Body position may influence the frequency of apnoea and hypopneas in 50–60% of patients (Cartwright, 1984). The AHI increases in a supine position and is lower in an elevated position (30–60°) and lateral position (McEvoy *et al.*, 1986). Some patients have predominantly positional apnoea (related to the supine posture), and attempts to avoid this position during sleep may help reduce the severity of OSA. However, positional therapy may not be effective in the obese patient. Positional therapy should however be considered in patients with OSA who have at least twice the number of respiratory events in the supine position compared with the lateral position and have an AHI of <10 events per hour. Nasal obstruction will worsen any tendency to snoring and OSA, and should be treated (usually pharmacologically); there is little evidence that nasal surgery is of any use in the treatment of OSA. The effects of external nasal dilator strips on snoring are variable, with some studies reporting success (Pevernagie *et al.*, 2000). These strips have no effect on OSA.

Continuous positive airway pressure

The application of nasal CPAP for the treatment of OSA was first described by Sullivan and colleagues (1981) and revolutionized the field of sleep-disordered breathing (Sullivan *et al.*, 1981). Nasal CPAP is the most effective treatment available for OSA. A CPAP machine works by delivering positive pressure to the upper airway via a nose (or face) mask, thus providing a pneumatic splint that prevents upper airway closure. The pressure is usually generated by an electromechanical blower that delivers air flow through wide-bore tubing to a nasal mask with a fixed expiratory resistance. Adjusting the air flow allows different pressures to be delivered at the nares. The optimal pressure required to prevent upper airway closure is determined by a sleep study. The required pressure can vary between 4 and 20 cmH$_2$O. Many patients show a rebound phenomenon during these treatment nights, with markedly increased amounts of REM and slow-wave sleep.

Treatment with nasal CPAP normalizes sleep architecture (Fig. 20.4), decreases upper airway oedema and significantly improves daytime sleepiness both subjectively and objectively (Sullivan *et al.*, 1994). Studies have shown that CPAP improves daytime alertness, cognitive function, mood and quality of life in patients with OSA of all degrees of severity, from mild (including *upper airway resistance syndrome*) through to severe (Engleman *et al.*, 1994; 1999; Jenkinson *et al.*, 1997; Ballester *et al.*, 1999). These studies include carefully controlled trials with either placebo tablets or subtherapeutic CPAP (Jenkinson *et al.*, 1999). There is also evidence that treatment with CPAP reduces the incidence of actual and near-miss traffic accidents in patients with OSA (Krieger *et al.*, 1997). As discussed previously, CPAP treatment reverses many of the adverse effects of OSA on blood pressure, pulmonary hypertension and various hormonal levels, including leptin, and mortality.

CPAP does not cure OSA. When treatment with CPAP is stopped, OSA recurs and symptoms return. However, regular use of CPAP may lead to a reduction in the underlying severity of OSA as assessed by sleep studies performed after a period of treatment. This reduction in severity is probably due to the effects of CPAP in reducing upper airway oedema and treating sleep deprivation. Recently, Barnes and colleagues (2002) reported in a randomized crossover study of CPAP vs. a placebo tablet in mild OSA that CPAP failed to improve measures of objective or subjective sleepiness in patients with mild OSA, and that placebo effect may account for some of the treatment responses previously reported (Barnes *et al.*, 2002).

The main problem limiting the efficacy of CPAP has been long-term compliance (Grunstein, 1995). Various studies of compliance indicate that somewhere between 40% and 70% of patients have difficulties with compliance (Krieger, 1992). On the whole, those centres that provide more intensive initial (within the first few weeks of treatment) assistance to patients have better long-term compliance than others; compliance with treatment in this initial period predicts long-term compliance. In addition, those patients who have the greatest symptomatic improvement with CPAP are, not surprisingly, the more compliant. The CPAP machine and mask remain fairly cumbersome and inconvenient. Side-effects related to the patient–mask interface are the most common and, although often minor, have a major impact on patient tolerance and use of the treatment. Poorly fitting masks can cause skin irritation and even ulceration. More importantly, poor mask fit can result in an air leak, either around the mask or through the mouth. Due to the high air flow generated by the CPAP machine, leaks can produce major effects on the mouth and nose, with dryness of the mouth and nasal congestion and rhinorrhoea. These problems can be effectively treated by improving mask fit, providing a chin-strap to prevent mouth-opening or humidifying and warming the air with humidifiers built into the circuit. The technology of mask and machine is constantly improving, with machines available now that ramp pressure up slowly at sleep onset and continuously adjust the required pressure through the night. These modifications may improve compliance in some patients. Those patients who require higher pressures or have milder disease are less likely to be compliant. Obese patients with OSA generally require higher pressures than patients who are not obese.

Despite these problems, CPAP remains highly effective for the treatment of all symptoms related to all degrees of OSA and should not be abandoned without intensive attempts to improve an individual's tolerance and compliance.

Newer generations of CPAP devices that provide automatic adjustments of positive airway pressure are widely available. The algorithms employed by these devices are not well known and are variable between various devices (Farre *et al.*, 2002). Auto-adjusting devices are generally just as effective as conventional fixed CPAP in OSA outcomes. There is also evidence that auto-adjusting devices are associated with lower mean pressures than conventional CPAP; however, this has not been shown to be associated with better compliance rates (Littner *et al.*, 2002).

Mandibular advancement devices

Mandibular advancement devices (MADs) are intraoral orthodontic devices that are designed to displace the mandible anteriorly, increasing the anteroposterior diameter of the upper airway and so reducing upper airway closure and collapse when worn at night. These devices are effective at reducing snoring, assessed both objectively and subjectively (Pasquali *et al.*, 1990). The effects of these devices in OSA are less clear. A number of uncontrolled studies have demonstrated significant reductions in the AHI with MADs, but many patients had significant residual apnoea and some patients had an increased AHI with these devices (Schmidt-Nowara *et al.*, 1995; Clark *et al.*, 1996). Controlled trials comparing MADs with CPAP have confirmed that MADs reduce the AHI by around 50% in some (not all) patients with mild to moderate OSA and significantly reduce daytime sleepiness (O'Sullivan *et al.*, 1995; Ferguson *et al.*, 1996). However, CPAP treatment results in a lower AHI and is successful in more patients. In 48 patients with OSA, randomized to 8 weeks of CPAP vs. 8 weeks of MAD (a crossover trial), there were significantly greater improvements in a number of sleep variables with CPAP than with the MAD. The authors of the study concluded that MAD did not represent first-line therapy for OSA patients (Engleman *et al.*, 2002).

These devices (MADs) require careful orthodontic attention to ensure that adequate anterior displacement of the mandible is achieved. The efficacy of these devices is likely to be reduced in the more obese patients as skeletal factors and maxillofacial abnormalities are less important in the genesis of upper airway obstruction in this group. In general, these devices tend to be less effective in those patients with more severe OSA. However, if a patient is intolerant of CPAP, it may be worthwhile trialling a MAD. There are few data available on compliance. Short-term side-effects are generally minor and are related to excessive salivation, jaw and tooth discomfort and occasional joint discomfort. Fortunately, serious complications are not common, but occlusal changes may occur.

The American Academy of Sleep Medicine has published guidelines about the use of oral appliances. Essentially, oral appliances are indicated as first-line therapy in simple snoring and mild OSA, and as second-line therapy for patients with moderate to severe OSA when other therapies have failed (American Sleep Disorders Association, 1995).

Tracheostomy

Prior to the advent of CPAP, tracheostomy was the only effective treatment for OSA (Standards of Practice Committee for the American Sleep Disorders Association, 1996). This operation is invasive, with significant morbidity, particularly in obese subjects, and is only partly effective in treating OHS. It should be reserved for those patients with very severe OSA, who are completely intolerant of any other treatment. Prior to any surgery, the patient should be reviewed in a specialist sleep centre, with intensive attempts to introduce nasal CPAP, including customized masks, humidification of inspired air and even ENT review/intervention to facilitate CPAP usage. With skilful surgery and close follow-up, tracheostomy may be a *last-resort* therapeutic option in some patients.

Uvulopalatopharyngoplasty and other upper airway surgery

Uvulopalatopharyngoplasty (UPPP) was originally described in Japan in the 1950s for the treatment of heavy snoring, and involves a careful surgical removal of the uvula and part of the soft palate (with or without tonsillectomy). The operation was introduced to the USA for the treatment of OSA in the early 1980s and was greeted with some enthusiasm. However, the efficacy of UPPP in the treatment of OSA is limited (Rodenstein, 1992). When treatment success is defined as a reduction in AHI of only 50%, a successful result is seen in less than 50% of patients. There are no preoperative tests that satisfactorily predict the response to surgery. There is a significant morbidity and even mortality. Excessive removal of palatal tissue can lead to velopharyngeal incompetence, with nasal regurgitation and speech changes. Subsequent use of CPAP may be more difficult following UPPP. Not surprisingly, many studies report particularly poor results in obese patients. Present-day guidelines state that the efficacy of UPPP is variable and that it should only be considered after non-surgical therapies have failed (Standards of Practice Committee for the American Sleep Disorders Association, 1996).

Modifications of the UPPP have been introduced where either a surgical laser is used to resect the palate (laser-assisted uvulopalatoplasty, LAUP) or high-frequency radio waves (somnoplasty) are used in an attempt to stiffen palatal tissue. The treatment response is variable and unpredictable. Ryan and Love (2000) studied 44 patients at baseline and 3 months after LAUP, and reported worsening of OSA (AHI increased by more than 100%) in 30% of their patient group, with a very poor relationship between subjective and objective measures of efficacy. There is clearly a placebo effect in snoring surgery, which has been demonstrated in other forms of surgical intervention. Recently, a randomized controlled study comparing temperature-controlled radiofrequency ablation to the tongue base and palate (TCRFTA) with CPAP and sham CPAP (ineffective CPAP) showed that treatment with TCRFTA and CPAP improved quality-of-life scores and sleepiness in mild to moderate OSA (Woodson *et al.*, 2002).

More complex maxillofacial surgery, usually performed in two phases, has been used with some success in the treatment of OSA. The first phase involves a UPPP in combination with genioglossus advancement, via a mandibular osteotomy, and hyoid myotomy. The Stanford group has reported overall success rates of around 60% with this procedure, but with less success in those patients with more severe disease (>60 events per hour and desaturation to 70%) and in the morbidly obese (Powell *et al.*, 1998). The second phase involves bimaxillary advancement, which was reported to be as successful as CPAP in treating a group of patients with severe OSA (AHI 68 per hour) and a mean BMI of 31 kg/m^2 (Riley *et al.*, 1993). In contrast, Bettega and colleagues (2000) found that phase I surgery was generally ineffective in OSA, with successful results in only 22% of patients. In their study, phase II surgery was successful in 75% of patients, but morbidity was significant. These complex surgical procedures are highly specialized and not widely available.

Pharmacological treatment

There are no placebo-controlled studies showing constant efficacy of any medication in OSA or OHS (Hedner and Grote, 2002). Obviously, weight-lowering drugs may be of benefit through weight loss but no drug has been found that alters the collapsibility of the upper airway during sleep. Studies looking at agents such as medroxyprogesterone, protriptyline and SSRIs as a primary therapy for OSA have been disappointing. A recent systematic review concluded that present data do not support the use of drugs as an alternative to CPAP in OSA (Smith *et al.*, 2002).

More recently, two randomized, double-blind placebo-controlled trials have shown that modafinil (non-amphetamine wakefulness promoter) may be useful as an adjunct therapy for OSA patients who are still sleepy despite CPAP use. Modafinil does not seem to affect sleep-disordered breathing (i.e. AHI) but improves measures of sleepiness compared with placebo (Kingshott *et al.*, 2001; Pack *et al.*, 2001).

Management of obstructive sleep apnoea with daytime respiratory failure (including obesity hypoventilation syndrome)

These patients should be managed in a specialist sleep and respiratory failure centre and, depending on the chronicity and the severity of their condition, many are best managed with a brief period of hospitalization. There is a wide range in the degree of hypercapnic hypoxic respiratory failure associated with the combination of OSA and obesity, and the management of these patients should be individualized. For example, the obese patient with severe OSA and a daytime P_aco_2 of 48 mmHg, normal pH and a P_ao_2 of 72 mmHg can usually be managed with CPAP alone; when the OSA is adequately treated, the daytime blood gases will improve.

Many of these patients come to medical attention with acute-on-chronic respiratory failure due to a superimposed condition, such as a respiratory tract infection, or even post-anaesthetic for an unrelated surgical procedure. In these decompensated patients, oxygen therapy alone should be used with caution with very close monitoring of hypercapnia and, as the main pathology in these patients is impaired respiratory

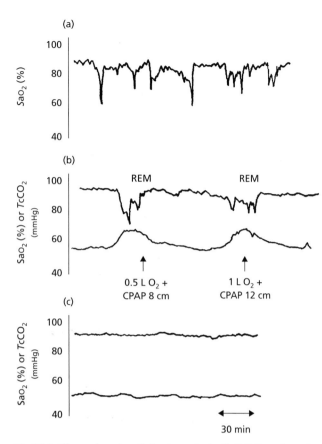

Fig 20.6 Efficacy of nasal ventilation in a patient with OHS. Recordings of oxygen saturation (S_aO_2, %) show marked falls in oxygen level during sleep (a). Addition of CPAP and low-flow oxygen (0.5 L = 0.5 L/min of supplemental oxygen; 1 L = 1 L/min) results in normal oxygen saturation in NREM sleep but persisting hypoxaemia in REM sleep (b). Use of nasal ventilation, either pressure support or volume cycled, will prevent oxygen desaturation in REM sleep (c) and prevent rises in $tcCO_2$ levels.

drive, sedatives or hypnotics should be avoided. Until recently, the only treatments available for these decompensated patients, and for those patients with severe chronic respiratory failure due to OHS, were very high CPAP pressures, CPAP plus added oxygen or, for the most unwell or obtunded patients, a short period of intubation and mechanical ventilation (Sullivan *et al.*, 1983; Piper and Sullivan, 1996).

New devices (modifications of CPAP) have become available for the treatment of respiratory failure (Fig. 20.6). These devices can deliver either volume-cycled ventilation or positive pressure ventilation to the upper airway via nose or facemask, effectively providing mechanical ventilation without the need for intubation. These devices can provide support to the patient's spontaneous respiratory efforts or deliver a set number of breaths as a back-up if the patient's inspiratory efforts are inadequate to trigger the machine. These devices are extremely effective in the treatment of both acute and chronic respiratory failure due to hypoventilation related to

obesity and OSA (Piper *et al.*, 1993; Piper and Sullivan, 1994), and are well tolerated by the patients.

When the acutely unwell patient has been stabilized, sleep studies can be performed to determine whether home use of non-invasive positive pressure ventilation (NIPPV) is required, at what pressures and whether added oxygen is needed. A similar approach is used in the treatment of patients with chronic severe OHS. After a period of treatment with NIPPV (months) some of these patients can be treated with CPAP alone. These patients are best managed in a specialist sleep unit with expertise in the long-term management of sleep-related respiratory failure.

Conclusion

Obesity can produce a measurable reduction in lung function and is very strongly associated with breathing disorders in sleep, such as OSA and hypoventilation.

Moderate to severe degrees of obesity can lead to a restrictive abnormality in lung function due to the mechanical effects of central body fat. Obese subjects may have reduced lung volumes and an increased work of breathing. Central fat deposition is also linked to upper airway collapsibility in sleep, and epidemiological data have identified obesity as a crucial risk factor in the development of OSA. Sleep-disordered breathing has a number of clinical consequences, including excess cardiovascular morbidity. The combination of obesity-induced reduced pulmonary function and sleep-disordered breathing can lead to progressive respiratory failure during sleep finally resulting in awake hypercapnic respiratory failure (OHS, central hypoventilation). This respiratory failure can occur without any intrinsic lung disease. Weight reduction can improve lung function and reduce the severity of sleep apnoea and OHS. Treatment of sleep-breathing disorders has been advanced greatly by the use of positive airway pressure devices and OHS can be reversed with the use of these devices.

References

Ambrogetti, A., Olson, L.G. and Saunders, N.A. (1991) Differences in the symptoms of men and women with obstructive sleep apnoea. *Australia and New Zealand Journal of Medicine* **21**, 863–866.

American Sleep Disorders Association (1995) Practice parameters for the treatment of snoring and obstructive sleep apnea with oral appliances. *Sleep* **18**, 511–513.

Bady, E., Achkar, A., Pascal, S., Orvoen-Frija, E. and Laaban, J.P. (2000) Pulmonary arterial hypertension in patients with sleep apnoea syndrome. *Thorax* **55**, 934–939.

Ballester, E., Badia, J.R., Hernandez, L., Carrasco, E., de Pablo, J., Fornas, C., Rodriguez-Roisin, R. and Montserrat, J.M. (1999) Evidence of the effectiveness of continuous positive airway pressure in the treatment of sleep apnea/hypopnea syndrome. *American Journal of Respiratory Care Medicine* **159**, 495–501.

Barnes, M., Houston, D., Worsnop, C.J., Neill, A.M., Mykytyn, I.J.I, Kay, A. and Trinder, J. (2002) A randomised controlled trial of continuous positive airway pressure in mild obstructive sleep apnea. *American Journal of Respiratory Care Medicine* **165**, 773–780.

Bearpark, H., Elliott, L., Grunstein, R., Cullen, s., Schneider, H., Althaus, W. and Sullivan, C. (1995) Snoring and sleep apnea. A population study in Australian men. *American Journal of Respiratory Care Medicine* **151**, 1459–1465.

Becker, H.F., Jerrentrup, A., Ploch, T., Grote, L. and Penzel, T. (2003) Effects of nasal continuous positive airway pressure treatment on blood pressure in patients with obstructive sleep apnoea. *Circulation* **107**, 68–73.

Beebe, D.W. and Gozal, D. (2002) Obstructive sleep apnea and the prefrontal cortex, towards a comprehensive model linking nocturnal upper airway: obstruction to daytime cognitive and behavioural deficits. *Journal of Sleep Research* **11**, 1–16.

Begle, R.L., Badr, S., Skatrud, J.B. and Dempsey, J.A. (1990) Effect of lung inflation on pulmonary resistance during NREM sleep. *American Review of Respiratory Disease* **141**, 854–860.

Berthon-Jones, M. and Sullivan, C.E. (1987) Time course of change in ventilatory response to CO_2 with long-term CPAP therapy for obstructive sleep apnea. *American Review of Respiratory Disease* **135**, 144–147.

Bettega, G., Pepin, J.L., Veale, D., Deschaux, C., Raphael, B. and Levy, P. (2000) Obstructive sleep apnea syndrome: fifty-one consecutive patients treated by maxillofacial surgery. *American Journal of Respiratory Care Medicine* **162**, 641–649.

Bixler, E., Vgontzas, A., Lin, H., Ten Have, T. and Rein, J. (2001) Prevalence of sleep-disordered breathing in women. *American Journal of Respiratory Care Medicine* **163**, 608–613.

Brooks, B., Cistulli, P.A., Borkman, M., Ross, G., McGhee, S., Grunstein, R.R., Sullivan, C.E. and Yue, D.K. (1994) Obstructive sleep apnea in obese non-insulin-dependent diabetic patients: effect of continuous positive airway pressure treatment on insulin responsiveness. *Journal of Clinical Endocrinology and Metabolism* **79**, 1681–1685.

Brooks, D., Horner, R.L., Kozar, L.F., Render-Teixeira, C.L. and Phillipson, E.A. (1997) Obstructive sleep apnea as a cause of systemic hypertension. Evidence from a canine model. *Journal of Clinical Investigation* **99**, 106–109.

Brooks, L.J. and Strohl, K.P. (1992) Size and mechanical properties of the pharynx in healthy men and women. *American Review of Respiratory Disease* **146**, 1394–1397.

Brown, I.G., Zamel, N. and Hoffstein, V. (1986) Pharyngeal cross-sectional area in normal men and women. *Journal of Applied Physiology* **61**, 890.

Carlson, J.T., Hedner, J., Elam, M., Ejnell, H., Sellgren, J. and Wallin, B.G. (1993) Augmented resting sympathetic activity in awake patients with obstructive sleep apnea. *Chest* **103**, 1763–1768.

Carlson, J.T., Rangemark, C. and Hedner, J.A. (1996) Attenuated endothelium-dependent vascular relaxation in patients with sleep apnoea. *Journal of Hypertension* **14**, 577–584.

Cartwright, R.D. (1984) Effect of sleep position on sleep apnea severity. *Sleep* **7**, 110–114.

Charuzi, I., Ovnat, A. and Peiser, J. (1985) The effect of surgical weight reduction on sleep quality in obese-related sleep apnea syndrome. *Surgery* **97**, 535–538.

Chin, K., Shimizu, K., Nakamura, T., Narai, N., Masuzaki, H., Ogawa, Y., Mishima, M., Nakamura, T., Nakao, K. and Ohi, M. (1999) Changes in intra-abdominal visceral fat and serum leptin levels in patients with obstructive sleep apnea syndrome following nasal continuous positive airway pressure therapy. *Circulation* **100**, 706–712.

Ciscar, M.A., Juan, G. and Martinez, V. (2001) Magnetic resonance imaging of the pharynx in OSA patients and healthy subjects. *European Respiratory Journal* **17**, 79–86.

Cistulli, P.A. and Sullivan, C.E. (1995) Sleep apnea in Marfan's syndrome. Increased upper airway collapsibility during sleep. *Chest* **108**, 631–635.

Cistulli, P., Barnes, D.J., Grunstein, R.R. and Sullivan, C.E. (1994) Effect of short-term hormone replacement in the treatment of obstructive sleep apnoea in postmenopausal women. *Thorax* **49**, 699–702.

Clark, G.T., Blumenfeld, I., Yoffe, N., Peled, E. and Lavie, P. (1996) A crossover study comparing the efficacy of continuous positive airway pressure with anterior mandibular positioning devices on patients with obstructive sleep apnea. *Chest* **109**, 1477–1483.

Davies, R.J. and Stradling, J.R. (1990) The relationship between neck circumference, radiographic pharyngeal anatomy, and the obstructive sleep apnoea syndrome. *European Respiratory Journal* **3**, 509–514.

Dixon, J.B., Schachter, L.M. and O'Brien, P.E. (2001) Sleep disturbance and obesity, changes following surgically induced weight loss. *Archives of Internal Medicine* **161**, 102–106.

Do, K.L., Ferreyra, H., Healy, J.F. and Davidson, T.M. (2000) Does tongue size differ between patients with and without sleep-disordered breathing? *Laryngoscope* **110**, 1552–1555.

Dyugovskaya, L., Lavie, P. and Lavie, L. (2002) Increased adhesion molecules expression and production of reactive oxygen species in leukocytes of sleep. *American Journal of Respiratory Care Medicine* **165**, 934–939.

Engleman, H.M., Martin, S.E., Deary, I.J. and Douglas, N.J. (1994) Effect of continuous positive airway pressure treatment on daytime function in sleep apnoea/hypopnoea syndrome. *Lancet* **343**, 572–575.

Engleman, H.M., Martin, S.E., Kingshott, R.N., Mackay, T.W., Deary, I.J. and Douglas, N.J. (1998) Randomised placebo controlled trial of daytime function after continuous positive airway pressure (CPAP) therapy for the sleep apnoea/hypopnoea syndrome. *Thorax* **53**, 341–345.

Engleman, H.M., Kingshott, R.N., Wraith, P.K., Mackay, T.W., Deary, I.J. and Douglas, N.J. (1999) Randomized placebo-controlled crossover trial of continuous positive airway pressure for mild sleep apnea/hypopnea syndrome. *American Journal of Respiratory Care Medicine* **159**, 461–467.

Engleman, H.M., McDonald, J.P., Graham, D., Lello, G.E., Kingshott, R.N. and Coleman, E.L. (2002) Randomised cross-over trial of two treatments for sleep apnea/hypopnea syndrome, continuous positive airway pressure and mandibular repositioning splint. *American Journal of Respiratory Care Medicine* **166**, 855–869.

Farre, R., Montserrat, J.M., Rigau, J. and Trepat, X. (2002) Response of automatic continuous positive airway pressure devices to different sleep breathing patterns, a bench study. *American Journal of Respiratory and Critical Care Medicine* **166**, 469.

Ferguson, K.A., Ono, T., Lowe, A.A., Ryan, C.F. and Fleetham, J.A. (1995) The relationship between obesity and craniofacial structure in obstructive sleep apnea. *Chest* **108**, 375–381.

Ferguson, K.A., Ono, T., Lowe, A.A., Keenan, S.P. and Fleetham, J.A. (1996) A randomized crossover study of an oral appliance vs nasal-continuous positive airway pressure in the treatment of mild-moderate obstructive sleep apnea. *Chest* **109**, 1269–1275.

Findley, L.J., Fabrizio, M.J., Knight, H., Norcross, B.B., LaForte, A.J. and Suratt, P.M. (1989) Driving simulator performance in patients with sleep apnea. *American Review of Respiratory Disease* **140**, 529–530.

Findley, L., Smith, C., Hooper, J., Dineen, M. and Suratt, P.M. (2000) Treatment with nasal CPAP decreases automobile accidents in patients with sleep apnea. *American Journal of Respiratory Care Medicine* **161**, 857–859.

Fleetham, J.A. (1992) Upper airway imaging in relation to obstructive sleep apnea. *Clinical Chest Medicine* **13**, 399–416.

Fleetham, J.A., Arnup, M.E. and Anthonisen, N.R. (1984) Familial aspects of ventilatory control in patients with chronic obstructive pulmonary disease. *American Review of Respiratory Disease* **129**, 3–7.

Fletcher, E.C., Bao, G. and Li, R. (1999) Renin activity and blood pressure in response to chronic episodic hypoxia. *Hypertension* **34**, 309–314.

George, C.F., Boudreau, A.C. and Smiley, A. (1997) Effects of nasal CPAP on simulated driving performance in patients with obstructive sleep apnoea. *Thorax* **52**, 648–653.

Grunstein, R.R. (1995) Sleep-related breathing disorders. 5. Nasal continuous positive airway pressure treatment for obstructive sleep apnoea. *Thorax* **50**, 1106–1113.

Grunstein, R.R. and Sullivan, C.E. (1988) Sleep apnea and hypothyroidism: mechanisms and management. *American Journal of Medicine* **85**, 775–779.

Grunstein, R.R., Handelsman, D.J., Lawrence, S.J., Blackwell, C., Caterson, I.D. and Sullivan, C.E. (1989) Neuroendocrine dysfunction in sleep apnea, reversal by continuous positive airways pressure therapy. *Journal of Clinical Endocrinology and Metabolism* **68**, 352–358.

Grunstein, R.R., Ho, K.Y. and Sullivan, C.E. (1991) Sleep apnea in acromegaly. *Annals of Internal Medicine* **115**, 527–532.

Grunstein, R., Wilcox, I., Yang, T.S., Gould, Y. and Hedner, J. (1993a) Snoring and sleep apnoea in men: association with central obesity and hypertension. *International Journal of Obesity and Related Metabolic Disorders* **17**, 533–540.

Grunstein, R.R., Handelsman, D.J., Stewart, D.A. and Sullivan, C.E. (1993b) Growth hormone secretion is increased by nasal CPAP treatment of sleep apnoea. *American Review of Respiratory Disease* **147**, A686.

Grunstein, R.R., Stenlof, K., Hedner, J. and Sjostrom, L. (1995a) Impact of obstructive sleep apnea and sleepiness on metabolic and cardiovascular risk factors in the Swedish Obese Subjects (SOS) Study. *International Journal of Obesity and Related Metabolic Disorders* **19**, 410–418.

Grunstein, R.R., Stenlof, K., Hedner, J.A. and Sjostrom, L. (1995b) Impact of self-reported sleep-breathing disturbances on psychosocial performance in the Swedish Obese Subjects (SOS) Study. *Sleep* **18**, 635–643.

Guilleminault, C., Stoohs, R., Clerk, A., Simmons, J. and Labanowski, M. (1992) From obstructive sleep apnea syndrome to upper airway resistance syndrome, consistency of daytime sleepiness. *Sleep* **15**, S13–16.

Gyulay, S., Olson, L.G., Hensley, M.J., King, M.T., Allen, K.M. and Saunders, N.A. (1993) A comparison of clinical assessment and home oximetry in the diagnosis of obstructive sleep apnea. *American Review of Respiratory Disease* **147**(1), 50–53.

Harman, E.M., Wynne, J.W. and Block, A.J. (1982) The effect of weight loss on sleep-disordered breathing and oxygen desaturation in morbidly obese men. *Chest* **82**, 291–294.

He, J., Kryger, M.H., Zorick, F.J., Conway, W. and Roth, T. (1988) Mortality and apnea index in obstructive sleep apnea. Experience in 385 male patients. *Chest* **94**, 9–14.

Hedner, J. (2001) Editorial. *American Journal of Respiratory Care Medicine* **163**, 5–6.

Hedner, J. and Grote, L. (2002) Pharmacological therapy in sleep apnea. In: McNicholas, W.T., Phillipson, E.A. eds. *Breathing Disorders in Sleep*. London: WB Saunders, 149–156.

Hedner, J., Ejnell, H. and Caidahl, K. (1990) Left ventricular hypertrophy independent of hypertension in patients with obstructive sleep apnoea. *Journal of Hypertension* **8**, 941–946.

Hedner, J.A., Wilcox, I., Laks, L., Grunstein, R.R. and Sullivan, C.E. (1992) A specific and potent pressor effect of hypoxia in patients with sleep apnea. *American Review of Respiratory Disease* **146**, 1240–1245.

Hoffstein, V. and Szalai, J.P. (1993) Predictive value of clinical features in diagnosing obstructive sleep apnea. *Sleep* **16**, 118–122.

Horner, R.L., Innes, J.A., Murphy, K. and Guz, A. (1991) Evidence for reflex upper airway dilator muscle activation by sudden negative airway pressure in man. *Journal of Physiology* **436**, 15–29.

Hung, J., Whitford, E.G., Parsons, R.W. and Hillman, D.R. (1990) Association of sleep apnoea with myocardial infarction in men. *Lancet* **336**, 261–264.

Ip, M.S., Lam, B., Ng, M.N., Lam, W.K., Tsang, K.W. and Lam, K.S. (2002) Obstructive sleep apnea is independently associated with insulin resistance. *American Journal of Respiratory and Critical Care Medicine* **165**, 670–676.

Jenkinson, C., Stradling, J. and Petersen, S. (1997) Comparison of three measures of quality of life outcome in the evaluation of continuous positive airways pressure therapy for sleep apnoea. *Journal of Sleep Research* **6**, 199–204.

Jenkinson, C., Davies, R.J., Mullins, R. and Stradling, J.R. (1999) Comparison of therapeutic and subtherapeutic nasal continuous positive airway pressure for obstructive sleep apnoea, a randomised prospective parallel trial. *Lancet* **353**, 2100–2105.

Juniper, M., Hack, M.A., George, C.F., Davies, R.J. and Stradling, J.R. (2000) Steering simulation performance in patients with obstructive sleep apnoea and matched control subjects. *European Respiratory Journal* **15**, 590–595.

Kansanen, M., Vanninen, E. and Tuunainen, A. (1998) The effect of very low-calorie diet-induced weight loss on the severity of obstructive sleep apnea and autonomic nervous function in obese patients with obstructive sleep apnea syndrome. *Clinical Physiology* **18**, 377–385.

Kato, M., Roberts-Thompson, P., Philips, B.G. and Haynes, W.G. (2000) Impairment of endothelium-dependent vasodilation of resistance vessels in patients with obstructive sleep apnoea. *Circulation* **102**, 2607–2610.

Katz, I., Stradling, J., Slutsky, A.S., Zamel, N. and Hoffstein, V. (1990) Do patients with obstructive sleep apnea have thick necks? *American Review of Respiratory Disease* **141**, 1228–1231.

Kingshott, R.N., Vennelle, M. and Coleman, E.L. (2001) Randomized, double-blind, placebo-controlled crossover trial of modafinil in the treatment of residual excessive sleepiness in the sleep apnea/hypopnea syndrome. *American Journal of Respiratory Care Medicine* **163**, 918–923.

Koenig, J.S. and Thach, B.T. (1988) Effects of mass loading on the upper airway. *Journal of Applied Physiology* **64**, 2294–2299.

Krieger, J. (1992) Long-term compliance with nasal continuous positive airway pressure (CPAP) in obstructive sleep apnea patients and non-apneic snorers. *Sleep* **15**, S42–46.

Krieger, J., Meslier, N., Lebrun, T., Levy, P., Phillip-Joet, F., Sailly, J.C. and Racineux, J.L. (1997) Accidents in obstructive sleep apnea patients treated with nasal continuous positive airway pressure: a prospective study. The Working Group ANTADIR, Paris and CRESGE, Lille, France. Association Nationale de Traitement a Domicile des Insuffisants Respiratoires. *Chest* **112**, 1561–1566.

Larsson, H., Carlsson-Nordlander, B., Lindblad, L.E., Norbeck, O. and Svanborg, E. (1992) Temperature thresholds in the oropharynx of patients with obstructive sleep apnea syndrome. *American Review of Respiratory Disease* **146**, 1246–1249.

Lavie, P., Herer, P., Peled, R., Berger, I., Yoffe, N., Zomer, J. and Rubin, A.H. (1995) Mortality in sleep apnea patients, a multivariate analysis of risk factors. *Sleep* **18**, 149–157.

Leech, J.A., Onal, E., Baer, P. and Lopata, M. (1987) Determinants of hypercapnia in occlusive sleep apnea syndrome. *Chest* **92**, 807–813.

Littner, M., Hirshkowitz, M., Davila, D., Anderson, W.M. and Kushida, C.A. (2002) Practice parameters for the use of auto-titrating continuous positive airway pressure devices for titrating pressures and treating adult patients with obstructive sleep apnea syndrome: an American Academy of Sleep Medicine report. *Sleep* **25**, 143.

Lofaso, F., Coste, A., d'Ortho, M.P, Zerah-Lancner, F., Delclaux, C., Goldenberg, F. and Harf, A. (2000) Nasal obstruction as a risk factor or sleep apnoea syndrome. *European Respiratory Journal* **16**, 639–643.

Lopata, M. and Onal, E. (1982) Mass loading, sleep apnea, and the pathogenesis of obesity hypoventilation. *American Review of Respiratory Disease* **126**, 640–645.

McEvoy, R.D., Sharp, D.J. and Thornton, A.T. (1986) The effects of posture on obstructive sleep apnea. *American Review of Respiratory Disease* **133**, 662–666.

McNamara, S.G., Grunstein, R.R. and Sullivan, C.E. (1993) Obstructive sleep apnoea. *Thorax* **48**, 754–764.

Mezzanotte, W.S., Tangel, D.J. and White, D.P. (1992) Waking genioglossal electromyogram in sleep apnea patients versus normal controls (a neuromuscular compensatory mechanism). *Journal of Clinical Investigation* **89**, 1571–1579.

Montplaisir, J., Bedard, M.A., Richer, F. and Rouleau, I. (1992) Neurobehavioral manifestations in obstructive sleep apnea syndrome before and after treatment with continuous positive airway pressure. *Sleep* **15**, S17–19.

Nelson, S. and Hans, M. (1997) Contribution of craniofacial risk factors in increasing apneic activity among obese and non-obese habitual snorers. *Chest* **111**, 154–162.

Nieto, F.J., Young, T.B., Lind, B.K., Shahar, E., Samet, J.M., Redline, S., D'Agostino, R.B., Newman, A.B., Lebowitz, M.D. and Pickering, T.G. (2000) Association of sleep-disordered breathing, sleep apnea, and hypertension in a large community-based study. Sleep Heart Health Study. *Journal of the American Medical Association* **283**, 1829–1836.

Nowbar, S., Burkart, K.M. and Zwillich, C.W. (2000) Hypoventilation

among obese patients, a common and under-diagnosed problem. *American Journal of Respiratory Care Medicine* **161**, A890.

O'Donnell, C.P., Schaub, C.D., Haines, A.S., Berkowitz, D.E., Tankersley, C.G., Schwartz, A.R. and Smith, P.L. (1999) Leptin prevents respiratory depression in obesity. *American Journal of Respiratory Care Medicine* **159**, 1477–1484.

O'Sullivan, R.A., Hillman, D.R., Mateljan, R., Pantin, C. and Finucane, K.E. (1995) Mandibular advancement splint, an appliance to treat snoring and obstructive sleep apnea. *American Journal of Respiratory Care Medicine* **151**, 194–198.

Pack, A.I., Black, J.E. and Schwartz, J.R. (2001) Modafinil as adjunct therapy for daytime sleepiness in obstructive sleep apnea. *American Journal of Respiratory Care Medicine* **164**, 1675–1681.

Palomaki, H., Partinen, M., Erkinjuntti, T. and Kaste, M. (1992) Snoring, sleep apnea syndrome, and stroke. *Neurology* **42**, 75–81, discussion 82.

Parra, O., Arboix, A., Bechich, S., Garcia-Eroles, L., Montserrat, J.M., Lopez, J.A., Ballester, E., Guerra, J.M. and Sopena, J.J. (2000) Time course of sleep-related breathing disorders in first-ever stroke or transient ischemic attack. *American Journal of Respiratory and Critical Care Medicine* **161**, 375–380.

Pasquali, R., Colella, P. and Cirignotta, F. (1990) Treatment of obese patients with obstructive sleep apnea syndrome: effect of weight loss and interference otorhinolaryngoiatric pathology. *International Journal of Obesity* **14**, 207–217.

Peker, Y., Hedner, J., Norum, J., Kraiczi, H. and Carlson, J. (2002) Increased incidence of cardiovascular disease in middle-aged men with obstructive sleep apnoea: a 7-year follow up. *American Journal of Respiratory Care Medicine* **165**, 1395–1399.

Peppard, P.E., Young, T., Palta, M., Dempsey, J. and Skatrud, J. (2000a) Longitudinal study of moderate weight change and sleep-disordered breathing. *Journal of the American Medical Association* **284**, 3015–3021.

Peppard, P.E., Young, T., Palta, M. and Skatrud, J. (2000b) Prospective study of the association between sleep-disordered breathing and hypertension. *New England Journal of Medicine* **342**, 1378–1384.

Pepperell, J.C., Ramdassingh-Dow, S., Crosthwaite, N. and Mullins, R. (2002) Ambulatory blood pressure after therapeutic and subtherapeutic nasal continuous positive airway pressure for obstructive sleep apnoea, a randomised parallel trial. *Lancet* **359**, 204–210.

Pevernagie, D., Hamans, E., Van Cauwenberge, P. and Pauwels, R. (2000) External nasal dilation reduces snoring in chronic rhinitis patients: a randomized controlled trial. *European Respiratory Journal* **15**, 996–1000.

Phillips, B.G., Kato, M., Narkiewicz, K., Choe, I. and Somers, V.K. (2000) Increases in leptin levels, sympathetic drive, and weight gain in obstructive sleep apnea. *American Journal of Physiology and Heart Circulation Physiology* **279**, H234–237.

Phipps, P.R., Starritt, E., Caterson, I. and Grunstein, R.R. (2002) Association of serum leptin with hypoventilation in human obesity. *Thorax* **57**, 75–76.

Pillar, G., Peled, R. and Lavie, P. (1994) Recurrence of sleep apnea without concomitant weight increase 7.5 years after weight reduction surgery. *Chest* **106**, 1702–1704.

Piper, A.J. and Sullivan, C.E. (1994) Effects of short-term NIPPV in the treatment of patients with severe obstructive sleep apnea and hypercapnia. *Chest* **105**, 434–440.

Piper, A.J. and Sullivan, C.E. (1996) Effects of long-term nocturnal nasal ventilation on spontaneous breathing during sleep in neuromuscular and chest wall disorders. *European Respiratory Journal* **9**, 1515–1522.

Piper, A.J., Laks, L. and Sullivan, C.E. (1993) Effectiveness of short-term NIPPV in the management of patients with severe OSA and REM hypoventilation. *Sleep* **16**, S115–116, discussion S116–117.

Powell, N.B., Riley, R.W. and Robinson, A. (1998) Surgical management of obstructive sleep apnea syndrome. *Clinical Chest Medicine* **19**, 77–86.

Punjabi, N.M., Sorkin, J.D., Katzel, L.I., Goldberg, A.P., Schwartz, A.R. and Smith, P.L. (2002) Sleep-disordered breathing and insulin resistance in middle-aged and overweight men. *American Journal of Respiratory and Critical Care Medicine* **165**, 677–682.

Redline, S. and Strohl, K.P. (1998) Recognition and consequences of obstructive sleep apnea hypopnea syndrome. *Clinical Chest Medicine* **19**, 1–19.

Redline, S., Kump, K., Tishler, P.V., Browner, I. and Ferrette, V. (1994) Gender differences in sleep disordered breathing in a community-based sample. *American Journal of Respiratory Care Medicine* **149**, 722–726.

Remmers, J.E., deGroot, W.J., Sauerland, E.K. and Anch, A.M. (1978) Pathogenesis of upper airway occlusion during sleep. *Journal of Applied Physiology* **44**, 931–938.

Riley, R.W., Powell, N.B. and Guilleminault, C. (1993) Obstructive sleep apnea syndrome: a review of 306 consecutively treated surgical patients. *Otolaryngology Head and Neck Surgery* **108**, 117–125.

Rodenstein, D.O. (1992) Assessment of uvulopalatopharyngoplasty for the treatment of sleep apnea syndrome. *Sleep* **15**, S56–62.

Rosenow, F., McCarthey, V. and Caruso, A.C. (1998) Sleep apnoea in endocrine diseases. *Journal of Sleep Research* **7**(1), 3–11.

Rubinstein, I., Colapinto, N., Rotstein, L.E., Brown, I.G. and Hoffstein, V. (1988) Improvement in upper airway function after weight loss in patients with obstructive sleep apnea. *American Review of Respiratory Disease* **138**, 1192–1195.

Rubinstein, I., Bradley, T.D., Zamel, N. and Hoffstein, V. (1989) Glottic and cervical tracheal narrowing in patients with obstructive sleep apnea. *Journal of Applied Physiology* **67**, 2427–2431.

Ryan, C.F. and Love, L.L. (2000) Unpredictable results of laser assisted uvulopalatoplasty in the treatment of obstructive sleep apnoea. *Thorax* **55**, 399–404.

Sajkov, D., Cowie, R.J., Thornton, A.T., Espinoza, H.A. and McEvoy, R.D. (1994) Pulmonary hypertension and hypoxemia in obstructive sleep apnea syndrome. *American Journal of Respiratory Care Medicine* **149**(1), 416–422.

Sajkov, D., Wang, T., Saunders, N.A., Bune, A.J., Neill, A.M. and McEvoy, R.D. (1999) Daytime pulmonary hemodynamics in patients with obstructive sleep apnea without lung disease. *American Journal of Respiratory Care Medicine* **159**, 1518–1526.

Sampol, G., Munoz, X. and Sagales, M.T. (1998) Long term efficacy of dietary weight loss in sleep apnoea/hypopnoea syndrome. *European Respiratory Journal* **12**, 1156–1159.

Sanner, B.M., Konermann, M., Tepel, M., Groetz, J., Mummenhoff, C. and Zidek, W. (2000) Platelet function in patients with obstructive sleep apnoea syndrome. *European Respiratory Journal* **16**, 648–652.

Schmidt-Nowara, W., Lowe, A., Wiegand, L., Cartwright, R., Perez-Guerra, F. and Menn, S. (1995) Oral appliances for the treatment of snoring and obstructive sleep apnea: a review. *Sleep* **18**, 501–510.

Schwab, R.J., Gefter, W.B., Hoffman, E.A., Gupta, K.B. and Pack, A.I. (1993) Dynamic upper airway imaging during awake respiration in normal subjects and patients with sleep disordered breathing. *American Review of Respiratory Disease* **148**, 1385–1400.

Schwab, R.J., Gupta, K.B., Gefter, W.B., Metzger, L.J., Hoffman, E.A. and Pack, A.I. (1995) Upper airway and soft tissue anatomy in normal subjects and patients with sleep-disordered breathing. Significance of the lateral pharyngeal walls. *American Journal of Respiratory Care Medicine* **152**, 1673–1689.

Schwab, R.J., Pasirstein, M., Pierson, R. and Mackley, A. (2003) Identification of upper airway anatomic risk factors for obstructive sleep apnoea with volumetric magnetic resonance imaging. *American Journal of Respiratory Care Medicine* **168**, 522–530.

Schwartz, A.R., Gold, A.R. and Schubert, N. (1991) Effects of weight loss on upper airway collapsibility in obstructive sleep apnea. *American Review of Respiratory Disease* **144**, 494–498.

Series, F., Cormier, Y. and Desmeules, M. (1990) Influence of passive changes of lung volume on upper airways. *Journal of Applied Physiology* **68**, 2159–2164.

Shahar, E., Whitney, C.W., Redline, S., Young, T., Boland, L.L., Baldwin, C.M., Nieto, F.J., O'Connor, G.T., Rapoport, D.M. and Robbins, J.A. (2001) Sleep-disordered breathing and cardiovascular disease cross sectional results of the Sleep Heart Health Study. *American Journal of Respiratory Care Medicine* **163**, 19–25.

Shahar, E., Redline, S., Young, T., Boland, L. and Baldwin, C. (2003) Hormone replacement therapy and sleep-disordered breathing. *American Journal of Respiratory Care Medicine* **167**, 1186–1192.

Shamsuzzamam, A.S., Winnicki, M., Lanfranchi, P., Wolk, R. and Kara, T. (2002) Elevated C-reactive protein in patients with obstructive sleep apnoea. *Circulation* **105**, 2462–2464.

Sin, D.D., Fitzgerald, F., Parker, J.D., Newton, G., Floras, J.S. and Bradley, T.D. (1999) Risk actors for central and obstructive sleep apnea in 450 men and women with congestive heart failure. *American Journal of Respiratory Care Medicine* **160**, 1101–1106.

Smith, P.L., Gold, A.R., Meyers, D.A., Haponik, E.F. and Bleecker, E.R. (1985) Weight loss in mildly to moderately obese patients with obstructive sleep apnea. *Annals of Internal Medicine* **103**, 850–855.

Smith, I., Lasserson, T. and Wright, J. (2002) Drug treatments for obstructive sleep apnea. Cochrane Database of Systematic Reviews 2002.

Somers, V.K., Mark, A.L., Zavala, D.C. and Abbound, F.M. (1989) Contrasting effects of hypoxia and hypercapnia on ventilation and sympathetic activity in humans. *Journal of Applied Physiology* **67**, 2095–2100.

Standards of Practice Committee for the American Sleep Disorders Association. (1996) Practice parameters for the treatment of obstructive sleep apnea in adults: the efficacy of surgical modifications of the upper airway. Report of the American Sleep Disorders Association. *Sleep* **19**, 152–155.

Stradling, J.R. and Crosby, J.H. (1991) Predictors and prevalence of obstructive sleep apnoea and snoring in 1001 middle aged men. *Thorax* **46**, 85–90.

Sugerman, H.J., Fairman, R.P. and Sood, R.K. (1992) Long-term effects of gastric surgery for treating respiratory insufficiency of obesity. *American Journal of Clinical Nutrition* **55**, 597S–601S.

Sullivan, C.E. and Grunstein, R.R. (1994) Continuous positive airway pressure. In: Kryger, M.H., Dement, W.C., Roth, T.P. eds. *Sleep*

Disordered Breathing: Principles and Practice of Sleep Medicine. Philadelphia: WB Saunders, 559–570.

Sullivan, C.E., Issa, F.G., Berthon-Jones, M. and Eves, L. (1981) Reversal of obstructive sleep apnoea by continuous positive airway pressure applied through the nares. *Lancet* **1**, 862–865.

Sullivan, C.E., Berthon-Jones, M. and Issa, F.G. (1983) Remission of severe obesity-hypoventilation syndrome after short-term treatment during sleep with nasal continuous positive airway pressure. *American Review of Respiratory Disease* **128**(1), 177–181.

Sullivan, C.E., Marrone, O. and Berthon-Jones, M. (1990) Sleep apnea—pathophysiology, upper airway and control of breathing. In: Guilleminault, C.P.M. ed. *Obstructive Sleep Apnea Syndrome: Clinical Research and Treatment*. New York: Raven Press.

Suratt, P.M., McTier, R.F., Findley, L.J., Pohl, S.L. and Wilhoit, S.C. (1992) Effect of very-low-calorie diets with weight loss on obstructive sleep apnea. *American Journal of Clinical Nutrition* **56**, 182S–184S.

Van de Graaff, W.B. (1988) Thoracic influence on upper airway patency. *Journal of Applied Physiology* **65**, 2124–2131.

Wade, A.J., Marbut, M.M. and Round, J.M. (1990) Muscle fibre type and aetiology of obesity. *Lancet* **335**, 805–808.

Weitzenblum, E., Krieger, J., Apprill, M., Vallee, E., Ehrhart, M., Ratomaharo, J., Oswald, M. and Kurtz, D. (1988) Daytime pulmonary hypertension in patients with obstructive sleep apnea syndrome. *American Review of Respiratory Disease* **138**, 345–349.

Wolk, R., Kara, T. and Somers, V.K. (2003) Sleep-disordered breathing and cardiovascualr disease. *Circulation* **108**, 9–12.

Woodson, T., Stewart, D., Wraver, E. and Javaheri, S. (2002) A randomised trial of temperature-controlled radiofrequency ablation, continuous positive airway pressure and placebo for obstructive sleep apnea. *Ototolaryngology* **128**, 848–861.

Working Group on OSA and Hypertension (1993) Obstructive sleep apnea and blood pressure elevation: what is the relationship? *Blood Press* **2**, 166–182.

Worsnop, C.J., Naughton, M.T., Barter, C.E., Morgan, T.O., Anderson, A.I. and Pierce, R.J. (1998) The prevalence of obstructive sleep apnea in hypertensives. *American Journal of Respiratory and Critical Care Medicine* **157**, 111–115.

Yokoe, T., Minoguchi, K., Matsuo, H., Oda, N., Minoguchi, H., Yoshino, G., Hirano, T. and Adachi, M. (2003) Elevated levels of C-reactive protein and interleukin-6 in patients with obstructive sleep apnea syndrome are decreased by nasal continuous positive airway pressure. *Circulation* **107**, 1129–1134.

Young, T., Palta, M., Dempsey, J., Skatrud, J., Weber, S. and Badr, S. (1993) The occurrence of sleep-disordered breathing among middle-aged adults. *New England Journal of Medicine* **328**, 1230–1235.

Management

21 An overview of obesity management

Peter G. Kopelman and Ian D. Caterson

Introduction, 319

How much weight loss?, 319

Aims of obesity treatment, 320

Assessment of the overweight and
obese patient, 321
  General, 321
  Specific weight history, 321
  Physical examination and
  investigations, 321
  Assessment of risk, 323

Assessment of motivation to lose
weight, 323

Obesity management
programmes, 323
  Eating (diet intervention), 324
  Physical activity (exercise
  programme), 324
  Behaviour modification, 324
  Lifestyle programme, 324
  Maintenance programme, 324

Monitoring and longer term
follow-up, 324

Audit and outcome measures, 325
  Adjunctive therapies, 325
  Low-calorie/energy diets, 325
  Pharmacotherapy, 325
  Selection of patients for
  pharmacotherapy, 325
  Obesity surgery, 326

Summary, 326

References, 326

Introduction

Obesity management is perceived as a challenge: it requires considerable time usually in a busy practice, skills in which a therapist may not have been trained and a feeling that successful outcome is unlikely. Such a situation tends to make many health professionals unprepared to become involved in obesity management.

There are reasons for the perceived lack of success, which include lack of training, few long-term maintenance programmes, little understanding of the pathophysiology of weight control and often a prejudice about obesity ('all it takes is self-control and will power'). In addition, few health professionals have been taught about nutrition and physical activity, or realistic weight loss goals. Obesity treatment is frequently instituted without the benefit of an integrated lifestyle management programme.

Modern obesity treatment programmes aim to improve health and well-being and this needs to be emphasized. Obesity treatment by health professionals should be seen to be for health benefit and not as a response to the dictates of modern-day fashion. Not all of those who seek weight loss treatment require it. It is important for the therapist to recognize this and to let such individuals know when they do *not* need to lose weight. Although most will accept such advice, in some cases it may be necessary to refer for specific counselling or therapy for an eating disorder.

Obesity therapy today is based on clinical assessment and the assessment of associated medical risks (such as metabolic and locomotor disease). For some patients, general advice on eating and activity may be all that is required. For others, in need of therapy for health reasons, it is advisable to include a lifestyle programme and, when necessary, to consider adjunctive therapy. Treatment requires sufficient consultation time and, once adequate weight loss (or other goal) has been achieved, an ongoing weight maintenance programme to be provided. The need for long-term follow-up cannot be stressed too firmly: successful long-term weight maintenance depends on continuing follow-up. This chapter summarizes such an approach to weight management.

How much weight loss?

There are few long-term studies of intentional weight loss and its effect on mortality. Some studies are under way at present and other larger studies are planned. It appears that intentional weight loss in women results in a reduction of mortality in the first 2 years, and that this reduction is particularly explained by cancer deaths. There are additionally improvements in medical risk factors and complications from other diseases.

Many individuals have unrealistic expectations about weight loss and set themselves, or their patients, unachievable weight loss goals. It is not necessary to reach the *ideal* or *healthy* weight because health benefits can be obtained first from maintaining weight (not gaining more) and second from los-

Table 21.1 Health benefits of moderate weight loss (5–10% of presenting body weight).

Mortality
20% decrease in overall
30% decrease in diabetes-related deaths
40% decrease in cancer-related deaths
Blood pressure
10 mmHg decrease
Lipids
15% decrease in cholesterol
Reductions in other lipids
Diabetes
Better blood glucose control

Table 21.2 Possible goals of obesity management.

These will be individual and need to be negotiated with each patient.
Body weight
Loss (5–10% of body weight)
Possible maintenance of present weight (especially in the older patient)
Waist reduction
(? Change in body composition)
Metabolic disease – better control and/or less medication
Diabetes
Dyslipidaemia
Hypertension
Mechanical disease – better control, less intensive therapy
OSA
Arthritis
Activity
Control of mechanical disease
More able, less short of breath
Less restriction
Feeling of well-being
Fewer medications overall
Quality of life, well-being and psychosocial functioning
Fertility (important for IVF programmes)
Individual goal
'The special dress'
Occupational reasons, etc.

ing a moderate amount of weight, between 5% and 10% of presenting weight. This amount of weight loss produces reduction of risk and health benefit. A list of potential benefits is given in Table 21.1.

Recent studies confirm that mild to moderate weight loss can be achieved by lifestyle intervention and be maintained for up to 4 years. There have been several major trials on diabetes prevention in Scandinavia, China and the USA. The Diabetes Prevention Programme study from the USA studied the effects of placebo, metformin and a reasonably intensive lifestyle intervention in diabetes prevention. At the end of 4 years there was a 58% reduction in the incidence of diabetes. This was produced by a maintained mean weight loss of 4.6 kg. The other studies, which had, in general, less intensive lifestyle interventions, produced similar results. A seemingly small weight loss of a few kilograms may have major benefits. Initial patient management should be a moderate weight loss of 5–10%. If successful then later treatment can set a new target or goal for further weight loss.

Because of the difficulties in understanding appropriate and necessary weight loss, and in the absence of training and experience of weight management, many organizations and health departments have produced (and occasionally update) best-practice guidelines. Examples of such guidelines are those of the Scottish Intercollegiate Guidelines Network (1996), the NIH (1998), the Royal College of Physicians of London (2003) and the National Health and Medical Research Council of Australia (2003).

Such guidelines, with their evidence-based approach, highlight areas of difficulty. For example, the body mass index (BMI) cut-off points for obesity, which were derived from largely Caucasian (indeed US) data, are probably inappropriate for other ethnic groups. Some organizations (including the World Health Organization, WHO) and countries have suggested lower BMI cut-off points for individuals from Asia and possibly higher values for those of Pacific Islands descent. A further problem with such guidelines is their potential rigidity. It is essential to realize that with increasing risk factors or disease, or possibly with those of Asian origin, treatment needs to be instituted or intensified at the earliest stage and/or lower BMI level.

Aims of obesity treatment

With this in mind, what are the aims of obesity treatment? A 5–10% weight loss is one. However, weight loss should not be the sole objective for obesity treatment. Additional aims are to reduce risk to health and complications from associated disease that may be present. Furthermore, treatment is not just for the short term, but rather for a lifetime. A list of possible aims are given in Table 21.2. If weight loss cannot be achieved, an aim of no additional weight gain may be practical, achievable and of benefit. In some patients who find weight loss difficult due to mechanical complications (such as osteoarthritis), or emotional or psychological factors, prevention of further weight gain may be more appropriate than actual weight loss.

All such goals should be negotiated with the patient and documented. When the goals are achieved the patient must be congratulated and given credit for their success. New goals

Table 21.3 Essential elements for an appropriate setting for the management of overweight and obesity.

Trained staff directly involved in the running of the weight loss programme. These staff (medical, nursing and other health-care professionals) should have attended courses on the management of obesity and must be provided with opportunities to continue their education.

A printed programme for weight management, which includes clearly outlined dietary advice, behavioural modification techniques, physical exercise and strategies for long-term lifestyle change. Such a programme may include a family and/or group approach.

Suitable equipment, in particular accurate and regularly calibrated weighing scales take measure and stadiometer.

Specified weight loss goals, with energy deficits being achieved through moderating food intake and increasing physical expenditure.

Documentation of individual patients' health risks. This will include BMI, waist circumference, blood pressure, blood lipids, cigarette smoking and other comorbid conditions.

A clearly defined follow-up procedure, which involves collaboration between the different settings of care, provides regular monitoring and documentation of progress and includes details of criteria for judging the success of weight loss. This will allow a weight loss programme to be properly supported, medical conditions to be monitored, and problems or issues to be addressed at the earliest opportunity.

(which may include further loss or weight maintenance) should then be negotiated.

Overall, weight loss should be approached incrementally with new weight loss goals being set when the original target has been reached. It is likely that goals for older patients (> 65 years) will be different from those who are young. There is a suggestion that although a population becomes heavier with age, the risk from obesity does not increase proportionately.

Assessment of the overweight and obese patient

General

For most health professionals, patients will be seen in a consulting room/area. Necessary equipment should include weighing scales that measure up to 200 kg or more, large blood pressure cuffs, a long tape measure for waist circumference and larger width chairs. A list of the requirements that are appropriate for a clinic treating obese individuals is given in Table 21.3.

Specific weight history

There are a number of specific factors that should be sought and a brief list is given in Table 21.4. The history of weight gain should be obtained to elucidate possible causative factors and to determine the patient's insight and understanding of the factors underlying their weight gain. Such questions might include: 'At what stage did you gain weight?', 'Do you know of specific reasons for your weight gain?' and 'Can you describe your eating patterns and what activity you do?'. It is helpful to decide whether childhood-onset obesity is due to a particular life event or a specific syndrome. The latter is rare and may be identified by the length of history and specific associated clinical features. Specific single gene disorders are associated with

the early onset of massive obesity, usually a strong family history and often characteristic clinical features such as hypogonadism.

A number of diseases may be associated with weight gain, although uncommonly with massive obesity, and clinical features of these should be sought. The diseases include endocrine diseases (hypothyroidism, acromegaly, Cushing's syndrome and diabetes), various types of arthritis or injury that may be associated with immobility, and cardiac disease, which may also reduce activity. There are particular drugs that are associated with weight gain and a history of the use of such drugs should be obtained. Examples of such drugs are given in Table 21.5.

Physical examination and investigations

A detailed physical examination should always be performed. Weight and height should be measured, and BMI calculated. (BMI cut-off points are shown in Table 21.6.) It is worth recording the distribution of fat tissue by measuring the waist circumference. (The waist measurement is taken as the narrowest circumference midway between the lower border of the ribs and the upper border of the iliac crest.) Examination of the skin is important. Thin, atrophic skin (together with abdominal adiposity and relatively thinner extremities) is a feature of excess use or secretion of glucocorticoids; acanthosis nigricans (pigmented, 'velvety' skin creases especially in the axillae or around the neck) is associated with insulin resistance; hirsutism in women may indicate polycystic ovary syndrome or simply obesity per se. A neck circumference of greater than 43 cm indicates the likelihood of obstructive sleep apnoea (OSA) and the pharynx should be examined to exclude evidence of obstruction from tonsils or other cause of narrowing. Blood pressure and cardiovascular function should be noted.

Some investigations are useful but care should be taken to choose those appropriate for the individual. In addition to as-

Table 21.4 Points that should be elucidated in any clinical history taken from a patient prior to obesity management.

Medical history
Risk factors
Presence of established complications of obesity (remember to ask about snoring, sleep and daytime somnolence)

Body weight history
When was weight gained (e.g. puberty, stopping sport, employment, marriage, pregnancies, etc.)?
Previous treatment(s) for obesity (including successes and failures)

Family history of obesity, and related diseases and risk factors
Type 2 diabetes, hypertension, premature coronary heart disease

Diet history
Eating pattern and amount (compared with friends)
Hunger
Stress or emotional eating, binges
Alcohol intake

Regular physical activity pattern

Relevant social history
Cigarette smoking and cessation (did the patient gain weight then?)

Drug history
Anti-psychotics
Anti-depressants
Steroids
Anti-convulsants
Lithium
Beta-blockers

Reproductive history
Irregular periods
Polycystic ovary syndrome

Table 21.5 Drug treatment (class of drug and examples) that may be associated with weight gain.

Anti-psychotic (olanapine, clozapine, risperidone)

Anti-depressants (tricyclic antidepressants)

Lithium

Anti-epileptic drugs (valproate, carbamazepine, gabapentin)

Diabetic medications (insulin, sulphonylureas, thiazolidinediones)

Steroid hormones (glucocorticoids, possibly oral contraceptives)

Beta-blockers

Antihistamines

Table 21.6 WHO classification of overweight and obesity in adults according to BMI.

Classification	BMI (kg/m^2)	Risk of co-morbidities
Underweight	<18.5	Low (but risk of other clinical problems increased)
Normal range	18.5–24.9	Average
Pre-obese	25.0–29.9	Mildly increased
Obese	≥30.0	
Class I	30.0–34.9	Moderate
Class II	35.0–39.9	Severe
Class III	≥40.0	Very severe

sessing for risk factors (see below), it may be useful to measure plasma thyroid stimulating hormone (TSH) and testosterone; the latter is often low, particularly in those men with OSA, whereas it may be elevated in obese women. Liver transaminases (alanine and aspartate) may be elevated, particularly in those with abdominal adiposity and/or the metabolic syndrome. This may reflect associated non-alcoholic steatohep- atitis (NASH). Often in the early stages of weight loss, these liver enzymes rise but they usually settle as weight stabilizes. The measurement of serum leptin is not recommended as a routine but it may be required in patients with extreme early-onset obesity. Although the rare leptin-deficient syndrome can be treated, the serial measurement of leptin in simple or spontaneous obesity may prove to be a useful marker of fat loss.

Assessment of risk

An initial risk measure is the presence of abdominal adiposity. The WHO has suggested the measures shown in Table 21.7, but for those of Asian origin, these measures may be 90 cm or greater in males and 80 cm or greater in females.

As well as the presence of hypertension, assessment must be made of the presence of cardiac disease and of diabetes. OSA (as determined by sleep history, examination of the pharynx and neck circumference) is an added risk. Dyslipidaemia [(classically hypertriglyceridaemia, with low HDL-cholesterol (< 1 mmol/L) and elevated LDL-cholesterol (> 3.5 mmol/L)] confers additional risk. Cigarette smoking is a major risk factor.

These risks may need to be quantified by specific investigations such as an exercise electrocardiograph (ECG) or sleep studies.

Table 21.7 Abdominal circumference (waist) at which risk increases.

Risk	Increased	Substantial increase
Men	94 cm (OR 2.2)	102 cm (OR 4.6)
Women	80 cm (OR 1.6)	88 cm (OR 2.6)
Asian men		90 cm
Asian women		80 cm

OR, odds ratio, which is the increase in risk associated with this situation, compared with a lower waist circumference.
The values are those suggested by the World Health Organization in its technical report.

Assessment of motivation to lose weight

Not all patients are prepared or are ready to lose weight despite a medical requirement. Sometimes it may be advisable to assess the patient's readiness and motivation by direct questioning or using the *stages of change* model. It may be necessary to suggest that rather than embarking on an intensive programme at the present time, the patient should return at a later stage for reassessment and review, when they are prepared and motivated to lose weight.

Obesity management programmes

The therapies and degree of intensity of any weight loss programme should be based on an assessment of the degree of adiposity (anthropometry) and the presence or absence of medical risk factors. A suggested approach is outlined in Table 21.8. Mild to moderate *uncomplicated* overweight and obesity may require advice with a specific eating and physical activity programme. Greater degrees of obesity and risk, or the presence of disease, require more intensive lifestyle interventions, the use of pharmacotherapy, possibly very low-calorie/ energy diets (meal replacements) or surgery. Although all of these aspects of obesity treatment will be considered in detail in other chapters, it is worthwhile briefly reviewing each modality.

It also needs be underlined that any weight programme must provide a weight maintenance component. This is the most time-consuming component, but regular and long-term follow-up visits and intervention are part of the management of any chronic disorder.

The components of a weight management programme are:

Table 21.8 Practical approach to obesity treatment – clinical assessment and rational management outline.

BMI	Risk rating	Interventions						
		General advice	Eating	Activity	Lifestyle programme	Anti-obesity drugs	VLCDs	Surgery
18.5–24.9	Low	Use						
	High		Use	Use				
25–29.9	Low				Use			
	High				Use	Consider*		
30–34.9	Low				Use	Consider/use		
	High				Use	Use		
35–39.9	Low				Use	Use		
	High				Use	Use	Consider	Consider
40+	High				Use	Use	Use	Consider

Risk rating: low, waist <102 cm in men and <88 cm in women and no risk factors present; high, waist greater than the above measures *or* the presence of risk factors.
Risk factors: type 2 diabetes/impaired glucose tolerance, hypertension, coronary heart disease, dyslipidaemia, obstructive sleep apnoea.
*Pharmacotherapy should be considered at a BMI >27 with the presence of disease when there has been no weight loss in 12 weeks of a lifestyle programme.
Pharmacotherapy might be considered earlier in those with greater BMI or with more risk factors and diseases.

- general advice;
- eating (diet intervention);
- physical activity;
- behaviour modification;
- lifestyle programme; and
- maintenance programme—monitoring and longer term follow-up.

In addition, it may be necessary to consider adjunctive therapies for some patients.

General advice should be given in all circumstances and will include aspects of eating, physical activity and behaviour modification. However, for most individuals with increased adiposity and/or medical risk an additional planned programme of intervention is necessary. Such a programme usually involves a number of visits (10–12 over a period of 3–6 months) with specific tasks for each one. If weight loss is insufficient during this time then consideration should be given to drug treatment or other therapies.

Eating (diet intervention)

Although energy (calorie) restriction produces good weight loss, some individuals may find this irksome and impossible to maintain. For such patients, a low-fat eating plan may prove effective: such plans may be maintained for several years. Fat intake can be reduced to less than 40 g/day (or lower for women) with the remainder of the diet being *ad libitum*. Greater losses may be obtained by additionally reducing energy intake. Men may also need to reduce energy intake by limiting their alcohol intake.

The major discussion of diet and obesity is in Chapter 22.

Physical activity (exercise programme)

Emphasis should be placed on increasing total daily activity to between 60 and 90 min each day (Saris *et al.*, 2003). Although exercise and fitness are important, the initial emphasis should be on increasing the activities of daily living, in particular more walking. A formal written exercise prescription has been shown to increase effectiveness in general practice. Giving patients the opportunity to use or purchase a pedometer and then setting the number of steps they need do in a day may prove an effective method of increasing activity. For patients with arthritis or other disabilities, hydrotherapy (exercising in water) may be a way of initiating movement and this type of activity can assist weight loss. A more detailed discussion is provided in Chapter 24.

Behaviour modification

This therapy is important and central to any weight loss programme and it is discussed in Chapter 23. There are many components to behaviour modification, but one simple one is the use of a food and exercise diary. This allows habit recognition and change. All subjects, but most particularly those who are overweight or obese, under-report food intake and over-report the activity they undertake. A diary provides an important starting point for discussion and suggests possible interventions. Additional behavioural therapies include discussion about habits, change and alternative ways of approaching situations. Other techniques involve stress management, improving self-esteem and, occasionally, more specific counselling or psychiatric intervention.

Lifestyle programme

Programmes for lifestyle change usually have a number of initial intensive visits (e.g. 10 or 12) and then, depending on the patient's response, further visits may be scheduled or, in addition, drugs or other treatment initiated (see Chapters 22, 25 and 26). When goals are reached then the visits are extended. Such a lifestyle programme should involve a range of health professionals (dietitians, physiotherapists, nurses, psychologists). Good results (and satisfaction for the treatment group) are usually obtained by the involvement of multidisciplinary teams.

Because of this partial abrogation of obesity treatment by health professionals and because of community perceptions, many organizations and groups have been established to *fill the gap*. Some commercial groups use conventional therapy (e.g. Weight Watchers or programmes used in some gyms), whereas others rely on alternative or natural therapies and still others use *magic* treatments that sound plausible but which really have neither scientific basis nor effectiveness. Examples of the *magic* type of therapy would be total-body wrapping, some herbal concoctions and bulking agents. Few have been tested rigorously and many are costly, but the very existence of such programmes and therapies shows that many individuals desire to lose weight but need to be guided into the correct approach and provided with effective therapy.

Maintenance programme

This is an essential part of any weight loss programme and the most neglected. Follow-up programmes are essential and effective (Chapter 27).

Monitoring and longer term follow-up

Patients involved in an obesity treatment programme require the following:
- monitoring of weight (ideally monthly, no greater than 2-monthly);
- monitoring of pulse rate and blood pressure;
- monitoring of obesity-related risks and diseases (e.g. dyslipidaemia, type 2 diabetes).

Table 21.9 Process measures to judge the success of anti-obesity treatment.

Measures	Immediate benefits	Longer term benefits
Physical	Weight loss Reduction in waist circumference Improvement in comorbidities	Reduced breathlessness, decreased sleep apnoea, reduced angina, reduced blood pressure
Metabolic	Decreased fasting blood glucose and plasma insulin Improvement in fasting lipid profile Decreased HbA1c (if diabetic)	Reduction in doses of concomitant medications
Functional	Increased mobility Decreased symptoms Increased well-being and mood Increased health-related quality of life	Reduced time away from work, improved involvement in social activities, decreased number of consultations with health professionals

The treatment plan should be recorded for each patient and incorporated into local audit data-recording systems. As weight loss progresses, adjustments may be necessary of medications taken by the patient for obesity-related or obesity-responsive diseases and risks. For example, the dose of an oral hypoglycaemic agent may need to be reduced as insulin sensitivity increases with weight loss.

Audit and outcome measures

Table 21.9 lists the process measures that may be used to judge the success or otherwise of an obesity management programme. Ultimately, the success of anti-obesity drugs must be judged by a reduction in outcome measures, which includes myocardial infarction, cerebrovascular accidents, physical disability and death.

Adjunctive therapies

Adjunctive therapies, or more intensive treatments (discussed in Chapters 25 and 26) should be considered for those patients who are at medical risk from their obesity when primary interventions have failed to achieve adequate weight loss after a sustained period of time (not less than 12 weeks). Such patients may include those who have a BMI of:

- > 35;
- > 25, with two or more risks;
- > 30 or < 35, and who have been treated with a lifestyle programme for 12 weeks without success or reaching goals (this is particularly important if they have risk factors);
- > 27, and who have not lost weight on a lifestyle programme after 24 weeks, especially with risk factor(s).

For patients of Asian background, at particular risk of medical complications, it may be important to consider this type of adjunctive therapy earlier or at lower BMIs.

Low-calorie/energy diets

Milk provides most of the essential macro- and micronutrients. A diet based on 1220 mL (2 pints) of milk is effective in inducing substantial weight loss. It may be used for several weeks as essentially the only form of food for 3 or 4 days each week.

Commercially produced very low-calorie diets (VLCDs), may also be effective. They contain between 400 and 800 kcal/day, usually as protein, with added necessary vitamins and minerals. Such diets can be commenced after a period on a lifestyle programme. There should be a definite protocol for their use, which includes behaviour modification. The initial lifestyle programme is necessary to provide a base therapy to which a patient may return after the most *drastic* VLCD. It is important not to prescribe VLCDs for patients with liver or renal disease. However, with appropriate treatment modifications and precautions they can be used for diabetic patients, even if treated with insulin. Insulin and sulphonylurea doses may need to be reduced substantially during the VLCD treatment programme. Once treatment is completed, a maintenance programme is essential. Subsequent weight regain may suggest a period of retreatment with VLCDs.

Pharmacotherapy

This treatment may prove effective, as an adjunct to lifestyle intervention in selected patients: a detailed discussion is provided in Chapter 25. The newer drugs available (worldwide) are orlistat (Xenical) and sibutramine (Reductil, Meridia).

Selection of patients for pharmacotherapy

It is important that doctors who prescribe such drugs are fully familiar with either the primary literature or an authoritative summary.

The criteria applied to the use of an anti-obesity drug are similar to those applied to the treatment of other relapsing disorders. It is important to avoid offering anti-obesity drug therapy to patients who are seeking a *quick fix* for their weight problem. The initiation of drug treatment will depend on the clinician's judgement concerning the risks to an individual from continuing obesity.

Obesity surgery

This is the most effective, but most drastic, form of treatment available for obesity. The Swedish Obese Study has shown that, with appropriate follow-up, a substantial weight loss can be maintained for at least 10 years. Some surgical procedures are designed to reduce intake or absorption, but the more recent, such as gastric banding (laparoscopic) or gastric stapling and gastric bypass, have fewer side-effects and excellent results. Both an experienced surgical team and a dedicated long-term follow-up team are required. This treatment is discussed more fully in Chapter 26.

Summary

Obesity treatment is necessary and possible. The proper assessment of patients, goal setting and a planned intervention programme (eating, activity and behaviour modification) are the critical components. A weight maintenance programme is an essential ingredient. In those individuals in whom primary intervention fails to achieve medically satisfactory weight loss, additional intervention, such as VLCD, drugs or surgery, may be justified.

References

Angulo, P. (2002) Non-alcoholic fatty liver disease. *New England Journal of Medicine* **346**, 1221–1231.

Bjorvell, H. and Rossner, S. (1987) Long-term effects of commonly available weight reducing programmes in Sweden. *International Journal of Obesity* **11**, 67–71.

Bjorvell, H. and Rossner, S. (1992) A ten-year follow-up of weight change in severely obese subjects treated in a combined behavioural modification programme. *International Journal of Obesity* **16**, 623–625.

Diabetes Prevention Program Group (2002) Reduction in the incidence of type 2 diabetes with lifestyle intervention or metformin. *New England Journal of Medicine* **346**, 393–403.

Grunstein, R.R., Handelsman, D.J., Lawrence, S.J., Blackwell, C., Caterson, I.D. and Sullivan, C.E. (1989) Neuroendocrine dysfunction in sleep apnea: reversal by continuous nasal positive airway pressure. *Journal of Clinical Endocrinology and Metabolism* **68**, 352–358.

National Health and Medical Research Council (2003) Clinical practice guidelines for the management of overweight and obesity in adults. Canberra: National Health and Medical Council of Australia.

National Institutes of Health (1998) Clinical Guidelines on the Identification, Evaluation, and Treatment of Overweight and Obesity in Adults: The Evidence Report. National Institutes of Health. *Obesity Research* **6** (Suppl. 2), 51S–209S.

Royal College of Physicians (2003) *Anti-obesity drugs: Guidance on appropriate prescribing and management.* A report of a working party of the Nutrition Committee of the Royal College of Physicians. London: Royal College of Physicians.

Saris, W.H.M., Blair, S.N., *et al.* (2003) How much physical activity is enough to prevent unhealthy weight gain? Outcome of the IASO 1st Stock Conference and consensus statement. *Obesity Reviews* **4**, 101–114.

Scottish Intercollegiate Guidelines Network (1996) *Obesity in Scotland: A National Clinical Guideline Recommended for Use in Scotland.* Glasgow: Scottish Intercollegiate Guidelines Network, 1–71.

Sjostrom, C.D., Lissner, L., Wedel, H. and Sjostrom, L. (1999) Reduction in incidence of diabetes, hypertension and lipid disturbances after intentional weight loss induced by bariatric surgery: the SOS Intervention Study. *Obesity Research* **7**, 477–484.

Swinburn, B.A., Walter. L.G., Arroll, B., Tilyard, M.W. and Russell, D.G. (1998) The green prescription study: a randomised controlled trial of written exercise advice provided by general practitioners. *American Journal of Public Health* **88**, 288–291.

Toubro, S. and Astrup, A. (1994) Dietary weight maintenance: low-fat, high-carbohydrate ad libitum versus calorie counting. *International Journal of Obesity* **18** (Suppl. 2), 123.

Toubro, S. and Astrup, A.V. (1998) A randomized comparison of two weight-reducing diets. Calorie counting versus low-fat carbohydrate-rich *ad libitum* diet. *Ugeskr Laeger* **160**, 816–820.

Tuomilehto, J., Lindstrom, J., Eriksson, J.G., Valle, T.T., Hamalainen, H., Ilanne-Parikka, P., Keinanen-Kiukaanniemi, S., Laakso, M., Louheranta, A., Rastas, M., Salminen, V. and Uvsitupa, M. The Finish Diabetes Prevention Study Group. (2001) Prevention of type 2 diabetes mellitus by changes in lifestyle among subjects with impaired glucose tolerance. *New England Journal of Medicine* **344**, 1343–1350.

Williamson, D.F., Pamuk, E., Thun, M., Flanders, D., Byers, T. and Heath, C. (1995) Prospective study of intentional weight loss and mortality in never-smoking overweight US white women aged 40–64 years. *American Journal of Epidemiology* **141**, 1128–1141.

World Health Organization. (2000) *Obesity: Preventing and Managing the Global Epidemic.* Technical Report 894. Geneva: WHO, 256.

World Health Organization, International Obesity Task Force and International Association for the Study of Obesity. (2000) *The Asia-Pacific Perspective: Redefining Obesity and its Treatment.* Sydney: Health Communications.

22 Dietary management of obesity: eating plans

Janet Franklin and Carolyn Summerbell

Changing face of treatment, 327

Dietary treatment of obesity, 328
   Energy-deficit approaches, 328

The range of dietary treatments used by the private sector, 336
   Slimming clubs, 336
   Special diets, 337
   Quackery and 'health foods' that claim to aid weight loss, 337
   Guidelines to evaluate diets, 337

Basic principles, 337
   Assessment of dietary intake, 337
   How the information collected in diet diaries may be used in the dietary treatment of obesity, 337
The problems associated with under-reporting of energy intake by obese clients, 338
Is it worth assessing food intake in obese clients?, 338
Setting goals and rate of weight loss, 339
The impact of information from other sources, 339

Nutrition in practice, 339
   Eating patterns, 339
   Type of food and cooking methods, 340
   Behavioural habits, 340

Prader–Willi syndrome: special dietary needs, 341

Maintenance/success, 342

Sources of recommendations or clinical guidelines on the management of obesity, 343

Conclusion, 343

References, 343

Appendix, 348

Changing face of treatment

Obesity was once revered, as it was associated with wealth and fertility. However, around 400 BC, Hippocrates observed that the incidence of sudden death increased, as did menstrual irregularities and infertility, in the obese compared with the lean. He prescribed treatment consisting of hard labour, sleeping on a hard bed, eating only once daily, eating fatty food for greater satiation and walking naked for as long as possible. Hippocrates and his successor Galen believed it to be due to personal weaknesses. During the twelfth to the fifteenth centuries, treatment consisted of taking lots of baths and eating bulky foods with few calories. Over the next two centuries, a more scientific approach to obesity was adopted and, conversely, the empirically based moralistic view declined in popularity. At that time, it was widely believed that obesity resulted from an imbalance in body chemicals or a mechanical malfunction.

In the eighteenth and nineteenth centuries, eating and activity patterns were still the focus of treatment. However, this period witnessed a resurgence of the moralistic view, albeit with more focus on eating habits and physical activity. Obesity treatment generally consisted of advising patients to limit their food choices and to leave the dining area while still hungry. The aetiology of obesity concentrated on two main areas:

1 obesity being the consequence of a physical malfunction such as Prader–Willi syndrome, and
2 obesity being developed from a personality weakness.

During this period physical anthropometry was performed. A formula was developed for ideal weight, (height adjusted) — the Quetelet index, subsequently known as the body mass index (BMI).

During the twentieth century, the incidence of overweight and obesity spiralled out of control. This was accompanied by a significant increase in obesity research, with specific focus on genetics, regulation of food intake and behavioural treatments for obesity.

Worldwide treatment followed similar lines of advice, i.e. urging people to reduce their food intake and increase their physical activity. At this time, psychiatry entered the field of obesity and offered new ideas about its aetiology. One theory was that obesity resulted from acting out unconscious impulses, which reflected disturbed personality development. However, this has never been tested and there seems little evidence to support it. In the 1960s and 1970s, psychological assessment was included in the management of obesity. Behavioural treatment targeted lifestyle changes (based on the learning theory) and dominated treatment. It achieved reasonable success. Today, psychology remains a useful adjunct in weight management programmes (Bray, 1990).

Pharmaceutical preparations, very low-energy diets (VLEDs) and surgery all emerged as treatments during this period. Surgery for the very obese provided slightly better success but had attendant risks.

Dietary treatment of obesity

Energy-deficit approaches

An energy-deficit diet can be achieved by many means. A 2- to 4-MJ (500–1000 kcal) deficit from daily intake (i.e. intakes that are weight maintaining, rather than weight increasing) is thought to lead to approximately 0.5–1 kg of weight loss per week (Anonymous, 1998).

Fixed-energy diets

A *fixed energy level diet* is one way to achieve an energy deficit. Intake is limited by controlling portion sizes, menu choice and composition. These diets are often around 5 MJ (1200 kcal) for women and 7.5 MJ (1800 kcal) for men and are considered a moderate hypocaloric diet. There is minimal self-monitoring, choice and freedom. Lack of variety and difference from normal eating patterns often contribute to a lack of compliance. Commercial weight loss companies with pre-packaged foods often use this method. Long-term results are often similar to, if not better than, those of other well-controlled trials (Lowe *et al.*, 2001).

Self-limiting

Another method is to *self-limit* one or all dietary constituents, for example maintaining 55% of the diet as carbohydrate, 30% as fat and 15% as protein no matter what the caloric intake. This allows dieters to choose their food and monitor their intake. The diet offers freedom and variety and is often referred to as an *ad libitum* diet. A well-known example of this diet is the National Cholesterol Education Step 1 and Step 2 programmes developed by the American Heart Association. These diets usually lead to a weight loss ranging from 2 to 6 kg and decrease of 2–5 cm in waist measurement over a 1- to 2-year period (Astrup *et al.*, 2002). However, the amount of weight loss depends on the pretreatment weight; higher weights before treatment lead to greater weight loss.

It is suggested that *ad libitum* diets may be better at maintaining weight loss than more restrictive diets, particularly if intensively monitored over the long term. It is also postulated that adherence to an *ad libitum* diet slows the progression of chronic diseases such as diabetes (Toubro and Astrup, 1997; Tuomilehto *et al.*, 2001; Knowler *et al.*, 2002).

Low-energy diets

Low-energy diets (LEDS) provide between 3.5 and 5 MJ (800–1200 kcal) per day. They are not recommended without medical supervision. With the ingestion of so few kilojoules, it is almost impossible to meet ideal micronutrient requirements and, consequently, supplementation is recommended. This supplementation can be either through addition of vitamins and minerals in tablet form or through fortification of food (see Table 22.1 for examples of these diets). LEDs achieve better weight loss than the *ad libitum*, low-fat type of diets. Over a 14-week period, 7–13 kg of weight loss and a 10-cm reduction in waist measurement can be achieved. However, after 1 year, weight loss of approximately 6–7 kg is common, and after 2 years the norm is a 3.5-kg weight reduction. At 5 years, there is often very little change from baseline.

One advantage of these diets is that when eaten in total or as part of meal replacement therapy, the food choices are limited. This often makes it easier for the individual to maintain the diet, as it reduces the need for decision-making and reliance on willpower. However, if the individual cannot maintain most of the restrictive practices, weight gain will recur (Glenny *et al.*, 1997).

Very low-energy (calorie) diets

Very low-energy diets (VLEDs or VLCDs) are diets that provide approximately 1.7–3.4 MJ (400–800 kcal) per day. These are below an individual's resting metabolic rate (RMR).

In addition to the energy level, other determinants of a VLED are that it must:

1 contain all the RDI for minerals and vitamins, electrolytes and fatty acids.
2 provide between 0.8 and 1.5 g of high-quality protein;
3 be over a fixed time period;
4 be different from usual intake.

VLEDs need to be carefully formulated to prevent complications, and should also be medically supervised with the client being followed up regularly. There are several potential complications associated with the use of VLED, for example (Anonymous, 1993):

- ketosis (common);
- lethargy, weakness, fatigue (common);
- light-headedness, dizziness (common);
- constipation (common);
- menstrual irregularity (common);
- gastrointestinal upset (common);
- cold intolerance (common);
- dry skin (common);
- electrolyte imbalances;
- dehydration;
- decrease in exercise tolerance;
- decreased voluntary physical activity;
- cardiac changes;
- nutrient deficiencies;
- feeling faint on standing;
- anaemia;

Table 22.1 Menu plans for different dietary calorie-controlled eating.

Meal	3350 kJ (800 kcal)	5000 kJ (1200 kcal)
Breakfast	Cereal 45 g 180 mL of skimmed milk Multivitamin that contains fat-soluble vitamins and iron	90 g of cereal 180 mL of skimmed milk
Morning tea Lunch	Apple One piece of bread Salad 100 g of chicken	Apple Two pieces of wholemeal bread 75 g of chicken plus salad 200 g of diet yoghurt
Afternoon tea Dinner	Banana 250 mL of low-fat vegetable soup 200 g of diet yoghurt	15 g of nuts 90 g of meat Small potato Four broccoli florets One medium carrot 1 cup of fruit salad
Supper	Tea	Tea/milk/coffee plus biscuit

- perhaps hair loss;
- muscle cramping;
- nausea;
- diarrhoea;
- gout;
- gall bladder disease;
- brittle nails;
- oedema.

The VLED was established after it was found that although fasting led to large losses of body weight and reduced hunger, people often died suddenly. Subsequently, it was found that if a small amount of food was consumed then the likelihood of death was greatly reduced. It was determined that minimal intake stopped death but still led to considerable weight loss, and importantly did not increase hunger (Anonymous, 1993). VLEDs were originally protein-sparing modified fasts (PSMF) with whole foods, mostly in the form of game and other lean meats, being used. Now VLEDs are mostly found in a liquid form, and are based on either milk or egg protein.

The VLED should only be used in highly motivated patients who have tried many other methods or who are at a high medical risk. VLED should never be attempted by self-initiated dieters. Their use should be limited in children, people recovering from severe wound healing, those who have a wasting condition and pregnant or lactating women. People who suffer from psychotic episodes are also unlikely to be able to cope with the restrictions involved with a VLCD (see Table 22.2 for contraindications) (Anonymous, 1993).

Children should only be prescribed VLEDs in extreme circumstances, and under medical supervision (Willi *et al.*, 1998a). When VLEDs are used, it is imperative that optimum protein and caloric consumption occurs in order to maintain

growth. VLEDs have been used successfully in adolescents, but restricted to those who can be medically supervised (Willi *et al.*, 1998b). Use of VLED in elderly people is cautiously recommended, as decreased lean muscle mass and the difficulty of balancing consumption of prescribed medications and eating may hinder the potential benefits.

There appears little benefit in VLED less than 3.2 MJ (800 kcal). The commercially produced VLED may only provide 1.6 MJ (400 kcal). The addition of a calorie-controlled meal may actually reduce the incidence of bingeing (which can occur in some patients), after stopping the VLED, without compromise to weight loss.

Typically, a programme including a VLED comprises:
- an initial 4-week programme of 1200 kcal (range 1000–1500 kcal), which helps the client prepare for the restriction and lessens the amount of electrolytes lost;
- 8–16 weeks on a VLED consisting mostly of three or four drinks of commercially prepared VLED, some vegetables each day, plus 2 L of fluid combined with behavioural therapy and an exercise programme;
- 4 weeks on two meals of the VLED preparation plus one normal meal of low-calorie content;
- 4 weeks on one meal of the VLED preparation plus two meals of healthy eating;
- then a maintenance phase with follow-up (Wadden, 1993).

These recommendations are based on the assumption that less severe energy restriction and the inclusion of a daily meal of conventional foods will produce robust weight losses, while avoiding the dietary deprivation and other factors that are associated with weight rebound following VLEDs (Anonymous, 1993).

Results are rarely as impressive as the calorie deficit should

Table 22.2 Contraindications for VLED.

Increased requirements
Pregnancy
Lactation
Illness
Wasting conditions: Cushing's syndrome, cancer, burns, cachexia

Increased medical risk
Recent cardiac disease
Cerebrovascular disease: due to recent accident, recent ischaemic heart disease, transient ischaemic heart disease
Underlying renal disease
Underlying hepatic disease
Eating disorders

Used with consultation
Elderly people
Children
Type 1 diabetes

suggest. The RMR normally drops and the voluntary energy output during physical activity commonly falls, thus the difference is not as great as anticipated. However, during the active stage 90% of patients generally achieve greater than 10 kg of weight loss compared with LED, with which only 60% generally achieve this result. The average weight loss of those who maintain the programme is approximately 22–32 kg for women and men. The average weight loss of those who drop out of the programme is approximately 14–20 kg. Patients normally regain about 35–50% of their lost weight within 1 year, 10–20% regain all their weight and about the same amount maintain their weight loss. Long-term results are no better than other methods of weight loss, but cost is substantially greater. The benefit comes from the rapidity of the weight loss, which may be necessary prior to surgery, to enhance mobility or for other medical reasons. The average weight loss per week is 1.5–2.0 kg for women and 2.0–2.5 kg for men (Anonymous, 1993).

If the VLED is repeated, the amount of weight loss achieved is reduced even if weight regain is close to or above the original weight. Weight loss has been achieved for up to 45 months after starting the VLED, but weight loss diminishes dramatically after 12 weeks. For this reason, it is recommended to stop the VLED at this point.

Although attrition rates are reported to be similar to those of other programmes, in free-living conditions it could be higher than 50% (Anonymous, 1993; Lantz *et al.*, 2003).

VLED can be useful for weight maintenance. For example, it has been trialled intermittently for 2 weeks every 3 months or on demand, i.e. when weight reaches a certain level, for a period of 2 years resulting in slower weight regain compared with control subjects (Lantz *et al.*, 2003). These methods showed that although it slowed progression it did not stop overall weight gain (Lantz *et al.*, 2003). Other groups have used it as either 1 day per week for 15 weeks or 5 consecutive days

every 5 weeks. Both methods showed improved weight loss over a 1500- to 1800-kcal diet and achieved better glycaemic control (Williams *et al.*, 1998). The best maintenance results are achieved when there is large weight loss during treatment and follow-up that includes behavioural therapy and exercise (Astrup and Rossner, 2000; Saris, 2001).

Other benefits of VLED include improvements in the following (Anonymous, 1993):
- metabolic syndrome;
- glycaemic control (within 1 week of starting);
- blood pressure (8–13%);
- serum cholesterol (5–25%);
- triglycerides (15–50%).

Some clients report an improvement in mood but this seems to be more related to the behavioural therapy that should accompany the programme rather than the diet per se.

Total fasting

Total fasting is not recommended as a method for weight loss as it can lead to large losses of protein, diuresis (fluid loss), kaliuresis (potassium loss) and saluresis (sodium loss), and to other nutrient deficiencies. The loss in muscle mass and the large energy deficit leads to a greater decline in RMR and voluntary physical activity (as lethargy is common). Thus, weight regain is likely. There is a high risk of the refeeding syndrome when eating is resumed. Refeeding syndrome can be defined as a severe and potentially fatal electrolyte and fluid shift associated with metabolic abnormalities in malnourished patients undergoing refeeding after a period of limited or no intake.

American Dietetic Association recommendations

The American Dietetic Association (ADA) recommendations are that 80–90% of energy intake should be consumed as carbohydrate and fat. Previously, they recommended 55% carbohydrate and 30% fat (Fig. 22.1). This modification allows greater flexibility so that glucose and lipid levels, eating patterns, taste preference and desired weight change can be considered. These recommendations will require individuals to generally increase carbohydrate intake and reduce their fat and/or protein intake (Norton, 1995). In particular, a dietary reduction of saturated fat seems most beneficial in patients suffering from a chronic disease. If a patient has high triglycerides or VLDL, the new and flexible plan allows for slightly higher fat intake, in the form of monounsaturated fat and a slightly lower carbohydrate intake. The bottom line is that a person needs to maintain the diet in the long term in order to sustain the benefits achieved by the improved diet.

Low-fat diets

The relationship between *fat and weight* gain remains controversial, as evidence from various studies is inconsistent. The message to eat less fat has been around for decades and

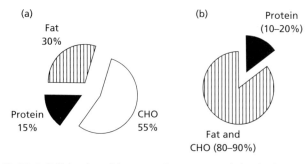

(a)
Fat
30%

Protein
15%

CHO
55%

(b)
Protein
(10–20%)

Fat and
CHO (80–90%)

Fig 22.1 Old (a) and new (b) macronutrient recommendations by the American Dietetic Association (ADA).

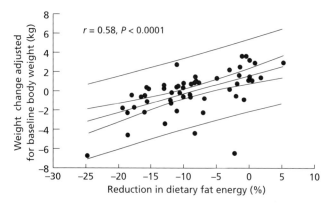

$r = 0.58$, $P < 0.0001$

Fig 22.2 A meta-analysis of weight loss in 48 *ad libitum* low-fat diet intervention studies. The relationship between the reduction in dietary fat and weight change is adjusted for pretreatment body weight. Each dataset represents a study group. (Reproduced with permission from Astrup, 1998.)

National Nutritional surveys like those done in Australia show a reduction in fat intake. However, weight is increasing. Whether fat intake in the diet leads to weight gain seems to be dependent on:

1 the activity patterns of the individual (Stubbs *et al.*, 1995);

2 the individual's genetic predisposition to obesity (Heitmann *et al.*, 1995).

These factors may explain why the relationship between weight and fat is not as strong as one would expect, given the properties of fat (Pirozzo *et al.*, 2002).

At best, it seems that a small weight loss (2–5 kg) for a brief period can be expected, with higher values achieved by the people with initially heavier weights (Lissner and Heitmann, 1995; Astrup *et al.*, 2000; Willett, 2002). A meta-analysis demonstrated a dose-dependent relationship between decreased fat intake and weight loss (Astrup, 1998) (Fig. 22.2). For every 1% decrease in energy from fat there was a 0.28-kg decrease in body weight (Yu-Poth *et al.*, 1999; Astrup *et al.*, 2002). Focusing on fat intake rather than counting calories does not seem to produce greater weight loss. However, there have been reports that it is a more palatable way to lose weight, and can often be advantageous with binge eaters (Jeffery *et al.*, 1995). However, long-term studies (18 or more months) have not shown any additional benefits (Pirozzo *et al.*, 2002; Willett, 2002). Reducing both calories and fat seems to produce significantly greater weight loss than just counting calories (Glenny *et al.*, 1997).

In some instances, the decreased fat intake can cause a rise in triglycerides, particularly if the fat has been substituted by carbohydrate. This occurrence appears to be dependent on the types of fat and carbohydrate consumed. By consuming carbohydrates with a low glycaemic load [glycaemic index, GI, × amount of carbohydrate present] and/or having the main fat sources as mono- (MUFAs) and polyunsaturated fats (PUFAs), this effect seems to disappear or at least improve (Hung *et al.*, 2003). A decreased fat intake per se can lead to an improvement in triglycerides, particularly if the decreased fat intake is accompanied by a reduction in weight (Noakes and Clifton, 2000; Hung *et al.*, 2003). In the long term, there is some evidence to suggest that a low-fat diet helps maintain weight or limits weight gain (Kuller *et al.*, 2001; Pirozzo *et al.*, 2002).

Therefore, low-fat diets are as good as other interventions at reducing weight, not better.

Moderate-fat diets

Moderate-fat diets can improve an individual's enjoyment of a diet, particularly if the type of fat is manipulated to increase MUFA or PUFA consumption. It can also improve their serum lipid profile, but has minimal impact on weight unless a calorie restriction is also in place (Fleming, 2002; Hung *et al.*, 2003). For instance, when a low-fat, high-carbohydrate diet was compared with a diet of equal hypocaloric value but of higher MUFA content, weight loss was the same. The increased MUFA diet did, however, lead to improvements in blood lipids and fasting insulin, even in normolipidaemic obese women (Golay *et al.*, 1996; Low *et al.*, 1996; Zambon *et al.*, 1999).

Fat has a hedonistic appeal (Drewnowski and Greenwood, 1983). By allowing people to eat slightly more fat than was historically the case, enjoyment and sustainability of a diet is enhanced. The mitigating factor is that less food will need to be consumed in order to lose weight. Eating patterns and compliance become important issues, and it again reminds clinicians of the need to tailor dietary programmes to suit individual needs. *To date, there is no evidence to suggest that a high-MUFA diet is superior to a low-fat diet in promoting weight loss or the prevention of weight gain. Its benefit is the favourable impact on cardiovascular risk factors* (Astrup *et al.*, 2002).

High-protein diets

A diet is *high protein* if it contains over 20% of total energy consumed as protein, and is very high protein if the protein content is greater than 30% of the total energy. A low-carbohydrate diet contains less than 40% of total energy from carbohydrate (St Jeor *et al.*, 2001). A popular example of a high-protein diet is the Atkins diet.

When consuming lower energy diets, adequate amounts of protein are needed to spare nitrogen and maintain muscle mass. Often the patient's normal diet exceeds the recommended protein intake, even at this higher level of consumption, and a reduced protein intake is required.

High-protein, low-calorie diets are attractive as they induce ketogenesis and initially produce larger weight loss due to fluid depletion, and the formation of ketones, which helps to suppress appetite. This in turn promotes reduced caloric intake. *It appears that the calorie content, and not necessarily the macronutrient composition, is the major weight loss-inducing factor in a high-protein diet* (St Jeor *et al.*, 2001; Bravata *et al.*, 2003).

There have been concerns that if the protein intake were increased then blood lipid levels would be disrupted or further exaggerated. However, recent studies have shown that a slightly increased protein intake within a *controlled environment* can improve blood lipid levels. A *controlled environment* is when the percentage of energy contributed by each nutrient is constant, for example protein is kept between 15% and 35% although calories are not constant. Other concerns are that the increased protein would lead to increased purines (amino acids) that increase uric acid levels, which may cause gout in susceptible people. Studies have shown that high-protein diets can speed the progression of renal disease in diabetics, even if the high-protein diet is only used in the short term (St Jeor *et al.*, 2001). More immediate adverse effects may be fatigue (due to a depletion of glycogen), dizziness, headaches or nausea (thought to be caused by sodium loss). Many of these diets restrict the intake of fruit, vegetables and wholegrains, which provide essential mineral and vitamins and are likely to prevent the formation of cancers. Most of the benefits of high-protein diets are short term, as few data exist on long-term outcomes. They also present a risk of deficiency in vitamins E, A and B$_6$, thiamine, folate, calcium, magnesium, iron, potassium and dietary fibre (Klauer and Aronne, 2002).

A meta-analysis by Bravata and colleagues (2003) of 38 studies that compared high- and low-carbohydrate diets, conducted for 15 days or less, demonstrated that lower carbohydrate diets produced absolute greater weight loss (16.9 kg vs. 1.9 kg) than higher carbohydrate diets. However, the diets were very heterogeneous. When only the randomized control trials and randomized crossover trials were compared the difference in weight indicated a trend towards the lower carbohydrate studies leading to greater weight loss, but it was no longer significantly different (3.6 kg vs. 2.1 kg) (Bravata *et al.*, 2003). It would appear that the calorie content, the starting weight and the duration of the programme are better predictors of weight loss than the carbohydrate content of the diet (Bravata *et al.*, 2003).

With a reduced carbohydrate content, many people fear a rise in blood lipids; however, no change was seen in the meta-analysis; none reported on lipid levels of hyperlipidaemic subjects (Bravata *et al.*, 2003). There was no effect on insulin, glucose or blood pressure (Bravata *et al.*, 2003). The heterogeneity was a problem with this meta-analysis, therefore a strong conclusion could not be drawn.

One study looked at the progression of coronary artery disease in 10 subjects being treated for cardiovascular problems when they consumed high-protein diets for 1 year. Weight loss was 0.6 kg with worsened total cholesterol, LDL, VLDL, TG and fibrinogen levels. An increase in C-reactive protein occurred, indicating an inflammatory or infectious process. Therefore, it appeared that the high-protein diet was increasing the progression of coronary heart disease in these high-risk patients (Fleming, 2000). However, a high-protein ketogenic diet used in obese males showed a reduction in lipid values (Tapper-Gardzina *et al.*, 2002).

High-protein diets may also lead to increased calcium loss. A study conducted on premenopausal women showed that there was no effect on calcium retention or biomarkers under controlled conditions (Roughead *et al.*, 2003). However, another study in adolescents indicated that a short-duration, high-protein diet led to increased urinary calcium excretion. Over 3 months, bone mineral density decreased, even with vitamin D and calcium supplementation (Tapper-Gardzina *et al.*, 2002).

There is much information in the popular press about high-protein diets; this leads clinicians to be concerned that in the wider community individuals may be less vigilant about their consumption of fibre and other nutrients (see later for information on popular diets).

Glycaemic index

The glycaemic index is a way of ranking food according to that food's 0- to 2-h effect on postprandial blood glucose levels (BGL). The GI is determined by measuring the area under a blood glucose curve, which is created by the digestion of a quantity of food equivalent to 50 g of carbohydrate (see Fig. 22.3). This area is compared with that created by a reference food, either glucose or white bread of equal carbohydrate content. This ratio is expressed as a percentage and is the GI of a food (Wolever *et al.*, 1991).

The GI of a food will vary depending on the rate of digestion. The faster the digestion of a food, the higher the GI value. There are many factors that will affect the digestion of a food (Table 22.3), but the only way to determine the GI of a food is to measure it (Table 22.4).

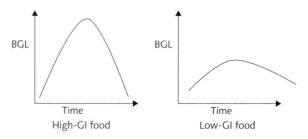

Fig 22.3 The difference in blood glucose level (BGL) after a food with a high glycaemic index (GI) and one with a low GI.

Table 22.3 Factors that influence the glycaemic index (GI) of a food.

Factors affecting GI	Comments
Type of starch	Different starches have different structures, which are digested at different rates. Amylose is slowly digested, whereas amylopectin is rapidly digested (Jenkins *et al.*, 1998; Kabir *et al.*, 1998; Bjorck *et al.*, 2000)
Type of sugar	Lactose, fructose, sucrose and glucose have variable rates of digestion, giving GIs from 23 to 100
Cooking	Cooking food changes its structure; gelatinization occurs to the carbohydrate after cooking and cooling, and this lowers the GI of a food (Ross *et al.*, 1987; Jenkins *et al.*, 1994; Granfeldt *et al.*, 2000)
Processing	Processing foods breaks down the food into small particles, which makes the food more easily digested, for example white flour (Brand *et al.*, 1985; Ross *et al.*, 1987; Morris and Zemel, 1999; Granfeldt *et al.*, 2000)
Other macronutrients	The presence of other nutrients such as fat and protein can lower the GI of a food by slowing its digestion (Trout *et al.*, 1993)
Acidity	Acidity affects gastric emptying and hence the GI of a food; the addition of vinegar, citric acid or other fruits will therefore lower the GI (Liljeberg and Bjorck, 1998; Trout and Behall, 1999)
Fibre	Has been shown to slow the rate of digestion, particular soluble fibre
Food type	Adding certain food groups, for example fruit, legumes or whole grains, can all lower the GI of the meal, as well as the effects of the following meal (Wolever and Jenkins, 1985; 1986; Wolever, 1987; Wolever *et al.*, 1988)

Table 22.4 Quick guide to classifying GI of food.

GI classification
Low < 50
Medium 50–70
High > 70

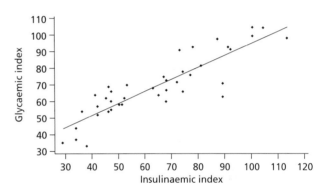

Fig 22.4 Correlation between GI and insulinaemic index (II) for 43 starchy foods. The II is the ratio of the area under the insulin curve 90–120 min after eating a test food compared with the reference food's response. (Reproduced with permission from Bjorck *et al.*, 2000.)

The obese population is at the greatest risk of the *metabolic syndrome*. This includes hyperlipidaemia, hyperinsulinaemia or severe insulin resistance (Ascott-Evans, 2002). It has been demonstrated that there is benefit from the use of low-GI foods in offsetting these risk factors. Low-GI foods appear to improve blood lipid profile by decreasing LDL levels and increasing HDL levels concurrently. Additionally, improved fibrinolytic activity and reduced risk of myocardial infarct has been demonstrated (Frost *et al.*, 1996; 1998, 1999; Jarvi *et al.*, 1999; Liu *et al.*, 2000).

Many studies have shown that blood insulin levels closely track BGL in most individuals (Bjorck *et al.*, 2000) (Fig. 22.4). Significantly, a low-GI diet improves insulin sensitivity in both diabetics and non-diabetics (Frost *et al.*, 1999). One study of obese women showed that a low-GI diet decreased fasting insulin levels in parallel with weight loss (Slabber *et al.*, 1994). However, it has subsequently been found that not all low-GI foods lead to a predicted lower insulin response (Gannon *et al.*, 1986; Liljeberg *et al.*, 1996; Bjorck *et al.*, 2000). Clearly, more work is required before any strong conclusions can be drawn.

There appear to be many benefits from using GI to help control BGL and to improve the cardiovascular profile in people whose BMI is greater than 23 (Liu *et al.*, 2000). However, it remains controversial as to whether or not GI should be used in weight loss programmes per se. A meta-analysis of the data has shown that low-GI meals lead to non-significantly lower energy intake (3.5 MJ) compared with (4.1 MJ) high-GI meals, and this did not lead to a significant difference in weight loss (Raben, 2002). In animal studies using a low-GI diet, a decrease in fat deposition can be demonstrated, and is not accompanied by depletion of lean muscle mass. However, this has not yet been replicated in humans (Raben, 2002).

Foods need to be tested to determine their GI and, as we have discussed, there are many variables that influence the GI. Therefore, before GI can be recommended for use in long-term weight management programmes, a more extensive list of foods and their GIs is necessary (Bjorck *et al.*, 2000; Raben, 2002).

The less restrictive dieting approach

Dieting is typically defined by restrictive practices. Most people who seek help from professional bodies, particular tertiary institutions, have had a long history of dieting and weight swings. Repeated attempts to lose weight often end in failure when the individual cannot maintain their weight using highly restrictive practices. It is suggested that dieting and being 'weight obsessed' is contributing to their obesity rather than helping them to solve it. Others argue that sometimes the detrimental effects of dieting are worse than the weight per se and a non-dieting approach to health would be of benefit (Garner and Wooley, 1991). One of these approaches has coined the title 'health at any size (H@AS)'. This is based on the premise that the overweight person wants to eat healthily and be active, and that if restrictions and pressures are eliminated, they would naturally adopt healthier patterns. This would ultimately lead to a weight change that was genetically right for them. The H@AS system also assumes that health is a result of behaviours that are independent of body weight. The person using the system is encouraged to give up dieting and instead let the body guide them to what it wants and needs. This would lead to a weight that might not be what the medical profession or individual initially would determine ideal but would lead to an improved quality of life.

The supporters of H@AS suggest that dieting has led to unhealthy practices that have caused people to ignore or not recognize their own hunger cues. Satiety, desire and exercise were seen in the context of weight loss cues, rather than for enjoyment (Gaesser and Miller, 1999). The work by Mellin and co-workers (1997), summarized by Miller, outlines the aims of the programme (Miller and Jacob, 2001). The aim of this non-dieting approach is predicated on three main areas, i.e. mind, body and lifestyle. For example, mind skills might involve increasing one's knowledge of their feelings and needs, developing appropriate goals, expectations and positive cognitions. Body skills might include decreasing negative thoughts about their body weight, understanding their body's weight loss threshold and making sure that they attend to total body self-care. Lifestyle skills would probably include learning hunger and satiety signals and responding appropriately to these cues. Participation in daily physical activity for both fulfillment and self-restoration, and other programmes, have been used to identify the tastes of foods, assess how a person feels after consumption of foods and to identify healthy eating habits (Miller and Jacob, 2001; Kausman et al., 2003).

Psychological improvements tend to be the main outcomes measured with H@AS, which makes it hard to compare it to other treatment methods, as their outcomes are mostly based on biochemical or anthropometric measurements (Miller and Jacob, 2001). However, the evidence that traditional methods of weight loss (that focus on weight loss for better health and physical activity for weight loss alone) cause psychological harm is fairly sketchy and as of yet unfounded (Miller and Jacob, 2001). In fact, many studies showing weight loss have also shown an improvement in quality of life (Wing et al., 1984; Lopez de la Torre Casares, 1999; Weiner et al., 1999; Burns et al., 2001; Dixon et al., 2001; Dixon and O'Brien, 2002). It seems to be generally excepted that weight loss can lead to improvements

in many medical problems (Pi-Sunyer, 1993). It is also well known that there are some medical problems that are increased with weight loss (Pi-Sunyer, 1993). But the risk of complication from weight loss does not outweigh the risk of obesity-related comorbidities (Pi-Sunyer, 1993). Brownell (1993) suggests that the failure of programmes that are run at tertiary institutions should not tar all programmes, as those seeking help from these groups may actually have more specific needs and medical problems, and are therefore more likely to fail.

The American National Weight Control Registry records details of people who have maintained 13 kg or more weight loss for greater than 1 year (Klem et al., 1997). The average intake was approximately 5.5 MJ (1300 kcal) (which is considered hypocaloric/restrictive) and they exercised to expend at least 1.7 MJ (400 kcal) per day, more than that which is recommended for general health. This would suggest that these people do not find this as deprivation as they are able to maintain it in the long term (Klem et al., 1997).

In some cases the non-dieting approach (involving less restrictive practices and choices of food and exercise) combined with a higher caloric guide (1800 kcal) created less weight loss in the short term (2.5 kg vs. 5.6 kg), but larger weight losses in the long term (10 kg vs. 4.5 kg—1 year), compared with more traditional methods of weight loss (involving restrictive practices, strict 5-MJ (1200-kcal) diet, exercise prescription, stimulus control, self-monitoring and behavioural substitution) (Sbrocco et al., 1999). Another study, with a small sample size and no control, used the non-dieting approach and showed that the participants, who were followed up periodically for 2 years, experienced weight loss over the total period rather than initial weight loss, followed by weight gain (Mellin et al., 1997). Other studies that compared highly restrictive practices, e.g. VLED and conventional higher calorie diets, showed that although the weight loss was slower, it was better maintained (Paisey et al., 2002) (Fig. 22.5).

It is said that to maintain the drastic weight loss achieved with the traditional methods, unrealistic amounts of exercise are needed (Tremblay et al., 1999; Miller and Jacob, 2001). The H@AS method advocates exercising only to levels that are maintainable in the long term and hence a weight that reflects these levels (Miller and Jacob, 2001). A benefit of the H@AS approach is that people do not feel as though they are on a diet (Kausman et al., 2003). They are encouraged to listen to their bodies and eat to their needs and wants rather than just eating to the calorie restriction. Experience shows that, in the long term, people often consume fewer calories than when they are trying to follow a strict diet plan (Miller and Jacob, 2001).

Other factors should also be considered when looking at these programmes. For instance, the assumption that all obese patients know how to eat a healthy diet once the restrictions are removed is really unproven and for some people, rapid weight loss is essential in order to improve their medical conditions (Miller and Jacob, 2001).

Whether weight loss is shown to occur in these patients

or not, other eating-related psychopathology tends to decline. Factors such as restraint eating, bingeing, self-image and even depression and anxiety scores are often improved (Mellin *et al.*, 1997; Goodrick *et al.*, 1998; Tanco *et al.*, 1998).

It therefore can be an effective programme for a certain type of person. It is probably most suitable for people with the following characteristics:

* highly restrictive practices in the past;
* failed weight loss;
* eating reasonably well at present day;
* good nutritional knowledge;
* long-term dieters;
* preoccupied by body weight and eating behaviour;
* no longer think that they can achieve weight loss;
* think that they are already doing everything right;
* highly emotional or non-hungry eaters.

It seems to work especially well when combined with a liberal caloric guide, for example approximately 1800 kcal. Often these clients have been 'trapped' in the diet cycle (Fig. 22.6) for most of their lives, and this method can help them to break that pattern of repeated attempts and failure. It is probably not suitable for individuals who have little concept of good nutrition, who love high-fat, high-sugar or protein foods, who think that normal eating involves extremely large portions and who re-

port extreme hunger signals. Other methods might be needed first to correct these behaviours before the benefits of this method would be seen.

Emotional eating or eating for reasons other than hunger is a common sabotage of weight loss efforts (Schlundt *et al.*, 1989). This programme can help emotional eaters as it allows them to identify their hunger and satiety cues and helps them to nurture themselves in other more productive ways that do not necessarily involve food.

It should also be noted that this method has not been tested on culturally diverse groups. Women of Caucasian background make up the majority of test populations (Miller and Jacob, 2001). The other downside is that it needs a trained professional who can administer an effective cognitive–behavioural programme, as the H@AS is strongly dependent on cognitive restructuring. This may prove difficult in many medical weight loss settings (Miller and Jacob, 2001).

Meal frequency

The impact of meal frequency on weight is not as clear as might be expected. Observational data suggest, but are not conclusive, that an inverse relationship exists between weight and food frequency (Bellisle *et al.*, 1997). It has also been suggested that people who eat frequently have better internal hunger–satiety regularity systems (Westerterp-Plantenga *et al.*, 2002). A recent study showed, however, that obese women ate more often and ate most of their meals in the afternoon period compared with lean counterparts (Berteus Forslund *et al.*, 2002). Intervention studies suggest that a single meal leads to greater consumption at a subsequent *ad libitum* meal compared with the same amount spread over several meals, despite a lack of difference between hunger ratings and total insulin secretion (although insulin fluctuations were less in the multimeal group) (Speechly and Buffenstein, 1999; Speechly *et al.*, 1999). Thus, the authors suggest that the reduced consumption could perhaps be explained through the reduced insulin fluctuations (Speechly and Buffenstein, 1999, Speechly *et al.*, 1999).

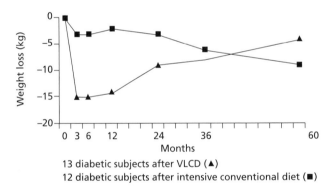

Fig 22.5 Mean weight loss over 5 years after intensive self-selected diet treatments of highly restricted or moderately restricted intakes. (Reproduced with permission from Paisey *et al.*, 2002.)

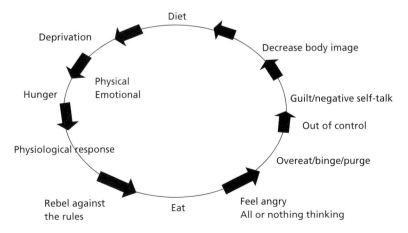

Fig 22.6 The diet cycle. People start on a diet because they want to change their body in some way; subsequently, they start to feel deprived both physically and emotionally. This deprivation leads them to have increased thoughts about food and display food-seeking behaviour; often they feel like they are missing out. Finally, they eat. At this point, the 'all-or-nothing thinking' starts and they feel guilty. These feelings may lead to overconsumption of food and in some purging behaviour. Negative self-talk ensues, with statements such as 'I am such a bad person' and 'I have no will power'. A decrease in body image occurs, which starts the whole cycle again. The person vows that it will be better this time.

Meal frequency does not seem to be of any benefit in terms of lowering total insulin secretion although it may reduce fluctuations) or total energy expenditure (even diet-induced thermogenesis does not appear to be increased with higher meal frequency in most studies) (Wolfram *et al.*, 1987; Verboeket-van de Venne and Westerterp, 1991; Bellisle *et al.*, 1997; Thomsen *et al.*, 1997).

Changing meal frequency so that the same amount of food is eaten over several meals may be harder than we think, as it appears there is strong genetic predisposition to an individual's pattern of eating. De Castro (1993) investigated the genetic component to meal size, meal frequency and meal composition. The study demonstrated that the genetic component explained 44–65% of the variance (de Castro, 1993). However, other factors also increase food frequency, such as food availability (Stubbs *et al.*, 2001) and enforced eating restrictions (Frost and Pirani, 1987; Lamberg, 2000); both of these have been shown to lead to increased food intake and, in some individuals, to weight gain.

In conclusion, there is limited evidence to suggest that meal frequency plays a role in weight loss, unless calorie intake is altered to form a deficit from normal. Frequent food intake, which is consumed at regular intervals, compared with a single intake, however, may lead to better intake regulation. *The key is for people to eat less food several times per day, at regular intervals, rather than consuming big meals infrequently.*

The range of dietary treatments used by the private sector

Slimming clubs

The dietary treatments offered by *slimming clubs* are conventional reducing diets with a 'twist'. Some clubs, such as Weight Watchers, use a form of calorie counting to help the patients control their energy intake. Foods are given 'points' on the basis of their energy value and their fat content, and there are no 'forbidden' foods. The client is allowed to eat foods up to the value of a given number of 'points', which is calculated on the basis of their body weight (heavier clients being allowed more points). Clients following a Weight Watchers diet are advised to eat a healthy diet, are allowed a number of 'free' foods per day and get 'bonus' points for exercise. Other slimming clubs, such as Slimming World (UK), do not use calorie counting. Clients are advised to follow a diet plan that is made up of different coloured days, in which, for example, a green day is made up of fruit and vegetables. Each coloured day contains a list of 'free' foods, healthy extras (which are allowed in moderation) and 'sins'. Clients are allowed between 5 and 15 'sins' per day; a chocolate bar such as a Mars Bar constitutes 15 'sins', whereas a glass of wine is 5 'sins'.

It is difficult to assess the efficacy of the advice offered by slimming clubs as there is little evidence from controlled trials. However, there is no reason to believe that the dietary treatments advocated by slimming clubs are less effective than those advocated by health professionals. When Biesalski (1994) compared the results from a Weight Watchers study with a clinical study (both performed in Sweden), he found that the Weight Watchers group had lost significantly more weight than the clinical group at 24 months. This does not prove that obese people who attend slimming clubs fare better than those who attend hospital obesity clinics (as different 'types' of people attend different 'types' of treatment), but it does show that slimming clubs can be effective for some.

Special diets

There is a myriad of special diets that are purported to aid weight loss (Liebermeister, 1994). They often suggest combining certain foods, placing restrictions on certain food types during special times of the day or eliminating whole food groups. They all work on the principle that consuming a low-calorie diet will stimulate weight loss, but few admit to such a simple claim. The diets are usually explained in paperback books and are widely available in bookshops. They claim to be offering something 'different', perhaps even an as yet unknown metabolic pathway, which the diet can disturb in the favour of weight loss. Whatever the claim, it is always compelling. Perhaps what is most distressing is that some of these books claim that weight loss, using their diets, will not be difficult. All clients find losing weight by dieting difficult, and sometimes impossible, but rarely easy.

Perhaps the most popular diet over recent years has been the Atkins diet. The diet does not involve calorie counting and encourages the consumption of high-fat and high-protein foods, but severely limits carbohydrate-rich foods, such as bread, pasta, rice and breakfast cereals. It is clear why the diet can cause weight loss—diets that restrict food choice are liable to also result in a decrease in energy intake (Rolls, 1986). However, the high-protein Atkins diet has a number of side-effects of concern, specifically hyperlipidaemia and the potential for harm resulting from a low intake of fibre and various minerals. However, in recent years the Atkins diet has evolved so that it addresses some of these concerns. It now contains an active weight loss phase and a maintenance programme. In the maintenance programme, fruit and vegetable consumption is encouraged. In a recent multicentre randomized trial looking at the difference between a conventional calorie-controlled diet and the Atkins diet, a greater net loss was achieved by the Atkins diet. However, the difference was not significant at the end of 12 months, indicating that regain was greater in the Atkins diet group. However, the controversial decline in lipid profile did not occur nor was insulin secretion or glucose levels (Foster *et al.*, 2003) effected and, in fact, there was a significant improvement in triglyceride and HDL-cholesterol concentrations in the Atkins diet group. It should be noted that the participants had no comorbidities at baseline.

Quackery and 'health foods' that claim to aid weight loss

'Health foods' constitute a group of products, which, as far as the consumer is concerned, fall on the boundary between foods and medicines. In many cases, their advertising usually includes the implication that the consumption of the product will confer health benefits on the consumer. Of particular relevance to this chapter are the health claims made about products which are purported to aid weight loss.

A case in point that was reported in the *Healthwatch Newsletter* (Garrow, 1995) related to a slimming product named Autoslim, which was advertised in 1993 in a UK national newspaper. The advert claimed that the product would 'cause steady weight loss day after day'. As a result of taking this preparation 'your body's metabolism will activate and actually start to burn off excess calories and fat'. The metabolic situation created was described as a 'fat furnace'. The product was supplied by mail order only but with a money-back guarantee. The product came with a sheet describing 'Newton's special diet plan', on which the customer was allowed to eat unlimited amounts of fresh fruit and vegetables, lean meat and fish, but no white bread, cakes, nuts, sugar, sweets, milk, cheese or fat in any form.

After the trading standards officer was alerted to the existence of Autoslim, the product was analysed and was found to contain trivial amounts of some amino acids, but these were in any case supplied in far greater amounts by the normal diet and would cause no significant change in metabolic rate. The company was prosecuted for supplying goods to which a false description was applied because Autoslim had no effect on body weight or weight reduction. The defence was that the diet advice supplied with the product would cause weight reduction if followed, and the product might motivate customers to keep to the diet. The defendants were found guilty on all charges, fined a total of £6000 and ordered to pay the costs of prosecution, estimated at about £5000.

There are many other products on the market such as 'Autoslim' and the health professional who treats obese patients needs to keep abreast of such products so that they can give sound advice on them if needed. As highlighted above, information from other sources may be more compelling than the advice offered by the health professional but, regardless of its credibility, it should be treated seriously. If you have any concerns about slimming products, which you believe are untrue, you should notify the relevant authorities.

Guidelines to evaluate diets

For decades the scientific community has been trying to determine the perfect 'weight loss' diet; perhaps this is an unrealistic expectation, given that the aetiology of obesity is multifactorial. It logically follows that effective treatment of obesity should be as diverse as its causes. In clinical practice, it is highly likely that different approaches will be implemented for different people at different stages of their lives.

In 1990, in reaction to the plethora of commercially available weight loss programmes, a task force was established in Michigan, USA, which developed guidelines to better inform the public. Some of these guidelines included the following advice:
- The weight goal for a client should be based on personal and family history and not exclusively on height and weight charts.
- The calories consumed per day should not be lower than 1000 kcal without medical supervision.
- Protein intake should be between 0.8 and 1.5 g/kg of goal body weight but no more than 100 g of protein per day.
- In total, 10–30% of the energy of the diet should come from fat.
- There should be at least 100 g/day of carbohydrate without medical supervision and at least 50 g/day with medical supervision.

However, these guidelines permit wide interpretations in weight loss treatment.

Basic principles

Assessment of dietary intake

A first step in making changes is a shared awareness and understanding of the client's present position. In order to begin education on new eating habits, one must be aware of old habits, regardless of the type of dietary treatment used. Although there are a number of tools that will assess dietary intake (Bingham, 1987), the most common methods used in this setting are the diet history and the 7-day unweighed diet diary methods. The 7-day unweighed diet diary is deemed to be the most useful method in this context (British Dietetic Association, 1996), and is best obtained by asking the client to keep a food diary for 1 week. The client must be given clear instructions on how to complete the diary, either verbally, or preferably in written format, in the diary provided. Although foods do not need to be weighed, a reasonable description of the types of foods and quantities consumed, in household measures, needs to be given.

How the information collected in diet diaries may be used in the dietary treatment of obesity

The completed diary then becomes the basis for discussion of eating habits. Any changes must be (as far as possible) acceptable to the client in terms of palatability and practicality, otherwise the client will not comply with the dietary advice. An understanding of the client's lifestyle, including financial and time constraints, and cultural issues if appropriate, is also important. The health professional should ensure that any advice does not compromise other aspects of healthy eating (Gibney, 1992), such as micronutrient intake and protein–energy ratio to achieve better nitrogen retention and minimize loss of fat-free mass (Garrow, 1991).

The diary may indicate an erratic eating pattern, with problems such as irregular meals, periods of fasting, excessively restrained eating, frequent snacking, grazing or binge eating.

It may be useful to ask for additional information in the diet diary, such as relating mood or circumstances to eating, or monitoring physical activity, to help identify areas for behaviour change. Many of these factors can be helped by the health professional, in particular a dietitian, but sometimes referral to a clinical psychologist may be appropriate if the eating pattern is deemed to be abnormal or is being affected excessively by psychological/emotional issues. Often in these cases the additional confounders need to be dealt with before weight loss can be attempted (Haus *et al.*, 1994).

As well as providing a record of reported food intake and eating behaviour at baseline, the diet diary can be used throughout treatment to review and plan for future treatment. A diet diary encourages the client to be actively involved in treatment, and to take responsibility for making dietary and other behaviour changes. It may also provide an indication of the client's motivation, and ways of improving motivation and implementing change.

The problems associated with under-reporting of energy intake by obese clients

Predictive equations for obese individuals have been reviewed by Heshka and colleagues (1993), who recommend using those formulated by Fleisch (1951) or Robinson and Reid (1952). A common problem in developing dietary advice for the obese client on the basis of the reported food and drink consumed in a food diary is that the energy intake of the reported diet is significantly less than that estimated from predictive equations for that obese person in energy balance.

There is a wealth of evidence that shows that energy intakes reported by obese people are significantly lower than would be feasible if they were to maintain their level of obesity (Black *et al.*, 1991). Many authors have concluded from this evidence that obese people under-report their habitual energy intake during the study period. This may well be the case, but there is also the possibility that obese clients actively diet when asked to record their food intake and report a true intake of their dieting behaviour. Support for this explanation is provided by the frequent (but not published) observation that people often lose weight when they are asked to record their food intake, even when these people are students studying for a nutrition degree. If the low-energy intakes reported by obese clients are a result of true dieting behaviour, one might predict that if the obese client were asked to record their food intake for long enough they would either lose weight (and on this basis one may use continuous recording of food intake in a diary as an adjunct to therapy—see below) or report food intake associated with relapse. Unfortunately, little work around the

use of long-term continuous food records in obese clients has been carried out.

Regardless of the explanation for the low-energy intakes reported by obese clients, the health professional must accept that it may not be possible to obtain a comprehensive record of their food intake from a 7-day diary. If the obese client is reporting true dieting behaviour then the diet that they consume during relapse will remain a mystery, and may be completely different in terms of foods eaten, quantities consumed and eating behaviour compared with the diet they consume while losing weight. If the low-energy intakes reported by the obese client are a result of under-reporting then it may be possible to predict true dietary intake if the client is under-reporting the quantity of all foods and drinks consumed by the same degree (as one could simply multiply the amount of food eaten by the same factor required to obtain the estimated energy intake from the reported energy intake), i.e. non-specific under-reporting. However, the limited evidence on under-reporting suggests that the obese tend to under-record food from snacks compared with meals (Heitmann and Lissner, 1995; Summerbell *et al.*, 1996), and particularly from snacks consumed during the evening (Beaudoin and Mayer, 1953), compared with individuals of ideal weight, i.e. specific under-reporting. Therefore, as snacks tend to be made up of different foods and drinks and have a different macronutrient composition compared with meals (Summerbell *et al.*, 1995), specific under-reporting means that it is impossible to predict true dietary intake from a 7-day diet diary.

Is it worth assessing food intake in obese clients?

Even with these caveats, it is still useful to use a 7-day diary to assess food intake in obese clients (BDA, 1996). Apart from gleaning an insight into any possible behavioural problems it also reduces the reliance on memory and is a written learning tool.

However, the health professional should also calculate the client's energy intake from predictive equations, as having an estimate of energy intake is useful in calculating the true energy intake that will be required to lose weight; 1000 kcal per day below the estimated requirement will normally produce a weight loss of 0.5–1.0 kg per week (Garrow, 1988). A possible scenario (and one which is not uncommon in obesity clinics) may arise whereby the health professional advises the obese client to consume a diet that contains more energy than that which the obese person reports to consume. Although some clients may be alarmed at such advice, published outcomes (Frost *et al.*, 1991) have shown that this approach to formulating dietary advice works well.

In an attempt to improve (i.e. get nearer to the truth) the diet reported in a 7-day diary by obese clients, the health professional could ask additional questions about food intake. This may be seen as validating their reported food intake, but equally it may be viewed as attempting to 'trick' the client into revealing the truth. Although there are no standard questions or questionnaires that are designed for this specific purpose, one could ask about the frequency (say, per week) of consumption of certain types of foods, for example energy-dense foods and takeaways, and cross-reference this information with that in the diet diary. Questions around eating behaviour may also be useful, and a question that has been found to be particularly useful is 'Do you normally lose weight or gain weight when on holiday?' as many obese clients report losing weight on holiday. The answers to this question can then be used in helping the obese client to identify triggers for overeating and alter behaviour to reduce food intake at home. The obese client may have reduced their intake as they tend not to overeat with other people around, perhaps they were preoccupied with other interests and therefore not focusing on food or perhaps they undertook more exercise on holidays than at home. Indeed, there is evidence to show that many obese individuals do not overeat in public places (Coll *et al.*, 1979), but do so in private, particularly at home during the evening (Brandon, 1987).

Hope for a useable tool to assess true dietary intake comes from two published studies that have developed food-frequency questionnaires which appear to capture realistic energy intakes (Fricker *et al.*, 1989; Lindroos *et al.*, 1993).

Setting goals and rate of weight loss

Setting goals is also an important part of the weight loss process but these goals must be realistic. Goals should be time specific, measurable, achievable and behaviour based. In terms of weight goals, the clients need to have realistic expectations of what they can achieve. For clients who have 20 kg or more to lose, intermediate weight targets should be set, to reduce the chance of the client giving up due to the seemingly long and difficult task they have set themselves.

The obese person should also be clear about the expected rate of weight loss. As stated above, if a person consumes 1000 kcal per day less than they would normally eat, then they should lose between 0.5 and 1.0 kg per week. But, some people will be disappointed with a weight loss of less than 1 kg per week, and the obese person may give up on a diet because in their view it is not working, whereas in fact it is. Indeed, it has been shown that clients who have unrealistically high initial expected weight loss do not lose weight and consequently drop out of the programme (Bennett, 1986). It is important to help clients accept moderate, achievable expectations of weight loss, and to discourage unrealistic goals for the rate of loss and target weight.

The impact of information from other sources

It is easy to forget that the dietary advice given by the health professional is only part of the information that the client uses to change eating behaviour. Clients present with a wide variation in their baseline knowledge of the energy value of foods; some are real experts and know much more than most health professionals. The advice given by the health professional will be combined with the knowledge that the client already has, rather than overriding the client's baseline knowledge, and it is this combined knowledge that will form the basis of change to the diet. The constant and often more compelling background information on dieting from other sources, particularly from media, friends and family, will influence the changes to eating behaviour immediately and in the future. Indeed, the client may request advice from the health professional regarding a specific diet or food that they have heard will enhance their weight loss or make it easier. Regardless of the credibility of reported claims for such diets or foods, it is important that the health professional addresses them seriously and does not dismiss them as *'simply ridiculous'*; if the client thought that these claims were ridiculous they would not have asked for advice on them in the first place.

Nutrition in practice

Individual habits, lifestyle, personal needs and health status need to be taken into consideration, as does a person's access to food, their financial situation and their motivation. The American Dietetic Association (ADA) position paper emphasizes the need to think about the long-term management of weight rather than short-term losses, paying particular attention to sustainable changes while focusing on overall well-being, not just treatment or prevention of disease: they believe that the programme should include 'training in lifestyle modification with (a) a gradual change to a healthful eating style with increased intake of whole grains, fruit and vegetables; (b) a non-restrictive approach to eating based on internal regulation of food (hunger and satiety); and (c) a gradual increase to at least 30 min of enjoyable physical activity each day'.

Changing lifestyle factors still remain the most effective long-term treatment and although the clinician can help with this it is still the responsibility of the client to maintain changes and achieve the desired outcome (Poston and Foreyt, 2000).

The aim is to help create an energy deficit that achieves weight loss. Therefore, given the above information certain areas should be the focused on (a) eating patterns, (b) types of food and cooking methods, (c) behaviour patterns and (d) exercise, all of which can be gleaned from the food diary.

Eating patterns

Eating patterns involve the distribution of food, portion sizes, timing and speed of eating. Often the distribution of food is uneven. People will leave large time gaps between meals or skip meals altogether, leading to extreme hunger and food-seeking behaviour. The food sought at this time is often convenient, i.e. it is easily accessible, it gives instant gratification and comes in prepackaged containers. Convenience foods are mostly of low satiety, high energy and high fat value. When these foods are combined with increased hunger it predisposes the individual to overconsumption, i.e. eating beyond energy requirements. If a meal is eaten at this time, larger portions than normal are often consumed in a hurry, with no adjustment to body satiety cues. Although the number of meals in a day might be low, the total energy intake is often high. Therefore, the energy deficit created by skipping a meal or lengthening the time between meals is not achieved. It is best to eat regularly, leaving enough time to become hungry in between meals but not ravenous. Eating slowly can help one to notice hunger and satiety cues earlier and ultimately leads to decreased consumption. Slowing down eating techniques include putting knife and fork down in between bites, pausing during the meal and chewing food well before swallowing (Wadden, 1993).

Other people might eat regularly but consume large portions. An energy deficit could be achieved by reducing the size or composition of the meals. For instance, less food fits on a butter plate compared with a dinner plate, but the plate still looks full. Also, it is harder to overconsume bread that has many grains in it than it is to overconsume white bread, owing to its texture and density.

The variety of foods consumed has mixed implications for weight. Variety can help with compliance as it provides interest, reduces boredom and the feelings of restriction, as well as helping a person meet their nutrient requirements. On the other hand, increased variety can lead to overconsumption. For example, it has been shown that cafeteria-style eating leads to greater consumption of food and increased weight (Garner and Wooley, 1991; Raynor and Epstein, 2001).

Structured meal plans or meal replacements can help with weight loss. They may help the individual comprehend appropriate portion sizes and reduce confusion around food choice, thus aiding compliance and producing early results, which is motivating (Khaodhiar and Blackburn, 2002). Giving grocery lists can have a similar outcome (Glenny *et al.*, 1997).

Type of food and cooking methods

The type of food, where it is obtained and how it is cooked are important. The place of origin gives some indication of the composition of the food, for example take-away foods are often extremely high in fat, salt and energy, whereas home-cooked meals have a greater potential to be of lower energy as the cooking method can be manipulated.

Carbohydrate is needed to maintain blood sugar levels and fluid balance. Observationally, higher carbohydrate intake leads to lower BMI and waist–hip ratio (Toeller *et al.*, 2001). The best type of carbohydrate to consume is high in fibre, in the form of wholegrains and has a low GI (Hung *et al.*, 2003). Sugar

consumed in the form of sugary drinks is more likely to lead to weight gain than sugar ingested in solid forms (Astrup *et al.*, 2002). Fibre and water are two other important components of any weight loss diet, especially if protein has been increased. They help avoid constipation (a common side-effect from increased protein and reduced intake), and the fibre adds bulk to the meal. In Australia, it is recommend that approximately 30 g of fibre is consumed per day.

Many dieters restrict dairy and meat produce, believing it will help them with weight loss. However, a high proportion of women are anaemic and are not meeting their recommended dietary intakes for calcium; there is no need to eliminate either as they can be included by choosing lower fat versions. In fact, it has been shown that calcium consumption (dairy food being the major source in Western countries) leads to a lower weight in a dose–response manner, with each 300-mg increment in calcium intake being associated with 1 kg less of body fat in children and 2.5–3.0 kg of lower body weight in adults (Heaney *et al.*, 2002). *In vitro* studies have demonstrated that calcium results in stimulation of lipogenesis and inhibition of lipolysis. Preliminary results suggest that it might even aid in weight loss (Shi *et al.*, 2001).

Alcohol can also play a role in a person's weight. Alcohol has no storage capacity within the body and therefore any that is consumed must be oxidized. If energy requirements are met through alcohol alone then anything else that is eaten with it will be stored. Alcohol can also cause someone to eat more in a two-prong effect. Alcohol can affect restrictive dietary practices, by reducing resolve to limit intake as well as making people hungry. Often the only food available when consuming alcohol is high-energy, high-fat food, such as fried foods, crisps and nuts (Astrup, 1999a).

The food groups that need to be reduced include full-fat dairy products (including ice creams), meats, pastries, snacks/convenient foods, biscuits, cakes, confectionery, deep fried or fried foods, oils, spreads and take-aways.

National guides to healthy eating are a sound reference for healthy eating and weight loss. In Australia it is recommended that approximately two servings of low-fat dairy foods, two servings of fruits, five servings of vegetables, one or two servings of protein and 4–9 servings of carbohydrate are consumed daily, depending on sex, age and activity patterns.

Behavioural habits

Self-monitoring and reducing stimuli are two of the most effective dietary behavioural techniques used in obesity treatment today. Self-monitoring helps the client become more aware of the type, quantity and pattern of eating (Poston and Foreyt, 2000), for example the food/exercise/mood diary. Stimulus control involves first identifying and then modifying the environmental cues that are associated with a client's overeating or inactivity (Poston and Foreyt, 2000). In the short term, people avoid or manipulate problems in their immediate environment; however, over time, living in an obesogenic society, stimulus control in the wider community may be near to impossible (Khaodhiar and Blackburn, 2002).

Compliance with the programme is more important than the programme itself. Factors such as flavour, palatability and texture influence client compliance (Willett, 2002). Keeping changes close to the present practice ensures that the client will like what they are eating. Gradual change leads to better results in the long term than large changes made all at once (Foreyt and Goodrick, 1991). For example, if a person enjoys meat then teaching appropriate cooking techniques (in which the meat is trimmed and cooked with no added fat) can reduce energy intake without removing meat from the diet. Adapting frequently used recipes so they contain fewer calories is vital. Helping people focus on the foods they can eat rather than on the food they should perhaps limit can reassure clients that they have options and still achieve weight loss (Lyon *et al.*, 1995; Crombie, 1999).

Prader–Willi syndrome: special dietary needs

Prader–Willi syndrome (PWS) was named after Prader, Labhart and Willi in 1956. It is caused by an anomaly on the long arm of chromosome 15. Characterized by failure to thrive in infancy, neonates are hypotonic with insufficient suck and swallow reflexes. An increased appetite occurs during the toddler years. Affected individuals are developmentally delayed, with intelligence varying between moderate and borderline. They are short in stature, have low lean muscle mass and a high percentage of body fat, particularly in their distal limbs and trunk. Their RMR can be reduced by 20–50% if compared with height and weight respectively. Although they have the ability to expend as much energy as a non-PWS person, they tend to be less active. Their appetite becomes insatiable and non-selective. It is therefore not surprising that obesity is a consistent characteristic of this condition (Butler, 1990).

Their dietary requirements in infancy should follow normal infancy requirements. However, as their appetite grows, restrictions are needed. If a person with PWS consumes the same amount of calories as other individuals of the same age and height they will gain weight. Therefore, people with PWS require a low-energy diet to prevent obesity. To lose weight an individual with PWS requires a diet of 7–9 kcal/cm of height per day and for weight maintenance an energy intake of 8–14 kcal/cm per day is sufficient (Pipes and Holm, 1973; Ho and Pipes, 1976; Hoffman *et al.*, 1992). This applies for the child and the adult affected by Prader–Willi syndrome. This often translates into approximately 600–800 kcal per day for children and 800–1300 kcal for adolescents and adults. To start with, weighing food is probably necessary so that quantity is determined. Carers need a good understanding of the calorie content of food.

It is generally recommended that the macronutrient composition follows that of a healthy diet. The quality of food is important as quantity is limited, for example the protein eaten should be of high biological value, the carbohydrates high in fibre and the fats mostly in the form of mono- or polyunsaturates that are rich in omega 3. If a person with PWS follows the diet closely it is important that they take a multivitamin to meet micronutrient requirements. However, dietary compliance is often jeopardized as a person with PWS will seek out food from all sorts of sources such as bins, ground, people, shops (bought or stolen), open bags, unlocked cupboards or refrigerators and well-meaning acquaintances. The more supervision a person with PWS receives and the more consistent their routine, the lower the incidence of these behaviours.

A person with PWS likes routine and structure. Having meals at the same time every day can help limit tantrums and fights over food, which occur even in adulthood. Having very low-energy foods available can help deal with eating times but amounts should not vary drastically from meal to meal. Fortunately, people with PWS seem to prefer high-carbohydrate foods to high-fat foods, which helps when trying to find enjoyable low-energy foods for their consumption. If a person with PWS has diabetes, better diabetic control can be achieved by using low-GI carbohydrate choices. This tends to be successful if the person already has a regular, tightly controlled intake of carbohydrate of even distribution (which, if they are well managed, should be occurring).

A person with PWS has a constant preoccupation with food, even when they appear to be concentrating on something else. They will often scope out rooms to see if someone has been forgetful and left something out that they can reach. They can be very sneaky and will often hide food. Given the insatiable appetite and their need to seek food, locking cupboards and fridges in a home, supervising food preparation areas when in use and clearing away food (even scraps) immediately after finishing are important. This is often hard if there are people without PWS also living in the home. However, the person with PWS cannot control their desire to eat and no matter how hard you or they try, they will eat food if it is available to them. This also extends to the school or work environment, where rooms with bags should be locked and bins made inaccessible, and access to tearooms and to lockers should be limited. The PWS person appreciates these restrictions/strategies as they are often ostracized for their food-seeking actions. Other students may also give PWS students food, particularly if they are not well supervised. Restricting access to food in this way seems to contradict basic human rights of freedom of choice; however, someone with PWS eats not because they lack willpower or a weak character but because they have a genetic abnormality that leads to an uncontrollable and incurable hyperphagia (Pipes and Holm, 1973). These kinds of restriction help them to lead a healthy and happy life. Most deaths with PWS are due to complications of obesity. Money should also be restricted and not managed by the person with PWS as they will generally spend it on food.

Normal, low-energy cooking techniques should be used for this group of people. It again reduces tantrums if everyone at the dinner table is eating the same food. Perhaps portion sizes need to be predetermined. People with PWS love to eat large portions but will eat any food offered to them. For this reason, calories should be reduced in as many foods as possible so that quantity of food offered remains realistic.

It is important for every person that comes in contact with the individual with PWS to understand the need to restrict food. This can often be difficult particularly for grandparents and well-meaning adults. Giving these people information on PWS can help them to understand. If they are still having difficulties, a list of suitable food can help, for example diet versions of soft drinks or air-popped popcorn.

Appetite suppressants do not tend to work in this population. There has been some success with the use of VLED, but, as with any other person, the normal restrictive practices need to be in place to keep the weight off in the long term (Bistrian *et al.*, 1977).

People with PWS also want independence as they become older but unfortunately the nature of their condition does not allow them to be able to handle the freedom. This can be a very difficult time for both the family and the person with PWS. Linking in with PWS services, PWS-specific group homes and other community-based programmes can make this transition a lot easier.

The basic programme to follow from childhood (Pipes and Holm, 1973) is:

1 Determine baseline data of the child's caloric intake in relation to weight gain, and express as kcal per cm of height.
2 Educate child's primary carer on Prader–Willi syndrome, for example suitable diets/foods, caloric content, cooking methods, etc.
3 Involve immediate and extended family in the programme and necessary changes.
4 Control the environment, for example locking cupboards, fridges, etc.
5 Educate others who are involved with the child, for example teachers and peers.
6 Frequently monitor growth and intake.
7 Train the child to accept a food pattern that is compatible with a low-caloric diet and regular exercise.
8 Maintain changes and programmes throughout the child's life.

Maintenance/success

In today's obesogenic society, relapses are common particularly when people place unrealistic expectations on themselves. We know that weight maintenance is harder after weight loss, and that frequent weight cycling can be damaging to long-term maintenance (National Task Force on the Prevention and Treatment of Obesity, 1994).

Given that the goals during weight maintenance are slightly different from those of weight loss, it is not surprising that a different approach should be taken (Wadden, 1993). Requirements after weight loss are lower than the new body weight might suggest (Garner and Wooley, 1991). People believe that if they have been able to maintain their weight at the higher level then they will have no problems maintaining it at a lower level. This is not so. People need to change their habits for life, which often means adhering to certain levels of caloric restriction indefinitely (Garner and Wooley, 1991). Weight gain seems to occur even if the fat content of the diet remains low (Garner and Wooley, 1991).

What is success? Some have defined success as maintenance of all initial weight loss, or at least 9–11 kg of the original weight loss [a degree of weight loss associatied with significant improvement of obesity-related complications (Goldstein, 1992)]. The National Weight Control Registry in the USA defines success as at least 10% loss of initial body weight and which is maintained for at least 1 year (Wing and Hill, 2001).

The experience of the people from the registry can help to design appropriate maintenance programmes. It was found that 88% of participants in the registry reported restricting intake of certain types of food, 44% limited total quantity, 44% counted calories and 55% of the group used a commercial weight loss programme (Wing and Hill, 2001) (Fig. 22.7). They consumed on average 1381 kcal. Only 1% of the group ate diets that were low in carbohydrate. The total group ate approximately 4.9 meals/snacks per day and ate out 3.5 times per week, only once from a fast-food outlet. They avoided high-fat, fried foods and used low-fat substitutes. Other studies have shown that if cheese, butter, high-fat snacks, fried foods and desserts were eaten less than once per week then participants were more successful at long-term weight control (Holden *et al.*, 1992). French showed that reduced consumption of fried potato, dairy products, sweets and meat was positively correlated with weight loss and weight maintenance (French *et al.*, 1994). Characteristics of a small group of successful and unsuccessful dieters were compared in the UK

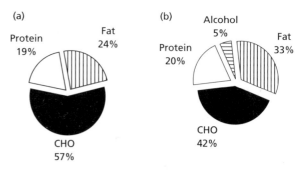

Fig 22.7 Macronutrient composition of successful 'dieters'. (a) Average diet composition from the National Weight Control Register in the USA. (b) Diet compositions of successful dieters in the UK.

(Fig. 22.7). The dietary factors that were significantly different from the unsuccessful dieters were the decreased total energy (achieved through decreased quantity of carbohydrate and fat) and the percentage of energy from protein. Also, the successful dieters had less emotional eating, were more restrained and less likely to eat in response to external cues (Kirk, 1997). Another interesting result from this study was that successful dieters found their 'allowed food' was good tasting, whereas the unsuccessful dieters did not always find this.

It is widely recognized that people find it hard to stick to changes in the long term. There is a period of high motivation at the beginning of the programme but motivation often wanes over time. Clinicians have to be realistic and acknowledge that it is unlikely that dietary intervention alone will maintain weight loss in obese subjects over a period of 2 or more years (Jakicic *et al.*, 2001).

Sources of recommendations or clinical guidelines on the management of obesity

A number of the reviews have provided recommendations or guidelines for management of obesity in adults (Scottish Intercollegiate Guidelines Network (SIGN) 1996; The National Heart, Lung, and Blood Institute (NHLBI), 1998, Douketis *et al.*, 1999). SIGN have also published useful guidance on the management of obesity in adults (SIGN, 1996). A US expert committee has published recommendations for the management of childhood obesity (Barlow and Dietz, 1998). A number of agencies have also published clinical guidelines for the management of childhood obesity [SIGN (available at http://www.sign.ac.uk); Royal College of Paediatrics, London]. The National Health and Medical Research Council of Australia has developed guidelines for the management of overweight and obesity in adults and children (http://www.health.gov.au/hfs/nhmrc/advice/mgtobsty.htm). The National Audit Office (NAO) published an important report on obesity in 2001 and has made a number of health policy recommendations (NAO, 2001).

Conclusion

Although there is little dispute that obesity is due at least in part to an excess energy intake, best results are usually achieved when both energy in and energy out are considered in the weight loss programme (Hirsch *et al.*, 1998; Astrup, 1999b; Holtmeier and Seim, 2000).

References

Anonymous (1993) Very low-calorie diets. National Task Force on the Prevention and Treatment of Obesity, National Institutes of Health.comment]. *Journal of the American Medical Association* **270**, 967–974.

Anonymous (1998) Clinical guidelines on the identification, evaluation, and treatment of overweight and obesity in adults: executive summary. Expert Panel on the Identification, Evaluation, and Treatment of Overweight in Adults. *American Journal of Clinical Nutrition* **68**, 899–917.

Ascott-Evans, B. (2002) The metabolic syndrome, insulin resistance and cardiovascular disease. *Cardiovascular Journal of Southern Africa* **13**, 187–188.

Astrup, A. (1998) The American paradox: the role of energy-dense fat-reduced food in the increasing prevalence of obesity. *Current Opinion in Clinical Nutrition and Metabolic Care* **1**, 573–577.

Astrup, A. (1999a) Dietary approaches to reducing body weight. *Best Practice and Research Clinical Endocrinology and Metabolism* **13**, 109–120.

Astrup, A. (1999b) Macronutrient balances and obesity: the role of diet and physical activity, *Public Health Nutrition* **2**, 341–347.

Astrup, A. and Rossner, S. (2000) Lessons from obesity management programmes: greater initial weight loss improves long-term maintenance. *Obesity Reviews* **1**, 17–19.

Astrup, A., Grunwald, G.K., Melanson, E.L., Saris, W.H. and Hill, J.O. (2000) The role of low-fat diets in body weight control: a meta-analysis of ad libitum dietary intervention studies. *International Journal of Obesity and Related Metabolic Disorders/Journal of the International Association for the Study of Obesity* **24**, 1545–1552.

Astrup, A., Buemann, B., Flint, A. and Raben, A. (2002) Low-fat diets and energy balance: how does the evidence stand in 2002? *Proceedings of the Nutrition Society* **61**, 299–309.

Barlow, S.E. and Dietz, W.H. (1998) Obesity evaluation and treatment: Expert Committee recommendations. The Maternal and Child Health Bureau, Health Resources and Services Administration and the Department of Health and Human Services. *Pediatrics* **102**, E29.

Beaudoin, R. and Mayer, J. (1953) Food intake of obese and non-obese women. *Journal of the American Dietetic Association* **29**, 29–34.

Bellisle, F., McDevitt, R. and Prentice, A.M. (1997) Meal frequency and energy balance. *British Journal of Nutrition* **77**, S57–70.

Bennett, G.A. (1986) Expectations in the treatment of obesity. *British Journal of Clinical Psychology* **25**, 311–312.

Berteus Forslund, H., Lindroos, A.K., Sjostrom, L. and Lissner, L. (2002) Meal patterns and obesity in Swedish women — a simple instrument describing usual meal types, frequency and temporal distribution. *European Journal of Clinical Nutrition* **56**, 740–747.

Biesalski, H.K. (1994) In: Ditschuneit, H., Gries, F.A., Hauner, H., Schusdziarra, V., Wechsler, J.G. eds. Essential requirements of long-term treatment of obesity. *Obesity in Europe 1993*. London: John Libbey and Co, 219–226.

Bingham, S. (1987) The dietary assessment of individuals; methods, accuracy, new techniques and recommendations. *Nutrition Abstracts and Reviews* **57**, 705–742.

Bistrian, B.R., Blackburn, G.L. and Stanbury, J.B. (1977) Metabolic aspects of a protein-sparing modified fast in the dietary management of Prader-Willi obesity. *New England Journal of Medicine* **296**, 774–779.

Bjorck, I., Liljeberg, H. and Ostman, E. (2000) Low glycaemic-index foods. *British Journal of Nutrition* **83**, S149–155.

Black, A.E., Goldberg, G.R., Jebb, S.A., Livingstone, M.B.E., Cole, T.L. and Prentice, A.M. (1991) Critical evaluation of energy intake using fundamental principles of energy physiology: 2. Evaluating the results of published surveys. *European Journal of Clinical Nutrition,* **45**, 583–599.

Brand, J.C., Nicholson, P.L., Thorburn, A.W. and Truswell, A.S. (1985) Food processing and the glycemic index. *American Journal of Clinical Nutrition* **42**, 1192–1196.

Brandon, J.E. (1987) Differences in self-reported eating and exercise behaviours and actual self-concept congruence between obese and non-obese individuals. *Health Values* **11**, 22–23.

Bravata, D., Sanders, L., Huang, J., Krumholz, H., Olkin, I., Gardner, C.D. and Bravata, D. (2003) Efficacy and safety of low-carbohydrate diets: a systematic review. *Journal of the American Medical Association* **289**, 1837–1850.

Bray, G.A. (1990) Obesity: historical development of scientific and cultural ideas. *International Journal of Obesity* **14**, 909–926.

British Dietetic Association (1996) *Position Paper on the Treatment of Obesity.* London: British Dietetic Association.

Brownell, K.D. (1993) Whether obesity should be treated. *Health Psychology* **12**, 339–341.

Burns, C.M., Tijhuis, M.A. and Seidell, J.C. (2001) The relationship between quality of life and perceived body weight and dieting history in Dutch men and women. *International Journal of Obesity and Related Metabolic Disorders/International Journal of Obesity* **25**, 1386–1392.

Butler, M.G. (1990) Prader-Willi syndrome: current understanding of cause and diagnosis. *American Journal of Medical Genetics* **35**, 319–332.

Case, C.C., Jones, P.H., Nelson, K. and Ballantyne, C.M. (2002) Impact of weight loss on the metabolic syndrome. *Diabetes* **51**, A608–A609.

de Castro, J.M. (1993) Genetic influences on daily intake and meal patterns of humans. *Physiology and Behavior* **53**, 777–782.

Coll, M., Meyer, A. and Stunkard, A.J. (1979) Obesity and food choices in public places. *Archives of General Psychiatry* **36**, 795–797.

Crombie, N. (1999) Obesity management. *Nursing Standard* **13**, 43–46.

Davis, A.M., Giles, A. and Rona, R. (2000) *Tackling Obesity: a Toolbox for Local Partnership Action.* London: Faculty of Public Health Medicine.

Dixon, J.B. and O'Brien, P.E. (2002) Changes in comorbidities and improvements in quality of life after LAP-BAND placement. *American Journal of Surgery* **184**, 51S–54S.

Dixon, J.B., Dixon, M.E. and O'Brien, P.E. (2001) Quality of life after lap-band placement: influence of time, weight loss, and comorbidities, *Obesity Research* **9**, 713–721.

Douketis, J.D., Feightner, J.W., Attia, J. and Feldman, W.F. (1999) Periodic health examination, 1999 update: 1. Detection, prevention and treatment of obesity. Canadian Task Force on Preventive Health Care. *Canadian Medical Association Journal* **160**, 513–525.

Drewnowski, A. and Greenwood, M.R. (1983) Cream and sugar: human preferences for high-fat foods. *Physiology and Behavior* **30**, 629–633.

Fleisch, A. (1951) Le metabolisme basal standard et sa determination au moyen du "Metabocalculator". *Helvetica Medica Acta* **1**, 23–44.

Fleming, R.M. (2000) The effect of high-protein diets on coronary blood flow. *Angiology* **51**, 817–826.

Fleming, R.M. (2002) The effect of high-, moderate-, and low-fat diets on weight loss and cardiovascular disease risk factors. *Preventive Cardiology* **5**, 110–118.

Foreyt, J.P. and Goodrick, G.K. (1991) Factors common to successful therapy for the obese patient. *Medicine and Science in Sports and Exercise* **23**, 292–297.

Foster, G.D., Wyatt, H.R., Hill, J.O., McGuckin, B.G., Brill, C.,

Mohammed, B.S., Szapary, P.O., Rader, D.J., Edman, J.S. and Klein, S. (2003) A randomized trial of a low-carbohydrate diet for obesity [comment]. *New England Journal of Medicine* **348**, 2082–2090.

French, S.A., Jeffery, R.W., Forster, J.L., McGovern, P.G., Kelder, S.H. and Baxter, J.E. (1994) Predictors of weight change over two years among a population of working adults: the Healthy Worker Project. *International Journal of Obesity and Related Metabolic Disorders/Journal of the International Association for the Study of Obesity* **18**, 145–154.

Fricker, J., Fumeron, F., Clair, D. and Apfelbaum, M. (1989) A positive correlation between energy intake and BMI in a population of 1312 overweight subjects. *International Journal of Obesity* **13**, 673–681.

Frost, G. and Pirani, S. (1987) Meal frequency and nutritional intake during Ramadan: a pilot study. *Human Nutrition — Applied Nutrition* **41**, 47–50.

Frost, G., Masters, K., King, C., Kelly, M., Hasan, U., Heavens, P., White, R. and Standford, J. (1991) A new method of energy prescription to improve weight loss. *Journal of Human Nutrition and Dietetics* **4**, 369–373.

Frost, G., Keogh, B., Smith, D., Akinsanya, K. and Leeds, A. (1996) The effect of low-glycemic carbohydrate on insulin and glucose response *in vivo* and *in vitro* in patients with coronary heart disease. *Metabolism: Clinical and Experimental* **45**, 669–672.

Frost, G., Leeds, A., Trew, G., Margara, R. and Dornhorst, A. (1998) Insulin sensitivity in women at risk of coronary heart disease and the effect of a low glycemic diet. *Metabolism: Clinical and Experimental* **47**, 1245–1251.

Frost, G., Leeds, A.A., Dore, C.J., Madeiros, S., Brading, S. and Dornhorst, A. (1999) Glycaemic index as a determinant of serum HDL-cholesterol concentration [comment]. *Lancet* **353**, 1045–1048.

Gaesser, G.A. and Miller, W.C. (1999) Symposium: has body weight become an unhealthy obsession? *Medicine and Science in Sports and Exercise* **31**, 1118–1146.

Gannon, M.C., Nuttall, F.Q., Krezowski, P.A., Billington, C.J. and Parker, S. (1986) The serum insulin and plasma glucose responses to milk and fruit products in type 2 (non-insulin-dependent) diabetic patients. *Diabetologia* **29**, 784–791.

Garner, D.M. and Wooley, S.C. (1991) Confronting the failure of behavioral and dietary treatments for obesity. *Clinical Psychology Review* **11**, 729–780.

Garrow, J. and Summerbell, C. (2000) In: Stevens, A., Raftery, J. eds. Obesity. *Health Care Needs Assessment: the Epidemiologically Based Needs Assessment Reviews: 3rd Series.* Abingdon: Radcliffe Medical Press.

Garrow, J.S. (1988) *Obesity and Related Disease.* Edinburgh: Churchill Livingstone,.

Garrow, J.S. (1991) The safety of dieting. *Proceedings of the Nutrition Society* **50**, 493–499.

Garrow, J.S. (1995) Slimming products: a success in court. *Healthwatch* **18**, 8.

Gibney, M.J. (1992) Are there conflicts in dietary advice for prevention of different diseases? *Proceedings of the Nutrition Society* **51**, 35–45.

Glenny, A.M., O'Meara, S., Melville, A., Sheldon, T.A. and Wilson, C. (1997) The treatment and prevention of obesity: a systematic review of the literature. *International Journal of Obesity* **21**, 715–737.

Golay, A., Eigenheer, C., Morel, Y., Kujawski, P., Lehmann, T. and de Tonnac, N. (1996) Weight loss with low or high carbohydrate diet? *International Journal of Obesity and Related Metabolic Disorders/Journal of the International Association for the Study of Obesity* **20**, 1067–1072.

Goldstein, D.J. (1992) Beneficial health effects of modest weight loss. *International Journal of Obesity and Related Metabolic Disorders/Journal of the International Association for the Study of Obesity* **16**, 397–415.

Goodrick, G.K., Poston, I.W., Kimball, K.T., Reeves, R.S. and Foreyt, J.P. (1998) Non-dieting versus dieting treatment for overweight binge eating women. *Journal of Consulting and Clinical Psychology* **66**, 363–368.

Granfeldt, Y., Eliasson, A.C. and Bjorck, I. (2000) An examination of the possibility of lowering the glycemic index of oat and barley flakes by minimal processing. *Journal of Nutrition* **130**, 2207–2214.

Haus, G., Hoerr, S.L., Mavis, B. and Robison, J. (1994) Key modifiable factors in weight maintenance: fat intake, exercise, and weight cycling. *Journal of the American Dietetic Association* **94**, 409–413.

Heaney, R.P., Davies, K.M. and Barger-Lux, M.J. (2002) Calcium and weight: clinical studies. *Journal of the American College of Nutrition* **21**, 152S–155S.

Heitmann, B.L. and Lissner, L. (1995) Dietary underreporting by obese individuals: is it specific or non-specific? *British Medical Journal* **311**, 986–989.

Heitmann, B.L., Lissner, L., Sorensen, T.I. and Bengtsson, C. (1995) Dietary fat intake and weight gain in women genetically predisposed for obesity. *American Journal of Clinical Nutrition* **61**, 1213–1217.

Heshka, S., Feld, K., Yang, M.U., Allison, D.B. and Heymsfield, S.B. (1993) Resting energy expenditure in the obese: a cross-validation and comparison of prediction equations. *Journal of the American Dietetic Association* **93**, 1031–1036.

Hirsch, J., Hudgins, L.C., Leibel, R.L. and Rosenbaum, M. (1998) Diet composition and energy balance in humans. *American Journal of Clinical Nutrition* **67**, 551S–555S.

Ho, V.A. and Pipes, P.L. (1976) Food and children with Prader-Willi syndrome. *American Journal of Diseases of Childhood* **130**, 1063–1067.

Hoffman, C.J., Aultman, D. and Pipes, P. (1992) A nutrition survey of and recommendations for individuals with Prader-Willi syndrome who live in group homes. *Journal of the American Dietetic Association* **92**, 823–830, 833.

Holden, J.H., Darga, L.L., Olson, S.M., Stettner, D.C., Ardito, E.A. and Lucas, C.P. (1992) Long-term follow-up of patients attending a combination very-low calorie diet and behaviour therapy weight loss programme. *International Journal of Obesity and Related Metabolic Disorders/Journal of the International Association for the Study of Obesity* **16**, 605–613.

Holtmeier, K.B. and Seim, H.C. (2000) The diet prescription for obesity. What works? *Minnesota Medicine* **83**, 28–32.

Hughes, J. and Martin, S. (1999) The Department of Health's project to evaluate weight management services. *Journal of Human Nutrition and Dietetics* **12**, 1–8.

Hung, T., Sievenpiper, J.L., Marchie, A., Kendall, C.W.C. and Jenkins, D.J. (2003) Fat versus carbohydrate in insulin resistance, obesity, diabetes and cardiovascular disease. *Current Opinion in Clinical Nutrition and Metabolic Care* **6**, 165–176.

Hunt, P. (2000) *So You Want to Lose Weight . . . for Good: a Guide to Losing Weight for Men and Women*. Publication M3. British Heart Foundation.

Jakicic, J.M., Clark, K., Coleman, E., Donnelly, J.E., Foreyt, J., Melanson, E., Volek, J. and Volpe, S.L. (2001) Appropriate intervention strategies for weight loss and prevention of weight regain for adults. *Medicine and Science in Sports and Exercise* **33**, 2145–2156.

Jarvi, A.E., Karlstrom, B.E., Granfeldt, Y.E., Bjorck, I.E., Asp, N.G. and Vessby, B.O. (1999) Improved glycemic control and lipid profile and normalized fibrinolytic activity on a low-glycemic index diet in type 2 diabetic patients, *Diabetes Care* **22**, 10–18.

Jeffery, R., Hellerstedt, W.L., French, S.A. and Baxter, J.E. (1995) A randomized trial of counseling for fat restriction versus calorie restriction in the treatment of obesity. *International Journal of Obesity* **19**, 132–137.

Jenkins, D.J., Jenkins, A.L., Wolever, T.M., Vuksan, V., Rao, A.V., Thompson, L.U. and Josse, R.G. (1994) Low glycemic index: lente carbohydrates and physiological effects of altered food frequency. *American Journal of Clinical Nutrition* **59**, 706S–709S.

Jenkins, D.J., Vuksan, V., Kendall, C.W., Wursch, P., Jeffcoat, R., Waring, S., Mehling, C.C., Vidgen, E., Augustin, L.S. and Wong, E. (1998) Physiological effects of resistant starches on fecal bulk, short chain fatty acids, blood lipids and glycemic index. *Journal of the American College of Nutrition* **17**, 609–616.

Kabir, M., Rizkalla, S.W., Champ, M., Luo, J., Boillot, J., Bruzzo, F. and Slama, G. (1998) Dietary amylose-amylopectin starch content affects glucose and lipid metabolism in adipocytes of normal and diabetic rats. *Journal of Nutrition* **128**, 35–43.

Kausman, R., Murphy, M., O'Connor, T. and Schattner, P. (2003) Audit of a behaviour modification program for weight management. *Australian Family Physician* **32**, 89–91.

Khaodhiar, L. and Blackburn, G.L. (2002) Obesity treatment: factors involved in weight loss maintenance and regain. *Current Opinion in Endocrinology and Diabetes* **9**, 369–374.

Kirk, S.F.L. (1997) Exploring the food beliefs and eating behaviour of successful and unsuccessful dieters. *Journal of Human Nutrition and Dietetics* **10**, 331–341.

Klauer, J.M. and Aronne, L.J.M. (2002) Managing overweight and obesity in women. *Clinical Obstetrics and Gynecology* **45**, 1080–1088.

Klem, M.L., Wing, R.R., McGuire, M.T., Seagle, H.M. and Hill, J.O. (1997) A descriptive study of individuals successful at long-term maintenance of substantial weight loss [comment]. *American Journal of Clinical Nutrition* **66**, 239–246.

Knowler, W.C., Barrett-Connor, E., Fowler, S.E., Hamman, R.F., Lachin, J.M., Walker, E.A., Nathan, D.M. and Diabetes Prevention Program Research. (2002) Reduction in the incidence of type 2 diabetes with lifestyle intervention or metformin [comment]. *New England Journal of Medicine* **346**, 393–403.

Kuller, L.H., Simkin-Silverman, L.R., Wing, R.R., Meilahn, E.N. and Ives, D.G. (2001) Women's Healthy Lifestyle Project: A randomized clinical trial: results at 54 months. *Circulation* **103**, 32–37.

Lamberg, L. (2000) Psychiatric help may shrink some waistlines. *Journal of the American Medical Association* **284**, 291–293.

Lantz, H., Peltonen, M., Agren, L. and Torgerson, J. S. (2003) Intermittent versus on-demand use of a very low calorie diet: A randomized 2-year clinical trial. *Journal of Internal Medicine* **253**, 463–471.

Liebermeister, H. (1994) In: Ditschuneit, H., Gries, F.A., Hauner, H., Schusdziarra, V., Wechsler, J.G. eds. Novelties and curiosities: miracle diets in the treatment of obesity. *Obesity in Europe 1993*. London: John Libbey and Co, 263–267.

Liljeberg, H. and Bjorck, I. (1998) Delayed gastric emptying rate may explain improved glycaemia in healthy subjects to a starchy meal with added vinegar. *European Journal of Clinical Nutrition* **52**, 368–371.

Liljeberg, H.G., Granfeldt, Y.E. and Bjorck, I.M. (1996) Products based on a high fiber barley genotype, but not on common barley or oats, lower postprandial glucose and insulin responses in healthy humans. *Journal of Nutrition* **126**, 458–466.

Lindroos, A.K., Lissner, L. and Sjostrom, L. (1993) Validity and reproducibility of a self-administered dietary questionnaire in obese and non-obese subjects. *European Journal of Clinical Nutrition* **47**, 461–481.

Lissner, L. and Heitmann, B.L. (1995) Dietary fat and obesity: evidence from epidemiology. *European Journal of Clinical Nutrition* **49**, 79–90.

Liu, S., Willett, W.C., Stampfer, M.J., Hu, F.B., Franz, M., Sampson, L., Hennekens, C.H. and Manson, J.E. (2000) A prospective study of dietary glycemic load, carbohydrate intake, and risk of coronary heart disease in US women [comment]. *American Journal of Clinical Nutrition* **71**, 1455–1461.

Lopez de la Torre Casares, M. (1999) [Obesity and quality of life.] *Nutricion Hospitalaria* **14**, 177–183.

Low, C.C., Grossman, E.B. and Gumbiner, B. (1996) Potentiation of effects of weight loss by monounsaturated fatty acids in obese NIDDM patients. *Diabetes* **45**, 569–575.

Lowe, M.R., Miller-Kovach, K. and Phelan, S. (2001) Weight loss maintenance in overweight individuals one to five years following successful completion of a commercial weight loss program. *International Journal of Obesity and Related Metabolic Disorders/ Journal of the International Association for the Study of Obesity* **25**, 325–331.

Lyon, X.-H., Di Vetta, V., Milon, H., Jequier, E. and Schutz, Y. (1995) Compliance to dietary advice directed towards increasing the carbohydrate to fat ratio of the everyday diet. *International Journal of Obesity* **19**, 260–269.

Mellin, L., Croughan-Minihane, M. and Dickey, L. (1997) The Solution Method: 2-year trends in weight, blood pressure, exercise, depression, and functioning of adults trained in development skills. *Journal of the American Dietetic Association* **97**, 1133–1138.

Miller, W.C. and Jacob, A.V. (2001) The health at any size paradigm for obesity treatment: the scientific evidence. *Obesity Reviews* **2**, 37–45.

Morris, K.L. and Zemel, M.B. (1999) Glycemic index, cardiovascular disease, and obesity [comment]. *Nutrition Reviews* **57**, 273–276.

National Audit Office (2001) *Tackling Obesity in England*. London: The Stationery Office.

National Heart, Lung, and Blood Institute (1998) *Clinical Guidelines on the Identification, Evaluation and Treatment of Overweight and Obesity in Adults. The Evidence Report*. Bethesda, MD: NIH.

National Heart, Lung, and Blood Institute (1999) *Aim for a Healthy Weight*. Bethesda, MD: NIH.

National Obesity Forum (2001) *National Obesity Forum Guidelines on Management of Adult Obesity and Overweight in Primary Care*. Nottingham: National Obesity Forum.

National Task Force on the Prevention and Treatment of Obesity (1994) Weight cycling. *Journal of the American Medical Association* **272**, 1196–1206.

Noakes, M. and Clifton, P.M. (2000) Weight loss and plasma lipids. *Current Opinion in Lipidology* **11**, 65–70.

Norton, R.A. (1995) 2000 diabetes. The right mix of diet and exercise, *RN* **58**, 20–24; quiz, 25.

Paisey, R.B., Frost, J., Harvey, P., Paisey, A., Bower, L., Paisey, R.M., Taylor, P. and Belka, I. (2002) Five year results of a prospective very low calorie diet or conventional weight loss programme in type 2 diabetes. *Journal of Human Nutrition and Dietetics* **15**, 121–127.

Pipes, P.L. and Holm, V.A. (1973) Weight control of children with Prader-Willi syndrome. *Journal of the American Dietetic Association* **62**, 520–524.

Pirozzo, S., Summerbell, C., Cameron, C. and Glasziou, P. (2002) Advice on low-fat diets for obesity[comment]. *Cochrane Database of Systematic Reviews*, CD003640.

Pi-Sunyer, F.X. (1993) National Institutes of Health Technology Assessment Conference: Short-term medical benefits and adverse effects of weight loss. *Annals of Internal Medicine* **119**, 722–726.

Poston, 2nd, W.S. and Foreyt, J.P. (2000) Successful management of the obese patient [erratum appears in *American Family Physician* 2000 Nov 1; 62(9): 1967]. *American Family Physician* **61**, 3615–3622.

Raben, A. (2002) Should obese patients be counselled to follow a low glycaemic index diet? NO. *Obesity Reviews* **3**, 245–256.

Raynor, H.A. and Epstein, L.H. (2001) Dietary variety, energy regulation, and obesity. *Psychological Bulletin* **127**, 325–341.

Robinson, J.D. and Reid, D.D. (1952) Standards for the basal metabolism of normal people in Britain. *Lancet* **1**, 940–943.

Rolls, B.J. (1986) Sensory-specific satiety. *Nutrition Reviews* **44**, 93–101.

Ross, S.W., Brand, J.C., Thorburn, A.W. and Truswell, A.S. (1987) Glycemic index of processed wheat products. *American Journal of Clinical Nutrition* **46**, 631–635.

Roughead, Z.K., Johnson, L.K., Lykken, G.I. and Hunt, J.R. (2003) Controlled high meat diets do not affect calcium retention or indices of bone status in healthy postmenopausal women, *Journal of Nutrition* **133**, 1020–1026.

Saris, W.H. (2001) Very-low-calorie diets and sustained weight loss. *Obesity Research* **9**, 295S–301S.

Sbrocco, T., Nedegaard, R.C., Stone, J.M. and Lewis, E.L. (1999) Behavioral choice treatment promotes continuing weight loss: preliminary results of a cognitive–behavioral decision-based treatment for obesity. *Journal of Consulting and Clinical Psychology* **67**, 260–266.

Schlundt, D.G., Sbrocco, T. and Bell, C. (1989) Identification of high-risk situations in a behavioral weight loss program: application of the relapse prevention model. *International Journal of Obesity* **13**, 223–234.

Scottish Intercollegiate Guidelines Network (1996) *Integrating Prevention with Weight Management*. Guideline no. 8. Edinburgh: Royal College of Physicians.

Shi, H., Dirienzo, D. and Zemel, M.B. (2001) Effects of dietary calcium on adipocyte lipid metabolism and body weight regulation in energy-restricted aP2-Agouti transgenic mice. *FASEB Journal* **15**, 291–293.

Slabber, M., Barnard, H.C., Kuyl, J.M., Dannhauser, A. and Schall, R. (1994) Effects of a low-insulin-response, energy-restricted diet on weight loss and plasma insulin concentrations in hyperinsulinemic obese females., *American Journal of Clinical Nutrition* **60**, 48–53.

Speechly, D.P. and Buffenstein, R. (1999) Greater appetite control associated with an increased frequency of eating in lean males. *Appetite* **33**, 285–297.

Speechly, D.P., Rogers, G.G. and Buffenstein, R. (1999) Acute appetite reduction associated with an increased frequency of eating in obese males. *International Journal of Obesity and Related Metabolic Disorders/Journal of the International Association for the Study of Obesity* **23**, 1151–1159.

St Jeor, S.T., Howard, B.V., Prewitt, T.E., Bovee, V., Bazzarre, T., Eckel, R.H., Nutrition Committee of the Council on Nutrition and Metabolism of the American Heart Association (2001) Dietary protein and weight reduction: a statement for healthcare professionals from the Nutrition Committee of the Council on Nutrition, Physical Activity, and Metabolism of the American Heart Association [comment]. *Circulation* **104**, 1869–1874.

Stubbs, R.J., Ritz, P., Coward, W.A. and Prentice, A.M. (1995) Covert manipulation of the ratio of dietary fat to carbohydrate and energy density: effect on food intake and energy balance in free-living men eating *ad libitum*. *American Journal of Clinical Nutrition* **62**, 330–337.

Stubbs, R.J., Johnstone, A.M., Mazlan, N., Mbaiwa, S.E. and Ferris, S. (2001) Effect of altering the variety of sensorially distinct foods, of the same macronutrient content, on food intake and body weight in men. *European Journal of Clinical Nutrition* **55**, 19–28.

Summerbell, C.D., Moody, R.C., Shanks, J., Stock, M.J. and Geissler, C. (1995) Sources of energy from meals versus snacks in 220 people in four age groups. *European Journal of Clinical Nutrition* **49**, 33–41.

Summerbell, C.D., Moody, R.C., Shanks, J., Stock, M.J. and Geissler, C. (1996) Relationship between feeding pattern and body mass index in 220 free-living people in four age groups. *European Journal of Clinical Nutrition* **50**, 513–519.

Tanco, S., Linden, W. and Earle, T. (1998) Well-being and morbid obesity in women: a controlled therapy evaluation. *International Journal of Eating Disorders* **23**, 325–339.

Tapper-Gardzina, Y., Cotugna, N. and Vickery, C.E. (2002) Should you recommend a low-carb, high-protein diet? [summary for patients in *Nurse Practitioner*. 2002 Apr; 27(4): 57; PMID: 12003009]. *Nurse Practitioner* **27**, 52–53, 55–56, 58–59.

Thomsen, C., Christiansen, C., Rasmussen, O.W. and Hermansen, K. (1997) Comparison of the effects of two weeks' intervention with different meal frequencies on glucose metabolism, insulin sensitivity and lipid levels in non-insulin-dependent diabetic patients. *Annals of Nutrition and Metabolism* **41**, 173–180.

Toeller, M., Buyken, A.E., Heitkamp, G., Cathelineau, G., Ferriss, B., Michel, G. and Group, E.I.C.S. (2001) Nutrient intakes as predictors of body weight in European people with type 1 diabetes. *International Journal of Obesity and Related Metabolic Disorders/Journal of the International Association for the Study of Obesity* **25**, 1815–1822.

Toubro, S. and Astrup, A. (1997) Randomised comparison of diets for maintaining obese subjects' weight after major weight loss: ad lib, low fat, high carbohydrate diet v fixed energy intake. *British Medical Journal* **314**, 29–34.

Tremblay, A., Doucet, E. and Imbeault, P. (1999) Physical activity and weight maintenance. *International Journal of Obesity and Related Metabolic Disorders/Journal of the International Association for the Study of Obesity* **23**, S50–54.

Trout, D. and Behall, K.M. (1999) Prediction of glycemic index among high-sugar, low-starch foods. *International Journal of Food Science and Nutrition* **50**, 135–144.

Trout, D.L., Behall, K.M. and Osilesi, O. (1993) Prediction of glycemic index for starchy foods. *American Journal of Clinical Nutrition* **58**, 873–878.

Tuomilehto, J., Lindstrom, J., Eriksson, J.G., Valle, T.T., Hamalainen, H., Ilanne-Parikka, P., Keinanen-Kiukaanniemi, S., Laakso, M., Louheranta, A., Rastas, M., Salminen, V., Uusitupa, M. and Finnish Diabetes Prevention Study. (2001) Prevention of type 2 diabetes mellitus by changes in lifestyle among subjects with impaired glucose tolerance [comment]. *New England Journal of Medicine* **344**, 1343–1350.

Verboeket-van de Venne, W.P. and Westerterp, K.R. (1991) Influence of the feeding frequency on nutrient utilization in man: consequences for energy metabolism. *European Journal of Clinical Nutrition* **45**, 161–169.

Wadden, T.A. (1993) In: Stunkard, A., Wadden, T. eds. The treatment of obesity: an overview. *Obesity: Theory and Therapy*. New York: Raven Press, 197–217.

Weiner, R., Datz, M., Wagner, D. and Bockhorn, H. (1999) Quality-of-life outcome after laparoscopic adjustable gastric banding for morbid obesity. *Obesity Surgery* **9**, 539–545.

Westerterp-Plantenga, M.S., Kovacs, E.M. and Melanson, K.J. (2002) Habitual meal frequency and energy intake regulation in partially temporally isolated men. *International Journal of Obesity and Related Metabolic Disorders/Journal of the International Association for the Study of Obesity* **26**, 102–110.

Willett, W.C. (2002) Dietary fat plays a major role in obesity: no [comment]. *Obesity Reviews* **3**, 59–68.

Willi, S.M., Wise, K.L., Welch, A.S. and Key, Jr, L.L. (1998a) A ketogenic very low calorie diet (VLCD) in the treatment of children with NIDDM + 500. *Pediatric Research Program Issue APS-SPR* **43**, 88.

Willi, S.M., Oexmann, M.J., Wright, N.M., Collop, N.A. and Key, Jr, L.L. (1998b) The effects of a high-protein, low-fat, ketogenic diet on adolescents with morbid obesity: body composition, blood chemistries, and sleep abnormalities. *Pediatrics* **101**, 61–67.

Williams, K.V., Mullen, M.L., Kelley, D.E. and Wing, R.R. (1998) The effect of short periods of caloric restriction on weight loss and glycemic control in type 2 diabetes. *Diabetes Care* **21**, 2–8.

Wing, R.R. and Hill, J.O. (2001) Successful weight loss maintenance. *Annual Review of Nutrition* **21**, 323–341.

Wing, R.R., Epstein, L.H., Marcus, M.D. and Kupfer, D.J. (1984) Mood changes in behavioral weight loss programs. *Journal of Psychosomatic Research* **28**, 189–196.

Wolever, T.M. (1987) Food glycaemic index or meal glycaemic response? *Human Nutrition — Applied Nutrition* **41**, 434–435.

Wolever, T.M. and Jenkins, D.J. (1985) Application of glycaemic index to mixed meals. *Lancet* **2**, 944.

Wolever, T.M. and Jenkins, D.J. (1986) The use of the glycemic index in predicting the blood glucose response to mixed meals. *American Journal of Clinical Nutrition* **43**, 167–172.

Wolever, T.M., Jenkins, D.J., Ocana, A.M., Rao, V.A. and Collier, G.R. (1988) Second-meal effect: low-glycemic-index foods eaten at dinner improve subsequent breakfast glycemic response. *American Journal of Clinical Nutrition* **48**, 1041–1047.

Wolever, T.M., Jenkins, D.J., Jenkins, A.L. and Josse, R.G. (1991) The glycemic index: methodology and clinical implications. *American Journal of Clinical Nutrition* **54**, 846–854.

Wolfram, G., Kirchgessner, M., Muller, H. L. and Hollomey, S. (1987) [Thermogenesis in humans after varying meal time frequency.] *Annals of Nutrition and Metabolism* **31**, 88–97.

Yu-Poth, S., Zhao, G., Etherton, T., Naglak, M., Jonnalagadda, S. and Kris-Etherton, P.M. (1999) Effects of the National Cholesterol Education Program's Step I and Step II dietary intervention programs on cardiovascular disease risk factors: a meta-analysis [comment]. *American Journal of Clinical Nutrition* **69**, 632–646.

Zambon, A., Sartore, G., Passera, D., Francini-Pesenti, F., Bassi, A., Basso, C., Zambon, S., Manzato, E. and Crepaldi, G. (1999) Effects of hypocaloric dietary treatment enriched in oleic acid on LDL and HDL subclass distribution in mildly obese women. *Journal of Internal Medicine* **246**, 191–201.

Appendix

Key documents and information sources on obesity	How to access
Toolkits/recommendations/clinical guidelines for health professionals on managing obesity, based on systematic reviews of the evidence	
The National Heart, Lung, and Blood Institute (NHLBI, 1998). Clinical Guidelines on the Identification, Evaluation, and Treatment of Overweight and Obesity in Adults. The Evidence Report	http://www.nhlbi.nih.gov/guidelines/obesity/ob_home.ht
The National Heart, Lung, and Blood Institute (NHLBI, 1998). A practical guide to The Evidence Report	http://www.nhlbi.nih.gov/guidelines/obesity/prctgd_c.pdf
The National Heart, Lung, and Blood Institute (NHLBI, 1999). Aim for a Healthy Weight is an excellent interactive website for both health professionals and patients. It lists a number of useful strategies to help treat obesity, based on the Evidence Report (NHLBI, 1998). Examples of weight goal records, food substitution ideas and food preparation leaflets, a guide to behavioural change strategies and exercise programmes for gradual build-up of activity/fitness are included. Consideration should be given to make this available to health professionals	http://www.nhlbi.nih.gov/health/public/heart/obesity/lose_wt/index.htm
Scottish Intercollegiate Guidelines Network Obesity in Scotland (SIGN, 1996). Integrating prevention with weight management	http://www.sign.ac.uk/
Douketis *et al.*, with the Canadian Task Force on Preventative Health Care (1999). Periodic health examination, 1999 update: 1. Detection, prevention and treatment of obesity	See reference
Barlow and Dietz (1998). Obesity evaluation and treatment: expert committee recommendations	www.pediatrics.org/cgi/content/full/102/3/e29
International Obesity Task Force (IOTF). Excellent website for international information regarding all areas of obesity on a global level	www.iotf.org
Australasian Society for the Study of Obesity (ASSO). The Asian Pacific region's scientific society, which reports on new developments in all areas of obesity research	www.asso.org.au
A comprehensive overview of obesity as part of the Health Care Assessment Series. It covers the epidemiological data, services available and the effectiveness of interventions of the prevention and treatment of obesity in adults and children (Garrow and Summerbell, 2000)	http://hcna.radcliffe-online.com/obframe.html
Toolkits/recommendations/clinical guidelines for health professionals on managing obesity, which are not based on systematic reviews of the evidence	
International Agency for Research on Cancer (IARC, 2001). Report of International Working Group — The role of weight control and physical activity in cancer prevention	http://www.iarc.fr/pageroot/UNITS/Chemoprevention2.html
Faculty of Public Health Medicine, London. Tackling obesity: a toolbox for local partnership action. (Davis *et al.*, 2000)	Tel: 0207 935 0243 email: enquiries@fphm.org.uk

Hunt, P. (2000). *So You Want to Lose Weight . . . For Good: a Guide to Losing Weight for Men and Women.* Publication No. M3. British Heart Foundation — http://www.bhf.org.uk/publications/secure/z_index.html

National Obesity Forum (NOF, 2001) Guidelines on management of adult obesity and overweight in Primary Care — http://www.nationalobesityforum.org.uk

Other useful resources

A directory of projects of weight management, compiled by the Department of Health, is available in each Regional Office. Three main themes emerged; that weight loss is rarely maintained, that multicomponent programmes are more successful and that regular follow-up is important (Hughes and Martin, 1999) — See reference

Clinical Evidence (2001). Relevant sections. A summary of the evidence from systematic reviews, where available, on various health related topics — Available via the NeLH website (http://www.nelh.nhs.uk/default.asp)

National Audit Office (NAO, 2001). Tackling Obesity in England — http://www.nao.gov.uk

World Health Organization (WHO, 1999). Obesity: Preventing and Managing the Global Epidemic — http://www.iotf.org/

Health Development Agency (HAD). Evidence Base — http://www.hda-online.org.uk/html/research/evidencebase.html

Cochrane Systematic Reviews on Obesity

Low-fat diets for the treatment of obesity (Pirrozo et al., 2002) — Available via the NeLH website (http://www.nelh.nhs.uk/default.asp)

Interventions for preventing obesity in childhood (Campbell et al., 2002)

Interventions for treating obesity in childhood (Summerbell et al., 2002)

Intervention for improving health professionals' management of obesity (Harvey et al., 2001)

Organizations dedicated to obesity

The International Obesity Task Force — http://www.iotf.org/

Association for the Study of Obesity — http://www.aso.org.uk

Patient-centred organizations/charities

National Association to Advance Fat Acceptance (NAFFA) — http://www.naafa.org/

The Obesity Awareness and Solutions Trust (TOAST) — http://www.toast-uk.org.uk/

Weight Concern — Brook House, 2–16 Torrington Place, London WC1E 7HN

23 Behavioural treatment of obesity: achievements and challenges

Thomas A. Wadden and Vicki L. Clark

Introduction, 350

Principles of behaviour therapy, 350
    Overview and defining
    features, 350
    Attending to consequences, 351
    Facilitating behaviour change, 351

Components of behavioural
treatment, 351
    Self-monitoring, 351
    Stimulus control, 352
    Cognitive restructuring, 352
    Dietary interventions, 352
    Physical activity, 354

Time-limited treatment delivery, 355

Group vs. individual treatment, 355

Treatment providers, 355

Short-term results, 355

Long-term results, 356

Improving the maintenance of
weight loss, 356
    Long-term treatment, 356
    High levels of physical
    activity, 357

Dietary options for long-term
    weight control, 357

New directions in behavioural
treatment, 358
    Internet and e-mail, 358
    Commercial programmes, 358
    Primary-care practice, 359

Tackling the toxic environment, 359

References, 359

Introduction

Modest weight loss may improve many of the health complications of obesity, as demonstrated recently by the Diabetes Prevention Program (DPP) (Diabetes Prevention Program Research Group, 2002). In this randomized controlled trial, 3200 overweight individuals with impaired glucose tolerance were assigned to: (a) a lifestyle intervention consisting of diet, exercise and behaviour modification; (b) metformin (850 mg b.i.d.); or (c) placebo. Patients in the lifestyle intervention lost an average of 7 kg in the first year and were found at 2.8 years to have reduced their risk of developing type 2 diabetes by 58% compared with placebo-treated participants. Other studies have shown improvements in hypertension, sleep apnoea and other weight-related health complications with a loss of 5–10% of initial weight (Goldstein, 1992; Blackburn, 1995).

The National Heart, Lung, and Blood Institute (NHLBI) has provided an algorithm to guide the treatment of obesity (see Table 23.1). Individuals with a body mass index (BMI) of 25–29.9 kg/m², who have no risk factors, are encouraged to take steps to prevent weight gain. Those of similar BMI, with two or more risk factors, are advised to lose weight, as are persons with a BMI ≥ 30 kg/m² (regardless of other risk factors). A programme of diet, exercise and behaviour modification is indicated as a first course of treatment for all overweight and obese individuals. This chapter describes behaviour modification for obesity, which can be used to facilitate adherence to a variety of diet and exercise regimens. We review the components of behaviour therapy for obesity, examine its short- and long-term results and discuss new directions for intervention.

Principles of behaviour therapy

The principles are outlined below.

Overview and defining features

Behaviour therapy provides a set of principles and techniques to help people modify their eating and activity habits. This approach recognizes that obesity is influenced by metabolic and genetic factors (Ravussin et al., 1988; Stunkard et al., 1990; Campfield et al., 1995), but believes that recent increases in the prevalence of obesity are attributable primarily to changes in our nation's eating and activity habits (Wadden et al., 2002). Behavioural treatment seeks to teach patients to modify these habits, in part by examining the antecedents and consequences of their behaviours. This approach incorporates principles of classical conditioning, which hold that two events will become linked together if they are paired repeatedly (Brownell, 2000; Wing, 2002). Moreover, the more frequently

Table 23.1 A guide to selecting treatment.

Treatment	BMI category					
	< 24	25–26.9	27–29.9	30–35	35–39	> 40
Diet, exercise, behaviour therapy	–	With comorbidities	With comorbidities	+	+	+
Pharmacotherapy	–	–	With comorbidities	+	+	+
Surgery	–	–	–	–	With comorbidities	+

Guidelines provided by the National Heart, Lung, and Blood Institute (NHLBI) utilize BMI category and the presence of comorbidities to aid in treatment selection.

they are paired, the stronger the association between them, until eventually the presence of one event automatically triggers the other. Eating popcorn at the movies is an example. If these events are paired repeatedly, simply entering a movie theatre will trigger a craving for popcorn. Behaviour therapy seeks to identify and control cues associated with unwanted eating and activity habits (Table 23.1).

Attending to consequences

Another goal of treatment is to identify the consequences of behaviours. Behaviours that are rewarded (i.e. reinforced) are more likely to be repeated (Brownell, 2000). For example, an individual who loses 2 lb (approximately 1 kg) during the week as a result of recording her food intake will be positively reinforced to continue recording. On the other hand, behaviours that are punished (or followed by negative consequences) are less likely to be repeated. An individual, for example, who increases her activity level by 200 min in 1 week may feel exhausted and fatigued. As a result, she may feel discouraged from continuing her exercise programme. If she began with a more modest exercise regimen (e.g. 10 min of exercise, 5 days per week) and gradually increased her activity level, she would be less likely to experience negative effects (Sbrocco *et al.*, 1999).

Facilitating behaviour change

Behaviour therapy provides a very goal-oriented approach to weight loss. Patients are encouraged to set concrete, tangible goals with measurable outcomes (Brownell, 2000; Wadden and Butryn, 2003); they should leave each session with a strategy for how to achieve their goals. This includes devising a detailed plan of what they will do, when and where they will do it and how often. For example, helping patients develop a plan to walk around the neighbourhood for 15 min on Monday, Wednesday, Thursday and Saturday evenings, immediately after dinner, is more helpful than simply telling them to increase their physical activity. Patients should set small goals which they can attain in order to maximize feelings of success. Small successes build upon each other until patients reach their ultimate goals (Brownell, 2000).

Components of behavioural treatment

Behavioural treatment incorporates multiple components including self-monitoring, stimulus control, diet, exercise, cognitive restructuring, social support, problem-solving, slowing the rate of eating and relapse prevention. Detailed descriptions of these components are available elsewhere (Brownell, 2000; Wadden and Foster, 2000; Wing, 2002). The present discussion describes self-monitoring, stimulus control, cognitive restructuring, diet and exercise. The last two sections are described at length because they offer more options for intervention.

Self-monitoring

Self-monitoring is the cornerstone of behavioural treatment for obesity (Brownell, 2000; Wing, 2002; Wadden and Butryn, 2003). Patients keep detailed records of their food intake, activity and weight. Initially, they record foods eaten, including the types and amounts, as well as their caloric value. Self-monitoring facilitates weight loss. Several studies found that individuals who regularly kept their food records lost significantly more weight than those who recorded inconsistently (Wadden *et al.*, 1997a; Boutelle and Kirshenbaum, 1998; Berkowitz *et al.*, 2003). Monitoring food intake helps patients reduce their tendency to underestimate how much they eat (Lichtman *et al.*, 1992). It also increases their awareness of eating habits and identifies behaviours that need to be changed. For example, an individual may notice a tendency to 'taste' while preparing food. These tastings may add several hundred calories per day.

Over time, patients increase their self-monitoring to include times, places and feelings associated with eating (Brownell, 2000). This additional information helps to identify problem areas. An individual, for example, may notice that he snacks excessively in the evenings. Another may realize that she often makes poor food choices when upset. Once problem areas have been identified, the patient and practitioner work together to develop a plan to overcome the obstacle.

Stimulus control

Patients are instructed in stimulus control techniques to make their environments more conducive to eating less (and more healthily) and exercising more. As described previously, an event can become a cue to eat when it is repeatedly paired with eating. For example, walking into the kitchen often elicits a desire to eat because this room is so strongly associated with food. People rarely experience a food craving when in the attic because of the absence of cues in this area. Many events can prompt a desire to eat. The most obvious are the sight and smell of food. There is truth to the old adage 'out of sight, out of mind'. Patients learn strategies, such as storing foods out of sight, to reduce unwanted eating by limiting exposure to problem foods. Additional eating cues include places, times and events. Patients are encouraged to limit the places at home in which they eat to the kitchen or dining room, and to eat at regular times of day. They also learn not to eat while engaging in other activities, such as watching television or talking on the phone. Food cues are neutralized by disconnecting them from eating.

Cues can also promote healthy eating and activity habits. The sight, for example, of a fruit basket, rather than a dish of sweets or candies, may encourage consumption of a healthy snack. Similarly, the sight of walking shoes by the front door might prompt patients to exercise. Behavioural treatment aims to decrease negative cues while increasing positive ones (Brownell, 2000).

Cognitive restructuring

In behavioural treatment, patients learn to identify, challenge and correct irrational thoughts that may undermine their weight loss efforts. For example, a participant who overeats on just one occasion during the week might think 'I've blown my diet' (i.e. catastrophizing). This self-statement is likely to lead to additional negative thoughts such as 'What's the use of trying? I'll never lose weight'. Such sentiments usually elicit more overeating and more negative thoughts, perpetuating a vicious cycle. Cognitive restructuring teaches patients to identify their negative, irrational thoughts and to replace them with more realistic statements. Rational responses such as 'just because I ate an extra 300 calories tonight doesn't mean I won't be able to lose weight' are more likely to elicit positive eating and activity habits. Through cognitive restructuring, patients learn to view a setback as a temporary lapse. The ultimate goal is to determine how lapses occurred and to develop strategies to prevent them.

Cognitive restructuring may also be useful in helping patients cope with unmet weight loss expectations. Obese individuals often begin treatment expecting to lose up to 25% of their initial weight (Foster *et al.*, 1997; Wadden *et al.*, 2003). Failure to meet their expectations may cause patients to feel disappointed or to discontinue treatment prematurely. To minimize these risks, providers should help patients set reasonable goals and expectations, and focus on the health benefits of modest weight losses.

Dietary interventions

Weight loss requires the induction of a negative energy balance (i.e. fewer calories are consumed than are expended). It is easier to achieve negative energy balance by reducing calorie intake than by increasing physical activity. For example, most patients would have to walk approximately 4 miles (6.4 km) to induce an energy deficit of 500 kcal. By contrast, the same 500 kcal deficit could be achieved by simply eliminating two 20-oz (600-mL) sugared soft drinks. Most people find the latter task easier.

Behaviour modification historically has encouraged patients to consume foods of their liking but to decrease their intake by 500–1000 kcal per day by reducing serving sizes or excess fat and sugar. Behavioural principles, however, can be used to facilitate adherence to a variety of different dietary approaches, including low-calorie diets, low-carbohydrate plans and low-energy density diets. This section provides a brief description of each of these approaches.

Low-calorie diets

The NHLBI expert panel recommended that obese individuals reduce their energy intake by 500–1000 kcal per day to induce a weight loss of 0.5–1 kg/week (NHLBI, 1998). Approximately 15% of calories should be derived from protein, " 30% from fat and ≥ 55% from carbohydrate. The *food guide pyramid* offers a convenient method of following a diet with this general macronutrient composition (Agricultural Research Service, 1995). The panel also recommended consumption of 20–30 g of fibre per day and 1000–1500 mg of calcium per day. For simplicity, patients are often given a predetermined calorie goal, rather than subtracting 500–1000 kcal per day from their daily energy requirements. (It is difficult to calculate daily requirements with accuracy.) Women, for example, are typically instructed to consume 1200–1500 kcal per day and men 1500–1800 kcal per day (Wing, 2002).

Portion-controlled foods

Obese individuals tend to underestimate their food intake by 30–50% when eating a diet of conventional foods (Lichtman *et al.*, 1992). This is attributable to misjudging portion sizes, failing to recognize hidden sources of fat or sugar or forgetting about some foods eaten. The use of portion-controlled foods, such as frozen food dishes (main courses), takes the guesswork out of calorie counting by providing patients with a fixed amount of food with a known energy content. Jeffery and colleagues (1993) compared the weight loss of patients who were prescribed a conventional diet of self-selected foods with that of individuals who were provided with actual foods for five breakfasts and five dinners per week. Although both groups were prescribed the same calorie goal (approximately 1000 kcal per day), the second group lost approximately 2.5 kg more than the first after 6 months of treatment. The provision of fixed portions of food appeared to facilitate patients' adherence to their calorie goals.

In a follow-up study, Wing and colleagues (1996a) randomly assigned women to standard behaviour modification plus: (a) no additional treatment; (b) detailed meal plans and grocery lists; (c) meal plans with food provided at reduced cost; and (d) meal plans with free food provision. Results showed that the last three groups lost more weight than the first group. There were, however, no differences among the three groups that received meal plans. Thus, it appears that the structure alone provided by detailed meal plans may be sufficient to improve outcome.

Liquid meal replacements

Liquid meal replacements are a popular form of a portion-controlled diet. Shakes, such as SlimFast, OPTIFAST and Ensure, provide patients a fixed quantity of food with a known calorie amount (i.e. 160–220 kcal per serving). They are convenient, easy to serve and are generally low in cost compared with a meal of conventional foods. A randomized controlled trial by Ditschuneit and colleagues (1999) compared the prescription of a self-selected diet of 1200–1500 kcal per day to one with the same calorie goal but which included a liquid meal replacement (i.e. SlimFast) for two meals and two snacks per day. Participants who consumed the meal replacement lost 7.8% of initial weight after 3 months, compared with a significantly smaller 1.5% for patients assigned to the conventional diet. A recent meta-analysis of six randomized controlled trials found that patients who consumed meal replacements lost an average of 2.5 kg more after 3 months (and 2.6 kg more after 1 year) than participants who consumed diets of conventional foods (Heymsfield *et al.*, 2003). In addition, the drop-out rate after 1 year was significantly lower in participants in the meal replacement group. Meal replacements may be particularly helpful in facilitating the maintenance of weight loss, as discussed later.

Low-carbohydrate diets

Popular low-carbohydrate plans, such as the Atkins diet (Atkins, 1998), induce weight loss, in part, by simplifying food choices. During the initial weeks, dieters consume the majority of their calories from protein and fat, limiting carbohydrate to less than 20 g per day. Elimination of an entire class of macronutrients facilitates weight loss, whereas the large amounts of dietary protein may satisfy appetite. The high fat content of these diets has raised concerns about the health consequences of low-carbohydrate approaches.

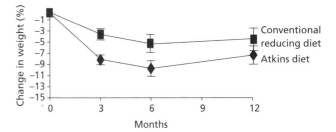

Fig 23.1 Percentage reduction in initial weight over 12 months on a low-fat vs. low-carbohydrate diet. (Reproduced from Foster *et al.*, 2003.)

A recent study revealed surprisingly favourable short-term findings. Foster and colleagues (2003) provided participants with a copy of *Dr. Atkins' New Diet Revolution* (Atkins, 1998) or *The Learn Program for Weight Management 2000*, the latter recommending a traditional balanced deficit diet (BDD) of 1200–1500 kcal per day (Brownell, 2000). Participants had minimal contact with professionals, consistent with the manner in which most dieters lose weight. Assessments were conducted at baseline and 3, 6 and 12 months. As shown in Fig. 23.1, the low-carbohydrate group lost significantly more weight at 6 months (7.0 kg vs. 3.2 kg) than did the BDD group. Both groups regained weight from months 7 to 12, such that differences in weight loss were not statistically significant at the end of the year. The low-carbohydrate group also had significantly greater reductions in triglycerides at months 3 and 12, as well as greater improvements in high-density lipoprotein (HDL) cholesterol at months 3, 6 and 12. Decreases in low-density lipoprotein (LDL) and total cholesterol were significantly more in the high-carbohydrate group at month 3, but there were no differences thereafter. The mechanisms underlying these favourable changes are not fully known (Foster *et al.*, 2003). Additional research is needed to evaluate the long-term safety and efficacy of such low-carbohydrate diets.

Low-energy density diets

The underlying principle of low-energy density diets is that the volume of food consumed, not calorie content, influences satiety (Rolls and Bell, 1999). Low-energy density diets aim to minimize the amount of energy (i.e. calories) in a given weight (g) of food. Energy density can be reduced by replacing fat (i.e. 9 kcal/g) with carbohydrate or protein (i.e. each 4 kcal/g) or by increasing the fibre or water content in foods (Melanson and Dwyer, 2002). To enhance satiety, water must be incorporated into food, rather than being drunk with the meal (Rolls *et al.*, 1999). Other examples of reducing energy density include encouraging patients to eat grapes rather than raisins or to add vegetables to a pasta dish.

Bell and Rolls (2001) found that a low-energy density diet reduced caloric intake in both lean and obese women compared with a high-energy dense meal. In another study, participants were fed meals varying in energy density and were instructed to eat until they felt full (Duncan *et al.*, 1983). Participants in the low-energy density group consumed only one-half as many calories as those in the high-energy density group (i.e. 1570 vs. 3000 kcal). A low-energy density diet, rich in fruits and vegetables, could be an excellent option for patients who feel hungry when dieting. This approach would let them eat more food while probably decreasing their calorie intake.

Summary

In summary, dieters can select from a variety of dietary interventions to facilitate the induction of weight loss. The choice of a particular approach depends, in large measure, on personal preferences. As a general rule, a portion-controlled diet will induce weight loss faster than a traditional balanced deficit diet (Heymsfield *et al.*, 2003). Rapid weight loss, however, may not be an important consideration for some individuals.

Physical activity

Increasing physical activity is another important goal of behavioural treatment. Exercise alone, in the absence of caloric restriction, induces modest weight loss of only 2–3 kg in 4–6 months (Miller *et al.*, 1997; NHLBI, 1998). There are, however, several reasons why obese individuals should increase their physical activity. First, exercise improves cardiovascular fitness independent of weight loss (Lee *et al.*, 1999). Lee and colleagues (1999) found that individuals who were fat but fit (as judged by a treadmill test) had lower rates of cardiovascular mortality than those who were lean but unfit. Second, exercise minimizes the loss of fat-free mass that occurs with diet-induced weight loss (Ballor and Poehlman, 1994). Finally, as discussed later, increased physical activity is critical for long-term weight control (Klem *et al.*, 1997).

At present, we emphasize the positive cardiovascular effects of exercise and explicitly tell patients not to expect to lose weight as a result of increasing their walking or other aerobic activity. In addition, we emphasize that exercise should not be boring, painful or otherwise aversive. This is emphasized while discussing the differences between programmed and lifestyle activity.

Programmed activity

Programmed activity refers to planned bouts of aerobic activity, such as walking, swimming or cycling, usually at a moderate intensity level (i.e. 60–80% of maximum heart rate) for at least 20–30 min at a time. The ultimate goal is for patients to exercise at least 180 min per week (i.e. 30 min per day, 6 days per week), although they are expected to work gradually towards this goal (Blair and Leermakers, 2002). They might begin by walking 10 min daily, three days of the week, until

their endurance improves. Resistance training may be added to the exercise regimen, given its favourable effects in preserving muscle strength and bone mass (Blair and Leermakers, 2002). The most important consideration in patients selecting an activity is to choose one they enjoy.

Patients keep records of their exercise, noting the type, time, location and duration of their activity (Brownell, 2000). This information is used to assess progress and to identify barriers to regular activity, of which lack of time is a common one. Jakicic and colleagues (1995) have studied the benefits of short vs. long bouts of activity to address this problem. Patients were randomly assigned to either one long (40-min) bout of exercise or four short (10-min) bouts. Exercise adherence was significantly better in the latter group (Jakicic *et al.*, 1995) and these patients tended to lose more weight than those in the long-bout condition. Additional studies have shown that exercise adherence is facilitated by having patients walk at home rather than participating in supervised, on-site walking programmes (King *et al.*, 1995; Perri *et al.*, 1997; Jakicic *et al.*, 1999). Although exercising at a health club is fine for those who enjoy it, exercising at home reduces common barriers, including lack of time or the need for transport or childcare.

Lifestyle activity

Lifestyle activity involves increasing energy expenditure throughout the day by methods including walking rather than riding or using stairs rather than escalators. The goal is to increase any type of movement, without concern for the intensity of the activity (Brownell, 2000). Lifestyle activity, as combined with diet, produces weight loss similar to that induced by programmed exercise plus diet (Andersen *et al.*, 1999; Dunn *et al.*, 1999). In a study by Andersen and colleagues (1999), all patients participated in a 16-week behavioural treatment programme. Those who were randomly assigned to the programmed activity group attended a 1-h step-aerobics class three times per week. Participants in the lifestyle activity group were instructed to increase their lifestyle activity by 30 min per day. At the end of 16 weeks, both groups had lost approximately 8 kg (as shown in Fig. 23.2). At a 1-year follow-up, participants in the lifestyle group tended to maintain their weight loss better than those in the original step-aerobics class ($P < 0.06$). The authors speculated that this was attributable to the superior maintenance of physical activity in the former group.

The use of pedometers to monitor participants' daily steps is an easy and inexpensive method of increasing lifestyle activity. Before treatment, participants typically walk 3000–4000 steps per day. Each week, they increase their step goal until they walk approximately 8000–10 000 steps per day. Pedometers are very reinforcing to patients because they provide a clear indicator of progress (Brownell, 2000).

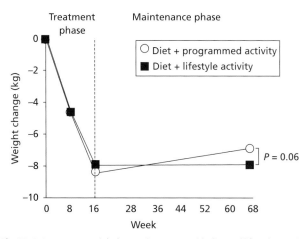

Fig 23.2 Long-term weight loss maintenance with diet and lifestyle activity vs. diet and programmed activity. (Reproduced from Andersen *et al.*, 1999.)

Time-limited treatment delivery

An initial course of behavioural treatment usually consists of 16–26 weekly sessions. Treatment has a clear starting and ending date, which seems to help participants pace their efforts. Once this initial phase of treatment is completed, patients are encouraged to participate in a weight loss maintenance programme, as discussed later.

Group vs. individual treatment

Treatment is typically delivered to groups of 10–20 people who start and end treatment together. This 'closed-group' approach ensures a high level of social support and continuity of care. Participants assist each other in their efforts to modify eating and activity habits. Groups may also provide participants with a healthy dose of competition. Patients take note of members who are losing weight or exercising regularly and often decide that they too want to be successful.

A recent randomized trial demonstrated the superiority of group over individual treatment for inducing weight loss, regardless of patients' preferred method of treatment (Renjilian *et al.*, 2001). Those with a clear preference for group or individual care were randomly assigned to one out of four treatment groups: (a) preferred group treatment and received group; (b) desired group treatment but received individual; (c) preferred individual therapy and received it; or (d) desired individual treatment and received group therapy. Participants who received group treatment lost significantly more weight than those assigned to individual therapy (Renjilian *et al.*, 2001). This was true even in cases in which participants preferred individual treatment and received it. Persons who desired and received individual therapy lost significantly less weight (i.e. about 2 kg) than persons who wanted in-

dividual treatment but were assigned to group sessions. We believe that group treatment was superior because of its provision of both social support and competition, as described previously.

Treatment providers

Group behavioural treatment typically is provided by dietitians, psychologists, exercise specialists or health educators. There has been surprisingly little research on the credentials or training experiences that are required to successfully provide behavioural treatment (Wang *et al.*, 2003). Results of several studies suggest that laypersons can be effective treatment providers. Most commercial weight loss programmes are, in fact, staffed by persons without professional training. Further research is needed to identify the professional training or personal characteristics required to provide effective weight management.

Short-term results

Table 23.2 presents the results of behavioural treatment from 1974 to 2002, as determined from randomized controlled trials published in four journals—*Addictive Behaviours*, *Behaviour Research and Therapy*, *Behaviour Therapy* and *Journal of Consulting and Clinical Psychology*. Only studies representative of standard behavioural treatment are included in the table. No interventions prescribed a diet providing fewer than 900 kcal per day (Wadden and Butryn, 2003).

The data show that patients treated at present by a comprehensive group, behavioural approach lose approximately 10.7 kg (about 10–12% of initial weight) in 30 weeks of treatment. In addition, about 80% of patients who begin treatment complete it. Thus, behaviour therapy yields very favourable results as judged by the current criteria for success (i.e. a 5–10% reduction in initial weight) proposed by the NHLBI (1998), the World Health Organization (WHO) (1998) and the Dietary Guidelines for Americans (Agricultural Research Service, 1995).

A comparison of early (i.e. 1974) and more recent studies (1996–2002) reveals that weight losses have more than doubled over the past 25 years, as treatment duration has increased more than threefold. Thus, for example, in 1974 treatment of 8.4 weeks was associated with a mean loss of 3.8 kg, whereas treatment from 1996 to 2002 averaged 31.6 weeks and produced a mean loss of 10.7 kg. Although several new components, including cognitive restructuring, have been added to the behavioural approach since 1974, the most parsimonious explanation for the larger weight losses is the longer duration of treatment and the use of portion-controlled diets in some studies. The rate of weight loss has remained constant at about 0.4–0.5 kg per week.

Table 23.2 Summary of behaviour therapy for obesity.

	1974	1985–1987	1991–1995	1996–2002*
Number of studies	15	13	5	9
Sample size	53.1	71.6	30.2	28.0
Initial weight (kg)	73.4	87.2	94.9	92.2
Length of treatment (weeks)	8.4	15.6	22.2	31.4
Weight loss (kg)	3.8	8.4	8.5	10.7
Loss per week (kg)	0.5	0.5	0.4	0.4
Attrition (%)	11.4	13.8	18.5	21.2
Length of follow-up (weeks)	15.1	48.3	47.7	41.8
Loss at follow-up (kg)	4.0	5.3	5.9	7.2

*Studies included in 1996–2002 samples are found in Meyers *et al.* (1996), Perri *et al.* (1997), Wadden *et al.* (1997a,b), Fuller *et al.* (1998), Harvey-Berino (1998), Sbrocco *et al.* (1999), Wing and Jeffery (1999), Perri *et al.* (2001) and Ramirez and Rosen (2001).

All studies sampled were published in the following four journals: *Addictive Behaviours*, *Behaviour Therapy*, *Behaviour Research and Therapy* and *Journal of Consulting and Clinical Psychology*.

All values, except for number of studies, are weighted means; thus, studies with larger sample sizes had a greater impact on mean values than studies with smaller sample sizes. The data are adapted and updated from Brownell and Wadden (1991).

Long-term results

Without continued treatment, patients typically regain 30–35% of their lost weight in the year following treatment (Wadden and Osei, 2002; Wadden and Butryn, 2003). Moreover, 5 years post treatment, 50% or more of patients regain all of their weight (Wadden *et al.*, 1989). Factors responsible for weight regain have not been fully identified, despite the frequency with which this problem is observed. Contributors to weight regain are likely to include compensatory metabolic responses that include reductions in resting energy expenditure and leptin, as well as increases in ghrelin (a gut peptide associated with reports of hunger) (Cummings *et al.*, 2002; Rosenbaum *et al.*, 2002). In addition, patients are confronted daily by a 'toxic' environment that explicitly encourages them to consume large quantities of high-fat, high-sugar foods (Brownell and Horgan, 2003). Weight gain (or regain) appears to be a nearly ineluctable response to this environment.

Inadequate treatment also contributes to weight regain. Short-term treatment of 16–26 weeks clearly is no match for what for most obese individuals is a chronic disorder (Wadden and Butryn, 2003). Obesity cannot be cured by 6 months of therapy, any more than type 2 diabetes or hypertension can be controlled lifelong by such brief intervention. The long-term results of obesity management have begun to improve with the recognition that obesity is a chronic disorder that requires long-term care (Perri and Corsica, 2002).

Improving the maintenance of weight loss

Long-term treatment

Several studies have demonstrated the benefits of patients continuing to attend weight maintenance classes after completing an initial 16–26 week weight loss programme (Perri *et al.*, 1988; Perri and Corsica, 2002). Perri and colleagues (1988), for example, found that individuals who attended every-other-week group maintenance sessions for the year following weight reduction maintained 13.0 kg of their 13.2-kg end-of-treatment weight loss, whereas those who did not receive such therapy maintained only 5.7 kg of a 10.8-kg loss. Maintenance sessions appear to provide patients with the support and motivation needed to continue to practise weight control skills, such as keeping food records and exercising regularly. In reviewing 13 studies on this topic, Perri and Corsica (2002) found that patients who received extended treatment, which averaged 41 sessions over 54 weeks, maintained 10.3 kg of their initial 10.7-kg weight loss. Figure 23.3 illustrates the difference in weight loss produced by standard and long-term treatment, as determined from three randomized trials in which all participants received behavioural weight control for the first 20 weeks. Thereafter, one-half of the participants continued to have every-other-week treatment for 1 year, whereas the other half received no further care.

The figure shows a clear limitation of long-term behavioural treatment—it appears only to delay rather than to prevent weight regain (Perri and Corsica, 2002). Patients maintain their full end-of-treatment weight loss as long as they participate in biweekly maintenance sessions. In fact, they lose additional weight during the first 6 months of extended treatment but regain the additional loss during the second 6 months of therapy (Perri *et al.*, 1988). Weight gain continues with the termination of maintenance therapy. The optimal frequency of maintenance therapy is not known. Patients eventually tire of attending sessions twice monthly (and may drop out) but monthly visits do not appear to be sufficient to maintain end-of-treatment weight loss (Jeffery *et al.*, 1993).

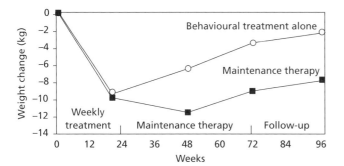

Fig 23.3 Long-term results of standard behavioural treatment with or without biweekly maintenance therapy. (Data taken from Perri *et al.*, 1986; 1988; 2001.). Note: data for week 98 are available for Perri *et al.*, 1986 and 1988 studies only.

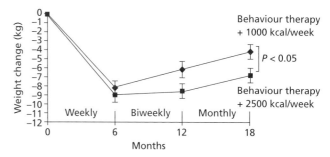

Fig 23.4 Participants prescribed high-activity goals (2500 kcal per week) maintained their weight loss significantly better than those in the low-activity group (1000 kcal per week) after 18 months. (Reproduced from Jeffery *et al.*, 2003).

Telephone and mail contact

Long-term contact may also be provided by telephone or mail. Perri and colleagues (1984) demonstrated that therapist contact by either of these modalities significantly improved weight maintenance, compared with no further intervention. When using telephone calls, the same therapist optimally should contact the patient on each occasion. A study in which patients were contacted by staff members unknown to them failed to improve weight maintenance beyond the results of a no-contact group (Wing *et al.*, 1996b).

High levels of physical activity

Data from case studies, correlational investigations and randomized trials have all concluded that high levels of physical activity facilitate long-term weight control (Schoeller *et al.*, 1986; Klem *et al.*, 1997; McGuire *et al.*, 1998; Jeffery *et al.*, 2003). Findings, for example, from the National Weight Control Registry clearly emphasize this point. Members of the Registry have lost an average of 32.4 kg and maintained their loss for 5.5 years. Women report expending approximately 2825 kcal per week, the equivalent of walking about 28 miles per week (or 75–90 min per day) (Klem *et al.*, 1997).

Based on these findings, Jeffery *et al.* (2003) recently compared, in a randomized controlled trial, the benefits of low versus high levels of physical activity. Participants in the high-activity group were instructed to expend 2500 kcal per week, whereas those in the low group were prescribed a goal of 1000 kcal per week. As shown in Fig. 23.4, weight losses of the two treatment conditions did not differ significantly at the end of 6 months during which participants attended weekly group meetings. Participants, however, in the high-activity group maintained their losses significantly better at both the 12- and 18-month follow-up assessments than did patients in the low-activity group. Jakicic and colleagues (1999) similarly found, in secondary analyses of results of a randomized trial, that obese individuals who exercised 200 or more minutes per

week achieved significantly greater weight losses at 18 months than persons who exercised less than 150 min per week.

The mechanisms by which exercise facilitates weight maintenance are not well understood (Wadden *et al.*, 1997b). The simplest explanation is that increased physical activity helps to keep patients in energy balance. Walking 2 or 3 miles (3 or 5 km) per day may help to compensate for occasional dietary indiscretions that are associated with weight regain (in persons who do not exercise regularly). Alternatively, exercise spares the loss of fat-free mass during diet-induced weight loss, an occurrence that could help minimize undesired reductions in resting energy expenditure (Wadden *et al.*, 1997b). Increased physical activity could also be associated with improved mood which, in turn, could facilitate long-term adherence to a low-calorie diet (Wadden *et al.*, 1997b). Regardless of the mechanism of action, the message remains the same: patients should increase their physical activity by whatever means possible, including increasing lifestyle activity and decreasing sedentary behaviours. Decreasing sedentary behaviours has proven particularly effective in overweight children (Epstein *et al.*, 2000).

Dietary options for long-term weight control

As discussed previously, the use of meal replacements significantly improves the induction of weight loss. This approach may also facilitate the maintenance of lost weight, as shown in Fig. 23.5. During the first 3 months of their randomized trial, Ditschuneit *et al.* (1999) instructed one-half of their participants to replace two meals and two snacks per day with SlimFast products. These individuals lost significantly more weight than patients who consumed a diet of conventional foods (7.8% vs. 1.5% respectively). Thereafter, participants in both groups replaced one meal and one snack per day with a liquid shake or meal bar. Individuals in the original (3-month) meal replacement group maintained a loss of 11% of initial weight 2 years after treatment and 8.4% at a 4-year follow-

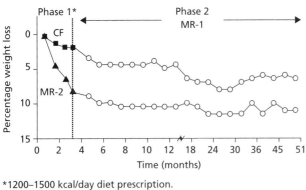

*1200–1500 kcal/day diet prescription.
CF = conventional foods.
MR-2 = replacements for two meals, two snacks daily.
MR-1 = replacements for one meal, one snack daily.

Fig 23.5 Long-term maintenance of weight loss using meal replacements versus conventional foods. (Reproduced from Fletchner-Mors *et al.*, 2000.)

up (Fletchner-Mors *et al.*, 2000). Patients who were originally treated by the conventional diet but were switched to meal replacements maintained a loss of 3.2% of initial weight. These are the most successful long-term findings to date for the dietary management of obesity. The study has limitations including the use of a non-randomized design after the first 3 months and the examination of a relatively small sample (i.e. 100 participants). If, however, the results were replicated in a large randomized controlled trial, they would have major implications for the long-term management of obesity.

Other dietary approaches for weight maintenance include consuming a low-fat diet that is high in complex carbohydrates, as reported by individuals in the National Weight Control Registry. In a 1-year weight maintenance study, participants randomly assigned to a low-fat, *ad libitum* carbohydrate diet, following initial weight loss, regained significantly less weight during the year than persons instructed to consume a low-calorie diet al.one (0.3 kg vs. 4.1 kg) (Toubro and Astrup, 1997). At 2 years after initial weight loss, participants assigned to the low-fat, *ad libitum* carbohydrate diet continued to show superior weight maintenance. Further assessment is needed of the optimal energy level and macronutrient content to facilitate long-term weight control.

New directions in behavioural treatment

This review has shown that behavioural treatment clearly is effective in inducing a loss of approximately 10% of initial weight and that losses of this size are associated with significant improvements in health (Diabetes Prevention Program Research Group, 2002). In addition to its successes, the behavioural treatment of obesity faces several challenges at present. First among these is making treatment more available to the

millions of Americans who need to lose weight. We briefly discuss three avenues for increasing access to behavioural weight control.

Internet and e-mail

Recent studies suggest that the Internet and e-mail are potentially effective methods for facilitating weight management. In an initial study, Tate and colleagues (2001) assigned participants to one of two 6-month weight loss programmes delivered over the Internet. An education intervention provided a directory of Internet resources for weight control. A behaviour therapy intervention provided this component, as well as 24 weekly lessons conducted by e-mail, weekly submission of self-monitoring diaries and an on-line bulletin board. The behaviour therapy participants lost significantly more weight at 6 months (4.1 kg vs. 1.6 kg respectively). In a subsequent study of 12 months' duration, Tate and colleagues (2003) randomly assigned individuals at risk for type 2 diabetes to an Internet weight loss programme or to the same intervention with the addition of weekly behavioural counselling, delivered by e-mail. Participants in the latter group lost significantly more weight at 1 year (4.4 kg vs. 2.0 kg respectively).

These studies, taken together, underscore the importance of participants keeping records of their food intake and physical activity, as well as completing other behavioural assignments. Educational instruction alone is not sufficient to induce clinically significant weight loss. The studies also suggest that even the most effective Internet interventions are likely to produce only half of the weight loss of traditional on-site behavioural programmes. However, from a public health perspective, the greater availability of Internet programmes may result in this approach having a greater impact on obesity management than traditional clinic- or hospital-based programmes that serve so few individuals.

Commercial programmes

Commercially provided weight loss programmes now include many of the components of behavioural treatment described above. Of these, Weight Watchers is by far the largest treatment provider. In 2002, clients attended 30.8 million weekly visits at approximately 3600 sites in the USA (Weight Watchers, 2002). The programme provides dietary education and group support in 1-h weekly meetings at a cost of approximately $12 per visit. Treatment groups may include as many as 100 individuals. Unlike the closed groups used in academic medical centres, in which the same patients attend treatment together each week, Weight Watchers meetings are open to whoever wishes to attend on a given evening or afternoon. This practice makes for ease of enrolment in the programme (although it may dilute the continuity of care).

Heshka and colleagues (2003) recently conducted a randomized controlled trial of 426 individuals who were assigned to Weight Watchers or a self-help intervention. Persons in the former group attended weekly Weight Watchers meetings in their local community. (Group leaders did not know that participants were enrolled in a research study.) Those in the self-help condition were provided two 20-min visits with a registered dietitian, as well as printed materials and other resources. At 1 year, 82% of the participants remained in the study, with no differences in attrition between the two groups. Participants assigned to Weight Watchers lost 5.4% of initial weight, compared with 1.6% in the self-help group (*P* < 0.0001). At 2 years, losses declined to 3.2% and 0.1% respectively (*P* < 0.0001; 73% of participants remained in treatment at this time with no differences in attrition between groups.

These findings suggest that Weight Watchers might be an appropriate first step of treatment for individuals who had failed to reduce on their own with diet and exercise. A substantial minority of individuals could be expected to lose 5% or more of their initial weight, a loss that could prevent or ameliorate health complications. There are other commercial and self-help programmes from which to choose. None, however, has evaluated its results of treatment in the same rigorous manner as Weight Watchers.

Primary-care practice

Aronne (2002) has described the role of primary-care physicians in preventing and treating obesity. This includes monitoring patients' weight (and BMI) on a regular basis, providing literature on healthy eating and activity habits, and assessing and managing weight-related health complications. Some physicians may wish to provide more intensive weight management, potentially by giving patients a structured treatment manual, having a registered dietitian consult in the office or establishing an afternoon or evening clinic to provide brief check-in visits (i.e. to measure weight, collect food records, etc.)

Primary-care physicians often report that they feel ill prepared to treat overweight individuals, whether because of lack of adequate training, poor reimbursement or a sense of futility—a feeling 'that nothing works' (Frank, 1993; Aronne, 2002). Patients may well sense their physician's lack of involvement. Nearly three-quarters of participants in a recent study reported that they looked to their doctors only a 'slight amount' or 'not at all' for advice about weight management (Wadden *et al.*, 2000). Nearly 45% indicated that their doctor had not prescribed any of 10 common weight loss methods. These data suggest that physicians and their obese patients may have landed in a weight management stalemate: no one talks about the problem. On a more positive note, fewer than 10% of patients reported that they were treated disrespectfully by their doctors concerning their weight. Moreover, most respondents were quite satisfied with the medical care they received for their general health.

It is challenging for most primary-care physicians to provide effective diet and exercise counselling in traditional office practice because they are not equipped to meet with their patients on a weekly or biweekly basis—the frequency of care that is likely to produce the best results (at least in the short term). Nevertheless, physicians can play an important role in the management of overweight and obesity by providing an atmosphere in which patients can discuss their concerns and frustrations about their weight. Moreover, they can provide a valuable service by familiarizing themselves with treatment options available in their community and using these resources (Aronne, 2002). This includes identifying a registered dietitian with whom to establish a consultative relationship. Physicians can similarly support their patients' participation in self-help or commercial programmes by enquiring at office visits about satisfaction with these programmes and congratulating patients on weight loss or behaviour change.

Tackling the toxic environment

Far greater resources and efforts also must be devoted to the prevention of obesity if we are to halt the progression of this epidemic, let alone reverse it (Brownell and Horgan, 2003). Our best hope for prevention may lie with children and adolescents. Efforts should be devoted to improving meals and snacks that are served at schools, providing more opportunities for physical activity at school and at home and educating youth about the importance of diet, activity and a healthy body weight. Ultimately, we must tackle what Brownell has referred to as a 'toxic environment', which explicitly encourages the consumption of supersized servings of high-fat, high-sugar foods, while implicitly discouraging physical activity, as a result of sedentary work and leisure habits (Horgan and Brownell, 2002; Wadden *et al.*, 2002). Changing this environment will require public policy initiatives, as were needed, for example to reduce cigarette smoking and to increase seat belt use (Mercer *et al.*, 2003). Although behavioural treatment can assist those who are already obese, there is a pressing need for wide-scale environmental interventions that will reduce the number of individuals who require such treatment.

References

Agricultural Research Service (1995) Report of Dietary Guidelines Advisory Committee on the dietary guidelines for Americans. *Nutrition Review* **53**, 376–379.

Andersen, R.E., Wadden, T.A., Bartlett, S.J., Zemel, B.S., Verde, T.J. and Franckowiak, S.C. (1999) Effects of lifestyle activity vs. structured aerobic exercise in obese women: A randomized trial. *Journal of the American Medical Association* **281**, 335–340.

Arrone, L.J. (2002) Treatment of obesity in the primary care setting. In:

Wadden, T.A., Stunkard, A.J. eds. *Handbook of Obesity Treatment*. New York: Guilford Press, 383–394.

Atkins, R.C. (1998) *Dr. Atkins' New Diet Revolution*. New York: Avon Books.

Ballor, D.L. and Poehlman, C.T. (1994) Exercise training enhances fat-free mass preservation during diet-induced weight loss: A meta-analytical finding. *International Journal of Obesity* **18**, 35–40.

Bell, E.A. and Rolls, B.J. (2001) Energy density of foods affects energy intake across multiple levels of fat content in lean and obese women. *American Journal of Clinical Nutrition* **73**, 1010–1018.

Berkowitz, R.I., Wadden, T.A., Tershakovec, A.M. and Cronquist, J.L. (2003) Behavior therapy and sibutramine for the treatment of adolescent obesity: a randomized controlled trial. *Journal of the American Medical Association* **289**, 1805–1812.

Blackburn, G.L. (1995) Effect of degree of weight loss on health benefits. *Obesity Research* **3**, 211S–216S.

Blair, S.N. and Leermakers, E.A. (2002) Exercise and weight management. In: Wadden, T.A., Stunkard, A.J. eds. *Handbook of Obesity Treatment*. New York: Guilford Press, 283–300.

Boutelle, K.N. and Kirschenbaum, D.S. (1998) Further support for consistent self-monitoring as a vital component of successful weight control. *Obesity Research* **6**, 219–224.

Brownell, K.D. (2000) *The LEARN Program for Weight Management 2000*. Dallas: American Health Publishing.

Brownell, K.D. and Wadden, T.A. (1991) The heterogeneity of obesity: Fitting treatments to individuals. *Behavior Therapy* **22**, 153–177.

Brownell, K.D. and Horgan, K.B. (2003) *Food Fight: The Inside Story of the Food Industry, America's Obesity Crises, and What We Can Do About It*. Chicago: Contemporary Books.

Campfield, L.A., Smith, F.J., Guisez, Y., Devos, R. and Burn, P. (1995) Recombinant mouse OB protein: Evidence for a peripheral signal linking adiposity and central neural networks. *Science* **269**, 475–476.

Cummings, D.E., Weigle, D.S., Frayo, R.S., Breen, P.A., Ma, M.K., Dellinger, E. and Purnell, J.Q. (2002) Plasma ghrelin levels after diet-induced weight loss or gastric bypass surgery. *New England Journal of Medicine* **346**, 1623–1630.

Diabetes Prevention Program Research Group (2002) Reduction in the incidence of type 2 diabetes with lifestyle intervention or metformin. *New England Journal of Medicine* **346**, 393–403.

Ditschuneit, H.H, Flechtner-Mors, M., Johnson, T.D. and Adler, G. (1999) Metabolic and weight loss effects of long-term dietary intervention in obese subjects. *American Journal of Clinical Nutrition* **69**, 198–204.

Duncan, K.H., Bacon, J.A. and Weinsier, R.L. (1983) The effects of high and low energy density diets on satiety, energy intake, and eating time of obese and nonobese subjects. *American Journal of Clinical Nutrition* **37**, 763–767.

Dunn, A.L., Marcus, B.H., Kampert, J.B., Garcia, M.E., Kohl, H.W. and Blair, S.N. (1999) Comparison of lifestyle and structured interventions to increase physical activity and cardiorespiratory fitness. *Journal of the American Medical Association* **281**, 327–334.

Epstein, L.H., Paluch, R.A., Gordy, C.C. and Dorn, J. (2000) Decreasing sedentary behaviors in treating pediatric obesity. *Archives of Pediatric and Adolescent Medicine* **154**, 220–226.

Flechtner-Mors, M., Ditschuneit, H.H., Johnson, T.D., Suchard, M. and Adler, G. (2000) Metabolic and weight loss effects of long-term intervention in obese patients: Four-year results. *Obesity Research* **8**, 399–402.

Foster, G.D., Wadden, T.A., Vogt, R.A. and Brewer, G. (1997) What is a reasonable weight loss? Patients' expectations and evaluations of obesity treatment outcomes. *Journal of Consulting and Clinical Psychology* **65**, 79–85.

Foster, G.D., Wyatt, H.R., Hill, J.O., McGuckin, B.G., Brill, C., Mohammed, B.S., Szapary, P.O., Rader, D.J., Edman, J.S. and Klein, S. (2003) A randomized trial of a low-carbohydrate diet for obesity. *New England Journal of Medicine* **348**, 2082–2090.

Frank, A. (1993) Futility and avoidance: Medical professionals in the treatment of obesity. *Journal of the American Medical Association* **269**, 2132–2133.

Goldstein, D.J. (1992) Beneficial effects of modest weight loss. *International Journal of Obesity* **16**, 397–416.

Fuller, P.R., Perri, M.G., Leermakers, E.A., Guyer, L.K. (1998) Effects of a personalized system of skill acquisition and an educational program in the treatment of obesity. *Addictive Behaviors* **23**, 97–100.

Harvey-Berino, J. (1998) Changing health behavior via telecommunications technology: using interactive television to treat obesity. *Behavior Therapy* **29**, 505–519.

Heshka, S., Anderson, J.W., Atkinson, R.L., Greenway, F.L., Hill, J.O., Phinney, S.D., Kolotkin, R.L., Miller-Kovach, K. and Pi-Sunyer, F.X. (2003) Weight loss with self-help compared with a structured commercial program: a randomized trial. *Journal of the American Medical Association* **289**, 1792–1798.

Heymsfield, S.B., van Mierlo, C.A., van der Knaap. H.C., Heo, M. and Frier, H.I. (2003) Weight management using a meal replacement strategy: meta and pooling analysis from six studies. *International Journal of Obesity* **27**, 537–549.

Horgan, K.B. and Brownell, K.D. (2002) Confronting the toxic environment: Environmental and public health actions in a world crisis. In: Wadden, T.A., Stunkard, A.J. eds. *Handbook of Obesity Treatment*. New York: Guilford, 95–106.

Jakicic, J.M., Butler, B.A. and Robertson, R.J. (1995) Prescribing exercise in multiple short bouts versus one continuous bout: Effects on adherence, cardiorespiratory fitness, and weight loss in overweight women. *International Journal of Obesity* **19**, 382–387.

Jakicic, J.M., Winters, C., Lang, W. and Wing, R.R. (1999) Effects of intermittent exercise and use of home exercise equipment on adherence, weight loss, and fitness in overweight women: A randomized trial. *Journal of the American Medical Association* **16**, 1554–1560.

Jeffery, R.W., Wing, R.R., Thornson, C., Burton, L.R., Raether, C., Harvey, J. and Mullen, M. (1993) Strengthening behavioral interventions for weight loss: a randomized trial of food provision and monetary incentives. *Journal of Consulting and Clinical Psychology* **61**, 1038–1045.

Jeffery, R.W., Wing, R.R., Sherwood, N.E. and Tate, D.F. (2003) Physical activity and weight loss: does prescribing higher physical activity goals improve outcome? *American Journal of Clinical Nutrition* **78**, 684–689.

King, A.C., Haskell, W.L., Young, D.R., Oka, R.K. and Stefanick, M.L. (1995) Long-term effects of varying intensities and formats of physical activity on participation rates, fitness, and lipoprotein levels in men and women aged 50 to 65 years. *Circulation* **15**, 2596–2604.

Klem, M.L., Wing, R.R., McGuire, M.T., Seagle, H.M. and Hill, J.O. (1997) A descriptive study of individuals successful at long-term maintenance of substantial weight loss. *American Journal of Clinical Nutrition* **66**, 239–246.

Lee, C.D., Blair, S.N. and Jackson, A.S. (1999) Cardiorespiratory fitness, body composition, and all-cause and cardiovascular disease mortality in men. *American Journal of Clinical Nutrition* **69**, 373–380.

Lichtman, S.W., Pisarka, K., Berman, E.R., Pestone, M., Dowling, H., Offenbacher, E., Weisel, H., Heshka, S. and Matthews, D.E. (1992) Discrepancy between self-reported and actual caloric intake and exercise in obese subjects. *New England Journal of Medicine* **327**, 1893–1898.

McGuire, M.T., Wing, R.R., Klem, M.L., Seagle, H.M. and Hill, J.O. (1998) Long-term maintenance of weight loss: Do people who lose weight through various weight loss methods use different behaviors to maintain their weight? *International Journal of Obesity* **22**, 572–577.

Melanson, K. and Dwyer, J. (2002) Popular diets for treatment of overweight and obesity. In: Wadden, T.A., Stunkard, A.J. eds. *Handbook of Obesity Treatment*. New York: Guilford, 249–275.

Mercer, S.L., Green, L.W., Rosenthal, A.C., Husten, C.G., Khan, L.K. and Dietz, W.H. (2003) Possible lessons from the tobacco experience for obesity control. *American Journal of Clinical Nutrition* **77**, 1073S–1082S.

Meyers, A.W., Graves, T.J., Whelan, J.P. and Barclay, D.R. (1996) An evaluation of a television-delivered behavioral weight loss program: are the ratings acceptable. *Journal of Consulting and Clinical Psychology* **64**, 172–178.

Miller, W.C., Koceja, D.M. and Hamilton, E.J. (1997) A meta-analysis of the past 25 years of weight loss research using diet, exercise or diet plus exercise intervention. *International Journal of Obesity* **21**, 941–947.

National Heart, Lung, and Blood Institute (NHLBI) (1998) Clinical guidelines on the identification, evaluation, and treatment of overweight and obesity in adults: The evidence report. *Obesity Research* **6** (Suppl.), 51S–210S.

Perri, M.G. and Corsica, J.A. (2002) Improving the maintenance of weight lost. In: Wadden, T.A., Stunkard, A.J. eds. *Handbook of Obesity Treatment*. New York: Guilford, 357–379.

Perri, M.G., Shapiro, R.M., Ludwig, W.W., Twentyman, C.T. and McAdoo, W.G. (1984) Maintenance strategies for the treatment of obesity: An evaluation of relapse prevention training and posttreatment contact by mail and telephone. *Journal of Consulting and Clinical Psychology* **52**, 404–413.

Perri, M.G., McAdoo, W.G., McAllister, D.A., Lauer, J.B. and Yancey, D.Z. (1986) Enhancing the efficacy of behavior therapy for obesity: Effects of aerobic exercise and a multicomponent maintenance program. *Journal of Consulting and Clinical Psychology* **54**, 670–675.

Perri, M.G., McAllister, D.A., Gange, J.J., Jordan, R.C., McAdoo, W.G. and Nezu, A.M. (1988) Effects of four maintenance programs on the long-term management of obesity. *Journal of Consulting and Clinical Psychology* **56**, 529–534.

Perri, M.G., Martin, A.D., Leermakers, E.A. and Sears, S.F. (1997) Effects of group versus home-based exercise training in healthy older men and women. *Journal of Consulting and Clinical Psychology* **65**, 278–285.

Perri, M.G., Nezu, A.M., McKelvey, W.F., Shermer, R.L., Renjilian, D.A., Viegener, B.J. (2001) Relapse prevention training and problem-solving therapy in the long-term management of obesity. *Journal of Consulting and Clinical Psychology* **69**, 722–726.

Ramirez, E.M. and Rosen, J.C. (2001) A comparison of weight control and weight control plus body image therapy for obese men and women. *Journal of Consulting and Clinical Psychology* **69**, 440–446.

Ravussin, E., Lillioja, S., Knowler, W.C., Christin, L., Freymond, D., Abbott, W.G., Boyle, V., Howard, B.V. and Bogardus, C. (1988) Reduced rate of energy expenditure as a risk factor for body weight gain. *New England Journal of Medicine* **318**, 467–472.

Renjilian, D.A., Perri, M.G., Nezu, A.M., Mckelvey, W.F., Shermer, R.L. and Anton, S.D. (2001) Individual vs. group therapy for obesity: Effects of matching participants to their treatment preference. *Journal of Consulting and Clinical Psychology* **69**, 717–721.

Rolls, B.J. and Bell, E.A. (1999) Intake of fat and carbohydrate: Role of energy density. *European Journal of Clinical Nutrition* **53S**, S166–S173.

Rolls, B.J., Bell, E.A., Thorwart, M.L. (1999) Water incorporated into a food but not served with a food decreases energy intake in lean women. *American Journal of Clinical Nutrition* **70**, 448–455.

Rosenbaum, M., Murphy, E.M., Heymsfield, S.B., Matthews, D.E. and Leibel, R. (2002) Low dose leptin administration reverses effects of sustained weight reduction on energy expenditure and circulating concentrations of thyroid hormones. *Journal of Clinical Endocrinology and Metabolism* **87**, 2391–2394.

Sbrocco, T., Nedegaard, R.C., Stone, J.M. and Lewis, E.L. (1999) Behavioral choice treatment promotes continuing weight loss: Preliminary results of a cognitive–behavioral decision-based treatment for obesity. *Journal of Consulting and Clinical Psychology* **67**, 260–266.

Schoeller, D.A., Ravussin, E., Schutz, Y., Acheson, K.J., Baertschi, P. and Jequier, E. (1986) Energy expenditure by doubly labeled water: Validation in humans and proposed calculation. *American Journal of Physiology* **250**, R823–R830.

Stunkard, A.J, Harris, J.R., Pederson, N.L. and McClearn, G.E. (1990) The body-mass index of twins who have been reared apart. *New England Journal of Medicine* **322**, 1483–1487.

Tate, D., Wing, R.R. and Winett, R. (2001) Development and evaluation of an Internet behavior therapy program for weight loss. *Journal of the American Medical Association* **285**, 1172–1177.

Tate, D.F., Jackvoney, E.H. and Wing, R.R. (2003) Effects of internet behavioral counseling on weight loss in adults at risk for type 2 diabetes. *Journal of the American Medical Association* **289**, 1833–1836,

Toubro, S. and Astrup, A. (1997) Randomized comparison of diets for maintaining obese subjects' weight after major weight loss: ad lib, low fat, high carbohydrate diet vs. fixed energy intake. *British Medical Journal* **314**, 29–34.

Wadden, T.A. and Foster, G.D. (2000) Behavioral treatment of obesity. *Medical Clinics of North America* **84**, 441–461.

Wadden, T.A. and Osei, S. (2002) The treatment of obesity: An overview. In: Wadden, T.A., Stunkard, A.J. eds. *Handbook of Obesity Treatment*. New York: Guilford Press, 229–248.

Wadden, T.A. and Butryn, M.L. (2003) Behavioral treatment of obesity. *Endocrinology and Metabolism Clinics of North America* **32**, 981–1003.

Wadden, T.A., Sternberg, J.A., Letizia, K.A., Stunkard, A.J. and Foster, G.D. (1989) Treatment of obesity by very-low-calorie diet, behavior therapy, and their combination: a five-year perspective. *International Journal of Obesity* **51**, 167–172.

Wadden, T.A., Berkowitz, R.I., Vogt, R.A., Steen, S.N., Stunkard, A.J. and Foster, G.D. (1997a) Lifestyle modification in the pharmacologic treatment of obesity: a pilot investigation of a potential primary care approach. *Obesity Research* **5**, 218–226.

Wadden, T.A., Vogt, R.A., Andersen, R.E., Bartlett, S.J., Foster, G.D., Kuehnel, R.H., Wilk, J.E., Weinstock, R.S., Buckenmeyer, P., Berkowitz, R.I. and Steen, S.N. (1997b) Exercise in the treatment of obesity: Effects of four interventions on body composition, resting energy expenditure, appetite, and mood. *Journal of Consulting and Clinical Psychology* **65**, 269–277.

Wadden, T.A., Anderson, D.A., Foster, G.D., Bennett, A., Steinberg, C. and Sarwer, D.B. (2000) Obese women's perceptions of their doctor's weight management attitudes and behaviors. *Archives of Family Medicine* **9**, 854–860.

Wadden, T.A., Brownell, K.B. and Foster, G.D. (2002) Obesity: responding to the global epidemic. *Journal of Consulting and Clinical Psychology* **70**, 510–525.

Wadden, T.A., Womble, L.G., Sarwer, D.B., Berkowitz, R.I., Clark, V.L. and Foster, G.D. (2003) Great expectations: "I'm going to lose 25% of my weight no matter what you say". *Journal of Consulting and Clinical Psychology* **71**, 1084–1089.

Wang, S.S., Wadden, T.A., Womble, L.G. and Nonas, C.A. (2003) What consumers want to know about commercial weight loss programs: a pilot investigation. *Obesity Research* **11**, 48–53.

Weight Watchers (2002) 2002 Annual Report (Available at: www.weightwatchers.com). Assessed Oct. 2, 2003.

Wing, R.R. (2002) Behavioral treatment of obesity. In: Wadden, T.A., Stunkard, A.J. eds. *Handbook of Obesity Treatment*. New York: Guilford Press, 301–316.

Wing, R.R. and Jeffery, R.W. (1999) Benefits of recruiting participants with friends and increasing social support for weight loss and maintenance. *Journal of Consulting and Clinical Psychology* **67**, 132–138.

Wing, R.R., Jeffery, R.W., Burton, L.R., Thorson, C., Nissinoff, K. and Baxter, J.E. (1996a) Food provisions vs. structured meal plans in the behavioral treatment of obesity. *Journal of Consulting and Clinical Psychology* **20**, 56–62.

Wing, R.R., Jeffery, R.W., Hellerstedt, W.L. and Burton, L.R. (1996b) Effect of frequent phone contacts and optional food provision on maintenance of weight loss. *Annals of Behavioral Medicine* **18**, 172–176.

World Health Organization (2000) *Obesity: Preventing and Managing the Global Epidemic Technical Report 894*. Geneva: WHO.

24   Exercise and obesity

Marleen A. van Baak and Wim H. M. Saris

Summary, 363

Exercise and body weight, 364
  Physical activity and prevention of
  weight gain, 364
  Exercise and weight
  reduction, 365
  Combined effects of exercise
  and dietary restriction on body
  weight, 365
  Exercise and weight loss
  maintenance, 365

Exercise and energy balance, 366
  Exercise and energy
  expenditure, 366
  Exercise and energy intake, 368

Exercise and substrate
utilization, 369
  Substrate utilization during
  exercise, 369
  Substrate utilization during
  exercise in obesity, 371
  Exercise and 24-h substrate
  utilization, 371
  Training and substrate utilization
  during exercise, 371
  Training and 24-h substrate
  utilization, 372

Exercise and obesity-related
morbidity and mortality, 372
  Insulin resistance and type 2
  diabetes, 373
  Blood lipids, 373

Blood pressure, 373
Other comorbidities associated
  with obesity, 373
Mental health and health-related
  well-being, 374
Aerobic fitness, 374
Mortality, 374

Summary of benefits of exercise in
obesity, 374

Exercise recommendations for
weight management, 374
  Exercise mode, 375
  Exercise prescription, 375
  Exercise adherence, 376
  Exercise risk, 376

References, 376

Summary

Exercise is recommended as an important strategy for prevention of obesity and as an effective adjunct to its treatment. Not only the weight loss effects are important in this respect, but also the weight loss-independent beneficial health effects of exercise in obesity. This chapter focuses on the effects of acute and regular exercise (training) in obesity and exercise recommendations for obese patients:

• Prospective epidemiological studies support the notion that a high level of physical activity protects against increases in weight and obesity.

• Endurance exercise training alone induces modest weight and fat loss, which may be slightly more pronounced in overweight than in lean individuals. Resistance training has little effect on weight, but increases fat-free mass. In combination with an energy-restricted diet, endurance exercise training results in some additional weight loss, which is small, however, compared with the diet-induced weight loss. Fat-free mass is reduced less than with diet alone for the same weight loss. Resistance exercise training may preserve fat-free mass more effectively during dietary restriction than endurance training.

• Regular exercise is an important determinant of successful weight maintenance after a period of weight loss. Evidence mainly comes from observational studies. Results of randomized controlled trials are inconsistent, which may be related to insufficient amounts of exercise.

• Energy expenditure is increased above resting levels during and after an exercise bout. Energy expended during exercise depends on the type, intensity and duration of the exercise bout, and the weight of the individual. The net energy cost of exercise may vary roughly between 2 and 20 kcal/kg/h. The magnitude of the post-exercise increase in energy expenditure (EPOC) also depends on duration and intensity of exercise. EPOC is small in comparison with the energy expended during the exercise bout itself.

• Exercise training does not lead to significant changes of resting metabolic rate (RMR) in lean or obese individuals. The addition of an exercise programme to a period of dietary restriction in obese individuals, on the other hand, may reduce the decrease in RMR accompanying a negative energy balance.

• Diet-induced thermogenesis (DIT) is not affected by exercise training in lean subjects, neither at rest nor after an acute bout of exercise. In obese people, training may increase DIT after acute exercise. However, the absolute increment of total energy expenditure owing to this effect is small.

• Exercise training increases average daily energy expenditure in lean individuals. Part of the increase may be due to an increase in non-exercise training activities. Similar trends are found in obese individuals.

• Adaptation of energy intake to increases in energy expenditure by exercise is slow. Lean subjects compensate the energy expended during exercise to a larger extent than obese individuals by increasing energy intake. A larger compensation, and even overcompensation, takes place on a high-fat diet compared with a high-carbohydrate diet.

• The composition of the substrate mix that is utilized during exercise depends on the intensity and duration of the exercise and the training status of the subject. At moderate exercise intensity (65% $\dot{V}o_{2max}$) utilization of fatty acids increases and that of carbohydrates decreases with time. At very low exercise intensity (25% $\dot{V}o_{2max}$) plasma free fatty acids are the main energy source. As intensity increases, the contribution of plasma glucose and muscle glycogen increases, and that of plasma fatty acids decreases. The contribution of intramuscular triglycerides is most pronounced at moderate exercise intensity. Obese individuals have a higher fat oxidation at the same relative exercise intensity than lean individuals.

• Endurance exercise training increases fat oxidation during exercise in lean and obese individuals. The main source of the increased fat oxidation is the intramuscular triglyceride stores. Training also increases post-exercise and basal fat oxidation. The effects of training on 24-h substrate oxidation are not clear.

• Epidemiological data suggest that moderate and high levels of cardiorespiratory fitness or physical activity reduce the risk of premature mortality in each category of body weight or adiposity. Moreover, regular exercise improves glucose tolerance, reduces blood pressure and improves aerobic fitness, independent of reductions in body weight.

• The question of which amount and type of exercise training is optimal for obese people probably does not have a single answer. It will depend on the goal(s) of the training programme. Effects on weight are related to the total amount of energy expended: 45–60 min of moderate-intensity exercise per day is necessary to prevent the transition from overweight to obesity, and 60–90 min per day to prevent weight regain after weight reduction in obese people. Exercise intensity may have an effect that is independent of the total amount of energy expended with respect to aerobic fitness, glucose tolerance, blood pressure and coronary heart disease risk reduction.

• Dynamic exercise with large muscle groups is recommended for weight management. Resistance training will increase muscle mass and improve muscular strength and endurance, but is less effective in reducing body weight.

• Degree of overweight is an important predictor of drop-out from exercise programmes. Strategies to improve exercise adherence in obese people need to be developed.

• A gradual increase in intensity and amount of exercise and the adoption of low-impact activities will contribute to the prevention of exercise-related injuries in obese people.

Exercise and body weight

Traditionally, exercise has been recommended as an important strategy for prevention of obesity and as an effective adjunct to its treatment. Much evidence has been accumulated over the past years to strengthen this recommendation, not only with respect to weight management, but also concerning the beneficial effects of exercise on obesity-related morbidities. This chapter will focus on the effects of acute and regular exercise (training) in obesity and its underlying mechanisms, and will address recommendations for exercise in overweight and obese individuals.

Exercise is every planned, structured and repetitive body movement done to improve or maintain one or more components of physical fitness. Because weight and many of the health parameters that will be discussed in this chapter can be regarded as components of physical fitness, the term exercise will be used throughout this chapter. The term *exercise* is nowadays often replaced by physical activity. Physical activity is any bodily movement produced by the skeletal muscles that results in a substantial increase in energy expenditure over the resting energy expenditure. It includes not only exercise (undertaken with the deliberate intent of improving health or physical performance) and sport, but also equivalent energy expenditure in other types of active leisure, occupational work and domestic chores. Using the term *physical activity* rather than exercise reflects the notion that activities of normal daily life can also contribute to the increased energy expenditure that is crucial for weight management, and this should be kept in mind when reading this chapter.

Physical activity and prevention of weight gain

Cross-sectional population-based studies usually show a negative correlation between level of physical activity and body mass, but this cannot be taken as proof that less active people gain more weight, because a low level of physical activity may be the consequence rather than the cause of weight gain. The question of cause or consequence is better answered by prospective studies. Reviews of prospective observational studies indicated that studies using baseline physical activity do not show a consistent association between the level of physical activity at baseline and weight gain. Those that used physical activity at follow-up are more consistent in their outcome, showing that a higher level of physical activity at follow-up is associated with less weight gain. Those studies that looked at changes in physical activity from baseline to follow-up tend to show reduced weight gain with increased physical activity (Fogelholm and Kukkonen-Harjula, 2000; Erlichman et al., 2002).

These large epidemiological studies support the notion that a high level of physical activity protects against increases in body weight and obesity. In addition, inactive behaviours, such as television watching, have been shown to be associated with increased risk of obesity in a large prospective study, independent of exercise levels (Hu *et al.*, 2003). However, long-term, randomized controlled trials to further substantiate this are lacking for obvious reasons.

Exercise and weight reduction

Numerous experimental studies have shown that adults on average lose a very modest amount of weight when they increase their physical activity by exercise. Wilmore (1995) reviewed a total of 53 studies on weight changes with exercise training without prescribed changes in diet. Although the variation between individual studies was large, a 6-month period of training resulted in an average loss of 1.6 kg of body mass, a loss of 2.6 kg of fat mass and a gain of 1.0 kg of fat-free mass. Garrow and Summerbell (1995) did a meta-analysis of the effect of exercise on weight changes in overweight subjects. The average body mass index (BMI) of subjects in the eight studies that were included in the analysis varied between 25 and 30 kg/m^2, indicating that the results are from overweight or mildly obese persons. Endurance exercise training without dietary restriction caused an average weight loss of 3 kg over 30 weeks in men and of 1.4 kg over 12 weeks in women, with little effect on fat-free mass.

The most recent review by Ross and Janssen (2001), including nine randomized controlled trials and 22 non-randomized trials on exercise and weight change in overweight and obese individuals (BMI > 25 kg/m^2), showed that the amount of energy expenditure by physical activity is positively associated with a reduction of body weight and total body fat in studies with a duration of 16 weeks or less. The range of energy expenditures varied between 500 and 5500 kcal per week. If the range of energy expenditures is limited to 500–2000 kcal per week, which is the range in which most exercise studies are found, a dose–response relationship is not very apparent, due to the large variation in body weight reductions. It is therefore not surprising that some studies have concluded that no dose–response relationship exists. The same review showed that there was no dose–response relationship in studies of longer duration (26 weeks or more). Abdominal fat was also reduced by exercise, although a dose–response relationship could not be established owing to limited data (Ross and Janssen, 2001).

Resistance exercise training has little effect on weight, but tends to increase fat-free mass and reduce fat mass (Ballor and Keesey, 1991; Garrow and Summerbell, 1995; Hunter *et al.*, 2000; Poehlman *et al.*, 2002).

These experimental results indicate that endurance exercise training induces moderate weight loss, which consists mainly of fat mass loss, and which may be slightly more pronounced in overweight than in lean subjects. The weight loss is usually less than might be expected from the increase in exercise-induced energy expenditure, suggesting that part of the increased energy expenditure is compensated for by increased energy intake.

Combined effects of exercise and dietary restriction on body weight

Although exercise alone results in modest weight loss, exercise is almost always prescribed as an adjunct to dietary restriction in weight reduction programmes. The combined effects of dietary restriction and exercise training on body weight have been reviewed extensively. Donnelly and colleagues (1991) showed that the average weight loss over seven studies with a duration varying between 21 and 112 (mean 62) days was approximately 1 kg higher when exercise training was added to a very low-calorie diet (500–800 kcal/day) than with the diet alone (9.7 vs. 8.6 kg). Garrow and Summerbell (1995) found a 1.5-kg difference in weight loss between low-calorie diets (< 1000 kcal/day, duration 8–16 weeks) and the same diet plus exercise (12.7 vs. 11.2 kg; mean of 11 studies). In less severe energy restriction (diets > 1000 kcal/day, duration 5–26 weeks) the difference was 0.8 kg (7.6 vs. 6.8 kg; mean of 10 studies).

From these studies it is clear that adding exercise training to an energy-restricted diet results in a modest extra weight loss that is small compared with the weight loss attained by the dietary treatment alone. Despite this modest extra weight loss, at the 1-year follow-up diet plus exercise appears to be the most successful weight management programme (Miller *et al.*, 1997; Wing, 1999).

Most reviews also addressed the question of whether adding exercise to an energy-restricted diet reduces or prevents the reduction of fat-free mass accompanying such diets. Although the results are not fully conclusive, the majority of studies indeed suggest that this is the case. The meta-analysis by Garrow and Summerbell (1995) indicates that for every 10 kg of weight loss by diet alone, the expected loss of fat-free mass is 2.9 kg in men and 2.2 kg in women. When the same weight loss is achieved by exercise combined with dietary restriction, the expected loss of fat-free mass is reduced to 1.7 kg in men and women. Resistance exercise may result in a more effective preservation of fat-free mass during a period of energy restriction than endurance training (Ballor *et al.*, 1996).

Exercise and weight loss maintenance

Although exercise training results in only modest (extra) reductions of body weight when prescribed alone or in combination with dietary restriction, regular exercise is considered of crucial importance for successful weight loss maintenance after a period of weight reduction. Most of the evidence comes from non-randomized weight reduction studies with an observational follow-up. Successful weight loss maintainers are characterized by high levels of physical activity, low dietary fat and high dietary carbohydrate intake, and regular self-monitoring of weight (Wing and Hill, 2001).

A review of weight maintenance studies showed that at present there is very little evidence from randomized controlled trials to support this. When weighted mean weight changes were calculated for the 11 randomized weight loss or weight maintenance studies with an average follow-up duration of 20 months (range 12–42 months), the weight regain during follow-up amounted to 0.28 kg/month in the exercise groups and 0.33 kg/month in the control groups in weight reduction programmes (Fogelholm and Kukkonen-Harjula, 2000). The reason for this lack of efficacy in randomized controlled trials may be that the amount of physical activity prescribed in these studies is insufficient and that the adherence to the exercise programmes is low.

In an 18-month weight loss maintenance study, using a combination of drug treatment, dietary and exercise advice, the most important predictors of successful weight loss maintenance were drug treatment during the weight maintenance phase, the magnitude of body weight loss during the weight loss phase and the level of leisure time physical activity during the weight maintenance phase (Van Baak *et al.*, in press).

Exercise and energy balance

In the previous section it was shown that regular exercise reduces body weight or prevents weight gain. It therefore creates a negative energy balance or prevents a positive energy balance. How is this accomplished? Energy expenditure and energy intake represent the two sides of the energy balance equation. Does exercise affect energy balance through effects on energy expenditure or on energy intake, or a combination of the two?

Exercise and energy expenditure

Total daily energy expenditure (24-h EE) can be divided into several components: resting metabolic rate (RMR), which accounts for approximately 60–70% of 24-h energy expenditure; the diet-induced thermogenesis (DIT), approximately 10% of 24-h EE; and the energy expenditure induced by physical activity or exercise, which is the most variable component and may vary from 15% of 24-h EE in sedentary people to 30–40% in active people to even 400% in professional cyclists under extreme circumstances. Acute exercise may affect all three components of 24-h EE. Apart from the acute effects, regular exercise or training may have additional effects.

Energy expenditure during exercise in lean and obese individuals

Energy expenditure increases during exercise. During activities such as walking or running, energy expenditure at a

Table 24.1 Energy cost of various physical activities expressed as METs (ratio of work metabolic rate to resting metabolic rate).

Activity	METs
Aerobics	6.5
Bicycling, 12–13.9 mph, leisure, moderate effort	8.0
Bicycling, 100-W stationary bicycle ergometer	5.5
Rowing ergometer, general	7.0
Running, jogging	7.0
Running, 6 mph	10.0
Soccer, casual	7.0
Stair-treadmill ergometer	9.0
Tennis, singles	8.0
Tennis, doubles	6.0
Walking, 3 mph, level, firm surface	3.3
Walking, brisk, 3.5 mph, level, firm surface	3.8

From Ainsworth *et al.* (2000).

certain speed increases with body mass. There are indications that obese individuals have an inefficient locomotor pattern and thus their energy expenditure at a certain speed is higher than predicted from their body mass. Those who are obese probably have to do more mechanical work during walking to overcome friction between thighs and between the arms and torso, and the arms and legs have to swing more widely to move around thighs and torso (Foster *et al.*, 1995). Weight changes may also affect muscle work efficiency: weight increase reduced work efficiency, whereas weight reduction increased muscle work efficiency (Rosenbaum *et al.*, 2003).

Table 24.1 gives a selection of total energy expenditure (resting energy expenditure plus the additional energy cost of exercise) during a number of recreational physical activities. A more detailed list of activities can be found in the work of Ainsworth and colleagues (2000). To obtain the extra energy expended during the activity, resting energy expenditure, 1 MET (or approximately 1 kcal/kg/h), has to be subtracted from the values in the table. The net energy cost of exercise (total—resting energy expenditure) varies roughly between 2 (leisure walking) and 20 METs (kcal/kg/h) (cross-country skiing). It should be realized that these are average values applicable under average conditions, applied to the average (non-obese) person.

Training and energy expenditure during exercise

Regular exercise or training may lead to more efficient movement patterns: the energy cost of running at a certain speed is approximately 15% lower in trained than in untrained runners, and elite swimmers use up to 50% less energy at a particular swimming speed than untrained swimmers. Whether obese individuals also expend less energy after training has not been studied.

Table 24.2 Causes of excess post-exercise oxygen consumption (EPOC).

Resynthesis of ATP and CP
Resynthesis of glycogen from lactate
Oxidation of lactate
Replenishment of oxygen stores (haemoglobin and myoglobin)
Thermogenic effects of elevated body temperature
Thermogenic effects of noradrenaline and adrenaline
Elevated heart rate, respiration and other physiological functions
Increased triglyceride fatty acid cycling

Post-exercise energy expenditure

Energy expenditure may remain elevated for up to 48 h during recovery from acute exercise. A number of different processes appear to be responsible for the excess post-exercise oxygen consumption (EPOC) (Table 24.2). The total magnitude of EPOC depends on intensity and duration of the exercise performed, with little EPOC when exercise intensity is below 70% of maximal oxygen consumption ($\dot{V}o_{2max}$). Values of up to 32 L (or 150 kcal) over 12 h post exercise have been reported. Dietary restriction appears to lower EPOC (Fukuba *et al.*, 2000). An exercise prescription of low to moderate exercise, aimed at the general public, would result in an EPOC of maximally 30 kcal per exercise bout (Poehlman *et al.*, 1991). EPOC has not been studied in obese individuals.

Training and resting metabolic rate

Several studies have addressed the question whether regular exercise affects RMR, independent of the acute effects of exercise (EPOC) described above and independent of changes in fat-free mass, which are known to affect resting metabolic rate. The results of cross-sectional studies, comparing untrained and trained individuals, are inconclusive. Of longitudinal training studies in lean as well as obese men and women, the majority show no effect on RMR adjusted for fat-free mass, measured between 12 and 96 h after the last training session. However, because exercise training, and especially resistance exercise training, in many cases increases fat-free mass, the absolute RMR is increased after exercise training in those cases.

Another issue is whether exercise training reduces or even prevents the fall in RMR that is associated with energy-restricted diets. Although the majority of studies suggest a positive effect, the evidence is not very strong. Those studies that do find less reduction of RMR usually conclude that the mechanism is partly a reduced loss of fat-free mass and partly an elevation of metabolic activity per unit of fat-free mass (Prentice *et al.*, 1991).

In conclusion, exercise training programmes generally do not lead to an increase in RMR in lean or obese individuals. The addition of a training programme during a period of dietary restriction in obese individuals, on the other hand, may reduce the decrease in RMR that accompanies a negative energy balance, most probably through a more favourable ratio between fat mass and fat-free mass loss.

Diet-induced thermogenesis

Considerable inconsistency exists regarding the acute effects of exercise on the thermic effect of a meal ingested after an exercise bout in either lean or obese subjects. Cross-sectional studies that compared DIT in trained and untrained subjects have also yielded conflicting results. Apart from the difficulty of measuring DIT, inconsistencies may be related to meal size and composition, the timing of the meal and exercise, the intensity and duration of the exercise, and differences in the characteristics of the subjects (Segal, 1995).

Well-controlled longitudinal training studies, in which the effect of exercise training was studied independent of changes in body mass and body fat in lean and obese subjects matched for fat-free mass, suggest that DIT is not affected by training in lean subjects, neither at rest nor after an acute bout of exercise. In obese subjects, who showed a blunted DIT, DIT was increased roughly 40% by acute exercise after training, although under resting conditions DIT was not affected by training (Segal, 1995). However, the absolute increment of total energy expenditure due to this effect is small.

24-h energy expenditure

As discussed in the preceding paragraphs, exercise increases energy expenditure during the exercise bout itself and may elevate post-exercise energy expenditure. Effects on RMR and DIT, if any, are probably small. However, from this it cannot be concluded automatically that exercise also elevates 24-h EE, as it is possible that non-exercise physical activity changes due to an exercise bout or training, either in a positive or in a negative direction.

Studies in a respiration chamber have shown that 24-h EE increases on a day with exercise (Melanson *et al.*, 2002a,b). Studies that have measured 24-h EE under free-living conditions with the doubly labelled water technique show that 24-h EE is usually higher during than before endurance training, although the change is not always statistically significant (Toth and Poehlman, 1996; Westerterp, 1998). The increase is often greater than expected from the training-related energy expenditure, thus suggesting increased non-exercise energy expenditure (Westerterp, 1998). Studies in overweight and obese subjects show similar trends (Blaak *et al.*, 1992; Donnelly *et al.*, 2003). Resistance training has also been found to increase 24-h EE in elderly people, both through an increase in fat-free mass and RMR and an increase in physical activity (Hunter *et al.*, 2000). The increase in 24-h EE is not maintained after stopping the exercise training (Poehlman *et al.*, 2002).

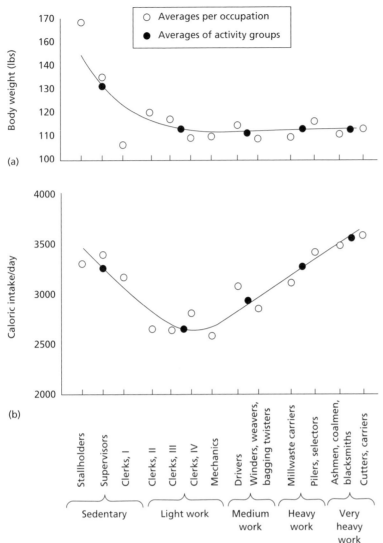

Fig 24.1 Body weight and caloric intake as a function of level of physical activity at work, in an industrial male population in West Bengal. (From Mayer *et al.*, 1956.)

Exercise and energy intake

In the preceding section, the effects of acute and regular exercise on the energy expenditure side of the energy balance equation have been described. In this section, interaction of exercise with energy intake will be discussed. This aspect has been less extensively studied, probably because of the difficulties associated with the accurate measurement of energy intake.

The classical study by Mayer and colleagues (1956) in 213 men employed at a jute mill in West Bengal, India, with a wide range of physical activity during work, showed that energy intake was more tightly coupled to the energy demand of the job above the level described as 'light work' (Fig. 24.1). In sedentary employees, food intake was increased inappropriately, resulting in increased body mass. Although this study has major shortcomings in design and analysis, the general conclusion is supported by animal research (Oscai, 1973). The studies that have actually measured the effect of increasing physical activ-

ity on energy intake experimentally will be discussed in the next paragraphs.

Acute post-exercise energy intake

Studies on the effects of exercise on energy intake during a post-exercise meal are scarce. In lean men, hunger ratings were reduced immediately after a 50-min endurance exercise session at 70% $\dot{V}o_{2max}$. This exercise-induced anorexia had disappeared within 15 min, and food intake during the test meal given 15 min after the exercise bout was unaffected by the previous exercise. In lean women, the transient anorectic effect was absent and food intake was also unaffected by the preceding exercise bout (King *et al.*, 1994; King and Blundell 1995). Other studies showed that non-dieting overweight women with low dietary restraint status tend to increase their energy intake after an exercise bout, whereas overweight highly restrained and normal-weight women show the reverse ten-

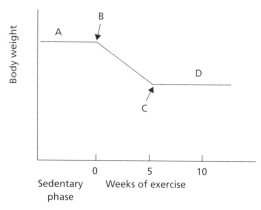

Fig 24.2 Hypothetical impact of exercise on body weight. 'A' indicates the initial steady state, 'B' represents the start of exercise, 'B to C' represents the adjustment period when a higher energy expenditure is not compensated by energy intake and 'C' represents the time at which new forces (behavioural and metabolic) interact to induce a new steady state ('D'). (From Blundell and King, 2000.)

dency. Highly restrained, dieting women showed the largest increase in energy intake after an exercise bout (Visona and George, 2002; George and Morganstein, 2003).

The physiological mechanism of the acute anorectic effect of exercise is unknown, but may involve stimulation of the noradrenergic, serotonergic and corticotrophin-releasing hormone systems in the brain, which are known to cause anorexia (Richard, 1995; Rowland *et al.*, 1996).

Adaptation of energy intake to increased energy expenditure

Blundell and King (2000) postulate that initially no tight coupling exists between increased energy expenditure by exercise and energy intake and that weight is lost, but gradually a new balance between energy expenditure and energy intake is attained by a combination of behavioural and physiological adaptations, thus stabilizing body weight (Fig. 24.2). The regulatory system that controls body (fat) mass and links energy intake to energy expenditure in the long term is not fully known. However, hormones such as leptin and insulin provide afferent input to the central nervous system about the energy stores of the body. Regular exercise lowers plasma insulin levels. Although it appears to have no effect on fasting plasma leptin concentration in humans, changes in energy balance induced by exercise influence the 24-h profile of leptin (Hickey and Calsbeek, 2001). Decreases in leptin and insulin concentrations induced by regular exercise will suppress anorexigenic signals, such as alpha-melanocyte stimulating hormone (α-MSH), and stimulate orexigenic signals, such as neuropeptide Y (NPY) and Agouti-related protein (AgRP), in the arcuate nucleus of the hypothalamus (Schwartz *et al.*, 2000), thus providing a mechanism for the adaptation of energy intake to a negative energy balance induced by exercise.

Lean subjects compensate for the energy expended during exercise more readily than obese subjects and body weight reduction with exercise training is therefore more pronounced in obese than in lean persons. However, the variability appears to be large. One of the factors responsible for this variability may be the degree of dietary restraint or disinhibition (Keim *et al.*, 1990). Moreover, women tend to adapt energy intake more readily to increases in energy expenditure due to exercise than men (Blundell and King, 2000).

Another factor that appears to have significant influence is the composition of the diet. Several studies show that larger compensation and even overcompensation of the exercise-induced increase in energy expenditure takes place on a high-fat diet than on a high-carbohydrate diet (Tremblay *et al.*, 1994; King and Blundell, 1995; King *et al.*, 1996). These observations are in agreement with the notion that carbohydrate balance is rather tightly regulated and that replenishment of the carbohydrate stores after exercise requires a larger energy intake on a high-fat diet than on a high-carbohydrate diet (Flatt, 1987). This finding underlines the importance of a relatively low-fat diet during weight loss and weight maintenance.

Cross-sectional studies indicate that trained individuals consume a larger proportion of carbohydrates in their diet than untrained people (Horber *et al.*, 1996) and that total daily energy intake is positively correlated with the carbohydrate-derived energy content of the diet (Saris, 1989).

Exercise and substrate utilization

Any intervention aimed at inducing weight loss in overweight persons should promote a negative fat balance. Exercise increases energy expenditure and substrate oxidation in skeletal muscles. Fatty acids are an important energy source for the exercising muscles. Moreover, due to the depletion of glycogen stores during exercise, fat oxidation is favoured following exercise. These combined effects result in increased fat oxidation. Exercise therefore allows fat oxidation to be in balance with fat intake at a lower body fat content (Flatt, 1995).

Substrate utilization during exercise

During exercise, oxygen consumption rises and increased amounts of substrates have to be made available to be used as fuels in the exercising muscles. Increased activity of the sympathetic nervous system plays an important role in the mobilization of substrates from their stores in the body (Fig. 24.3). Hormonal changes (insulin, glucagon, growth hormone, adrenaline) support the actions of the sympathetic nervous system. In addition, the sympathetic nervous system regulates the cardiovascular adaptations necessary for the transport of oxygen and substrates to, and waste products from, the exercising muscles.

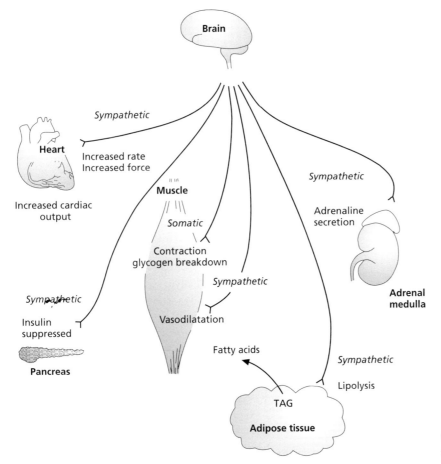

Fig 24.3 Coordination of metabolism by the nervous system during endurance exercise. (From Frayn, 1996.)

During the first minute of submaximal aerobic exercise, muscle glycogen breakdown is the main source of energy. As exercise continues, blood-borne substrates (glucose and non-esterified fatty acids, NEFAs) become more important (Fig. 24.4). Although blood glucose concentration usually does not change during non-exhaustive exercise, the turnover of blood glucose is increased. The liver provides the extra glucose by increased hepatic glycogenolysis and gluconeogenesis. The blood concentration of NEFAs initially falls but gradually increases during prolonged exercise above resting levels, indicating that adipose tissue lipolysis is not strictly matched to muscle NEFA utilization. Another source of fatty acids during exercise is the triglyceride stores present within the skeletal muscles. At moderate exercise intensity (65% $\dot{V}o_{2max}$) utilization of fatty acids increases and that of carbohydrates decreases with time (Romijn *et al.*, 1993) (Fig. 24.4), which is reflected by a gradual decrease of the respiratory quotient during prolonged exercise at this intensity.

The composition of the substrate mix utilized during exercise depends not only on duration but also on the intensity of exercise and the training status of the subject. The absolute fat oxidation (in g/min) is maximal at an exercise intensity of around 65% $\dot{V}o_{2max}$ but remains close to maximal at exercise intensities between 55% and 75% $\dot{V}o_{2max}$. At exercise inten-

sities above 75% $\dot{V}o_{2max}$, fat oxidation drops rapidly (Achten *et al.*, 2002). At very low exercise intensity (25% $\dot{V}o_{2max}$, similar to walking) plasma NEFAs are the main energy source. As intensity increases, the absolute contribution of plasma glucose and muscle glycogen increases and that of plasma NEFA decreases (Romijn *et al.*, 1993) (Fig. 24.5). The contribution of intramuscular triglycerides is largest at moderate exercise intensity (65% $\dot{V}o_{2max}$). At this exercise intensity, all four of the major substrates (plasma NEFA and glucose, muscle glycogen and triglycerides) contribute substantially to energy production. This is the exercise intensity generally chosen to improve fitness. At the high intensity of 85% $\dot{V}o_{2max}$, the absolute oxidation of fat is reduced and muscle glycogen becomes the most important substrate. This appears to be due not only to reduced fatty acid availability, but also to a limited capacity for fat oxidation in the muscle (Coyle, 1995).

It should be realized that these data have been collected in endurance-trained men under fasting circumstances. Although the general pattern of substrate utilization will be similar, less well-trained people will oxidize less fat and will utilize more muscle glycogen at a given percentage of $\dot{V}o_{2max}$ than with endurance-trained subjects. Pre-exercise carbohydrate-containing meals reduce fat oxidation and increase carbohydrate oxidation during exercise (Coyle,

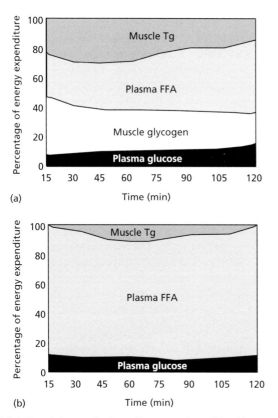

(a)

(b)

Fig 24.4 The relative contributions of intramuscular and blood-borne substrates to fuel utilization during prolonged exercise at 65% (a) and 25% (b) $\dot{V}o_{2max}$ in endurance-trained men. (From Romijn *et al.*, 1993.)

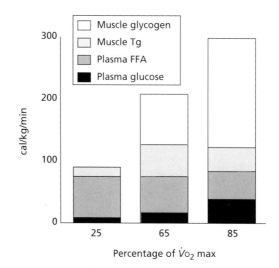

Fig 24.5 Maximal contribution to energy expenditure derived from glucose and free fatty acids (FFAs) taken up from blood and minimal contribution of muscle triglyceride (Tg) and glycogen stored after 30 min of exercise, expressed as function of exercise intensity. Total amount of calories derived from the plasma does not change in relation to exercise intensity. (From Romijn *et al.*, 1993.)

1995). Women demonstrate greater fat oxidation during exercise at the same relative intensity than equally trained men, which may be related to their higher fat mass (Carter *et al.*, 2001; Mittendorfer *et al.*, 2002).

Substrate utilization during exercise in obesity

Obese men and women derive a greater proportion of their energy from fat during 30 min to 1 h of exercise at 50–70% $\dot{V}o_{2max}$ than age- and aerobic capacity-matched lean men and women (Kanaley *et al.*, 2001; Goodpaster *et al.*, 2002). The extra fat oxidized is mainly derived from non-plasma sources. With longer exercise duration, this difference between lean and obese individuals may disappear. Formerly obese women have similar or lower fat oxidation during exercise than age-, weight- and aerobic capacity-matched control women (Ranneries *et al.*, 1998; Guesbeck *et al.*, 2001). A defect in fat oxidation may predispose individuals to obesity.

Exercise and 24-h substrate utilization

It is often claimed that the amount of fat oxidized is highest with low-intensity exercise. Although the proportion of fat oxidation of total energy expenditure is indeed highest during low-intensity exercise, the total amount of fat oxidized de-

pends on both the duration and the intensity of exercise. At higher intensities, the absolute fat oxidation per minute may be higher because the total energy expenditure is higher; at very high intensities, fat oxidation per minute may be lower, as indicated before. On the other hand, fat oxidation after exercise, which is increased in lean as well as obese individuals (Marion-Latard *et al.*, 2003), may be stimulated most after high-intensity exercise. Exercise also has the ability to alter the post-exercise partitioning of dietary fat between oxidation and storage towards increased oxidation of certain types of fatty acids (Votruba *et al.*, 2002).

To establish the most optimal exercise intensity for maximum total fat oxidation, 24-h fat oxidation needs to be studied. Data on this topic are relatively scarce. Exercise, either aerobic or resistance, performed during a 24-h stay in a respiration chamber increased 24-h energy expenditure and carbohydrate oxidation, but had no effect on 24-h fat oxidation in lean subjects (Melanson *et al.*, 2002a,b). There was no difference between aerobic exercise performed at 40% or 70% $\dot{V}o_{2max}$ with the same total energy expenditure (400 kcal) (Melanson *et al.*, 2002a). No data are available for obese subjects.

Training and substrate utilization during exercise

Training, even at exercise intensities as low as 40% $\dot{V}o_{2max}$, reduces utilization of both muscle glycogen and blood glucose during exercise at a given absolute submaximal exercise intensity. This training-induced reduction in carbohydrate oxidation during exercise is compensated for by an increase in fat oxidation. Studies indicate that the main source of this increased fat oxidation at a certain absolute exercise intensity

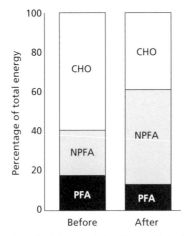

Fig 24.6 Percentage of total energy derived from carbohydrate (CHO), non-plasma fatty acid (FA) and plasma FA (PFA) fuel sources during prolonged exercise at 63% $\dot{V}o_{2\,max}$ before and after 12 weeks of endurance training. (From Martin *et al.*, 1993.)

may not be adipose tissue lipolysis, but rather intramuscular triglyceride stores (Hurley *et al.*, 1986; Martin *et al.*, 1993; Coyle 1995; Schrauwen *et al.*, 2002) (Fig. 24.6).

The underlying mechanisms for these training-induced adaptations probably involve changes in muscle respiratory capacity and hormonal adaptations. Increases in the skeletal muscle content of mitochondria, enzymes involved in activation, transfer into mitochondria and beta-oxidation of fatty acids, increases in cytosolic fatty acid-binding protein and change in activity of regulatory molecules such as 5'-AMP-activated protein kinase (AMPK), malonyl-CoA and acetyl-CoA carboxylase-2 (ACC2) occur with training (Henriksson 1995; Simoneau, 1995; Schrauwen *et al.*, 2002; Tunstall *et al.*, 2002; Nielsen *et al.*, 2003). Training also increases the capacity to store triglycerides in muscle in humans. The effects of endurance exercise on the glycolytic capacity of the skeletal muscle are modest, although high-intensity intermittent exercise training can induce increases in the enzymes of the glycolytic pathways. Training generally reduces the magnitude of the hormonal response to a standard exercise load. This is associated with improved target tissue sensitivity and/or responsiveness to a given quantity of hormone.

Data on the effects of exercise training on substrate utilization in obese people are rather scarce. Van Aggel-Leijssen and co-workers (2001a; 2002) performed a number of studies on the effects of training on substrate utilization during exercise in obese subjects, independent of changes in body or fat mass. They reported an increase in fat oxidation during exercise (at the same absolute intensity before and after training) in obese men and in obese women with an upper body fat distribution after 12 weeks of low-intensity exercise training (40% $\dot{V}o_{2\,max}$). The increased fat oxidation was due to an increase in non-plasma fatty acid oxidation, similar to what is found in lean individuals. However, no change in exercise fat oxidation was found in obese men after high-intensity training (70%

$\dot{V}o_{2\,max}$) or in lower body obese women after low-intensity training at 40% $\dot{V}o_{2\,max}$. Low-intensity training also prevented the reduction in fat oxidation induced by weight loss through an energy-restricted diet (Van Aggel-Leijssen *et al.*, 2001b).

Kanaley and colleagues (2001) found no change in fat oxidation during exercise (at the same relative exercise intensity before and after training) after training for 16 weeks at 70% $\dot{V}o_{2max}$ in obese women. Instead, carbohydrate oxidation was increased. There was no difference between upper and lower-body obese women. Crampes and colleagues (2003), on the other hand, reported an increase in fat oxidation during exercise (at the same relative exercise intensity before and after training) in obese men after training for 16 weeks at 50–85% $\dot{V}o_{2max}$ in the fasting but not in the fed state. In this study, body and fat mass of the subjects was reduced after training.

Thus, exercise training is able to increase the capacity for fat oxidation in obese individuals as in lean individuals. However, the optimal training intensity to produce this effect under different conditions remains to be established.

Training and 24-h substrate utilization

Because exercise training is associated with structural and enzymatic adaptations, training may not only affect substrate utilization during exercise but also in the non-exercising state. Many studies have shown that fat oxidation is increased during the first hours after exercise (Bielinski *et al.*, 1985; Bahr *et al.*, 1990). Cross-sectional studies in which substrate oxidation has been measured at least 24 h after the last exercise bout give ambiguous results: similar and increased fasting respiratory quotients (RQs) have been found when comparing trained and untrained subjects (Tremblay and Buemann, 1995). On the other hand, endurance as well as resistance training have been shown to increase fasting fat oxidation (Poehlman *et al.*, 1994; Calles-Escandón *et al.*, 1996; Hunter *et al.*, 2000), although not in all studies (Kanaley *et al.*, 2001).

Resistance training increased 24-h fat oxidation in a respiration chamber independent of a change in 24-h EE (Treuth *et al.*, 1995). Buemann and colleagues (1992), on the other hand, found no change in 24-h RQ after a training programme in post-obese women.

In conclusion, exercise training has the potential to increase fat oxidation at rest and during exercise in lean as well as obese individuals. This may be an important contributing factor in the prevention and treatment of obesity (Flatt, 1987; 1995; Tremblay and Buemann, 1995).

Exercise and obesity-related morbidity and mortality

Obesity has been associated with an increased premature mortality and increased risks for chronic diseases, such as type 2 diabetes, cardiovascular disease associated with dyslipidaemia and hypertension, osteoarthritis and sleep apnoea (National Institutes of Health, 1998). Regular exercise is known to have beneficial effects on most of these risks.

Insulin resistance and type 2 diabetes

Insulin resistance is an important feature in the development of glucose intolerance and type 2 diabetes. Exercise increases post-exercise insulin sensitivity, an effect that is maintained for 48–72 h. The molecular mechanisms underlying this increased insulin sensitivity have not been fully unravelled (Henriksen 2002; Wojtaszewski *et al.*, 2002). Insulin sensitivity is increased in those skeletal muscles that have been active during the exercise bout. The lowered glycogen content of these muscles probably plays an important role in determining the insulin response of glucose transport and glycogen synthesis. Incoming glucose is used mainly for glycogen synthesis and incoming fatty acids mainly for oxidation, which explains the increased fat oxidation reported after exercise.

Exercise training improves skeletal muscle insulin sensitivity of glucose transport in insulin-sensitive as well as insulin-resistant individuals with obesity or type 2 diabetes. This is associated with increased expression of the glucose transporter GLUT4 and insulin receptor substrate 1 in insulin-resistant muscle (Henriksen, 2002). Improvement in glucose tolerance after exercise training in these groups is a less consistent observation and may be related to exercise intensity, changes in fat mass, the interval between exercise and testing of glucose tolerance and the severity of glucose intolerance (Kelley and Goodpaster, 1999). The general conclusion seems justified that regular exercise can reduce insulin resistance and improve glucose intolerance in obesity, even in the absence of changes in weight and/or body composition.

Blood lipids

Obese individuals are characterized by high plasma total cholesterol and triglyceride concentrations, low high-density lipoprotein (HDL) cholesterol concentrations and normal to elevated low-density lipoprotein (LDL) cholesterol concentrations, with increased levels of the particularly atherogenic small, dense LDL particles, especially in the abdominally obese (National Institutes of Health, 1998).

Reductions in postprandial triglyceride levels are already apparent after a single exercise bout. A slow postprandial metabolism of triglycerides enhances the exchange of lipids between triglyceride-rich particles [chylomicrons and very low-density (VLDL) lipoproteins] and cholesterol-rich particles (HDL and LDL). This depletes HDL of cholesterol and leads to the formation of atherogenic small, dense LDL. Previous exercise will stimulate postprandial triglyceride metabolism, thus reducing this exchange. This translates into an increase in HDL-cholesterol if exercise is performed regularly

(Gill *et al.*, 2002). Endurance exercise training of sufficient volume (> 1200 kcal/week) lowers plasma triglycerides and increases plasma HDL-cholesterol, without changing LDL-cholesterol, which is more responsive to dietary changes (Durstine *et al.*, 2002).

Weight loss has been advocated for the treatment of obesity-associated dyslipidaemias and regular exercise has been recommended to promote weight loss in obese people and thereby favourably affect blood lipids (National Institutes of Health, 1998), although at present there is little conclusive evidence from randomized controlled trials that exercise can raise low HDL-cholesterol and lower high triglycerides and LDL-cholesterol levels in overweight and obese individuals, independent of weight loss (Stefanick, 1999).

Blood pressure

In epidemiological studies, higher levels of physical activity are associated with lower incidence of hypertension. This relationship is independent of baseline BMI or body fat, although in the Harvard alumni study the inverse relationship between exercise and the incidence of hypertension was more pronounced in the overweight individuals (Fagard, 1999).

Longitudinal studies show that regular exercise reduces high blood pressure and that this effect is similar in lean and overweight individuals, but larger in hypertensive than in normotensive persons. A meta-analysis on blood pressure changes associated with exercise training in hypertensive patients indicates systolic and diastolic blood pressure reductions averaging 7 and 6 mmHg respectively (3 and 2 mmHg, respectively, in normotensive individuals). These changes were independent of changes in body mass (Fagard, 1999). Several mechanisms have been proposed to explain the blood pressure-lowering effect of exercise, such as reduction of sympathetic nervous system activity, improvement of endothelium-mediated vasodilatation, increased systemic arterial compliance and changes in baroreflex control of skeletal muscle vascular resistance (Van Baak, 1998).

Weight reduction also lowers blood pressure in obesity. When exercise is added to an energy-restricted diet, no additional reduction of blood pressure is found (Fagard, 1999).

Other comorbidities associated with obesity

A review of the literature on the effects of exercise on obesity-related disorders including different types of cancer, gallstones, osteoarthritis, back pain, sleep apnoea, reproductive abnormalities and impaired health-related quality of life showed a lack of randomized controlled trials in obese subjects. Less rigorously controlled studies suggest positive effects of exercise on risk of colon cancer, hormone-sensitive cancers and gallstones. Whether these effects are independent of weight loss is unclear. There are insufficient data for the other disorders (Rissanen and Fogelholm, 1999).

Mental health and health-related well-being

It is not fully clear whether obesity is associated with psychopathology or emotional distress in the general population. However, obese patients seeking weight loss treatment often show emotional disturbances, such as depression, binge eating disorder and disturbed body image (National Institutes of Health, 1998).

Exercise helps to improve mental health in individuals reporting mood disturbances, including symptoms of anxiety and depression, and in patients with diagnosed depression (Surgeon General's Report, 1996; Dunn et al., 2001). There are few data to confirm whether this is also the case in obesity. An observational study suggests that higher levels of physical activity and increases in physical activity are associated with improvements in depression and well-being in obese individuals (Foreyt et al., 1995). A randomized study found no effect of exercise training on psychological well-being or mood states in obese women in the absence of weight loss. Weight loss induced by a combination of diet and exercise significantly improved well-being (Nieman et al., 2000).

Aerobic fitness

Obese individuals have lower aerobic fitness than lean individuals, when fitness is expressed as $\dot{V}O_{2max}$ per kilogram of body weight. When $\dot{V}O_{2max}$ is adjusted for fat-free mass, the difference between lean and obese usually disappears. However, the oxygen consumption during exercise at a submaximal load, such as walking at a certain speed, is higher in obese than in lean when expressed as $\%\dot{V}O_{2max}$, thus representing a higher physical stress (Goran et al., 2000). Improving aerobic fitness in obese people will therefore have beneficial effects on the physical stress of daily activities.

Regular exercise increases aerobic fitness in lean (Surgeon General's Report, 1996) and obese individuals, independent of changes in body weight (Van Aggel-Leijssen et al., 2001a; 2002) and there are no indications that the fitness response to exercise training is modified by adiposity.

Mortality

Although some controversy exists whether fatness is an independent predictor of mortality, epidemiological studies quite consistently show that, within each BMI or adiposity category, men and women with a higher aerobic fitness or higher level of physical activity have a lower all-cause mortality risk (Blair and Brodney, 1999; Haapanen-Niemi et al., 2000; Crespo et al., 2002; Farrell et al., 2002; Stevens et al., 2002).

Summary of benefits of exercise in obesity

From the studies described in the previous sections, the health benefits of regular exercise for the obese individual are evident, even in the absence of significant weight loss effects. Even though only part of the evidence comes from randomized controlled trials and more of these trials need to be performed, the results of these trials and of observational studies give strong support for an important place for regular exercise in the prevention and management of obesity. Exercise will prevent weight gain, improve weight loss maintenance, reduce the risk of chronic diseases such as type 2 diabetes and cardiovascular diseases, improve mental health and well-being, increase fitness and reduce the risk of premature mortality. Physicians and other health-care professionals should therefore counsel obese patients to engage in regular exercise as part of their routine practice.

Exercise recommendations for weight management

Specific exercise recommendations for weight control have emerged since the 1990s. Initially, exercise programmes that were conducted at least 3 days per week, of at least 20-min duration and of sufficient intensity to expend approximately 300 kcal per session were suggested as a threshold level for total body mass and fat mass loss by the American College of Sports Medicine (1990). If the exercise frequency was increased to 4 days per week the expenditure per session might be reduced to 200 kcal. A high frequency and long duration of exercise sessions for effective weight control was stressed; a minimal level of intensity appeared less important.

In 1998, the National Institutes of Health report on identification and treatment of obesity in adults concluded that all adults should set a long-term goal to accumulate at least 30 min, or more, of moderate-intensity physical activity on most, and preferably all, days of the week, for weight management. The World Health Organization also adopted this recommendation. These recommendations have been questioned and recently two publications have appeared that indicate that the amount of physical activity required for weight gain prevention is probably higher than recommended at present (Erlichman et al., 2002; Saris et al., 2003). It is estimated that 45 to 60 minutes of moderate-intensity exercise per day are necessary to prevent the transition from overweight to obesity, and 60 to 90 min of moderate-intensity exercise daily, or lesser amounts of more vigorous activity, to prevent weight regain after weight reduction in obese people (Saris et al., 2003).

At present, there is no evidence that exercise intensity has an effect on weight reduction or weight maintenance independent of its contribution to total energy expenditure. However, more vigorous exercise will allow the individual to attain a certain energy expenditure in a shorter time. Two caveats are important: more vigorous exercise is associated with a higher injury risk and it may lead to higher drop-out rates. A careful balance between time restraints and attainment of a sufficiently high total energy expenditure therefore needs to be sought in each individual. This also stresses the importance of improving aerobic fitness, because this will enable the obese individual to perform a higher workload with less physical stress.

A significant dose–response relationship between amount of exercise, expressed as energy expenditure per week, and body weight reduction has been demonstrated (Ross and Janssen, 2001). Suggestions for dose–response relationships with the total amount of exercise have also been found for several other health parameters (Kesaniemi *et al.*, 2001). Although the effects of exercise on body weight are related to total energy expenditure rather than exercise intensity, exercise intensity may be important for other health effects of exercise. For instance, it is well-known that a minimal exercise intensity is required to improve cardiovascular fitness and that a relationship exists between change in $\dot{V}o_{2max}$ and exercise intensity. Whether this is also the case for other health effects of exercise is unclear. The blood pressure-lowering effects of exercise appear to be more pronounced at moderate ($< 70\%$ $\dot{V}o_{2max}$) than at higher ($\geq 70\%$ $\dot{V}o_{2max}$) exercise intensities (Hagberg *et al.*, 2000), although it is not fully clear whether this is independent of the total amount of exercise. No independent effect of exercise intensity has been found with respect to lipoprotein profile (Kraus *et al.*, 2002), but exercise intensity appears to be inversely associated with risk of coronary heart disease, independent of total amount of exercise (Tanasescu *et al.*, 2002; Lee *et al.*, 2003). Glucose tolerance in obese individuals has been reported to be improved after 1 week of exercise training at 70% $\dot{V}o_{2max}$, but not after training at 50% $\dot{V}o_{2max}$ with the same total energy expenditure (Kang *et al.*, 1996).

Thus, the question of which type of exercise training is optimal for obese people probably does not have one single answer. The answer depends on the ultimate goal(s) of the training programme: is it body weight reduction, fat mass reduction, increased fat oxidation, risk factor reduction or improvement of general fitness, psychological well-being and health? How fast does one want to attain a certain goal? Interindividual differences in response to training programmes are also likely.

Exercise mode

Dynamic aerobic exercise is usually recommended to improve cardiorespiratory fitness and health, and in weight control programmes. To attain the high levels of energy expenditure that are important for weight management, activities that use a large muscle mass are preferred. For obese people, non-weight-bearing activities, such as swimming or cycling, may be particularly appropriate. Addition of rhythmical resistance exercise, performed at a moderate to slow speed, through the full range of motion, not impeding normal breathing, is recommended for improvement of muscular mass, strength and endurance (American College of Sports Medicine, 1990).

Exercise prescription

Prescriptions of frequency and duration of exercise sessions are simple and straightforward. The more difficult aspect of exercise prescription is defining and monitoring the intensity of exercise. The intensity of exercise can be prescribed as an absolute intensity, an absolute workload, but usually a relative intensity is prescribed, such as a percentage of the maximal oxygen uptake ($\dot{V}o_{2max}$). Relative intensities can be classified as shown in Table 24.3. As $\dot{V}o_{2max}$ is difficult to measure in non-laboratory exercise settings, prescription of exercise intensity is usually based on heart rate [(as a percentage of measured, but usually estimated, maximal heart rate (HR$_{max}$) or heart rate reserve (HRR, i.e. maximal heart rate–resting heart rate)] or subjective feelings of exertion (RPE, rating of perceived exertion). This is based on the linear relationship between %HRmax or %HRR and RPE on the one hand and %$\dot{V}o_{2max}$ on the other hand.

The relation between %HR$_{max}$ or %HRR and %$\dot{V}o_{2max}$ has been found to be similar in lean and obese adults (Miller *et al.*, 1991). However, HRmax was lower in obese than in lean subjects: in normal-weight subjects HRmax can be predicted by '220−age'; in obese subjects the equation '200−0.5 × age' was found to be more accurate (Miller *et al.*, 1991). However, in another study the relation between %HRR and %$\dot{V}o_{2max}$ in obese women changed with weight loss. Following weight loss, the same %HRR represented a higher level of intensity than before (Jakicic *et al.*, 1995a). This discrepancy may be due to differences in the severity of obesity in these studies. A certain RPE corresponding with the same $\dot{V}o_{2max}$ before and after weight loss was consistent with existing guidelines (70% $\dot{V}o_{2max}$

Table 24.3 Classification of intensity of exercise based on 20–60 min of endurance training.

Relative intensity (%)			Intensity classification
%HR$_{max}$	%$\dot{V}o_{2max}$ or %HRR	RPE	
< 35	< 30	< 10	Very light
35–59	30–49	10–11	Light
60–79	50–74	12–13	Moderate (somewhat hard)
80–89	75–84	14–16	Heavy
≥ 90	≥ 85	> 16	Very heavy

HR$_{max}$ = maximal heart rate; HRR = heart rate reserve (maximal heart rate – resting heart rate); RPE = rating of perceived exertion (20-point Borg scale); $\dot{V}o_{2max}$ = maximal oxygen uptake.
Adapted from American College of Sports Medicine (1990).

= 13–14 RPE) (Jakicic *et al.*, 1995a). RPE can therefore be used as a subjective marker of exercise intensity in obese individuals.

Exercise adherence

Overweight and obesity are negatively correlated with overall level of physical activity in adults (Trost *et al.*, 2002). Moreover, drop-out rates from exercise programmes are relatively high, and the degree of overweight is one of the most consistent predictors of drop-out from exercise programmes (Dishman *et al.*, 1985; King *et al.*, 1997). Unsupervised programmes with vigorous-intensity exercise show lower adherence rates (King *et al.*, 1997; Cox *et al.*, 2003).

Cognitive factors regarding exercise are of critical importance for the success of exercise in weight management. Analysis of prevailing cognitive rules and schemas and, if necessary, intervention should be components of exercise prescription (Brownell, 1995).

Several studies have been performed in order to identify factors that might improve exercise adherence in obese people. A 20-week training programme consisting of short bouts of exercise (multiple 10-min exercise bouts per day) improved adherence and tended to improve weight loss, without importantly affecting the changes in cardiorespiratory fitness, compared with a single daily long exercise bout (Jakicic *et al.*, 1995b). However, a similar study of 18 months' duration did not show any differences in long-term weight loss or weight maintenance between multiple short bouts and one long exercise bout. A third group that performed multiple short bouts and was provided with home exercise equipment, on the other hand, showed better weight loss and maintenance. This may have been related to the better exercise participation over the last 6 months of the study (Jakicic *et al.*, 1999).

Exercise risk

Apart from the benefits, exercise may also have risks. The most serious, but relatively infrequent risk is that of sudden cardiac death, usually as a result of underlying atherosclerotic coronary artery disease. Exercise also transiently increases the risk of acute myocardial infarction. The relative risk of both exercise-related myocardial infarction and sudden death is greatest in individuals who are the least physically active and perform unaccustomed vigorous exercise. Sedentary individuals should avoid isolated bouts of vigorous exercise and gradually increase physical activity levels over time (Thompson *et al.*, 2003).

Although less serious, the risk of falls and musculoskeletal injuries is much larger. Risk of injury increases with obesity, volume of exercise and participation in vigorous exercise, whereas higher fitness and gradual increases in volume over time are associated with reduced injury risk (Thompson *et al.*, 2003).

In the context of risk reduction, obese (and other) individuals with known or suspected cardiovascular, respiratory, metabolic, orthopaedic or neurological disorders are advised to consult their physician before beginning or significantly increasing physical activity, especially when activities with a higher intensity than walking are chosen.

References

Achten, J., Gleeson, M. and Jeukendrup, A.E. (2002) Determination of the exercise intensity that elicits maximal fat oxidation. *Medicine and Science in Sports and Exercise* **34**, 92–97.

Ainsworth, B.E., Haskell, W.L., Whitt, M.C., Irwin, M.L., Swartz, A.M., Strath, S.J., O'Brien, W.L., Bassott, Jr, D.R., Schmitz, K.H., Emplaincourt, P.O., Jacobs, Jr, D.R. and Leon, A.S. (2000) Compendium of physical activities: an update of activity codes and MET intensities. *Medicine and Science in Sports and Exercise* **32** (Suppl.), S498–S504.

American College of Sports Medicine (1990) The recommended quantity and quality of exercise for developing and maintaining cardiorespiratory and muscular fitness in healthy adults. *Medicine and Science in Sports and Exercise* **22**, 265–274.

Bahr, R., Hansson, P. and Sejersted, O.M. (1990) Triglyceride/fatty acid cycling is increased after exercise. *Metabolism* **39**, 993–999.

Ballor, D.L. and Keesey, R.E. (1991) A meta-analysis of the factors affecting exercise-induced changes in body mass, fat mass and fat-free mass in males and females. *International Journal of Obesity* **15**, 717–726.

Ballor, D.L., Harvey-Berino, J.R., Ades, P.A., Cryan, J. and Calles-Escandon, J. (1996) Contrasting effect of resistance and aerobic training on body composition and metabolism after diet-induced weight loss. *Metabolism* **45**, 179–183.

Bielinski, R., Schutz, Y. and Jéquier, E. (1985) Energy metabolism during the postexercise recovery. *American Journal of Clinical Nutrition* **42**, 69–82.

Blaak, E.E., Westerterp, K.R., Bar-Or, O., Wouters, L.J.M. and Saris, W.H.M. (1992) Effect of training on total energy expenditure and spontaneous activity in obese boys. *American Journal of Clinical Nutrition* **55**, 777–782.

Blair, S.N. and Brodney, S. (1999) Effects of physical inactivity and obesity on morbidity and mortality: current evidence and research issues. *Medicine and Science in Sports and Exercise* **31** (Suppl.), S646–S662.

Blundell, J.E. and King, N.A. (2000) Exercise, appetite control, and energy balance. *Nutrition* **16**, 519–522.

Brownell, K.D. (1995) Exercise and obesity treatment: Psychological aspects. *International Journal of Obesity* **19** (Suppl. 4), S122–S125.

Buemann, B., Astrup, A. and Christensen, N.J. (1992) Three months aerobic training fails to affect 24-hour energy expenditure in weight-stable, post-obese women. *International Journal of Obesity* **16**, 809–816.

Calles-Escandón, J., Goran, M.I., O'Connell, M., Nair, K.S. and Danforth, E. (1996) Exercise increases fat oxidation at rest unrelated to changes in energy balance or lipolysis. *American Journal of Physiology* **270**, E1009–E1014.

Carter, S.L., Rennie, C. and Tarnapolsky, M.A. (2001) Substrate utilization during endurance exercise in men and women after endurance training. *American Journal of Physiology* **280**, E898–E907.

Coyle, E.F. (1995) Substrate utilization during exercise in active people. *American Journal of Clinical Nutrition* **61** (Suppl.), 968S–979S.

Cox, K.L., Burke, V., Gorely, T.J., Beilin, L.J. and Puddey, I.B. (2003) Controlled comparison of retention and adherence in home vs. center-initiated exercise interventions in women aged 40–65 years: the S.W.E.A.T. study (Sedentary Women Exercise Adherence Trial). *Preventative Medicine* **36**, 17–29.

Crampes, F., Marion-Latard, F., Zakaroff-Girard, A., De Glisezinski, I., Harant, I., Thalamas, C., Stich, V., Riviere, D., Lafontan, M. and Berlan, M. (2003) Effects of a longitudinal training program on responses to exercise in overweight men. *Obesity Research* **11**, 247–256.

Crespo, C.J., Garcia Palmieri, M.R., Perez Perdomo, R. *et al.* (2002) The relationship of physical activity and body weight with all-cause mortality: results from the Puerto Rico Heart Health Program. *Annals of Epidemiology* **12**, 543–552.

Dishman, R.K., Sallis, J.E. and Orenstein, D.R. (1985) The determinants of physical activity and exercise. *Public Health Report* **100**, 158–171.

Donnelly, J.E., Jakicic, J. and Gunderson, S. (1991) Diet and body composition. *Sports Medicine* **12**, 237–249.

Donnelly, J.E., Hill, J.O., Jacobsen, D.J., Potteiger, J., Sullivan, D.K., Johnson, S.L., Heelan, K., Hise, M., Fennessey, P.V., Sonko, B., Sharp, T., Jakicic, K.M., Blair, S.N., Tran, Z.V., Mayo, M., Gibson, C. and Washburn, R.A. (2003) Effects of a 16-month randomized controlled exercise trial on body weight and composition in young, overweight men and women. *Archives of Internal Medicine* **163**, 1343–1350.

Dunn, A.L., Trivedi, M.H. and O'Neal, H.A. (2001) Physical activity dose-response effects on outcomes of depression and anxiety. *Medicine and Science in Sports and Exercise* **33** (Suppl.), S587–S597.

Durstine, J.L., Grandjean, P.W., Cox, C.A. and Thompson, P.D. (2002) Lipids, lipoproteins, and exercise. *Journal of Cardiopulmonary Rehabilitation* **22**, 385–398.

Erlichman, J., Kerbey, A.L. and James, W.P.T. (2002) Physical activity and its impact on health outcomes. Paper 2: prevention of unhealthy weight gain and obesity by physical activity: an analysis of the evidence. *Obesity Reviews* **3**, 273–288.

Fagard, R.H. (1999) Physical activity in the prevention and treatment of hypertension in the obese. *Medicine and Science in Sports and Exercise* **31** (Suppl.), S624–S630.

Farrell, S.W., Braun, L., Barlow, C.E., Cheng, Y.J. and Blair, S.N. (2002) The relation of body mass index, cardiorespiratory fitness, and all-cause mortality in women. *Obesity Research* **10**, 417–423.

Flatt, J.P. (1987) Dietary fat, carbohydrate balance, and weight maintenance: effects of exercise. *American Journal of Clinical Nutrition* **45**, 296–306.

Flatt, J. (1995) Integration of the overall response to exercise. *International Journal of Obesity* **19** (Suppl.4), S31–S40.

Fogelholm, M. and Kukkonen-Harjula, K. (2000) Does physical activity prevent weight gain—a systematic review. *Obesity Reviews* **1**, 95–112.

Foreyt, J.P., Brunner, R.L., Goodrick, G.K., St-Jeor, S.T. and Miller, G.D. (1995) Psychological correlates of reported physical activity in normal-weight and obese adults: the Reno diet-heart study. *International Journal of Obesity* **19** (Suppl.4), S69–S72.

Foster, G.D., Wadden, T.A., Kendrick, Z.V., Letizia, K.A., Lander, D.P. and Conill, A.M. (1995) The energy cost of walking before and after significant weight loss. *Medicine and Science in Sports and Exercise* **27**, 888–894.

Frayn, K.N. (1996) *Metabolic Regulation. A Human Perspective.* London: Portland Press.

Fukuba, Y., Yano, Y., Murakami, H., Kan, A. and Miura, A. (2000) The effect of dietary restriction and menstrual cycle on excess post-exercise oxygen consumption (EPOC) in young women. *Clinical Physiology* **20**, 165–169.

Garrow, J.S. and Summerbell, C.D. (1995) Meta-analysis: effect of exercise, with or without dieting, on the body composition of overweight subjects. *European Journal of Clinical Nutrition* **49**, 1–10.

George, V.A. and Morganstein, A. (2003) Effect of moderate intensity exercise on acute energy intake in normal and overweight females. *Appetite* **40**, 43–46.

Gill, J.M.R., Herd, S.L. and Hardman, A.E. (2002) Moderate exercise and post-prandial metabolism: issues of dose-response. *Journal of Sports Science* **20**, 961–967.

Goodpaster, B.H., Wolfe, R.R. and Kelley, D.E. (2002) Effects of obesity on substrate utilization during exercise. *Obesity Research* **10**, 575–584.

Goran, M., Fields, D.A., Hunter, G.R., Herd, S.L. and Weinsier, R.L. (2000) Total body fat does not influence maximal aerobic capacity. *International Journal of Obesity* **24**, 841–848.

Guesbeck, N.R., Hickey, M.S., MacDonald, K.G. *et al.* (2001) Substrate utilization during exercise in formerly morbidly obese women. *Journal of Applied Physiology* **90**, 1007–1012.

Haapanen-Niemi, N., Miilunpalo, S., Pasanen, M., Vuori, I., Oja, P. and Malmberg, J. (2000) Body mass index, physical inactivity and low level of physical fitness as determinants of all-cause and cardiovascular disease mortality—16 year follow-up of middle-aged and elderly men and women. *International Journal of Obesity* **24**, 1465–1474.

Hagberg, J.M., Park, J. and Brown, M.D. (2000) The role of exercise training in the treatment of hypertension. *Sports Medicine* **30**, 193–206.

Henriksen, E.J. (2002) Effects of acute exercise and exercise training on insulin resistance. *Journal of Applied Physiology* **93**, 788–796.

Henriksson, J. (1995) Muscle fuel selection: effect of exercise and training. *Proceedings of the Nutrition Society* **54**, 125–138.

Hickey, M.S. and Calsbeek, D.J. (2001) Plasma leptin and exercise. *Sports Medicine* **31**, 583–589.

Horber, F.F., Kohler, S.A., Lippuner, K. and Jaeger, P. (1996) Effect of regular physical training on age-associated alteration of body composition in men. *European Journal of Clinical Investigation* **26**, 279–285.

Hu, F.B., Li, T.Y., Colditz, G.A., Willett, W.C. and Manson, J.E. (2003) Television watching and other sedentary behaviors in relation to risk of obesity and diabetes mellitus in women. *Journal of the American Medical Association* **289**, 1785–1791.

Hunter, G.R., Wetzstein, C.J., Fields, D.A., Brown, A. and Bamman, M.M. (2000) Resistance training increases total energy expenditure and free-living physical activity in older adults. *Journal of Applied Physiology* **89**, 977–984.

Hurley, B.F., Nemeth, P.M., Martin, III, W.H., Hagberg, J.M., Dalsky, G.P. and Holloszy, J.O. (1986) Muscle triglyceride utilization during exercise: effect of training. *Journal of Applied Physiology* **60**, 562–567.

Jakicic, J.M., Donnelly, J.E., Pronk, N.P., Jawad, A.F. and Jacobsen, D.J. (1995a) Prescription of exercise intensity for the obese patient: the relationship between heart rate, VO_2 and perceived exertion. *International Journal of Obesity* **19**, 382–387.

Jakicic, J.M., Wing, R.R., Butler, B.A. and Robertson, R.J. (1995b) Prescribing exercise in multiple short bouts versus one continuous bout: effects on adherence, cardiorespiratory fitness, and weight loss in overweight women. *International Journal of Obesity* **19**, 893–901.

Jakicic, J.M., Winters, C., Lang, W. and Wing, R.R. (1999) Effects of intermittent exercise and use of home exercise equipment on adherence, weight loss, and fitness in overweight women. *Journal of the American Medical Association* **282**, 1554–1560.

Kanaley, J.A., Weatherup-Dentes, M.M., Alvarado, C.R. and Whitehead, G. (2001) Substrate oxidation during acute exercise and with exercise training in lean and obese women. *European Journal of Applied Physiology* **85**, 68–73.

Kang, J., Robertson, R.J., Hagberg, J.M., Kelley, D.E., Goss, F.L., DaSilva, S.G., Suminski, R.R. and Utter, A.C. (1996) Effect of exercise intensity on glucose and insulin metabolism in obese individuals and obese NIDDM patients. *Diabetes Care* **19**, 341–349.

Keim, N.L., Barbieri, T.F. and Belko, A.Z. (1990) The effect of exercise on energy intake and body composition in overweight women. *International Journal of Obesity* **14**, 335–346.

Kelley, D.E. and Goodpaster, B.H. (1999) Effects of physical activity on insulin action and glucose tolerance in obesity. *Medicine and Science in Sports and Exercise* **31** (Suppl.), S619–S623.

Kesaniemi, Y.A., Danforth, Jr., E., Jensen, M.D., Kopelman, P.G., Lefebvre, P. and Reeder, B.A. (2001) Dose-response issues concerning physical activity and health: an evidence-based symposium. *Medicine and Science in Sports and Exercise* **33** (Suppl.), S351–S358.

King, N.A. and Blundell, J.E. (1995) High-fat foods overcome the energy expenditure due to exercise after cycling and running. *European Journal of Clinical Nutrition* **49**, 114–123.

King, N.A., Burley, V.J. and Blundell, J.E. (1994) Exercise-induced suppression of appetite: effects on food intake and implications for energy balance. *European Journal of Clinical Nutrition* **48**, 715–724.

King, N.A., Snell, L., Smith, R.D. and Blundell, J.E. (1996) Effects of short-term exercise on appetite responses in unrestrained females. *European Journal of Clinical Nutrition* **50**, 663–667.

King, A.C., Kiernan, M., Oman, R.R., Kraemer, H.C., Hull, M. and Ahn, D. (1997) Can we identify who will adhere to long-term physical activity? Signal detection methodology as potential aid to clinical decision making. *Health Psychology* **16**, 380–389.

Kraus, W.E., Houmard, J.A., Duscha, B.D., Knetzger, K.J., Wharton, M.B., McCartney, J.S., Bales, C.W., Henes, S., Samsa, G.P., Otvos, J.D., Kulkarni, K.R. and Slentz, C.A. (2002) Effects of the amount and intensity of exercise on plasma lipoproteins. *New England Journal of Medicine* **347**, 1483–1492.

Lee, I., Sesso, H., Oguma, Y. and Paffenbarger, R.S. (2003) Relative exercise intensity of physical activity and risk of coronary heart disease. *Circulation* **107**, 1110–1116.

Marion-Latard, F., Crampes, F., Zakaroff-Girard, A., De Glisezinski, I., Harant, I., Stich, V., Thalamas, C., Riviere, D., Lafontan, M. and Berlan, M. (2003) Post-exercise increase of lipid oxidation after a moderate exercise bout in untrained healthy obese men. *Hormone and Metabolic Research* **35**, 97–103.

Martin, 3rd, W.H., Dalsky G.P., Hurley, B.F., Matthews, D.E., Bier, D.M., Hagberg, J.M., Rogers, M.A., King, D.S. and Holloszy, J.O. (1993) Effect of endurance training on plasma free fatty acid turnover and oxidation during exercise. *American Journal of Physiology* **265**, E708–E714.

Mayer, J., Roy, P. and Mitra, K.P. (1956) Relation between caloric intake, body weight, and physical work: studies in an industrial male population in West Bengal. *American Journal of Clinical Nutrition* **4**, 169–175.

Melanson, E.L., Sharp, T.A., Seagle, H.M., Horton, T.J., Donahoo, W.T., Grunwald, G.K., Hamilton, J.T. and Hill, J.O. (2002a) Effect of exercise intensity on 24-h energy expenditure and nutrient oxidation. *Journal of Applied Physiology* **92**, 1045–1052.

Melanson, E.L., Sharp, T.A., Seagle, H.M., Donahoo, W.T., Grunwald, G.K., Peters, J.C., Hamilton, J.T. and Hill, J.O. (2002b) Resistance and aerobic exercise have similar effects on 24-h nutrient oxidation. *Medicine and Science in Sports and Exercise* **34**, 1793–1800.

Miller, W.C., Wallace, J.P. and Eggert, K.E. (1991) Predicting max HR and the HR-VO2 relationship for exercise prescription in obesity. *Medicine and Science in Sports and Exercise* **25**, 1077–1081.

Miller, W.C., Koceja, D.M. and Hamilton, E.J. (1997) A meta-analysis of the past 25 years of weight loss research using diet, exercise or diet plus exercise intervention. *International Journal of Obesity* **21**, 941–947.

Mittendorfer, B., Horowitz, J.F. and Klein, S. (2002) Effect of gender on lipid kinetics during endurance exercise of moderate intensity in untrained subjects. *American Journal of Physiology* **283**, E58–E65.

National Institutes of Health (1998) Clinical guidelines on the identification, evaluation, and treatment of overweight and obesity in adults. *Obesity Research* **6** (Suppl. 2), 51S–209S.

Nielsen, J.N., Mustard, K.J.W., Graham, D.A., Yu, H., MacDonald, C.S., Pilegaard, H., Goodyear, L.J., Hardie, D.G., Richter, E.A. and Wojtaszewski, J.F. (2003) 5′-AMP-activated protein kinase activity and subunit expression in exercise-trained human skeletal muscle. *Journal of Applied Physiology* **94**, 631–641.

Nieman, D.C., Custer, W.F., Butterworth, D.E., Utter, A.C. and Henson, D.A. (2000) Psychological response to exercise training and/or energy restriction in obese women. *Journal of Psychosomatic Research* **48**, 23–29.

Oscai, L.B. (1973) The role of exercise in weight control. *Medicine and Science in Sports and Exercise* **1**, 103–123.

Poehlman, E.T., Melby, C.L. and Goran, M.I. (1991) The impact of exercise and diet restriction on daily energy expenditure. *Sports Medicine* **11**, 78–101.

Poehlman, E.T., Gardner, A.W., Arciero, P.J., Goran, M.I. and Calles-Escandon, J. (1994) Effects of endurance training on total fat oxidation in elderly persons. *Journal of Applied Physiology* **76**, 2281–2287.

Poehlman, E.T., Denino, W.F., Beckett, T., Kinaman, K.A., Dionne, I.J., Dvorak, R. and Ades, P.A. (2002) Effects of endurance and resistance training on total daily energy expenditure in young women: a controlled randomized trial. *Journal of Clinical Endocrinology and Metabolism* **87**, 1004–1009.

Prentice, A.M., Goldberg, G.R., Jebb, S.A., Black, A.E., Murgatroyd, P. and Diaz, E.O. (1991) Physiological responses to slimming. *Proceedings of the Nutrition Society* **50**, 441–458.

Ranneries, C., Bülow, J., Buemann, B., Christensen, N.J., Madsen, J. and Astrup, A. (1998) Fat metabolism in formerly obese women. *American Journal of Physiology* **274**, E155–E161.

Richard, D. (1995) Exercise and the neurobiological control of food intake and energy expenditure. *International Journal of Obesity* **19** (Suppl. 4), S73–S79.

Rissanen, A. and Fogelholm, M. (1999) Physical activity in the prevention and treatment of other morbid conditions and impairments associated with obesity: current evidence and research issues. *Medicine and Science in Sports and Exercise* **31** (Suppl.), S635–S645.

Romijn, J.A., Coyle, E.F., Sidossis, L.S., Gastaldelli, A., Horowitz, J.F., Endert, E. and Wolfe, R.R. (1993) Regulation of endogenous fat and carbohydrate metabolism in relation to exercise intensity and duration. *American Journal of Physiology* **265**, E380–E391.

Rosenbaum, M., Vandenborne, K., Goldsmith, R., Simoneau, J.A., Heymsfield, S., Joanisse, D.R., Hirsch, J., Murphy, E., Matthews, D., Segal, K.R. and Leibel, R.L. (2003) Effects of experimental weight perturbation on skeletal muscle work efficiency in human subjects. *American Journal of Physiology* **285**, R183–R192.

Ross, R. and Janssen, I. (2001) Physical activity, total and regional obesity: dose-response considerations. *Medicine and Science in Sports and Exercise* **33** (Suppl.), S521–S527.

Rowland, N.E., Morien, A. and Li, B. (1996) The physiology and brain mechanisms of feeding. *Nutrition* **12**, 626–639.

Saris, W.H.M. (1989) Physiological aspects of exercise in weight cycling. *American Journal of Clinical Nutrition* **49**, 1099–1104.

Saris, W.H.M., Blair, S.N., van Baak, M.A., Eaton, S.B., Davies, P.S., Di Pietro, L., Fogelholm, M., Rissanen, A., Schoeller, D., Swinburn, B., Tremblay, A., Westerterp, K.R. and Wyatt, H. (2003) How much physical activity is enough to prevent unhealthy weight gain? Outcome of the IASO 1st Stock Conference and consensus statement. *Obesity Reviews* **4**, 101–114.

Schrauwen, O., van Aggel-Leijssen, D.P.C., Hul, G., Wagenmakers, A.J.M., Vidal, H., Saris, W.H.M. and van Baak, M.A. (2002) The effect of a 3-month low-intensity endurance training program on fat oxidation and acetyl-CoA carboxylase-2 expression. *Diabetes* **51**, 2220–2226.

Schwartz, M.W., Woods, S.C., Porte, Jr, D., Selley, R.J. and Baskin, D.G. (2000) Central nervous system control of food intake. *Nature* **404**, 661–671.

Segal, K.R. (1995) Exercise and thermogenesis in obesity. *International Journal of Obesity* **19** (Suppl.4), S80–S87.

Simoneau, J. (1995) Adaptation of human skeletal muscle to exercise-training. *International Journal of Obesity* **19** (Suppl.4), S9–S13.

Stefanick, M.L. (1999) Physical activity for preventing and treating obesity-related dyslipoproteinemias. *Medicine and Science in Sports and Exercise* **31** (Suppl.), S609–S618.

Stevens, J., Cai, J., Evenson, K.R. and Thomas, R. (2002) Fitness and fatness as predictors of mortality from all causes and from cardiovascular disease in men and women in the Lipid Research Clinics Study. *American Journal of Epidemiology* **156**, 832–841.

Surgeon General's Report (1996) *Physical Activity and Health.* Atlanta: U.S. Department of Health and Human Services.

Tanasescu, M., Leitzmann, M.F., Rimm, E.B., Willett, W.C., Stampfer, M.J. and Hu, F.B. (2002) Exercise type and intensity in relation to coronary heart disease in men. *Journal of the American Medical Association* **288**, 1994–2000.

Thompson, P.D., Buchner, D., Pina, I.L., Balady, G.J., Williams, M.A., Marcus, B.H., Berra, K., Blair, S.N., Costa, F., Franklin, B., Fletcher, G.F., Gordon, N.F., Pate, R.R., Rodriguez, B.L., Yancey, A.K. and Wenger, N.K.; American Heart Association Council on Clinical Cardiology Subcommittee on Exercise, Rehabilitation, and Prevention; American Heart Association Council on Nutrition, Physical Activity, and Metabolism Subcommittee on Physical Activity. (2003) Exercise and physical activity in the prevention and treatment of atherosclerotic cardiovascular disease: a statement from the Council on Clinical Cardiology (Subcommittee on

Exercise, Rehabilitation, and Prevention) and the Council on Nutrition, Physical Activity, and Metabolism (Subcommittee on Physical Activity). *Circulation* **107**, 3109–3116.

Toth, M.J. and Poehlman, E.T. (1996) Effects of exercise on daily energy expenditure. *Nutrition Reviews* **54**, S140–S148.

Tremblay, A. and Buemann, B. (1995) Exercise-training, macronutrient balance and body weight control. *International Journal of Obesity* **19**, 79–86.

Tremblay, A., Alméras, N., Boer, J., Kranenbarg, E.K. and Després, J.P. (1994) Diet composition and postexercise energy balance. *American Journal of Clinical Nutrition* **59**, 975–979.

Treuth, M.S., Hunter, G.R., Weinsier, R.L. and Kell, S.H. (1995) Energy expenditure and substrate utilization in older women after strength training: 24-h calorimeter results. *Journal of Applied Physiology* **78**, 2140–2146.

Trost, S.G., Owen, N., Bauman, A.E., Sallis, J.F. and Brown, W. (2002) Correlates of adults' participation in physical activity: review and update. *Medicine and Science in Sports and Exercise* **34**, 1996–2001.

Tunstall, R.J., Mehan, K.A., Wadley, G.D., Collier, G.R., Bonen, A., Hargreaves, M. and Cameron-Smith, D. (2002) Exercise training increases lipid metabolism gene expression in human skeletal muscle. *American Journal of Physiology* **283**, E66–E72.

Van Aggel-Leijssen, D.P.C., Saris, W.H.M., Wagenmakers, A.J.M., Hul, G.B. and van Baak, M.A. (2001a) The effect of low-intensity exercise training on fat metabolism in obese women. *Obesity Research* **9**, 86–96.

Van Aggel-Leijssen, D.P.C., Saris, W.H.M., Hul, G.B. and van Baak, M.A. (2001b) Short-term effect of weight loss with or without low-intensity exercise training on fat metabolism in obese men. *American Journal of Clinical Nutrition* **73**, 523–531.

Van Aggel-Leijssen, D.P.C., Saris, W.H.M., Wagenmakers, A.J.M., Senden, J.M. and van Baak, M.A. (2002) Effect of exercise training at different intensities on fat metabolism of obese men. *Journal of Applied Physiology* **92**, 1300–1309.

Van Baak, M.A. (1998) Exercise and hypertension: facts and uncertainties. *British Journal of Sports Medicine* **32**, 6–10.

Van Baak, M.A., van Mil, E., Astrup, A.V., Finer, N., Van Gaal, L.F., Hilsted, J., Kopelman, P.G., Rössner, S., James, W.P.T., Saris, W.H.M. for the STORM Study Group (2003) Leisure time physical activity is an important determinant of long-term weight maintenance after weight loss in the STORM trial. *American Journal of Clinical Nutrition* **78**, 209–214.

Visona, C. and George, V.A. (2002) Impact of dieting status and dietary restraint on postexercise energy intake in overweight women. *Obesity Research* **10**, 1251–1258.

Votruba, S.B., Atkinson, R.L., Hirvonen, M.D. and Schoeller, D.A. (2002) Prior exercise increases subsequent utilization of dietary fat. *Medicine and Science in Sports and Exercise* **34**, 1757–1765.

Westerterp, K.R. (1998) Alterations in energy balance with exercise. *American Journal of Clinical Nutrition* **68** (Suppl.), 970S–974S.

Wilmore, J.H. (1995) Variations in physical activity habits and body composition. *International Journal of Obesity* **19** (Suppl.4), S107–S112.

Wing, R.R. (1999) Physical activity in the treatment of adulthood overweight and obesity: current evidence and research issues. *Medicine and Science in Sports and Exercise* **31** (Suppl.), S547–S552.

Wing, R.R. and Hill, J.O. (2001) Successful weight loss maintenance. *Annual Review of Nutrition* **21**, 323–341.

Wojtaszewski, J.F.P., Nielsen, J.N. and Richter, E.A. (2002) Effect of acute exercise on insulin signaling and action in humans. *Journal of Applied Physiology* **93**, 384–392.

25 Management of obesity: pharmacotherapy

Richard L. Atkinson

Introduction, 380

Rationale for use of obesity drugs, 380

Indications and contraindications for obesity drugs, 381

Drugs available at present for obesity, 381
  Adrenergic drugs, 382
  Serotonergic drugs, 383
  Combined adrenergic–serotonergic drug, 383

Peripherally acting malabsorptive agent, 383
Non-approved drugs with potential for treating obesity, 384
Over-the-counter diet supplements, herbs and other agents, 386

Agents with potential for treating obesity, 386
  Rimonabart, 387

Combinations of drugs for obesity, 387
  Phenylpropanolamine–benzocaine, 387

Phentermine–fenfluramine combination, 387
Fenfluramine–fluoxetine combination, 388
Phentermine–fluoxetine combination, 388
Sibutramine–orlistat, 388
Phentermine–orlistat, 388

Practical aspects of drug therapy, 388

Summary and conclusions, 388

References, 389

Introduction

Obesity is a chronic disease of multiple aetiologies (Bray, 2003; Friedman, 2003). The realization that obesity is a disease rather than a failure of willpower or lack of self-discipline has led to better acceptance of the use of drugs in the treatment of obesity. Realization that obesity is a chronic disease that will require lifelong treatment may lead to acceptance of lifelong use of obesity drugs. Virtually all other chronic diseases are treated by pharmacotherapy and, for most diseases, more than one drug is used. If a single drug is not effective, combinations of therapies are instituted. It seems very likely that the future of the treatment of obesity will revolve around better drugs, used in combination. Unfortunately, there are few drugs on the market at present that are approved for obesity, and the use of combinations of drugs for obesity has been extremely limited. This chapter will discuss the rationale for use of obesity drugs, the indications and contraindications, the drugs available at present, side-effects, potential future agents and combinations of drugs for obesity.

Rationale for use of obesity drugs

Numerous studies over the last century have documented that diet, exercise and behaviour modification of lifestyle may be successful in reducing body weight initially, but are unsuc-

cessful over the long term (Andersen *et al.*, 1988; Wadden *et al.*, 1989; Perri, 1992; Wilson, 1993; Ayyad and Andersen, 2000). A review/meta-analysis by Ayyad and Andersen (2000) found that the long-term failure rate of this 'standard' therapy is about 85%. It is very difficult to not eat when hungry and to persistently eat less palatable foods when highly palatable foods are constantly available. It is also difficult to sustain the levels of exercise and activity required to maintain lost weight. These problems contribute to the high failure rate of 'standard' therapy. Many people have a genetic predisposition to obesity. Such people must develop behaviour patterns of diet and activity not required of thin people. To lose weight and maintain the loss, obese people have to do more than thin people. Animals with defects of the *ob/ob* or *db/db* genes are models for obese humans. If these animals are pair-fed to lean littermates, they remain obese (Coleman, 1979). To achieve similar weights as their lean littermates, they have to eat one-half of the intake of their lean littermates (Coleman, 1979). It is likely that obese humans with genetic differences from lean individuals will behave somewhat like these genetically obese animals.

The present-day US environment requires less activity and has many more highly palatable food choices immediately available than the environment of our primitive ancestors. Genetic characteristics that favoured survival now favour the development of obesity in many people. It is clear that the biochemistry of the bodies of obese people is different from that of lean people. Upon losing weight, differences between lean and obese remain, and these differences favour weight regain in obese people (Eckel and Yost, 1987; Eckel *et al.*, 1995). Obesity drugs change the physiology and biochemistry of the bodies of obese people towards those of lean people, as does obesity surgery. These more passive methods of weight loss are likely to be the 'standard' treatment of obesity in the future.

For the present, it is reasonable that if obesity drugs are started and found to produce acceptable weight loss, they need to be continued indefinitely. Perhaps future therapies, such as gene therapy, will allow a single course of treatment to promote permanent change.

Indications and contraindications for obesity drugs

If obesity drugs must be continued indefinitely, they must be used carefully and only with appropriate indications. An expert panel of the North American Association for the Study of Obesity recommended that drugs are acceptable for individuals with a body mass index (BMI) of 27 or above (Pi-Sunyer, 1995). The Food and Drug Administration (FDA), National Institutes of Health (NIH) and World Health Organization (WHO) established more conservative criteria for use of obesity drugs (FDA/NIH/WHO, 1998; WHO, 1998). Without complications of obesity, a BMI of 30 is an indication. With complications of obesity, a BMI of 27 is an indication. Most clinicians and governmental regulatory bodies (e.g. FDA) favour at present these more conservative criteria listed in Table 25.1. Use of obesity drugs in individuals who do not meet the BMI limits of the FDA/NIH criteria needs to be justified, and the reasons should be very carefully documented in the medical record. There are a number of factors that may justify use of obesity drugs in individuals below the BMI cut-off points. Individuals with weight-related complications of obesity such as hypertension, diabetes and hyperlipidaemia may be candidates. Excess intra-abdominal fat (visceral obesity) is a major risk factor for diabetes, heart disease and strokes (Kissebach *et al.*, 1982) that may occur with greater frequency in certain racial and ethnic groups, such as Asian and Hispanic people. These individuals deposit visceral fat at much lower BMIs than non-Hispanic white people (Misra, 2003; Stevens, 2003). There has been significant debate about whether the cut-off points for defining obesity should be based on racial identity (Misra, 2003; Stevens, 2003).

Individuals who have a past history of obesity, but who have lost weight and been able to maintain it only with great difficulty, may also be considered for treatment with obesity drugs. Having such individuals regain their lost weight before being treated with obesity drugs seems senseless.

Contraindications for use of obesity drugs are listed in Table 25.1. Major medical illnesses, particularly if unstable, may be contraindications to use of some of the obesity drugs, particularly adrenergic agents and those that act on the central

Table 25.1 Criteria, contraindications and cautions for the use of obesity drugs.

FDA, NIH, WHO* BMI criteria for use of obesity drugs
BMI ≥ 30 kg/m^2
BMI ≥ 27 kg/m^2, with complications

Contraindications for use
Pregnancy, breast-feeding
Unstable cardiac disease
Uncontrolled hypertension (SBP > 180 mmHg, DBP > 110 mmHg)
Unstable severe systemic illness
History of anorexia nervosa
Active severe psychiatric disorder
Other drug therapy, if incompatible (e.g. monoamine oxidase inhibitors, anti-migraine drugs, adrenergic agents, drugs with arrhythmia potential)

Cautions for use
Presence of any severe systemic illness
History of severe psychiatric disorder
Other drug therapy
Closed angle glaucoma
Age < 18 years or > 65 years

*US Food and Drug Administration, US National Institutes of Health (Clinical Guidelines on the Identification, Evaluation and Treatment of Overweight and Obesity in Adults – The Evidence Report. Obesity Research 6 (Suppl. 2): 51S–209S, 1998. Preventing and managing the global epidemic of obesity: report of a WHO Consultation on Obesity. Geneva, 3–5 June, 1997. WHO/NUT/NCD98.1, Geneva, 1998.

nervous system (CNS). Pregnancy and lactation are clear contraindications, and use in children and the elderly is passively or actively discouraged by many paediatricians and geriatricians respectively. A number of drugs interact with obesity drugs, so a good drug history and use of a drug interaction manual or website (e.g. Drug Digest®; http://www.drugdigest.org/DD/Interaction/ChooseDrugs/1,4109,00.html) is very useful if the patient is on other drugs.

Major psychiatric disorders such as schizophrenia, bipolar disorder or panic attacks are contraindications or severe cautions for most obesity drugs. Also, patients with significant psychological concerns regarding excess body weight may be at risk for eating disorders. The physician should carefully evaluate such patients before prescribing obesity drugs. In some cases, referral for psychological or psychiatric counselling to deal with these concerns may be necessary before prescribing obesity drugs. A history of anorexia nervosa perhaps is an absolute contraindication to obesity drugs until more research can identify the mechanisms of this disorder and ways to safely treat it.

Drugs available at present for obesity

The number of obesity drugs available at present is limited. Table 25.2 lists drugs that are approved for the treatment of

Table 25.2 Approved weight loss drugs and drug enforcement agency (DEA) schedules.

Adrenergic agonists
(a) Amphetamine,* methamphetamine,* phenmetrazine* (DEA II); (b) benzphetamine, chlorphentermine,* chlortermine,* phendimetrazine (DEA III); (c) diethylpropion, mazindol,* phentermine (DEA IV); (d) phenylpropanolamine[†] (over the counter)

Serotonin agonists
(a) D,L-Fenfluramine[†] (DEA IV); (b) D-fenfluramine[†] (DEA IV)
Combined adrenergic/serotonergic agonist
Sibutramine (DEA IV)

Drug affecting absorption
Orlistat

---

*Not marketed at present for the treatment of obesity in the USA.
[†]Withdrawn from market in USA.

Table 25.3 Marketed drugs not approved for the treatment of obesity.

Adrenergic agonist
Ephedrine, caffeine

Serotonin agonists
Citalopram
Fluoxetine
Sertraline

Drug affecting absorption
Acarbose

Other
Bromocriptine
Bupropion
Cimetidine
Diazoxide
Metformin
Nicotine
Topiramate
Zonisamide

---

obesity in the USA or elsewhere in the world. The list includes drugs that are approved by the FDA for the treatment of obesity and also drugs that have been approved previously but that are no longer available. Table 25.3 lists drugs that are FDA approved for purposes other than obesity and have been shown to reduce body weight. Most of the drugs on the market act on the CNS by binding to adrenergic or serotonergic receptors, producing appetite suppression, enhanced satiety or both. Malabsorptive agents block the digestion of fat or carbohydrate. A number of other drugs are available on the market for other indications, and act by different mechanisms to produce weight loss.

Adrenergic drugs

Adrenergic drugs raise noradrenaline and/or dopamine in specific areas of the brain that are involved in regulating food intake, satiety and energy expenditure (Bray, 2000; Hirsch *et al.*, 2000; Ryan, 2000). Adrenergic drugs have the potential for abuse, but those most commonly used (phentermine, diethylpropion, phendimetrazine and mazindol) have minimal or no evidence of abuse. Higher abuse-potential drugs such as dexamphetamine and methamphetamine have no role in the modern-day treatment of obesity. The adrenergic agonists that are used most frequently by prescription in the USA are phentermine and diethylpropion, both of which are in the lowest Drug Enforcement Agency (DEA) category, Schedule IV. Phentermine was found to be more effective than diethylpropion in one controlled trial (Valle-Jones *et al.*, 1983). Phentermine has been used for up to 36 weeks in two studies from Munro's laboratory (Munro *et al.*, 1973). In both of these studies, weight losses were 13% of initial body weight, despite the lack of a strong diet and exercise component to the weight loss programme.

There is little to distinguish diethylpropion, phendimetrazine and benzphetamine from each other. All stimulate central noradrenaline secretion, and weight losses with each are similar (Scoville, 1976; Silverstone, 1992; Hirsch *et al.*, 2000; Ryan, 2000; Bray, 2000; Halpern and Mancini, 2003). Benzphetamine and phendimetrazine are in DEA Schedule III, and theoretically have a greater abuse potential than diethylpropion. However, Griffiths and colleagues (1979) demonstrated that diethylpropion had a higher reinforcement potential in nonhuman primates than the other Schedule III and IV agents.

Mazindol is unique among the pure adrenergic agents for obesity because its structure is not derived from the phenylethylamine parent molecule (Enzi, *et al.*, 1976; Inoue *et al.*, 1992; Bray, 2000). Mazindol is no longer available in the USA, but is used in other countries, particularly Japan. Mazindol produced weight losses of 14.2 and 12.0 kg, the best results of any of the single obesity drugs tested for 1 year or more (Enzi *et al.*, 1994).

Phenylpropanolamine (PPA) was the major drug in over-the-counter diet aids in the USA until recently, when it was removed by the FDA because of concern that it increased the risk of strokes. PPA acts on alpha-adrenergic receptors in the brain and causes a weight loss that is somewhat less than the prescription adrenergic agents (Silverstone, 1992).

Side-effects of all of the adrenergic agents are dry mouth, constipation, insomnia, tachycardia, hypertension and, rarely, cardiac arrhythmias (Munro *et al.*, 1968; Enzi *et al.*, 1976; Steel *et al.*, 1973; Scoville, 1976; Valle-Jones *et al.*, 1983; Inoue *et al.*, 1992; Silverstone, 1992; Goldstein and Potvin, 1994; Bray, 2000; Hirsch *et al.*, 2000; Ryan, 2000; Halpern and Mancini, 2003).

Serotonergic drugs

Dexfenfluramine and D,L-fenfluramine increase serotonin in the brain by increasing production and inhibiting uptake in neurons that are involved in controlling food intake and body weight (Garattini *et al.*, 1992; Garattini, 1995; Rowland *et al.*, 2000; Rothman and Baumann, 2002). Weight loss on these drugs was about 10% of initial body weight (Guy-Grand *et al.*, 1989). These drugs were removed from the market in 1997 because they produced damage to the aortic and mitral heart valves (Connolly *et al.*, 1997; Gardin *et al.*, 2000; Tellier, 2001; Weissman, 2001). Follow-up studies demonstrated that the cardiac valve damage regressed or did not change after the drugs were stopped (Gardin *et al.*, 2000; Tellier, 2001). The mechanism of cardiac valve damage is postulated to be through binding to 5-hydroxytryptamine-2B receptors (5-HT-2B) (Fitzgerald *et al.*, 2000). These drugs also bind to 5-HT-2C receptors (Fitzgerald *et al.*, 2000), which may not affect cardiac valves, and thus are a target of pharmaceutical company development.

Selective serotonin reuptake inhibitors (SSRIs) such as fluoxetine and sertraline increase serotonin levels in the brain and are associated with an initial weight loss of about 10% or more of initial body weight followed by weight regain (Goldstein *et al.*, 1993; 1995; Wadden *et al.*, 1995; Dhurandhar and Atkinson, 1996; Ricca *et al.*, 1996). Harvey and Bouwer demonstrated that body weight after 1 year of treatment was similar in the fluoxetine group vs. placebo, but thereafter body weight increased on fluoxetine (Harvey and Bouwer, 2000). These drugs are not approved by the FDA for the treatment of obesity, but are being used by physicians in an off-label fashion alone or in combination with phentermine or other adrenergic agents (Dhurandhar and Atkinson, 1996; Anchors, 1997a; Anchors, 1997b; Griffen *et al.*, 1998), as described below.

Combined adrenergic–serotonergic drug

Sibutramine is the only obesity drug on the market in this class. It inhibits re-uptake of both serotonin and noradrenaline (Ryan *et al.*, 1995; Heal *et al.*, 2001; Lean, 2001). It has minimal dopamine agonist activity and does not appear to have abuse potential. Sibutramine produces a weight loss of about 6–8% of initial body weight in most trials (Ryan *et al.*, 1997; James *et al.*, 2000; Ryan, 2000; Wadden *et al.*, 2000; Appolinario *et al.*, 2003; van Baak *et al.*, 2003; Berkowitz *et al.*, 2003; Kim *et al.*, 2003; McNulty *et al.*, 2003; Padwal *et al.*, 2003a,b; Ersoz *et al.*, 2004). The STORM trial in Europe included intensive lifestyle intervention plus sibutramine, and found an average weight loss of about 13% at 1 year (James *et al.*, 2000; van Baak *et al.*, 2003). Wadden and colleagues (2000) found an average loss of 11.6% of initial body weight at 1 year. Padwal and colleagues (2003a) performed a Cochrane review of all studies of obesity drugs in the medical literature with at least 1 year of follow-up. Five sibutramine trials were included and the average weight loss was 4.3 kg (or 4.6%) more than in the placebo

group in these studies. All of these studies included a diet and exercise component.

Sibutramine has been used effectively in obese people with additional disorders. Appolinario and colleagues (2003) treated 60 obese subjects with binge eating disorder and found significant decreases in binge eating, depression score on the Beck Inventory and body weight compared with placebo. McNulty and colleagues (2003) found that sibutramine enhanced both weight loss and diabetes control in type 2 diabetics, compared with standard treatment and placebo. Berkowitz and colleagues (2003) used behavioural therapy (BT) along with sibutramine or placebo in 82 adolescents aged 13–17 years in a 12-month study, the first 6 months of which was double-blinded. They found that the sibutramine group had greater weight loss and less hunger than those on placebo and BT. However, 33 out of the 82 subjects had to decrease the dose or discontinue the trial due to side-effects.

The side-effect profile of sibutramine is generally moderate, but the most common complaints are dry mouth, headache, insomnia, constipation, tachycardia, hypertension and paradoxically increased appetite (Ryan *et al.*, 1995; Ryan, 2000; James *et al.*, 2000; Wadden *et al.*, 2000; Appolinario *et al.*, 2003; van Baak *et al.*, 2003; Berkowitz *et al.*, 2003; Kim *et al.*, 2003; McNulty *et al.*, 2003; Padwal *et al.*, 2003a,b; Ersoz *et al.*, 2004). Kim and colleagues (2003) noted an increase in both systolic and diastolic blood pressure despite a significant weight loss, and concluded that the drug should be used with careful follow-up of blood pressure. However, Ersoz and colleagues (Ersoz *et al.*, 2004) compared sibutramine with metoprolol to sibutramine alone and noted that the rise in blood pressure was blocked in the metoprolol group, but weight loss was similar in the two groups. There have been very few serious adverse reactions to sibutramine and, if hypertension or tachycardia occur, they generally respond promptly to reduction or discontinuation of the drug. One unusual side-effect is paradoxical increase in hunger. Subjects may actually gain weight and must discontinue the drug if this side-effect occurs.

Peripherally acting malabsorptive agent

Orlistat is the only obesity drug approved by the FDA at present for obesity treatment that does not act on the CNS. Orlistat is not absorbed and acts within the GI tract by inhibiting intestinal lipase, thus blocking digestion and absorption of dietary fat (Tonstad *et al.*, 1994; Drent and van der Veen 1995; James *et al.*, 1997; Hollander *et al.*, 1998; Sjostrom *et al.*, 1998; Lucas *et al.*, 2003; Tiikkainen *et al.*, 2004). About one-third of ingested fat is not absorbed and passes through to the colon, where it is metabolized by colonic bacteria or is excreted. Orlistat is taken with meals and has no long-term activity. Initial studies with orlistat reported a weight loss of about 5–12% of baseline body weight at 1–2 years (Tonstad *et al.*, 1994; Drent *et al.*, 1997; Hollander *et al.*, 1998; Sjostrom *et al.*, 1998; Lucas *et al.*, 2003; Tiikkainen *et al.*, 2004). Sjostrom and colleagues (1998) found a weight loss of about 10% at 1 year and 8% at 2 years in a large multicentre European trial. The Cochrane review by Padwal and colleagues (2003a,b) evaluated 11 orlistat studies. Average weight loss was 2.7 kg (or 2.9%) greater than placebo.

Orlistat reduces serum lipids and glucose through an independent effect on serum lipids (Tonstad *et al.*, 1994; Sjostrom *et al.*, 1998; Lucas *et al.*, 2003), but without an independent effect on serum glucose (Tonstad *et al.*, 1994; Hollander *et al.*, 1998; Sjostrom *et al.*, 1998; Lucas *et al.*, 2003;). Tonstad and colleagues (1994) treated patients who had hyperlipidaemia (cholesterol ≥ 6.2 mmol/L) with orlistat and noted reductions in serum total cholesterol and LDL by 11% and 10% respectively. Tiikkainen and colleagues (2004) treated obese patients with orlistat or placebo to achieve a standard 8% weight loss over 3–6 months of treatment. They ensured that weight losses were matched then measured glucose and lipid dynamics. Measures of glucose and insulin sensitivity were similar between groups. However, the ratio of intra-abdominal fat to subcutaneous fat was decreased significantly only in the orlistat group, suggesting a selective and independent reduction in intra-abdominal fat by orlistat.

The side-effects of orlistat are predominantly gastrointestinal complaints, including gas, abdominal pain, diarrhoea and, occasionally, faecal incontinence (Tonstad *et al.*, 1994; Drent *et al.*, 1998; Hollander *et al.*, 1998; Lucas *et al.*, 2003; Tiikkainen *et al.*, 2004). Side-effects are self-limited and may be avoided by reducing dietary fat. Of somewhat more concern is the malabsorption of fat-soluble vitamins, and the manufacturer recommends taking a multivitamin supplement each day.

Orlistat is approved by the FDA for use in children and adolescents. McDuffie and colleagues (2002a) performed an extensive 12-week study on 20 adolescents, mean age 14.6 years, mean BMI 44.1 kg/m^2, treating them with behaviour modification, diet and exercise, and orlistat. The subjects lost 4.1% of initial body weight and 1.9 BMI units. Serum cholesterol, LDL, glucose, insulin and insulin resistance all improved significantly. This same group evaluated serum fat-soluble vitamin levels in adolescents on orlistat with a single multivitamin capsule each day (McDuffie *et al.*, 2002b). They found a significant reduction from baseline in serum vitamin D levels and a reduction in absorption of vitamin E from the gastrointestinal tract, but no significant differences in serum levels of vitamins A and E.

Zhi and colleagues (2003) performed a metabolic balance study of six macro- and microminerals in adolescents treated with orlistat and found no evidence of malabsorption. Norgren and colleagues (2003) treated 11 severely obese prepubertal children (aged 8.3–12.3 years) with orlistat, and reported that they tolerated the drug well, decreased their consumption of dietary fat and lost about 4 kg. Psychological evaluation showed that the children improved their body shape preoccupation and oral control. The children complied with the regimen, evidenced by pill counts, and stated that they wished to continue the drug upon completion of the study.

In all of the above studies in children and adolescents, the authors concluded that additional trials were needed and that drugs should be used with caution. With the increasing epidemic of obesity and the appearance of type 2 diabetes and hypertension in children, the caution expressed by many paediatricians about the use of drugs for obesity seems unduly conservative, especially as there is no hesitation to use oral hypoglycaemics, insulin and anti-hypertensive agents in children who have the complications of obesity.

Non-approved drugs with potential for treating obesity

In addition to the selective serotonin reuptake inhibitors (SSRIs) mentioned above, several other centrally active agents are on the market and approved for other indications, but have potential to produce weight loss.

Bupropion is an aminoketone class antidepressant that is chemically related to the phenylethylamines, with a structure similar to diethylpropion. It has adrenergic and serotonergic re-uptake inhibitor activity. Anderson and colleagues (2002) reported weight loss of about 10% of initial body weight after 1 year of treatment. Side-effects include gastrointestinal complaints, dry mouth, drowsiness, dizziness, anxiety and, rarely, cardiac symptoms such as tachycardia and arrhythmias.

Topiramate is approved for epilepsy, but its mechanism of action to produce weight loss is unknown. Weight loss was first noticed as a side-effect of treatment in patients with epilepsy. In an uncontrolled study, Ben-Menachem and colleagues (2003) gave topiramate to 38 seizure patients for 1 year. Weight losses at 3 months and 1 year in the whole sample were 3.9% and 7.3% of initial weight. For individuals with a BMI ≥ 30 kg/m^2, weight losses were 4.3% and 11.0%, with essentially all of the loss being from body fat. A number of clinical trials are under way to determine if topiramate will be useful for treating obesity. Bray and colleagues (2003) reported a multicentre, 6-month, randomized trial that found a weight loss of about 6% of initial body weight.

McElroy and colleagues (2003) evaluated the effectiveness of topiramate in a placebo-controlled, double-blind, randomized trial in 61 patients who had binge eating disorder and obesity (BMI ≥ 30 kg/m^2). The mean weight loss on topiramate was 5.9 kg and there was a dramatic reduction in binge eating frequency and binge/day frequency compared with placebo. Also, there were significant improvements in two psychological instruments, the Clinical Global Impression severity scale and the Yale-Brown Obsessive Compulsive Scale (modified for binge eating).

Smathers and colleagues (2003) gave topiramate to seven children with Prader–Willi syndrome and noted that there were improvements in self-abusive behaviour, an improved mood, and that the weight gain that is a hallmark of this syndrome had stabilized.

There are a number of side-effects of topiramate, including

drowsiness, dizziness, headache, trouble concentrating, short-term memory loss, GI complaints, depression, fatigue and paraesthesiae (Bray 2003; McElroy *et al.*, 2003). The paraesthesiae are distinctive and occur in the fingers and toes and around the mouth, especially with higher doses (> 200 mg), although they may occur at lower doses. The drowsiness is sufficiently common that the manufacturer recommends that the drug be taken before going to bed to avoid problems during the day. The decreased mentation occurs in the higher doses and can be severe enough in some patients that the drug must be stopped. Anecdotal reports from private physicians suggest that doses as low as 25–50 mg may cause reduction of body weight, and the study by Bray (2003) reported significant weight losses at a dose of 64 mg per day.

Zonisamide is also approved for treatment of epilepsy. It has serotonergic and dopaminergic activity and blocks sodium and calcium channels. Gadde and colleagues (2003) performed a 16-week randomized, blinded trial followed by a 16-week open-label extension. Weight loss was about 6% of initial body weight. Side-effects include gastrointestinal complaints, drowsiness, dizziness, headache, trouble concentrating, short-term memory loss, depression and fatigue.

Ephedrine, in combination with caffeine, with or without the addition of aspirin, has been used in Europe for many years to treat obesity. Methylxanthines (caffeine, theophylline, theobromine, etc.) and/or aspirin enhance the effects of ephedrine and increase weight loss and metabolic rate by slowing metabolism of noradrenaline (Arner, 1993; Daly *et al.*, 1993; Dulloo, 1993; Toubro *et al.*, 1993). Ephedrine-caffeine stimulates noradrenaline secretion, which then stimulates activity of cyclic AMP. Caffeine inhibits phosphodiesterase, the enzyme that metabolizes cyclic AMP, and thereby enhances noradrenaline. Aspirin enhances noradrenaline activity by inhibiting adenosine, which is involved in noradrenaline inactivation. The combination may be associated with increases in heart rate, blood pressure and metabolic rate (Arner, 1993; Daly *et al.*, 1993; Dulloo AG, 1993; Toubro *et al.*, 1993; Boozer *et al.*, 2001; 2002). The increases in heart rate and blood pressure associated with ephedrine-caffeine appear to be short-lived, but the effect on thermogenesis persists (Toubro *et al.*, 1993).

Pure ephedrine and caffeine have been used very sparingly in the US for obesity treatment. However, numerous over-the-counter dietary supplements contain ephedra and a methylxanthine (usually caffeine) as extracts of plants. These preparations were probably the most commonly used antiobesity products in the US, dwarfing any of the single obesity prescription drugs. The FDA banned ephedra from use in dietary supplements for obesity in December 2003. This ban will not prohibit physicians from prescribing ephedrine, usually in combination with caffeine or other methylxanthine as pure prescription preparations. However, the legal vulnerability should side-effects occur markedly reduces enthusiasm for their use.

Weight losses with pure ephedrine and caffeine were as great as 16% of initial body weight at 1 year in a study by Toubro and colleagues (1993), which included a significant diet and exercise programme. Boozer and colleagues (2002) demonstrated in short-term studies with a herbal preparation that carefully selected subjects lost more weight and did not have a higher prevalence of significant side-effects, particularly cardiac side-effects than placebo (Boozer *et al.*, 2002). Common side-effects are dry mouth, tremor, tachycardia and headache. Rare side-effects are hypertension, anxiety, cardiac arrhythmias and strokes.

Metformin is a peripherally acting anti-diabetes drug that enhances insulin sensitivity and has been associated with weight losses of 5–10% of initial body weight (Fontbonne *et al.*, 1996; Lee and Morley, 1998; Kay *et al.*, 2001; Gokcel *et al.*, 2002). Like acarbose, it does not increase insulin secretion, but enhances insulin sensitivity. One of the side-effects of metformin is gastrointestinal distress, so this may help reduce food intake, especially early in the course of treatment. Metformin may be particularly helpful in patients with obesity and infertility due to polycystic ovary syndrome (Pasquali *et al.*, 2000). Side-effects of metformin are nausea, abdominal pain and, rarely, lactic acidosis, especially in patients with renal disease.

Acarbose is a malabsorptive agent approved for the treatment of diabetes. It is an amylase inhibitor that blocks absorption of complex carbohydrates (Berger, 1992), and may be associated with improved insulin sensitivity (Meneilly *et al.*, 2000; Delgado *et al.*, 2002; Josse *et al.*, 2003). Acarbose has not been shown to be effective in treating obesity when used as a single agent. However, anecdotal reports suggest that occasionally it may produce modest additional weight loss when used in combination with other obesity drugs. It is possible that there is a subgroup of obese people who might respond to acarbose, but more research must be done to test this hypothesis. Side-effects are predominantly gastrointestinal complaints, gas, abdominal pain and occasionally diarrhoea (Berger, 1992; Meneilly *et al.*, 2000; Delgado *et al.*, 2002; Josse *et al.*, 2003).

Cimetidine is a proton pump inhibitor used to treat peptic ulcer disease, gastritis and oesophageal reflux disease. Cimetidine was found to improve weight loss on an energy-restricted diet in one study (Sta-Birketvedt, 1993), but not in another (Rasmussen *et al.*, 1993). The mechanism of action was postulated to be a suppression of gastric acid secretion (Sta-Birketvedt, 1993). Side-effects include diarrhoea, constipation, muscle pain, headache, dizziness and drowsiness.

Alemzadeh and colleagues (Alemzadeh, 1998) gave diazoxide to obese adults on an energy-restricted diet and noted a weight loss of 9.5% of initial body weight over 8 weeks, compared with a loss of 4.6% in placebo subjects. Side-effects include increased hair growth, gastrointestinal complaints, CNS effects including headache, dizziness, anxiety and paraesthesiae.

Cincotta and Meier (1996) gave bromocriptine or placebo to subjects for 18 weeks and noted a loss of 6.3 kg vs. 0.9 kg, re-

Table 25.4 Dietary supplements and herbal preparations marketed for obesity or weight control.*

Aspartame
Chromium compounds
Conjugated linoleic acid
Creatine
Dehydroepiandrosterone
Dietary fibre supplements
Olestra
Pyruvate

---

*None of these agents is approved by the FDA or other agency for the treatment of obesity, and none has clinically significant effectiveness for obesity.

spectively, in the two groups. Body fat decreased significantly and glucose and insulin levels during an oral glucose tolerance test were significantly lower in the bromocriptine group. Side-effects include gastrointestinal complaints, cardiac arrhythmias and CNS complaints including headaches and confusion.

Nicotine produces weight loss and may be the mechanism of maintenance of a lower body weight in smokers (Jensen *et al.*, 1995). Use of nicotine gum after smoking cessation prevented weight loss in one study (Nides *et al.*, 1994). Gastrointestinal complaints and headache are the more common side-effects, but excess amounts can cause coronary and cerebral vasoconstriction, dyspnoea and seizures.

Over-the-counter diet supplements, herbs and other agents

For most of the large number of diet supplements and herbal preparations being sold to reduce body weight or enhance lean body mass (Table 25.4), no research has been done and only lay publications are available (Balch and Balch, 1997). For others research shows modest to no effects, including dietary fibre supplements (Life Sciences Research Office, 1987), aspartame (Blackburn *et al.*, 1997), olestra (Lawson *et al.*, 1997), chromium compounds (Trent and Thieding-Cancel, 1995; Grant *et al.*, 1997; Pasman *et al.*, 1997; Wasser *et al.*, 1997; Cerulli al., 1998), dehydroepiandrosterone (Vogiatzi *et al.*, 1996), pyruvate (Stanko *et al.*, 1994; Stanko and Arch, 1996), creatine (Kreider *et al.*, 1998) and conjugated linoleic acid (CLA) (Blankson *et al.*, 2000; Whigham *et al.*, 2000; Riserus *et al.*, 2001; Belury *et al.*, 2003; Kamphuis *et al.*, 2003a,b). CLA has been tested extensively because it has excellent effectiveness in reducing adipose tissue in animals (Whigham *et al.*, 2000). However, studies in humans show very little or no effect in reducing obesity in humans (Whigham *et al.*, 2000; Blankson *et al.*, 2000; Riserus *et al.*, 2001; Belury *et al.*, 2003; Kamphuis *et al.*, 2003a,b).

In contrast with the diet supplements noted above, preparations containing ephedra with a methylxanthine and/or as-

pirin have been shown to produce significant weight loss, as described above (Boozer *et al.*, 2001; 2002). Herbal preparations with this mixture have been removed from the market in the USA by the FDA, but are available in many other parts of the world.

Despite the lack of research and minimal or no evidence of efficacy for most of these dietary supplement preparations, a large industry is present to promote their use through direct advertising to consumers. The revenues from this industry are enormous. In 1999, the US FDA estimated that revenues for the dietary supplement industry was worth over six billion dollars [Center for Food Safety and Applied Nutrition; US Food and Drug Administration website (http://vm.cfsan.fda.gov/~comm/ds-econa.html)]. Governmental agencies, such as the FDA and US Federal Trade Commission (FTC), may intervene if false claims are made, but there has been little action to protect vulnerable obese people from charlatans selling worthless preparations.

Agents with potential for treating obesity

A wide variety of agents are being evaluated by pharmaceutical companies or academic investigators for usefulness for treating obesity. These include gut peptides, brain peptides, neurochemicals and other agents. Space does not permit a complete review of these substances, but some that appear to be of interest because they reduce food intake or produce weight or fat loss in humans or animals are adiponectin, anorectin, apolipoprotein A-IV, axokine, bombesin, cholecystokinin, corticotrophin-releasing hormone (CRH), enterostatin, glucagon-like peptide 1 (GLP-1), growth hormone, insulin-like growth factors, leptin, neurotensin, oxyntomodulin, pancreatic polypeptide (PP), peptide YY 3–36 (PYY 3–36) and vasopressin (Rudman *et al.*, 1990; Okada *et al.*, 1991; Bray, 1992; Leibowitz, 1995; Batterham *et al.*, 2003a,b; Cohen *et al.*, 2003; Ellacott *et al.*, 2004; Gavrila *et al.*, 2003; Naslund *et al.*, 2004; Tso *et al.*, 2004; Yang *et al.*, 2004) (Table 25.5). Agonists for β-3 adrenergic receptors reduce body fat and increase lean body mass in animals (Yen, 1995; Stock, 1996), but to date have not been effective and/or safe in humans. Several uncoupling proteins potentially produce energy wastage (Bao *et al.*, 1998; Snyder *et al.*, 2004), but none has yet been developed into obesity drugs.

Cannabinoid agonists, galanin, ghrelin, melanin-concentrating hormone (MCH) and neuropeptide Y (NPY) are CNS neurotransmitters that stimulate food intake (Bauer *et al.*, 1989; Leibowitz, 1991; 1995; Tritos and Maratos-Flier 1999; Wren *et al.*, 2001; Cummings *et al.*, 2002; Silva *et al.*, 2002; Wilding, 2002; Collins and Kym, 2003; Black, 2004) (Table 25.5), and a search is on for antagonists to these substances. The cannabinoid antagonist rimonabant is in clinical trials to evaluate its potential for obesity treatment (Black, 2004).

It is likely that many, if not most, of these agents will fail, but

Table 25.5 Substances with potential for treating obesity.

Adiponectin
Anorectin
Apolipoprotein A–IV
Axokine (ciliary neurotrophic factor)
Beta-adrenergic receptor agonists
Bombesin
Cannabinoid antagonists (e.g. rimonabant)
Cholecystokinin
Corticotrophin-releasing hormone (CRH)
Enterostatin
Galanin antagonists
Glucagon-like peptide 1 (GLP-1)
Ghrelin antagonists
Growth hormone
Insulin-like growth factors
Leptin
Melanin-concentrating hormone (MCH) antagonists
Neuropeptide Y (NPY) antagonists
Neurotensin
Oxyntomodulin
Pancreatic polypeptide (PP)
Peptide YY 3–36 (PYY 3–36)
Vasopressin

even if the response is modest, it is possible that combinations with each other or with current obesity drugs will lead to significant weight loss in subgroups of obese patients.

A large number of genes have been identified that are associated with human obesity, including several single gene defects (Snyder *et al.*, 2004). Most genetic types of human obesity are polygenic. Pharmaceutical companies are evaluating the potential for gene therapies if specific patterns of gene defects or differences can be identified for action.

Rimonabant

Rimonabant is a selective central cannaboid (CB1) receptor antagonist. It is an appetite suppressant in advanced development for obesity treatment. The rationale behind this drug is to reduce appetite by blocking cannaboid receptors in the hypothalamus. The central cannaboid (CB1) receptors are believed to play a role in controlling food consumption and the phenomena of dependence/habituation. Preliminary results from a two year international multicentre study confirm its effectiveness in weight reduction, reduction in waist circumference—a marker of the dangerous abdominal obesity—and improvements in lipids and glycaemic profiles (Sjostrom *et al.*, 2004). The study also confirmed its good safety profile. The side effects reported were mainly mild and transient and most frequently involved nausea, diarrhoea and dizziness. Rimonabant also has potential as a treatment for smoking cessation because the central cannaboid system is also involved in the body's response to tobacco dependence.

Combinations of drugs for obesity

Although most chronic diseases are treated with combinations of drugs, obesity is an exception. There have been very few combinations studies. Those that have been evaluated include ephedrine–methylxanthines–aspirin, phenylpropanolamine–benzocaine, fenfluramine–phentermine, fluoxetine–phentermine, dexfenfluramine–fluoxetine, sibutramine–orlistat and phentermine–orlistat (Weintraub *et al.*, 1984; Greenway, 1992; Weintraub, 1992; Arner, 1993; Daly *et al.*, 1993; Dulloo, 1993; Toubro *et al.*, 1993; Hartley *et al.*, 1995; Dhurandhar and Atkinson, 1996; Pedrinola *et al.*, 1996; Anchors, 1997a,b; Atkinson *et al.*, 1997; Griffen and Anchors, 1998; Greenway *et al.*, 1999; Bowen and Atkinson, 2000; Devlin *et al.*, 2000; Wadden *et al.*, 2000; Boozer *et al.*, 2001; 2002; Kolotkin *et al.*, 2001). The combination of ephedrine and caffeine is described above, but the data from a sampling of other combination studies are described below.

Phenylpropanolamine–benzocaine

Benzocaine is a local anaesthetic agent contained in some over-the-counter weight reduction aids, the action of which was reported to 'numb the taste buds'. Greenway and colleagues (Greenway, 1992; Greenway *et al.*, 1999) reported that the combination of phenylpropanolamine and benzocaine was no more effective than placebo.

Phentermine–fenfluramine combination

Fenfluramine and dexfenfluramine are no longer on the market but represented probably the most effective pharmacological treatment for obesity yet seen (Weintraub *et al.*, 1984; Weintraub, 1992; Atkinson *et al.*, 1997). Weintraub and colleagues (1992) used the combination of phentermine resin and fenfluramine on 121 subjects for up to 3.5 years. All of the subjects were treated with diet, exercise and behaviour modification. At 60 weeks, patients lost 15.8 kg. This was the first long-term study of drug combination therapy for obesity, and demonstrated that significant weight loss persisted as long as the drugs were given, up to 4 years. Upon discontinuing medications at the end of the study, weight regain was rapid. Atkinson and colleagues (Atkinson *et al.*, 1997) reported weight loss of 16.5% of initial body weight (17 kg) at 1 year, and about 8% at 3 years in patients on fenfluramine and phentermine HCl. Reductions in systolic and diastolic blood pressures in hypertensive patients (28 mmHg and 17 mmHg respectively) and in serum cholesterol and triglycerides (27 mg/dl and 79 mg/dl respectively) in hyperlipidaemic patients (Weintraub, 1992) were found. Hartley and colleagues (Hartley *et al.*, 1995; Kolotkin *et al.*, 2001) found a 17.6% weight loss on phentermine–fenfluramine.

Fenfluramine–fluoxetine combination

Pedrinola and colleagues (Pedrinola *et al.*, 1996) gave fluoxetine–fenfluramine vs. fluoxetine–placebo in 33 women for 8 months in a randomized, double-blind trial. The fluoxetine–fenfluramine group lost 13.4 kg and the fluoxetine–placebo group lost 6.2 kg.

Phentermine–fluoxetine combination

In a preliminary report, Dhurandhar and Atkinson (1996) found that the combination of fluoxetine (20–60 mg/day) and phentermine hydrochloride (18.75–37.5 mg/day) produced weight losses similar to fenfluramine (20–60 mg/day) and phentermine HCl (18.7–37.5 mg/day). Anchors and colleagues (1997a,b; Griffen and Anchors, 1998) provided anecdotal reports that fluoxetine–phentermine in doses of 10–20 mg per day and 30 mg per day, respectively, achieved weight losses of about 15% of initial body weight. Devlin and colleagues (2000) gave fluoxetine–phentermine to overweight females with binge eating disorder in an open-label trial and found significant weight loss for 18 months in subjects who continued medication.

Sibutramine–orlistat

Wadden and colleagues (2000) gave orlistat to 34 obese female subjects who had lost about 11% of initial body weight during treatment for 12 months on sibutramine and lifestyle modification. Orlistat produced no additional weight loss during a 16-week extension with the drug combination.

Phentermine–orlistat

In a preliminary study, Bowen and colleagues (Bowen and Atkinson, 2000) gave orlistat to patients who were weight stable after at least 3 months of treatment with phentermine. There was a minimal weight loss (< 1 kg) over the next 2 months.

The data on combinations of obesity drugs demonstrate that some combinations produce greater weight loss than is seen with single agents. More studies that are carefully controlled and monitored with different combinations are needed. Anecdotal reports from private physicians suggest that combinations of phentermine and topiramate, phentermine and zonisamide, fluoxetine and bupropion, fluoxetine and topiramate, and metformin with either phentermine or sibutramine can produce acceptable weight losses in some patients. More research is needed with these combinations and they must be used with extreme caution. For medicolegal reasons, written, informed consent should be obtained, which explains the potential adverse reactions and the off-label status of these combinations. It should be emphasised that drug combinations for obesity are not authorised by regulatory authorities and responsibility for their prescription lies with the prescriber.

Practical aspects of drug therapy

The experience with obesity drugs is very limited, so there are few practical guidelines for their use. Patients differ markedly in their response to single agents or combinations of obesity drugs, and responders cannot be identified in advance. Effective dosage levels vary widely among individuals, so a sensible treatment regimen may begin with low doses of single agents, and progress to larger doses of multiple agents if necessary. For example, this may mean a dose of 18.75 mg of phentermine HCl, 10 mg of sibutramine, or 25 mg of topiramate. For many agents, starting at full doses initially produces unacceptable side-effects that may be limited or eliminated by starting low and graduating to full levels over days to months. If an increase in dosage does not cause additional weight loss in a period of 4–8 weeks, the dosage should be reduced back to the previous level.

If adding a new drug does not enhance weight loss or reduce complications of obesity, it should be discontinued. There is debate about the length of the trial to determine efficacy. Several pharmaceutical manufacturers recommend discontinuing an obesity drug if weight loss does not reach 4 lb (or 2 kg) in the first month of treatment. This is quite arbitrary, and the author's data with phentermine–fenfluramine showed that in patients who lost less than 2 kg after 4 weeks, eventual mean weight loss at 6 months was 10% of initial body weight (Dhurandhar *et al.*, 1999). Rather than using a fixed formula, careful assessment of individual patients will be a better guide for the length of time drugs should be given if response is not optimal.

From the opposite perspective, it is difficult to know when to discontinue a drug when it is working well, but side-effects are present. Patients may be reluctant to discontinue drugs, even in the face of significant side-effects, because the drugs are effective and weight regain is very likely if the drug or combination is stopped. Physicians must ask about side-effects and unilaterally intervene as the situation demands. In every case, physicians must use best judgement and communicate to the patient the rationale for any decision.

Summary and conclusions

As obesity is a chronic disease of multiple aetiologies, treatment with drugs, once started, is likely to be indefinite, probably lifelong. Because obese people have an altered biochemistry, drugs are probably their best hope for long-term success in maintaining weight loss. The drugs available at present which are approved for the treatment of obesity are only modestly effective, but there has been little effort to evaluate combinations of drugs. Most chronic diseases require two or more drugs for severe cases, and it is likely that obesity will also. Many new drugs are in development, and the future is bright for treatment of obesity with drugs. Physicians who use drugs for obesity must individualize treatment for each patient and consider at regular follow-up intervals if the drugs are effective or the dose or type needs to be changed.

References

Alemzadeh, R., Langley,G., Upchurch, L., Smith, P. and Slonim, A.E. (1998) Beneficial effect of diazoxide in obese hyperinsulinemic adults. *Journal of Clinical Endocrinology and Metabolism* **83**, 1911–1915.

Anchors, M. (1997a) *Safer Than Phen-Fen*. Rocklin, CA: Prima Publishing.

Anchors, M. (1997b) Fluoxetine is a safer alternative to fenfluramine in the medical treatment of obesity. *Archives of Internal Medicine* **157**, 1270.

Andersen, T., Stokholm, K.H., Backer, O.G. and Quaade, F. (1988) Long-term (5-year) results after either horizontal gastroplasty or very-low calorie diet for morbid obesity. *International Journal of Obesity* **12**, 277–284.

Anderson, J.W., Greenway, F.L., Fujioka, K., Gadde, K.M., McKenney, J, O'Neil, P.M. (2002) Bupropion SR enhances weight loss: a 48-week double-blind, placebo-controlled trial. *Obesity Research* **10**, 633–641.

Appolinario, J.C., Bacaltchuk, J., Sichieri, R., Claudino, A.M., Godoy-Matos, A., Morgan, C., Zanella, M.T. and Coutinho, W. (2003) A randomized, double-blind, placebo-controlled study of sibutramine in the treatment of binge eating disorder. *Archives of General Psychiatry* **60**, 1109–1116.

Arner, P. (1993) Adenosine, prostaglandins and phosphodiesterase as targeted for obesity pharmacotherapy. *International Journal of Obesity* **17** (Suppl, 1), S57–S59.

Atkinson, R.L., Blank, R.C., Schumacher, D., Dhurandhar, N.V. and Ritch, D.L. (1997) Long term drug treatment of obesity in a private practice setting. *Obesity Research* **5**, 578–586.

Ayyad, C. and Andersen, T. (2000) Long-term efficacy of dietary treatment of obesity: a systematic review of studies published between 1931 and 1999. *Obesity Reviews* **1**, 113–119.

van Baak, M.A., van Mil, E., Astrup, A.V., Finer, N., Van Gaal,L.F., Hilsted, J., Kopelman, P.G., Rossner, S., James, W.P. and Saris, W.H.: STORM Study Group (2003) Leisure-time activity is an important determinant of long-term weight maintenance after weight loss in the Sibutramine Trial on Obesity Reduction and Maintenance (STORM trial). *American Journal of Clinical Nutrition* **78**, 209–214.

Balch, J.F. and Balch, P.A. (1997) *Prescription for Nutritional Healing*. Garden City Park: Avery Publishing Group, 64–79 and 406–412.

Bao, S., Kennedy, A., Wojciechowski, B., Wallace, P., Ganaway, E. and Garvey, W.T. (1998) Expression of mRNAs encoding uncoupling proteins in human skeletal muscle: effects of obesity and diabetes. *Diabetes* **47**, 1935–1940.

Batterham, R.L., Cohen, M.A., Ellis, S.M., Le Roux, C.W., Withers, D.J., Frost, G.S., Ghatei, M.A. and Bloom, S.R. (2003a) Inhibition of food intake in obese subjects by peptide YY3–36. *New England Journal of Medicine* **349**, 941–948.

Batterham, R.L., Le Roux, C.W., Cohen, M.A., Park, A.J., Ellis, S.M., Patterson, M., Frost, G.S., Ghatei, M.A. and Bloom, S.R. (2003b) Pancreatic polypeptide reduces appetite and food intake in humans. *Journal of Clinical Endocrinology and Metabolism* **88**, 3989–3992.

Bauer, F.E., Zintel, A., Kenny, M.J., Calder, D., Ghatei, M.A. and Bloom, S.R. (1989) Inhibitory effect of galanin on postprandial gastrointestinal motility and gut hormone release in humans. *Gastroenterology* **97**, 260–264.

Belury, M.A., Mahon, A. and Banni, S. (2003) The conjugated linoleic acid (CLA) isomer, t10c12–CLA, is inversely associated with changes in body weight and serum leptin in subjects with type 2 diabetes mellitus. *Journal of Nutrition* **133**(1), 257S–260S.

Ben-Menachem, E., Axelsen, M., Johanson, E.H., Stagge, A. and Smith, U. (2003) Predictors of weight loss in adults with topiramate-treated epilepsy. *Obesity Research* **11**, 556–562.

Berger M. (1992) Pharmacological treatment of obesity: digestion and absorption inhibitors—clinical perspective. *American Journal of Clinical Nutrition* **55**, 318S–319S.

Berkowitz, R.I., Wadden, T.A., Tershakovec, A.M. and Cronquist, J.L. (2003) Behavior therapy and sibutramine for the treatment of adolescent obesity: a randomized controlled trial. *Journal of the American Medical Association* **289**, 1805–1812.

Black, S.C. (2004) Cannabinoid receptor antagonists and obesity. *Current Opinions in Investigation of Drugs* **5**, 389–394.

Blackburn, G.L., Kanders, B.S., Lavin, P.T., Keller, S.D. and Whatley, J. (1997) The effect of aspartame as part of a multidisciplinary weight control program on short- and long-term control of body weight. *American Journal of Clinical Nutrition* **65**, 409–418.

Blankson, H., Stakkestad, J.A., Fagertun, H., Thom, E., Wadstein, J. and Gudmundsen, O. (2000) Conjugated linoleic acid reduces body fat mass in overweight and obese humans. *Journal of Nutrition* **130**, 2943–2948.

Boozer, C.N., Nasser, J.A., Heymsfield, S.B., Wang, V., Chen, G. and Solomon, J.L. (2001) An herbal supplement containing Ma Huang-Guarana for weight loss: a randomized, double-blind trial. *International Journal of Obesity and Related Metabolic Disorders* **25**, 316–324.

Boozer, C.N., Daly, P.A., Homel, P., Solomon, J.L., Blanchard, D., Nasser, J.A., Strauss R. and Meredith. T. (2002) Herbal ephedra/caffeine for weight loss: a 6-month randomized safety and efficacy trial. *International Journal of Obesity and Related Metabolic Disorders* **26**, 593–604.

Bowen, R.L. and Atkinson, R.L. (2000) Addition of orlistat to long term phentermine treatment for obesity. *Obesity Research* **8**, 118.

Bray, G.A. (1992) Peptides affect the intake of specific nutrients in the sympathetic nervous system. *American Journal of Clinical Nutrition* **55**, 265S–271S.

Bray, G.A. (2000) A concise review on the therapeutics of obesity. *Nutrition* **16**, 953–960.

Bray, G.A. (2003) Risks of obesity. *Primary Care* **30**, 281–299, v–vi.

Bray, G.A., Hollander, P., Klein, S., Kushner, R., Levy, B., Fitchet, M. and Perry, B.H. (2003) A 6-month randomized, placebo-controlled, dose-ranging trial of topiramate for weight loss in obesity. *Obesity Research* **11**, 722–733.

Center for Food Safety and Applied Nutrition; US Food and Drug Administration (website: http://vm.cfsan.fda.gov/~comm/dsecona.html).

Cerulli, J., Grabe, D.W., Gauthier, I., Malone, M. and McGoldrick, M.D. (1998) Chromium picolinate toxicity. *Annals of Pharmacotherapy* **32**, 428–431.

Cincotta, A.H. and Meier, A.H. (1996) Bromocriptine (Ergoset) reduces body weight and improves glucose tolerance in obese subjects. *Diabetes Care* **19**, 667–670.

Cohen, M.A., Ellis, S.M., Le Roux, C.W., Batterham, R.L., Park, A., Patterson, M., Frost, G.S., Ghatei, M.A. and Bloom, S.R. (2003) Oxyntomodulin suppresses appetite and reduces food intake in humans. *Journal of Clinical Endocrinology and Metabolism* **88**, 4696–4701.

Coleman, D.L. (1979) Obese and diabetes: two mutant genes causing diabetes-obesity in mice. *Diabetologia* **14**, 141–148.

Collins, C.A. and Kym, P.R. (2003) Prospects for obesity treatment: MCH receptor antagonists. *Current Opinion in Investigational Drugs* **4**, 386–394.

Connolly, H.M., Crary, J.L., McGoon, M.D., Hensrud, D.D., Edwards, B.S., Edwards, W.D. and Schaff, H.V. (1997) Valvular heart disease associated with fenfluramine-phentermine. *New England Journal of Medicine* **337**, 581–588.

Cummings, D.E., Weigle, D.S., Frayo, R.S., Breen, P.A., Ma, M.K., Dellinger, E.P. and Purnell, J.Q. (2002) Plasma ghrelin levels after diet-induced weight loss or gastric bypass surgery. *New England Journal of Medicine* **346**, 1623–1630.

Daly, P.A., Krieger, D.R., Dulloo, A.G., Young, J.B. and Landsberg, L. (1993) Ephedrine, caffeine and aspirin: safety and efficacy for treatment of human obesity. *International Journal of Obesity* **17** (Suppl. 1), S73–78.

Delgado, H., Lehmann, T., Bobbioni-Harsch, E., Ybarra, J. and Golay, A. (2002) Acarbose improves indirectly both insulin resistance and secretion in obese type 2 diabetic patients. *Diabetes and Metabolism* **28**, 195–200.

Devlin, M.J., Goldfein, J.A., Carino, J.S. and Wolk, S.L. (2000) Open treatment of overweight binge eaters with phentermine and fluoxetine as an adjunct to cognitive–behavioral therapy. *International Journal of Eating Disorders* **28**, 325–332.

Dhurandhar, N.V. and Atkinson, R.L. (1996) Comparison of serotonin agonists in combination with phentermine for treatment of obesity. *FASEB Journal* **10**, A561.

Dhurandhar, N.V., Blank, R.C., Schumacher, D. and Atkinson, R.L. (1999) Initial weight loss as a predictor of response to obesity drugs. *International Journal of Obesity and Related Metabolic Disorders* **23**, 1333–1336.

Drent, M.L. and van der Veen, E.A. (1995) First clinical studies with orlistat: a short review. *Obesity Research* **3** (Suppl. 4), 623S–625S.

Dulloo, A.G. (1993) Ephedrine, xanthines and prostaglandin-inhibitors: actions and interactions in the stimulation of thermogenesis. *International Journal of Obesity* **17** (Suppl. 1), S35–S40.

Eckel, R.H. and Yost, T.J. (1987) Weight reduction increases adipose tissue lipoprotein lipase responsiveness in obese women. *Journal of Clinical Investigation* **80**, 992–997.

Eckel, R.H., Yost, T.J. and Jensen, D.R. (1995) Sustained weight reduction in moderately obese women results in decreased activity of skeletal muscle lipoprotein lipase. *European Journal of Clinical Investigation* **25**, 396–402.

Ellacott, K.L. and Cone, R.D. (2004) The central melanocortin system and the integration of short- and long-term regulators of energy homeostasis. *Recent Progress in Hormone Research* **59**, 395–408.

Enzi, G., Baritussio, A., Marchiori, E. and Crepaldi, G. (1976) Short-term and long-term clinical evaluation of a non-amphetamine anorexiant (mazindol) in the treatment of obesity. *Journal of International Medical Research* **4**, 305–317.

Ersoz, H.O., Ukinc, K., Baykan, M., Erem, C., Durmus, I., Hacihasanoglu, A. and Telatar, M. (2004) Effect of low-dose metoprolol in combination with sibutramine therapy in normotensive obese patients: a randomized controlled study. *International Journal of Obesity and Related Metabolic Disorders* **28**, 378–383.

Fitzgerald, L.W., Burn, T.C., Brown, B.S., Patterson, J.P., Corjay, M.H., Valentine, P.A., Sun, J.H., Link, J.R., Abbaszade, I., Hollis, J.M., Largent, B.L., Hartig, P.R., Hollis, G.F., Meunier, P.C., Robichaud, A.J. and Robertson, D.W. (2000) Possible role of valvular serotonin 5-HT(2B) receptors in the cardiopathy associated with fenfluramine. *Molecular Pharmacology* **57**, 75–81.

Fontbonne, A., Charles, M.A., Juhan-Vague, I., Bard, J.M., Andre, P., Isnard, F., Cohen, J.M., Grandmottet, P., Vague, P., Safar, M.E. and Eschwege, E. (1996) The effect of metformin on the metabolic abnormalities associated with upper-body fat distribution. BIGPRO Study Group. *Diabetes Care* **19**, 920–926.

Food and Drug Administration/National Institutes of Health/World Health Organization (1998) Clinical Guidelines on the Identification, Evaluation, and Treatment of Overweight and Obesity in Adults—The Evidence Report. *Obesity Research* **6** (Suppl. 2), 51S–209S.

Friedman, J.M. (2003) A war on obesity, not the obese. *Science* **299**, 856–858.

Gadde, K.M., Franciscy, D.M., Wagner, 2nd, H.R. and Krishnan, K.R. (2003) Zonisamide for weight loss in obese adults: a randomized controlled trial. *Journal of the American Medical Association* **289**, 1820–1825.

Garattini S. (1995) Biological actions of drugs affecting serotonin and eating. *Obesity Research* **3** (Suppl. 4), 463S–470S.

Garattini, S., Bizzi, A., Codegoni, A.M., Caccia, S. and Mennini, T. (1992) Progress report on the anorexia induced by drugs believed to mimic some of the effects of serotonin on the central nervous system. *American Journal of Clinical Nutrition* **55** (Suppl. 1), 160S–166S.

Gardin, J.M., Schumacher, D., Constantine, G., Davis, K.D., Leung, C. and Reid, C.L. (2000) Valvular abnormalities and cardiovascular status following exposure to dexfenfluramine or phentermine/fenfluramine. *Journal of the American Medical Association* **283**, 1703–1709.

Gavrila, A., Chan, J.L., Yiannakouris, N., Kontogianni, M., Miller, L.C., Orlova, C. and Mantzoro, C.S. (2003) Serum adiponectin levels are inversely associated with overall and central fat distribution but are not directly regulated by acute fasting or leptin administration in humans: cross-sectional and interventional studies. *Journal of Clinical Endocrinology and Metabolism* **88**, 4823–4831.

Gokcel, A., Gumurdulu, Y., Karakose, H., Melek Ertorer, E., Tanaci, N., Bascil Tutuncu, N. and Guvener, N. (2002) Evaluation of the safety and efficacy of sibutramine, orlistat and metformin in the treatment of obesity. *Diabetes, Obesity and Metabolism* **4**, 49–55.

Goldstein, D.J. and Potvin, J.H. (1994) Long-term weight loss: the effect of pharmacologic agents. *American Journal of Clinical Nutrition* **60**, 647–657.

Goldstein, D.J., Rampey, Jr, A.H., Dornseif, B.E., Levine, L.R., Potvin, J.H. and Fludzinski, L.A. (1993) Fluoxetine: a randomized clinical trial in the maintenance of weight loss. *Obesity Research* **1**, 92–98.

Goldstein, D.J., Rampey, Jr, A.H., Roback, P.J., Wilson, M.G., Hamilton, S.H., Sayler, M.E. and Tollefson, G.D. (1995) Efficacy and safety of long-term fluoxetine treatment of obesity: maximizing success. *Obesity Research* **3** (Suppl. 4), 481S–490S.

Grant, K.E., Chandler, R.M., Castle, A.L. and Ivy, J.L. (1997) Chromium and exercise training: effect on obese women. *Medicine and Science in Sports and Exercise* **29**, 992–998.

Greenway, F.L. (1992) Clinical studies with phenylpropanolamine: a metaanalysis. *American Journal of Clinical Nutrition* **55** (Suppl. 1), 203S–205S.

Greenway, F., Herber, D., Raum, W., Herber, D. and Morales, S. (1999) Double-blind, randomized, placebo controlled clinical trials with non-prescription medications for the treatment of obesity. *Obesity Research* **7**, 370–378.

Griffen, L. and Anchors, M. (1998) The 'phen-pro' diet drug combination is not associated with valvular heart disease. *Archives of Internal Medicine* **158**, 1278–1279.

Griffiths, R.R., Brady, J.V. and Bradford, L.D. (1979) Predicting the abuse liability of drugs with animal drug self-administration procedures: psychomotor stimulants and hallucinogens. *Advanced Behavavioural Pharmacology* **2**, 163–208.

Guy-Grand, B., Apfelbaum, M., Crepaldi, G., Gries, A., Lefebvre, P. and Turner, P. (1989) International trial of long-term dexfenfluramine in obesity. *Lancet* **2**, 1142–1145.

Halpern, A. and Mancini, M.C. (2003) Treatment of obesity: an update on anti-obesity medications. *Obesity Reviews* **4**(1), 25–42.

Hartley, G.G., Nicol, S., Halstenson, C., Khan, M. and Pheley, A. (1995) Phentermine, fenfluramine, diet, behavior modification, and exercise for treatment of obesity. *Obesity Research* **3** (Suppl. 3), 340s.

Harvey, B.H. and Bouwer, C.D. (2000) Neuropharmacology of paradoxic weight gain with selective serotonin reuptake inhibitors. *Clinical Neuropharmacology* **23**, 90–97.

Heal, D.J., Aspley, S., Prow, M.R., Jackson, H.C., Martin, K.F. and Cheetham, S.C. (1998) Sibutramine: a novel anti-obesity drug. A review of the pharmacological evidence to differentiate it from D-amphetamine and D-fenfluramine. *International Journal of Obesity* **22** (Suppl. 1), S18–28.

Hirsch, J., Mackintosh, R.M. and Aronne, L.J. (2000) The effects of drugs used to treat obesity on the autonomic nervous system. *Obesity Research* **8**, 227–233.

Hollander, P.A., Elbein, S.C., Hirsch, I.B., Kelley, D., McGill, J., Tayler, T., Weiss, S.R., Crockett, S.E., Kaplan, R.A., Comstock, J., Lucas, C.P., Lodewick, P.A., Canovatchel, W., Chung, J. and Hauptman, J. (1998) Role of orlistat in the treatment of obese patients with type 2 diabetes. A 1-year randomized double-blind study. *Diabetes Care* **21**, 1288–1294.

Inoue, S., Egawa, M., Satoh, S., Saito, M., Suzuki, H., Kumahara, Y., Abe, M., Kumagai, A., Goto, Y., Shizume, K., Shimizu, N., Naito, C. and Onishi, T. (1992) Clinical and basic aspects of an anorexiant, mazindol, as an antiobesity agent in Japan. *American Journal of Clinical Nutrition* **55**, 199S–202S.

James, W.P., Avenel, A., Broom, J. and Whitehead, J. (1997) A one year trial to assess the value of orlistat in the management of obesity. *International Journal of Obesity* **21** (Suppl. 3), S24–S30.

James, W.P., Astrup, A., Finer, N., Hilsted, J., Kopelman, P., Rossner, S., Saris, W.H. and Van Gaal, L.F. (2000) Effect of sibutramine on weight maintenance after weight loss: a randomised trial. STORM Study Group. Sibutramine Trial of Obesity Reduction and Maintenance. *Lancet* **356**, 2119–2125.

Jensen, E.X., Fusch, C., Jaeger, P., Peheim, E. and Horber, F.F. (1995) Impact of chronic cigarette smoking on body composition and fuel metabolism. *Journal of Clinical Endocrinology and Metabolism* **80**, 2181–2185.

Josse, R.G., Chiasson, J.L., Ryan, E.A., Lau, D.C., Ross, S.A., Yale, J.F., Leiter, L.A., Maheux, P., Tessier, D., Wolever, T.M., Gerstein, H., Rodger, N.W., Dornan, J.M., Murphy, L.J., Rabasa-Lhoret, R. and Meneilly, G.S. (2003) Acarbose in the treatment of elderly patients with type 2 diabetes. *Diabetes Research and Clinical Practice* **59**(1), 37–42.

Kamphuis, M.M., Lejeune, M.P., Saris, W.H. and Westerterp-Plantenga, M.S. (2003a) Effect of conjugated linoleic acid supplementation after weight loss on appetite and food intake in overweight subjects. *European Journal of Clinical Nutrition* **57**, 1268–1274.

Kamphuis, M.M., Lejeune, M.P., Saris, W.H. and Westerterp-Plantenga, M.S. (2003b) The effect of conjugated linoleic acid supplementation after weight loss on body weight regain, body composition, and resting metabolic rate in overweight subjects. *International Journal of Obesity and Related Metabolic Disorders* **27**, 840–847.

Kay, J.P., Alemzadeh, R., Langley, G., D'Angelo, L., Smith, P. and Holshouser, S. (2001) Beneficial effects of metformin in normoglycemic morbidly obese adolescents. *Metabolism* **50**, 1457–1461.

Kim, S.H., Lee, Y.M., Jee, S.H. and Nam, C.M. (2003) Effect of sibutramine on weight loss and blood pressure: a meta-analysis of controlled trials. *Obesity Research* **11**, 1116–1123.

Kissebach, A.H., Vydelingum, N., Murray, R., Evans, D.J., Hartz, A.J., Kalkhoff, R.K. and Adams, P.W. (1982) Relation of body fat distribution to metabolic complications of obesity. *Journal of Clinical Endocrinology and Metabolism* **54**, 254–260.

Kolotkin, R.L., Crosby, R.D., Williams, G.R., Hartley, G.G. and Nicol, S. (2001) The relationship between health-related quality of life and weight loss. *Obesity Research* **9**, 564–571.

Kreider, R.B., Ferreira, M., Wilson, M., Grindstaff, P., Plisk, S, Reinardy, J., Cantler, E. and Almada, A.L. (1998) Effects of creatine supplementation on body composition, strength, and sprint performance. *Medicine and Science in Sports* and *Exercise* **30**(1), 73–82.

Lawson, K.D., Middleton, S.J. and Hassall, C.D. (1997) Olestra, a nonabsorbed, noncaloric replacement for dietary fat: a review. *Drug Metabolism Review* **29**, 651–703.

Lean, M.E. (2001) How does sibutramine work? *International Journal of Obesity and Related Metabolic Disorders* **25** (Suppl. 4), S8–11.

Lee. A. and Morley, J.E. (1998) Metformin decreases food consumption and induces weight loss in subjects with obesity with type II non-insulin-dependent diabetes. *Obesity Research* **6**, 47–53.

Leibowitz, S.F. (1991) Brain neuropeptide Y: an integrator of endocrine, metabolic and behavioral processes. *Brain Research Bulletin* **27**, 333–337.

Leibowitz, S.F. (1995) Brain peptides and obesity: pharmacologic treatment. *Obesity Research* **3** (Suppl. 4), 573S–589S.

Life Sciences Research Office (1987) *Physiological Effects and Health Consequences of Dietary Fiber*. Pilch, S.M. ed. Washington, DC: Federation of American Societies for Experimental Biology, Contract Number FDA 223–84–2059, 160.

Lucas, C.P., Boldrin, M.N. and Reaven, G.M. (2003) Effect of orlistat added to diet (30% of calories from fat) on plasma lipids, glucose, and insulin in obese patients with hypercholesterolemia. *American Journal of Cardiology* **15**, 961–964.

McDuffie, J.R., Calis, K.A., Uwaifo, G.I., Sebring, N.G., Fallon, E.M., Hubbard, V.S. and Yanovski, J.A. (2002a) Three-month tolerability of orlistat in adolescents with obesity-related comorbid conditions. *Obesity Research* **10**, 642–650.

McDuffie, J.R., Calis, K.A., Booth, S.L., Uwaifo, G.I. and Yanovski, J.A. (2002b) Effects of orlistat on fat-soluble vitamins in obese adolescents. *Pharmacotherapy* **22**, 814–822.

McElroy, S.L., Arnold, L.M., Shapira, N.A., Keck, Jr, PE, Rosenthal, N.R., Karim, M.R., Kamin, M. and Hudson, J.I. (2003) Topiramate in the treatment of binge eating disorder associated with obesity: a randomized, placebo-controlled trial. *American Journal of Psychiatry* **160**, 255–261.

McNulty, S.J., Ur, E., Williams, G: Multicenter Sibutramine Study Group. (2003) A randomized trial of sibutramine in the management of obese type 2 diabetic patients treated with metformin. *Diabetes Care* **26**, 125–131.

Meneilly, G.S., Ryan, E.A., Radziuk, J., Lau, D.C., Yale, J.F., Morais, J., Chiasson, J.L., Rabasa-Lhoret, R., Maheux, P., Tessier, D., Wolever, T., Josse, R.G. and Elahi, D. (2000) Effect of acarbose on insulin sensitivity in elderly patients with diabetes. *Diabetes Care* **23**, 1162–1167.

Misra, A. (2003) Revisions of cut-offs of body mass index to define overweight and obesity are needed for the Asian-ethnic groups. *International Journal of Obesity and Related Metabolic Disorders* **27**, 1294–1296.

Munro, J.F., MacCuish, A.C., Wilson, E.M. and Duncan, L.P.J. (1968) Comparison of continuous and intermittent anorectic therapy in obesity. *British Medical Journal* **1**, 352–354.

Naslund, E., King, N., Mansten, S., Adner, N., Holst, J.J., Gutniak, M. and Hellstrom, P.M. (2004) Prandial subcutaneous injections of glucagon-like peptide-1 cause weight loss in obese human subjects. *British Journal of Nutrition* **91**, 439–446.

Nides, M., Rand, C., Dolce, J., Murray, R., O'Hara, P., Voelker, H. and Connett, J. (1994) Weight gain as a function of smoking cessation and 2-mg nicotine gum use among middle-aged smokers with mild lung impairment in the first 2 years of the Lung Health Study. *Health Psychology* **13**, 354–361.

Norgren, S., Danielsson, P., Jurold, R., Lotborn, M. and Marcus, C. (2003) Orlistat treatment in obese prepubertal children: a pilot study. *Acta Paediatrica* **92**, 666–670.

Okada, S., York, D.A., Bray, G.A. and Erlanson-Albertsson, C. (1991) Enterostatin (Val-Pro-Asp-Pro-Arg), the activation peptide of procolipase selectively reduces fat intake. *Physiology and Behaviour* **49**, 1185–1189.

Padwal, R., Li, S.K. and Lau, D.C. (2003a) Long-term pharmacotherapy for obesity and overweight. Cochrane Database System Review, 2003, CD004094.

Padwal, R., Li, S.K. and Lau, D.C. (2003b) Long-term pharmacotherapy for overweight and obesity: a systematic review and meta-analysis of randomized controlled trials. *International Journal of Obesity and Related Metabolic Disorders* **27**, 1437–1446.

Pasman, W.J., Westerterp-Plantenga, M.S. and Saris, W.H. (1997) The effectiveness of long-term supplementation of carbohydrate, chromium, fibre and caffeine on weight maintenance. *International Journal of Obesity* **21**, 1143–1151.

Pasquali, R., Gambineri, A., Biscotti, D., Vicennati, V., Gagliardi, L., Colitta, D., Fiorini, S., Cognigni, G.E., Filicori, M. and Morselli-

Labate, A.M. (2000) Effect of long-term treatment with metformin added to hypocaloric diet on body composition, fat distribution, and androgen and insulin levels in abdominally obese women with and without the polycystic ovary syndrome. *Journal of Clinical Endocrinology and Metabolism* **85**, 2767–2774.

Pedrinola, F., Sztejnsznajd, C., Lima, N., Halpern, A. and Medeiros-Neto, G. (1996) The addition of dexfluramine to fluoxetine in the treatment of obesity, a randomized clinical trial. *Obesity Research* **4**, 549–554.

Perri, M.G. (1992) Improving maintenance of weight loss following treatment by diet and lifestyle modification. In: Wadden, T.A., VanItallie, T.B. eds. *Treatment of the Seriously Obese Patient*. New York: Guilford Press, 456–477.

Pi-Sunyer, X. (1995) Guidelines for the approval and use of obesity drugs. *Obesity Research* **3**, 473–478.

Rasmussen, M.H., Andersen, T., Breum, L., Gtzsche, P.C. and Hilsted, J. (1993) Cimetidine suspension as adjuvant to energy restricted diet in treating obesity. *British Medical Journal* **24**, 1093–1096.

Ricca, V., Mannucci, E., Di Bernardo, M., Rizzello, S.M., Cabras, P.L. and Rotella, C.M. (1996) Sertraline enhances the effects of cognitive–behavioral treatment on weight reduction of obese patients. *Journal of Endocrinological Investigation* **19**, 727–733.

Riserus, U., Berglund, L. and Vessby, B. (2001) Conjugated linoleic acid (CLA) reduced abdominal adipose tissue in obese middle-aged men with signs of the metabolic syndrome: a randomised controlled trial. *International Journal of Obesity and Related Metabolic Disorders* **25**, 1129–1135.

Rothman, R.B. and Baumann, M.H. (2002) Serotonin releasing agents. Neurochemical, therapeutic and adverse effects. *Pharmacology, Biochemistry, and Behavior* **71**, 825–836.

Rowland, N.E., Roth, J.D., McMullen, M.R., Patel, A. and Cespedes, A.T. (2000) Dexfenfluramine and norfenfluramine: comparison of mechanism of action in feeding and brain Fos-ir studies. *American Journal of Physiology. Regulatory, Integrative, and Comparative Physiology* **278**, R390–399.

Rudman, D., Feller, A.G., Nagraj, H.S., Gergans, G.A., Lalitha, P.Y., Goldbery, A.F., Schlenker, R.A., Cohn, L., Rudman, I.W. and Mattson D.E. (1990) Effects of human growth hormone in men over 60 years old. *New England Journal of Medicine* **323**, 1–6.

Ryan, D.H. (2000) Use of sibutramine and other noradrenergic and serotonergic drugs in the management of obesity. *Endocrinology* **13**, 193–199.

Ryan, D.H., Kaiser, P. and Bray, G.A. (1995) Sibutramine: a novel new agent for obesity treatment. *Obesity Research* **3** (Suppl. 4), 553S–559S.

Scoville, B.A. (1976) Review of amphetamine-like drugs by the Food and Drug Administration. In: Bray, G.A. ed. *Obesity in Perspective*. Fogarty International Center for Advanced Studies in the Health Sciences, Series on Preventive Medicine, vol. II. Washington, DC: US Government Printing Office, 441–443.

Silva, A.P., Cavadas, C. and Grouzmann, E. (2002) Neuropeptide Y and its receptors as potential therapeutic drug targets. *Clinica Chimica Acta* **326**(1–2), 3–25.

Silverstone, T. (1992) Appetite suppressants: a review. *Drugs* **43**, 820–836.

Sjostrom, L., Rissanen, A., Andersen, T., Boldrin, M., Golay, A., Koppeschaar, H.P. and Krempf, M. (1998) Randomised placebo-controlled trial of orlistat for weight loss and prevention of weight regain in obese patients. European Multicentre Orlistat Study Group. *Lancet* **352**, 167–172.

Sjostrom, L., Despres, J.P. and Golay, A. (2004) Weight loss in overweight obese dyslipidemia subjects treated with Rimonabant: the RIO-lipids Trial. *International Journal of Obesity* **28** (Suppl. 1), S28.

Smathers, S.A., Wilson, J.G. and Nigro, M.A. (2003) Topiramate effectiveness in Prader–Willi syndrome. *Pediatrics and Neurology* **28**, 130–133.

Snyder, E.E., Walts, B., Perusse, L., Chagnon, Y.C., Weisnagel, S.J., Rankinen, T. and Bouchard, C. (2004) The human obesity gene map: the 2003 update. *Obesity Research* **12**, 369–439.

Sta-Birketvedt, G. (1993) Effect of cimetidine suspension on appetite and weight in overweight subjects. *British Medical Journal* **306**, 1091–1093.

Stanko, R.T. and Arch, J.E. (1996) Inhibition of regain in body weight and fat with addition of 3-carbon compounds to the diet with hyperenergetic refeeding after weight reduction. *International Journal of Obesity and Related Metabolic Disorders* **20**, 925–930.

Stanko, R.T., Reynolds, H.R., Hoyson, R., Janosky, J.E. and Wolf, R. (1994) Pyruvate supplementation of a low-cholesterol, low-fat diet: effects on plasma lipid concentrations and body composition in hyperlipidemic patients. *American Journal of Clinical Nutrition* **59**, 423–427.

Steel, J.M., Munro, J.F. and Duncan, L.J. (1973) A comparative trial of different regimens of fenfluramine and phentermine in obesity. *Practitioner* **211**, 232–236.

Stevens, J. (2003) Ethnic-specific revisions of body mass index cutoffs to define overweight and obesity in Asians are not warranted. *International Journal of Obesity and Related Metabolic Disorders* **27**, 1297–1299.

Stock, M.J. (1996) Potential for β_3-adrenoceptor agonists in the treatment of obesity. *International Journal of Obesity* **20** (Suppl. 4), 4–5.

Tellier, P. (2001) Fenfluramines, idiopathic pulmonary primary hypertension and cardiac valve disorders: facts and artifacts. *Annales de Medicine Interne* (Paris) **152**, 429–436.

Tiikkainen, M., Bergholm, R., Rissanen, A., Aro, A., Salminen, I., Tamminen, M., Teramo, K. and Yki-Jarvinen, H. (2004) Effects of equal weight loss with orlistat and placebo on body fat and serum fatty acid composition and insulin resistance in obese women. *American Journal of Clinical Nutrition* **79**(1), 22–30.

Tonstad, S., Pometta, D., Erkelens, D.W., Ose, L., Moccetti, T., Schouten, J.A., Golay, A., Reitsma, J., Del Bufalo, A. and Posotti, E. (1994) The effect of the gastrointestinal lipase inhibitor, orlistat, on serum lipids and lipoproteins in patients with primary hyperlipidaemia. *European Journal of Clinical Pharmacology* **46**, 405–410.

Toubro, S., Astrup, A.V., Breum, L. and Quaade, F. (1993) Safety and efficacy of long-term treatment with ephedrine, caffeine, and an ephedrine/caffeine mixture. *International Journal of Obesity* **17** (Suppl. 1), S69–S72.

Trent, L.K. and Thieding-Cancel, D. (1995) Effects of chromium picolinate on body composition. *Journal of Sports Medicine and Physical Fitness* **35**, 273–280.

Tritos, N.A. and Maratos-Flier, E. (1999) Two important systems in energy homeostasis: melanocortins and melanin-concentrating hormone. *Neuropeptides* **33**, 339–349.

Tso, P., Sun, W. and Liu, M. (2004) Gastrointestinal Satiety Signals IV. Apolipoprotein A-IV. *American Journal of Physiology. Gastrointestinal and Liver Physiology* **286**, G885–890.

Valle-Jones, J.C., Brodie, N.H., O'Hara, H., O'Hara, J. and McGhie, R.L. (1983) A comparative study of phentermine and diethylpropion in the treatment of obese patients in general practice. *Pharmatherapeutica* **3**, 300–304.

Vogiatzi, M.G., Boeck, M.A., Vlachopapadopoulou, E., el-Rashid, R. and New, M.I. (1996) Dehydroepiandrosterone in morbidly obese adolescents: effects on weight, body composition, lipids, and insulin resistance. *Metabolism* **45**, 1011–1015.

Wadden, T.A., Sternberg, J.A., Letizia, K.A., Stunkard, A.J. and Foster, G.D. (1989) Treatment of obesity by very low calorie diet, behavior therapy, and their combination: a five year perspective. *International Journal of Obesity* **13** (Suppl. 2), 39–46.

Wadden, T.A., Bartlett, S.J., Foster, G.D., Greenstein, R.A., Wingate, B.J., Stunkard, A.J. and Letizia, K.A. (1995) Sertraline and relapse prevention training following treatment by very-low-calorie diet: a controlled clinical trial. *Obesity Research* **3**, 549–557.

Wadden, T.A., Berkowitz, R.I., Womble, L.G., Sarwer, D.B., Arnold, M.E. and Steinberg, C.M. (2000) Effects of sibutramine plus orlistat in obese women following 1 year of treatment by sibutramine alone: a placebo-controlled trial. *Obesity Research* **8**, 431–437.

Wasser, W.G., Feldman, N.S. and D'Agati, V.D. (1997) Chronic renal failure after ingestion of over-the-counter chromium picolinate. *Annals of Internal Medicine* **126**, 410.

Weintraub, M. (1992) Long-term weight control: The National Heart, Lung, and Blood Institute funded multimodal intervention study. *Clinical Pharmacology and Therapeutics* **51**, 581–646.

Weintraub, M., Hasday, J.D., Mushlin, A.I. and Lockwood, D.H. (1984) A double blind clinical trial in weight control: use of fenfluramine and phentermine alone and in combination. *Archives of Internal Medicine* **144**, 1143–1148.

Weissman, N.J. (2001) Appetite suppressants and valvular heart disease. *American Journal of Medical Science* **321**, 285–291.

Whigham, L.D., Cook, M.E. and Atkinson, R.L. (2000) Conjugated linoleic acid: implications for human health. *Pharmacological Research* **42**, 503–510.

Wilding, J.P. (2002) Neuropeptides and appetite control. *Diabetic Medicine* **19**, 619–627.

Wilson, G.T. (1993) Behavioral treatment of obesity: thirty years and counting. *Advances in Behaviour Research and Therapy* **16**, 31–75.

WHO (1998) Preventing and managing the global epidemic of obesity: report of a WHO Consultation on Obesity. Geneva, 3–5 June, 1997. WHO/NUT/NCD98.1, Geneva, 1998.

Wren, A.M., Seal, L.J., Cohen, M.A., Brynes, A.E., Frost, G.S., Murphy, K.G., Dhillo, W.S., Ghatei, M.A. and Bloom, S.R. (2001) Ghrelin enhances appetite and increases food intake in humans. *Journal of Clinical Endocrinology and Metabolism* **86**, 5992.

Yang, Y.K. and Harmon, C.M. (2003) Recent developments in our understanding of melanocortin system in the regulation of food intake. *Obesity Reviews* **4**, 239–248.

Yen, T.T. (1995) β-Agonists as antiobesity, antidiabetic and nutrient partitioning agents. *Obesity Research* **3** (Suppl. 4), 531S–536S.

Zhi, J., Moore, R. and Kanitra, L. (2003) The effect of short-term (21-day) orlistat treatment on the physiologic balance of six selected macrominerals and microminerals in obese adolescents. *Journal of the American College of Nutrition* **22**, 357–362.

26 The management of obesity: surgery

Paul E. O'Brien and John B. Dixon

Introduction, 394

The evolution of surgical
technique, 394
  The initial phase (1950–70)—small
  bowel bypass, 394
  The middle phase (1970–90)—
  stomach stapling, 394
  The current phase (1990–present)—
  minimally invasive and adjustable
  procedures, 396

Overview of outcomes from bariatric
procedures, 396
  Weight loss outcomes from
  bariatric surgery, 397
  Changes in health after bariatric
  surgery, 397

Characteristics of the ideal surgical
procedure, 400
  Roux-en-Y gastric bypass, 400
  Biliopancreatic diversion, 401

Laparoscopic adjustable gastric
banding, 402

Conclusions, 403

References, 404

Introduction

As obesity becomes identified as the most significant pathogen in the developed world and as obesity-related disease now challenges smoking as the principal contributor to premature death, seeking an effective solution to the obesity epidemic represents our greatest public health challenge at present. Prevention is clearly the optimal goal but, with present-day data indicating progression of the epidemic, effective preventive programmes that will impact on the broad community problem are still to come. At this time, there is no non-surgical method for predictably achieving major weight loss in obese people and maintaining that weight loss for an extended period. Programmes at present involving diet, behavioural modification, exercise and activity, with or without drug supplementation, are able, at best, to achieve a modest weight loss, which is generally sustained only for the duration of the programme.

Surgical methods have been known to achieve substantial and durable weight loss for half a century and yet they have not achieved a significant impact on community health. Only a small fraction of obese people have been prepared to seek the surgical approach to their problem because of the risks of death or complications, the invasiveness and the costs. With the introduction of new techniques, in particular laparoscopic adjustable gastric banding, and with the application of minimally invasive approaches to all forms of obesity surgery, it is timely to review the range of surgical options and their potential strengths and weaknesses.

The evolution of surgical technique

The initial phase (1950–70)—small bowel bypass

Surgical management of obesity began with the introduction of the jejuno-ileal bypass (JIB) in the 1950s. In this procedure, the proximal jejunum was diverted to a distal part of the gut, leaving a long segment of excluded small intestine and marked reduction in absorptive capacity. Many variations existed. A typical pattern is shown in Fig. 26.1, in which the proximal 35 cm of proximal jejunum was joined end-to-side to the last 10 cm of ileum (Fig. 26.1). The JIB procedures represented the best and the worst of bariatric surgery. Major and sustained weight loss was achieved and there were impressive health benefits, particularly in relation to lipid metabolism. However, it caused serious problems including copious offensive diarrhoea, electrolyte imbalances, oxalate calculi in the kidneys and progressive hepatic fibrosis with eventual liver failure and, for these reasons, was generally abandoned during the 1970s in favour of stomach-stapling procedures (Jorizzo et al., 1983; O'Leary 1983; Corrodi, 1984; DeWind and Payne, 1985; Parfitt et al., 1985).

The middle phase (1970–90)—stomach stapling

The Roux-en-Y gastric bypass (RYGB) operation was introduced by Edward Mason in 1960 (Mason and Ito, 1967). In this procedure, the stomach was completely partitioned into a small upper gastric pouch, draining into a Roux–en-Y limb of proximal jejunum of variable length, from 40 to 150 cm, and a

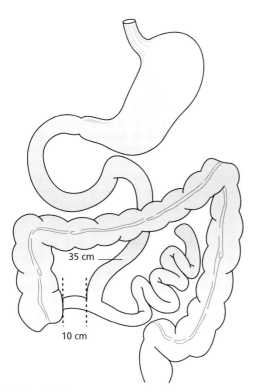

Fig 26.1 Jejuno-ileal bypass.

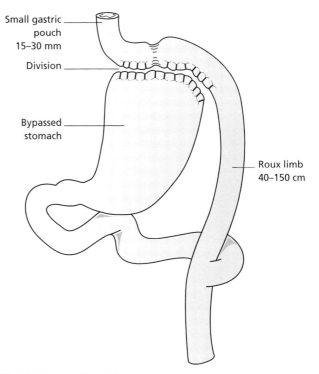

Fig 26.2 Roux-en-Y gastric bypass.

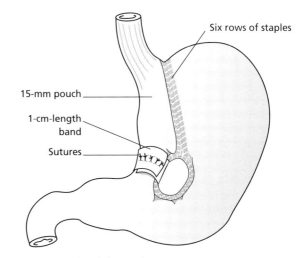

Fig 26.3 Vertical-banded gastroplasty.

distal excluded stomach (Fig. 26.2). This procedure provided a hybrid between the malabsorptive approach of JIB and later, more purely restrictive operations. It has undergone various modifications over the subsequent 40 years and still serves us well as an effective anti-obesity operation. However, its drawbacks of perioperative deaths and significant perioperative and late morbidity, although markedly less threatening than those of JIB, have nevertheless been sufficient to cause most obese people to stay away.

Dr Mason and his colleague Dr Printen (Printen and Mason, 1973) then introduced a purely restrictive operation of gastroplasty. The procedure involves partitioning the stomach into a small upper pouch draining through a narrow stoma into the remainder of the stomach. Numerous variations of this procedure have followed, the most significant variant being the vertical-banded gastroplasty (VBG), which was first described by Dr Mason in 1982 (Mason, 1982) and is shown in Fig. 26.3. It was hoped that this group of operations would provide greater short- and long-term safety and yet retain the power of gastric bypass. Unfortunately, both randomized controlled trials and observational studies have consistently shown that it has failed in both aspirations (Pories *et al.*, 1982; Sugerman *et al.*, 1987; Hall *et al.*, 1990).

In the meantime, there was a resurgence of malabsorptive surgery with the Italian surgeon Nicolo Scopinaro introducing the biliopancreatic diversion procedure (BPD) (Scopinaro *et al.*, 1979). It too has undergone change with time and experience. The basic procedure involves distal gastrectomy, leaving

a proximal pouch of 200–500 mL, a 200-cm length of terminal ileum anastomosed to the gastric pouch, and the biliopancreatic limb entering at 50 cm from the ileocaecal valve (Fig. 26.4) (Scopinaro *et al.*, 1996). The most notable remodelling of the procedure is the so-called duodenal switch variant (BPD-DS) proposed by Picard Marceau's group in 1995 (Marceau *et al.*, 1998), in which a longitudinal gastrectomy enabled retention of the gastric antrum with, hopefully, controlled gastric emptying, and the ileal limb was anastomosed to the proximal duodenum (Fig. 26.5). The benefit of this variation remains controversial.

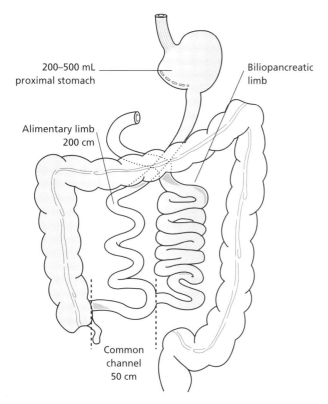

Fig 26.4 Biliopancreatic diversion.

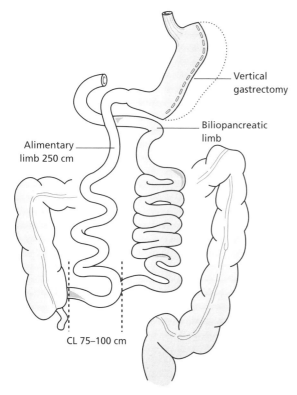

Fig 26.5 Biliopancreatic diversion with duodenal switch.

The current phase (1990–present)—minimally invasive and adjustable procedures

This phase is characterized by the advent of the laparoscopic adjustable gastric band (LAGB), with the particular features of minimal anatomical disturbance, adjustability and potential reversibility (Belachew *et al.,* 1994; 2001). Also there has been the introduction of a laparoscopic approach to gastric bypass (Wittgrove *et al.,* 1996) and biliopancreatic diversion (Ren *et al.,* 2000).

Adjustable gastric banding had first been proposed by two Austrian surgical researchers, Szinicz and Schnapka, in 1982 (Szinic and Schnapka, 1982). The idea was brought into clinical practice by Lubomyr Kuzmak in 1986 (Kuzmak *et al.,* 1991), but did not attract major interest until the advent of the technology that enabled the performance of complex laparoscopic surgical procedures became widespread in the early 1990s. The BioEnterics® Lap-Band® system (LAGB) was specifically designed for laparoscopic placement and was introduced into clinical practice by Mitiku Belachew from Huy, Belgium, in September 1993 (Fig. 26.6). Because of the dual attractions of a controlled level of effect through adjustability and of laparoscopic placement without resection of gut or anastomoses, this procedure has rapidly become the dominant bariatric procedure in all regions of the developed world except, thus far, the USA, where its introduction was delayed by regulatory requirements until June 2001.

Overview of outcomes from bariatric procedures

The most important single outcome in treating obesity is

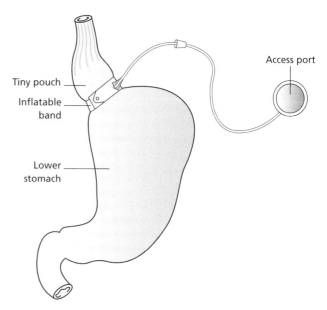

Fig 26.6 Laparoscopic adjustable gastric banding.

improvement in health. Second, we seek improvement in quality of life. Measuring weight loss itself is inappropriate as a single endpoint. It is measuring the means to the end. Without improvement in the comorbidities of obesity, the achieving of weight loss is not relevant to community health care. However, by tradition, weight loss has been and is still the first parameter that is examined and reported. We will stay with this tradition by first reviewing the effectiveness of bariatric surgical procedures in causing weight loss and then reviewing the effects on health and quality of life.

Weight loss outcomes from bariatric surgery

Weight loss can be described in different ways, each of which has its advantages and drawbacks. We will use the percentage of excess weight lost (%EWL) as our preferred method. Absolute weight change (in kilograms or body mass index (BMI) units or percentage of weight lost) fails to recognize the significance of initial weight as a variable in estimating or comparing effects. Percentage of BMI lost (%EBL) is arguably the most relevant to health status and may become preferred but at present lacks broad usage. Most reports provide %EWL, thus allowing comparison between studies.

Reports of short-term weight loss are not relevant when assessing a long-term effect. Ideally, weight loss as an outcome of bariatric surgery should not be considered at less than 5 years' follow-up. However, there are surprisingly few reports that can provide such data. We will restrict our examination to those reports that have included at least 100 patients and that provide at least 1 year of follow-up data, expressing the outcome in the terms of %EWL. In the tables, we have included all the studies we could find that provide the data that fulfil these requirements.

A number of significant observations can be drawn from these tables and figures:

1 All of the current surgical procedures result in major weight loss with mean values of between 50% and 80% of excess weight lost.

2 These levels of weight loss generate major improvement in health and quality of life. Therefore, the surgical treatment of obesity is seen to be effective and, as no other methods can achieve anything like these levels of weight loss, the surgical approaches are at present the only seriously effective methods available. The recognition of this overall effectiveness of the surgical approach is much more important than any debate about which of the surgical procedures provides the best balance of safety and effectiveness.

3 Biliopancreatic diversion produces the most weight loss and, although there are only a small number of reports, these reports indicate a durable effect well beyond 5 years.

4 Gastric stapling procedures show good initial weight loss at 1 and 2 years, followed by a fading effect that is clearly evident by 5 years. Interestingly, for a group of operations which have been in use for more than 30 years, and for which there are nu-merous publications, we could find only three reports that give outcome data beyond 5 years.

5 Laparoscopic adjustable gastric banding (LAGB) generates weight loss more slowly than the other procedures but is as effective as gastric stapling procedures at 4 and 5 years (Fig. 26.6). The adjustability is expected to allow maintenance of the weight loss over a longer period than the non-adjustable gastric stapling operations. As the LAGB procedures were only introduced in 1993, demonstration of the durability of weight loss will take more time.

Changes in health after bariatric surgery

Obesity generates a wide range of illnesses, to the point where it could now reasonably be regarded as the worst pathogen in the Western communities. The following are a summary of the changes in a selection of these comorbidities to illustrate the major health benefits that can be achieved by bariatric surgical procedures. The effects may have been achieved through weight loss per se, or as a result of changes in anatomy and function of the gut.

Type 2 diabetes

Type 2 diabetes is the paradigm of an obesity-related illness. Multiple studies have documented the benefit achieved by all the bariatric procedures available at present (Pories *et al.*, 1995; Smith *et al.*, 1996; Dixon and O'Brien, 2002a; Rubino and Gagner, 2002). We have studied 50 patients, who were followed for 1 year after Lap-Band placement (Dixon and O'Brien, 2002a). There was a significant improvement in all measures of glucose metabolism, with complete remission of diabetes in 32 patients (64%), improvement of control in 13 (26%) and 5 (10%) were relatively unchanged. Importantly, duration of time with diabetes was a predictor of outcome, indicating that early treatment of obesity is indicated in the newly diagnosed diabetic.

Weight loss protects obese subjects with or without impaired glucose tolerance from the development of diabetes. From a pool of 1300 severely obese subjects whom we have treated by LAGB, 85 patients had impaired fasting glucose. Greater than 90% were found to have normal fasting plasma glucose at 2 years after the operation. For the general community, it is expected that in those with impaired fasting glucose there will be an annual conversion rate of 5–6% to type 2 diabetes. However, none of our patients with insulin resistance has thus far developed diabetes. Furthermore, with a total of more than 4000 patient–years of follow-up of patients without diabetes preoperatively, there has been only a single patient develop type 2 diabetes. Thus, weight loss following surgery dramatically reduces the risk of developing the disease.

Importantly, the improvement in diabetes following weight loss is related to the dual effects of improvement in insulin sensitivity and pancreatic beta-cell function (Dixon *et al.*, 2003a).

As beta-cell function deteriorates progressively over time in those with type 2 diabetes, early weight loss intervention should therefore be a central part of initial therapy in severely obese subjects who develop type 2 diabetes. For obese patients with type 2 diabetes, weight loss provides benefit unequalled by any other therapy, and may prove to be the only therapy that substantially changes the natural history of the disease (Pories *et al.*, 1995; Pinkney *et al.*, 2001).

Dyslipidaemia of obesity

Increased fasting triglyceride and decreased high-density lipoprotein (HDL) cholesterol concentrations characterize the dyslipidaemia of obesity and insulin resistance (Despres, 1993). This dyslipidaemic pattern is highly atherogenic and is the most common pattern associated with coronary artery disease (Koba *et al.*, 2000). Weight loss surgery produces substantial decreases in fasting triglyceride levels, an elevation of HDL-cholesterol levels to normal and improved total cholesterol–HDL-cholesterol ratio (Busetto *et al.*, 2000; Bacci *et al.*, 2002; Dixon *et al.*, 2002). Although elevation of total cholesterol is not a feature of obesity, hypercholesterolaemia can be controlled by malabsorptive procedures such as BPD (Scopinaro *et al.*, 1998) and RYGB (Brolin *et al.*, 2000).

Hypertension

There is evidence of a reduction in both systolic and diastolic blood pressure (BP) following weight loss in association with a bariatric procedure (Sjostrom *et al.*, 1999). We have studied the outcome of 147 consecutive hypertensive patients at 12 months after LAGB. Preoperatively, only 17 of these patients had BP within the normal range, all were on therapy. Hypertension was present in 130 patients preoperatively; 101 of these were taking antihypertensive medications and the remaining 29 were not on therapy. Mean BP for these patients was 156/97 mmHg prior to surgery.

At 12 months after LAGB, 105 patients had normal BP, 42 remained hypertensive, and only 42 were taking any antihypertensive medication at that time. Mean BP was 127/76 mmHg. From these data, we found that 80 patients (55%) had resolution of the problem (i.e. normal BP and taking no antihypertensive therapy), 45 patients (31%) were improved (less therapy and easier control), and 22 patients (15%) were unchanged (Dixon and O'Brien, 2002b). We have demonstrated that the fall in blood pressure is sustained to at least 4 years after surgery but durability of blood pressure reduction over a longer period is uncertain (Sjostrom *et al.*, 2000).

Ovarian dysfunction, infertility and pregnancy

Obesity, especially central obesity, is associated with ovulatory dysfunction and infertility. In premenopausal women,

weight loss significantly reduces active testosterone by reducing total testosterone and increasing the proportion of bound testosterone due to increased sex hormone-binding globulin. This change usually restores normal ovulation and often fertility. Women are advised to use contraception during the very active weight loss phase following LAGB, usually for the first year. However, studies reporting pregnancy after LAGB report unexpected pregnancies in previously infertile women. These studies also report the value of the adjustability of the LAGB, enabling reduction of gastric restriction in early pregnancy to reduce the impact of any hyperemesis and to allow more favourable nutritional conditions for normal fetal development. Weight gain is advised in all pregnancies, with the advised weight gain based on prepregnancy BMI. The LAGB provides a mechanism during pregnancy to allow appropriate weight gain, and can be readjusted, if necessary, to prevent excessive weight gain (Dixon *et al.*, 2001a). The caesarean section rate and the incidence of gestational diabetes and hypertension is also seen to be reduced (Dixon *et al.*, 2001a).

Gastro-oesophageal reflux disease

Gastro-oesophageal reflux disease (GERD) is more than twice as prevalent in the morbidly obese (Dixon and O'Brien, 1999); 87 patients who had moderate or severe GERD have been followed for at least 12 months after LAGB; 73 (89%) have had total resolution of the problem, as defined by the absence of symptoms without treatment for the previous month. Preoperative and postoperative pH study and manometry have been performed on 12 of these patients who had severe symptoms preoperatively. The mean DeMeester score was 38 ± 15 preoperatively and 7.9 ± 8 at follow-up ($P < 0.001$). In all but one of these patients, symptoms had resolved completely. Others have also demonstrated that a correctly placed LAGB and RYGB reduces gastro-oesophageal reflux (Balsiger *et al.*, 2000a; Weiss *et al.*, 2000; Schauer *et al.*, 2001).

Asthma

There is a positive relationship between asthma and obesity (Young *et al.*, 2001). Certainly, the physiological changes of obesity on lung function would aggravate asthma. We have reported major improvement, even remission, of asthma following LAGB (Dixon *et al.*, 1999). Our study demonstrated improvement in all measured aspects of the disease, including symptoms, severity, need for asthma medications (including corticosteroids) and hospital admissions. The asthma severity score fell from 44.5 before operation to 14.3 at 12 months after operation ($P < 0.005$). It is hypothesized that improved respiratory mechanics and possibly a reduction in gastro-oesophageal reflux following LAGB may contribute to the improvement in asthma.

Obstructive sleep apnoea

A range of sleep disorders is associated with obesity. The most serious of these is obstructive sleep apnoea (OSA). Severe obesity is the greatest risk factor for the development of sleep apnoea, with a 10-fold increase in prevalence. Excessive daytime sleepiness, a disabling and potentially dangerous condition, is very common in the obese population and is not necessarily related to OSA (Vgontzas *et al.*, 2000). There are major improvements in sleep quality, excessive daytime sleepiness, snoring, nocturnal choking and observed OSA with weight loss following LAGB surgery (Dixon *et al.*, 2001b).

OSA and other sleep disturbances have been studied in 313 patients prior to LAGB and repeated at 1 year after operation in 123 of the patients. There was a high prevalence of significantly disturbed sleep in both men (59%) and women (45%). Observed sleep apnoea was decreased from 33% to 2%, habitual snoring from 82% to 14%, abnormal daytime sleepiness from 39% to 4% and poor sleep quality from 39% to 2%.

Depression

Depression is common in the morbidly obese. Does the presence of obesity cause the person to be depressed or does depression cause the person to eat too much? We have investigated the effect of weight loss induced by LAGB on depression as measured by the Beck Depression Inventory (BDI) (Dixon *et al.*, 2003b). Preoperative BDI on 487 consecutive patients was a mean of 17.7 ± 9.5, a level within the range for moderate depression. Weight loss was associated with a significant and sustained fall in BDI scores, with a mean score of 7.8 ± 6.5 ($n = 373$) at 1 year after surgery. By 4 years after surgery, the 134 patients studied had lost 54% of excess weight and had a BDI of 9.6 ± 7.7. Although a small number remained in the major depressive illness category, the shift of the majority to normal values for BDI strongly indicates that most of the depression of obesity is reactive to the problem of obesity rather than a cause of obesity and is resolved by weight loss.

Changes in quality of life after bariatric surgery

Improvement in QOL is one of the most gratifying outcomes of bariatric surgery. A number of studies clearly demonstrate major QOL improvements following LAGB and other procedures (Weiner *et al.*, 1999; Balsiger *et al.*, 2000b; Schok *et al.*, 2000; Dixon, 2001; Horchner *et al.*, 2001). We reported a large prospective study of QOL after LAGB, in which we employed the Medical Outcomes Trust Short Form-36 (SF-36). The SF-36 is a reliable, broadly used instrument that has been validated in obese people. In our study, 459 severely obese subjects had lower scores compared with community normal values for all eight aspects of QOL measured, especially the physical health scores. LAGB provided a dramatic and sustained improvement in all measures of the SF-36. Improvement was greater in those with more preoperative disability, and the extent of weight loss was not a good predictor of improved QOL. Mean scores returned to those of community normal values by 1 year after surgery, and remained in the normal range throughout the 4 years of the study. It is significant that patients who required revisional surgery during the follow-up period achieved the same improvement in measures of QOL. Similar improvements in QOL have been demonstrated in patients having LAGB for previously failed gastric stapling (O'Brien *et al.*, 2000).

Body image

Studies of appearance orientation and appearance evaluation indicate that the severely obese usually have quite normal pride and investment in their appearance and presentation but they evaluate their appearance as being very poor (Dixon *et al.*, 2002c). Weight loss following LAGB has been shown to produce major improvements in self-evaluation of appearance, although it does not return to community normal levels. The extent of the improvement in appearance is related to the percentage of excess weight loss. The discrepancy between one's pride and investment in appearance and presentation and one's self-evaluation of appearance is lower with weight loss, reducing psychological stress (Dixon *et al.*, 2002).

The Swedish Obese Subjects study

This study is of particular importance because of the large number of patients studied, the long follow-up and the focus on health and survival. It commenced in 1987, with matching of almost 2000 patients seeking obesity surgery with an equal group of severely obese patients who had medical therapy alone. The intention is to follow all patients for at least 10 years. Although the major endpoint of the study, a comparison of mortality, has not yet been released, several progress reports have indicated favourable effects in the surgically treated group. There has been a sustained reduction in incidence of type 2 diabetes (Torgerson and Sjostrom, 2001) and other cardiovascular risk factors, a reduction in medication needed to treat other cardiovascular risk factors (Agren *et al.*, 2002), improved health-related quality of life and a reduction in symptoms of depression (Torgerson, 2003). This study, which is still progressing, should provide valuable information regarding the risk to benefit balance of obesity surgery. However, the study has several significant weaknesses. It is not a randomized trial and, despite attempts to achieve good matching, there are many significant differences between the groups. Furthermore, gastroplasty, which was the principal surgical procedure used in the study, is now considered obsolete and has been replaced by more effective procedures.

Table 26.1 Attributes of an ideal bariatric operation.

Minimally invasive
Safe
Effective – weight loss, comorbidities, QOL
Durable – effective over time
Low reoperation rate
Minimal side-effects
Technically feasible broadly
Reversible
Controllable/adjustable

Characteristics of the ideal surgical procedure

Although no alternative treatment for their problem is yet available, very few obese people in our community are seeking surgical treatment at present. Over the past 10 years, in the USA, an average of less than 50 000 have undergone surgery for weight control each year. On the basis of a prevalence of morbid obesity (BMI > 40) of 8% (Calle *et al.*, 2003), we can calculate that less than one in 400 of those who have the problem of morbid obesity are seeking a surgical solution each year. Clearly, this is not solving a major public health problem and is almost irrelevant in the overall context of treatment strategies. For a surgical treatment of obesity to make an impact, it must become more broadly acceptable to the population at risk.

Table 26.1 lists the characteristics that should be present if surgical treatment is likely to become broadly acceptable.
• Bariatric procedures need to be performed laparoscopically. The patient will require it because they do not want the pain, the scars and the long recuperation. The surgeon will not be able to justify the higher perioperative complication rates.
• They need to be safe, very safe. There cannot be mortality. Even the 0.5–1.0% that is the norm for RYGB should be regarded as unacceptable.
• It must be effective, not only in achieving weight loss, but also improving in the comorbidities of obesity and in quality of life.
• The effects must be durable. They need to last for years—5, 10, 15 years—if they are to be considered worthwhile.
• There should be a low need for revisional surgery. There is no broadly accepted incidence that could be acceptable but possibly a revisional surgery rate of less than 5% during the first 10 years would be a reasonable target.
• There must be minimal side-effects. Particularly worrying are the late nutritional side-effects of RYGB and BPD. Why exchange one problem for another?
• With up to 20% of the adult population needing help, an operative procedure has to be able to be done by the broad general surgical group. It must be relatively straightforward or death or complications will ensue.

• Whatever we do today is unlikely to be the best treatment in 20 years' time so the procedure should be easily and totally reversible so future options are not excluded.
• Ideally, it needs to be controllable. If the day of the operation is the last chance we have for setting the parameters, it is likely that, with time, the settings of the procedure will be suboptimal. This does not allow for a durable outcome. The recidivism of the RYGB is a powerful demonstration of this issue.

Each of the surgical options at present will be examined with this list of attributes in mind.

Roux-en-Y gastric bypass (Fig. 26.2)

Over the past 20 years this operation has represented the gastric stapling procedures to which other gastric stapling procedures have been compared. There are more short- and medium-term data available on RYGB than other procedures. Several prospective randomized controlled trials have compared the operation with gastroplasty (Fig. 26.3) and consistently shown better outcomes (Pories *et al.*, 1982; Sugerman *et al.*, 1987; 1989; Hall *et al.*, 1990), and gastroplasty in its various forms should now be regarded as a superseded procedure. There have been no randomized trials to date comparing RYGB with LAGB or BPD.

Key technical features

The procedure has evolved significantly during the past 30 years (Fig. 26.2). Important aspects of the present-day technique include the following:
• *Laparoscopic approach.* Increasingly, this is becoming the standard approach. This approach presents a number of technical challenges for the surgeon resulting in a procedure that is considered to be equal to the most difficult laparoscopic procedure of oesophagectomy at present (Schauer *et al.*, 2001) and therefore has the potential for a higher mortality and morbidity than the open operation. Nevertheless, the laparoscopic approach is perceived by the patient to be less invasive and preferable. Nguyen and colleagues (2001) performed a prospective randomized trial of the open vs. laparoscopic approach to RYGB. They showed improved postoperative respiratory recovery and less wound problems in the laparoscopic group. Anastomotic leak rates were similar. Wound problems were more common after open surgery and anastomotic stricturing was more common after the laparoscopic approach.
• *Total division of the stomach into a very small upper pouch of 15–20 mL from the remainder using the linear cutter form of stapling device.* The divided stomach reduces the risk of staple line disruption but increases the opportunity for postoperative leaks.
• *A Roux-en-Y loop of proximal jejunum is formed by division of the proximal gut, side-to-side anastomosis of the proximal end to jejunum to create a Roux length of between 80 and 250 cm.* The optimal length of the Roux limb, and the benefit of tailoring the length to the individual patient's weight, remain to be defined.

Table 26.2 %EWL after Roux-en-Y gastric bypass – open and laparoscopic.

Study	Time (months)							
	n	12	18	24	36	48	60	Other
Linner (1982)	174				77			
Sugerman *et al.* (1989)	182	68						
Jones (2000)	312	78						62% at 10 years
Maclean *et al.* (2000)	106							55% at 10 years
Pories *et al.* (1995)	608	69					58	49% at 14 years
Capella and Capella (1996)	560							
Freeman *et al.* (1997)	121	66		74	71	58	62	
Smith *et al.* (1996)	205	72		70	66	56	62	
Balsiger *et al.* (2000b)	191	68		72	66	63		
Oh *et al.* (1997)	193	87		71	70	56		
Wittgrove and Clark (2000)	500	77						
Schauer *et al.* (2000)	275	69	72	83				
Higa *et al.* (2000b)	1040	70						
Choban	150	60	62	58	58			
Courcoulas *et al.* (2003)	160	67						

The table includes all studies reported to June 2003 in which more than 100 patients are involved and follow-up of at least 12 months is available.

- *The distal end is taken by either an antecolic or retrocolic path to be anastomosed to the gastric pouch.* The formation of this anastomosis may involve use of a circular stapler with a 21-mm anvil pass transorally (Wittgrove and Clark, 2000), a linear cutter to form a side-to-side anastomosis (Schauer *et al.*, 2000) or suturing a two-layer anastomosis (Higa *et al.*, 2000a).
- *The stoma size is a further variable, particularly with the laparoscopic approach.* With open surgery, a measured stoma of approximately 1 cm was planned. With the laparoscopic approach, there is less ability to set the stomal size because of the technical limitations. Discussion of technical details of the gastrojejunostomy and the avoidance or treatment of leaks from this anastomosis remains a major activity at meetings of bariatric surgeons, indicating an unresolved dilemma.

Effects and side-effects

Table 26.2 lists the outcomes from major reports of RYGB. Overall there has been a perioperative mortality of 0.5–1%, significant perioperative complications in 5–25% of patients, a median length of stay of 6 days, incisional hernia in up to 24% and a weight loss of 49–62% EWL at follow-up of between 5 and 15 years.

Nutritional problems are frequent and compliance with replacement therapy has been shown to be low, leaving the patient vulnerable to deficiency problems if he or she is lost to follow-up.

Biliopancreatic diversion (Figs 26.4 and 26.5)

Key technical features

The combination of partial gastrectomy and intestinal bypass without a blind loop was created by Nicola Scopinaro in 1979 (Scopinaro *et al.*, 1979).

- His technique involves standard transverse hemigastrectomy, closure of the duodenal stump, division of the small bowel at 200 cm from the ileocaecal junction, with anastomosis of the distal end to the gastric remnant and end-to-side anastomosis of the proximal end to the distal ileum at 50 cm from the ileocaecal junction.
- Since 1986, Scopinaro has tailored the size of the gastric remnant to be between 200 and 500 mL, depending on the preoperative weight and a number of patient characteristics and, more recently, has reported tailoring the intestinal lengths on similar grounds (Scopinaro *et al.*, 1998). Establishment of the precision or validity of these variations has not been reported.
- A prominent variation on the traditional technique is the duodenal switch (BPD-DS), in which there is preservation of normal gastric emptying by performing a longitudinal sleeve gastrectomy, anastomosis of the Roux limb to the proximal duodenum, and staple closure of the duodenum beyond this anastomosis (Lagace *et al.*, 1995).
- The BPD and its variant can be performed laparoscopically, although with difficulty, and high perioperative mortality has been reported in association with this approach, especially in the superobese (Ren *et al.*, 2000).

Effects and side-effects

Impressive and durable weight loss is achieved with all variants of the BPD (Table 26.3). Marceau *et al.* (1998) reported better weight loss with the BPD-DS than a previous series of BPD but the weight loss in their BPD-DS group is not different from that achieved by Scopinaro without duodenal switch. Recently reported data by Scopinaro relate to patients having the post-

Table 26.3 %EWL after biliopancreatic diversion with or without a duodenal switch.

Study	Time (months)								
	n	12	18	24	36	48	60	72	96
Scopinaro *et al.* (1998)	2241			74		75		75	76
Marceau *et al.* (BPD) (1998)	233								61
Marceau *et al.* (DS) (1998)	457					73			
Baltasar *et al.* (2001)	125	70							
Totte *et al.* (1999)	180	58	63		70				
Hess and Hess (1998)	440	74	78	81	80	80	74	75	76
Rabkin (1998)	105	64							

The table includes all studies reported to June 2003 in which more than 100 patients are involved and follow-up of at least 12 months is available.
BPD, biliopancreatic diversion; DS, duodenal switch.

1986 variation, which he calls the *ad hoc* stomach (AHS) type of BPD. He reports a remarkable constancy of weight lost with 74% EWL at 2 years (*n* = 1284) and 78% EWL at 12 years (*n* = 58) (Scopinaro *et al.*, 1998). Hess and Hess (1998) have studied multiple variations of intestinal length without establishing a clear difference in outcomes. The relevance of the technical differences with respect to weight loss remains to be established.

The primary mechanism of all forms of BPD is malabsorption, especially of fat. All patients will have foul-smelling stools, generally 2–4 per day, and excessive wind (Scopinaro *et al.*, 1998). Whereas fat malabsorption is the aim, malabsorption of protein and micronutrients are the side-effects. Scopinaro *et al.* (1998) measured protein loss in the stool to be an average of 30 g per day, five times the normal value (Scopinaro *et al.*, 1998), and recommended a daily protein intake of at least 90 g per day to compensate for this. Iron deficiency is expected to occur and anaemia occurs in up to one-third of patients at 4 years after surgery if prophylaxis is inadequate (Brolin *et al.*, 1991; Marceau *et al.*, 2001). All patients need supplemental iron. Because of the low compliance with oral regimens, parenteral replacement is recommended (Marceau *et al.*, 2001). In addition, supplements of calcium, the fat-soluble vitamins, A and D, and the water-soluble vitamins are important.

Laparoscopic adjustable gastric banding (Fig. 26.6)

Key technical features

This procedure has the potential to fulfil the role of ideal bariatric procedure as it satisfies or nearly satisfies all the attributes listed in Table 26.1.

• It has been designed as a laparoscopic procedure. It could be done by open technique, but the safety and the accuracy of placement would suffer as a result.
• It is safe, 10 times as safe as gastric bypass (Chapman *et al.*, 2002) and remarkably free of significant postoperative complications (O'Brien *et al.*, 2002).
• It is effective in achieving good weight loss, of the order of between 50% and 60% of excess weight (Table 26.2), and there

are major improvements in obesity-related comorbidities and quality of life (Dixon and O'Brien, 2002b). With up to 6 years of follow-up data and only 3.6% of patients lost to follow-up, the effectiveness appears to be durable (O'Brien *et al.*, 2002). There is not the progressive fading of effectiveness that was characteristic of gastric-stapling procedures. This is presumed to reflect the benefit of adjustability. However, longer follow-up and more studies are required to establish this feature more securely.

• The one weakness of the LAGB in the initial years of its application has been the need for revisional procedures because of late problems with prolapse, erosions and tubing problems. These have now been reduced markedly, with an expectation that less than 5% will need revisional procedures. However, this long-term freedom from the need for reoperation remains to be firmly established.
• The procedure is technically feasible for the surgeons with competence in laparoscopic abdominal surgery.
• The LAGB can be removed easily by laparoscopic approach, allowing the stomach to return to its normal configuration.
• The ability to control the degree of gastric restriction through the adjustability is a unique feature of the LAGB and arguably its most attractive feature.

Effects and side-effects

The LAGB is a very safe procedure, with perioperative mortality of less than one in 2000 and a perioperative complication rate of less than 2% (O'Brien and Dixon, 2002). Late problems of prolapse, erosions and tubing problems are becoming infrequent. In our series, there was prolapse of the stomach through the band in 31% in the first 400 patients treated, 11% in the next 400 and 2.4% in the last 500. Erosion of the band into the stomach has occurred in 3.2% of our patients but none has occurred in the last 800 patients treated. There have been no tubing breaks since the use of a modified-access port design was initiated in March 2001.

Almost all published reports are for the BioEnterics® Lap-Band® system (LAGB®) and weight loss data for this device are shown in Table 26.4. There are several other bands now avail-

Table 26.4 Weight loss after laparosopic adjustable gastric band expressed as %EWL.

Study	Months after LAGB® placement								
	n	12	18	24	36	48	60	72	84
Belachew *et al.* (2002)	763	40	47	54	73				
O'Brien *et al.* (2002)	706	47	51	52	53	52	54	57	
Cadiere *et al.* (2000)	652	58		68					
Zinzindohoue *et al.* (2003)	500			52	55				
Fox *et al.* (2003)	105	61		74	72	60			
Vertruyen (2002)	543	38		61	62	58	53		52
Dargent (1999)	500	56		65	64				
Toppino *et al.* (1999)	361	42							
Fielding *et al.* (1999)	335	52	62						
Paganelli *et al.* (2000)	156	43							
Weiner *et al.* (1999)	184	58		87					
Niville and Dams (1999)	126	48	58						
Berrevoet *et al.* (1999)	120	46	53						
Total	*4865*	*46.4*	*56.0*	*59.4*	*61.2*	*56.2*	*53.5*	**57**	**52**

The table includes all studies reported to June 2003 in which more than 100 patients are involved and follow-up of at least 12 months is available.
LAGB®, laparosopic adjustable gastric band.

Table 26.5 %EWL after the Swedish adjustable gastric band (SAGB®).

Study	Time (months)						
	n	12	18	24	36	48	60
Ceelen *et al.* (2003)	625	46		50	47		
Victorzen and Tolonen (2002)	110			52			
Steffen *et al.* (2003)	824	30		41	49	55	57
Mittermair *et al.* (2003)	454				72		

The table includes all studies reported to June 2003 in which more than 100 patients are involved and follow-up of at least 12 months is available.

able but the only other band for which there are any published data is the Swedish adjustable gastric band (SAGB®) and the weight loss reported after this band is shown in Table 26.5. It can be reasonably expected that patients will have lost between 50% and 60% EWL by 3 years after the operation and that the effect is stable for up to 6 years. The benefits to health and quality of life have been impressive and are reviewed above. Inevitably, there is some loss of patients to follow-up and it is best practice to assume that these are the least successful. In our study of 700 patients followed for up to 6 years (O'Brien *et al.*, 2002) there was a loss to follow-up of 3.6%.

With the LAGB we can offer a very safe procedure with no deaths, a perioperative complication rate of less than 2% and there is at present approximately 5% likelihood of needing revisional procedures in the future (O'Brien *et al.*, 2002). The LAGB has been shown to be effective in generating major weight loss and improvement in health and quality of life, and the effects are achieved gently through its safe laparoscopic placement and its adjustability.

Conclusions

All bariatric surgical procedures that are available at present are effective in achieving substantial loss of weight and improvement in health and quality of life. For the person with severe obesity (BMI > 35), the surgical approach is the only one that can offer a predictable benefit in the short and medium term, and should be considered if the obesity is a significant problem to the person.

It is likely that all bariatric procedures will be undertaken laparoscopically as the standard and, on the basis of present-day data, for safety, efficacy and acceptability, the LAGB is the preferred option as a primary bariatric procedure. More long-term data (> 5-year follow-up) are needed on all the options, and careful randomized controlled trials using each technique optimally and following the patients for at least 5 years would be very valuable.

References

Agren, G., Narbro, K., Naslund, I., Sjostrom, L. and Peltonen M. (2002) Long-term effects of weight loss on pharmaceutical costs in obese subjects. A report from the SOS intervention study. *International Journal of Obesity and Related Metabolic Disorders* **26**, 184–192.

Bacci, V., Basso, M.S., Greco, F., Lamberti, R., Elmore, U., Restuccia, A., Perrotta, N., Silecchia, G., and Bucci A. (2002) Modifications of metabolic and cardiovascular risk factors after weight loss induced by laparoscopic gastric banding. *Obesity Surgery* **12**, 77–82.

Balsiger, B.M., Murr, M.M., Mai, J. and Sarr, M.G. (2000a) Gastroesophageal reflux after intact vertical banded gastroplasty: correction by conversion to Roux-en-Y gastric bypass. *Journal of Gastrointestinal Surgery* **4**, 276–281.

Balsiger, B.M., Kennedy, F.P., Abu-Lebdeh, H.S., Collazo-Clavell, M., Jensen, M.D., O'Brien, T., Hensrud, D.D., Dinneen, S.F., Thompson, G.B., Que, F.G., Williams, D.E., Clark, M.M., Grant. J.E., Frick, M.S., Mueller, R.A., Mai, J.L. and Sarr, M.G. (2000b) Prospective evaluation of Roux-en-Y gastric bypass as primary operation for medically complicated obesity [see comments]. *Mayo Clinic Proceedings* **75**, 673–680.

Baltasar, A., Bou, R., Bengochea, M., Arlandis, F., Escriva, C., Miro, J., Martinez, R. and Perez, N. (2001) Duodenal switch: an effective therapy for morbid obesity—intermediate results. *Obesity Surgery* **11**, 54–58.

Belachew, M., Legrand, M.J., Defechereux, T.H., Burtheret ,M.P. and Jacquet, N. (1994) Laparoscopic adjustable silicone gastric banding in the treatment of morbid obesity. A preliminary report. *Surgery and Endoscopy* **8**, 1354–1356.

Belachew, M., Legrand, M.J. and Vincent ,V. (2001) History of Lap-Band: from dream to reality. *Obesity Surgery* **11**, 297–302.

Belachew, M., Belva, P.H. and Desaive, C. (2002) Long-term results of laparoscopic adjustable gastric banding for the treatment of morbid obesity. *Obesity Surgery* **12**, 564–568.

Berrevoet, F., Pattyn, P., Cardon, A., de Ryck, F., Hesse ,U.J. and de Hemptinne, B. (1999) Retrospective analysis of laparoscopic gastric banding technique: short-term and mid-term follow-up. *Obesity Surgery* **9**, 272–275.

Brolin, R.E., Gorman R.C., Milgrim L.M. and Kenler HA. (1991) Multivitamin prophylaxis in prevention of post-gastric bypass vitamin and mineral deficiencies. *International Journal of Obesity* **15**, 661–667.

Brolin, R.E., Gorman, J.H., Gorman, R.C., Petschenik, A.J., Bradley, L.J., Kenler, H.A. and Cody, R.P. (1998) Are vitamin B12 and folate deficiency clinically important after Roux-en-Y gastric bypass? *Journal of Gastrointestinal Surgery* **2**, 436–442.

Brolin, R.E., Bradley, L.J., Wilson, A.C. and Cody, R.P. (2000) Lipid risk profile and weight stability after gastric restrictive operations for morbid obesity. *Journal of Gastrointestinal Surgery* **4**, 464–469.

Busetto, L., Pisent, C., Rinaldi, D., Longhin, P.L., Segato, G., De Marchi, F., Foletto, M., Favretti, F., Lise, M. and Enzi, G. (2000) Variation in lipid levels in morbidly obese patients operated with the LAP-BAND adjustable gastric banding system: effects of different levels of weight loss. *Obesity Surgery* **10**, 569–577.

Cadiere, G.B., Himpens, J., Vertruyen, M., Germay, O., Favretti, F. and Segato, G. (2000) Laparoscopic gastroplasty (adjustable silicone gastric banding). *Seminars in Laparoscopic Surgery* **7**, 55–65.

Calle, E.E., Rodriguez, C., Walker-Thurmond, K. and Thun, M.J. (2003) Overweight, obesity, and mortality from cancer in a prospectively studied cohort of U.S. adults. *New England Journal of Medicine* **348**, 1625–1638.

Capella, J.F. and Capella, R.F. (1996) The weight reduction operation of choice: vertical banded gastroplasty or gastric bypass? *American Journal of Surgery* **171**, 74–79.

Ceelen, W., Walder, J., Cardon, A., Van Renterghem, K., Hesse, U., El Malt, M. and Pattyn, P. (2003) Surgical treatment of severe obesity with a low-pressure adjustable gastric band: experimental data and clinical results in 625 patients. *Annals of Surgery* **237**, 10–16.

Chapman, A., Kiroff, G., Game, P., Foster, B., O'Brien, P., Ham, J. and Maddern, G. (2002) *Systematic Review of Laparoscopic Adjustable Gastric Banding in the Treatment of Obesity*, ASERNIP-S Report No 31. Adelaide, South Australia: ASERNIP-S.

Choban, P.S., Onyejekwe, J. *et al.* (1999) A health status assessment of the impact of weight loss following Roux-en-Y gastric bypass for clinically severe obesity. *Journal of the American College of Surgeons* **188**, 491–497.

Corrodi, P. (1984) Jejunoileal bypass: change in the flora of the small intestine and its clinical impact. *Review of Infectious Diseases* **6** (Suppl. 1), S80–84.

Courcoulas, A., Perry, Y., Buenaventura, P. and Luketich, J. (2003) Comparing the outcomes after laparoscopic versus open gastric bypass: a matched paired analysis. *Obesity Surgery* **13**, 341–346.

Dargent, J. (1999) Laparoscopic adjustable gastric banding: lessons from the first 500 patients in a single institution. *Obesity Surgery* **9**, 446–452.

Despres, J. (1993) The insulin resistance-dyslipidemia syndrome: the most prevalent cause of coronary artery disease. *Canadian Medical Association Journal* **148**, 1339–1340.

DeWind, L.T. and Payne, JH. (1976) Intestinal bypass surgery for morbid obesity. Long-term results. *Journal of the American Medical Association* **236**, 2298–2301.

Dixon, J.B. (2001) Elevated homocysteine with weight loss. *Obesity Surgery* **11**, 537–538.

Dixon, J.B. and O'Brien, P.E. (1999) Gastroesophageal reflux in obesity: the effect of lap-band placement. *Obesity Surgery* **9**, 527–531.

Dixon, J.B. and O'Brien, P. (2002a) Health outcomes of severely obese type 2 diabetic subjects 1 year after laparoscopic adjustable gastric banding. *Diabetes Care* **25**, 358–363.

Dixon, J.B. and O'Brien, P.E. (2002b) Changes in comorbidities and improvements in quality of life after LAP-BAND placement. *American Journal of Surgery* **184**, S51–54.

Dixon, J. and O'Brien, P. (2002c) Ovarian dysfunction, androgen excess and neck circumference in obese women: Changes with weight loss (abstract). *Obesity Surgery* **12**, 193.

Dixon, J.B., Chapman, L. and O'Brien, P. (1999) Marked improvement in asthma after Lap-Band surgery for morbid obesity. *Obesity Surgery* **9**, 385–389.

Dixon, J.B., Dixon, M.E. and O'Brien, P.E. (2001a) Pregnancy after lap-band surgery: management of the band to achieve healthy weight outcomes. *Obesity Surgery* **11**, 59–65.

Dixon, J.B., Schachter, L.M. and O'Brien, P.E. (2001b) Sleep disturbance and obesity: changes following surgically induced weight loss. *Archives of Internal Medicine* **161**, 102–106.

Dixon, J.B., Dixon, M.E. and O'Brien, P.E. (2002) Body image:

appearance orientation and evaluation in the severely obese. Changes with weight loss. *Obesity Surgery* **12**, 65–71.

Dixon, J.B., Dixon, A.F. and O'Brien, P.E. (2003a) Improvements in insulin sensitivity and beta-cell function (HOMA) with weight loss in the severely obese. *Diabetic Medicine* **20**, 127–134.

Dixon, J.B., Dixon, M.E. and O'Brien, P.E. (2003b) Depression in association with severe obesity: changes with weight loss. *Archives of Internal Medicine* **163**, 2058–2065.

Fielding, G.A., Rhodes, M. and Nathanson, L.K. (1999) Laparoscopic gastric banding for morbid obesity. Surgical outcome in 335 cases. *Surgery and Endoscopy* **13**, 550–554.

Fox, S.R., Fox, K.M., Srikanth, M.S. and Rumbaut, R. (2003) The Lap-Band System in a North American population. *Obesity Surgery* **13**, 275–280.

Freeman, J.B., Kotlarewsky, M. and Phoenix, C. (1997) Weight loss after extended gastric bypass. *Obesity Surgery* **7**, 337–344.

Hall, J.C., Watts, J.M., O'Brien, P.E., Dunstan, R.E., Walsh, J.F., Slavotinek, A.H. and Elmslie, R.G. (1990) Gastric surgery for morbid obesity. The Adelaide Study. *Annals of Surgery* **211**, 419–427.

Hess, D.S. and Hess, D.W. (1998) Biliopancreatic diversion with a duodenal switch. *Obesity Surgery* **8**, 267–282.

Higa, K.D., Boone, K.B., Ho, T. and Davies, O.G. (2000a) Laparoscopic Roux-en-Y gastric bypass for morbid obesity: technique and preliminary results of our first 400 patients. *Archives of Surgery* **135**, 1029–1034.

Higa, K.D., Boone, K.B. and Ho, T. (2000b) Complications of the laparoscopic Roux-en-Y gastric bypass: 1,040 patients: what have we learned? *Obesity Surgery* **10**, 509–513.

Horchner, R., Tuinebreijer, M.W. and Kelder, P.H. (2001) Quality-of-life assessment of morbidly obese patients who have undergone a Lap-Band operation: 2-year follow-up study. Is the MOS SF-36 a useful instrument to measure quality of life in morbidly obese patients? *Obesity Surgery* **11**, 212–218; discussion 219.

Jones, Jr, K.B. (2000) Experience with the Roux-en-Y gastric bypass, and commentary on current trends. *Obesity Surgery* **10**, 183–185.

Jorizzo, J.L., Apisarnthanarax, P., Subrt, P., Hebert, A.A., Henry, J.C., Raimer, S.S., Dinehart, S.M. and Reinarz, J.A. (1983) Bowel-bypass syndrome without bowel bypass. Bowel-associated dermatosis-arthritis syndrome. *Archives of Internal Medicine* **143**, 457–461.

Koba, S., Hirano, T., Sakaue, T., Sakai, K., Kondo, T., Yorozuya, M., Suzuki, H., Murakami, M. and Katagiri, T. (2000) Role of small dense low-density lipoprotein in coronary artery disease patients with normal plasma cholesterol levels. *Journal of Cardiology* **36**, 371–378.

Kuzmak, L.I. (1991) A review of seven years' experience with silicone gastric banding. *Obesity Surgery* **1**, 403–408.

Lagace, M., Marceau, P., Marceau, S., Hould, F.S., Potvin, M., Bourque, R.A. and Biron, S. (1995) Biliopancreatic diversion with a new type of gastrectomy: some previous conclusions revisited. *Obesity Surgery* **5**, 411–418.

Linner, J.H. (1982) Comparative effectiveness of gastric bypass and gastroplasty: a clinical study. *Archives of Surgery* **117**, 695–700.

MacLean, L.D., Rhode, B.M. and Nohr, C.W. (2000) Late outcome of isolated gastric bypass. *Annals of Surgery* **231**, 524–528.

Marceau, P., Hould, F.S., Simard, S., Lebel, S., Bourque, R.A., Potvin, M. and Biron, S. (1998) Biliopancreatic diversion with duodenal switch. *World Journal of Surgery* **22**, 947–954.

Marceau, P., Hould, F.S., Lebel, S., Marceau, S. and Biron, S. (2001)

Malabsorptive obesity surgery. *Surgery Clinics of North America* **81**, 1113–1127.

Mason, E.E. (1982) Vertical banded gastroplasty for obesity. *Archives of Surgery* **117**, 701–706.

Mason, E.E. and Ito, C. (1967) Gastric bypass in obesity. *Surgery Clinics of North America* **47**, 1345–51.

Mittermair, R.P., Weiss, H., Nehoda, H., Kirchmayr, W. and Aigner, F. (2003) Laparoscopic Swedish adjustable gastric banding: 6-year follow-up and comparison to other laparoscopic bariatric procedures. *Obesity Surgery* **13**, 412–417.

Nguyen, N.T., Goldman, C., Rosenquist, C.J., Arango, A., Cole, C.J., Lee, S.J. and Wolfe, B.M. (2001) Laparoscopic versus open gastric bypass: a randomized study of outcomes, quality of life, and costs. *Annals of Surgery* **234**, 279–289; discussion 289–291.

Niville, E. and Dams, A. (1999) Late pouch dilation after laparoscopic adjustable gastric and esophagogastric banding: incidence, treatment, and outcome. *Obesity Surgery* **9**, 381–384.

O'Brien, P.E. and Dixon, J.B. (2002) Weight loss and early and late complications—the international experience. *American Journal of Surgery* **184**, S42–45.

O'Brien, P., Brown, W. and Dixon, J. (2000) Revisional surgery for morbid obesity—conversion to the lap-band system. *Obesity Surgery* **10**, 557–563.

O'Brien, P.E., Dixon, J.B., Brown, W., Schachter, L.M., Chapman, L., Burn, A.J., Dixon, M.E., Scheinkestel, C., Halket, C., Sutherland, L.J., Korin, A. and Baquie, P. (2002) The laparoscopic adjustable gastric band (Lap-Band): a prospective study of medium-term effects on weight, health and quality of life. *Obesity Surgery* **12**, 652–660.

O'Leary, J.P. (1983) Hepatic complications of jejunoileal bypass. *Seminars in Liver Disease* **3**, 203–215.

Oh, C.H., Kim, H.J. and Oh, S. (1997) Weight loss following transected gastric bypass with proximal Roux-en-Y. *Obesity Surgery* **7**, 142–147; discussion 148.

Paganelli, M., Giacomelli, M., Librenti, M.C., Pontiroli, A.E. and Ferla, G. (2000) Thirty months experience with laparoscopic adjustable gastric banding. *Obesity Surgery* **10**, 269–271.

Parfitt, A.M., Podenphant, J., Villanueva, A.R. and Frame, B. (1985) Metabolic bone disease with and without osteomalacia after intestinal bypass surgery: a bone histomorphometric study. *Bone* **6**, 211–220.

Pinkney, J.H., Sjostrom, C.D. and Gale, E.A. (2001) Should surgeons treat diabetes in severely obese people? *Lancet* **357**, 1357–1359.

Pories, W.J., Flickinger, E.G., Meelheim, D., Van Rij, A.M. and Thomas, F.T. (1982) The effectiveness of gastric bypass over gastric partition in morbid obesity: consequence of distal gastric and duodenal exclusion. *Annals of Surgery* **196**, 389–399.

Pories, W.J., Swanson, M.S., MacDonald, K.G., Long, S.B., Morris, P.G., Brown, B.M., Barakat, H.A., deRamon, R.A., Israel, G. and Dolezal, J.M. (1995) Who would have thought it? An operation proves to be the most effective therapy for adult-onset diabetes mellitus. *Annals of Surgery* **222**, 339–350; discussion 350–352.

Printen, K.J. and Mason, E.E. (1973) Gastric surgery for relief of morbid obesity. *Archives of Surgery* **106**, 428–441.

Rabkin, R.A. (1998) Distal gastric bypass/duodenal switch procedure, Roux-en-Y gastric bypass and biliopancreatic diversion in a community practice. *Obesity Surgery* **8**, 53–59.

Ren, C.J., Patterson, E. and Gagner, M. (2000) Early results of laparoscopic biliopancreatic diversion with duodenal switch: a case series of 40 consecutive patients. *Obesity Surgery* **10**, 514–523; discussion 524.

Rubino, F. and Gagner, M. (2002) Potential of surgery for curing type 2 diabetes mellitus. *Annals of Surgery* **236**, 554–559.

Schauer, P.R. and Ikramuddin S. (2001) Laparoscopic surgery for morbid obesity. *Surgery Clinics of North America* **81**, 1145–1179.

Schauer, P.R., Ikramuddin, S., Gourash, W., Ramanathan, R. and Luketich, J. (2000) Outcomes after laparoscopic Roux-en-Y gastric bypass for morbid obesity. *Annals of Surgery* **232**, 515–529.

Schauer, P., Hamad, G. and Ikramuddin, S. (2001) Surgical management of gastroesophageal reflux disease in obese patients. *Seminars in Laparoscopic Surgery* **8**, 256–264.

Schok, M., Geenen, R., van Antwerpen, T., de Wit, P., Brand, N. and van Ramshorst, B. (2000) Quality of life after laparoscopic adjustable gastric banding for severe obesity: postoperative and retrospective preoperative evaluations. *Obesity Surgery* **10**, 502–508.

Scopinaro, N., Gianetta, E., Civalleri, D., Bonalumi, U. and Bachi, V. (1979) Bilio-pancreatic bypass for obesity: II. Initial experience in man. *British Journal of Surgery* **66**, 618–620.

Scopinaro, N., Gianetta, E., Adami, G.F., Friedman, D., Traverso, E., Marinari, G.M., Cuneo, S., Vitale, B., Ballari, F., Colombini, M., Baschieri, G. and Bachi, V. (1996) Biliopancreatic diversion for obesity at eighteen years. *Surgery* **119**, 261–268.

Scopinaro, N., Adami, G.F., Marinari, G.M., Gianetta, E., Traverso, E., Friedman, D., Camerini, G., Baschieri, G. and Simonelli, A. (1998) Biliopancreatic diversion. *World Journal of Surgery* **22**, 936–946.

Sjostrom, C.D., Lissner, L., Wedel, H. and Sjostrom, L. (1999) Reduction in incidence of diabetes, hypertension and lipid disturbances after intentional weight loss induced by bariatric surgery: the SOS Intervention Study. *Obesity Research* **7**, 477–484.

Sjostrom, C.D., Peltonen, M., Wedel, H. and Sjostrom, L. (2000) Differentiated long-term effects of intentional weight loss on diabetes and hypertension. *Hypertension* **36**, 20–25.

Smith, S.C., Edwards, C.B. and Goodman, G.N. (1996) Changes in diabetic management after Roux-en-Y gastric bypass. *Obesity Surgery* **6**, 345–348.

Steffen, R., Biertho, L., Ricklin, T., Piec, G. and Horber, F.F. (2003) Laparoscopic Swedish adjustable gastric banding: a five-year prospective study. *Obesity Surgery* **13**, 404–411.

Sugerman, H.J., Starkey, J.V. and Birkenhauer, R. (1987) A randomized prospective trial of gastric bypass versus vertical banded gastroplasty for morbid obesity and their effects on sweets versus non-sweets eaters. *Annals of Surgery* **205**, 613–624.

Sugerman, H.J., Londrey, G.L., Kellum, J.M., Wolf, L., Liszka, T., Engle, K.M., Birkenhauer, R. and Starkey, J.V. (1989) Weight loss with vertical banded gastroplasty and Roux-Y gastric bypass for

morbid obesity with selective versus random assignment. *American Journal of Surgery* **157**, 93–102.

Szinicz, G. and Schnapka, G. (1982) A new method in the surgical treatment of disease. *Acta Chirurgica Austrica* (Suppl. 43).

Toppino, M., Morino, M., Bonnet, G., Nigra, I. and Siliquini, R. (1999) Laparoscopic surgery for morbid obesity: preliminary results from SICE registry (Italian Society of Endoscopic and Minimally Invasive Surgery). *Obesity Surgery* **9**, 62–65.

Torgerson, J.S. (2003) Swedish obese subjects—where are we now? *International Journal of Obesity* **27**, 19.

Torgerson, J.S. and Sjostrom, L. (2001) The Swedish Obese Subjects (SOS) study—rationale and results. *International Journal of Obesity and Related Metabolic Disorders* **25** (Suppl. 1), S2–4.

Totte, E., Hendrickx, L. and van Hee, R. (1999) Biliopancreatic diversion for treatment of morbid obesity: experience in 180 consecutive cases. *Obesity Surgery* **9**, 161–165.

Vertruyen, M. (2002) Experience with lap-band system up to 7 years. *Obesity Surgery* **12**, 569–572.

Vgontzas, A.N., Papanicolaou, D.A., Bixler, E.O., Hopper, K., Lotsikas, A., Lin, H.M., Kales, A. and Chrousos, G.P. (2000) Sleep apnea and daytime sleepiness and fatigue: relation to visceral obesity, insulin resistance, and hypercytokinemia. *Journal of Clinical and Endocrinological Metabolism* **85**, 1151–1158.

Victorzen, M. and Tolonen, P. (2002) Intermediate results following laparoscopic adjustable gastric banding for morbid obesity. *Digest of Surgery* **19**, 354–358.

Weiner, R., Datz, M., Wagner, D. and Bockhorn, H. (1999) Quality-of-life outcome after laparoscopic adjustable gastric banding for morbid obesity. *Obesity Surgery* **9**, 539–545.

Weiss, H.G., Nehoda, H., Labeck, B., Peer-Kuhberger, M.D., Klingler, P., Gadenstatter, M., Aigner, F. and Wetscher, G.J. (2000) Treatment of morbid obesity with laparoscopic adjustable gastric banding affects esophageal motility. *American Journal of Surgery* **180**, 479–482.

Wittgrove, A.C. and Clark, G.W. (2000) Laparoscopic gastric bypass, Roux-en-Y- 500 patients: technique and results, with 3–60 month follow-up. *Obesity Surgery* **10**, 233–239.

Wittgrove, A.C., Clark, G.W. amd Schubert, K.R. (1996) Laparoscopic gastric bypass, Roux-en-Y: technique and results in 75 patients with 3–30 months follow-up. *Obesity Surgery* **6**, 500–504.

Young, S.Y., Gunzenhauser, J.D., Malone, K.E. and McTiernan, A. (2001) Body mass index and asthma in the military population of the northwestern United States. *Archives of Internal Medicine* **161**, 1605–1611.

Zinzindohoue, F., Chevallier, J.M., Douard, R., Elian, N., Ferraz, J.M., Blanche, J.P., Berta, J.L., Altman, J.J., Safran, D. and Cugnenc, P.H. (2003) Laparoscopic gastric banding: a minimally invasive surgical treatment for morbid obesity: prospective study of 500 consecutive patients. *Annals of Surgery* **237**, 1–9.

27 Weight loss maintenance

Kristina Elfhag and Stephan Rössner

Some general considerations on
weight maintenance, 407
   Effects of weight loss, 407
   How should obesity be
   measured?, 408
   Natural weight development, 408
   The weight loss plateau, 409

Factors affecting weight loss
maintenance, 409
   Definition and prevalence of
   weight loss maintenance, 409
   Prevalence of weight
   maintenance, 410
   Weight loss goals, 410

Weight loss patterns, 410
Physical activity, 410
Dietary intake, 410
Eating patterns, 411
Binge eating, 411
Self-monitoring, 412
Stress and coping, 412
Attitudes, 412
Personality, 413
Depression, 413
Weight cycling, 413
Methodological considerations in
research on weight loss
maintenance, 413

The successful weight
   maintainer, 414

Treatment considerations, 415
   Obesity as a chronic condition, 415
   Targets in treatment, 416
   Strategies for the long-term
   treatment, 416
   Are long-term interventions
   necessary for weight
   maintenance?, 417
   Alternative medicine, 417

References, 418

Some general considerations on weight maintenance

Over the last few years, a paradigm shift has been observed as regards the feasibility of long-term weight loss. Clinicians were once satisfied if substantial weight loss could be introduced in patients, but realized that relapse was more the rule than the exception. In this early era, the famous quotation by Stunkard was made: 'Most of those who are obese will not go into obesity treatment, most of those who go into treatment will not lose weight and most of those who lose weight will regain it' (Stunkard, 1958). This extremely negative view was later challenged when it was realized that weight loss could generally be accomplished in a great number of obese individuals. It also became apparent that focus had to be shifted much more on to weight loss maintenance and prevention of weight regain after the initial treatment period.

Our own study in 1985 was actually one of the first to demonstrate that with standard conventional treatment tools, such as diet, exercise and behaviour modification, substantial weight loss could be achieved and maintained over a 4-year period (Björvell and Rössner, 1985).

When these patients were reinvestigated 10–12 years later, almost all weight loss achieved at the 4-year follow-up had been maintained 6–8 years later, as shown in Fig. 27.1 (Björvell and Rössner, 1992). Admittedly, this was a result obtained in a selected group, supervised by a PhD student with an interest, far more than what then could be expected in

a routine clinical setting, and without a control group. Nevertheless, the study still demonstrated that weight loss maintenance was possible.

Effects of weight loss

In the late 1980s, focus began to shift and it was realized that weight normalization was an impossible dream. Furthermore, weight loss normalization was not even necessary for important metabolic benefits to take place. The classical Goldstein meta-analysis from 1992 demonstrated that a 5–10% weight loss was enough to achieve significant improvement with regard to obesity-associated metabolic risk factors, with improved glycaemic control, reduced blood pressure and cholesterol levels (Goldstein, 1992). Several studies were summarized, demonstrating that as little as 5% weight loss also had beneficial health effects. It may indeed seem astonishing that such a small percentage of weight loss can improve health. An individual taking part in a weight loss programme, doing quite well, by most standards, and losing from 115 to 105 kg, will of course still remain obese and may not look much different in appearance, although the health status and metabolic risk factors have improved markedly.

A lowered obese body weight has furthermore been shown to affect the subjective experience of the health-related quality of life positively. Such effects include making daily tasks easier, with reduced obstacles in physical mobility and improvements in the person's general health perception (Karlsson *et al.*, 1998; Wing and Hill, 2001).

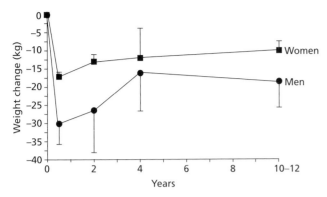

Fig 27.1 Long-term behavioural treatment of obesity (*n* = 49) (Source: Björvell and Rössner, 1992.)

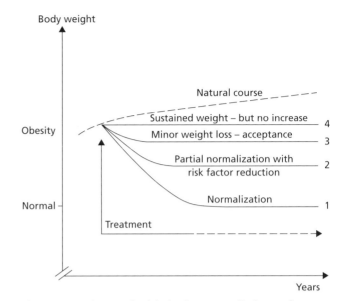

Fig 27.2 Natural course of weight development, and indicators of success in long-term weight reduction programmes.

Besides the positive health benefits of a lowered body weight, beneficial effects on psychosocial functioning and mental aspects of quality of life are also known. Psychosocial functioning has been shown to improve with weight loss. With a reduced body weight, less obstacles were perceived concerning activities such as social gatherings, buying clothes, going away for holidays, bathing in public and having intimate relations with a partner (Karlsson *et al.*, 1998). Mental aspects of quality of life, such as mental well-being, are also positively related to reduced body weights. Overall mood, anxiety and depression have been found to improve with long-term weight loss in various treatments according to some studies, although the size of the effect of some of these associations is small (Karlsson *et al.*, 1998; National Task Force on the Prevention and Treatment of Obesity, 2000).

How should obesity be measured?

Studies on the efficacy of long-term weight loss programmes have generally used the body mass index (BMI) with the World Health Organization (WHO) definitions for obesity as a tool to characterize the patients under study (WHO, 2000). Although this is a useful standard that has been applied in almost every study on obesity treatment for the last 20 years, more attention has been brought to the fact that measurement of abdominal fat may be more important.

Recently, it has been demonstrated that abdominal obesity, as measured by the waist–hip ratio (WHR) is an independent, potent risk factor for stroke in several ethnic groups and is an even stronger predictor than BMI (Suk *et al.*, 2003). The WHR has been used as a supplement to identify individuals at risk, but it has been questioned whether the introduction of the hip circumference in this ratio confuses the picture. A high WHR, indicating a propensity for metabolic risk, may actually not only be the result of an extended waist circumference, but also could reflect a reduced hip circumference, due to changes in muscle mass, effects of certain types of pharmacotherapy, etc.

Waist circumference is an easier and possibly more relevant way to assess the metabolic risk factors associated with the abdominal obesity (Han *et al.*, 1995; Lean *et al.*, 1998). Long-term mortality data suggest that waist circumference as an indicator of the risk associated with obesity may be more crucial than BMI (Bigaard *et al.*, 2003). Thus, when considering long-term evaluations, waist circumference may be even more relevant for assessing health risks than BMI.

Natural weight development

Figure 27.2 illustrates the clinical realities of long-term weight control. As basal metabolic rate decreases with age, in most societies an increase of body weight is observed over time. As an example, our cross-sectional Swedish data suggest an increase in body weight of 2–3 kg per decade (Kuskowska-Wolk and Rössner, 1990). If this is the situation for the general public, the weight development in obese subjects is even steeper.

Figure 27.3 demonstrates the weight trajectory in control subjects in the Gothenburg SOS study (Swedish Obese Subjects) (Sjöström *et al.*, 1992). As can be seen from this figure, the weight increase over time is quite pronounced for both men and women and all age groups. Taken together, this means that a therapist working with a patient who can maintain his weight for a significant period of time actually represents a degree of therapeutical success. A problem, however, is that although most therapists will see this as a treatment success, their patients will regard the lack of weight loss as a failure. What is often expected is weight normalization, something that would practically never happen in reality. The best therapists and patients can hope for is a result somewhere

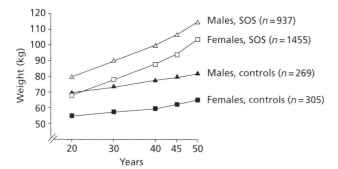

Fig 27.3 The weight trajectory in control subjects in the Gothenburg SOS study: self-reported weight, cross-sectional, SOS plus controls.

between the curves 2 and 3 in Fig. 27.2. In clinical reality, this would correspond to a weight loss of between 5% and 10%. Once the nadir has been achieved, it is reasonable to assume that unless more and more efforts are made, these curves will also start to slope upwards in parallel with the top line in the figure.

The weight loss plateau

It is interesting that irrespective of treatment (whether diet, exercise, behaviour modification or pharmacotherapy), most, although not quite all, treatment programmes result in continuous weight loss for about 6 months, after which weight loss will plateau. Thus, strategies, whatever method is being used, have to change from the initial weight loss period to the maintenance phase. Reassurance, support and acceptance are important components of the treatment, so that the patient understands and hopefully accepts that further weight loss may not take place. Although some individuals might find it difficult to accept that weight loss does not continue, the plateau can actually quite easily be explained on physiological grounds. With the reduction in lean body mass, which is an inevitable consequence of any weight loss, the basal metabolic rate will go down and the overall needs of the individual after weight loss are lower (James, 1984). Thus, intake and expenditure will balance at a lower level after successful weight loss, and when this takes place, no further weight loss can be expected.

Factors affecting weight loss maintenance

Identifying factors facilitating weight loss maintenance is of interest, as they can enhance our understanding of the behaviours and prerequisites that are crucial in sustaining a lowered body weight. Such knowledge has implications for what strategies should be entrained and encouraged in treatment and the advice given at the weight maintenance phase, as well as selecting persons who are likely to succeed for the longer

term in obesity treatments. The last strategy is a necessity for effective use of the limited resources available to treat the increasing numbers of obese persons today. It also enables a professional awareness of the risk of exposing a patient to additional aversive psychological consequences of experiencing failure in treatment (Wooley and Garner, 1991).

Definition and prevalence of weight loss maintenance

In looking at factors for weight loss maintenance, a definition of what constitutes weight maintenance should first be considered. Weight loss maintenance implies a sustained weight loss that had been accomplished by treatment interventions or by own efforts. This is the general definition shared across studies performed, although the specific criteria used differ. A more precise definition that has been suggested is: 'Achieving an intentional weight loss of at least 10% of initial body weight and maintaining this body weight for at least one year' (Wing and Hill, 2001).

This definition includes an initial amount of weight loss. There must first be some agreement on how much weight loss should be considered as a 'success' in treatment. The deliberate nature of weight loss is emphasized, as unintentional weight loss obviously has very different causes and effects. The definition also includes the duration of time for which the lowered weight has been sustained.

The time of assessment for evaluation of weight maintenance can also differ. Pretreatment factors determining later weight loss maintenance have the greatest informative value for treatment assignments. Another approach is to assess the patients at the time of admission, from active treatment, and predict further weight development from these characteristics. A last tactic is to retrospectively identify those who can be classified as successful weight loss maintainers and describe the behavioural characteristics of these persons as they manifest at the time of 'success'. The latter approach can give information on the behaviours and strategies that could be more focused and encouraged in treatment programmes, rather than on treatment assignment.

In our evaluation of factors affecting weight maintenance we have included studies with these different methodological approaches, and with a broad definition of weight maintenance implying intentional weight loss that has subsequently been maintained for at least 6 months. The studies include patient samples as well as general population samples. With this rather broad inclusion criterion, a fuller description of possible factors in weight maintenance could be derived, which enables a model of weight maintenance to be further considered.

Furthermore, as behavioural factors have been considered to be stronger predictors of weight maintenance and regain than physiological factors, we have focused on the former in favour of the latter (Wing and Hill, 2001).

Prevalence of weight maintenance

Quite optimistic results on weight loss maintenance are reported from a telephone survey in a US population sample. Weight loss maintenance for 5 years or more was reported by around 25% of those who had deliberately lost at least 10% of their maximum body weight (McGuire *et al.*, 1999a).

Looking at patient samples, a median of 15% could be identified as successful weight maintainers in a review of 17 clinical studies. In this review, weight maintenance was defined as maintenance of the entire weight loss or ≥ 9–11 kg of the initial weight loss at follow-up periods of at least 3 years (Ayyad and Andersen, 2000). The successful weight maintenance results in the studies reviewed ranged from 0% to 49%. If the patients lost to follow-up were considered to be failures, which is reasonable, the median success rate was 13%, with a range of 0–35% success (Ayyad and Andersen, 2000).

Weight loss goals

It is common for patients to have unrealistic expectations about the weight loss that will be achieved by treatment. In one study, none of the participants achieved the 'dream weight' for which they had hoped, and most of them ended up with a weight loss that they had considered as a failure before treatment, even though the standard treatment programme was well designed and executed (Foster *et al.*, 1997). Heavier patients and men had lower target weights (Foster *et al.*, 2001). The fact that expectations regarding the goal weight may be unrealistic has been confirmed in other studies (Linne *et al.*, 2002). However, according to these results, men were more realistic in their approach to what could be achieved with a weight loss regimen than women.

The weight goals may be one factor in determining if the person will succeed or fail at maintaining a lower body weight (Marston and Criss, 1984; Jeffery *et al.*, 1998). Those who later maintained their weight were more likely to have achieved their self-determined goal weight. It has been suggested that the failure to reach a self-determined weight may discourage the person's belief in their ability to control his or her weight and result in an abandonment of weight maintenance behaviours (Cooper and Fairburn, 2001). However, we have little scientific evidence that modifying weight loss goals would be important for subsequent results.

Weight loss patterns

Initial weight loss has been identified as a predictor for later weight loss, and also for weight loss maintenance in various treatments (Astrup and Rössner, 2000; van Baak *et al.*, 2003). The greater the initial weight loss, the better is the subsequent outcome. Such a predictor tells us that there is a consistent weight loss pattern from the beginning of the treatment. Initial weight loss can also reflect a better compliance with the treatment (van Baak *et al.*, 2003). However, information on initial weight loss provides little understanding of the underlying factors contributing to success or failure.

According to other results, larger weight losses during intentional weight loss have predicted more weight regain (McGuire *et al.*, 1999b). This suggests that greater weight lost can also imply there is more weight to be regained. It is still unclear how the early weight loss response that predicts long-term outcome should be defined. The complexity in evaluating the predictive value of weight loss patterns can be illustrated by a recent analysis of two long-term clinical trials with orlistat (Rissanen *et al.*, 2003). In this analysis, weight loss of > 5% body weight after 12 weeks of diet and orlistat was a good indicator of 2-year weight loss, whereas ≥ 2.5-kg initial weight loss during the 4-week lead-in (European guideline requirements) and ≥ 10% weight loss after 6 months did not add significantly to the prediction of the 2-year outcome.

Time of duration of weight loss has also been studied. The longer the weight loss has been maintained, the better are the chances for further continuation of a lower body weight (McGuire *et al.*, 1999b; Wing and Hill, 2001). The subjects who have maintained weight losses during a longer time report that they use less effort for continuing weight control (Klem *et al.*, 2000a). The pleasure derived from controlling weight was not changed over time, suggesting a shift in balance towards more pleasure overall, which can promote further maintenance of body weight.

Physical activity

Physical activity is related to long-term weight maintenance, according to many findings (Kayman *et al.*, 1990; Schoeller *et al.*, 1997; Wing and Hill, 2001). Physical activity facilitates weight maintenance through direct energy expenditure and improved physical fitness, which facilitates the amount and intensity of daily activities (Saris, 1998). Walking is one of the most frequent aspects of physical exercise reported; cycling and weight lifting also have some popularity (Wing and Hill, 2001). In the STORM study, leisure-time activity predicted weight maintenance in sibutramine treatment (van Baak *et al.*, 2003). Such leisure-time physical activity included time spent walking and cycling, and as a type of displacement effect less time spent watching television. It is suggested these factors can discriminate a sedentary life style from a more active one even better than a measure of sports activity.

Dietary intake

Weight loss maintenance is obviously associated with lower caloric intake (Kathan *et al.*, 1982) and reduced portion sizes (Jeffrey *et al.*, 1984). More specifically, weight maintenance is also associated with reduced frequency of snacks (Harris *et al.*, 1994; Westenhoefer, 2001) and less dietary fat (Harris *et al.*, 1994; Westenhoefer, 2001; Wing and Hill, 2001).

Reduction of particular food types such as French fries, dairy products, sweets and meat (French *et al.*, 1994) and cheese, butter, high-fat snacks, fried foods and desserts (Holden *et al.*, 1992) is also seen in persons maintaining their weight. The importance of high-quality foods such as fresh fruits and vegetables (Westenhoefer, 2001) and healthy eating (Ogden, 2000) has also been noted.

A regular meal rhythm has been identified as helpful in weight maintenance (Westenhoefer, 2001), and regularly eating breakfast has furthermore been reported among weight maintainers (Wyatt *et al.*, 2002). It is suggested that breakfast can reduce hunger, making the breakfast eaters chose less energy-dense foods during the rest of the day, as well as providing energy to perform physical activity during the day.

Eating patterns

Generally, eating behaviour has been evaluated during ongoing treatments. The most common measure for eating behaviours is the Three Factor Eating Questionnaire (TFEQ) (Stunkard and Messick, 1985), measuring eating restraint, disinhibition and hunger. Restraint means trying to resist from eating by conscious determination and control in order to control body weight. Disinhibition measures loss of control over eating, and the hunger scale shows the experience of hunger feelings and cravings for food.

Eating restraint is known to be associated with a lower amount of food intake (Lindroos *et al.*, 1997), and the restraint increases with successful weight loss in behaviour modification treatments (Björvell *et al.*, 1994; Karlsson *et al.*, 1994). This means restriction of food intake is accompanied by weight loss.

The contrary pattern, a decrease in eating restraint and increase in disinhibition have accordingly been found for those regaining their body weight (McGuire *et al.*, 1999b; Wing and Hill, 2001). Findings that more restraint is related to more weight loss are limited, however, in their informative value. These types of data merely tell us that restraint in food intake leads to less food consumed and thus more weight loss and that the control over food intake is crucial in behaviour modification programmes, emphasizing the participant's efforts to reduce food intake by will.

An attempt towards using data on eating patterns somewhat more prospectively, by comparing the eating patterns at the time of discharge from treatment in evaluating subsequent weight development, has also been used. In line with the earlier information on eating patterns, this revealed that reduction of disinhibited eating during active treatment was a positive predictor of post-treatment weight reduction (Cuntz *et al.*, 2001), and higher levels of dietary disinhibition, assessed after an intentional weight loss phase, accordingly predicted weight regain (McGuire *et al.*, 1999b). More hunger at discharge, according to the TFEQ, has also been shown to be a negative predictor of post-treatment weight development

(Cuntz *et al.*, 2001). This means that more intense hunger and disinhibited eating pose a problem for subsequent overconsumption.

Another study has analysed pretreatment data on eating behaviours as predictors of weight development after treatment. These results revealed that a high pretreatment score on the TFEQ hunger scale predicted weight regain at follow-up after VLCD treatment (Pasman *et al.*, 1999). With more intense hunger initially, a VLCD treatment has thus not provided a solution to the participant's eating behaviour on a more long-term basis. Often, however, the pretreatment TFEQ scores have not provided predictive information on subsequent weight loss (Björvell *et al.*, 1994; Karlsson *et al.*, 1994).

On the issue of control over eating behaviours, it has been suggested that a more flexible control over eating behaviour is associated with improved weight maintenance than with more rigid control (Westenhoefer, 2001). Although eating restraint is often reported to be associated with weight loss in behavioural treatments, such restraint has also been associated with periods of overeating, and is suggested to be a risk factor for the development of eating disorders (Tuschl, 1990). The rigid controls that could be considered as risk factors for such a subsequent total breakdown of controls can be described as a dichotomous 'all-or-nothing' approach to weight and eating; it implies extreme behaviours, such as attempts to totally avoid sweets and liked foods. The flexible controls are rather characterized by a 'more-or-less' approach that can be adopted as a longer term task (Westenhoefer, 2001). This suggests, that rigid controls should not be encouraged in the treatment of obese patients, although flexible controls should be supported.

Binge eating

Binge eating constitutes a more pronounced problem in obese eating behaviour, which has been recognized in the last few decades (Stunkard, 1959). The prevailing suggested definition of binge eating (binge eating disorder), although still not a formal diagnosis, includes the consumption of large quantities of food without being in control of this behaviour, and also experiencing distress about the binge eating (American Psychiatric Association, 1994).

Binge eating at entry has predicted greater subsequent weight regain (McGuire *et al.*, 1999b). Gainers had more binge episodes per month in the initial assessment, and had also increased their number of binge episodes at 1-year follow-up. A more profound disturbance in obese eating behaviour can thus pose a problem in weight maintenance. Binge eating has also been related to a history of weight cycling (Sherwood *et al.*, 1999), which would reflect prior failures in maintaining weight losses. In obesity surgery, the weight regain after 5 years has been found to be considerably higher in binge eaters than in the patients without binge eating (Pekkarinen *et al.*, 1994).

However, others conclude that binge eating status does seem to be a weak prognostic indicator of weight regain, but that this relationship can be mediated by psychological dysphoria (Sherwood *et al.*, 1999). In yet other studies, binge eating has not been related to long-term weight loss outcome (Gladis *et al.*, 1998). Such a finding would suggest that although binge eating obviously implies more profound difficulties with eating behaviour, the binge eaters could also benefit from standard obesity treatment programmes.

Self-monitoring

Self-monitoring means observing oneself and one's behaviour. Self-monitoring of body weight and food intake are important factors in weight loss as well as weight loss maintenance (Wing and Hill, 2001). Regularly weighing oneself is an example of self-monitoring, as is recording the food intake consumed. Self-monitoring of food intake is suggested to reflect one component of cognitive restraint known to be important for weight control. It could also be suggested that these persons continue to use self-monitoring strategies that have been learned during the treatment phase (Wing and Hill, 2001). In weight regainers, self-monitoring has been shown to decline with time (McGuire *et al.*, 1999b).

Stress and coping

Experiencing stressful life events has been associated with weight regain (Gormally *et al.*, 1980; Gormally and Rardin, 1981; Dubbert and Wilson, 1984). It may, more specifically, be the ability to cope with stress that is crucial for the person's possibility to maintain a weight, rather than the actual number of life changes and circumstances that are potential stressors (Gormally and Rardin, 1981; Grilo *et al.*, 1989; Drapkin *et al.*, 1995; Westenhoefer, 2001). Personality factors would contribute to the ability to find coping strategies for use in various life situations, rather than reverting to old eating habits.

The research findings on regainers describe poor coping strategies. A common characteristic identified in regainers is that they tend to eat in response to stressful life events and negative emotions, which can be evoked by stressors in everyday life (Gormally and Rardin, 1981; Kayman *et al.*, 1990). Rather than using direct ways to handle problems in life, it was further common to use escape–avoidance ways of coping, which included eating, sleeping more and passively wishing that the problem would vanish (Kayman *et al.*, 1990). Persons who are likely to regain their weight have also reported being more help-seeking as a way to cope with dietary lapse, such as seeking help from a friend, spouse or family member, or to start a weight loss programme (Dohm *et al.*, 2001). This finding was discussed as suggesting a lack of self-sufficiency or self-efficacy.

Overeating could thus be considered as a poor coping strategy, and as a reflection of the absence of a mobilization of more efficient coping. Being dependent on others for help and having a passive orientation also seem to represent a less successful approach than finding one's own solutions and being more active.

The maintainers were more prone to report using effective problem-solving to cope with demands in life, by finding new solutions to these situations or by using concepts taught in treatment (Gormally and Rardin, 1981). Others have likewise shown that maintainers, compared with regainers, reported being able to cope more easily with cravings (Ferguson *et al.*, 1992), and to use direct coping to counter relapse (Dohm *et al.*, 2001). Such direct coping included treating the relapse as a small mistake, recover and lose weight again, increase exercise and start controlling food intake (Dohm *et al.*, 2001). The weight maintainers were less likely to seek help from others as a way to handle their problem (Dohm *et al.*, 2001).

Attitudes

Persons who were less prone to attribute the reason for their obesity to medical factors have been shown to be more successful in later maintaining weight loss (Ogden, 2000). Moreover, the successful persons were more motivated to lose weight for reasons that related to having confidence in themselves, rather than pressures from others or medical reasons (Ogden, 2000). The confidence factors more specifically included increasing self-esteem—liking and feeling better with oneself.

Retrospective studies of successful weight maintainers have shown more concern with weight, shape and appearance in women successfully maintaining a lower body weight (Colvin and Olson, 1983). The women were described as having developed a 'healthy narcissism' about their appearance and physical condition. This suggests that caring about one's appearance and physical condition is important for the motivation to control body weight. The natural weight development in female adolescents has also been shown to be somewhat less with higher physical appearance self-esteem, as well as social self-esteem (French *et al.*, 1996). It is suggested these women can have higher levels of self-efficacy in weight-controlling behaviours.

Furthermore, the women who had maintained their achieved weight loss were more self-confident and capable of taking responsibility over their lives and were found to assume responsibility for their need to lose weight. They had developed their own personally individualized diets, exercise and maintenance plans, and had also became more active outside the home (Colvin and Olson, 1983). Finding such personally adjusted strategies in weight control could be considered as a sign of psychological strengths and coping abilities, as well as an awareness of one's own role in weight control.

Other results agreeing with the notion that taking responsibility for one's life is important for weight development have shown that maintainers attribute their success to their own determination and patience (Ferguson *et al.*, 1992). The specific responses given were often related to having a definitive commitment and making up one's mind. Autonomy seen in autonomous motivation has furthermore predicted more regular attendance at a weight loss programme, and also better weight loss maintenance (Williams *et al.*, 1996).

Personality

The psychological findings suggest these are important aspects to consider in understanding obesity-related behaviour. The underlying personality characteristics enabling a more comprehensive understanding of the various behavioural manifestations are, however, so far insufficiently studied in the research on weight development. According to a study that has used the personality inventory Karolinska Scale of Personality (KSP) (Schalling and Edman, 1993) related to treatment outcome, scores of *anxiety*, *monotony avoidance* and *suspiciousness* were negatively related to weight loss maintenance, whereas *socialization* positively related to weight loss maintenance (Jönsson *et al.*, 1986). Others have, however, concluded that the personality traits measured by KSP did not appear to be important predictors of weight loss or relapse in obesity treatment (Poston *et al.*, 1999). Considering the positive findings, such a trend would suggest that healthier personality traits imply better chances to maintain the weight loss, whereas traits reflecting more of a disturbance can imply somewhat worse prerequisites.

Other studies on personality specifically aiming at weight loss maintenance are sparse. The data from the self-report inventory, the Minnesota Multiphasic Personality Inventory (MMPI or MMPI-2) (Dahlstrom *et al.*, 1982), have generally given little or no predictive information about subsequent weight loss (Grana *et al.*, 1989; Lauer *et al.*, 1996). Some scant findings have been reported, such as hypochondria, predicting poorer treatment outcome in bariatric surgery, as rated by the surgeons 4 years later (Webb *et al.*, 1990).

Depression

Depression has sometimes been associated with weight regain. More self-reported depressive symptoms at an initial assessment after weight loss have been associated with weight regain, although it did not contribute as a predictor (McGuire *et al.*, 1999b), and lower levels of depression, have been associated with recovery from relapse (Phelan *et al.*, 2003). Others have shown no relationship between depression and weight maintenance, although there was a negative relationship to weight loss at the end of active treatment (Wadden *et al.*, 1992). Some negative impact of depression on weight loss maintenance could thus be considered. It could be suggested that the participants with depression at entry to a weight loss treatment have not received a treatment that is fully targeting their problems.

Weight cycling

Weight cycling refers to the repeated loss and regain of weight, although there is no standard definition for weight cycling (National Task Force on the Prevention and Treatment of Obesity, 1994). A history of weight cycling has been found to be associated with weight regain after obesity treatment (Haus *et al.*, 1994; McGuire *et al.*, 1999b). Likewise, patients reporting repeated dietary attempts that are related to weight cycling have been found to be more prone to regain weight (Pasman *et al.*, 1999). It has been suggested that weight maintenance behaviours, such as reduced dietary fat and physical exercise, should be trained before new weight reduction attempts for these patients (Haus *et al.*, 1994).

Weight cycling is important to consider here, as it represents failure in weight maintenance followed by renewed attempts to reduce weight. Weight cycling has sometimes been associated with mental distress and psychopathology (Brownell and Rodin, 1994; Foreyt *et al.*, 1995), although others have found no such relationship (Simkin-Silverman *et al.*, 1998). They conclude that weight cycling does not seem to impact on psychological health in an aversive way (Simkin-Silverman *et al.*, 1998). Considering the positive research findings, mental distress could, of course, also characterize the person being more prone to diet and also having more difficulties in sustaining the weight lost, rather than being a consequence.

More disturbed eating behaviours and a higher prevalence of binge eating have also been noted (Brownell and Rodin, 1994). The greater the number of weight loss efforts, the greater the occurrence or severity of binge eating. Whether weight cycling causes binge eating or the reverse could not, however, be concluded.

Furthermore, the body weight variability in weight cycling is more definitely related to negative health outcomes, such as cardiovascular disease and increased mortality (Brownell and Rodin, 1994). Some results also suggest short-term changes in weight may be related to long-term increase of body weight and more obesity (Jeffery *et al.*, 2002).

Methodological considerations in research on weight loss maintenance

The studies reported are not free from methodological objections. Furthermore, we have reported significant factors found in separate studies that have not always have been replicated in other studies. Physical activity is, for example, not always related to weight loss maintenance, or is not important in overall models including other factors (Dohm *et al.*, 2001). Furthermore, it has been claimed that very few dietary factors have been shown to be clearly associated with obesity using evidence-based principles and long-term evaluation of weight loss. Only fat and energy density have been firmly found to be positively associated with obesity (Astrup, 2003).

It has been suggested that there is a need for more trials to understand the strategies for successful long-term weight loss maintenance, using improved methodology. In most of the studies so far, the individual importance of each contributing factor has not been well isolated, and it is often difficult to understand whether fat reduction, high-fibre or -protein diets, physical activity or behavioural changes play the major role in achieving the desired effects. Astrup concludes that future clinical trials should take the following facts into consideration:

• Patient attention, food provision and visits must be standardized.
• Compliance must be checked by the use of biological markers.
• Intake of non-fat dietary components must be standardized.
• Lifestyle changes must be described in detail.
• Gene–nutrient interaction must be evaluated, the last issue clearly a question for future research once such genes have been better identified.

Furthermore, the role of different treatments and the patient–treatment interaction should be noted. Factors in weight loss and weight loss maintenance are mostly considered to be very general. This may be so with some factors, but other predictors of treatment outcomes in obesity may be more specifically related to the type of treatment evaluated. For example, obesity surgery creates quite a different situation for weight maintenance than does behaviour modification, and each of these situations may be better suited to patients with different characteristics. One study has shown that patients with substantial weight loss by means of surgery or non-surgical means did differ in their behaviours to maintain weight losses. The surgical group reported eating considerably more dietary intake of fat and less carbohydrate and protein than the non-surgical control subjects, and further had lower levels of physical activity (Klem *et al.*, 2000b). Different pretreatment characteristics of the patients succeeding in two such different treatment conditions would perhaps be even more intriguing. Behaviour modification programmes with therapeutic interventions helping the patient to recognize and deal with emotions would further help some patients to eat less, whereas receiving nutritional knowledge and help in creating more structure over eating and lifestyle behaviour will target the needs of others, manifested by different weight loss patterns. Pharmacological treatments also create very specific prerequisites for weight loss and weight maintenance if the drug is used on a more prolonged basis. A satiety-enhancing drug, for example, may give the most striking results for patients who are particularly vulnerable to the need for food and the influence of physical demand states such as hunger (Elfhag *et al.*, 2003a). A drug working locally by reducing the fat absorption may be more efficacious for others. As the drug creates aversive side-effects if dietary prescriptions are not adhered to, the forced necessity to pay more attention to food consumed and the adherence to better eating habits could perhaps provide help related to self-monitoring and meal structure. These are examples to illustrate how future research could more specifically consider the type of treatment interventions in relation to the individual characteristics. Increasing such knowledge may make optimal individual treatment choices possible, leading to better long-term results.

Thus, clearly, we need to better understand why weight maintenance is so difficult, and how it can be promoted. A key question may be if physiology, psychology or a combination of these factors can give us more understanding of the mechanisms of weight loss maintenance (Wing, 2003), and others suggest the psychological factors in weight maintenance can be of particular importance and should be more focused (Byrne, 2002). We also suggest the type of treatment evaluated should be more considered. One type of treatment approach may suit some persons well, whereas quite another approach would suit others, and this will lead to different patterns concerning the maintenance of weight loss.

The issue of measurement used to evaluate long-term outcomes in obesity should also be addressed. Abdominal fat was earlier described as being a possibly even more relevant measure of the health-related consequences of being obese, and could also be considered as a follow-up measure. Using waist circumference as a measure would also circumvent the misleading information provided by body weight for patients increasing their physical activity and thus muscle mass. Increase in muscle mass and decrease of fat tissue may lead to an unchanged total weight despite a dramatic metabolic improvement. Focusing on waist circumference will also spare some patients the disappointment in seeing no result on the scale.

The successful weight maintainer

To summarize the findings on factors affecting weight loss maintenance that we have described, a profile characterizing the 'successful weight maintainer' can be suggested. This ideal person starts losing weight successfully quite early in treatment and reaches the self-determined weight loss goal. Our ideal weight maintainer leads an active life, spending less time watching television and rather more time on activities such as walking and cycling. He or she is in control over eating behaviour and is not overly disturbed by hunger. Food intake is kept at a lower level, meal rhythm is regular, always including breakfast, and healthy foods are chosen in favour of high-fat food. Snacking is reduced. Cravings can somehow be dealt with. If experiencing a relapse though, our weight maintainer can manage to handle this in a balanced way without exaggerating this as a detrimental failure. Controls are flexible rather than rigid and there is a self-sufficiency and autonomy.

Although personality findings were sparse in the research on weight loss, some conclusions can be inferred from the overall findings in the literature. A consistent pattern emerges in which the person likely to succeed in maintaining a lower body weight has a personality functioning with more strengths and stability.

Such strengths include a capacity for control and flexible thinking and also the ability to cope with relapse rather than to revert to a dichotomous all-or-none thinking. The ability to create and sustain a meal structure and alter food habits can also imply psychological resources and capacities. Finding coping strategies to handle cravings and stressful situations in life reflect an ability to use creativity and thinking, and come up with one's own solutions. Self-monitoring suggests self-awareness, and self-sufficiency and autonomy would likewise constitute strengths.

Not surprisingly, this ideal weight maintainer has fewer inner afflictions and instability such as mental distress, binge eating and weight cycling, but instead more stability of weight patterns, eating and emotions. There may be more of an internal motivation for weight loss, with wishes to become more confident and feel better about oneself. A healthy narcissism implying that there is at least some energy invested in oneself, with caring for oneself, one's appearance and physical status, can also be considered as strength.

The regainer has instead more affliction and difficulties in self-management, and less efficient ways to handle obstacles in weight maintenance. It seems that a psychological view could give more understanding of obesity behaviours. More severe problems related to eating and obesity, as considered from a personality perspective, can contribute to an explanation of poorer weight loss results from traditional treatment programmes (Elfhag *et al.*, 2004). In accordance with this psychological pattern, research has shown that middle-aged women who had kept a lean body weight had better psychosocial adaptation and psychological health (Baghaei *et al.*, 2002).

The possibility of biological disturbances causing greater hunger that contributes to the factors found in the weight regainers should also be considered. Struggling with hunger would lead to some of the behavioural manifestations such as disinhibition, binge eating and cravings, and also to an overall discouragement and impaired self-confidence. For a listing of factors associated with weight loss maintenance and weight regain, see Tables 27.1 and 27.2.

Treatment considerations

Despite the encouraging health benefits from weight loss maintenance, there are great risks that weight regain will occur once intervention has ceased. Obesity is difficult to treat and the long-term weight loss outcome is generally modest in various types of treatment programmes (Wooley and Garner, 1991; Lean, 1998).

Just as with any other medication, obesity treatment, whether with diet or pharmacotherapy, will only work if the

Table 27.1 Suggested factors associated with weight loss maintenance as described in the text.

Has achieved the self-determined weight loss goal
More initial weight loss
Physically active lifestyle
Regular meal rhythm
Breakfast eating
Less dietary fat, more healthy foods
Reduced frequency of snacks
Flexible control over eating
Self-monitoring
Better coping strategies
Can find ways to handle craving
Self-efficacy
Autonomy
'Healthy narcissism'
Motivation for weight loss: becoming more confident
Socialization

Table 27.2 Suggested factors associated with weight regain as described in the text.

Fails to reach a self-determined weight goal
Attribution of obesity to medical factors
History of weight cycling
Sedentary lifestyle
Disinhibited eating
More hunger
Binge eating
Eating in response to negative emotions and stress
Depression
Distress
Poor coping strategies
Escape–avoidance to problem
Passive wishes
Help seeking
Motivation for weight loss: medical reasons, other persons
Personality traits indicating more disturbances

treatment interventions are incorporated and adhered to or the medication is taken. Realization of this problem leads to different views when considering the management of obesity. One view considers obesity as a chronic condition as a starting point, whereas another view is to regard the responsibility being with the patient. Some important targets in treatment that may aid long-term management of obesity are also suggested.

Obesity as a chronic condition

One trend in understanding the treatment principles for obesity emanates from the realization that obesity is a chronic disease, and that long-term treatment strategies are essential from the beginning. The characteristics of treatment from the 1980s was a programme lasting less than half a year. Maintenance programmes of longer duration, such as 1 or 2 years, are now more often recommended. Today many standard programmes, based on diet, exercise and behaviour modification, run for up to 2 years, and some of them for longer.

It has been claimed that behavioural change can only be achieved if treatment involves a long-lasting training process (Westenhoefer, 2001). Several programmes have taken into account the fact that obese patients need a long time to adjust to a new healthier lifestyle. In the behavioural modification process, changes are introduced one by one, and most patients start to make the changes in their lives with which it is easiest to comply. The experience of our day-care unit is that basic behavioural changes, such as re-establishing a proper eating pattern with breakfast, lunch and dinner, may take a long time to achieve. Training obese patients to eat according to the Swedish so-called plate model, where one-half of the plate is filled with vegetables (raw or cooked), one quarter with a carbohydrate portion (rice, potatoes, pasta, bread) and the last quarter with a protein component (meet, fowl, egg, fish, shellfish, etc.) as recommended by the Swedish food agency, may take considerable time to become an inherent part of a new eating style.

Targets in treatment

Eating more regular meals and making better food choices that result from behaviour modification programmes were also recognized as factors contributing to weight maintenance. Several of the other factors identified and described are also incorporated into standard behaviour modification programmes. Such treatments are based on restriction of calories and increased physical activity. Behavioural interventions targeting eating behaviour, cognitions and feelings that are related to food and eating, and self-monitoring of behaviours are also integrated parts of such programmes. Recording food intake for several days is an example of training self-monitoring behaviours. Learning to deal with emotions and cognitions that can lead to overeating require new coping strategies. The training of self-control and the handling of situations implying risk for overeating are also stressed (Wadden, 1993; Allison, 1995; Melin and Rössner, 2003).

This means that the standard programmes at present are already targeting some crucial factors that are important for weight maintenance. Some other factors that are not always integrated parts of treatment programmes should also be mentioned.

To start with, some pretreatment factors should be considered. Special attention may be warranted for patients with pretreatment characteristics such as depression, binge eating and a history of weight cycling, although there are conflicting research findings on the role of these factors in weight mainte-

nance. Excluding patients with these features would, however, not be warranted, as these patients could be in greater distress about their situation, having previously attempted to diet. This may mean that they are in even more need of help. It is a challenge to find the treatment interventions that do address the needs of such patients.

Striving for positive goals in weight loss, such as feeling better with oneself rather than starting treatment because of outer pressure, could also be addressed before starting treatment.

Modifying unrealistic weight loss goals may be an important initial task in treatment (Rössner, 1992). It is essential for patients and therapists to realize at the outset that weight loss will hardly ever be up to expectations. This is even more crucial when considering the importance of having achieved a self-determined weight loss goal when it comes to long-term results.

Furthermore, initial weight loss is often related to better long-term results, meaning that the patients who are likely to succeed can be identified quite early in treatment. A run-in period may even be suggested, and the patients who resist losing weight could be moved to other treatment interventions. This would be a cost-effective way, as well as sparing the patient disappointment later in time.

In treatment, it seems important for patients to learn how to handle stress in their life situations. Providing support for developing self-sufficiency and finding inner strengths, ideas and capacities would be essential for long-term results. Treatments putting the participant in a passive patient role should perhaps be particularly avoided in obesity treatments.

Feeling good about oneself seen in the 'healthy narcissism' should also be noted. This could be promoted by acknowledging the importance of feeling more attractive and liking oneself more, and recognizing the enjoyment in taking good care of body, appearance and health.

Other factors that have been less researched could, of course, prove to be equally or even more important in weight maintenance. For example, there are results showing that treatments combining diet with group therapy could be more successful than diet combined with more traditional interventions (Ayyad and Andersen, 2000). This would suggest that the patients who were given an opportunity to work with their underlying emotions, needs and thoughts have better resolved their problems with obesity behaviours. In our clinic, we have identified difficulties with emotions and an overall more complex psychological pattern that may be related to eating and staying obese in a subgroup of obese patients (Elfhag *et al.*, 2003b). Patients with such characteristics may need more therapeutically oriented interventions.

Strategies for the long-term treatment

Interventions providing a more long-term perspective would be of clinical interest. This does not necessarily mean that patients need to be continuously treated. It would, however, be a challenge to develop more longer term-based strategies and recommendations. Introduction of weight loss by any standard method such as diet, exercise, behaviour modification, very low-calorie diets or pharmacotherapy will always be a first step. Strategies that have been less tested in long-term programmes could include aspects such as weight loss maintenance with supervised booster sessions or other means. Possibly also by the addition of a pharmacological agent at a lower dose or given in repeated periods. The weight maintenance phase would also include strategies to immediately detect and treat weight relapse such as initiation of pharmacotherapy or other active interventions if weight exceeds a preset threshold. Risk situations may include patients facing a period in their lives when they may have less ability to comply with a strict new dietary regimen. Life changes such as starting a new job, getting married or having children, as well as diseases and long-term sick leave, are some examples of challenges in the life situation. Seasonal variations in food intake due to holidays or mood fluctuations, such as those related to seasonal affective disorder (SAD), may also make treatment compliance more difficult.

The role of pharmacotherapy in this long-term strategy is far from clear. Treatment could be given with standard doses when weight exceeds a preset threshold. Intermittent treatment has been found to be effective with sibutramine (Wirth and Krause, 2001) and could be used to lower the total exposure to a drug, which is to be used for several years ahead. Treatment combinations with drugs with various modes of action, possibly at lower doses, could form an alternative strategy (see Chapter 25).

Are long-term interventions necessary for weight maintenance?

As a consequence of the chronic condition approach, many standard programmes continue over longer periods of time. However, such considerable treatment interventions have also been questioned. It has been argued that such extended treatment periods are of little benefit to the patient. Finnish therapists have suggested that what is achieved during the first year is all that can be achieved, and with extended programmes only attrition problems arise, whereas little else can be gained other than frustration (Kaukua *et al.*, 2003).

Another crucial question is if these interventions actually can lessen patients' motivation to take responsibility for their lifestyle changes (Mustajoki and Pekkarinen, 1999). As treatment of longer durations demands considerable resources, and as the obesity epidemic implies, there are far from sufficient resources to treat the increasing number of obese patients referred to obesity clinics, the cost-effectiveness of programmes is becoming more and more crucial. It has been suggested that weight reduction programmes lasting 4–6 months can be developed to promote subsequent weight loss mainte-

nance. Supporting the patient's full responsibility for lifestyle changes is then one of the essential components from the onset of treatment.

A less costly weight loss maintenance intervention using the Internet has been compared to therapist-led interventions, and the results revealed there were no differences in weight loss between the groups, although the therapist-led group was more satisfied with their group assignment (Harvey-Berino *et al.*, 2002a). Such results suggest that there can be less costly and equally effective ways to promote a positive weight development. Long-term weight maintenance was, however, better for the patients in the in-person therapist support (Harvey-Berino *et al.*, 2002b).

Alternative medicine

As long-term weight loss maintenance may be difficult to achieve, numerous alternative approaches have been tried. A critical analysis using Cochrane methodology was recently presented by the Swedish Council of Technology Assessment in Health Care (The Swedish Council on Technology Assessment in Health Care, 2002). In this extensive analysis, searches were carried out in Medline, Cochrane library and M-base and, furthermore, Chinese databases were analysed. Applied search words were *obesity* and *alternative medicine*. In total, 517 papers were identified, out of which 81 were found to be original clinical studies. Out of these, only 11 fulfilled the minimal criteria for appropriate long-term treatment strategies with adequate methodology. Most studies on alternative therapies were found to be of short duration, and of those accepted three were of moderately high scientific value, whereas the others were regarded as poor. Two studies on hypnosis were among those considered to be scientifically acceptable with a follow-up period of up to 2 years. One of these studies showed positive effects of hypnosis, whereas the other did not (Goldstein, 1981; Cochrane and Friesen, 1986).

A couple of studies on acupuncture were not adequately designed scientifically or were of such low scientific value that no conclusions could be drawn. The interesting aspect of the Swedish analyses was that it was possible to receive access to Chinese databases, which are often omitted in meta-analyses for linguistic reasons. Here, 50 such references were scrutinized but no conclusions about the value of these alternative therapies could be drawn.

Alternative ways of approaching obesity are of interest for future attempts to broaden the choice of interventions. Given the importance of the patients' active role and self-sufficiency in long-term weight loss results, this may also be considered in the various alternative treatments. Whereas hypnosis, for example, implies the patient is assigned a passive role with something 'being done' to him or her, an intervention, for example transcendental meditation, which has been tried in areas including cardiovascular risks and stress (Alexander *et al.*, 1996; Roth and Creaser, 1997; Vyas and

Dikshit, 2002), suggests that the person will accomplish changes by their own means.

References

Alexander, C.N., Schneider, R.H., Staggers, F., Sheppard, W., Clayborne, B.M., Rainforth, M., Salerno, J., Kondwani, K., Smith, S., Walton, K.G. and Egan, B. (1996) Trial of stress reduction for hypertension in older African Americans. II. Sex and risk subgroup analysis. *Hypertension* **28**, 228–237.

Allison, D.B. (1995) *Handbook of Assessment Methods for Eating Behaviours and Weight-related Concerns*. Thousand Oaks, CA: Sage Publications.

American Psychiatric Association (1994) *Diagnostic and Statistical Manual of Mental Disorders. DSM-IV*. Washington, DC: APA.

Astrup, A. (2003) Dietary fat and obesity: still an important issue. *Scandinavian Journal of Nutrition* **47**, 50–57.

Astrup, A. and Rössner, S. (2000) Lessons from obesity management programmes: greater initial weight loss improves long-term maintenance. *Obesity Reviews* **1**, 17–19.

Ayyad, C. and Andersen, T. (2000) Long-term efficacy of dietary treatment of obesity: a systematic review of studies published between 1931 and 1999. *Obesity Reviews* **1**, 113–119.

van Baak, M.A., van Mil, E., Astrup, A.V., Finer, N., Van Gaal, L.F., Hilsted, J., Kopelman, P.G., Rössner, S., James, W.P. and Saris, W.H. (2003) Leisure-time activity is an important determinant of long-term weight maintenance after weight loss in the Sibutramine Trial on Obesity Reduction and Maintenance (STORM trial). *American Journal of Clinical Nutrition* **78**, 209–214.

Baghaei, F., Rosmond, R., Westberg, L., Hellstrand, M., Landen, M., Eriksson, E., Holm, G. and Bjorntorp, P. (2002) The lean woman. *Obesity Research* **10**, 115–121.

Bigaard, J., Tjonneland, A., Thomsen, B.L., Overvad, K., Heitmann, B.L. and Sorensen, T.I. (2003) Waist circumference, BMI, smoking, and mortality in middle-aged men and women. *Obesity Research* **11**, 895–903.

Björvell, H. and Rössner, S. (1985) Long term treatment of severe obesity: four year follow up of results of combined behavioural modification programme. *British Medical Journal (Clin Res Ed)* **291**, 379–382.

Björvell, H. and Rössner, S. (1992) A ten-year follow-up of weight change in severely obese subjects treated in a combined behavioural modification programme. *International Journal of Obesity and Related Metabolic Disorders* **16**, 623–625.

Björvell, H., Aly, A., Langius, A. and Nordström, G. (1994) Indicators of changes in weight and eating behaviour in severely obese patients treated in a nursing behavioural program. *International Journal of Obesity* **18**, 521–525.

Brownell, K.D. and Rodin, J. (1994) Medical, metabolic, and psychological effects of weight cycling. *Archives of Internal Medicine* **154**, 1325–1330.

Byrne, S.M. (2002) Psychological aspects of weight maintenance and relapse in obesity. *Journal of Psychosomatic Research* **53**, 1029–1036.

Cochrane, G. and Friesen, J. (1986) Hypnotherapy in weight loss treatment. *Journal of Consulting and Clinicial Psychology* **54**, 489–492.

Colvin, R.H. and Olson, S.B. (1983) A descriptive analysis of men and women who have lost significant weight and are highly successful at maintaining the loss. *Addictive Behaviour* **8**, 287–295.

Cooper, Z. and Fairburn, C.G. (2001) A new cognitive–behavioural approach to the treatment of obesity. *Behaviour Research and Therapy* **39**, 499–511.

Cuntz, U., Leibbrand, R., Ehrig, C., Shaw, R. and Fichter, M.M. (2001) Predictors of post-treatment weight reduction after in-patient behavioral therapy. *International Journal of Obesity and Related Metabolic Disorders* **25** (Suppl. 1), S99–S101.

Dahlstrom, W.G., Welsh, G.S. and Dahlstom, L.E. (1982) *An MMPI Handbook. Vol. 1. Clinical Interpretation*. Minneapolis, MN: University of Minnesota Press.

Dohm, F.A., Beattie, J.A., Aibel, C. and Striegel-Moore, R.H. (2001) Factors differentiating women and men who successfully maintain weight loss from women and men who do not. *Journal of Clinical Psychology* **57**, 105–117.

Drapkin, R.G., Wing, R.R. and Shiffman, S. (1995) Responses to hypothetical high risk situations: do they predict weight loss in a behavioral treatment program or the context of dietary lapses? *Health Psychology* **14**, 427–434.

Dubbert, P.M. and Wilson, G.T. (1984) Goal-setting and spouse involvement in the treatment of obesity. *Behaviour Research and Therapy* **22**, 227–242.

Elfhag, K., Rössner, S., Carlsson, A.-M. and Barkeling, B. (2003a) Sibutramine treatment in obesity: predictors of weight loss including Rorschach personality data. *Obesity Research* **11**, 1391–1399.

Elfhag, K., Carlsson, A.-M. and Rössner, S. (2003b) Subgrouping in obesity based on Rorschach personality characteristics. *Scandinavian Journal of Psychology* **44**, 399–407.

Elfhag, K., Rössner, S., Lindgren, T., Andersson, I. and Carlsson, A.-M. (2004) Rorschach personality predictors of weight loss with behavior modification in obesity treatment. *Journal of Personality Assessment* **3**, 293–305.

Ferguson, K.J., Brink, P.J., Wood, M. and Koop, P.M. (1992) Characteristics of successful dieters as measured by guided interview responses and Restraint Scale scores. *Journal of the American Dietetic Association* **92**, 1119–1121.

Foreyt, J.P., Brunner, R.L., Goodrick, G.K., Cutter, G., Brownell, K.D. and St Jeor, S.T. (1995) Psychological correlates of weight fluctuation. *International Journal of Eating Disorders* **17**, 263–275.

Foster, G.D., Wadden, T.A., Vogt, R.A. and Brewer, G. (1997) What is a reasonable weight loss? Patients' expectations and evaluations of obesity treatment outcomes. *Journal of Consulting and Clinical Psychology* **65**, 79–85.

Foster, G.D., Wadden, T.A., Phelan, S., Sarwer, D.B. and Sanderson, R.S. (2001) Obese patients' perceptions of treatment outcomes and the factors that influence them. *Archives of Internal Medicine* **161**, 2133–2139.

French, S.A., Jeffery, R.W., Forster, J.L., McGovern, P.G., Kelder, S.H. and Baxter, J.E. (1994) Predictors of weight change over two years among a population of working adults: the Healthy Worker Project. *International Journal of Obesity and Related Metabolic Disorders* **18**, 145–154.

French, S.A., Perry, C.L., Leon, G.R. and Fulkerson, J. A. (1996) Self-esteem and change in body mass index over 3 years in a cohort of adolescents. *Obesity Research* **4**, 27–33.

Gladis, M.M., Wadden, T.A., Vogt, R., Foster, G., Kuehnel, R.H. and Bartlett, S. J. (1998) Behavioral treatment of obese binge eaters: do they need different care? *Journal of Psychosomatic Research* **44**, 375–384.

Goldstein, D.J. (1992) Beneficial health effects of modest weight loss. *International Journal of Obesity* **16**, 397–415.

Goldstein, Y. (1981) The effect of demonstrating to a subject that she is in a hypnotic trance as a variable in hypnotic interventions with obese women. *International Journal of Clinical and Experimental Hypnosis* **29**, 15–23.

Gormally, J. and Rardin, D. (1981) Weight loss and maintenance and changes in diet and exercise for behavioral counseling and nutrition education. *Journal of Counselling Psychology* **28**, 295–304.

Gormally, J., Rardin, D. and Black, S. (1980) Correlates of successful response to a behavioral weight control clinic. *Journal of Counselling Psychology* **27**, 179–191.

Grana, A.S., Coolidge, F. L. and Merwin, M.M. (1989) Personality profiles in the morbidly obese. *Journal of Clinical Psychology* **45**, 762–765.

Grilo, C.M., Shiffman, S. and Wing, R.R. (1989) Relapse crises and coping among dieters. *Journal of Consulting and Clinical Psychology* **57**, 488–495.

Han, T.S., van Leer, E. M., Seidell, J.C. and Lean, M.E. (1995) Waist circumference action levels in the identification of cardiovascular risk factors: prevalence study in a random sample. *British Medical Journal* **311**, 1401–1405.

Harris, J.K., French, S.A., Jeffery, R.W., McGovern, P.G. and Wing, R.R. (1994) Dietary and physical activity correlates of long-term weight loss. *Obesity Research* **2**, 307–313.

Harvey-Berino, J., Pintauro, S., Buzzell, P., DiGiulio, M., Casey Gold, B., Moldovan, C. and Ramirez, E. (2002a) Does using the Internet facilitate the maintenance of weight loss? *International Journal of Obesity and Related Metabolic Disorders* **26**, 1254–1260.

Harvey-Berino, J., Pintauro, S. J. and Gold, E.C. (2002b) The feasibility of using Internet support for the maintenance of weight loss. *Behaviour Modification* **26**, 103–116.

Haus, G., Hoerr, S.L., Mavis, B. and Robison, J. (1994) Key modifiable factors in weight maintenance: fat intake, exercise, and weight cycling. *Journal of the American Dietetic Association* **94**, 409–413.

Holden, J.H., Darga, L.L., Olson, S.M., Stettner, D.C., Ardito, E.A. and Lucas, C.P. (1992) Long-term follow-up of patients attending a combination very-low calorie diet and behaviour therapy weight loss programme. *International Journal of Obesity and Related Metabolic Disorders* **16**, 605–613.

James, W.P. (1984) Dietary aspects of obesity. *Postgraduate Medical Journal* **60** (Suppl. 3), 50–55.

Jeffrey, R.W., Bjornson-Benson, W.M., Rosenthal, B.S., Kurth, C.L. and Dunn, M.M. (1984) Effectiveness of monetary contracts with two repayment schedules on weight reduction in men and women from self-referred population samples. *Preventative Medicine* **15**, 273–279.

Jeffery, R.W., McGuire, M.T. and French, S.A. (2002) Prevalence and correlates of large weight gains and losses. *International Journal of Obesity and Related Metabolic Disorders* **26**, 969–972.

Jönsson, B., Björvell, H., Levander, S. and Rössner, S. (1986) Personality traits predicting weight loss outcome in obese patients. *Acta Psychiatrica Scandinavica* **74**, 384–387.

Karlsson, J., Hallgren, P., Kral, J., Lindroos, A.K., Sjöström, L. and Sullivan, M. (1994) Predictors and effects of long-term dieting on mental well-being and weight loss in obese women. *Appetite* **23**, 15–26.

Karlsson, J., Sjöstrom, L. and Sullivan, M. (1998) Swedish obese subjects (SOS): an intervention study of obesity. Two-year follow-up of health-related quality of life (HRQL) and eating behavior after gastric surgery for severe obesity. *International Journal of Obesity and Related Metabolic Disorders* **22**, 113–126.

Kathan, M., Pleas, J., Thackery, M. and Wallston, K.A. (1982) Relationship of eating activity self-reports to follow-up weight maintenance of obesity. *Behaviour Therapy* **13**, 521–528.

Kaukua, J., Pekkarinen, T., Sane, T. and Mustajoki, P. (2003) Health-related quality of life in obese outpatients losing weight with very-low-energy diet and behaviour modification: a 2-year follow-up study. *International Journal of Obesity and Related Metabolic Disorders* **27**, 1072–1080.

Kayman, S., Bruvold, W. and Stern, J. S. (1990) Maintenance and relapse after weight loss in women: behavioral aspects. *American Journal of Clinical Nutrition* **52**, 800–807.

Klem, M.L., Wing, R.R., McGuire, M.T., Seagle, H.M. and Hill, J.O. (1998) Psychological symptoms in individuals successful at long-term maintenance of weight loss. *Health Psychology* **17**, 336–345.

Klem, M.L., Wing, R.R., Lang, W., McGuire, M.T. and Hill, J.O. (2000a) Does weight loss maintenance become easier over time? *Obesity Research* **8**, 438–444.

Klem, M.L., Wing, R.R., Chang, C.C., Lang, W., McGuire, M.T., Sugerman, H.J., Hutchison, S.L., Makovich, A.L. and Hill, J.O. (2000b) A case-control study of successful maintenance of a substantial weight loss: individuals who lost weight through surgery versus those who lost weight through non-surgical means. *International Journal of Obesity and Related Metabolic Disorders* **24**, 573–579.

Kuskowska-Wolk, A. and Rössner, S. (1990) Body mass distribution of a representative adult population in Sweden. *Diabetes Research and Clinical Practice* **10** (Suppl. 1), S37–41.

Lauer, J.B., Wampler, R., Lantz, J.B. and Madura, J.A. (1996) MMPI profiles of female candidates for obesity surgery: A cluster analytical approach. *Obesity Surgery* **6**, 28–37.

Lean, M.E. (1998) Obesity: what are the current treatment options? *Experimental and Clinical Endocrinology and Diabetes* **106** (Suppl. 2), 22–26.

Lean, M.E., Han, T.S. and Seidell, J.C. (1998) Impairment of health and quality of life in people with large waist circumference. *Lancet* **351**, 853–856.

Lindroos, A.K., Lissner, L., Mathiassen, M.E., Karlsson, J., Sullivan, M., Bengtsson, C. and Sjöström, L. (1997) Dietary intake in relation to restrained eating, disinhibition, and hunger in obese and nonobese Swedish women. *Obesity Research* **5**, 175–182.

Linne, Y., Hemmingsson, E., Adolfsson, B., Ramsten, J. and Rössner, S. (2002) Patient expectations of obesity treatment—the experience from a day-care unit. *International Journal of Obesity and Related Metabolic Disorders* **26**, 739–741.

McGuire, M.T., Wing, R.R. and Hill, J.O. (1999a) The prevalence of weight loss maintenance among American adults. *International Journal of Obesity and Related Metabolic Disorders* **23**, 1314–1319.

McGuire, M.T., Wing, R.R., Klem, M.L., Lang, W. and Hill, J.O. (1999b) What predicts weight regain in a group of successful weight losers? *Journal of Consulting and Clinical Psychology* **67**, 177–185.

Marston, A.R. and Criss, J. (1984) Maintenance of successful weight loss: incidence and prediction. *International Journal of Obesity* **8**, 435–439.

Melin, I. and Rössner, S. (2003) Practical clinical behavioral treatment of obesity. *Patient Education and Counseling* **49**, 75–83.

Mustajoki, P. and Pekkarinen, T. (1999) Maintenance programmes after weight reduction: how useful are they? *International Journal of Obesity and Related Metabolic Disorders* **23**, 553–555.

National Task Force on the Prevention and Treatment of Obesity. (1994) Weight cycling. *Journal of the American Medical Association* **272**, 1196–1202.

National Task Force on the Prevention and Treatment of Obesity. (2000) Dieting and the development of eating disorders in overweight and obese adults. *Archives of Internal Medicine* **160**, 2581–2589.

Ogden, J. (2000) The correlates of long-term weight loss: a group comparison study of obesity. *International Journal of Obesity and Related Metabolic Disorders* **24**, 1018–1025.

Pasman, W.J., Saris, W.H. and Westerterp-Plantenga, M.S. (1999) Predictors of weight maintenance. *Obesity Research* **7**, 43–50.

Pekkarinen, T., Koskela, K., Huikuri, K. and Mustajoki, P. (1994) Long-term results of gastroplasty for morbid obesity: binge eating as a predictor of poor outcome. *Obesity Surgery* **4**, 248–255.

Poston, 2nd, W.S., Ericsson, M., Linder, J., Nilsson, T., Goodrick, G.K. and Foreyt, J.P. (1999) Personality and the prediction of weight loss and relapse in the treatment of obesity. *International Journal of Eating Disorders* **25**, 301–309.

Rissanen, A., Lean, M., Rössner, S., Segal, K.R. and Sjöstrom, L. (2003) Predictive value of early weight loss in obesity management with orlistat: an evidence-based assessment of prescribing guidelines. *International Journal of Obesity and Related Metabolic Disorders* **27**, 103–109.

Roth, B. and Creaser, T. (1997) Mindfulness meditation-based stress reduction: experience with a bilingual inner-city program. *Nurse Practitioner* **22**, 150–152, 154, 157 passim.

Rössner, S. (1992) Factors determining the long-term outcome of obesity. In: Björntorp, P., Brodoff, B.N. eds. *Obesity*. Philadephia: J.B. Lippincott Co., 712–719.

Saris, W.H. (1998) Fit, fat and fat free: the metabolic aspects of weight control. *International Journal of Obesity and Related Metabolic Disorders* **22** (Suppl. 2), S15–S21.

Schalling, D. and Edman, G. (1993) *The Karolinska Scales of Personality (KSP) Manual: An Inventory for Assessing Temperament Dimensions Associated with Vulnerability for Psychosocial Deviance*. Stockholm, Sweden: Department of Psychiatry, Karolinska Institutet.

Schoeller, D.A., Shay, K. and Kushner, R.F. (1997) How much physical activity is needed to minimize weight gain in previously obese women? *American Journal of Clinical Nutrition* **66**, 551–556.

Sherwood, N.E., Jeffery, R.W. and Wing, R.R. (1999) Binge status as a predictor of weight loss treatment outcome. *International Journal of Obesity and Related Metabolic Disorders* **23**, 485–493.

Simkin-Silverman, L.R., Wing, R.R., Plantinga, P., Matthews, K.A. and Kuller, L.H. (1998) Lifetime weight cycling and psychological health in normal-weight and overweight women. *International Journal of Eating Disorders* **24**, 175–183.

Sjöström, L., Larsson, B., Backman, L., Bengtsson, C., Bouchard, C., Dahlgren, S., Hallgren, P., Jonsson, E., Karlsson, J., Lapidus, L., Lindroos, A.-K., Lindstedt, S., Lissner, L., Narbro, K., Näslund, I., Olbe, L., Sullivan, M., Sylvan, A., Wedel, H. and Ågren, G. (1992) Swedish obese subjects (SOS). Recruitment for an intervention study and a selected description of the obese state. *International Journal of Obesity and Related Metabolic Disorders* **16**, 465–479.

Stunkard, A.J. (1958) The management of obesity. *New York State Journal of Medicine* **58**, 79–87.

Stunkard, A.J. (1959) Eating patterns and obesity. *Psychiatric Quarterly* **33**, 284–292.

Stunkard, A.J. and Messick, S. (1985) The Three Factor Eating Questionnaire to measure dietary restraint, disinhibition and hunger. *Journal of Psychosomatic Research* **29**, 71–83.

Suk, S.-H., Sacco, R.L., Boden-Albala, B., Cheun, J.F., Pittman, J.G., Elkind, M.S. and Paik, M.C. (2003) Abdominal obesity and risk of ischemic stroke. The Northern Manhattan Stroke Study. *Stroke* **34**, 1586.

The Swedish Council on Technology Assessment in Health Care. (2002) *Obesity — Problems and Measures (Fetma — problem och åtgärder)*. Göteborg: Elanders Graphic Systems.

Tuschl, R.J. (1990) From dietary restraint to binge eating: some theoretical considerations. *Appetite* **14**, 105–109.

Vyas, R. and Dikshit, N. (2002) Effect of meditation on respiratory system, cardiovascular system and lipid profile. *Indian Journal of Physiology and Pharmacology* **46**, 487–491.

Wadden, T. A. (1993) The treatment of obesity. In: Stunkard, A.J., Wadden T.A. eds. *Obesity: Theory and Therapy*. New York: Raven.

Wadden, T.A., Foster, G.D., Wang, J., Pierson, R.N., Yang, M.U., Moreland, K., Stunkard, A.J. and VanItallie, T.B. (1992) Clinical correlates of short- and long-term weight loss. *American Journal of Clinical Nutrition* **56**, 21S–24S.

Webb, W.W., Morey, L.C., Castelnuvo-Tedsco, P. and Scott, H.W. (1990) Heterogenity of personality traits in massive obesity and outcome prediction of bariatric surgery. *International Journal of Obesity* **14**, 13–20.

Westenhoefer, J. (2001) The therapeutic challenge: behavioral changes for long-term weight maintenance. *International Journal of Obesity and Related Metabolic Disorders* **25** (Suppl. 1), S85–88.

Williams, G.C., Grow, V.M., Freedman, Z.R., Ryan, R.M. and Deci, E.L. (1996) Motivational predictors of weight loss and weight loss maintenance. *Journal of Personality and Social Psychology* **70**, 115–126.

Wing, R.R. (2003) Behavioral interventions for obesity: recognizing our progress and future challenges. *Obesity Research* **11** (Suppl.), 3S–6S.

Wing, R.R. and Hill, J.O. (2001) Successful weight loss maintenance. *Annual Review of Nutrition* **21**, 323–341.

Wirth, A. and Krause, J. (2001) Long-term weight loss with sibutramine: a randomized controlled trial. *Journal of the American Medical Association* **286**, 1331–1339.

Wooley, S. C. and Garner, D. M. (1991) Obesity treatment: the high cost of false hope. *Journal of the American Dietetic Association* **91**, 1248–1251.

World Health Organization (2000) *Obesity: Preventing and Managing the Global Epidemic*. Report of a WHO consultation. World Health Organization Technical Report Series **894**, i–xii, 1–253.

Wyatt, H.R., Grunwald, G.K., Mosca, C.L., Klem, M.L., Wing, R.R. and Hill, J.O. (2002) Long-term weight loss and breakfast in subjects in the National Weight Control Registry. *Obesity Research* **10**, 78–82.

28 Educating and training health-care professionals

Peter G. Kopelman

Introduction, 421

Why is it important to educate
health professionals about
nutrition?, 421

Where to start?, 422
   Education and training in
   nutrition, 422
   Undergraduate or preregistration
   training, 422

Postgraduate and post-registration
training – continuing professional
development, 423
Training in the management of
overweight and obese patients, 423
Long-term weight
maintenance, 424

Summary, 424

Further reading, 424

Appendix, 424
   Knowledge and understanding
   of obesity, 424
   Diet and nutrition, 424
   Physical activity, 425
   Counselling skills, 426
   Principles of behaviour
   change, 426
   Assessment skills, 426
   Therapeutic intervention, 426

Introduction

The dramatic increase in the prevalence of overweight and obesity has not been matched by an increase in the amount of education and training provided for health professionals, irrespective of their discipline. Too often, health professionals ignore the obvious signs or symptoms of a nutritional disorder within a patient and, if they are overweight, simply instruct the patient to go on a diet. It is therefore not surprising that intervention only comes when medical complications have become apparent. This oversight reflects a poor understanding of nutritional issues and a lack of knowledge and skills about their management. There is limited information provided in both undergraduate and postgraduate training programmes and scant attention in specialist medical training. The medical profession's appreciation of the medical consequences of obesity is reflected by the absence of specialist units in most regional hospitals and reluctance to consider pharmacotherapy or surgery for patients most at risk. As clinical teachers have had little or no training in the subject, they tend not to teach it. As a result, many doctors neglect clinical nutrition through unawareness of its potential benefits in the prevention and treatment of disease.

This chapter will focus first on the education of health professionals in nutritional care and then address the deficiencies in training for the management of overweight and obese patients.

Why is it important to educate health professionals about nutrition?

A health professional's primary role is, by definition, to care for his or her patients. As a consequence, they need to fully understand the fundamentals of nutritional science and be able to apply these in clinical practice. This will facilitate the following associated professional roles:

- *Educational.* Health-care professionals are held in regard by the public as providers of authoritative information and advice on food, health and nutrition. Health-care professionals need to ensure that they remain familiar with up-to-date information concerning nutritional health. This should be regarded as an essential element of their continuing professional development.
- *Advisory.* Health professionals can influence food and nutrition policy in their own hospital setting and within the local community. They should be encouraged to nominate a lead for nutrition and, where appropriate, be involved in nutrition management and the nutrition team. Job plans should reflect the importance of nutrition as a part of weekly duties.
- *Organizational.* Health professionals should be encouraged to initiate or contribute to programmes on nutrition by working as individuals, through professional societies or other health-care organizations. Training must include the management of this kind of work.
- *Investigatory.* Health professionals should be encouraged to consider research into nutritional topics as part of their work.

This should include both applied basic and molecular science as well as clinical investigations. Governments, through the provision of research funding for nutrition, should acknowledge the importance of such research.

Where to start?

Education and training in nutrition

Nutrition fits into every medical discipline. Medical curricula contain a wealth of information that is relevant to diet and nutrition but which generally represents a classical approach through biochemistry and physiology. It remains uncommon for nutrition to be taught as metabolism at the whole body level, thereby enabling health professionals to understand how function is maintained in health and disturbed by disease. However, it is generally acknowledged that many recently trained health professionals still have an inadequate knowledge of the nutritional aspects of health promotion and disease treatment.

The need for better training in human nutrition is now recognized in all disciplines of health care. In the UK, the Government's Nutrition Task Force, created under the Health of the Nation initiative, published in 1994 a 'Core Curriculum for Nutrition in the Education of Health Professionals', which is globally applicable. The curriculum identifies a minimum core of essential knowledge for all health professionals:

The Core Curriculum is divided into three sections:

• *A. Principles of Nutritional Science,* including foods and nutrient, metabolic processes, physical activity, effect of diet and nutrient status on biochemistry and organ function.

• *B. Public Health Nutrition,* including the average diet, lifestyle and risk factors, dietary reference values, nutritional surveillance, education and motivation, food policies and composition.

• *C. Clinical Nutrition and Nutritional Support*:
 – assessment of clinical and functional metabolic state, effect of functional state on nutritional intake and status, effect of status on clinical outcomes;
 – anorexia and starvation, response to injury, infection and stress;
 – altered nutritional requirements in relevant disease states, unusual requirements;
 – general principles of nutritional support, routes of support;
 – basis of nutrition-related diseases, therapeutic diets, weight reduction;
 – drug–nutrient interactions.

The aims of the Core Curriculum were to enable health professionals to:

• appreciate the importance and relevance of nutrition to the promotion of good health, and prevention and treatment of disease;

• describe the basic scientific principles of human nutrition;

• identify nutrition-related problems in individuals and the community;

• give consistent and sound dietary advice;

• provide appropriate and safe clinical nutritional support, and know how and when to refer to a specialist in clinical nutrition.

To implement the Core Curriculum, training of health professionals needs to start at an undergraduate/preregistration level and then continue through into professional training and development.

Undergraduate or preregistration training

Every opportunity should be taken to introduce nutritional concepts into undergraduate training. Nutrition is a key component of health and illness and should be identified as such by students. There is every reason for students to feel engaged with the science and application of nutrition because good nutrition should be a principle followed by themselves. There have been advances in teaching nutrition. However, the time allocated to nutritional issues remains difficult to identify, and information is not available regarding how well nutrition is incorporated into curricula using problem-based learning as the core method of medical education. This needs to be addressed in the following ways:

• Nutrition should be promoted as a model subject for teaching across the entire undergraduate curriculum, and the nutrition being taught should be what a health professional needs to know. Human nutrition can be incorporated as an integrated theme to link basic sciences, clinical and public health aspects of health and disease in the core curriculum.

• Nutrition offers the potential of 'horizontal integration' across disciplines as a component of problem-based approaches. Problem-based learning engages students in small groups to investigate and solve clinically based problems that are presented as case scenarios.

• Nutrition is well suited to project work, particularly for public health nutrition.

• Nutritional screening and assessment should be included as part of the teaching of clinical skills, and students should be instructed about relevant practical skills, such as the assessment of swallowing.

• Nutritional topics should be assessed at all levels throughout undergraduate/preregistration training—the objective-structured clinical examination (OSCE) provides a practical examination format. OSCEs are a series of examination stations in which the student's skills at tackling a common clinical problem are observed at each station by an examiner, who marks the student's performance using a structured mark sheet.

• An agreed procedure for clinical assessment of the nutritional status of patients should be included as a core skill; this should be part of any routine examination.

• Teaching of nutrition should draw widely on available skills across disciplines, including medicine, pharmacy, dietitians and nursing.

Nutritional education must not stop at the time of graduation but continue through the post-graduation period and into continuing professional development.

Postgraduate and post-registration training — continuing professional development

Postgraduate nutritional training should form a continuum with undergraduate training and lead to an appreciation that nutrition is important in all disciplines of medicine. Health professionals should be motivated to regard nutrition as important in the prevention and management of disease. Much of nutritional learning, whether acquiring knowledge or skills, will be acquired in a work-based setting. The major elements will include:

• assessment of nutritional state and its effect on clinical outcomes;
• nutritional requirements in illness and the metabolic effect of injury and infection;
• general principles of nutritional support and routes of support;
• principles of the dietetic management of nutrition-related disorders.

Regular multiprofessional teaching sessions on nutrition should be included as part of training programmes—this should include guidance on nutritional assessment and nutritional requirements in health and disease, and an appreciation of nutrition as a determinant of risk. Topics that should be addressed include:

• *undernutrition*—identification of underlying factors and their management;
• *overweight and obesity*—identification of patients requiring weight reduction and their management;
• *nutritional risk states*—competences in the recognition of suboptimal nutrition, which may contribute to the risk of ill health;
• general principles of nutritional support and the management of starvation.

Health professionals must ensure that a written statement is always made in the clinical notes of patients about their nutritional state as part of the history and physical examination of every new patient. They should be aware of the influence of nutritional status on susceptibility to illness. Every discipline should include an appropriate reference to nutrition in their core curriculum, and questions on nutrition should be included in examinations for higher qualifications. Inclusion of questions on nutrition in professional examinations, and incorporation into assessment procedures, is the key to the acceptance of nutrition by teachers and students as an important and valued subject area.

Crucially, clinical teachers must be encouraged to attend training courses on nutrition—education and training in nutrition will only become successful when a multidisciplinary core of staff is established with the necessary experience and teaching skills.

Training in the management of overweight and obese patients

An increasingly critical element of nutritional care is the management of overweight and obese patients. At present, literature suggests that many health professionals have inadequate and confused knowledge of best practice in obesity management. Among the nursing and dietetic professions, research has highlighted the limited confidence of these health-care workers in their ability to assist patients in their attempts to lose weight. Family doctors often fail to recognize obesity as a serious medical condition, and commonly recommend weight management only when an accompanying comorbidity is evident. Although the assessment of attitudes towards obesity has been limited, available evidence suggests a very negative approach to obese people, with many health professionals believing its management to be frustrating, time consuming and pointless.

Health professionals should understand the aetiology and pathophysiology of increasing body fatness, and appreciate the importance of prevention and intervention when the condition is established. They should also acknowledge the familial basis to obesity and bear this in mind when managing the individual patient. Obesity management may be divided into a modular training programme to enable health professionals to gain knowledge and skills in a stepwise manner. Importantly, this should also facilitate the acquisition of appropriate attitudes towards patients with the condition.

Such programmes will include the following topics:
• knowledge and understanding of overweight and obesity;
• diet and nutrition;
• physical activity;
• counselling skills and principles of behaviour change;
• assessment skills;
• therapeutic interventional skills.

An outline of such a modular programme is provided as an appendix to this chapter.

The aim of such a programme is to better equip health professionals with the knowledge, skills and confidence to help obese and overweight patients to implement lifestyle change. Additionally, it is essential that health professionals are fully aware of when, how and to whom to refer within or outside their multidisciplinary team. Likewise, special groups such as *adolescent and childhood obesity*, *obesity during pregnancy* and *morbid obesity* generally require more specialist input.

Long-term weight maintenance

Patients who lose and maintain significant amounts of lost weight engage in four behavioural patterns:
- They exercise regularly (1500 kcal or more weekly).
- They weigh themselves regularly (daily).
- They eat a low-fat, low-calorie diet.
- They monitor their food intake.

Continuous vigilance appears to be the key. To foster such vigilance, long-term contact by health professionals or support groups is important. Such contact helps maintain motivation, provides encouragement, protects against relapse and provides further opportunities to learn new skills. Ongoing contact with health professionals can help monitor changes and lapses, provide opportunities to change direction when necessary and allow referral to new therapeutic options if required. Continuing contact with a well-motivated and trained multidisciplinary health team is the key to long-term success.

Summary

Successful management of overweight and obesity requires a structured education programme that involves all health professionals and commences at the outset of their training. Health professionals need to be appropriately knowledgeable about the principles of nutrition and nutritional care and be able to apply these principles in practice when managing overweight or obese patients. The implementation of education and training will necessarily involve universities, training colleges for professions allied to medicine, nursing and medical schools, postgraduate medical institutions, health services and governments. However, their longer term success is dependent on the commitment and enthusiasm of present health professionals and all others who are involved in patient care.

Further reading

Centres for Obesity Research and Education (www.uchsc.edu/core).
Department of Health (1995) Nutrition: core curriculum for nutrition in the education of health professionals. In: *Health of the Nation* series. London: Department of Health.
The Intercollegiate Course on Human Nutrition (Royal Medical Colleges, UK) (www.icgnutrition.org.uk).
The Learn® Program for Weight Management 2000 (www.thelifestylecompany.com).

Appendix

Knowledge and understanding of obesity

This covers physiology, genetics, psychobiology, pathophysiology, categorization of obesity types and treatment types of obesity.

Aims

- To enhance awareness and understanding of obesity as a serious medical condition.
- To extend knowledge and understanding of the aetiology of obesity and the physiological consequences of excess weight.
- To recognize the medical importance of modest weight loss and maintenance.

Learning objectives

- To be aware of worldwide and local obesity prevalence and probable trends for the future.
- To understand the definition and classification of obesity/overweight by body mass index.
- To recognize obesity as a chronic disease and to be aware of the medical importance and consequences of overweight/obesity in terms of morbidity and mortality.
- To be aware of the medical complications of obesity and recognize obesity as a risk factor for various comorbidities.
- To understand the influence of abdominal obesity: definition, visceral fat distribution, subcutaneous fat distribution, clinical assessment.
- To understand the direct and indirect costs of obesity.
- To enhance awareness of the social implications of obesity.
- To consider why obesity should be treated and who should be treated.
- To understand the medical benefits of modest weight loss.
- To increase knowledge of the physiology of weight control and the implication of endocrine, neurological and gastrointestinal systems.
- To be aware of the multifactorial aetiology of obesity.
- To be aware of the importance of realistic weight goals and the concept of weight cycling.
- To understand the roles of pharmacotherapy and surgery as adjuncts to lifestyle management in certain selected individuals.
- To increase knowledge of the various local commercial slimming programmes.

Skills training

- To be able to calculate and classify body mass index.
- To know how to measure and classify waist circumference.
- To know how to assess health risks, cardiovascular risk factors and status.
- To be able to determine realistic weight goals for patients
- To appreciate importance of involvement of a multiprofessional team.

Diet and nutrition

This covers nutrition knowledge, dietary manipulation, eating behaviour and eating disorders.

Aims

- To facilitate understanding and awareness of the role of dietary advice in the management of obesity.
- To provide a foundation in the dietary knowledge and skills required for best practice in the dietary management of obesity.

Learning objectives

- To increase awareness of the role different macronutrients play in the aetiology and treatment of obesity.
- To increase awareness of how patterns of food intake and eating behaviour have changed over the last few decades.
- To enhance knowledge of the energy requirements of obese subjects and develop the ability to estimate energy requirements for individual patients.
- To gain insight and understanding into the appropriate non-judgemental approach in helping patients make the required lifestyle changes (linking in with the behavioural change components of the programme).
- To understand the function, sources and recommended intakes of macronutrients and relevant micronutrients, and how they should ideally be balanced in a healthy diet.
- To be aware of the various dietary assessment methods in use.
- To understand the phenomenon of energy intake under-reporting and the practical implications this may have in the management of such patients.
- To understand the importance of, and practical strategies to use in, the self-monitoring of food intake.
- To be aware of the importance of matching and tailoring dietary strategies to individual patients and practical techniques to determine such individualized management.
- To increase knowledge of alternative dieting practices, diet trends, myths and misconceptions and the nutritional implications of such practices.
- To understand and develop dietary strategies for eating out, special occasions, etc.
- To enhance knowledge and understanding of food labels in relation to weight management.
- To be aware of the energy content of common foods.
- To increase awareness of dietary considerations among various ethnic groups and vegetarians; knowledge of the nutritional content of various ethnic and vegetarian foods; practical acceptable strategies for manipulating such diets.
- To understand the importance of eating behaviour on energy intake and strategies to manage eating behaviour (link in with behaviour change sessions).
- To be aware of the diagnostic criteria for eating disorders, with particular reference to binge eating disorder, and to have an understanding of appropriate referral strategies.

Skills training

- To develop the necessary skills for appropriate assessment of dietary intake in obese individuals.
- To be able to calculate energy requirements of overweight and obese individuals.
- To gain practical experience of how to translate nutritional aims into realistic food changes that are tailored to the individual patient.
- To be able to interpret the nutritional information on a food label.
- To be able to identify rich food sources of various macro- and micronutrients
- To be able to judge when a client may be presenting with a significant eating disorder and who requires further referral.

Physical activity

Aims

- To facilitate understanding and awareness of the role of physical activity in the management of obesity.
- To provide a foundation in the knowledge and skills required to safely, competently and effectively advise on physical activity in the overweight and obese populations.

Learning objectives

- To understand how activity trends have changed over time.
- To understand the beneficial effect of exercise on risk factors associated with obesity—blood lipids, blood pressure, insulin resistance.
- To be aware of the beneficial psychological effects of physical activity on mood, self-efficacy, self-esteem and body image.
- To be aware of the lack of importance ascribed by many patients to the role of physical activity in weight management.
- To understand the important role physical activity plays in the prevention of obesity and the maintenance of reduced weight.
- To understand the role of physical activity in weight reduction programmes and the combined effects with diet.
- To gain insight into the common barriers to physical activity change and practical strategies for tackling such barriers (link with behavioural management section).
- To increase knowledge of the effects of exercise on 24-hour energy expenditure and post-exercise energy expenditure.
- To understand the effects of physical activity on 24-hour energy intake, post-exercise energy intake and macronutrient selection.
- To understand the effects of exercise on substrate utilization.

- To be aware of the effects of physical activity on body mass and body composition.
- To understand the different exercise intensities and their effect on metabolism and weight change.

Skills training

- To enhance skills in assessing habitual physical activity in obese individuals.
- To enhance skills in recommending a physical activity programme — factors to consider, adherence, risks.

Counselling skills

There is widespread agreement that the interpersonal skills of the health professional, in the way they introduce and recommend behavioural change, contribute significantly to the success of cognitive–behavioural treatment (CBT). These generic, interpersonal communication skills help the health professional to maximize the therapeutic effect as they guide, motivate and support the overweight patients in changing their lifestyle. Communication skills are also known as counselling skills, as they are a major feature of counselling training, but it is important to recognize that in the case of CBT, interpersonal skills provide the background for providing treatment and not the treatment itself.

Aim

- To increase awareness and effectiveness of interpersonal interactions in the clinical setting.

Learning objectives

- To be able to create rapport, so that clients feel comfortable and able to communicate their concerns.
- To understand and empathize with the client's position.
- To be able to give advice and guidance in an acceptable, comprehensible and engaging fashion.
- To manage the treatment sessions so that appropriate progress is achieved, and terminating treatment appropriately and sympathetically.
- To maintain or increase clients' self-esteem and self-efficacy, even when treatment outcomes are modest.
- To be able to manage clients in group settings so that participants experience the critical elements of a CBT programme, while also profiting from insights and support from other group members.

Skills training

- To increase social interaction skills.
- To enhance communication skills.
- To develop treatment management skills.
- To enhance group work skills.

Principles of behaviour change

CBT programmes are based on psychological research that suggests that certain practices are helpful in achieving behaviour change. In the classic CBT treatment programme, the approach should be educational, cooperative and empirical, with the therapist and patient working together to discover how best to apply CBT principles in the individual's circumstances.

Learning objectives

- To be aware of the importance of self-monitoring.
- To understand the concept of functional analysis.
- To be aware of the importance of goal setting.
- To understand the value of self-reinforcement.
- To understand the importance of cognitive restructuring.
- To be aware of the role of learned self-control.
- To understand the need for the clients to adopt a problem-solving perspective.
- To be aware of the value of recruiting social support for change.

Assessment skills

Aims

- To be able to make a comprehensive assessment of overweight and obese subjects in order to facilitate individualized management.
- To understand when implementation of treatment may not be appropriate.

Learning objectives

- To be able to assess the client's psychosocial history.
- To be aware of specific issues that should be addressed related to weight loss — e.g. motivation, goals for change, treatment expectations.
- To be able to carry out a comprehensive assessment of dietary intake and eating patterns (linking with nutrition and diet module).
- To be able to assess physical activity.
- To be aware of behavioural contraindications to treatment — bulimia nervosa, psychiatric disorders, major life crisis.

Therapeutic intervention

Aims

- To be able to identify the appropriate patient, the appropriate time and type of medical and/or surgical intervention.
- To be aware of the importance of monitoring patients before, during and after therapeutic intervention.

Learning objectives

- To be aware of the actions of anti-obesity drugs, appropriate prescribing and potential adverse reactions.
- To understand the indications and contraindications to the use of anti-obesity drugs.
- To understand the principles of drug responsiveness and non-responsiveness and risk–benefit analysis for the use of anti-obesity drugs.
- To be aware of the potential for weight regain after cessation of drug treatment and the need to reinforce lifestyle measures to maintain weight loss.

- To understand the principles of surgical treatment for obesity.
- To be aware of the criteria for suitability of obese patients for surgical treatment.
- To understand the preoperative assessment and perioperative monitoring for patients undergoing bariatric surgery.
- To be aware of the need to follow up patients following bariatric surgery on a lifetime basis in a multidisciplinary clinic.
- To be aware of the longer term consequences of bariatric surgery.

PART 7

Environmental and policy approaches

29 Obesity in Asian populations

Timothy P. Gill

Introduction, 431

The global problem of obesity, 431

Obesity in the Asian region, 431
    Adults, 431
    Children, 433

Relationship between weight and
health in Asians, 434

Potential reasons for a varying
relationship between BMI and health
risk in Asians, 435
    Methodological issues, 435
    Variations in body
    composition, 436
    Frame size/proportions, 436
    Body fat distribution, 436
    Rate of weight gain, 437

Rapid changes in diet and physical
activity, 438
Stunting/low birth weight: the
potential impact of fetal
undernutrition and later obesity, 439

Summary and conclusion, 439

References, 440

Introduction

Although the level of obesity, as defined by the standard WHO classification, remains low in most Asian countries, many Asian races appear to be especially susceptible to the development of obesity-related illness, even at low levels of body mass index (BMI). In addition, the health consequences of weight gain appear to be more intense than in those of European origin. The exact reasons for these variations in the relationship between BMI and health risk remain unclear, but they have led to a debate about the need for ethnic-specific BMI cut-off points to define overweight and obesity within Asia. This chapter examines the nature of the relationship between markers of adiposity and health status in Asians, and explores possible reasons for the apparent variation between Asian and Caucasian populations.

The global problem of obesity

Other chapters have highlighted the rise of the obesity epidemic to the point where obesity can now be considered one of the major public health problems facing the world today. It appears that prevalence rates are increasing in all parts of the world in both men and women and also in children. Indeed, overweight, obesity and health problems associated with them are now so common that they are replacing the more traditional public health concerns such as undernutrition and infectious disease as the most significant contributors to global ill health (World Health Organization, 1998). In 2002, noncommunicable diseases accounted for 60% of total mortality worldwide and 46% of the global burden of disease (WHO, 2002). The major cause of death throughout the world is now coronary heart disease.

At the physiological level, obesity can be defined as a condition of 'abnormal or excessive fat accumulation in adipose tissue to the extent that health may be impaired' (WHO, 2000). However, it is difficult to measure body fat directly and so surrogate measures such as the BMI are commonly used to indicate overweight and obesity in adults. Additional tools are available for identification of individuals with increased health risks due to 'central' fat distribution, and for the more detailed characterization of excess fat in special clinical situations and research.

In the new graded classification system developed by the WHO (2000), a BMI of 30 kg/m^2 or above denotes obesity. There is a high likelihood that individuals with a BMI at or above this level will have excessive body fat. However, the health risks associated with overweight and obesity appear to rise progressively with increasing BMI from a value below 25 kg/m^2, and it has been demonstrated that there are benefits to having a BMI measurement nearer 20–22 kg/m^2, at least within industrialized countries. To highlight the health risks that can exist at BMI values below the level of obesity, and to raise awareness of the need to prevent further weight gain beyond this level, the first category of overweight included in the new WHO classification system is termed 'preobese' (BMI 25–29.9 kg/m^2).

Obesity in the Asian region

Adults

The WHO estimates that around one billion people throughout the world are overweight and that over 300 million of these

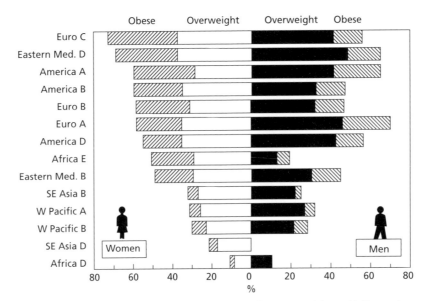

Fig 29.1 Estimates of the prevalence of overweight and obesity in 45- to 59-year-olds in different parts of the world. (Source: James *et al.*, 2001. Reprinted with permission of the North American Association for the Study of Obesity). Note that 191 countries are included in the subregional groupings, which have been constructed on the basis of the observed infant mortality rates and life expectancies of the different countries. To illustrate the nature of the regions specified, the three countries in each subregion with the biggest populations are defined below. Afr D: Nigeria, Algeria and Ghana; Afr E: Ethiopia, Congo and South Africa; Amr A: USA, Canada and Cuba (all of the countries in region); Amr B: Brazil, Mexico and Colombia; Amr D: Peru, Ecuador and Guatemala; Emr B: Iran, United Arab Emirates and Saudi Arabia; Emr D: Pakistan, Egypt and Sudan; Eur A: Germany, France and UK; Eur B: Turkey, Poland and Uzbekistan; Eur C: Russian Federation, Ukraine and Kazakhstan; Sear B: Indonesia, Thailand and Sri Lanka (all of the countries in region); Sear D: India, Bangladesh and Myanmar; Wpr A: Japan, Australia and Singapore; and Wpr B: China, Vietnam and the Philippines.

Table 29.1 Rates of overweight (%) and obesity within Asia.

Country	Source	Year	Age	Men		Women	
				BMI 25–29.9	BMI ≥ 30	BMI 25–29.9	BMI ≥ 30
Australia	Dunstan *et al.* (2000)	2000	25+	48.3	19.1	30.2	21.8
New Zealand	NZ Ministry of Health (1999)	1997	15+	40.4	14.7	30.1	19.2
Taiwan	Lin *et al.* (2003)	1993–96	19+	22.3	2.3	19.9	5.6
China	Wang *et al.* (2001)	1995–97	20–74	21.3	2.1	21.7	3.7
Hong Kong	Ko *et al.* (1997)	1997	18+	28.3	2.5	23.5	3.8
Japan	Yoshiike *et al.* (1998)	1990–94	35–64	24.3	1.9	20.2	2.9
Korea	Kim *et al.* (2004)	1998	19+	24.3	1.7	23.5	3.0
Malaysia	Ismail *et al.* (2002)	1996	18+	20.1	4.0	20.4	7.6
The Philippines	Villavieja *et al.* (2001)	1998	20+	14.9	2.1	18.9	4.4
Singapore	Ministry of Health, Singapore (1999)	1998	18–69	28.6	5.3	20.3	6.7
Thailand	Department of Health, Thailand (1995)	1991	20+	12.0	1.7	19.5	5.6

are obese (WHO, 2002). However, despite contributing almost one-half of the world's population the number of people defined as having obesity within Asia using the official WHO criteria is disproportionately low. The prevalence of overweight and obesity for men and women aged 45–59 years within different WHO regions is shown in Fig. 29.1. The lowest rates of overweight and obesity are found within the countries of sub-Saharan Africa but the South-East Asia region of WHO, together with the Western Pacific region, which includes many

countries within Asia, also reported low levels of overweight and obesity.

Unfortunately, there are no comprehensive data on the weight status of all countries within Asia, and when data are available the quality can be variable. Not all countries undertake national surveys that measure weight and height and, even if this is undertaken, the data are not always reported in a format consistent with the WHO BMI cut-off points. However, there are sufficient nationally representative studies to pro-

Table 29.2 The prevalence of overweight and obesity in children within Asia.

Country	Prevalence of overweight and obesity (M/F)	Age range (years)	Sample size	Definition used	Date and data source	Source
Australia	M 19.5%, F 21.1%	2–18	2962	IOTF	National Nutrition Survey 1995, 2–18 years	Magarey *et al.* (2001)
China	M 8.4%, F 7.0%	6–18	2688	IOTF	The 1997 China Health and Nutrition Survey	Wang *et al.* (2002)
Hong Kong	M 13.4%, F 10.5%		25 000	> 120% of median weight for height	1996 Survey of Schools	Leung *et al.* (1996)
Malaysia	M 10.9%, F 8.0%	7–16	6239	NCHS > +2SD	1994/95 Multiethnic study of children from 22 schools in Kuala Lumpur	Kasmini *et al.* (1997)
The Philippines	M 1.1%, F 0.8%	0–5, 6–10		NCHS > +2SD	1998 National survey	Food and Nutrition Research Institute, Manila (2001)
South Korea	M 10.6%, F 10.6%	5–16	54 813	Reference centiles	Representative national data	Korean Association for the Study of Obesity (1998)
Thailand	M 17.5%, F 17.7% M 9.2%, F 10.8%	0–5 6–14		%W/H > 120%, BMI for age for sex above P95	1995 National nutrition survey Thai growth reference	Department of Health, Thailand (1995)
Taiwan	28.0%, 21.32%	12–15	1500	110–120% of IBW for overweight, ≥ 120% IBW for obesity	Taipei only	Chu (2001)

IOTF, International Obesity Task Force; NCHS, National Center for Health Statistics.

vide a reliable guide to the true levels of overweight and obesity within the region. A selection of these data are presented in Table 29.1 and compared with national data collected in Australia and New Zealand.

All countries within Asia had national rates of overweight and obesity well below that of Australia and New Zealand. However, it is interesting to note that although there is an enormous difference in rates of obesity between Asia and Australasia, the differential in rates of overweight is considerably less. The Philippines and Thailand had the lowest reported rates of overweight and obesity. In Thailand, the 1998 National Nutrition Survey showed that only 17% of men and 23% of women were overweight or obese, with obesity rates very low. However, these figures were an increase from the same national survey 5 years previously. Both Japan and Korea reported very low obesity rates but the levels of overweight were well above 20% for both men and women. The rates of overweight and obesity for Taiwanese men are similar to those of mainland China, but women in Taiwan tended to be heavier. In contrast, substantially more men and women from Hong Kong were overweight. The ethnically diverse countries of Singapore and Malaysia had the highest levels of overweight and obesity within the region. Surveys of ethnic variation within both

countries showed that subjects of Malay ethnic origin had significantly higher body weights than those of Chinese or Indian background. Comparisons of the weight status of urban and rural populations consistently reveal significantly lower levels of overweight and obesity in rural areas.

Children

Data on the weight status of children within Asia are still incomplete and suffer from the additional problems associated with the lack of a universally agreed way of measuring and defining overweight and obesity in children. A collection of large-scale surveys of child weight status within Asian countries is presented in Table 29.2. However, care must be taken in comparing the figures for different countries as vastly different assessment approaches have been utilized. It is also important to consider the age of the children surveyed as this also influences the levels of overweight and obesity experienced.

The prevalence of overweight varied from 0.9% in The Philippines to 15% in Australia (Table 29.2). In addition, the prevalence of combined overweight and obesity was reported to be around 19.5–21.1% in Australia on the basis of the definition by Cole and colleagues (2000), and as high as 21.3–28.0%

Table 29.3 Countries with the highest estimates of number of cases of diabetes in 2000 and 2030.

Rank	2000 Country	People with diabetes (millions)	2030 Country	People with diabetes (millions)
1	India	31.7	India	79.4
2	China	20.8	China	42.3
3	USA	17.7	USA	30.3
4	Indonesia	8.4	Indonesia	21.3
5	Japan	6.8	Pakistan	13.9
6	Pakistan	5.2	Brazil	11.3
7	Russian Federation	4.6	Bangladesh	11.1
8	Brazil	4.6	Japan	8.9
9	Italy	4.3	The Philippines	7.8
10	Bangladesh	3.2	Egypt	6.7

Source: Wild *et al.* (2004).

when a standard of more than 120% of ideal body weight (IBN) was applied to a survey in Taiwan. The differences in the rates of overweight and obesity among Asians compared with Caucasians are less obvious in children than in adults. Although it is often difficult to compare results obtained using different definitions of overweight and obesity, it is clear that overweight is a serious issue within the children of Asia, with all populations having at least one in ten children in this category.

Despite this, undernutrition remains a major problem in some countries in the region. In The Philippines, for example, among 6- to 10-year-old children, 41% were stunted as defined by the WHO classification for height-for-age and 30% were underweight on the basis of the definition of the WHO classification for weight-for-age (Food and Nutrition Research Institute, 2001). In China, the proportion of underweight was 9% among children aged 6–9 years and 15% among adolescents aged 10–18 years (Wang *et al.*, 2002)

Relationship between weight and health in Asians

The levels of coronary heart disease, diabetes, stroke and certain cancers have been rising steadily throughout the Asia–Pacific region for the last two decades, and cardiovascular diseases are now the most common cause of mortality (Western Pacific Regional Office of the World Health Organization, 1999). Asia already accounts for a sizeable proportion of the world's population with diabetes, and the number of people with diabetes is expected to treble by the year 2030 (Wild *et al.*, 2004). Table 29.3 shows the extraordinary high proportion of cases of diabetes found in Asian countries such as India, China, Pakistan, Indonesia, Japan and Bangladesh, despite the seemingly low rates of obesity detected in these countries.

A number of studies have compared the relationship between increasing BMI or waist circumference and risk of

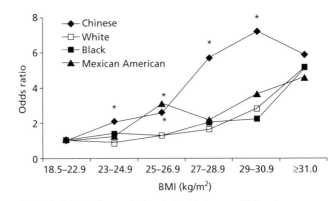

Fig 29.2 Ethnic difference in the relationship between BMI and hypertension prevalence (*$P < 0.05$). (Source: Bell *et al.*, 2002a. Reprinted with the permission of Oxford University Press.)

ill health in populations of Asian or Caucasian origin, and reached a conclusion that the level of risk rises much more steeply in the Asian populations. A recent study by Bell and colleagues (2002a) analysed cross-sectional data within adults aged 35–65 years from China, the Philippines and the USA, and found variations in the relationship between BMI and blood pressure in different ethnic groups. They found that as BMI increased, the risk of hypertension increased for each ethnic group. However, at BMI levels below 25 kg/m^2 the relationship between BMI and hypertension was significantly stronger among Chinese adults compared with Mexican Americans, non-Hispanic white people and black people (see Fig. 29.2).

Ramachandran and colleagues (1997) used epidemiological data from an Indian population in Madras, from Mexican Americans and non-Hispanic white people to examine the relationship between anthropometric measurements and the prevalence of type 2 diabetes in these ethnic groups. They found that although white Americans had the highest rates of obesity, they had the lowest levels of diabetes. The Madras Indians and Mexican Americans had equivalent rates of diabetes, occurring at much lower levels of BMI among the Asian subjects.

In addition, a recent study by Shiwaku and colleagues (2004) compared metabolic risk factors in Japanese men and women to a matched group of Mongolians. They found that the Mongolians had a higher prevalence of obesity and a higher body fat percentage but a weaker relationship between BMI and dyslipidaemia than the BMI-matched Japanese.

Numerous studies have also demonstrated the high levels of metabolic risk factors at relatively low levels of BMI among Asian populations. A very large collaborative study within mainland China, involving some 240 000 subjects from across China, revealed that levels of hypertension, diabetes, dyslipidaemia and risk factor clusters begin to increase rapidly at levels of BMI and waist circumference below current recommendations for action in Caucasians (Zhou, 2002).

A smaller study by Jia and colleagues (2002) among a middle-income community in Shanghai showed very high rates of metabolic risk factors at low levels of BMI. This study on 2776 adults (aged 20–94 years) found that the prevalence of obesity was only 4.3%, but more than one-third of the subjects had dyslipidaemia, 9.8% had type 2 diabetes and 58.4% of the population had hypertension. Deurenberg-Yap and colleagues (2001) studied the relationship between BMI and waist circumference in the multiethnic population of Singapore. They found a very high absolute risk of having one or more metabolic risk factors in all ethnic groups at BMI levels between 22 and 24 kg/m^2, and waist circumference between 75 and 80 cm for women and 80–85 cm for men. These are well below the cut-off points recommended for Caucasians by the WHO (WHO, 2000). Similar findings have been reported for Korea (Moon *et al.*, 2002), Japan (Liu *et al.*, 1999) and Hong Kong (Ko *et al.*, 1997). In addition Shen and colleagues (2003) recently demonstrated high levels of fatty liver among administrative officers in Shanghai at relatively low levels of BMI.

However, Stevens (2003) shows that the relationship between all-cause mortality and increasing BMI differs very little between different Asians populations and is very similar to that of Caucasians.

Potential reasons for a varying relationship between BMI and health risk in Asians

Methodological issues

A wide variety of studies have examined the relationship between adiposity and health in Asian populations. An objective analysis of these studies suggests that a range of methodological issues including how adiposity is defined, how study populations were selected and defined as being Asian, how health risk outcome was defined and how the relationship between health risk and adiposity was measured, all have potential to influence the definition of the relationship between adiposity

and health risk in Asians. It is possible that the application of inappropriate methodology may create or magnify, or conversely hide or weaken, any true difference that may exist in the relationship between adiposity and health in different ethnic groups.

Many discussions of the relationship between obesity and ill health in Asia treat all Asian populations as a single ethnic entity. Asia makes a major contribution to the world's land mass as well as its total population. It is an enormously diverse region that is populated by peoples of vastly different racial and ethnic backgrounds. Within most countries of Asia there are peoples from a range of historical and ethnic backgrounds, often with their own language, culture and religious practices. In China today there are at least 56 different ethnic groups, and although the Han peoples make up 92% of the total population, their racial background, physical appearance, language and culture varies in different regions of China (China Internet Information Center, 2004). In addition, there continues to be significant migration within Asia itself, which has created substantial populations of people of Chinese and Indian descent throughout many Asian countries. These issues raise questions as to whether all racial and ethnic groups within Asia can be treated as a homogeneous group or alternatively whether a single ethnic or national group can be used to defined the relationship between adiposity and health in all Asians.

Stevens and colleagues (2002) have highlighted the influence that the choice of outcomes and the measure of risk assessment applied has on determining the relationship between BMI and health risk in different ethnic groups. In their analysis they compared the associations of BMI with health risk in African-American and Caucasian women in the USA using four different outcomes (mortality, diabetes, hypertension and hypertriglyceridaemia) and three different risk estimates (absolute risk, relative risk and risk difference). When attempting to define a BMI that produced an equivalent level of risk in African-American women to that found in white women at a given BMI, the values ranged from extremely low to extremely high levels of BMI, depending on the outcome and risk assessment method used. For example, the relationship between mortality and BMI was much stronger in African-American women, whereas the relationship between hypertriglyceridaemia and BMI was much stronger in white women. Stevens argues that mortality should be the risk marker of choice as it is definite and easy to measure and because the association between risk factors and disease events may vary between ethnic groups (Stevens, 2003). However, mortality does have limitations as it reflects exposure to a wide range of factors, apart from BMI, over a long period of time.

In many parts of Asia, increases in BMI have only become significant in recent years. In recognition of these issues, the WHO Expert Consultation on Appropriate Body Mass Index for Asian Populations indicated that research should focus on markers of adiposity in Asian populations and their relationship to risk of developing comorbidities such as hypertension, type 2 diabetes and hyperlipidaemias (WHO Expert Consultation, 2004). The consultation also suggested that the rate difference was the best measure for defining the relationship between BMI and health outcome as relative risk can be greatly influenced by variations in baseline rates of the risk factor being studied. These methodological considerations may give cause to re-examine some of the evidence put forward to support ethnic-specific variations in the relationship between BMI and health risk in Asians. Some comparisons of health risk have used all-cause mortality as the outcome measure but many more have used metabolic risk factors such as hypertension and diabetes. However, most of these studies have also defined the relationship in terms of relative risk or rate ratios making true comparisons between ethnic groups difficult.

Variations in body composition

Other chapters in this book (see Chapters 1 and 2) have indicated that BMI is a relatively simple and useful measure of adiposity in humans that correlates relatively highly with percentage of body fat determined by more comprehensive techniques. However, it is important to understand that BMI is merely a proxy measure of fatness that is based on weight adjusted for height and that its relationship to body fatness is influenced by variations in overall levels of lean tissues as well as body build and proportions.

There is a growing body of evidence that indicates that the proportion of fat-free mass varies between peoples of different ethnic or racial backgrounds. Studies comparing the body composition of different ethnic groups in the USA found that bone mineral mass and skeletal muscle mass were greater in African-Americans compared with whites (Ortiz et al., 1992). Similar studies of the Pacific Islanders found that Polynesians from Samoa and Maori people within New Zealand had a higher lean muscle mass than New Zealand Caucasians (Rush et al., 1997; Swinburn et al., 1999). In contrast, studies of the body composition of Asians have consistently revealed a lower lean mass and a higher proportion of body fat than Caucasians. Gurrici and colleagues (1998) and Werkman and colleagues (2000) compared the body composition of Dutch Caucasians to Indonesian and Chinese subjects of the same age and sex, and found a significantly lower proportion of lean muscle tissue in the Asian subjects.

In addition, a significant number of studies have reported a relatively higher level of body fat within Asian subjects than Caucasians. However, the methods used to measure body composition in these trials have varied greatly and some of the less rigorous techniques, such as bioelectrical impedance, can be subject to considerable bias. Regardless of these limitations, the findings of these studies have been very consistent, with almost all studies showing a higher level of body fat at a lower BMI in Asians. This finding has been demonstrated in Chinese,

Malay and Indians in Singapore (Deurenberg-Yap et al., 2000), Hong Kong Chinese (Ko et al., 2001), Taiwan Chinese (Chang et al., 2003), Indians within India (Dudeja et al., 2001) and Indonesians (Gurrici et al., 1998). Recently, a metaanalysis of body composition studies conducted within different ethnic groups showed that American black people have a 1.3-kg/m^2 higher BMI and Polynesians have a 4.5-kg/m^2 higher BMI for the same level of body fat, age, and gender when compared to Caucasians. By contrast, the same analysis showed that for the same level of body fat, age and gender, BMIs in Chinese, Ethiopians, Indonesians and Thais were shown to be 1.9, 4.6, 3.2 and 2.9 kg/m^2 lower than in Caucasians (Deurenberg et al., 1998).

It would be tempting to believe that the association between lower levels of BMI and higher risk of ill health in Asians is due to the higher relative level of overweight among Asians. However, the direct connection between higher proportions of body fat in Asians and increasing levels of obesity-related illness is yet to be determined.

Frame size/proportions

Some researchers believe that much of the ethnic variation in the relationship between BMI and body fatness is explained by differing body proportions and frame sizes. This issue was first raised by Norgan (1994) when he demonstrated that the high levels of body fat at low BMIs found in Australian Aboriginal people could be explained by their high relative leg length. Long legs distort the relationship between BMI (which, after all, is a ratio of weight to height squared) and body fat, which means that for the same level of fatness Aborigines have a lower BMI. Body proportions also explained the difference in relative body fatness between Malay and Chinese Indonesians (Gurrici et al., 1999). In this study, frame size (as indicated by knee and wrist breadth) was also seen to be an influence on the BMI–adiposity relationship, with a larger frame size being equated with a lower level of body fatness for the same BMI. In another study by Deurenberg and colleagues (1999), the significant difference in body fatness at the same BMI that existed between Chinese in Singapore and Chinese in Beijing could almost all be accounted for when relative leg length and frame size were controlled. Conversely, Craig and colleagues (2001) used elbow breadth to indicate that Tongans had a larger skeletal size, which led to a lower estimated body fat mass at the same BMI than Caucasians from Australia.

Body fat distribution

Over the last two decades, important new information concerning the relationship between obesity and many chronic diseases has emerged, which highlights the importance of body fat distribution as a more important determinant of risk than BMI alone. Early studies by Larsson and colleagues (1984) and Lapidus and colleagues (1984) demonstrated a strong association between waist–hip ratio (WHR) and myocardial infarction, stroke and death. Subsequent studies have indicated that it is a high level of intra-abdominal or visceral fat that carries the greatest health risks. Although the WHR has now been shown to be a poor quantifier of total visceral fat deposits, it does allow the differentiation between those obese persons with large central fat stores and those who store fat peripherally. More recent studies have also found strong associations between central obesity and hypertension, hypertriglyceridaemia, hypercholesterolaemia, hyperglycaemia, hyperinsulinaemia, low HDL levels, type 2 diabetes, elevated clotting risk and hyperuricaemia (see Chapters 12 and 17). More importantly, the risk imposed by central obesity was independent of total BMI and was found in those who would not be classified as obese based on their BMI alone.

The first indication that peoples of Asian origin were more prone to visceral obesity and cardiovascular disease (CVD) at low levels of BMI came from studies involving migrants from South Asia. McKeigue and colleagues (1991) found that migrants from India, Pakistan and Bangladesh who settled in England had very much higher rates of coronary heart disease (CHD) than the general population, even though they had lower BMI. Assessment of their CVD risk factors revealed that they had all the markers of the metabolic syndrome, and both men and women had more central distribution of body fat for a given BMI compared with European control subjects. Similar results have been found for South Asian immigrants in the USA (Klatsy and Armstrong, 1991) and Australia (Lear *et al.*, 2003). This relationship was also confirmed in native South Asians, with central obesity being shown to have a more important association with hyperglycaemia than generalized obesity (Shelgikar *et al.*, 1991).

Very few countries within Asia have undertaken a systematic collection and analysis of an indicator of abdominal obesity such as WHR or waist circumference. However, a number of large studies of central adiposity have been suggested as representative of the national situation. Ko and colleagues (2001) collected waist circumference measures on 1513 Hong Kong Chinese, and comparing these data against the WHO criteria for Caucasians found that 4.5% of men and 22.5% of women were above the at-risk level. They found central adiposity was a more sensitive indicator of risk of ill health than BMI. Lee *et al.* (2002) also found similar results in another group of Hong Kong Chinese. In Korea, the levels of abdominal obesity were assessed using data from the 1998 National Health and Nutrition Survey. A total of 18.5% of men and 38.5% of women were found to be abdominally obese, whereas only 1.7% of men and 3% of women were classified as obese, and 24% of men and 25% of women were classified as overweight by BMI. A raised waist circumference was found to be associated with a clustering of cardiovascular risk factors (Park *et al.*, 2003).

Central obesity is already emerging as a serious problem in India, even at low relative weight (Gopalan, 1998). Among non-overweight urban middle-class residents with BMI < 25 kg/m², nearly 20% of men and 22% of women had a high WHR. In overweight subjects with a BMI over 25 kg/m², abdominal obesity was found in a striking 68% of men and 58% of women (Table 29.4).

The relationship between increased central adiposity and increased levels of metabolic risk factors is strong and graded in Asian populations, and appears to explain a proportion of the increased risk of ill health at lower BMI. However, some studies have indicated that the strong association between abdominal obesity and CVD in Asians cannot be totally explained by increased rates of central obesity (Lim *et al.*, 2002)

There is a range of measures that have been proposed as the most useful proxy of abdominal obesity including waist circumference, WHR, conicity index and waist–height ratio. There remains considerable debate over which of these measures of abdominal obesity best predicts risk of ill health. Patel and colleagues (1999) studied the relationship between a range of measures of abdominal obesity and metabolic risk factors in Chinese, European and South Asian adults. They found that not all of the proxy measures of abdominal obesity were related to features of the metabolic syndrome consistently across the ethnic groups studied. However, waist circumference and waist–height ratio were the most consistent, and WHR the least, when comparing across the ethnic groups. Waist–height ratio was also identified as the best predictor of cardiovascular disease risk factors in a study of Hong Kong Chinese. Ho and colleagues (2003) found that the optimal waist to height cut-off value for predicting risk was 0.48 for both men and women. However, Jia and colleagues (2003) used magnetic resonance imaging (MRI) to measure the total visceral fat stores in 690 Chinese adults and found that although waist circumference, BMI and WHR were all predictive of visceral fat stores, waist circumference was the best predictor.

Rate of weight gain

Over the last two decades, important new information concerning the relationship between obesity and CVD has emerged, and it highlights the importance of weight gain and duration of overweight and abdominal fat distribution. These factors (gain and duration) are more important determinants of CVD risk than BMI alone. Both the Health Professionals

Table 29.4 Subjects with high WHR (abdominal obesity) by grades of BMI in urban Indians (%).

Details	Grades of BMI	Males	Females
Underweight	< 18.5	1.8	1.75
Normal	18.5–24.9	17.8	20.0
Overweight	≥ 25	68.1	58.0

Source: Gopalan (1998).

Study and the Nurses Health Study have shown that an association between weight gain and CVD is independent of total BMI. Those who had gained the most weight in adulthood and who had the longest duration of overweight had the highest level of risk for type 2 diabetes and CVD (Willett *et al.*, 1999).

This association of weight gain, duration of adiposity, and CVD risk is of importance to Asia as populations are gaining weight. In Japan, although overall rates of obesity remain below 3%, obesity prevalence increased by a factor of 2.4 in the adult male population and by a factor of 1.8 in women aged 20–29 years (Yoshiike *et al.*, 2002). The level of obesity among Chinese adults remains low, but the marked shifts in diet, activity and overweight suggest that major increases in overweight and obesity will occur. The data of the National China Health and Nutrition Survey (CHNS), an ongoing longitudinal survey of eight provinces in China, show a consistent increase in adult obesity in both urban and rural areas (Ge *et al.*, 1994; Popkin *et al.*, 1995). Changes in diet and activity patterns are rapid in urban residents of all incomes but are even more rapid in middle- and high-income rural residents. Data from Thailand suggest that obesity rates are increasing, at least in affluent urban populations. In 1996, the overall prevalence of overweight and obesity was 28.3% and 6.8%, respectively, with 8.8% of women and 3.5% of men being classified obese. This has almost doubled from 1991 when only 3.8% of women and 3% of men were classified as obese (Kosulwat, 2002).

However, the most alarming aspect of the epidemiological transition in Asia is the rapid increases in the prevalence of childhood overweight and obesity. In Australia, the prevalence of overweight and obesity doubled both in boys and girls over the period 1985–97 (Magarey *et al.*, 2001). Childhood and adolescent obesity was reported to have increased twofold during the last decade in Korea. In Hong Kong, however, smaller increases were reported in recent surveys: from 7.6% to 10.4% for boys and from 7.8% to 8.9% for girls at the age of 7 years between 1993 and 1996 (Leung *et al.*, 2000), and from 12.1% to 14.1% among school children from 1997 to 2001. The increases in the prevalence of overweight and obesity in Taiwan were also not as prominent as those reported in Australia and Korea (Chu, 2001).

In China, a moderate shift from a situation of under- to overnutrition was shown over a 6-year period from 1991 to 1997. This phenomenon was more prominent in urban than in rural areas (Wang *et al.*, 2002). However, in The Philippines, the prevalence of underweight decreased from 34.5% to 30.6% in 0- to 5-year-old children and from 34.2% to 32.9% in 6- to 10-year-old children from the late 1980s to early 2000s. The prevalence of overweight increased from 0.6% to 1.1% and from 0.1% to 0.8% respectively.

Rapid changes in diet and physical activity

Modernization has brought many social, economic and health benefits to developing countries throughout the world. However, the rapid economic growth, urbanization and occupational restructuring have also resulted in dramatic changes in diet and physical activity levels that have led to rapid increases in population mean body weight. Many countries in the Asia–Pacific region are becoming reliant on nontraditional food sources and there has been a shift towards diets higher in both animal and vegetable fats (particularly vegetable oils) and sugars (Drewnowski and Popkin, 1997). This has been proposed as a major factor driving the increase in body weight (Popkin and Doak, 1998; WHO, 2000). Escalating levels of obesity together with alcohol abuse and cigarette smoking are associated with high rates of type 2 diabetes, hypertension, dyslipidaemia and CVD. This has been described as the 'New World syndrome' and is responsible for the disproportionately high rates of mortality in developing nations and among the disadvantaged ethnic minority groups in developed countries.

This situation has arisen as a result of changing dietary patterns, which have created diets that are more energy dense and higher in fat, together with the rising urbanization that has brought about a more sedentary lifestyle.

Popkin and colleagues (2001) examined the per capita total dietary energy available for consumption in a range of Asian countries, and found that the total available energy had increased substantially over the last few decades. In high-income countries, including Singapore, Hong Kong and South Korea, the contribution of dietary fat to total energy increased from 8.8% in 1962 to 23.7% in 1996. In lower income Asian countries, including Vietnam, Laos and Cambodia, the increase was not as great, at around 13.0–15.9%. At the same time, the contribution of carbohydrate to total energy decreased proportionately. The amount of cereals available for consumption in high-income Asian countries actually diminished on a per capita basis from 1962 to 1996, although in middle- and low-income countries, the amount increased slightly. In contrast, the amount of meat/poultry, fish/seafood, animal fat and added sugar available for consumption in high-income countries increased greatly during this period. Smaller increases in the consumption of these foods were also found among middle-income countries, including Malaysia, Thailand and The Philippines. Increases for such foods in low-income countries were significantly less.

At the same time, rapid urbanization has occurred in most of the countries within the Asian region. A high percentage of the population now resides in urban areas, particularly within high-income countries, but also to a lesser extent among the middle- and lower income countries. Urbanization is generally associated with higher income and therefore higher energy intake from a greater use of energy-dense foods and fat. At the same time, urbanization brings about a change in physical activity, with a shift away from labour-intensive agricultural activities towards a more sedentary lifestyle. The association between dietary and environmental factors and obesity was investigated by Popkin and colleagues (1995) using data from

Table 29.5 Proposed classification of weight by BMI and waist circumference in adult Asians.

Classification	BMI (kg/m²)	Risk of comorbidities Waist circumference	
		< 90 cm (men) < 80 cm (women)	≥ 90 cm (men) ≥ 80 cm (women)
Underweight	< 18.5	Low (but risk of other clinical problems increased)	Average
Normal range	18.5–24.9	Average	Increased
Overweight	≥ 23.0		
At risk	23.0–24.9	Increased	Moderate
Obese class I	25.0–29.9	Moderate	Severe
Obese class II	≥ 30.0	Severe	Very severe

Source: WHO, IASO, IOTF (2000).

the 1989 and 1991 China Health and Nutrition Surveys. They found that higher fat and energy intake was associated with increased BMI. Household income and physical activity level were also significantly associated with BMI. There were differences between urban and rural residents with urban residents having a lower energy intake, higher fat intake and lower physical activity level.

Bell and colleagues (2002b) examined the association between motor vehicle ownership and weight status in China. The acquisition of cars is a relatively new option for most Chinese people, and 26% of adults owned a car in 1997. However, the odds of being obese were 80% higher for men and women in households who owned a motorized vehicle than those who did not. In addition, men who had recently acquired a motor vehicle experienced a 1.8-kg greater weight gain than those whose vehicle status remained the same, and they had twice the risk of becoming obese.

Stunting/low birth weight: the potential impact of fetal undernutrition and later obesity

In countries undergoing transition, where overnutrition coexists with undernutrition, the shift in population weight status has been linked to exaggerated problems of obesity and associated non-communicable diseases in adults. Recent studies have shown that infants who were undernourished *in utero* and then born small have a greater risk of obesity-related morbidity as adults if they gain weight (Ravelli *et al.*, 1976; Jackson *et al.*, 1996). In particular, poor intrauterine nutrition appears to predispose some groups to abdominal obesity, and results in an earlier and more severe development of comorbid conditions such as hypertension, CHD and diabetes (Law *et al.*, 1992; Barker, 1999). The apparent impact of intrauterine nutrition on the later structure and functioning of the body has become known as 'programming' and is often referred to as the 'Barker hypothesis'. In many parts of Asia, women enter pregnancy malnourished and the problem

of undernutrition *in utero* may be further exacerbated by the low-protein, rice-based diets common in the region (James, 1997).

The ramifications of programming are immense for countries such as India and China, where a large proportion of infants are still born undernourished. If these children are later exposed to the high-fat diets and sedentary lifestyles associated with economic transition, and develop into obese adults, it is likely that they will suffer severe consequences in the form of early heart disease, hypertension and diabetes.

Summary and conclusion

It does appear that Asian countries and populations have elevated levels of weight-related illness despite the apparently low levels of overweight and obesity found in surveys at present. The reasons for this paradox have not been clearly elucidated. It may be that the present-day WHO definition using BMI is inappropriate, that Asians are fatter for a given BMI, that Asians have a greater tendency to deposit abdominal fat or that they are born small and are subjected to a high-fat, high-energy diet and reduced activity as they become more affluent. Whatever the reason, Asians are becoming more obese and as they do so CVD and diabetes (among other diseases) are becoming more prevalent.

It is necessary to determine whether Asians are more susceptible to metabolic disease, have a greater tendency to deposit abdominal adipose tissue, and whether the present-day definitions of obesity and health risk need to be revised for Asian populations. However, while we wait for the necessary studies to be planned and performed, it is important not to neglect the existing problems arising from the increasing weight of people within this region. Strategies need to be developed to treat those with an existing weight problem and the associated diseases, and to prevent more Asians becoming overweight and obese.

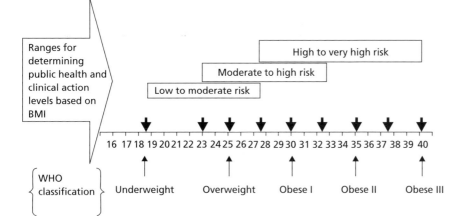

Fig 29.3 WHO BMI cut-off points for public health action. (Source: WHO, 2004. Reprinted with permission from Elsevier.)

The WHO Expert Consultation on Appropriate Body Mass Index assessed the issue of defining appropriate BMI action points for addressing overweight and obesity for Asian populations, but they found that insufficient information was available to make specific recommendations. Instead, the Consultation proposed that the existing definitions of obesity be maintained but also identified a series of BMI cut points that should be used for reporting population BMI distributions or defining specific action levels for addressing obesity in populations or individuals (see Fig. 29.3). It may be in the interim that the suggested cut-off points for Asians [WHO, International Association for the Study of Obesity (IASO), International Obesity Task Force (IOTF), 2000] (Table 29.5) could be used as an interim measure to guide both studies and clinical management. There is little doubt that overweight/obesity is becoming one of the major health problems for the Asian region.

References

Barker, D.J.P. (1999) Foetal undernutrition and obesity in later life. In: Guy-Grand, B., Ailhaud, G. eds. *Progress in Obesity Research* 9. London: John Libbey.

Bell, A.C., Adair, L.S., Popkin, B.M. (2002a) Ethnic differences in the association between body mass index and hypertension. *American Journal of Epidemiology* **155**, 346–353.

Bell, A.C., Ge, K. and Popkin, B.M. (2002b) The road to obesity or the path to prevention: motorized transportation and obesity in China. *Obesity Research* **10**, 277–283.

Chang, C.J., Wu, C.H., Chang, C.S., Yao, W.J., Yang, Y.C., Wu, J.S. and Lu, F.H. (2003) Low body mass index but high percent body fat in Taiwanese subjects: implications of obesity cutoffs. *International Journal of Obesity* **27**, 253–259

China Internet Information Center (CIIC) (2004) China's population

mix–website (http://www.china.org.cn/). Accessed March 12, 2004.

Chu, N.F. (2001) Prevalence and trends of obesity among school children in Taiwan: the Taipei Children Heart Study. *International Journal of Obesity* **25**, 170–176.

Cole, T.J., Bellizzi, M.C., Flegal, K.M. and Dietz, W.H. (2000) Establishing a standard definition for child overweight and obesity worldwide: international survey. *British Medical Journal* **320**, 1240–1243.

Craig, P., Halavatau, V., Comino, E. and Caterson, I. (2001) Differences in body composition between Tongans and Australians: time to rethink the healthy weight ranges? *International Journal of Obesity* **25**, 1806–1814.

Department of Health, Thailand (1995) *The Fourth National Nutrition Survey of Thailand, 1995.* Bangkok: Ministry of Public Health.

Deurenberg, P., Yap, M. and van Staveren, W.A. (1998) Body mass index and percent body fat: a meta analysis among different ethnic groups. *International Journal of Obesity* **22**, 1164–1171.

Deurenberg, P., Deurenberg Yap, M., Wang, J., Lin, F.P. and Schmidt, G. (1999) The impact of body build on the relationship between body mass index and percent body fat. *International Journal of Obesity* **23**, 537–542.

Deurenberg-Yap, M., Schmidt, G., van Staveren, W.A. and Deurenberg, P. (2000) The paradox of low body mass index and high body fat percentage among Chinese, Malays and Indians in Singapore. *International Journal of Obesity* **24**, 1011–1017.

Deurenberg-Yap, M., Chew, S.K., Lin, V.F., Tan, B.Y., van Staveren, W.A. and Deurenberg, P. (2001) Relationships between indices of obesity and its co-morbidities in multi-ethnic Singapore. *International Journal of Obesity* **25**, 1554–1562.

Drewnowski, A. and Popkin, B.M. (1997) The nutrition transition, new trends in the global diet. *Nutrition Review* **55**, 31–43.

Dudeja, V., Misra, A., Pandey, R.M., Devina, G., Kumar, G. and Vikram, N.K. (2001) BMI does not accurately predict overweight in Asian Indians in northern India. *British Journal of Nutrition* **86**, 105–112.

Dunstan, D., Zimmet, P.Z., Welborn, T.A., Cameron, A.J., Shaw, J., de

Courten, M., Jolley, D. and McCarty, D.J. *Diabesity and Associated Disorders in Australia 2000. The Accelerating Epidemic.* Melbourne: IDI.

Epidemiology and Disease Control Department (1999) *National Health Survey 1998.* Singapore: Ministry of Health Singapore.

Food and Nutrition Research Institute (2001) *Philippine Nutrition: Facts and Figures.* Manila: Department of Science and Technology.

Ge, K., Weisell, R., Guo, X., Cheng, L., Ma, H., Zhai, F. and Popkin, B.M. (1994) Body mass index of Chinese adults in 1980s. *European Journal of Clinical Nutrition* **48**, 148–154.

Gopalan, C. (1998) Obesity in Indian urban 'middle class'. *Bulletin of the Nutrition Foundation of India* **19**, 1–5.

Gurrici, S., Hartriyanti, Y., Hautvast, J.G. and Deurenberg, P. (1998) Relationship between body fat and body mass index: differences between Indonesians and Dutch Caucasians. *European Journal of Clinical Nutrition* **52**, 779–783.

Gurrici, S., Hartriyanti, Y., Hautvast, J.G. and Deurenberg, P. (1999) Differences in the relationship between body fat and body mass index between two different Indonesian ethnic groups: the effect of body build. *European Journal of Clinical Nutrition* **53**, 468–472.

Ho, S.Y., Lam, T.H. and Janus, E.D. (2003) Waist to stature ratio is more strongly associated with cardiovascular risk factors than other simple anthropometric indices. *Annals of Epidemiology* **13**, 683–691.

Ismail, M.N., Chee, S.S., Nawawi, H., Yusoff, K., Lim, T.O. and James, W.P. (2002) Obesity in Malaysia. *Obesity Reviews* **3**, 203–208.

Jackson, A.A., Langley-Evans, S.C., McCarthy, H.D. (1996) Nutritional influences on early life upon obesity and body proportions. In: Chadwick, D.J. and Cardew, G.C. eds. *The Origins and Consequences of Obesity.* Chichester: Wiley, 118–137 (Ciba Foundation Symposium 201).

James, W.P.T. (1997) Long term fetal programming of body composition and longevity. *Nutrition Reviews* **55**, S31–S34.

James, P.T., Leach, R., Kalamara, E. and Shayeghi, M. (2001) The worldwide obesity epidemic. *Obesity Research* **9**, 2285–2335.

Jia, W.P., Xiang, K.S., Chen, L., Lu, J.X. and Wu, Y.M. (2002) Epidemiological study on obesity and its comorbidities in urban Chinese older than 20 years of age in Shanghai, China. *Obesity Reviews* **3**, 157–165.

Jia, W.P., Lu, J.X., Xiang, K.S., Bao, Y.Q., Lu, H.J. and Chen, L. (2003) Prediction of abdominal visceral obesity from body mass index, waist circumference and waist-hip ratio in Chinese adults: receiver operating characteristic curves analysis. *Biomedical and Environmental Science* **16**, 206–211.

Kasmini, K., Idris, M.N., Fatimah, A., Hanafiah, S., Iran, H. and Asmah Bee, M.N. (1997) Prevalence of overweight and obese school children aged between 7 to 16 years among the major 3 ethnic groups in Kuala Lumpur, Malaysia. *Asia Pacific Journal of Clinical Nutrition* **6**, 172–174.

Kim, Y., Suh, Y.K. and Choi, H. (2004) BMI and metabolic disorders in South Korean adults: 1998 Korea National Health and Nutrition Survey. *Obesity Research* **12**, 445–453.

Klatsky, A.L. and Armstrong, M.A. (1991) Cardiovascular risk factors among Asian Americans living in northern California. *American Journal of Public Health* **81**, 1423–1428.

Ko, G.T.C., Chan, J.C.N., Woo, J., Lau, E., Yeung, V.T.F., Chow, C.-C., Wai, H.P.S., Li, J.K.Y., So, W.-Y. and Cockram, C.S. (1997) Simple anthropometric indexes and cardiovascular risk factors in Chinese. *International Journal of Obesity* **21**, 995–1001.

Ko, G.T., Tang, J., Chan, J.C., Sung, R., Wu, M.M., Wai, H.P. and Chen, R. (2001) Lower BMI cut-off value to define obesity in Hong Kong Chinese: an analysis based on body fat assessment by bioelectrical impedance. *British Journal of Nutrition* **85**, 239–242.

Korean Association for the Study of Obesity. (1998) *Growth Charts of Children and Adolescents in South Korea.* Seoul: KASO.

Kosulwat, V. (2002) The nutrition and health transition in Thailand. *Public Health Nutrition* **5**(1A), 183–189.

Lapidus, L., Bengston, C., Laarson, C., Pennert, K., Rybo, E. and Sjostrom, L. (1984) Distribution of adipose tissue and risk of cardiovascular disease and death: A 12 year follow up of participants in a population study of women in Gothenburg, Sweden. *British Medical Journal* **289**, 1257–1261.

Larsson, B., Svardsudd, K., Welin, L., Wilhelmsen, L., Bjorntorp, P. and Tibblin, G. (1984) Abdominal adipose tissue distribution, obesity and risk of cardiovascular disease and death: 13-year follow of participants in a study of men born in 1913. *British Medical Journal* **288**, 1401–1404.

Law, C.M., Barker, D.J., Osmond, C., Fall, C.H. and Simmond, S.J. (1992) Early growth and abdominal fatness in adult life. *Journal of Epidemiology and Community Health* **46**, 184–186.

Lear, S.A., Toma, M., Birmingham, C.L. and Frohlich, J.J. (2003) Modification of the relationship between simple anthropometric indices and risk factors by ethnic background. *Metabolism* **52**, 1295–1301.

Lee, Z.S., Critchley, J.A., Ko, G.T., Anderson, P.J., Thomas, G.N., Young, R.P., Chan, T.Y., Cockram, C.S., Tomlinson, B. and Chan, J.C. (2002) Obesity and cardiovascular risk factors in Hong Kong Chinese. *Obesity Reviews* **3**, 173–182.

Leung, S.S., Lau, J.T., Xu, Y.Y., Tse, L.Y., Huen, K.F., Wong, G.W., Law, W.Y., Yeung, V.T., Yeung, W.K. and Leung, N.K. (1996) Secular changes in standing height, sitting height and sexual maturation of Chinese: the Hong Kong Growth Study, 1993. *Annals of Human Biology* **23**, 297–306.

Leung, S.S., Chan, S.M., Lui, S., Lee, W.T. and Davies, D.P. (2000) Growth and nutrition of Hong Kong children aged 0–7 years. *Journal of Paediatrics and Child Health* **36**, 56–65.

Lim, S.C., Tan, B.Y., Chew, S.K. and Tan, C.E. (2002) The relationship between insulin resistance and cardiovascular risk factors in overweight/obese non-diabetic Asian adults: the 1992 Singapore National Health Survey. *International Journal of Obesity* **26**, 1511–1516.

Lin, Y.-C., Yen, L.-L.,Chen, S.-Y., Kao, M.D., Tzeng, M.S. and Huang, P.C. (2003) Prevalence of overweight and obesity and its associated factors: findings from the National Nutrition and Health Survey in Taiwan, 1993–1996. *Preventive Medicine* **37**, 233–241.

Liu, L. Choudhury, S.R. Okayama, A. Hayakawa, T. Kita, Y., and Ueshima, H. (1999) Changes in body mass index and its relationships to other cardiovascular risk factors among Japanese population: results from the 1980 and 1990 national cardiovascular surveys in Japan. *Journal of Epidemiology* **9**, 163–174.

McKeigue, P.M., Shah, B. and Marmot, M.G. (1991) Relation of central obesity and insulin resistance with high diabetes prevalence and cardiovascular risk in South Asians. *Lancet* **337**, 382–386.

Magarey, A.M., Daniels, L.A., and Boulton, T.J. (2001) Prevalence of overweight and obesity in Australian children and adolescents: reassessment of 1985 and 1995 data against new standard international definitions. *Medical Journal of Australia* **174**, 561–564.

Moon, O.R., Kim, N.S., Jang, S.M., Yoon, T.H. and Kim, S.O. (2002)

The relationship between body mass index and the prevalence of obesity-related diseases based on the 1995 National Health Interview Survey in Korea. *Obesity Reviews* **3**, 191–196.

Norgan, N.G. (1994) Interpretation of low body mass indices: Australian aborigines. *American Journal of Physical Anthropology* **94**, 229–237.

NZ Ministry of Health (1999) *NZ Food: NZ People. Key Results of the 1997 National Nutrition Survey.* Wellington: MOH.

Ortiz, O., Russell, M., Daley, T.L., Baumgartner, R.N., Waki, M., Lichtman, S., Wang, J., Pierson, R.N. and Heymsfield, S.B. (1992) Differences in skeletal muscle and bone mineral mass between black and white females and their relevance to estimates of body composition. *American Journal of Clinical Nutrition* **55**(1), 8–13.

Park, H.S., Yun, Y.S., Por, J.Y., Kim, Y.S. and Choi, J.M. (2003) Obesity, abdominal obesity and clustering of cardiovascular risk factors in South Korea. *Asia Pacific Journal of Clinical Nutrition* **12**, 411–418.

Patel, S., Unwin, N., Bhopal, R., White, M., Harland, J., Ayis, S.A., Watson, W. and Alberti, K.G. (1999) A comparison of proxy measures of abdominal obesity in Chinese, European and South Asian adults. *Diabetic Medicine* **16**, 853–860.

Popkin, B.M. and Doak, C.M. (1998) The obesity epidemic is a worldwide phenomenon. *Nutrition Reviews* **56**, 106–114.

Popkin, B.M., Paeratakul, S.,. Zhai, F., and Ge, K. (1995) Body weight patterns among the Chinese: Results from 1989 and 1991 China Health and Nutrition Surveys. *American Journal of Public Health* **85**, 690–694.

Popkin, B., Horton, S. and Kim, S. (2001) *The Nutrition Transition and Prevention of Diet-Related Chronic Diseases in Asia and the Pacific.* ADB Nutrition and Development Series no. 6. Manila: Asian Development Bank.

Ramachandran, A., Snehalatha, C., Viswanathan, V., Viswanathan, M. and Haffner, S.M. (1997) Risk of non-insulin-dependent diabetes mellitus conferred by obesity and central adiposity in different ethnic groups: a comparative analysis between Asian Indians, Mexican Americans and Whites. *Diabetes Research and Clinical Practice* **36**, 121–125.

Ravelli, G.P., Stein, Z.A. and Susser, M. (1976) Obesity in young men after famine exposure in utero and early infancy. *New England Journal of Medicine* **295**, 349–353.

Rush, E.C., Plank, L.D., Laulu, M.S. and Robinson, S.M. (1997) Prediction of percentage body fat from anthropometric measurements: comparison of New Zealand European and Polynesian young women. *American Journal of Clinical Nutrition* **66**(1), 2–7.

Shelgikar, K.M., Hockaday, T.D. and Yajnik, C.S. (1991) Central rather than generalized obesity is related to hyperglycaemia in Asian Indian subjects. *Diabetic Medicine* **8**, 712–717.

Shen, L., Fan, J.G., Shao, Y., Zeng, M.D., Wang, J.R., Luo, G.H., Li, J.Q. and Chen, S.Y. (2003) Prevalence of nonalcoholic fatty liver among administrative officers in Shanghai: an epidemiological survey. *World Journal of Gastroenterology* **9**, 1106–1110.

Shiwaku, K., Anuurad, E., Enkhmaa, B., Nogi, A., Kitajima, K., Shimono, K., Yamane, Y. and Oyunsuren, T. (2004) Overweight Japanese with body mass indexes of 23.0–24.9 have higher risks for obesity-associated disorders: a comparison of Japanese and Mongolians. *International Journal of Obesity* **28**, 152–158.

Stevens, J. (2003) Ethnic-specific revisions of body mass index cutoffs to define overweight and obesity in Asians are not warranted. *International Journal of Obesity* **27**, 1297–1299.

Stevens, J., Juhaeri, Cai, J. and Jones, D.W (2002) The effect of decision rules on the choice of a body mass index cutoff for obesity: examples from African American and white women. *American Journal of Clinical Nutrition* **75**, 986–992.

Swinburn, B.A., Ley, S.J., Carmichael, H.E. and Plank, L.D. (1999) Body size and composition in Polynesians. *International Journal of Obesity* **23**, 1178–1183.

Villavieja, G.M., Constantino, A.S., Laña, R.D., Nones, C.A., España, N. and Pine, C.R. (2001) Anthropometric assessment of adolescents, adults, pregnant and lactating women: Philippines, 1998: reports of the Fifth National Nutrition Survey 1998 (part 1). Food and Nutrition Research Institute, Department of Science and Technology. *Philippines Journal of Nutrition* **48**, 1527.

Wang, W., Wang, K. and Li, T. (2001) A study on the epidemiological characteristics of obesity in Chinese adults. *Zhonghua Liu Xing Bing Xue Za Zhi* **22**, 129–32 (In Chinese with English abstract).

Wang, Y., Monteiro, C. and Popkin, B.M. (2002) Trends of obesity and underweight in older children and adolescents in the United States, Brazil, China, and Russia. *American Journal of Clinical Nutrition* **75**, 971–977.

Werkman, A., Deurenberg-Yap, M., Schmidt, G. and Deurenberg, P. (2000) A comparison between composition and density of the fat-free mass of young adult Singaporean Chinese and Dutch Caucasians. *Annals of Nutrition and Metabolism* **44**, 235–242.

Western Pacific Regional Office, WHO. (1999) *Western Pacific Regional Databank on Socioeconomic and Health Indicators.* Manila: WHO, WPRO.

Western Pacific Regional Office of the World Health Organization, The International Association for the Study of Obesity and The International Obesity Task Force (2000) *The Asia-Pacific Perspective: Redefining Obesity and its Treatment.* Sydney: Health Communications Australia Pty.

Wild, S., Roglic, G., Green, A., Sicree, R. and King, H. (2004) Global prevalence of diabetes. Estimates for the year 2000 and projections for 2030. *Diabetes Care* **27**,1047–1053.

Willett, W.C., Dietz, W.H. and Colditz, G.A. (1999) Guidelines for healthy weight. *New England Journal of Medicine* **6**, 427–434.

World Health Organization (1998) *Life in the 21st Century.* World Health Report 1998. Geneva: WHO.

World Health Organization (2000) *Obesity: Preventing and Managing the Global Epidemic.* Geneva: WHO.

World Health Organization (2002) *Reducing Risks — Promoting Healthy Life.* World Health Report 2002. Geneva: WHO.

World Health Organization Expert Consultation (2004) Appropriate body-mass index for Asian populations and its implications for policy and intervention strategies. *Lancet* **363**, 157–163.

Yoshiike, N., Matsumura, Y., Zaman, M.M. and Yamaguchi, M. (1998) Descriptive epidemiology of body mass index in Japanese adults in a representative sample from the National Nutrition Survey 1990–94. *International Journal of Obesity* **22**, 684–687.

Yoshiike, N., Seino, F., Tajima, S., Arai, Y., Kawano, M., Furuhata, T. and Inoue, S. (2002) Twenty-year changes in the prevalence of overweight in Japanese adults: the National Nutrition Survey 1976–95. *Obesity Reviews* **3**, 183–190.

Zhou, B.F. (2002) Predictive values of body mass index and waist circumference for risk factors of certain related diseases in Chinese adults: study on optimal cut-off points of body mass index and waist circumference in Chinese adults. *Biomedical and Environmental Science* **15**, 83–96.

Environmental and policy approaches: alternative methods

Garry Egger and Anne Thorburn

Introduction, 443

Host, 444
  Traditional weight loss
  treatments, 444
  Traditional treatment
  delivery, 444
  Alternative weight loss
  treatments, 446
  Alternative treatment
  delivery, 450

Environment, 451
  Traditional approaches, 451
  Alternative approaches, 451

Vectors and agents, 452
  Traditional approaches, 452
  Alternative approaches, 452

Summary, 453

References, 453

Introduction

That obesity is an epidemic throughout many parts of the world is now beyond question (World Health Organization, 2000). Yet the current approaches to managing the problem generally do not reflect this. Typically, epidemics are dealt with by considering all three points of an epidemiological triad; host, vector and environment (Fig. 30.1), the host being the sufferer of the disease, the vector being the deliverer of an infective agent and the environment being the situation in which the vector is allowed to flourish.

In the case of infectious diseases, these are clearly defined. With non-communicable diseases (NCDs) on the other hand, an epidemic is often considered as something different, and the host is usually the only component treated. Recognition of the importance of vectors and environments when this has occurred has usually led to big improvements in epidemic outcomes (Egger *et al.*, 2003a). Haddon's (1980) reassessment of motor vehicle accidents, for example, led to a paradigm shift in dealing with injury with consequent big improvements in motor vehicle injury rates (e.g. Mathers *et al.*, 2000). Similarly, big inroads into the smoking epidemic did not happen until changes occurred in the cultural environment, making smoking less socially acceptable in the workplace and public places (Chapman, 1993).

Recourse to the epidemiological triad highlights the need to combine both population and individual approaches for successful interventions into epidemics. Data on cardiovascular disease trends in Finland accentuate the importance of this (WHO, 2003a). From Fig. 30.2, for example, it can be seen that a general shift in cholesterol levels to the left occurred in men in Finland after the introduction of public health campaigns aimed at public education and modifying the environment (particularly decreasing the availability of high-fat dairy products) in North Karelia in the mid-1970s. Specific shifts at the upper end of the curve, however, did not occur until the advent of the statin drugs in the 1980s and 1990s, resulting in a tightening of the curve to the right, suggesting added reductions in high-risk cases. As might be expected, these shifts have been mirrored in cardiovascular disease death rates.

The population approach includes all three corners of the epidemiological triad. The individual, or 'high-risk,' approach is concentrated primarily on medical and other intensive interventions with the host alone. To date, the obesity epidemic has been dealt with largely in the latter fashion. Services are generally based around the clinical management of overweight and obese individuals. And although this is *necessary*, it is obviously not *sufficient* for dealing with big shifts in body weight in large populations. A more holistic approach incorporating 'traditional' approaches to each corner of the triad has been considered previously (Egger and Swinburn, 1997). In this chapter we expand this to include other, 'alternative' treatments and treatment deliveries, both existing and potential, to each of the three points of the triad, in an attempt to maximize resources at the population, as well as the individual level. Our use of 'alternative' here is confined to '*those approaches to obesity management not involving modifications of energy balance in individual or populations through generally accepted and traditional scientific means*'. We consider these along-

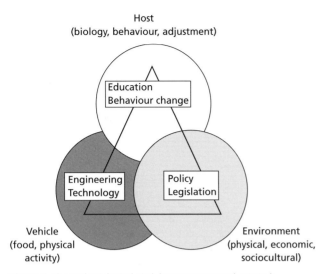

Fig 30.1 The epidemiological triad. (Source: Egger *et al.*, 2003a.)

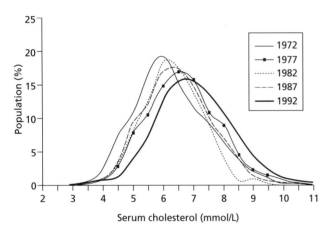

Fig 30.2 Cholesterol distribution in men of 30–59 years of age, North Karelia, Finland, 1972–92. [Source: National Public Health Institute, Helsinki, Finland (WHO, 1992).]

side the better known traditional approaches for each corner of the triad.

Host

Traditional weight loss treatments

A number of standard treatments are now available for dealing with obesity and overweight, many of which are dealt with elsewhere in this book. A meta-analysis of the success of these as part of the development of the National Clinical Practice Guidelines for Management of Overweight and Obesity in Australia (National Health and Medical Research Council, 2003) shows a variable and somewhat disappointing level of effectiveness. A summary of findings giving average weight losses for each technique is shown in Table 30.1.

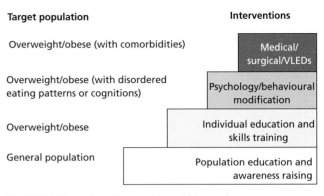

Fig 30.3 A 'stepped-care' approach to weight control management. (Source: Egger and Binns, 2002.)

Success rates vary from relatively minor with lifestyle change alone to extremely significant, using the more intensive surgical approach as an adjunct to lifestyle change. There are, however, some key points to note about these findings. In the first place they represent reported results from largely academic research studies carried out in groups. It is likely that many people can lose significant amounts of weight by undertaking personal changes in dietary and exercise habits without recourse to established programmes. Second, although the reported losses are small, these can be highly significant in terms of metabolic benefits. Several studies have now shown that a 5–10% loss of body weight can result in a significant improvement in metabolic risk factors (Dhabuwala *et al.*, 2000; Peppard *et al.*, 2000). Third, as Rossner (1999) has shown, there are a number of possible scenarios resulting from a weight loss programme. As the normal course of body weight in modern societies is a steady gain, even stable weight over the long term can represent a degree of success. Partial normalization, with a 5–10% loss can result in metabolic improvements, but total normalization is likely to be the exception rather than the rule. Treatment goals therefore need to be realistic and include both health improvements (e.g. lowered blood pressure, blood lipids and blood sugars) and behaviour change as well as weight loss.

Traditional treatment delivery

Delivery of weight control interventions at the host level is an important aspect of treatment. A stepped-care model (see Fig. 30.3) for doing this in the clinical setting has been described elsewhere (Egger and Binns, 2002).

The rapid rise of the obesity epidemic has meant rapidly changing demands in the areas of nutrition, physical activity and weight management, for which many health professionals have had little formal training. This has led to a need for dynamic, interactive and mobile sources of up-skilling and networking, which are highly adaptive to changing and evolving knowledge.

Table 30.1 The effects of weight loss treatments in overweight or obese adults: a summary.

Treatment	Weight loss/gain (kg) over 1–2 years*	Weight loss/gain (kg) over >2 years*	Ability to prevent regain?
No treatment†	−0.2	+1.9 over 3–6 years	No
Diet			
Ad lib low-fat diet	−3.9 (−2.3 to −6.1) −4.4%	−2.7 (−3.6 to −1.8) over 3–6 years	Yes, to some degree
Low-energy diet	−6.7 (−12.2 to +0.4) −6.9%	−1.1 (−4.1 to +2.7) over 4–5 years	No
Very low-energy diet	−16.3 (−8.6 to 25.6)‡ −14.7%‡ ¶ −4.2 (−8.6 to +0.5)§ −4.0%§ −11.8 (−9.2 to −14.2)¶ −11.0%¶	−4.1 (−7.9 to +1.0) over 3–5 years	Yes, to some degree in some individuals if combined with a lifestyle modification programme
Meal replacement	−5.5 (−3.0 to −7.7) −6.0%	−6.5 (−4.2 to −9.5) over 4–5 years	Yes, based on limited evidence
Low glycaemic index, high-protein or high-monounsaturated fatty acid diets	Not known	Not known	Not known
Physical activity	−1.8 (−5.8 to +0.7) −2.1%**	−1.3 (−3.1 to +1.0) over 2–6 years	Yes, if 80 min or more of daily activity
Diet plus activity	−7.5 (−15.2 to −4.2) −8.1%	−3.1 (−9.9 to 0) over 2–6 years	Yes, to some degree
Behaviour	−4.7 (−12.9 to −0.2) −5.1%	−2.8 (−9.6 to −0.2) over 3–5 years	Yes, to some degree
Pharmacological			
Diethylpropion	−6.5 (−1.9 to −13.1)	Not known	Yes, while drug is taken
Phentermine	−6.3 (−3.6 to −8.8)	Not known	Yes, while drug is taken
Sibutramine	−5.6 (−7.9 to −3.8) 6.0%	Not known	Yes, while drug is taken
Sibutramine plus lifestyle modification	−10.8 (−16.6 to −5.2) 10.7%	Not known	Yes, while drug is taken
Orlistat plus a mildly hypocaloric diet	−8.4 (−13.1 to −6.2)** −8.6%	−6.9‡‡	Yes, while drug is taken with a normal energy diet
Surgery			
Gastric bypass	−46 (−53 to −35) −36%	−42 (−62 to −29) over 3–14 years	Yes
Biliopancreatic bypass	−53 (−62 to −42) −38%	−54 (−84 to −37) over 3–8 years	Yes
Non-adjustable gastroplasty	−41 (−63 to −25) −32%	−25 (−39 to −17) over 3–8 years	Some weight regain
Adjustable gastric banding	−31 (−46 to −22) −24%	−34 (−43 to −28) over 3–4 years	Yes

*Results expressed as mean weight loss, with range of weight loss in parentheses and % weight loss in italics.

†Based on the placebo arms of 31 treatment studies lasting 1–2 years and 8 studies lasting more than 2 years.

‡After 4–20 weeks.

§After 1–2 years without diet or behavioural therapy.

¶After 1–2 years with diet or behavioural therapy.

**With 3–5 h of moderate or vigorous activity per week.

††Weight loss due to orlistat alone is 2.8 kilograms.

‡‡Not yet published in peer-reviewed literature (abstract only).

Source: National Health and Medical Research Council (2003).

In Australia, over 4000 general practitioners and 3000 exercise and nutrition workers have been involved in training in weight control and obesity management as part of out-service Post- and Pre-Graduate Certificates, conducted by Sydney University since 1997. A survey carried out with 266 participating doctors and 607 overweight patients in 1999 showed that 96% said they felt more confident in helping patients lose weight, and 28% claimed to have lost weight themselves after the training programme (Egger *et al.*, 2003b). In New Zealand, over 50% of GPs are now using written exercise ('green') prescriptions (Wilson *et al.*, 2001) on a regular basis with a reasonable level of medium-term success. As over 80% of people visit their GPs in these countries each year, there is substantial potential for population as well as individual changes through these strategies, particularly if they are combined with other corners of the epidemiological triad.

The development of clinical guidelines for nutrition, physical activity and weight control and obesity management in several countries has also assisted in providing professionals with principles of treatment operations.

Commercial weight loss programmes

Data from some countries suggest that up to 13% of women and 5% of men participate in commercial weight loss programmes (Latner, 2001), and that these may be more successful than other approaches (Heshka *et al.*, 2000). However, few randomized controlled trials of commercial programmes have been carried out. One recent trial compared the effects of a self-help programme (brief counselling and provision of printed materials) with a commercial programme (Weight Watchers) in overweight and obese men and women (Heshka *et al.*, 2000).

Table 30.2 Popular alternative approaches to weight loss.

Host approaches	*Environmental approaches*
Ingestible treatments	Environmental diagnosis (e.g. ANGELO)
Herbal substances: whole plants (e.g. brindleberry), ingredients (e.g. HCA)	Lay support groups
Non-herbal supplements (e.g. chromium picolinate)	School canteen modifications
Natural non-herbal substances (e.g. chitosan)	Exercise/fitness facilities for children/older adults
Food components (e.g. capsaicin, caffeine, pectin)	New building codes
Single foods (e.g. grapefruit, cabbage)	Radical taxing initiatives
Non-ingestible treatments	Vehicle restricted localities
Topical creams/soaps	Signage (e.g. stair alternatives)
Acupuncture/acupressure	Modified town planning
Hypnosis	Intersectoral involvement
Electrical stimulation	Environmental modification (e.g. biosphere)
Psychotherapy	Subsidize cost of exercise facilities and low-energy foods
Body wraps	Target worksites, e.g. employee activity incentive programmes
Passive exercise devices	Target sociocultural aspects of environment not just physical aspects
Yoga/t'ai chi, etc.	Intervene in restaurant environment (e.g. educate chefs, nutritional information on menu)
Massage	
Aromatherapy	*Vector approaches*
Alternative forms of treatment delivery	Movement-activated electronic games and entertainment devices
Correspondence	Active commuting
Mass media/multimedia	Pet ownership
Internet	New (active) sports development
Shared care	Virtual reality devices
Group therapy	Electronic prompts

After 26 weeks, subjects in the commercial programme had greater decreases in body weight (–4.8 vs. –1.4 kg) and waist circumference (–4.3 vs. –0.7 cm) than those in the self-help programme.

There is also evidence of successful long-term maintenance of weight loss from commercial programmes. Lowe *et al.* (2001), for example, have shown that 5 years following successful completion of a commercial weight loss programme (Weight Watchers) 43% of subjects maintained a weight loss of 5% or more, and 19% maintained a weight loss of at least 10%. Similarly, Gosselin and Cote (2001), have shown that 5–11 years after women had participated in a popular commercial programme based on Canada's Food Guide, 29% maintained a weight loss of at least 5%, and 14% maintained a weight loss of at least 10%. It seems, therefore, that in some individuals, commercial weight loss programmes can lead to effective weight maintenance long after the individuals have left the programme.

In summary, there is a range of traditional treatments and treatment deliveries for weight loss, with variable degrees of success. In general, it can be said that success rates are not high and that all successful approaches involve a long-term lifestyle change, but delivery of these and adjunctive treatments, such as surgery, drug treatments, and behaviour modification, can add to their success.

Alternative weight loss treatments

Although there are a significant number of traditional treatment options, as seen above, there is obviously widespread disillusionment with their success. Surveys indicate that although up to 72% of men and 85% of women in some countries are trying to lose, or at least not gain, weight at any one particular time (Kottke *et al.*, 2002), less than 30% of those trying to lose and 20% of those trying not to gain report using 'traditional' treatments to do so (Khan *et al.*, 2001), 'Alternative' treatments at the host level are often more widely used, although their effectiveness has yet to be established. A summary of the major alternative options, within the points of the triad, is shown in Table 30.2.

The approaches considered in more detail below are: (a) ingestible substances; (b) non-ingestible treatments; and (c) alternative treatment delivery.

Ingestible substances

As many as 7% of the US population (Allison *et al.*, 2001), and up to 28% of young, obese women (Blanck *et al.*, 2001), regularly use non-prescription, over-the-counter substances for weight loss. Although the range of these products is extensive and being added to constantly, there are a number of ingredients that recur constantly. A number of these, their theoretical rationale and level of supporting evidence are shown in Table 30.3 (National Health and Medical Research Council, 2003).

In a number of recent reviews of the efficacy of these products (Egger *et al.*, 1999; 2003b; Morelli and Zoorob, 2000; Allison *et al.*, 2001; National Health and Medical Research Council, 2003), the authors have concurred that although several products do have a reasonable physiological rationale, claims of effectiveness are usually not based on well-controlled studies that are published in reliable peer-reviewed literature. An exception to this is a caffeine–ephedrine combination that has been shown to have short-term weight loss benefits, but which has been discontinued as a weight loss product in most countries because of the potential addictive and tolerance effects (Astrup *et al.*, 1992). Attempts to emulate this with chemically similar substances, such as guarana or ephedra, or plant products such as the Chinese herb Ma Huang, have not been successful. Side-effects and some deaths have led the US Food and Drug Administration (FDA) to take action in 2002 against marketers of this product, and its continued availability and long-term safety is under question at present.

Another food ingredient with suggestions for weight loss is pectin from dietary fibre. Foods high in fibre are filling and can lead to early satiation during meals and snacks. This should have a beneficial effect in treating obesity by decreasing total energy intake. Foods high in dietary fibre also have a lower energy density as dietary fibre contributes fewer kilojoules than other carbohydrates (Livesey, 1995). Indeed, a diet high in fibre-rich foods has been shown to have a positive effect for weight loss (Catellanos and Rolls, 1997). Whether particular types of fibre added to dietary supplements in small amounts have any direct effect on weight loss, however, is unclear. Longer term studies have so far shown no effects on weight loss from fibre supplements (Pasman *et al.*,1997).

Three other commonly used over-the-counter supplements are worth considering in more detail, based on their popularity in weight loss concoctions and their theoretical or physiological actions.

Hydroxycitric acid

There have been seven studies examining the effects of hydroxycitric acid (HCA, contained in brindleberry) and weight loss in humans reported in the literature to date (Conte, 1993; Badmaev and Majeed, 1995; Girola *et al.*, 1996; Thom, 1996; Rothacker and Waitman, 1997; Heymsfield *et al.*, 1998). Of these studies, five reported some positive results, but all suffered serious experimental inadequacies such as lack of a control group, insufficient numbers, inadequate testing period or the combination of HCA with other substances (for a more detailed review, see Allison *et al.*, 1998). Two studies were from industry publications and two are unpublished. In the first rigorous, randomized control study of HCA and weight

loss, no difference was found between one group of obese individuals who were given 1500 mg of HCA per day and another group who were given a placebo over a 12-week period (Allison *et al.*, 1998). Rat studies that claim HCA may reduce food intake were partly supported by a 2-week single-blind crossover trial in humans in the Netherlands, which reported a 5–30% decrease in 24-h energy intake, although without changes in appetite profile or dietary restraint (Westerterp-Plantenga and Kovacs, 2002). However, another study of 89 mildly obese women found no effects of HCA on appetite variables and no satiety effect (Mattes and Bormann, 2002). Hence there appears to be no convincing evidence of the effects of HCA in weight loss.

Capsaicin

Capsaicin is the major pungent ingredient of hot chillies and peppers, which is marketed as an ingredient to increase metabolism and increase the power of other herbal products. Capsaicin activates neurons and neuropeptides that are thought to suppress food intake (Buck and Burks, 1986). It may also increase secretion of adrenaline, which stimulates gluconeogenesis and lipolysis (MacLean, 1985). A recent study on capsaicin has shown that an entrée of spicy food may reduce the intake of food in a main meal by approximately 200 kcal (Tremblay, 1998). Studies in rats suggest that doses of capsaicin that are obtainable in a highly spiced diet can increase body temperature and oxygen consumption (Watanabe *et al.*, 1988; Cameron-Smith *et al.*, 1990). In humans, there is some evidence of a sustained increase in oxygen consumption following a meal containing a chilli extract (Cameron-Smith *et al.*, 1990). However, some studies were unable to show any changes in oxygen consumption, fat utilization or body temperature (Edwards *et al.*,1992; Glickman-Weiss *et al.*, 1998). Capsaicin in low-fat spicy foods may add variety to a low-energy diet, with some possible benefits on energy balance. There is no support, however, for taking the substance as a supplement.

Chitosan

Chitosan is an amino polysaccharide derived from the powdered shells of marine crustaceans, such as prawns and crabs, which is thought to bind to dietary fat, preventing digestion and storage. Because this action is similar to that of the approved prescription medication orlistat, a similar weight loss outcome might be expected. However, the available evidence to date fails to support this. Some human studies have shown lipid lowering (Ventura, 1996) as well as weight loss with chitosan (Maezaki *et al.*, 1993; Abelin and Lassus, 1994; Veneroni *et al.*, 1996), although none has been published in peer-reviewed journals and all are limited by methodological flaws, including small numbers, high drop-out rate and lack of adherence to a high-fat diet. Trials have shown a weight loss effect when chitosan is given with a hypocaloric diet for up to 4 weeks (Abelin and Lassus, 1994; Giustina and Ventura, 1995; Sciutto and Columbo, 1995), but a meta-analysis of these

Table 30.3 Identification and assessment of common ingredients in popular weight loss supplements.

Constituent	Active ingredient	Source	Proposed action	Theoretical rationale[a]	Supporting evidence[b]	Potential risks
Brindleberry	Hydroxycitric acid (HCA)	Rind of a type of citrus fruit	Inhibits lipogenesis from CHO; reduces appetite through gluconeogenesis	x	Negative	No
Peppers	Capsaicin	Spicy foods; chilli	Increases energy expenditure	**	* (in food)	Yes
Caffeine/guarana	Caffeine	Seeds of a climbing shrub from Brazil and Uruguay	Increases metabolic rate	**	* (caffeine)	Yes
L-Carnitine	L-Carnitine	Synthesized from lysine	Fat 'metabolizer'	**	–	No
Fibre/pectin	Water-soluble dietary fibre—polymer of galacturonic acid	Fruit/jams	Increases satiety	**	* (in food)	No
Fucus vesiculosus kelp	Iodine	Seawrack or bladderwrack (types of seaweed)	Increases metabolic rate through increased activity of thyroid gland	*	–	No
Chitosan	Deacetylated chitin (amino polysaccharide)	Marine crustacean shells	Inhibits fat absorption	* (with low-energy diet)	*	Yes
Chromium picolinate	Soluble chromium	Supplement	Improves insulin sensitivity	*	Negative	Yes
Gingko biloba EGb761	Flavonoid, terpenes	Extract from maidenhair	Stress reduction, prevents oedema	–	–	Yes
Grapeseed extract	Bioflavonoids	Extract from seeds	Antioxidant; benefits circulation	–	–	No
Soy lecithin	Phospholipid	Soy beans	Increases fat transport	*	–	No
Horse chestnut	Saponins	Seeds, flowers and bark of tree	Antioxidant; benefits circulation by decreasing oedema, increased 'flushing'	–	–	No
Dried sweet clover	Isoflavine	Extract from plant	Oestrogenic properties; increases circulation	–	–	No
Inositol	Vitamin-like compound	Component of liver/muscle	Prevents fat accumulation in liver	*	–	No
St John's wort	Not clear	Perennial herb	Antidepressant	–	–	Yes

a. x, theory is inaccurate/disproved; –, no evidence supporting theoretical rationale in weight loss; * or **, level of evidence supporting rationale in weight loss (high level of evidence = ***).
b. Negative, scientific evidence against claims; –, no scientific evidence supporting claims; * or **, level of evidence supporting claims.
Source: National Health and Medical Research Council (2003).

(Ernst and Pittler, 1998) shows discrepancies in the data, suggesting that the studies are flawed. In a recent randomized control trial, no effect of chitosan was found without a reduction in food intake (Pittler *et al.*, 1999). However, this study involved only 17 people over 1 month. Malabsorption of fat in the digestive tract may theoretically affect energy uptake, but there is no long-term evidence showing the effectiveness of this strategy for weight loss with a substance such as chitosan.

Other supplements

A number of compounds including bissey nut extract, citrus aurantium, coleus forskolin, ephedra alkaloids, ginseng, green tea extract, L-tyrosine, magnesium stearate, gymnema sylvestre and pyruvate have been promoted as weight loss substances. However, to date, there is no acceptable evidence supporting any of these for weight loss in humans. More detailed future research may show advantages for these and other non-prescribed substances and the possible benefits of synergistic effects between ingredients cannot be ruled out, and needs further study. Average long-term weight losses, even with proven prescribed medications, are poor and only exist while a drug is being taken. If non-prescribed substances are to be successful, lifetime use may be needed, as with other chronic disorders.

Non-ingestible treatments

As well as ingestible substances, there is a wide range of alternative non-ingestible treatments claiming benefits for weight loss. Some of the more enduring include the following.

Skin creams

Most skin creams claiming weight loss properties are focused on 'cellulite' reduction (Rosenbaum *et al.*, 1998). Cellulite creams are diverse, with 32 products that were surveyed containing 263 ingredients (Sainio *et al.*, 2000). Caffeine is commonly reported as an active ingredient, although no published evidence supports a role for topically applied caffeine in cellulite reduction. In their review of thigh creams, Allison and colleagues (2001) conclude that any changes resulting from these are at most cosmetic, and there is no evidence for medical/health benefits of these treatments. Slimming soaps that contain seaweed extract as the active ingredient have also been claimed to have weight loss effects (Marshall, 1995), but again there is no published supporting evidence or physiological basis for these claims.

Acupuncture and acupressure

Acupuncture, acupressure and related oriental techniques are frequently cited as strategies to curb appetite and lower body weight. At least four controlled studies have found no such effect (Allison *et al.*, 1995), although improved psychological

status has been observed in a recent randomized, placebo-controlled trial (Mazzoni *et al.*, 1999). In one controlled study, combined acupressure and transcutaneous electrical stimulation (TENS) of the auricular branch of the vagal nerve, using an AcuSlim device, suppressed appetite and body weight (-3.0 ± 1.4 kg) when applied twice weekly for 4 weeks (Richard and Marley, 1998). However, auricular acupressure without electrical stimulation has not been found to have any effect (Allison *et al.*, 1995). Further studies are required to provide data on the longer term effectiveness of acupressure techniques in weight loss.

Electrical stimulation

Electronic muscle stimulation (EMS) or TENS apparatus is used as a supplementary treatment option in the management of selected muscular rehabilitation and conditioning. At least one study has shown significant weight loss with TENS compared with a control group (Richard and Marley, 1995) prompting a suggestion for further independent research on this process. However, no impact of EMS on body weight has been demonstrated (Porcari *et al.*, 2002).

Hypnosis

Hypnotherapy is often used as an adjunct treatment in weight loss, although few controlled studies exist on its effectiveness. A meta-analysis of five controlled studies using hypnosis for weight loss demonstrated a small non-significant effect, but a further review of the same dataset, with the inclusion of one additional study, suggested a small significant effect (2.6 kg) (Kirsh, 1996). In more recent studies, a slight benefit (mean loss of 2 kg) occurred with hypnosis plus overt aversion (electric shock, disgusting tastes and smells) compared with hypnosis alone (Johnson, 1997), although a similar study did not confirm this (Johnson and Karkut, 1996). In another study, 60 obese patients with obstructive sleep apnoea were randomized to receive two forms of hypnosis (directed at stress reduction or reducing energy intake reduction) compared with standard dietary advice alone. After initial weight loss in all groups, the hypnotherapy for stress reduction was the only intervention to achieve persistent weight loss (mean 3.8 kg) (Sreadling *et al.*, 1998).

Several other alternative treatment approaches including massage, body wrapping and strapping, Eastern stress management techniques such as yoga and t'ai chi, and a range of passive exercise devices have been proposed for weight loss, but at present none has any reliable evidence supporting its use for weight loss.

In summary, a caffeine–ephedrine mix is the only alternative non-prescription ingestible product with convincing evidence of weight loss success. However, the short-term nature of this approach and adverse side-effects have led to it being banned in most countries. Other substances such as HCA, capsaicin and chitosan, although claiming success, have not consistently demonstrated success in controlled studies. At present, there are no convincing data available for herbal mixes. Minor weight loss benefits have been reported with alternative non-ingestible treatments such as hypnosis, and possibly acupressure with electrical stimulation in some situations, suggesting a possible justification for further research. Other treatments such as skin creams, body wrapping and passive exercise devices have no reliable evidence for their support.

Alternative treatment delivery

Perhaps more interesting than alternative therapeutic treatments are alternative forms of delivery of otherwise traditional treatments and preventative methods. These are now becoming of interest to orthodox researchers, and a recent workshop on innovative approaches has now considered many of the available options (for a workshop report, see http://www.niddk.nih.gov/fund/other/obesity_report.pdf). Four main methods of delivery are considered here.

Correspondence

Correspondence programmes offer a cost-effective means of delivering weight control programmes to a large number of people. Consumer preferences indicate that this approach may also be more desirable for many than face-to-face formats, particularly in higher education and income level groups (Sherwood et al., 1998). Programmes can range from being totally self-help with minimal contact to adding a component to a shared-care programme. They have also been offered at no cost, at commercial rates or with different forms of cost incentives. Reported success rates are generally higher with some level of payment, perhaps indicating a level of self-selection through commitment. Telephone-based interventions have also been found to have reasonable success in some cases. Correspondence may be more effective in some groups than others and may depend on the type of intervention required. King and colleagues (1989) found that exercise is easier to maintain by men who are using minimal-contact strategies than dietary approaches focusing on modification of energy intake.

Internet

The development of the Internet provides unique opportunities for delivery of weight loss programmes. However, at present there is a huge variation in relevance and quality of sites, with probably less than 5% providing sound weight loss advice (Miles et al., 2000). Also, despite the wide proliferation of services, there is almost a complete lack of evidence of the effects of the Internet on health outcomes (Bessell et al., 2002). One study comparing passive website education with more intensive Internet behaviour therapy did find positive short-term (6-month) effects on weight loss, with bigger effects in the more intensive group (Tate et al., 2001). Other studies are being

tested with physical activity (Napolitano et al., 2003) and overweight teenagers (Williamson, 2003).

Mass media/multimedia

Mass media programmes in lifestyle change were initially tested in the 1970s with limited success. More recently, mass media in community interventions have been found to increase awareness but have limited impact on weight loss at the population level (Jeffrey, 1995; Miles et al., 2001). The development of multimedia systems presents a new and expanded opportunity for programme delivery. Some existing correspondence programmes have used elements of this such as videos, audio tapes and print. However, the current availability of computer-based audio and video CDs and e-mail, and Internet delivery of these strategies provides promising new opportunities to satisfy the requirements of many people for minimal-contact interactive services. At present there is no evidence of the benefits of such systems.

Shared care

Shared care has been used as an effective delivery option for many health-related programmes, ranging from asthma to pregnancy. Because weight control ideally calls for multidisciplinary input, the idea of shared care between disciplines is a logical approach to service delivery. Shared care is often referred to in principle, although surprisingly few evaluative studies have been reported. However, there is some evidence of better weight loss than in conventional single disciplinary interventions (Richman et al., 1996). Options that optimize use of the practitioner's time by combining developed programmes with correspondence courses may be a logical direction for the future.

Combined approach

Although each of the delivery services discussed here has the potential for improving outcomes in weight control, a combination of these approaches would seem to have logical advantages over any single approach. Some attempts have been made at this with programmes such as GutBusters in Australia (Egger et al., 1996), which was developed as a shared-care correspondence course, carried out in conjunction with trained GPs. As a result of the appeal of the programme, and the availability of new technology, the GutBuster programme has now been modified and expanded to include a range of weight loss programmes at different levels of intervention, using multimedia materials in a correspondence pack, connecting participants to an interactive Internet site (www.professortrim.com) and shared care with over 1000 GPs and 100 specially trained 'personal weight coaches'. Prospective evaluation is being established to monitor the ongoing effectiveness of the programme.

Environment

Traditional approaches

Although changes to the environment are considered a vital part of managing infectious disease epidemics, attention has only recently been paid to the environment in relation to non-communicable disease (NCD) epidemics. Theoretical propositions have been put forward in relation to obesity management, including the use of a diagnostic tool (Swinburn *et al.*, 1999). However, at least one group of experts concedes that major environmental changes aimed at obesity reduction will be difficult in modern societies (Peters and Hill, 2002). Traditional approaches such as advocacy and legislation have worked in the case of smoking (Chapman, 1993), and structural changes, such as dividing of roads and fencing requirements for swimming pools, have reduced traffic injuries and drowning (Mathers *et al.*, 2000). However, the general failure to consider population approaches to obesity has so far resulted in few policies or environmental strategies being used directly for obesity management. Restriction of fast-food advertising to children, mandated food labelling, modification of school canteens, community exercise facilities, tax incentives on reduced energy foods and trade policy could all presumably be brought to the fore in a concerted environmental approach to obesity. A number of these have been suggested previously (Swinburn and Egger, 2002). For a more comprehensive approach, however, we may need to look to alternative, more radical and more long-term solutions to the problem.

Alternative approaches

In almost all countries, standard environmental approaches to obesity management have yet to be considered as part of a mainstream attack on obesity. Suggestions for alternative approaches are therefore theoretical and have little evidential support. Some of these have been suggested previously (Swinburn and Egger, 2002) and some are being researched at present (e.g. see http://www.niddk.nih.gov/fund/other/obesityreport.pdf). As an additional 'wish list', the following could be seen as a starting point for public debate.

Encouragement of fitness centres for children and older adults

Although health clubs and gymnasiums have existed for many years, the development of new fitness forms, such as aerobics to music, led to a revitalization of the fitness industry in the late 1970s and early 80s. Typically, however, modern fitness centres are economically driven, and hence cater to the more fit and affluent in the community. Tax or other incentives to encourage exercise facilities for children and older adults could lead to more active involvement by these groups.

Development of new building codes

Building codes and town planning changes have the potential to influence activity levels in large sectors of the community. These are long-term rather than short-term measures and require a level of acceptance by the community that obesity is a key issue. Building codes encouraging use of stairways, open areas for active commuting and town planning restricting the use of motor vehicles, such as the Central London vehicle restriction plan, are potential opportunities.

Encouragement of advocacy groups

Self-help groups are common in most forms of illness. In general, these are aimed at providing a service and support for sufferers. Advocacy groups, on the other hand, such as FOE (Fighting the Obesity Epidemic), which exists in New Zealand, contribute to advocacy services aimed at increasing public awareness and action against obesity. Such groups are usually self-funded but could benefit from government support on the basis of decreasing health costs.

Radical taxing initiatives

Although taxing of excess body fatness has discriminatory overtones, there are opportunities for tax incentives in people who are prepared to accept low-cost approaches to dealing with the problem. Incentives for individuals with impaired glucose tolerance, which would normally progress to full diabetes, to reduce their risk through non-drug approaches like lifestyle change and weight loss could well be considered within present-day government medical support systems.

Pet ownership

There is mounting evidence to suggest that those who keep pets are likely to benefit from various improvements in health. Although it is not known whether pet ownership influences body weight, such a relationship is likely to exist as pets can stimulate exercise, reduce anxiety and provide an external focus of attention. On the other hand, stray dogs in indigenous cultures often restrict the motivation of people to walk (Egger *et al.*, 1999), and hence public health measures to license or eliminate stray animals may be an effective environmental approach typical activity.

Improving active opportunities

As part of a WHO obesity control project in Tonga, businesses have contributed to the development of a footpath in a main thoroughfare region, which traditionally discouraged walking because of dust in the dry season and mud in the wet (WHO, 2002b). The intention of this approach is to enable individuals to become more active rather than rely on automated transport.

Electronic prompts

Consumers could more easily identify low-energy food choices if the energy content of serving sizes was more obvious. For example, this information could be stored electronically in the product's bar code and could be displayed at the checkout register or at 'energy' checkpoints throughout supermarkets. This would be much more informative for consumers than 'tick' systems for low-fat foods, and would eliminate some of the confusion that exists over the energy density of foods that are labelled 'no cholesterol', 'baked not fried', 'extra lean' or 'lite'.

Changing activity choice in children

Two recent studies have shown that physical activity increases in obese children when access to sedentary activities is contingent on some form of exercise. In one study, obese children who accumulated 750 pedometer counts to earn 10 min of access to video games or movies engaged in more physical activity than children in a control group who had unrestricted access to sedentary behaviours (Goldfield *et al.*, 2000). Similarly, children who were only allowed to watch video movies and play video games after riding a stationary bicycle increased their physical activity and decreased their TV activities compared with children in a control group who were able to freely engage in sedentary activities (Saelens and Epstein, 1998). In African-American girls, taking up after-school dance classes has also been shown to reduce television viewing (Robinson *et al.*, 2003).

Vectors and agents

Traditional approaches

Typically, dealing with vectors and their agents makes up a large part of the treatment of any infectious disease epidemic. This is generally accomplished through either engineering or technology. Mosquito-borne disease, for example, is dealt with by spraying insecticides to kill mosquitoes and their infective agent. The agent of obesity is positive energy balance and its vectors are high-energy dense foods and modern technology, particularly effort-reducing (time-saving) and effort-sparing (time-consuming) machines. The standard technological approach to dealing with obesity to date has been to reduce the energy density of foods and engineer a wide range of exercise machines. There is potential to improve on this approach by modifying foods and the preparation of foods without changing taste, or at least changing it minimally. An example is the ability to dramatically change the fat content of chips according to deep-frying practices (Morley-John *et al.*, 2002). Further development of specially prepared food and meal replacements by food technologists may prove useful as these products enable people to easily control their food environment, and recent data show that once-a-day meal substitution is surprisingly effective (see Table 30.1). However, there are limited opportunities for expanding these traditional approaches, and lateral thinking to develop alternative approaches may have some benefits.

Alternative approaches

There are a limited number of alternative options for modifying the vectors of energy balance. Some of these are shown below.

Active commuting to school

New initiatives such as 'walking buses' can encourage physical activity in children by providing a safe, creative and enjoyable way for children to walk to and from school with parental supervision.

Development of new sporting activities

New sports can encourage participation in physical activity. These are continually being invented or reinvented. For example, snowboarding, kite surfing, bocce ball and even riding scooters have been popular in recent years.

Virtual reality devices

These devices use virtual environments for health care and have been developed for many purposes, including preventative medicine and patient education. As a tool in clinical psychology, they may be useful in promoting healthy eating and encouraging physical activity in people who are obese or have binge eating disorders (Riva *et al.*, 2001).

Active electronic games

Electronic devices in game parlours, which require movement, such as foot pads, mean that players are required to be active, rather than passive, as is usually the case in most electronic games. These can result in considerable expenditure of energy. An automated system that makes television and small screen entertainment contingent upon physical activity also has the potential for modifying activity in the treatment of obesity. For example, entertainment devices could be invented, which only operate when physical activity is being performed e.g. electronic games that are only activated by movement, or TVs that only operate when motion is detected on a pedometer or exercise bike.

Summary

Obesity is a multifaceted problem with no single treatment solution. In considering its epidemic nature in modern societies, a holistic approach, involving host, vector and environment would seem to be necessary to limit its spread and reduce the growth of associated metabolic diseases. Environmental and policy approaches that involve professional and lay groups as well as new and alternative programmes and sources of delivery may be necessary as part of the gamut of solutions offered to overweight and obese individuals in order to limit the huge potential increases in treatment costs expected to occur in the immediate future.

References

Abelin, J. and Lassus, A.L. (1994) *112 Bipolymer—Fat [binder] as a Weight Reducer in Patients with Moderate Obesity*. Medical Research Report. A study performed at Ars Medicina, Helsinki, August–October, 1994.

Allison, D.B., Kreibich, K., Heshka, S. and Heymsfield, S.B. (1995) A randomised placebo-controlled clinical trial of an acupressure device for weight loss. *International Journal of Obesity* **19**, 653–658.

Allison, D.B., Fonatine, K.R., Heshka, S., Mentore, J. and Heymsfield, S.B. (2001) Alternative treatments for weight loss: A critical review. *Critical Review of Food Science and Nutrition* **41**, 1–28.

Astrup, A., Breum, L. and Toubro, S. (1992) The effect and safety of an ephedrine/caffeine compound compared to ephedrine, caffeine and placebo in obese subjects on an energy restricted diet. A double blind trial. *International Journal of Obesity* **16**, 269–277.

Badmaev, V. and Majeed, M. (1995) Open field, physician controlled, clinical evaluation of botanical weight loss formula citrin. Presented to Nutracon 1995, Nutriceutical, Dietary Supplements and Functional Foods and reported in Heymsfield et al. (below).

Bessell, T.L., McDonald, S., Silagy, C.A., Anderson, J.N., Hiller, J.E. and Sansom, L.N. (2002) Do Internet interventions for consumers cause more harm than good? A systematic review. *Health Expectations* **5**, 28–37.

Blanck, H.M., Khan, L.K. and Serdula, M.K. (2001) Use of non-prescription weight loss products: results from a multi-state survey. *Journal of the American Medical Association* **286**, 930–935.

Buck, S.H. and Burks, T.F. (1986) The neuropharmacology of capsaicin: review of some recent observations. *Pharmacology Review* **38**, 179–226.

Cameron-Smith, D., Colquhoun, E.Q., Ye, J.M., Hettiarachchi, M. and Clark, M.G. (1990) Capsaicin and dihydrocapsaicin stimulate oxygen consumption in the perfused rat hindlimb. *International Journal of Obesity* **14**, 259–270.

Catellanos, V. and Rolls, B. (1997) Diet composition and the regulation of food intake and body weight. In: Dalton, S. ed. *Overweight and Weight Management*. Gaithersburg, MD: Aspen Publications.

Chapman, S. (1993) Unwrapping gossamer with boxing gloves. *British Medical Journal* **307**, 429–432.

Conte, A.A. (1993) A non-prescription alternative on weight reduction therapy. *American Journal of Bariatric Medicine* **3**, 17–19.

Dhabuwala, A., Cannan, R.J. and Stubbs, R.S. (2000) Improvement in co-morbidities following weight loss from gastric bypass surgery. *Obesity Surgery* **10**, 428–435.

Edwards, S.J., Montgomery, I.M., Colquhoun, E.Q., Jordan, J.E. and Clark, M.G. (1992) Spicy meal disturbs sleep: an effect of thermoregulation? *International Journal of Psychophysiology* **13**, 97–100.

Egger, G. and Swinburn, B. (1997) An ecological approach to the obesity pandemic. *British Medical Journal* **315**, 477–480.

Egger, G. and Binns, A. (2002) *The Expert's Weight Loss Guide*. Sydney: Allen and Unwin.

Egger, G., Bolton, A., O'Neill and Freeman, D. (1996) Effectiveness of an abdominal obesity reduction programme in men: the GutBuster 'waist loss' programme. *International Journal of Obesity* **23**, 564–569.

Egger, G., Stanton, R. and Cameron-Smith, D. (1999) The effectiveness of popular, non-prescription, weight loss supplements. *Medical Journal of Australia* **171**, 604–608.

Egger, G., Swinburn, B. and Rossner, S. (2003a) Dusting off the epidemiological triad: could it work with obesity. *Obesity Reviews* **4**, 115–119.

Egger, G., Stanton, R. and Cameron-Smith, D. (2003b) Alternative treatments for weight loss: range, rationale and effectiveness. In: Medieros-Neto, G., Halpern, A., Bouchard, C. eds. *Progress in Obesity Research*: 9. London: Eurotext Ltd., John Libbey, 922–926.

Ernst, E. and Pittler, M.H. (1998) A meta-analysis of chitosan for body weight reduction. *Perfusion* **11**, 461–465.

Girola, M., De Bernardi, M. and Conti, S. (1996) Dose effect in lipid lowering activity of a new dietary intetrator (chitosan, Garcinia cambogia extract, and chrome). *Acta Toxicologica Therapiae* **17**, 25–40.

Giustina, A. and Ventura, P. (1995) Weight-reducing regimens in obese subjects: effects of a new dietary fibre integrator. *Acta Toxicologica Therapiae* **16**, 199–214.

Glickman-Weiss, E., Hearon, C.M., Nelson, A.G., Nelson, A.G. and Day, R. (1998) Does capsaicin affect physiologic and thermal responses of males during immersion in 22 degrees C? *Aviation, Space and Environmental Medicine* **69**, 1095–1099.

Goldfield, G.S., Kalakanis, L.E., Ernst, M.M. and Epstein, L.H. (2000) Open-loop feedback to increase physical activity in obese children. *International Journal of Obesity* **24**, 888–892.

Goldstein, D. (1992) Beneficial health effects of modest weight loss. *International Journal of Obesity* **16**, 397–415.

Gosselin, C. and Cote, G. (2001) Weight loss maintenance in women two to eleven years after participating in a commercial program: a survey. *BMC Womens Health* **1**, 2.

Haddon, W. (1980) Advances in the epidemiology of injuries as a basis for public policy. *Public Health Reports* **95**, 411–420.

Heshka, S., Greenway, F., Anderson, J.W., Atkinson, R.L., Hill, J.O., Phinney, S.D., Millar-Kovach, K. and Pi-Sunyer, X. (2000) Self-help weight loss versus a structured commercial program after 26 weeks: a randomized controlled study. *American Journal of Medicine* **109**, 282–287.

Heymsfield, S.B., Allison, D.B., Vasselli, J.R., Pietrobelli, A., Geenfield, D. and Nunez, C. (1998) Garcinia cambogia (hydroxycitric acid) as a potential antiobesity agent: a randomised controlled trial. *Journal of the American Medical Association* **11**, 1596–1600.

Jeffery, R.W. (1995) Community programs for obesity prevention: the

Minnesota Heart Health Program. *Obesity Research* **3** (Suppl. 2), 283S–288S.

Johnson, D.L. (1997) Weight loss for women: studies of smokers and nonsmokers using hypnosis and multicomponent treatments with and without overt aversion. *Psychology Reports* **30**, 931–933.

Johnson, D.L. and Karkut, R.T. (1996) Participation in multicomponent hypnosis treatment programs for women's weight loss with and without overt aversion. *Psychology Reports* **79**, 659–668.

Khan, L.K., Serdula, M.K., Bowman, B.A. and Williamson, D.F. (2001) Use of prescription weight loss pills among U.S. adults in 1996–1998. *Annals of Internal Medicine* **134**, 282–286.

King, A.C., Frey-Hewitt, B., Dreon, D.M. and Wood, P.D. (1989) Diet vs. exercise in weight maintenance. The effects of minimal intervention strategies on long-term outcomes in men. *Archives of Internal Medicine* **149**, 2741–2746.

Kirsh, I. (1996) Hypnotic enhancement of cognitive–behavioral weight loss treatments another meta-reanalysis. *Journal of Consultation and Clinical Psychology* **64**, 517–519.

Kottke, T.E., Clark, M.M., Aase, L.A., Brandel, C.L., Brekke, M.J., Brekke, L.N., DeBoer, S.W., Hayes, S.N., Hoffman, R.S., Menzel, P.A. and Thomas, R.J. (2002) Self-reported weight, weight goals, and weight control strategies of a midwestern population. *Mayo Clinic Proceedings* **77**, 114–121.

Latner, J. (2001) Self-help in the long-term treatment of obesity. *Obesity Reviews* **2**, 87–97.

Livesey, G. (1995) Fibre as energy in man. In: Kritchevsky, D., ed. *Dietary Fibre in Health and Disease*. Minnesota: Eagan Press, 46–57.

Lowe, M.R., Miller-Kovach, K. and Phelan, S. (2001) Weight loss maintenance in overweight individuals one to five years following successful completion of a commercial weight loss program. *International Journal of Obesity* **25**, 325–331.

MacLean, D.B. (1985) Abrogation of peripheral cholecystokinin-satiety in the capsaicin treated rat. *Regulatory Peptides* **11**, 321–333.

Maezaki, Y., Tsuji, K., Nakawa, N., Naguchi, K. and Fuji, H. (1993) Hypocholesterolaemic effect of chitosan in adult males. *Bioscience, Biochemistry and Biotechnology* **57**, 1439–1444.

Marshall, S. (1995) It's so simple: Just lather up, watch the fat go down the drain. *Wall Street Journal (Eastern Ed)* **226**, B1.

Mathers, C., Vos, T. and Stevenson, C. (2000) *The Burden of Disease and Injury in Australia*. Canberra: Australian Institute of Health and Welfare.

Mattes, R.D. and Bormann, L. (2002) Effects of (-)-hydroxycitric acid on appetitive variables. *Physiological Behaviour* **71**, 87–94.

Mazzoni, R., Mannucci, E., Rizzello, S.M., Ricca, V. and Rotella. (1999) Failure of acupuncture in the treatment of obesity: a pilot study. *Eating and Weight Disorders* **4**, 198–202.

Miles, J., Petrie, C. and Steel, M. (2000) Slimming on the Internet. *Journal of the Royal Society of Medicine* **93**, 254–257.

Miles, A., Rapoport, L., Wardle, J., Afuape, T. and Duman, M. (2001) Using the mass-media to target obesity, an analysis of the characteristics and reported behaviour change of participants in the BBC's 'Fighting Fat, Fighting Fit' campaign. *Health and Education Research* **16**, 357–372.

Morelli, V. and Zoorob, R.J. (2000) Alternative therapies. Part I: depression, diabetes, obesity. *American Family Physician* **62**, 1051–1060.

Morley-John, J., Swinburn, B.A., Metcalf, P.A. and Raza, F. (2002) Fat content of chips, quality of frying fat and deep-frying practices in New Zealand fast food outlets. *Australia and New Zealand Journal of Public Health* **26**, 101–106.

Napolitano, M.A., Fotheringham, M., Tate, D., Sciamanna, C., Leslie, E., Owen, N., Bauman, A. and Marcus, B. (2003) Evaluation of an internet-based physical activity intervention: a preliminary investigation. *Annals of Behavioural Medicine* **25**, 92–99.

National Health and Medical Research Council (2003) *National Clinical Practice Guidelines for Management of Overweight and Obesity in Australia*. Canberra: Australian Government Press.

Pasman, W.J., Westerterp-Plantenga, M.S., Muls, E., Vansant, G., van Ree, J. and Saris, W.H. (1997) The effectiveness of long-term fibre supplementation on weight maintenance in weight-reduced women. *International Journal of Obesity* **21**, 548–555.

Peppard, P., Young, T., Palta, M., Dempsey, J. and Skatrud, J. (2000) Longitudinal study of moderate weight change and sleep-disordered breathing. *Journal of the American Medical Association* **284**, 3015–3020.

Peter, J.C., Wyatt, H.R., Donahoo, W.T. and Hill, J.O. (2002) Viewpoint: from instinct to intellect: the challenge of maintaining healthy weight in the modern world. *Obesity Reviews* **3**, 69–74.

Pittler, M.H., Abbot, N.C., Harkness, E.F. and Ernst, E. (1999) Randomized, double-blind trial of chitosan for body weight reduction. *European Journal of Clinical Nutrition* **53**, 379–381.

Porcari, J.P., McLean, K.P., Foster, C., Kernozek, T., Crenshaw, B. and Swenson, C. (2002) Effects of electrical muscle stimulation on body composition, muscle strength, and physical appearance. *Journal of Strength Condition Research* **16**, 165–172.

Richard, D. and Marley, J. (1998) Stimulation of auricular acupuncture points in weight loss. *Australian Family Physician* **27** (Suppl. 2), S73–77.

Richman, R.M., Webster, P., Salgo, A.R., Mira, M., Steinbeck, K.S. and Caterson, I.D. (1996) A shared care approach in obesity management: the general practitioner and a hospital based service. *International Journal of Obesity* **20**, 413–419.

Riva, G., Alcaniz, M., Anolli, L., Bacchetta, M., Banos, R., Beltrame, F., Botella, C., Galimberti, C., Gamberini, L., Gaggioli, A., Molinari, E., Mantovani, G., Nugues, P., Optale, G., Orsi, G., Perpina, C. and Troiani, R. (2001) The VEPSY updated project: virtual reality in clinical psychology. *Cyberpsychology and Behaviour* **4**, 449–455.

Robinson, T.N., Killen, J.D., Kraemer, H.C., Wilson, D.M., Matheson, D.M., Haskell, W.L., Pruitt, L.A., Powell, T.M., Owens, A.S., Thompson, N.S., Flint-Moore, N.M., Davis, G.J., Emig, K.A., Brown, R.T., Rochon, J., Green, S. and Varady, A. (2003) Dance and reduced television viewing to prevent weight gain in African American girls: the Stanford GEMS pilot study. *Ethnicity and Disease* **13**, S65–77.

Rosenbaum, M., Prieto, V., Hellmer, J., Boschmann, M., Krueger, J., Leibel, R.L. and Ship, A.G. (1998) An exploratory investigation of the morphology and biochemistry of cellulite. *Plastic and Reconstructive Surgery* **101**, 1934–1939.

Rossner, S. (1999) Integrated obesity management. *International Journal of Obesity* **23** (Suppl. 4), S1–S2.

Rothacker, D.Q. and Waitman, B.E. (1997) Effectiveness of a Garcinia cambogia and natural caffeine combination in weight loss: a double-blind placebo-controlled pilot study. *International Journal of Obesity* **21** (Suppl. 2), 53.

Saelens, B.E. and Epstein, L.H. (1998) Behavioural engineering of activity choice in obese children. *International Journal of Obesity* **22**, 275–277.

Sainio, E.L., Rantanen, T. and Kanerva, L. (2000) Ingredients and safety of cellulite creams. *European Journal of Dermatology* **10**, 596–603.

Sciutto, A.M. and Columbo, P. (1995) Lipid-lowering effect of chitosan dietary integrator and hypocaloric diet in obese patients. *Acta Toxicologica Therapiae* **16**, 215–230.

Sherwood, N.E., Morton, N., Jeffery, R.W., French, S.A., Neumark-Sztainer, D. and Falkner, N.H. (1998) Consumer preferences in format and type of community-based weight control programs. *American Journal of Health Promotion* **13**, 12–18.

Sreadling, J., Roberts, D., Wilson, A. and Lovelock, F. (1998) Controlled trial of hypnotherapy for weight loss in patients with obstructive sleep apnoea. *International Journal of Obesity* **28**, 278–281.

Swinburn, B. and Egger, G. (2002) Prevention strategies against weight gain and obesity. *Obesity Reviews* **3**, 299–301.

Swinburn, B., Egger, G. and Raza, F. (1999) Dissecting obesogenic environments: The development and application of a framework for identifying and prioritizing environmental interventions for obesity. *Preventative Medicine* **29**, 563–570.

Tate, D.F., Wing, R.R. and Winett, R.A. (2001) Using Internet technology to deliver a behavioral weight loss program. *Journal of the American Medical Association* **285**, 1172–1177.

Thom, E. (1996) *Hydroxycitrate (HCA) in the Treatment of Obesity.* Paper presented to the European Conference on Obesity, Barcelona, 1996.

Tremblay, A. (1998) *Physical Activity and Weight Maintenance.* Paper presented to the 8th World Congress on Obesity, Satellite Symposium on Physical Activity and Weight Loss, Maastricht, Holland, September 1998.

Veneroni, G., Veneroni, F. and Contos, S. (1996) Effect of a new chitosan on hyperlipidaemia and overweight in obese patients. In: Muzzarelli, R.A.A. ed. *Chitin Enzymology, Vol. 2.* Italy: Atec Edizioni, 63–67.

Ventura, P. (1996) Lipid lowering activity of chitosan, a new dietary integrator. In: Muzzarelli, R.A.A. ed. *Chitin Enzymology, Vol. 2.* Italy: Atec Edizioni, 55–62.

Watanabe, T., Kawada, T., Kurosawa, M., Sato, A. and Iarai, K. (1988) Adrenal sympathetic efferent nerve and catecholamine secretion excitation caused by capsaicin in rats. *American Journal of Physiology* **255**, E23–27.

Westerterp-Plantenga, M.S. and Kovacs, E.M. (2002) The effect of (-)-hydroxycitrate on energy intake and satiety in overweight humans. *International Journal of Obesity* **26**, 870–872.

Williamson, D. (2003) HIP Teenagers study (unpublished). For details, see website (http://www.niddk.nih.gov/fund/other/obesity_report.pdf).

Wilson, B., Wilson, N. and Russell, D. (2001) Obesity and body fat distribution in the New Zealand population. *New Zealand Journal of Medicine* **114**, 127–130.

World Health Organization (2000) *Obesity: Preventing and Managing the Global Epidemic.* Report of a WHO consulation. WHO Technical Report Series 2000; 894, i–xii. Geneva: WHO.

World Health Organization (2002a) *Reducing Risks, Promoting Healthy Life.* World Health Report 2002: Geneva: WHO.

World Health Organization (2002b) *Obesity Prevention in Tonga.* A Technical Report to the Western Pacific Region, Manila, 2002.

31 A comprehensive approach to obesity prevention

Boyd Swinburn and Colin Bell

Treating obesity as an epidemic, 456

Lessons from other epidemics, 458

What is a comprehensive approach?, 458

Priority target groups, 460

Role of clinical management programmes in reducing obesity prevalence, 460

Community-based action in Colac, 461

Influencing homes and parents, 462

The school (and pre-school) setting, 463

Active neighbourhoods, 463

Fast-food outlets, 464

Other community settings, 464

The built environment, 465
   Food distribution and pricing, 466
   Food-labelling interventions, 466

Food marketing targeting young children, 466
   Mass-media campaigns, 467
   Unpaid media, lobbying, 467

What type of evidence is needed?, 467

How much evidence is needed for action?, 468

Role of monitoring in obesity prevention, 468

Research needed to build the evidence on prevention, 468

Conclusions, 469

References, 469

Treating obesity as an epidemic

Taking a step back from people with obesity problems to look at populations with obesity problems gives one a very different view of the likely causes of and solutions to this major health challenge. For populations, the role of genes fades into the background and the role of the environmental and social changes becomes dominant. The patterns of change of obesity prevalence within a population over time and between populations tell us a great deal about the nature of the epidemic.

In the high-income countries of Western Europe, the USA and Australasia, the epidemic started to increase rapidly over the 1980s and 1990s, whereas in middle-income countries, it has increased more recently. Even in some of the poorer countries, it is overtaking undernutrition in prevalence rates (World Health Organization, 2000). In the early stages of the epidemic, the effects are seen predominantly in middle-aged people, women, urban dwellers and the higher socioeconomic (SES) groups. These are the first population subgroups influenced by the environmental drivers of obesity—cars, labour-saving devices, passive entertainment and recreation choices, high-fat foods and high-sugar drinks.

As the time passes (and the population's economic prosper-ity increases), the obesity prevalence rates in men increase to match those in women in parallel with reductions in occupational physical activity due to mechanization. The SES gradient reverses (especially in women) as lower income people gain access to the 'obesogenic' forces in the environment and education about the need for healthy eating and regular physical activity slows the rate of weight gain in the higher SES groups. The urban–rural gradient also reverses as agriculture and horticulture become mechanized and the urban populations take on healthier eating and activity patterns.

The major trend now being seen in many countries is increasing prevalence rates among children. The specific obesogenic factors for children that are on the increase include marketing of energy-dense foods and beverages to children, concerns about the safety of neighbourhoods, both parents (or the solo parent) working so that children spend their after-school time inside the house (so called 'latch key' kids) and electronic and computer games.

One way of viewing obesity at a population level is through the classic epidemiological triad (see Chapter 30). The triad was originally used as a model for combating infectious diseases and was later applied to injuries and some non-communicable diseases (Haddon, 1980). It is eminently applicable to obesity and helps to define the different nature of the determinants of obesity and potential strategies for action (Egger and Swinburn, 1997). All corners of the triad are, of course, interconnected.

The 'agent' is the final common pathway and for infectious diseases it is the infecting organism. For obesity, it is chronic positive energy imbalance. The energy intake 'vectors' or carriers of passive overconsumption of total energy (Blundell and King, 1996) are largely energy-dense foods (mainly high-fat foods), energy-dense beverages (high sugar, fat or alcohol) and large portion sizes (Rolls *et al.*, 2000; 2002). The vectors of low energy expenditure are two types of machines—those that reduce the energy cost of work or transport (e.g. electric appliances, cars) and those that promote passive recreation (e.g. television, videos).

The 'host' factors include age, gender, genetic make-up, physiological factors (e.g. hormonal status, metabolic rate), behaviours and personal attitudes and beliefs. The 'environmental' factors can be considered in four different categories— the physical environment (what is available), the economic environment (what are the financial factors, both income and costs), the policy environment (what are the rules) and the sociocultural (what are society's attitudes, beliefs, perceptions and values) (Swinburn *et al.*, 1999).

The real drivers of the present obesity epidemic are the changing environments and vectors, and many of these changes make life easier, more convenient and more enjoyable for people. They also make a lot of money for the producers of obesogenic vectors (such as cars, televisions, fast food) and this is a powerful force in market-driven economies. This model helps to explain the changing obesity prevalence in the following way: changes in the environments and vectors are driven by powerful motives of improving people's lives and making money. People respond to these changes by largely changing their 'default' behaviour choices based on what is easy, what is desirable (which is influenced by marketing) and what everyone else is doing. These changes are creating the *increasing prevalence of obesity over time*. On top of that, the natural variation in host characteristics (mainly biology and behaviour) creates most of the *differences between individuals*.

The concept of genetic susceptibility to weight gain would be familiar to most people—a person with a 'high dose of fat genes' will gain more weight than a person with more 'lean genes' in an obesogenic environment. The classic experiment that demonstrated this was the Quebec overfeeding study in identical twins (Bouchard *et al.*, 1990). Over a period of 3 months, participants were overfed by 1000 kcal per day for 6 days per week for 3 months. Under these identical, closely controlled obesogenic conditions, all participants gained weight (not surprising), but some gained much more than others (the range was +4.3 kg to +13.3 kg, Fig. 31.1). Identical twins tended to gain similar amounts of weight, suggesting that much of this variation in weight gain could be genetically based.

Building on this concept of susceptible individuals in obesogenic environments, one could also consider some cultures to

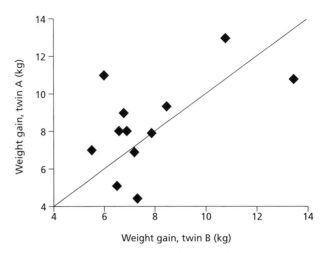

Fig 31.1 Weight gain in response to an identical overfeeding dose (6000 kcal/week for 3 months) in identical male twins. (Source: Bouchard *et al.*, 1990.)

be more susceptible than others. A particular culture might have hospitality traditions that place a high value on hosts overproviding foods (especially high status, fatty foods) and on guests overeating the offered food. There may also be a low cultural value placed on adults (especially women) being physically active. Therefore, a person from this cultural background would be more predisposed to weight gain than someone from another culture with different traditions such as a high vegetable-based diet and belief systems about the benefits of regular physical activity and overall balance in life.

Furthermore, people may be socioeconomically predisposed to weight gain. In high-income countries, there is a consistent trend, especially in women, for people with low income or low educational attainment to have higher prevalence rates of obesity (Stunkard, 1996). In addition, there is some evidence for a vicious cycle between socioeconomic status and obesity such that one begets the other (Stunkard, 1996). Therefore, people from low-income families could be considered economically and/or educationally predisposed to obesity.

These broader concepts of predisposition to obesity (genetic, cultural, economic, educational) help to explain the wide variation in body sizes between individuals when they all seem to have dietary and physical activity habits that are not particularly extreme. People generally make similar default behavioural choices to those around them, but put on weight at different rates. This is why it is important to tackle both the behaviours and the wider environment in its broadest sense.

Therefore, reversal of the obesity epidemic will require both individual and population-based approaches. The individual approaches focus on the host and are largely educational, with some medical and surgical options for those with established obesity. The population-based approaches try to influence the vectors and environments as well as the hosts (mainly through public education and information).

What are the main drivers for making the environment less obesogenic? The economic driver of making a profit can make some aspects of the environment less obesogenic, such as making low-fat food items and private gyms more readily available. However, this will only achieve so much. For more major and sustained changes, the drivers will need to be enlightened policy and public attitudes and beliefs. Policies that promote active transport over car transport, reduce the heavy marketing of energy-dense foods to young children, change the foods available at school canteens and increase the recreation space in neighbourhoods will create sustainable environmental changes.

Changes in the public's knowledge, attitudes and beliefs will translate into consumer demands for less energy-dense foods and beverages, housing in neighbourhoods with good public transport and recreation spaces, improved school food and so on. Such changes in public demand may take a long time, but when they do occur they tend to be long-lasting and powerful. A parallel example has been the increasing public demand and expectations for smoke-free public environments.

Lessons from other epidemics

A degree of success has been achieved in controlling several epidemics of infectious and non-infectious causes of death in many high-income countries, and some general principles can be extracted and applied to the obesity epidemic (Swinburn, 1995). The key components of the control of these epidemics can be classified as host (h), vector (v) and environment (e).

Reductions in morbidity and mortality from tobacco have been achieved through a multipronged approach, including taxation (e), smoke-free legislation (e), education and quit lines (h), regulations (e) and labelling and warnings (v). Cardiovascular diseases have also decreased in response to improved health care (h), reduced saturated fat content of meats and low-fat dairy options (v), education on diet and physical activity (h), regulatory framework (e) for nutrient labelling on foods (v) and tobacco control (above).

The road toll has been reduced by advertising campaigns and driver education (h), regulations and laws on drink-driving, seat belts, driver licences (e), median barriers and improved roads (e), improved car safety (v) and changes in public attitudes (e). Reduced mortality from cervical cancer has mainly involved population screening programmes and surgical treatment (h) plus education measures about safe sex (h). Reductions in sudden infant death syndrome (SIDS) have been achieved mainly through education (h). Control of the HIV AIDS epidemic has involved substantial education (h), medical care (h and v), changes in social attitudes (e), increased availability of condoms and needle exchange/

disposal systems, (v) and blood screening (v). The melanoma mortality rates are no longer rising in countries like Australia, probably due to the increased awareness of the need for sun protection (h), local authority policies on shade provision (e), school policies on hats (e) and the widespread availability of devices like sunscreen and hats with neck protection, and shade cloth to block UV light (v).

The successes in controlling these epidemics have been achieved in the face of substantial barriers including: strong commercial interests (tobacco, dairy industries), social taboos (advertisements about sex), fashion (sun-tanned skin), unknown cause (SIDS), huge and increasing rates (heart disease), addiction (smoking), traditions and habits (butter and full-fat milk) and social attitude norms (drinking and driving, smoking in enclosed public spaces) (Swinburn, 1995). The barriers for preventing obesity are no less formidable, but the strategies for surmounting them have been well tested in these other epidemics.

The main lessons learned from these prevention programmes that could be applied to the obesity/diabetes epidemic are: taking a more comprehensive approach by addressing all corners of the triad; increasing the environmental (mainly policy-based) initiatives; increasing the 'dose' of interventions through greater investment in programmes; exploring opportunities to further influence the energy density of manufactured foods (one of the main vectors for increased energy intake); developing and communicating specific, action messages; and developing a stronger advocacy voice so that there is greater professional, public and political support for action (Swinburn, 1995).

What is a comprehensive approach?

A comprehensive approach to obesity prevention is one that simultaneously addresses as many of the underlying behavioural and environmental causes of obesity as possible. The underlying premise is that single strategy approaches such as public education about healthy choices (Jeffery and French, 1999), or single setting approaches such as a school-based programme (Sahota et al., 2001a,b) are going to be insufficient to achieve the 'intervention' dose required to reverse the present-day trends in obesity. Theoretically, the approach with the greatest likelihood of effect is one that encompasses multiple strategies (such as social marketing, policy change, environmental change, management of overweight and obesity), in multiple settings and sectors and across both sides of the energy balance equation.

Within such a comprehensive approach, influencing the environment to make healthy choices the easy choices has to be central. The environmental causes of obesity are often difficult to conceptualize and therefore influence. To support this process, we have previously described a systematic approach to classifying and scanning obesogenic environments

Environment size — Environment type	Microenvironment (settings) Food	PA	Macroenvironment (sectors) Food	PA
Physical	What is available?			
Economic	What are the financial factors?			
Policy	What are the rules?			
Sociocultural	What are the attitudes, beliefs, perceptions and values?			

Fig 31.2 The ANGELO framework (Analysis Grid for Environments Linked to Obesity) used to 'scan' the environment for barriers and facilitators to healthy eating and regular physical activity (PA).

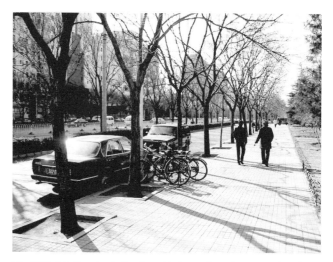

Fig 31.3 A Beijing street, showing wide footpaths and a separate lane for bicycles and parked cars only.

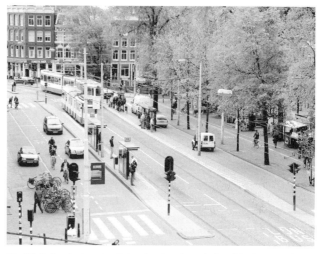

Fig 31.4 Amsterdam street showing that the majority of the lanes are for 'active transport'—walking, cycling, public transport—with only one lane for cars.

(Swinburn *et al.*, 1999; Egger *et al.*, 2003). The ANGELO framework (Analysis Grid for Environments Linked to Obesity) is shown in Fig. 31.2.

Large or macroenvironments that can influence obesity include industries, services or infrastructures such as transport systems, the media, and food production, manufacturing, distribution and marketing industries. Microenvironments are the settings where people gather, particularly those involving food and/or physical activity. Examples include homes, schools, churches, clubs and neighbourhoods. Within both macro- and microenvironments, different types of environment can be identified. We define these environments as physical (what is available), economic (what are the financial factors), policy (what are the rules) and sociocultural (what are society's attitudes, perceptions, beliefs and values) (Swinburn *et al.*, 1999). Using this ANGELO framework, a group of informed stakeholders can readily 'scan' the relevant environments and identify specific elements for prevention strategies. Adding the social marketing strategies to these environmental ones provides the basis for a comprehensive approach.

Exactly what combination of these potential interventions should be included in a multisetting, multistrategy prevention programme is determined by local relevance, likely impact, changeability and resource constraints. Setting-specific delivery is also pragmatic and needs to be guided by those with the expertise. For example, teachers know most about schools and what they can deliver, parents know about home-based strategies and their local environment.

To be effective, obesity prevention strategies require government support at a national level to combat macro-environmental influences that are obesity promoting and to encourage those that are obesity preventing. For example, countries such as China (Fig. 31.3) and the Netherlands (Figs 31.4 and 31.5) have a tradition of active transport with a transport infrastructure and culture that promotes bicycles and public transport as well as cities with mixed land use and high population densities (Bell *et al.*, 2002). Their challenge is to pre-serve and extend these structures and cultures in the face of an increasing pressure for private car transport.

Countries such as the USA, on the other hand, are faced with the monumental long-term task of trying to retro-fit their car-dominated culture and infrastructure towards an environment that is more conducive to active transport (Craig *et al.*, 2002). For example, most suburbs that have been built in the last 50 years have been designed for car travel almost exclusively with poorly interconnected looping street patterns (Fig. 31.6).

The characteristics of a comprehensive approach then include support for obesity prevention at a macroenvironment level (in most cases through international, national and state initiatives), engaging multiple settings at a community level,

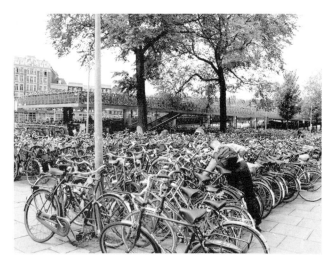

Fig 31.5 Bicycle parking in Amsterdam, showing a large area and multilevel parking building next to the railway station for parking bicycles.

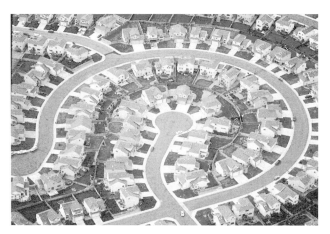

Fig 31.6 Modern suburban planning with streets designed for car transport. Very few intersections or cross-connections between streets means that a pedestrian has to walk long distances between places that are physically relatively close.

applying multiple strategies within each setting and focusing on populations who have most to gain from prevention efforts (e.g. children) and the most to lose from non-intervention (e.g. low-income and other high-risk groups). Supporting activities for interventions are also needed such as: ongoing monitoring of overweight and obesity and its determinants; training programmes to increase the capacity of the public health workforce to manage obesity prevention; coordination of activities and demonstration projects; and a national communication campaign to promote consistent action-orientated messages to the public.

The demonstration areas should be well-defined communities in which obesity prevention efforts can be concentrated and quantified. Within these communities, schools, early-childhood care centres, neighbourhoods, fast-food environments, sport and recreation clubs, religious organizations,

individual households and other settings would all make realistic changes to their policy, economic, physical or socio-cultural environment designed to prevent obesity. Of course the impact and cost effectiveness of each of these actions need to be closely evaluated. Complementing these activities would be a range of obesity management options for those children who are already overweight and obese.

Priority target groups

Who should be the priority groups for obesity prevention action? Once obesity becomes well established in the adult population, one could argue that it is too late for prevention efforts. However, these people will be contributing the most to the obesity-related burden in the short and medium term, and obesity management should be focused on the high-risk individuals and subpopulations (such as those at risk of diabetes; Knowler *et al.*, 2002). The primary prevention efforts, on the other hand, should be targeted to populations prior to the expected large increases in obesity prevalence. This includes those living in low-income countries (Bell and Popkin, 2001) and children and adolescents (Robinson, 2001). Additional reasons for focusing on children are: they have less control over their own food and physical activity choices; they are more dependent on their environments and are more susceptible to its influences (e.g. television advertising); they are at the formative stage of life in which many lifelong habits are being developed; and there is a duty of care for adults and society to provide the best possible environment for children. This last point is an important argument for gaining political and community support for obesity prevention programmes.

Role of clinical management programmes in reducing obesity prevalence

The evidence for the effectiveness of obesity management programmes, particularly for children, has not kept up with the obesity epidemic. Available studies in school and clinical settings suggest conventional behavioural modification approaches to reducing energy intake (dietary changes), increasing energy expenditure (physical activity) or reducing inactivity that involve the child's family have the best chance of success (Epstein *et al.*, 1990; Berkowitz *et al.*, 2001). Pharmacological treatment may be an option in some situations but experience is understandably limited in this area. Theoretically, if an obesity management programme is integrated into a comprehensive community-based programme (as outlined above) it would increase the chances of long-term success but this has not been tested. The constraints of the systems that govern clinical care (especially the funding systems) usually do not allow clinicians sufficient time to fully manage overweight children and their families even if they have the skills and training to do so. Community-based management programmes run by other health professionals could provide clinicians with the 'effector arm' to deliver much of the education, counselling and follow-up.

Rose and Day (1990) have suggested that the best way to reduce the prevalence of conditions like obesity was to shift the whole distribution curve of body mass index (BMI) to the left. Evidence that such a population approach works comes from efforts to reduce blood cholesterol levels in North Karelia, Finland, between 1972 and 1992 (WHO, 2002) (refer to Fig. 30.2). The whole distribution curve of cholesterol levels shifted to the left and corresponded with substantial declines in coronary heart disease mortality. Since 1992 and the advent of widespread prescribing of lipid-lowering drugs, the high-cholesterol end of the distribution has been remarkably flattened, further shifting the population mean levels to the left. This indicates the potential of combined population approaches and effective clinical management to substantially reduce the incident rates of disease. Unfortunately, tackling obesity is at about the same stage that tackling high cholesterol levels was 30 years ago—few proven long-term strategies exist at both population and clinical levels.

We are therefore at the stage where research into effective prevention and treatment options is paramount. However, there are already many people with overweight and obesity who are in need of treatment. This is particularly true for two groups of patients: those who already have (or are at high risk of) obesity complications such as diabetes and sleep apnoea, and children and adolescents because of the associated psychosocial problems, strong tracking of obesity into adulthood (Magarey *et al.*, 2003) and long-term health outcomes associated with obesity (Berkowitz *et al.*, 2001).

There are multiple potential sources of information and support for weight management (Fig. 31.7). Apart from commercial organizations, most options are not well developed. Settings-based promotion of nutrition and physical activity (in schools, workplaces, etc.) and communication programmes (social marketing) from government agencies, which would form the basis of a comprehensive obesity prevention programme, are in their infancy. Community-based weight management programmes led by trained professionals such as school nurses, practice nurses or teachers are also an option that needs to be developed, especially for the management of overweight and obesity in children and adolescents for whom there is a reluctance by parents to medicalize the problem. As the prevention programmes and community-based management options develop, the need for strong linkages between the provider groups will become paramount (Fig. 31.7). In particular, general practitioners will need to link with community-based management programmes as part of their referral network. Specialist services are clearly important for difficult cases in which significant medical or psychological problems are part of the cause or consequence of obesity.

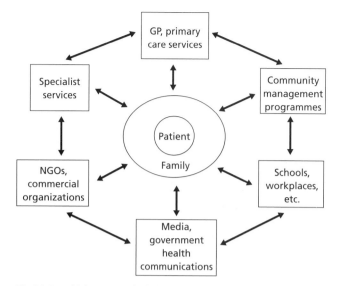

Fig 31.7 Multiple sources of information and support for overweight patients and their families.

Community-based action in Colac

By focusing funding, training programmes, management programmes, research expertise and other resources into a whole community as a demonstration site, programmes can be developed and the evidence gathered about effectiveness and sustainability. This protects the intervention activities from becoming so big that they are unwieldy and difficult to manage, and maximizes the chances of achieving a sufficient intervention dose. We are evaluating such community-based action in Colac, South-western Victoria, Australia. Colac is a rural township with a population of approximately 11 000 people, 2 hours by car from Melbourne.

Mobilizing Colac for action took over a year from the establishment of a working group to starting the implementation of an action and social marketing plan. The first step was to establish networks between community workers, teachers, health professionals, local government and others with an interest in obesity prevention. These networks took shape around a local steering committee, which included representatives from local government, Colac Area Health, and Deakin University (which was providing intervention and evaluation support). A series of training workshops was held to build the knowledge and skills of physical activity and nutrition promotion in the networks and increase their capacity to plan, market, run and evaluate intervention programmes. A key feature of the planning process was using the ANGELO framework (see section What is a comprehensive approach?) to help members of the community identify opportunities for change in their own settings and prioritize these based on likely impact, relevance and changeability (Swinburn *et al.*, 1999). This formed the basis of a 10-point action plan, which included ob-

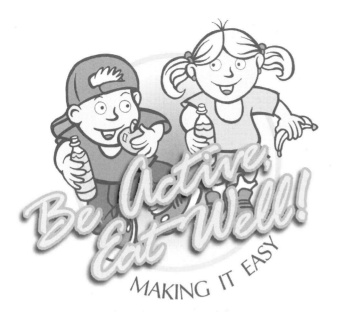

Fig 31.8 Logo from the 'Be Active, Eat Well' project in Colac, Victoria.

jectives around capacity building, communications and specific behavioural changes such as reducing television viewing and increasing fruit consumption. To increase the sustainability of the interventions, the communities developed, owned and actually did the interventions. The university team provided the community with the best international evidence about which interventions were most likely to work, supported the community team and evaluated the process and outcomes.

Having reached a critical mass of 'obesity prevention' capacity (resources secured, key stakeholders engaged and trained, a community action group operating successfully), the action plan could be implemented. The target population selected was children aged 2–12 years and their parents and carers, and the target settings were homes, schools, preschools, neighbourhoods, primary-care and fast-food outlets. A social marketing plan was developed following a specific training workshop on the topic. The programme brand 'Be Active, Eat Well' (Fig. 31.8) provided the umbrella under which four linked messages were developed to coincide with the action plan—more active play after school, less TV; more fruit everyday, less packaged snacks; more water, less sweet drinks; more active transport to and from school, less car transport. The strategies to publicize the messages included paid and unpaid coverage in the local paper, school newsletters, local radio, and so on.

Close evaluation is essential for these demonstration programmes. Each objective of the action plan has an associated evaluation outcome and each strategy is linked with process evaluation measures. There are four linked surveys undertaken before and after 3 years of intervention: *children*—weight, height, waist and lunchbox contents; *parents*—telephone interview on the child's eating and physical activity patterns, as-

pects of the home environment (e.g. family television-viewing patterns), aspects of the local neighbourhood (e.g. perceived safety for children riding bikes and walking); *school*—an environmental audit of the school in relation to physical activity and nutrition; and *town*—an environmental audit of the town in relation to physical activity and nutrition (e.g. fat content of hot chips, available playgrounds, etc.).

The comparison group is a group of similar schools randomly selected from the rest of the Barwon-South Western region as a part of a regional monitoring programme (see Role of monitoring in obesity prevention).

Two other whole-of-community interventions are being established in the region as part of an overall 'Sentinel Site for Obesity Prevention' and, ideally, a number of similar sites will be developed and linked into a collaborative network across the country that develops and shares instruments, designs, methodologies and results. The advantages of such a network lie not only in economies of scale, but also in getting the necessary variation across communities to measure effectiveness, ensuring it is the local experts who are the main contributors to the design and implementation of the interventions and achieving broader monitoring of secular trends in obesity prevalence. Other advantages are that it allows local innovative ideas to be evaluated and it contributes to a groundswell of public action to reduce childhood obesity. Within a country, therefore, a set of networked whole-of-community demonstration projects could be a vital catalyst and advocate for broader national action on reducing childhood obesity.

Influencing homes and parents

Many of a child's physical activity and eating behaviours are learned in the home, making the home or family environment a vital setting for preventing childhood obesity. Children's eating patterns are shaped in the family environment by food availability and accessibility, parental role modelling, television viewing and child–parent interactions (Campbell and Crawford, 2001). Children's activity patterns and sedentary behaviours are also shaped by the family environment (Davison and Birch, 2001). For example, parent participation in physical activity has been positively related to activity in children, particularly in girls (Sallis *et al.*, 1988). Children in Australia watch an average of 23 hours of television per week at home (Zuppa *et al.*, 2003) and other studies have shown children's television viewing to be associated with both parental viewing practices and their monitoring of their children's viewing hours (Davison and Birch, 2001).

Opportunities for influencing the family environment are limited, however, because it is difficult to access. There is also a danger that interventions directed only at the home may encourage the prevailing but counterproductive attitude that parents and children should be held solely responsible for childhood obesity. Mass media is probably the most important

Table 31.1 School-based interventions with successful reductions in weight (reported as changes in mean BMI or prevalence).

Study	Duration	Intensity	Weight outcome
Flores (1995)	Short (3 months)	High	−1.1 kg/m² BMI
Robinson (1999)	Medium (6–12 months)	High	−0.42 kg/m² BMI
Manios and Kafatos (1999)			−1.0 kg/m² BMI
Simonetti *et al.* (1986)			−4.9% overweight and obesity
Gortmaker *et al.* (1999)	Long (> 12 months)	Lower	−5.5% obesity BMI plus triceps skinfold > 85th percentile (girls)

way to access parents and families and to deliver action messages in relation to making the home environment less obesogenic. Other opportunities to influence homes are through the contact that schools, pre-schools, sports clubs, churches and other settings have with parents and families. The best evidence for reducing obesity through a home setting is with programmes that promote reductions in television viewing (Robinson, 1999).

The school (and pre-school) setting

Schools, and increasingly pre-schools and daycare, are a key setting for promoting healthy weight because they have contact with virtually all children throughout a substantial part of childhood and adolescence. This includes children at the highest risk of obesity, for example those from low-income families. One approach that can be used for school-based obesity prevention is the Health Promoting Schools model (WHO, 1996) that employs multiple strategies across the whole school environment. For obesity prevention, this could include: policies on physical activity and nutrition; physical structures and spaces that promote active play and sport; incorporating nutrition and expanding physical education in the curriculum; teacher training; parent and community support; linking with local government to promote active play; increased availability of healthy choices in school food services; water fountain provision; and an expanded use of specialist teachers, especially for physical education in primary schools.

Many studies contribute to the evidence for school-based obesity prevention, including a limited number of randomized controlled trials (Campbell *et al.*, 2001). In general, school-based programmes are eminently achievable, the programmes are well received by stakeholders, and they have proven successful in influencing dietary/physical activity knowledge and behaviour as well as health behaviours beyond those that were originally planned. Few, however, have demonstrated any long-term impact on weight. Short- to medium-term studies have produced decreases in childhood obesity of up to 5% and over 1.1 BMI units (Flores, 1995; Manios and Kafatos, 1999; Robinson, 1999) (Table 31.1). Longer term trials have also shown a reduction of around 5%

in obesity rates. The largest impact resulted from programmes that reduced television viewing time at home. Two major US school-based studies have successfully implemented such programmes (Gortmaker *et al.*, 1999; Robinson, 1999).

An explanation for some studies that show changes in physical activity and eating behaviour but little change in weight is likely to be that children do not spend all their time in school. A significant proportion of their energy intake and energy expenditure occurs in other settings. For example, in Australia, 37% of children's daily energy intake is consumed in the school environment on a school day, but only 16% of energy is consumed in the school environment over the period of a year when holidays and weekends are taken into account (Bell and Swinburn, 2004).

Schools are attractive as a setting for interventions for a variety of reasons: they provide access to most children for an extended period; synergies are possible between education goals and health promotion; they provide an avenue through which parents can be reached; and they are highly symbolic for the community and can take a lead in creating healthy behaviour patterns in children. The limitations are that schools often have enough on their plates without stretching their resources to accommodate interventions and they are only one of many settings that influence children's weight.

Active neighbourhoods

There has been a sharp decline in children's physical activity outside the structured school or sports environment, and strategies are needed that promote physical activity in neighbourhood settings that are integral to children's daily lives. The benefits of such strategies are enormous. An estimate from a recent systematic review (Kahn *et al.*, 2002) indicates that exposure to an environment that supports physical activity could produce a 20–25% increase in the number of people exercising for at least 30 minutes three or more times each week.

Environmental factors that influence physical activity at a neighbourhood level include access to recreation facilities, safety, street design, housing density, land use mix, availability of public transport, and pedestrian and bicycle facilities. Interventions focusing on these areas may include policies, regulations and guidelines that support and promote active recreation and transportation, awards and funding support for local governments, facility improvements, programmes such as 'walking school buses', monitoring programmes and communications to increase active transport, active play and recreation. With appropriate support, local governments have the structures, skills and experience in working with the community and the environment to be able to implement many of these activities.

In Britain, 50% of children aged 4–11 years were driven less than a mile to school on a regular basis, a distance that is easily walked (Sleap and Warburton, 1993). Similarly, most children at a New Zealand school travelled to school by car even though their most preferred method of travel was walking (Collins and Kearns, 2001). Therefore, one strategy that can be adopted relatively quickly is promoting active transport (walking, cycling), especially to and from school (Tudor-Locke et al., 2001).

Fast-food outlets

A growing body of evidence links rising obesity prevalence with increasing fast-food consumption (Binkley et al., 2000). Australian household expenditure on takeaways and snacks increased from 10.5% to 18% between 1984 and 1994 (Jones, 2000), and increasing alongside expenditure has been the size of the fast-food meal. Chain outlets practise 'supersizing,' which is likely to promote overconsumption of high-fat foods and high-sugar drinks [a large Big Mac meal (4796 kJ) contains 37.6% more energy and 29% more fat than a small Big Mac meal (3485 kJ) but costs only 20.6% more]. Moreover, fast-food outlets tend to cluster in low-income areas, potentially promoting increased consumption among those most at risk of obesity. Reidpath and colleagues (2002) found that the density of fast-food outlets in low-income neighbourhoods was 2–3 times that of high-income neighbourhoods.

Fast food also has a higher total fat and saturated fat content than food prepared at home (Lin et al., 1999; Ashton and Hughes, 2000). In Australia this is largely because the deep-frying oils that are high in saturated fatty acids (SFAs) (tallow and palm oil) are the least expensive.

Significant reductions in fat intake can be achieved simply by modifying deep-frying practices, and this has important implications at a population level (Morley-John et al., 2002). Components of interventions aimed at reducing saturated and total fat consumption include training programmes for best practice deep frying, regulations on training as well as monitoring the amount and type of fat in fast foods (similar to food safety regulations), communication of the nutrition content of fast food to customers (i.e. extending food-labelling regulations to include fast food), levying of the SFA content of frying fats (to neutralize the price incentive of high SFA fats), collaboration with industry to reduce supersizing and in-

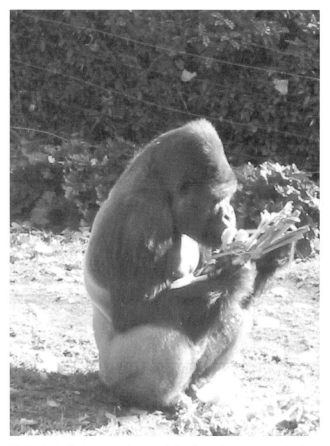

Fig 31.9 Gorilla in a zoo eating a specially tailored diet to ensure optimal health.

crease healthy options and limiting the density of fast-food outlets. It is interesting to note that McDonald's in Australia is now vigorously promoting their nutrition information pamphlets and posters and in the USA, Kraft Foods recently put a cap on portion sizes.

Of course, fast-food outlets are not the only source of energy-dense foods outside the home. A typical 362-item vending machine, for example, contains 5.5 kg of sugar, 4.4 kg of fat and more than 380 MJ (unpublished data). Banning vending machines in schools will therefore reduce children's exposure to energy-dense foods and beverages. The foods most prominently displayed at cafés also tend to be energy dense. This is graphically illustrated at a zoo, where the Western lowland gorilla consumes an appropriate diet of fruit, leafy green vegetables, skimmed milk and protein-rich 'primate' cake (grains, cereals, peanuts), whereas the primates visiting the zoo are served an inappropriate diet of energy-dense snacks and fried foods at the zoo cafeteria (Figs 31.9 and 31.10).

Other community settings

A comprehensive approach to obesity prevention should also encompass interventions in other settings or areas, as appro-

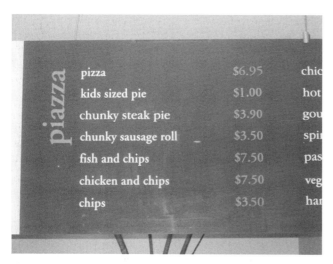

pizza	$6.95	chic
kids sized pie	$1.00	hot
chunky steak pie	$3.90	gou
chunky sausage roll	$3.50	spi
fish and chips	$7.50	pas
chicken and chips	$7.50	veg
chips	$3.50	han

Fig 31.10 Cafeteria menu in the zoo to feed visiting primates with highly inappropriate food.

priate. Other settings include early childhood care and education settings, clubs and churches or other religious communities. Interventions to increase breast-feeding rates across a variety of settings are also important.

Interventions in early childhood care settings aim to provide environments and education activities that promote healthy food choices and regular physical activity and to increase parents' and carers' knowledge and skills in nutrition and physical activity. Components of the intervention may include policies on food and active play, curriculums on nutrition and motor skills, staff training and guidelines and monitoring on food service and environments for active play. Some evaluated trials have been conducted in childcare centres and pre-schools (but not in out-of-school-hours care); however, limited outcomes have been reported. The effect of food policy improvements on behaviour change has not been quantified but curriculum-based approaches have been associated with increased familiarity with and consumption of fruits and vegetables (Edmunds, 2002).

For many people, churches and other religious institutions are the centre of community life, and churches have been successfully used as a setting for weight loss in Pacific Islands and African American communities (Kumanyika and Charleston, 1992; Simmons *et al.*, 2001). We found that a nutrition and exercise intervention programme was successful in arresting weight gain in adult members of a Samoan church community in New Zealand, but that in the absence of wider environmental change, the weight was regained in the long term (Bell *et al.*, 2001).

The settings that support antenatal/post-natal care are important for promoting breast-feeding, which is protective against unhealthy weight gain and a number of other childhood illnesses (Oddy, 2000). Several large-scale, longitudinal

studies have demonstrated a strong protective effect of exclusive breast-feeding against the development of obesity in later childhood (Dietz, 2001; Armstrong and Reilly, 2002). Dietz (2001) reported a population-attributable fraction of 15% for breast-feeding in the development of obesity, although some of this effect size may be due to confounding factors such as the body size and socioeconomic status of the mothers. In Australia, breast-feeding rates are well below the national targets set in 1996: only 18.6% of infants are fully breast-fed at 6 months compared with the target of 50%. Components of breast-feeding interventions might include increased antenatal education for parents, the adoption and promotion of Baby Friendly hospitals, increased support for existing professional and trained volunteers to support breast-feeding in the 6-month post-natal period. Increased rates of breast-feeding (both initiation and duration) have been demonstrated through such programmes (Fairbank *et al.*, 2000).

The built environment

Within the built environment, the land development patterns (i.e. public transport- and pedestrian-oriented vs. car-oriented) and the mode of transport investment (i.e. public transport, walking and cycling paths vs. highways) are closely inter-related and between them they have a profound effect on physical activity levels (Frank and Engleke, 2001). Public transport can be categorized, with walking and cycling as 'active transport' because of the regular short walking trips included in the use of public transport. In car-dominated societies, only a minority of trips are walking or cycling (for example, in the USA it is about 10%) and then most of them are for recreation purposes rather than transportation to a destination, whereas in several European countries, walking plus cycling trips equal or exceed car trips (Frank and Engleke, 2001). This probably explains part of the differences in obesity prevalence rates between the continents. In a study from China, where cycling is still the most common form of transportation, the acquisition of a motorized vehicle doubled the odds of becoming obese (Bell *et al.*, 2002).

Although there is an opportunity (largely unrealized) to ensure that the new urban/suburban developments are conducive to active transport and active recreation, so much of the present-day built environment is car oriented. For these existing communities, a long and expensive process of 'retro-fitting' the appropriate structures and urban forms to promote physical activity will be needed. Higher density developments, greater mix of land use (a balance between residential and commercial), pedestrian- and cycle-friendly street design, greater investment in public transport and the designation of streets and areas in the central business districts as car-free are all options to achieve this (Crawford, 2000; Frank and Engleke, 2001). Influencing attitudes towards active transport is also an important part of gaining shifts in modes of transport use because attitudes may be as strongly associated with car transport as land use characteristics (Kitamura *et al.*, 1997).

If the environment is conducive to active transport, a mass-marketing approach appears to be able to influence long-term behaviours. In a pilot study in Perth, Australia, simple marketing of the active transport options to each household in a suburb resulted in 14% less car travel and increased use of walking, cycling and public transport (Western Australian Government, 2002). Changes were most marked for short journeys and were sustained over 2 years. Modest shifts in transport mode multiplied by the large volumes of short journeys for which active transport is an option can result in important increases in physical activity for the population.

The design of buildings also influences incidental activity. In particular, stairs seem to have evolved from a design feature (often with central prominence) and a means of moving between floors to a hidden, locked security risk for use as a fire escape only. Several studies have shown that when stairs are a viable option to taking a lift or an escalator, a prompt sign at the bottom increases the use of the stairs (Kerr, 2004).

Food distribution and pricing

Food supply interventions aim to increase or decrease the availability and accessibility of certain types of foods. Some programmes aim to improve access to healthy food choices in targeted populations, for example the provision of free or subsidized fruit to children in schools (UK Department of Health, 2001). The wider development and promotion of energy-dilute, micronutrient-dense products or the gradual reformulation of existing high-volume, energy-dense snack foods, such as potato crisps, are options for promoting healthy eating that are under the control of the food industry. Small changes in the fat content of high-volume products have significant potential to provide health benefits at a population level.

Fiscal strategies such as levies can be used to modify prices to influence consumption. Levies are rarely applied to improve population health but this potential exists. A substantial levy on energy-dense foods or drinks, for example soft drink, that resulted in a 20% increase in soft drink price could result in a 10% reduction in consumption (based on a price elasticity of 0.5); 18 states in the USA apply soft drink levies that are too small to affect consumption but raise substantial revenue for consolidated revenue (Jacobson and Brownell, 2000), and in Australia, levies apply at present to milk and sugar to raise revenue to support primary producers in the dairy and sugar cane industries (Gordon, 2002). Revenue raised through levies could potentially be used to fund public health nutrition programmes.

Food-labelling interventions

Full nutrition information panels on foods have been or are being introduced by regulation in many countries (Neuhouser

et al., 1999). In the US, about two-thirds of people report using nutrition panels (French *et al.*, 2001), and this appears to significantly influence food choices (Weimer, 1999). The impact of mandatory nutrition panels on the formulation and reformulation of manufactured foods may also be significant but it is not well documented. Mandatory nutrition information panels are a key strategy to improve the nutrition status of populations; however, they need to be complemented by other strategies that will influence the food choices of low-income and less-educated consumers (Wang *et al.*, 1995).

Nutrition 'signposts' are signals (such as logos) at point of choice, which indicate to the consumer that a food meets certain nutrition standards. An example is the 'Pick the Tick' symbol programme run by the National Heart Foundations in Australia and New Zealand (Noakes and Crawford, 1991). They make identifying healthier food choices simpler for consumers and are frequently used by shoppers when choosing products (Noakes and Crawford, 1991). In addition, the nutrition criteria for the products serve as '*de facto*' standards for product formulation and many manufacturers will formulate or reformulate products to meet those standards (Young and Swinburn, 2002). Energy density criteria are needed for low-fat products.

Health and nutrition claims are closely regulated because of the potential for misleading information. In the USA, over the last 10 years, between 20% and 37% of new products that were launched into the market each year carried a nutrition claim with over one-half of those claims in recent years being for reduced or low fat (Weimer, 1999). The claims clearly provide information about some aspect of the content of the food but for some restrained eaters, 'low-fat' or 'low-calorie' claims can become an unconscious message to eat more of the product (Miller *et al.*, 1998). In some manufactured products, the fat is removed so that a low-fat claim can be made, but it is replaced with sugar such that the energy density remains unchanged (Seidell, 1999). This negates the impact of low-fat products for preventing weight gain.

Food marketing targeting young children

Heavy marketing of energy-dense foods and beverages to children, especially through television advertising, has been implicated as a causal factor in increasing obesity. The fat, sugar and energy content of foods advertised to children is extremely high compared with their daily needs and most of the foods advertised fall into the 'eat least' sections of the recommended dietary guidelines (Dibb and Castwell, 1995; Hill and Radimer, 1997; Wilson *et al.*, 1999). Exposure to advertising has been shown to increase children's requests for advertised products (Borzekowski and Robinson, 2001; Robinson *et al.*, 2001) and young children have a limited ability to understand advertising intent (Oates *et al.*, 2001).

Television advertising to children under 12 years has not

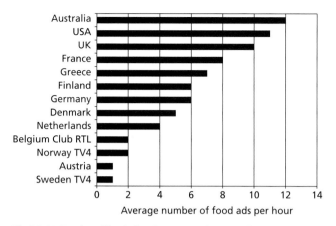

Fig 31.11 Number of food advertisements per hour on television in selected countries. (Source: Dibb and Castwell, 1995.)

been permitted in Sweden since commercial television began over a decade ago, although children's television programmes from other countries and through satellite television probably dilute the impact of the ban in Sweden. Norway, Austria, Ireland, Australia, Greece, Quebec and Denmark also have restrictions on television advertising to young children (International Association of Consumer Food Organizations, 2003). There is a wide range of frequency of food advertisements, with Australia topping the list of several Organization for Economic Cooperation and Development (OECD) countries (Fig. 31.11).

The justification for policies or regulations to restrict food marketing directed at young children cannot rest on a proven cause-and-effect link between such marketing and childhood obesity, because no such direct evidence exists. There is, however, a substantial amount of indirect evidence of an important linkage, including the continued huge investment in marketing (especially through television advertising) by companies selling fast food, soft drinks and other energy-dense products (Hastings *et al.*, 1996). Advertising to young children relies on 'pester power' to work and this undermines parents' attempts to provide healthy food choices for their children. A groundswell of parental opposition to advertising targeting young children and enlightened government policies and regulations will be needed to counter the obvious commercial attraction of this type of marketing, and this is yet to happen to any significant extent in any country.

Mass-media campaigns

Social marketing of healthy eating and physical activity lifestyles is an essential element of any comprehensive programme for obesity prevention. Although information, education and communication strategies alone generally do not change behaviour over the long term (Owen *et al.*, 1995), they are vital for raising awareness, increasing knowledge and changing intentions (Taylor *et al.*, 1991; Cavill, 1998; Miles *et al.*, 2001). Some changes in behaviour can be seen from mass-media campaigns in certain circumstances, such as during a campaign on physical activity participation (Booth *et al.*, 1992) or if the message is highly specific and action oriented, such as changing from high- to low-fat milk (Reger *et al.*, 1999) or if it is closely linked to accessing a service that can then influence behaviour, such as the Quit advertisements and the Quitline.

A sustained media campaign backed by programmes, policies and other sources of information and support would be a central component of a comprehensive approach to obesity prevention. Experience from campaigns on road safety, quitting smoking, sun protection, safe sex, etc. can be translated into a similar programme for obesity prevention.

Unpaid media, lobbying

The most cost-effective way to influence change is through lobbying decision-makers (usually politicians). Lobbying is big business in the corporate world and public health advocates are merely neophytes with tiny budgets. However, the issues promoted by public health advocates often resonate with the community and the opportunities to get significant unpaid press coverage are often substantial. A well-organized public lobby group can keep an issue bubbling in the media and put pressure on decision-makers in this way. The anti-smoking group, ASH, was a particularly successful model of public health advocacy, which started as a 'ginger group' with radical agendas and a modus operandi that was designed to grab the headlines. As smoke-free has become more widespread, the ASH position became less radical and more mainstream. For childhood obesity, there is little in the way of such public movements, although individually most parents are anxious to provide healthy environments for children (including safer streets, less advertising of junk foods and better school food).

What type of evidence is needed?

There is no shortage of evidence on obesity. Unfortunately, most of it is related to genes, metabolism and biochemistry or it is descriptive epidemiology. The evidence that is desperately needed is around the effectiveness of interventions. There appears to be almost an inverse relationship between the volume of evidence available and its utility to decision-makers (Fig. 31.12). The monitoring of data to show comparative trends in obesity and its determinants plus data on cost-effectiveness or cost utility (i.e. the cost per disability-adjusted life-year saved) to show where future investments should be made are probably the two most useful types of information for decision-makers.

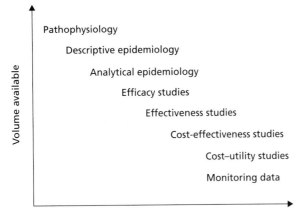

Fig 31.12 The relationship between the volume of evidence available and its value to policy-makers.

How much evidence is needed for action?

Evidence-based medicine (EBM) has been developed as an aid to decision-making at the clinical level by making the evidence upon which decisions are made explicit, transparent and as unbiased as possible. The EBM movement has moved into other areas so that evidence-based health promotion, health policy and health communication are now being demanded, but the processes and models for reaching the population equivalent of EBM are not well developed. Randomized controlled trials (the backbone of EBM) are rarely available or even possible at the population level. The processes for taking the evidence and adding in other issues such as feasibility, cost, acceptability and equity to develop priorities for action are not well developed. These are the equivalent processes for clinical medicine that take place inside the doctor's head (the evidence is weighed up with other patient factors, costs and external factors to reach a clinical action decision).

In many instances, action is needed before sufficient evidence of effectiveness is available and in these instances, it is extremely important to fully evaluate any programmes or policies. With a vulnerable population, such as children, there is a strong case to take a highly precautionary approach so that there is a low threshold for action to prevent harm. The precautionary principle has been borrowed from environmental action when considering potential action to protect the environment in circumstances of high uncertainty of outcome (Tickner *et al.*, 1996). The battle over the high volume of television advertising for junk foods that is targeted at children is a classic case for invoking the precautionary principle so that regulations are put in place to reduce the advertising, even in the absence of unequivocal evidence that it is doing any harm.

Role of monitoring in obesity prevention

Very few countries have systems in place for regularly monitoring the height and weight of children, and most rely on widely spaced national surveys or occasional local surveys for trend information. Monitoring is the process of measuring a set of key indicators for a known risk and systematically following their progress over time. The value of monitoring lies in the ability to assess prevalence and to show trends. For obesity prevention, the key indicators should include obesity prevalence data as well as determinants at the individual level (such as knowledge, attitudes and behaviours) and the environmental level (such as school food policies and canteen sales, funding for active transport options and the presence of footpaths and bicycle tracks). Ultimately, regular monitoring would not only provide trend data, but also allow appropriate benchmarking with which a jurisdiction, such as a local government authority, can compare its results with other similar jurisdictions.

The monitoring data could also be used to evaluate the impact of community interventions and health promotion programmes in demonstration areas. This would, in the long term, be a key strategy for the sustainability of programmes and actions by schools, local governments, regions, states and other participants. Strong policy backing and funding would be essential for such a monitoring programme so that it eventually becomes a regular part of the activities of local and state governments as well as key settings such as schools.

Research needed to build the evidence on prevention

The research base underpinning population-based obesity prevention is very small. A substantial investment is needed to boost knowledge in this area so that strategies are much better informed. The foundational research needs to be evaluation of community-based demonstration programmes that test multiple prevention strategies in varied environments. The outcome of interest should be BMI and other individual characteristics and behaviours, along with household, neighbourhood, school and community factors, which should be measured as explanatory variables. Recognizing that factors beyond the control of the community also influence obesity, policy-relevant research on the macroenvironmental and sociocultural influences is also needed. For example, we do not fully understand the influence of food advertising on obesity nor are we well informed about how cultural practices in the home, community or business may influence food choice or physical activity. The economic case for obesity prevention needs to be researched in a much more complete way so that we are able to present to government with a balance sheet that outlines the cost of the obesity epidemic and also the savings if particular interventions are introduced. We also need to carefully consider how to fund this type of evidence building, and taxing energy-dense foods and technology that promotes sedentary behaviour should be considered a realistic option.

Other key areas of research include the relationships between social and environmental factors (including socioeconomic status) and physical activity and nutrition behaviours, the needs and issues of at-risk populations (such as low-income groups, indigenous communities) and effective options for management of children who are overweight at present.

Conclusions

Single-strategy or single-setting interventions are unlikely to achieve the dose required for obesity prevention, so multiple strategies (educational, policy, fiscal, environmental changes, social marketing) in multiple settings (homes, schools, workplaces, neighbourhoods, etc.) are needed, along with enlightened policies at the macro level (regulation of television advertising directed at young children, policies promoting active transport, etc.). Integrating obesity management programmes with prevention programmes is also likely to achieve the synergies needed to deal with both the current and future problem of overweight and obesity.

References

Armstrong, J. and Reilly, J. J. (2002) Breastfeeding and lowering the risk of childhood obesity. *Lancet* **359**, 2003–2004.

Ashton, B. and Hughes, R. (2000) *Takeaway food project report number. 1: A review of public health nutrition intelligence of the takeaway food sector.* Queensland Health, The Heart Foundation (Queensland Division), Griffith University, 1–47.

Bell, A. C. and Popkin, B. M. (2001) The epidemiology of obesity in developing countries. In: Johnston, F.E., Foster, G.D. eds. *Obesity Growth and Development.* London: International Association for Human Auxology.

Bell, A. C. and Swinburn, B. (2004) What are the key food groups to target for preventing obesity and improving nutrition in schools? *European Journal of Clinical Nutrition* **58**, 258–263.

Bell, A. C., Swinburn, B. A., Amosa, H. and Scragg, R. (2001) A nutrition and exercise intervention program for controlling weight in Samoan communities in New Zealand. *International Journal of Obesity* **25**, 920–927.

Bell, A. C., Ge, K. and Popkin, B.M. (2002) The road to obesity or the path to prevention: motorized transportation in China. *Obesity Research* **10**, 277–283.

Berkowitz, R. I., Lyke, J. A. and Wadden, T. A. (2001) Treatment of child and adolescent obesity. In: Johnston, F.E., Foster, G.D. eds. *Obesity Growth and Development.* London: International Association for Human Auxology.

Binkley, J. K., Eales, J. and Jekanowski, M. (2000) The relation between dietary change and rising US obesity. *International Journal of Obesity and Related Metabolic Disorders* **24**, 1032–1039.

Blundell, J. E. and King, N. A. (1996) Over-consumption as a cause of weight gain: behavioural-physiological interactions in the control of food intake (appetite). *Ciba Foundation Symposium* **201**, 138–154; discussion 154–158, 188–193.

Booth, M., Bauman, A., Oldenburg, B., Owen, N. and Magnus, P. (1992) Effects of a national mass-media campaign on physical activity participation. *Health Promotion International* **7**, 241–247.

Borzekowski, D. L. and Robinson, T. N. (2001) The 30-second effect: an experiment revealing the impact of television commercials on food preferences of preschoolers. *Journal of the American Dieticians Association* **101**, 42–46.

Bouchard, C., Tremblay, A., Despres, J. P., Nadeau, A., Lupien, P. J., Theriault, G., Dussault, J., Moorjani, S., Pinault, S. and Fournier, G. (1990) The response to long-term overfeeding in identical twins. *New England Journal of Medicine* **322**, 1477–1482.

Campbell, K. and Crawford, D. (2001) Family food environments as determinants of preschool-aged children's eating behaviours: implications for obesity prevention policy: a review. *Australian Journal of Nutrition and Diet* **58**, 19–25.

Campbell, K., Waters, E., O'Meara, S. and Summerbell, C. (2001) Interventions for preventing obesity in childhood. A systematic review. *Obesity Reviews* **2**, 149–157.

Cavill, N. (1998) National campaigns to promote physical activity: can they make a difference? *International Journal of Obesity* **22**, S48–S51.

Collins, D. C. and Kearns, R. A. (2001) The safe journeys of an enterprising school: negotiating landscapes of opportunity and risk. *Place* **7**, 293–306.

Craig, C. L., Brownson, R. C., Cragg, S. E. and Dunn, A. L. (2002) Exploring the effect of the environment on physical activity: a study examining walking to work. *American Journal of Preventive Medicine* **23**, 36–43.

Crawford, J. (2000) *Carfree Cities.* Utrecht: International Books.

Davison, K. K. and Birch, L. L. (2001) Childhood overweight: a contextual model and recommendations for future research. *Obesity Reviews* **2**, 159–171.

Dibb, S. and Castwell, A. (1995) Easy to swallow, hard to stomach: The results of a survey of food advertising on television. London: The National Food Alliance.

Dietz, W. H. (2001) Breastfeeding may help prevent childhood overweight. *Journal of the American Medical Association* **285**, 2506–2507.

Edmunds, L. (2003) Evaluation of the Grab 5! project to increase fruit and vegetables in primary school age children: summary. May 2003, University of Oxford: http://www.grab5.com.

Egger, G. and Swinburn, B. (1997) An 'ecological' approach to the obesity pandemic. *British Medical Journal* **315**, 477–480.

Egger, G., Swinburn, B. and Rossner, S. Dusting off the epidemiological trial: could it work with obesity. *Obesity Reviews* **4**, 115–120. (In press)

Epstein, L. H., Valoski, A., Wing, R. R. and McCurley, J. (1990) Ten-year follow up of behavioural family based treatment for obese children. *Journal of the American Medical Association* **264**, 2519–2523.

Fairbank, L., O'Meara, S., Renfrew, M. J., Woolridge, M., Sowden, A. J. and Lister-Sharp, D. (2000) A systematic review to evaluate the effectiveness of interventions to promote the initiatioin of breastfeeding. *Health and Technology Assessment* **4**, 1–171.

Flores, R. (1995) Dance for health: improving fitness in African American and Hispanic adolescents. *Public Health Reports* **110**, 189–193.

Frank, L. D. and Engleke, P. (2001) How land use and transportation systems impact on public health: A literature review of the relationship between physical activity and the built form. *Report to the Centers for Disease Control and Prevention, Georgia Institute of Technology.*

French, S. A., Story, M. and Jeffery, R. W. (2001) Environmental influences on eating and physical activity. *Annual Review of Public Health* **22**, 309–335.

Gordon, J. (2002) Bevy of levies. In: *The Sunday Age.* Melbourne: Fairfax Publishers.

Gortmaker, S. L., Peterson, K., Wiecha, J., Sobol, A. M., Dixit, S., Fox, M. K. and Laird, N. (1999) Reducing obesity via a school-based interdisciplinary intervention among youth: Planet Health. *Archives of Pediatric and Adolescent Medicine* **153**, 409–418.

Haddon, Jr, W. (1980) Advances in the epidemiology of injuries as a basis for public policy. *Public Health Reports* **95**, 411–421.

Hill, J. M. and Radimer, K. L. (1997) A content analysis of food advertisements in television for Australian children. *Journal of Nutrition and Dietetics* **54**, 174–181.

International Association of Consumer Food Organisations (2003) IACFO website (www.foodcomm.org.uk).

Jacobson, M. F. and Brownell, K. D. (2000) Small taxes on soft drinks and snack foods to promote health. *American Journal of Public Health* **90**, 854–857.

Jeffery, R. W. and French, S. A. (1999) Preventing weight gain in adults: the pound of prevention study. *American Journal of Public Health* **89**, 747–751.

Jones, V. (2000) Takeaway Food Project Triennial Report (1996–1999). Heart Foundation of Australia (NSW Division), 1–48.

Kahn, E. B., Ramsey, L. T., Brownson, R. C., Heath, G. W., Howze, E. H., Powell, K. E., Stone, E. J., Rajab, M. W. and Corso, P. (2002) The effectiveness of interventions to increase physical activity. A systematic review. *American Journal of Preventive Medicine* **22**, 73–107.

Kerr, N. A., Yore, M. M., Ham, S. A. and Dietz, W. H. (2004) Increasing stair use in a worksite through environmental changes. *American Journal of Health Promotion* **18**, 312–315.

Kitamura, R., Mokhtarian, P. L. and Laidet, L. (1997) A micro-analysis of land use and travel in five neighborhoods in the San Francisco Bay area. *Transportation* **24**, 125–158.

Knowler, W. C., Barrett-Connor, E., Fowler, S. E., Hamman, R. F., Lachin, J. M., Walker, E. A. and Nathan, D. M. (2002) Reduction in the incidence of type 2 diabetes with lifestyle intervention or metformin. *New England Journal of Medicine* **346**, 393–403.

Kumanyika, S. K. and Charleston, J. B. (1992) Lose weight and win: a church-based weight loss program for blood pressure control among black women. *Patient Education and Counselling* **19**, 19–32.

Lin, B.-H., Frazao, E. and Guthrie, J. (1999) Away-from-home foods increasingly important to quality of American diet. Food and Rural Economics Division, Economic Research Service. Washington, DC: US Department of Agriculture.

Magarey, A. M., Daniels, L. A., Boulton, T. J. and Cockington, R. A. (2003) Predicting obesity in early adulthood from childhood and parental obesity. *International Journal of Obesity and Related Metabolic Disorders* **27**, 505–513.

Manios, Y. and Kafatos, A. (1999) Health and nutrition education in elementary schools: changes in health knowledge, nutrient intakes and physical activity over a six year period. *Public Health and Nutrition* **2**, 445–448.

Miles, A., Rapoport, L., Wardle, J., Afuape, T. and Duman, M. (2001) Using the mass-media to target obesity: an analysis of the characteristics and reported behaviour change of participants in the BBC's 'Fighting Fat, Fighting Fit' campaign. *Health Education Research* **16**, 357–372.

Miller, D. L., Castellanos, V. H., Shide, D. J., Peters, J. C. and Rolls, B. J. (1998) Effect of fat-free potato chips with and without nutrition labels on fat and energy intakes. *American Journal of Clinical Nutrition* **68**, 282–290.

Morley-John, J., Swinburn, B., Metcalf, P., Raza, F. and Wright, H. (2002) Fat content of chips, quality of frying fat and deep-frying practices in New Zealand fast food outlets. *Australia and New Zealand Journal of Public Health* **26**, 101–107.

Morton, H. (1996) In: *Multidisciplinary Approaches to Food Choice.* Adelaide: Adelaide Conference on Food Choices.

Neuhouser, M. L., Kristal, A. R. and Patterson, R. E. (1999) Use of food nutrition labels is associated with lower fat intake. *Journal of the American Dietetics Association* **99**, 45–53.

Noakes, M. and Crawford, D. (1991) The National Heart Foundation's 'Pick the Tick' Program. Consumer awareness, attitudes and interpretation. *Food Australia* **43**, 262–266.

Oates, C., Blades, M. and Gunter, B. (2001) Children and television advertising: When do they understand persuasive intent? *Journal of Consultation and Behaviour* **1**, 238–245.

Oddy, W. H. (2000) Breastfeeding and asthma in children: findings from a West Australian study. *Breastfeeding Review* **8**, 5–11.

Owen, N., Bauman, A., Booth, M., Oldenburg, B. and Magnus, P. (1995) Serial mass-media campaigns to promote physical activity: reinforcing or redundant? *American Journal of Public Health* **85**, 244–224.

Reger, B., Wootan, M. G. and Booth-Butterfield, S. (1999) Using mass media to promote healthy eating: A community-based demonstration project. *Preventive Medicine* **29**, 414–421.

Reidpath, D. D., Burns, C., Garrard, J., Mahoney, M. and Townsend, M. (2002) An ecological study of the relationship between social and environmental determinants of obesity. *Place* **8**, 141–145.

Robinson, T. N. (1999) Reducing children's television viewing to prevent obesity: a randomized controlled trial. *Journal of the American Medical Association* **282**, 1561–1567.

Robinson, T. N. (2001) Population-based prevention for children and adolescents. In: Johnston, F. E., Foster, G. D. eds. *Obesity Growth and Development.* London: International Association for Human Auxology.

Robinson, T. N., Saphir, M. N., Kraemer, H. C., Varady, A. and Haydel, K. F. (2001) Effects of reducing television viewing on children's requests for toys: a randomized controlled trial. *Journal of Developmental Behaviour and Pediatrics* **22**, 179–184.

Rolls, B. J., Engel, D. and Birch, L. L. (2000) Serving portion size influences 5-year-old but not 3-year-old children's food intakes. *Journal of the American Dietetics Association* **100**, 232–234.

Rolls, B. J., Morris, E. L. and Roe, L. S. (2002) Portion size of food affects energy intake in normal-weight and overweight men and women. *American Journal of Clinical Nutrition* **76**, 1207–1213.

Rose, G. and Day, S. (1990) The population mean predicts the number of deviant individuals. *British Medical Journal* **301**, 1031–1034.

Sahota, P., Rudolf, M. C., Dixey, R., Hill, A. J., Barth, J. H. and Cade, J. (2001a) Evaluation of implementation and effect of primary school based intervention to reduce risk factors for obesity. *British Medical Journal* **323**, 1027.

Sahota, P., Rudolf, M. C., Dixey, R., Hill, A. J., Barth, J. H. and Cade, J. (2001b) Randomised controlled trial of primary school based intervention to reduce risk factors for obesity. *British Medical Journal* **323**, 1029–1032.

Sallis, J. F., Patterson, T. L., McKenzie, T. L. and Nader, P. R. (1988) Family variables and physical activity in preschool children. *Journal of Developmental Behaviour and Pediatrics* **9**, 57–61.

Seidell, J. C. (1999) Prevention of obesity: the role of the food industry. *Nutrition, Metabolism and Cardiovascular Disease* **9**, 45–50.

Simonetti D'Arca, A., Tarsitani, G., Cairella, M., Siani, V., De Filippis, S., Mancinelli, S., Marazzi, M.C. and Palombi, L. (1986) Prevention of obesity in elementary and nursery school children. *Public Health* **100**, 166–173.

Simmons, D., Thompson, C. F. and Volklander, D. (2001) Polynesians: prone to obesity and Type 2 diabetes mellitus but not hyperinsulinaemia. *Diabetic Medicine* **18**, 193–198.

Sleap, M. and Warburton, P. (1993) Are primary school children gaining heart health benefits from their journeys to school? *Child Care, Health and Development* **19**, 99–108.

Stunkard, A. J. (1996) Socioeconomic status and obesity. In: Chadwick, D.J., Cardew, G. eds. *The Origins and Consequences of Obesity.* Chichester: Wiley, 174–193.

Swinburn, B. A. (1995) Insulin resistance and low metabolic rate: do they cause obesity? *Asia-Pacific Journal of Clinical Nutrition* **4**, 343–344.

Swinburn, B., Egger, G. and Raza, F. (1999) Dissecting obesogenic environments: the development and application of a framework for identifying and prioritizing environmental interventions for obesity. *Preventive Medicine* **29**, 563–570.

Taylor, C. B., Fortmann, S. P., Flora, J., Kayman, S., Barrett, D. C., Jatulis, D. and Farquhar, J. W. (1991) Effect of long-term community health education on body mass index. The Stanford Five-City Project. *American Journal of Epidemiology* **134**, 235–249.

Tickner, J., Raffensperger, C. and Myers, N. (1996) The Precautionary Principle in Practice, Lowell Centre for Sustainable Production, Science and Environmental Health Network: Lowell, 1–23.

Tudor-Locke, C., Ainsworth, B. E. and Popkin, B. M. (2001) Active commuting to school: an overlooked source of children's physical activity? *Sports Medicine* **31**, 309–313.

UK Department of Health (2001) The National School Fruit Scheme. London: Department of Health, 1–17.

Wang, G., Fletcher, S. M. and Carley, D. H. (1995) Consumer utilization of food labeling as a source of nutrition information. *Journal of Consumer Affairs* **29**, 368.

Weimer, J. (1999) Accelerating the trend toward healthy eating. In: *America's Eating Habits: Changes and Consequences* Washington, DC: USDA/Econ. Res. Serv., 385–401.

Western Australian Government (2002) Government of Western Australia website (www.travelsmart.transport.wa.gov.au).

Wilson, N., Quigley, R. and Mansoor, O. (1999) Food ads on TV: a health hazard for children? *Australia and New Zealand Journal of Public Health* **23**, 647–650.

World Health Organization (1996) Development of health promoting schools—a framework for action. In: *Health Promoting Schools.* Geneva: WHO, Regional Office for the Western Pacific.

World Health Organization (2000) Obesity: preventing and managing the global epidemic. Geneva: WHO, 253.

World Health Organization (2002) Reducing risks, promoting healthy life. Geneva: WHO.

Young, L. R. and Swinburn, B. (2002) The impact of the Pick the Tick food information programme on the salt content of food in New Zealand. *Health Promotion International* **17**, 13–19.

Zuppa, J. A., Morton, H. and Metha, K. P. (2003) Television food advertising: Counterproductive to children's health? A content analysis using the Australian Guide to Healthy Eating. *Nutrition and Diet* **60**, 78–84.

Index

Page numbers in **bold** refer to tables and page numbers in *italics* refer to figures.

abdomen
  adipose tissue *see* visceral adipose tissue
  diameter *see* waist circumference
  obesity *see* visceral obesity
acanthosis nigricans, 238–239, 321
acarbose, 262, **382**, 385
'accelerated starvation', 285
acne, polycystic ovary syndrome, 281
acromegaly, 301
active electronic games, 452
active neighbourhoods, obesity prevention,
    463–464
active transport infrastructure
  obesity prevention, 459, *459*, 465–466
  promotion, 464
activity *see* physical activity
'activity diaries'
  food pattern monitoring, 128
  weight management, 324
acupressure, 449
acupuncture, 417, 449
AcuSlim device, 449
acylation-stimulation protein (ASP), 113
adaptive reproductive suppression
    hypothesis, 50, **51**
adaptive thermogenesis
  energy expenditure, 76
  models for body composition regulation, 78
addiction, hedonic processes of appetite
    control, 145–146
adenosine triphosphate (ATP)
  energy expenditure, 149
  synthesis in skeletal muscle, **105**, 105–107,
    106
  thermogenesis mechanism, 77
adipokines, insulin resistance, 186, 257–258
adiponectin, 386, **387**
  adipose tissue release, 103, 205
  insulin resistance, 186–187, 258
  obesity, 206
adipose tissue, *111*, 111–115
  brown, 77, 103

carbohydrate metabolism, 111
daily energy fluxes, role in, 104, *105*
distribution, 4
  abdominal, vascular disease risk, 271
  Asian population, 436–437, **437**
  childhood obesity, 21, 224–225,
    232–233
  epidemiological associations, 253, *253*
  evolution and culture, 48
  gender differences, 165, *166*
  growth pattern association, 95
  measurement, 4, **4**, 12, 19–21, *20*
  endocrine function, 174, 198, *199*, 205, **205**,
    205–206
  genetic abnormality in metabolic
    syndrome, 174
  infancy, 98
  inflammatory mediators, 272
  measurement, 12
  metabolic importance, 102–104
  metabolism
    disturbances and obesity development,
      113–114
    obesity, *114*, 114–115
  non-esterified fatty acid release, 111–112
  paracrine function, 174
  percentage estimation
    body mass index *see* body mass index
    (BMI)
    equation, 3
  steroid metabolism, 203
  thermogenesis control, 78
  triacylglycerol clearance, 112–113
adipose tissue–brain axis, 205
adiposity signals
  hunger-satiety, 73–74
  insulin, 74
adjunctive therapies in weight management,
    325
ad libitum diets, 328, **445**
adolescent obesity *see* childhood/adolescent
    obesity

adoption studies, heritability of fat mass, 82
adrenal androgens, fat distribution effect, 201
adrenal crisis, pro-opiomelanocortin
    deficiency, 88
adrenaline
  energy expenditure, 156
    mediation, 157
  obesity hypertension, 273
  psychological thermogenesis, 70
adrenergic drugs, 382, **382**, 383
β-adrenoceptors
  energy expenditure mediation, 157
  resting metabolic rate effect, 154
adrenocorticotrophic hormone (ACTH)
    deficiency, 88–89
adult obesity, childhood obesity consequence,
    231–232
adult stigmatism of children, 36
aerobic exercise, 375
aerobic fitness, 374
aerobic metabolic pathways, physical activity,
    155
Aerobics Centre Longitudinal Study, 269
age
  body mass index, 12–13, *13*
  food intake control effects, 127–128
  risk factors, 5, *5*
  visceral adipose tissue differences, 165–166
  see also childhood/adolescent obesity;
    children
agriculturalists, 47
agriculture development, 124
Aim for a Healthy Weight, 348
air displacement plethysmography, 24
  body volume measurement, 14
  children, **216**
Albright hereditary osteodystrophy, 84
alcohol
  dietary interventions, consumption in, 340
  drug-induced thermogenesis, 70
  risk factors of consumption, 5
  weight loss diets, 133

Alstrom's syndrome, **83**
  Bardet–Biedl syndrome *vs.*, 84
  childhood obesity, 225
alternative compartmentalization, 70–71, *71*
alternative medicine, **446**, 446–450
  weight loss maintenance, 417–418
American College of Sports Medicine,
    physical activity recommendations, 374
American diabetes prevention study, 263
American Dietetic Association (ADA), 330,
    331
American Harvard Growth Study
    (1922–1935), 233
American National Education Program, 169
American Weight Control Registry, 334
amino acid(s)
  oxidation, 105
  pregnancy, 285
  skeletal muscle metabolism, 102
aminostatic signals, hunger-satiety, 73
amphetamines, **382**
amylin *see* islet amyloid polypeptide (IAPP)
anaemia, pregnancy, 288
anaerobic metabolism, physical activity, 155
androgen production, female obesity, 203
android obesity *see* visceral obesity
androstenedione
  fat distribution effect, 201
  obesity cause, 202–203
Angelman syndrome, 84
ANGELO framework, 461
  obesity prevention, 459, *459*
angiotensin, adipose tissue release, 205
angiotensin-converting enzyme (ACE)
    inhibitors, salt intake, 133
angiotensinogen, 206
animal proteins, dietary composition, 123–125
anorectin, 386, **387**
anorexia, exercise-induced, 368–369
anorexia nervosa, 381
anthropometry
  body composition measurement, 16–17
  children, 217
  fat distribution measurement, 21
    following weight loss, 23
anti-smoking group (ASH), 467
anxiety, 33
  children, 244
  physical activity effect, 374
apnoea, **297**
  see also obstructive sleep apnoea (OSA)
apnoea-hypopnoea index (AHI), 278, **297**
apolipoprotein A-IV, 386, **387**
apolipoprotein B
  ischaemic heart disease risk, 171, *171*
  visceral adipose tissue effect, 164, 166–167,
    168
apolipoprotein(s)
  coronary heart disease risk, 164

genetic abnormality in metabolic
    syndrome, 174
appetite, 71
  lifestyle factors, 71
  programming, fetal origins of obesity, 99
  regulation, programming during infancy,
    98
appetite control, 137
  amylin, 141
  cholecystokinin, 139–140
  conceptualization of the control system,
    138, 138–139
  episodic signals, 139–142
  genetics *see* genetics
  glucagon-like peptide -1, 140–141
  hedonic processes, 144–146
  homeostatic processes, *138*, *140*, 144–146
  hunger-pleasure interaction, 144–145
  individual variability, 146–147
  leptin, 142
  obesity management, 137–138
  peptide YY, 141
  risk factors, 146, **146**
  satiety cascade, 139
    peptides, 141–142
  satiety signals, 139
  tonic signals, 139–142, *140*, 142
appetite suppressants, 342
arcuate (ARC)-PVN pathway, 72
arcuate nucleus, 206
arthritis, obesity impact, 9
Asian populations and obesity, 431–442
  adults, 431–433, *432*, **432**
  body composition variations, 436
  body fat distribution, 436–437, **437**
  body mass index and health risk
    relationship, 435–439
  children, **433**, 433–434
  dietary changes, 438–439
  fetal undernutrition, 439
  frame size/proportions, 436
  health and weight relationship, *434*, **434**,
    434–435
  methodological issues, 435–436
  physical activity changes, 438–439
  prevalence, **432**, 432–434, **433**, 438
  stunting/low birth weight, 439
  weight gain rate, 437–438
aspartame, 386, **386**
aspirin, 385, 386
  cardiovascular disease prevention, 272
assessment (of obesity), 3–4, 321–323
  body composition *see* body composition
    measurement
  body mass index *see* body mass index (BMI)
  children *see* childhood/adolescent obesity,
    assessment
  environment, 321, **321**
  fat distribution, 4, **4**

investigations, 321–322
  of motivation to lose weight, 323
  physical examination, 321–322, **322**
  of risk, 323
  weight history, 321, **322**
  see also body composition measurement
associated diseases, 8–10
Association for the Study of Obesity, 349
association studies, 83
asthma
  childhood obesity, 238
  surgery for obesity effect, 398
atenolol, obese diabetic patient, 262
atherosclerosis
  adiponectin effect, 187
  physical activity risk, 376
  plaque formation, metabolic syndrome,
    257
  risk from childhood obesity, 233
  vascular disease in obesity, 272
Atkins diet, 132–133, 331–332, 353
  side effects, 336
ATP *see* adenosine triphosphate (ATP)
'at-risk-for-overweight', US terminology, 223
attribution theory to weight stigma, 37
atypical antipsychotics, weight gain role, 259
Australasian Society for the Study of Obesity
    (ASSO), 348
autoregulatory adjustments, energy
    expenditure *see* energy expenditure,
    autoregulatory adjustments
Autoslim, 337
autosomal dominant pleiotropic obesity
    syndromes, **83**
autosomal recessive pleiotropic obesity
    syndromes, **83**
aversion therapy, 449
Avon Longitudinal Study of Pregnancy and
    Childhood, 95
axokine, 386, **387**

Baby Friendly hospitals, breast feeding, 465
balanced deficit diet (BDD), 353, *353*
Baltic states, prevalence, 8
Bardet–Biedl syndrome (BBS), 85
  childhood obesity, 225
bariatric procedures *see* surgery; *specific
    procedures*
Barker hypothesis, 439
basal metabolic rate (BMR), 152
  energy demand, 128, *129*
  energy expenditure, 69, *69*
  leptin therapy effect, 86, *88*
  menstrual cycle effects, 127
  pregnancy effects, 283
  weight loss effects, 131
'battle of the sexes' hypothesis, 50, **51**
'Be Active, Eat Well' campaign, 462, *462*
behavioural problems, children, 244

behavioural risk factors, 5–6
  appetite control, 146, *146*
Behavioural Risk Factor Surveillance System
    (BRFSS), 6, *6*
behavioural therapy, 350–362, **351**, **356**, **445**
  appetite control, 138, *138*
  cognitive restructuring, 352, 355
  commercial programmes, 358–359
  dietary *see* dietary interventions
  family readiness in childhood obesity
    management, 226
  group interventions, 355
  Internet and e-mail interventions, 358
  modification programmes, 324
  physical activity *see* physical activity
  primary care provision, 359
  principles, 350–351
  professional education/training, 426
  results
    long-term, 356–358, *357*, 407–408, *408*
    short-term, 355–356
  self-monitoring, 340, 351
  stimulus control, 339, 340–341, 352
  weight loss maintenance role, 414, 416
  see also counseling
behaviours, childhood obesity, 245
belief's (inappropriate) on the cause of
    obesity, 35
benign intracranial hypertension, childhood
    obesity, 241
Benn index, children, 217
benzocaine, 387
benzphetamine, 382, **382**
beta-cells, insulin synthesis/secretion, 254
beta-cells, dysfunction/failure, 258–259
  diabetes mellitus, 188
    type 2, 255–256
  fetal malnutrition, 259
  islet amyloid polypeptide, 259
  lipotoxicity, 259
bias, 34–37
  reduction methods, 37–38
'bicarbonate-urea' method, 150
bicep skinfold, 16
Biemond's syndrome, 11
  Bardet–Biedl syndrome *vs.*, 84
  childhood obesity, 225
Big Mac meal, 464
bigness preference, cultural differences, 49–50
biliopancreatic diversion (BPD), 401–402, **445**
  duodenal switch variant (BPD-DS)
    evolution, 395, *396*
    technique, 401
  effects, 401–402, **402**
    dyslipidemia effects, 398
  evolution, 395, *396*
  side-effects, 401–402
  technical features, 401
  weight loss outcomes, 397

binge eating disorder
  children, 225, 245
  phentermine-fluoxetine therapy, 388
  silbutramine therapy, 383
  weight regain association, 411–412, 413, 416
bioelectrical impedance analysis (BIA), 24
  body composition measurement, 17–18
  children, 19, 216–217, 221
  commercial machines, 17
  fat distribution measurement, 21
  foot-to-foot systems, 17
  health risk analysis, 23
BioEnterics® Lap-Band® system, 396, 402, **403**
bioflavonoids, **448**
biological risk factors, 5
birth size, adult body weight association,
    93–95, *94*
bissey nut extract, 449
blood flow, role in obesity development, 114
blood glucose levels (BGLs), high GI foods,
    332
blood pressure, weight loss benefits, 260
Blount's disease, 240
BMI-for-age
  assessment, **223**, 223–224, *224*
  children, 217
    percentile charts, *221*, 223
  classification, 215, 217–220, *218–219*
  percentile charts, 215
    subscapular skinfold measurement
      association, 223
  skinfold thickness correlation, 221
Bodpod™
  body volume measurement, 14
  children, 19
body composition
  adaptive thermogenesis, 78
  Asian population variation, 436
  changes with massive weight loss, 16, *16*
body composition measurement, 12–28
  applications, 21–24
    categorization of obesity, 21–22
    health risk assessment, 23
    obesity management, *22*, 22–23
    research, 23–24, *24*
  body fat, 12
  body mass index *see* body mass index
    (BMI)
  children, 18–19
  gross, 13–24
  multicompartment models, 15–16
  prediction techniques, 16–18
  reference methods, 13–15
  weight, 12
  see also assessment (of obesity); *specific*
    techniques
body density, 13–14
body esteem
  children, 36–37

culture effect, 55
  psychological outcome influence, 34
body fat *see* adipose tissue
body image, surgery for obesity effect, 399
body maintenance, culture, health and fitness,
    60
body mass index (BMI), 327, 408
  age related changes, 217
    see also BMI-for-age
  alternative causes, 12
  Asian population *see* Asian populations and
    obesity
  centile curves, 222
  centile points, 221
  children, 217
    categorization of obesity, 21–22
    centiles, 221
  cut-off points, 221–222, *222*, 320, 321, **322**
    adults, 215
    Asian population, **439**, 440, *440*
    children, 221–222
    ethnic specificity, 431
    global differences, **222**
  diabetes development risk, 252, *252*
  dyslipidaemia association, ethnic
    differences, 435
  ethnic differences, 22, 436
    hypertension association, 434, *434*
    size preference, 53, **53**, *54*
  ethnicity, migrant population changes, 82
  fat-free mass accumulation limit effects, 130
  genetic contribution, 82
  inappropriate use, 3
  leg length effect, 436
  limitations, 12–13, 22
  mortality association, 8, *8*
  obesity measurement, 3
  optimal, 4
  overweight classification, **4**
  SD scores, 21–22
  stroke association, 275
  'tracking' through life, 93
  see also body weight
body size, BMR determination, 69
body volume measurement, 14
body weight
  birth size association, 93–95, *94*
  body composition measurement, 12
  children, 217
    growth association, *95*, 95–96
  difference to height percentile, 220, *221*
  fluctuation, 67
  gain
    adult life, diabetes development risk, 252,
      252
    appetite control, 146
    food intake control adjustments, 131–134
    individual variability in susceptibility,
      146–147

normal, 130
physical activity, 364–365
rate, 437–438
resistance, 146–147
history, 321, **322**
homeostasis, 67–80
energy expenditure *see* energy
expenditure
food intake control *see* food intake,
control
food intake patterns, 68–69
human energetics, basic concepts and
principles, 67–71
integrating intake and expenditure,
78–79, *79*
thermodynamics laws, 67–68, *68*
timescale, 71
instability, mortality, 8–9
loss *see below*
maintenance, 323
physical activity, 363
management
childhood obesity, family involvement,
227
physical activity *see* physical activity
physical activity combined with diet,
365
motor vehicle ownership, 439
physical activity, 364–366
regulation, 126
see also body mass index (BMI)
body weight loss
abdominal magnetic resonance imaging
scan, 20, *20*
amount, planning in management,
319–320
benefits, 260–261
best-practice guidelines, 320
body composition changes, 16, *16*
factors influencing, 22–23
body mass index changes, 13, *13*
diabetes, 261
diabetes prevention, 263
diets, 131–134
alcohol, 133
carbohydrates, 133
fats and fatty acids, effect on, 132–133
fructosans, 133
glycaemic index, 133
prescription of, 131–132, *132*
protein intakes, 133
salt, 133–134
expectations, 319
extremely obese individuals, time span,
130
following obesity surgery, 397
goals, **320**, 320–21
hypertension effect, 273, 275
leptin therapy *see* leptin

maintenance, 407–420
alternative medicine role, 417–418
attitudes to, 412–413
behavioural interventions role, 414, 416
definition and prevalence, 409–410
factors affecting, 409–415, **415**
health benefits, 407–408
liquid meal replacements, 357–358, *358*
natural weight trajectory, 408, *409*
pharmacotherapy role, 414
physical activity, 365–366
physical activity role, *355, 357, 357*, 410,
413
professional education/training, 424
research, 413–414
treatment considerations, 415–418
metabolic risk profile improvement, 176
moderate, 320, **320**
motivation assessment, 323
physical activity, 365
plateau, 409
programme, diabetes, 261
Bogalusa Heart Study, 233
bombesin, 386, **387**
Bonaparte, Napoleon, 49
Börjeson–Forssman–Lehmann syndrome, **83**,
225
bottle feeding, appetite and satiety in later life,
97
brachiofemoral-adipomuscular ratio, 4
breast cancer, obesity/overweight impact, 9
breast-feeding, **287**, 288
appetite and satiety in later life, 97–98
energy intake control, 127
obesity prevention role, 465
protective effect, 97
breathlessness
childhood obesity, 235
intraabdominal pressure, 277
lung function, 277
brindleberry, **448**
bromocriptine, **382**, 385–386
brown adipose tissue (BAT), 77, 103
built environment, obesity prevention,
465–466
bulimic eating disorders, 225
bullying, 36
bupropion, **382**, 384, 388
'business of thinness', 57
Busselton Sleep Survey, 300, *301*

caesarian sections, **287**, 288
cafeteria food, 464
caffeine, 385, **446**
drug-induced thermogenesis, 70
skin creams, 449
caffeine-ephedrine, **382**, 385, 447, 449
caffeine-guarana, **448**
calcium loss, high-protein diets, 332

calipers, body composition measurement, 16
calorie-restricted diets *see* low-energy diets
(LEDs)
calorimetry, 106, 149
energy expenditure measurement,
149–150
Cambridge diet, 132
Canada's Food Guide, 446
cancer, 9
cannabinoid antagonists, 386, 387
capsaicin, **446**, 447, **448**, 449
carbohydrate-rich diets, 133
carbohydrates
Asian population consumption, 438
dietary interventions, 340
energy intake adaption to energy
expenditure, 369
evolution of obesity, 48
handling in obese people, 129
high intensity activity requirement, 155
intake restriction diets, 132–133
metabolism/oxidation
adipose tissue, 111
ATP synthesis energy source, 105
energy expenditure measurement, 150
insulin resistance effect, 255, *256*
during physical activity, 372
skeletal muscle, 107
overfeeding, 128
quantity, 153
skeletal muscle, 102
weight loss diets, 133
carbon dioxide production, 149
cardiac diseases/disorders
childhood obesity, 237
physical activity, 375, 376
risk factors in children, 225
weight management effect, 241–242
see also specific diseases/disorders
cardiac failure
children, 237
sleep-disordered breathing association,
301–302
cardiac hypertrophy, *274*, 274–275
obesity, 274–275
cardiomyopathy of obesity, 274
cardiorespiratory disease, 276–279
cardiovascular disease (CVD)
age related risk in obesity, 166
Asian population, 434, 437–438
'cheap food' policy, 125
childhood obesity risk factors, *233*, 233–234
epidemic reduction, 458
metabolic syndrome, 189
obesity consequence, 269–280
cardiorespiratory disease, 276–279
children, 236–237, **237**
intra-abdominal pressure, 276–277
lung function, 277–278

physical fitness as mortality risk
predictor, 269
sudden death, 269–271
obstructive sleep apnoea association,
303–305
see also specific diseases/disorders
L-Carnitine, **448**
car oriented environment, 465
β-carotene, cardiovascular disease
prevention, 272
Carpenter syndrome, 225
catecholamine-induced thermogenesis, 156
catecholamines, energy expenditure, 156
cellulite reduction products, 449
central apnoea, 297–298
congestive heart failure in obesity, 276
'central motive state', appetite control, 143
central obesity *see* visceral obesity
cephalic phase of appetite, 139
cerazette, 291
cerebral infarction *see* strokes
cerebrovascular disease
obesity/overweight impact, 9
sleep-disordered breathing association,
302
see also strokes
cervical cancer, 458
charities, patient-centred, 349
'cheap food' policy, 124–125
chemical maturation in children, 18
dual energy X-ray absorptiometry, 19
chemoreceptors
appetite control, 139
hunger-satiety signals, 72
Cheyne–Stokes respiration
comorbid conditions, 301–302
congestive heart failure in obesity, 276
definition, **297**, 298
childhood/adolescent obesity, 213–248
aetiology
disordered eating association, 245
genetic defects, 241
psychiatric disorders, 244
self-esteem, 243
self-perception, 243–244
see also infant origins of obesity
Asian population, **433**, 433–434
assessment, 216–217, 216–223, 216t,
223–227, 225–226
global comparisons, 222, **222**
guidelines, **223**, *224*
incorrect diagnosis, 222
lifestyle, 226
regional adiposity, 224–225
sensitivity, 222–223
skinfolds, 224
specificity, 222–223
BMI-for-age *see* BMI-for-age
classification, 215–223

clinical examination, *244*
clinician deportment, 227
complications, **235**, 235–242, **237**
breathlessness, 235
cardiovascular, 236–237, *237*, **237**
cutaneous striae, 236
discrimination, 243
endocrine, **237**, 238–239
gastrointestinal, **237**, 240–241
heat intolerance, 235
heat rash, 235
hypertension risk, 272–273
musculoskeletal discomfort, 236
neurological, **237**, 241
orthopaedic, **237**, 240
physical, 235–236
pseudogynaecomastia in males, 236
psychosocial, *242*, 242–245
during puberty, 239
puberty staging, 236
reproductive, 239–240
respiratory, **237**, 237–238
skin lesions, 235
small genitalia in males, 236
stereotyping, 242–243
stigmatization, 242–243
tiredness, 235–236
consequences of, 231–235, **232**
adult morbidity increase, *233*, 233–234,
234
adult mortality increase, 233–234
adult obesity, 231–232
adverse adult psychological outcomes,
235
belonging to an obese family, 232
fat distribution, 232–233
health-care provision disadvantages,
234
puberty, risk time of further weight gain,
232
cut-off point selection, 221–222, *222*
definition, 215–223
management
comorbidities, effect on, 241–242
family readiness, 226
psychological effect, 244
prevalence increase factors, 456
terminology use, 227
children activity patterns, 462
driven to school, 464
eating patterns, 462
food marketing targets, 466–467
growth
adult body weight association, *95*,
95–96
adult obesity, 93–96
physical activity decline, 463
physical activity interventions, 452
target groups for obesity prevention, 460

China
fat intake, 124
obesity prevention, 459, *459*
sugars, 125
chitosan, **446**, 447–448, **448**, 449
chlorphentermine, **382**
chlortermine, **382**
CHNS *see* National China Health and
Nutrition Survey (CHNS)
cholecystokinin (CCK), 386, **387**
appetite control, 139–140
gastrointestinal hunger-satiety signals, 73
cholelithiasis, 241
cholesterol levels
dyslipidaemia, 163
environmental intervention effects, 443, *444*
pregnancy, 284
vascular disease risk, 272
see also low-density lipoprotein (LDL)-
cholesterol
chromium compounds, 386, **386**
chromium picolinate, **448**
chromosomes, obesity loci, 83, **83**
chronic obstructive pulmonary disease
(COPD), 305
churches, obesity prevention role, 465
chylomicrons
dyslipidaemia, 163
pregnancy, 284
cimetidine, **382**, 385
cirrhosis, 251, 263, 264
citalopram, **382**
citrus aurantium, 449
'civilization syndromes', 48
*Civil Service Commission v. Pennsylvania
Human Relations Commission*, 1991, 30
classical conditioning, 350–351
classification
International Classification of Diseases, 58
overweight, 3
WHO graded system for obesity, 431
climate at birth, 98, *98*
climate hypothesis, cultural body size
preference, 50, **51**
clinical management programme, 460–461,
461
clinical research needs, research
recommendations, 40, **40**
clinician deportment, childhood obesity, 227
clover, sweet, **448**
coactivator protein PGC-1, 89–90
Cochrane Systematic Reviews on Obesity, 349
cognitive-behaviocral model, 38–39
cognitive restructuring
behavioural therapy, 352, 355
H@AS approach, 335
Cohen's syndrome, **83**, 225
cold-induced thermogenesis, 70, 153
coleus forskolin, 449

college admission, 31
college dismissal due to weight, 31
college student attitudes, 33
combination therapy, 262
combined oral contraceptive pills, 291
commercial weight loss programmes, 355, 358–359, 445–446
community-based programmes, 460–461, 464–465
    action in Colac, 461–462, *462*
compartmentalization, children, 216
computerized tomography (CT), 19–20
    children, 216, **216**, 225
    visceral adipose tissue measurement, 166, *167*, 176, 225
Confidential Enquiry into Maternal Deaths in the United Kingdom, 288
congenital abnormalities, 290
congenital leptin deficiency, 86, 90
congestive heart failure (CHF), 275–276, *277*
    hypertension effect, 273
conjugated linoleic acid, 386, **386**
constipation, 340
continuing professional development, 423
continuous positive airway pressure (CPAP), *303*, 305, 307–308, *310*
    new devices, 310, *310*
    obese hypoventilation syndrome treatment, *310*
contraception, 291–292
Core Curriculum, 422, 424–427
corn syrups, dietary composition, 125
coronary artery disease (CAD)
    high-protein diets, 332
    hypertriglyceridaemia, 256
coronary heart disease (CHD), 3
    Asian population, 434, 437
    'cheap food' policy effect, 125
    dyslipidaemia, 163–165
    metabolic syndrome, 170–172, *171*
    obesity/overweight impact, 9, **9**
    prevention through physical activity, 156
    sudden death in obesity, 270
coronary syndromes, acute, 271
cor pulmonale, 297
correspondence programmes, 450
corticotrophin-releasing hormone (CRH), 386, **387**
cortisol, insulin resistance, 257
cosmetics industry, 57
cosmetic surgeons, 57
counseling, 176
    professional education/training, 426
    see also behavioural therapy
craniopharyngioma, 208
cravings, appetite control, 145
C-reactive protein (CRP)
    adiposity relationship, 170
    high-protein diets, 332

ischaemic heart disease risk, 171
    metabolic syndrome, 169–170, 190
    obstructive sleep apnoea, 305
creatine, 386, **386**
cultural competence, 60
culture, 46–64
    body maintenance, health and fitness, 60
    control and surveillance of the body, 57
    cultural competence, 60
    definitions, 46–47
    differences between societies, 49–52
        bigness preference, 49–50
        ideal female body shape, cultural predictors, 50–52, **51**
        smallness preference, 50
    differences within societies, 52–55
        ethnic differences, 53, **53**, *54*
        poverty, 52–53
        social factors, 52
        Westernization, process of, 53, 55
    environment, 48–59
    evolution of fat storage and distribution, 48
    evolution over time, 47–48
    influence on medical definitions of obesity, 57–58
    medicalization of obesity, 58–59
    normalizing process, resistance to, **59**, 59–60
    slim ideal emergence, 55, **56**, 57
    social and environmental orientation on obesity, 60
    social/biological body divide, 55
    susceptibility to weight gain, 457
    twenty-first century, in the, 60–61
    weight attitudes, 37
    Western societies in the twentieth century, 55–59
    see also ethnicity
Cushing's syndrome
    central obesity, *200*, 200–201
    children, 225, 236
    endocrine testing, 207, 208
    obesity cause, 198–199
cutaneous striae, 236
cycle-friendly street design, 465

dairy produce consumption, 340
DASH trials, 130
deep subcutaneous fat compartment, insulin resistance, 172–173
deep vein thrombosis (DVT), 291
deficit diet scheme, inappropriateness, 131–132, *132*
definitions
    obesity, 3
    overweight, 3
dehydroepiandrosterone (DHEA), 386, **386**
    fat distribution effect, 201
demedicalization attempts, 59

demographic risk factors, 5
depoprovera, 291
depression, 33
    children, 36, 225, 244
    physical activity effect, 374
    surgery for obesity effect, 399
    weight regain association, 413, 416
desogestrel, 291
deuterium isotope
    energy expenditure measurement, 150
    total body water measurement, 14
dexamphetamine, 382
dexfenfluramine, 383
diabetes mellitus, 3, 188–189, *189*
    aetiology
        Asian population, 434, **434**
        childhood obesity, 225
        obesity/overweight impact, 9, **9**
        Prader–Willi syndrome, 84
    anti-obesity drug use, 262, *262*
    heart failure coexistence, 276
    pregnancy *see* gestational diabetes
    prevention
        physical activity, 156
        weight loss, 263, 320
    screening, 208
        children, 208
    Task Force on Obesity target group, 10
    treatment of obesity *see* management (of obesity)
    weight loss, 261
diabetes mellitus, type 2, 251
    adiponectin, 187
    childhood obesity, 238–239
    comorbidity, 260
    epidemiological associations, *252*, 252–253, *254*
    ethnic differences, 434–435
    fatty acid oxidation role, 108
    following surgery for obesity, 397–398, 399
    interleukin 6 effect, 187
    management of obesity, 260
    metabolic syndrome association, 254, *254*
    pathogenesis, 255–256
    physical activity effect, 373
Diabetes Prevention Program (DPP), 320, 350
Dianette, 291
diaries (of food intake) *see* food diaries
diazoxide, **382**, 385
dietary composition, 123–136
    animal protein, 123–125
    energy density and food intake, 125–128, *126*
    energy intake adaption to energy expenditure, 369
    essential fatty acids, 123–125
    evolutionary perspective, 123–125
        corn syrups, 125
        dietary availability, 124

fat intakes, 124
food supply transformation, macronutrient intake effects, 124–125
fructosans, 125
sugars, 125
macronutrient intake, optimum, **130**, 130–131
weight loss diets *see* body weight loss
dietary fibre supplements, 386, **386**, 447, **448**
dietary interventions, 324, 352–354
eating plans, 327–349
fixed-energy diets, 328
high-protein diets, 331–332
less restrictive approach, 333–335, *335*
low-calorie diets *see* low-energy diets (LEDs)
low-carbohydrate diets, 353, *353*
low-energy density diets, 353–354
meal frequency, 335–336
moderate-fat diets, 331
self-limiting (*ad libitum*) diets, 328
see also specific named diets
effects, **445**
evaluation guidelines, 337
medical, concept, 57
physical activity combination, 365
Prader–Willi syndrome *see* Prader–Willi syndrome
principles, 337–340
private sector, 336–337
professional education/training, 424–425
psychological harm, 59, **59**
supplements, 386, **386**
under-reporting of food intake, 338
as way of life, 55
weight loss maintenance, 342–343
Dietary Intervention Study in Hypertension (DISH), 260
'diet cycle', 335, *335*
'diet diaries', 337–339
'diet–heart hypothesis', 270
diethylpropion, 382, **382**
effects, **445**
diet-induced thermogenesis (DIT), 70
energy expenditure, 128, 366
exercise/physical activity, 363, 367
interindividual variation, 76
obese people, 129
during pregnancy, 284
resting energy expenditure, 152, 153
dieting industry, annual turnover, 57
diffuse capacity for carbon monoxide (DLCO), 277
discrimination, childhood obesity, 243
disordered eating, childhood obesity, 245
diuretic use, long QT syndrome, 270
dizygotic twin studies, 82
dopamine, addiction in appetite control, 145, 146

doubly labelled water (DLW), 150
Down's syndrome
childhood obesity, 225
obstructive sleep apnoea, 301
Dr. Atkins' New Diet Revolution, 353
DRD2 receptors, 146
'drive for food defect', 143
drosperinone, 291
drugs
diabetes mellitus type 2 cause, 259–260
induced thermogenesis, 70
weight gain, **259**, 259–260, 321, **322**
dual energy X-ray absorptiometry (DXA), 24
birth weight and adult body size, 94
body composition measurement, 13, 14–15, *15*
children, 19, 216, **216**, 221, 225
fat distribution measurement, 20–21
measurement difficulties in obese subjects, 15
dynamic equilibrium model, energy expenditure, 75–76
dynamic thermogenesis, 70
dyslipidaemia, 163–183
body mass index association, 435
coronary heart disease risk, 163–165
lipid metabolism, 163
lipoprotein metabolism, 163, *164*
metabolic syndrome *see* metabolic syndrome
physical activity effect, 373
surgery, 398
therapeutic implications, 175–176
visceral adipose tissue, 165–166, *166*
dyspnoea, *278*

East Flanders Prospective Twin Study, 94
eating behaviour, 137–148
patterns, 137
see also appetite control
eating (diet intervention) programmes *see* dietary interventions
eccentric ventricular hypertrophy, 274
economic factors
aetiology of obesity, 47, 48
employment, 29
for obesity prevention, 468–469
education, 31–32, 34, 35
bias reduction by, 37–38
childhood obesity effects, 235
professional *see* professional education/training
risk factor, 5, *5*
electronic games, active, 452
electronic muscle stimulation (EMS), 449
electronic prompts, use in consumer food choice, 452
e-mail resources, weight loss interventions, 358

emotional/external cued eating, 335, *335*, 343
childhood obesity, 245
employment, 29–30, 34
bias, 34
childhood obesity effects, 235
negative stereotypes, 34
termination, wrongful, 30
endocrine diseases/disorders, 198–200, **199**, *199*
childhood obesity, 225, **237**, 238–239
obstructive sleep apnoea association, 305–306
endocrine function of adipose tissue, *205*, **205**, 205–206
endocrine testing, 206–209
children, 208–209
interpretation in obese patients, 207–208
endometrial cancer, 9
endometritis, 288
end-stage renal disease, hypertension, 273
endurance training, 363, 364, 365
energy balance, 67–80
physical activity, 366–369
and body weight, 156
time trend cause, 8
see also body weight
energy density
dietary composition, 125–128
food intake, 125–128, *126*
gene-environment interactions, 81–82
impact on daily food intake, 125–126
physical activity *see* physical activity
taxation, 469
energy exchanges, *150*
energy expenditure, 68–71, 149–160, 366
autoregulatory adjustments, 75–78, 79
adaptive thermogenesis, 76, 78
dynamic equilibrium model, 75–76
physical activity thermogenesis, 76–77
thermogenesis mechanisms, 77–78
components, 69–71, 151, *151*
alternative compartmentalization, 70–71, *71*
basal metabolic rate, 69, *69*
physical activity, due to, 69–70
thermogenic stimuli, response to, 70
definitions, 149
exercise training effect, 363
genes, 89–90
integration with food intake, 78–79, *79*
measurements, 128–130, 149–151
food pattern monitoring, 128
metabolic efficiency *see* metabolic efficiency
prediction as an index of normal food intake, 128–129
resting metabolic rate prediction, 151, **151**
obesity, **157**, 157–158

physical activity *see* physical activity, energy expenditure
resting energy expenditure *see* resting energy expenditure (REE)
thermogenesis *see* thermogenesis
time trend cause, 8
white adipose tissue role, 103
energy homeostasis, genetics, 85–86
energy intake
  adaption to energy expenditure, 364
  leptin therapy effect, 86, *88*
  physical activity associated *see* physical activity, energy intake
  time trend cause, 7, 8
  weight loss composition influence, 23
Ensure, 353
enterostatin, 386, **387**
entropy, 68
environment, 48–59, 60, 456
  childhood obesity, 227
  culture in the twenty-first century, 60
  gene interactions, 81–82
  interventions, 356, 359, 451–452
    effect on cholesterol levels, 443, *444*
  mechanisms, 98–99
  obesity development, 48
  obesity prevention, 457
  physical activity influence at neighbourhood level, 463–464
  temperature, 98, *98*
  of weight management assessment, 321, **321**
ephedra alkaloids, 385, 386, 447, 449
ephedrine, **382**, 385
ephedrine-caffeine, **382**, 385, 447
epidemic (of obesity), 99
  prevention, 456–458
  requirements for reversal, 457–458
epidemiology (in obesity), 3–11, 252–254, 456–457
episodic signals, 139–142, *140*
essential fatty acids, dietary composition, 123–125
ethnicity
  body mass index, 22, 436
    association with hypertension differences, 434, *434*
    cut-off point specificity, 431
  culture, 53, **53**, *54*
  diabetes mellitus type 2, 253, 434–435
    children, 238
  employment, 30
  fat-free mass, 436
  genetic susceptibility to obesity, 82
  risk factor, 5
  see also culture
Europe, prevalence, 6, **7**
European Prospective Investigation into Nutrition and Cancer (EPIC), 6

evidence-based medicine (EBM), 468
excessive daytime sleepiness (EDS), 302, 303
exercise
  aerobic exercise, 375
  induced anorexia, 368–369
  see also physical activity
external cued eating *see* emotional/external cued eating

'facilitated anabolism', 285
facultative diet-induced thermogenesis, 70
Faculty of Public Health Medicine, 348
falls, 376
families
  childhood obesity management, 226
  involvement in weight management, 227
  relationships, 33
'fast-foods'
  advertising, 451
  consumption, 60
  energy density, 125
  obesity prevention, 464, *464, 465*
fasting, 330
  resting energy expenditure, 152
fat, body *see* adipose tissue
fat-free mass (FFM)
  accumulation limit, 130
  children, 19
    hydration, 18, 19
  ethnic differences, 436
  resting metabolic rate, effect on, 152
  two compartment model of body composition, 13
  weight loss effects, 131
fat-free tissue hydration
  accurate measurement, 16
  obese subjects, 14
fats
  malabsorption, anti-obesity drugs, 262
  storage
    evolution and culture, 48
    regulation, 75
fats, consumption
  Asian populations, 438
  CCK effect, 140
  coronary heart disease, 270
  energy density, 125, *126*
  evolutionary perspective, 124
  food intake control bypass, 127
  handling in obese people, 129
  intake restriction diets, 133
  low intake diets, 134
  sudden death, 270
  thermogenesis increase, 128
  time trend cause, 7
  weight loss diets, 132–3
  World Health Organization recommended limit, 130

fats, oxidation
  energy expenditure measurement, 150
  physical activity, 364, 369, 370
    gender differences, 371
    intensity, 370
    training effect, 371–372
  rates, 129
fatty acids
  coronary heart disease, 270
  oxidation
    ATP synthesis energy source, 105
    impairment in obese subjects, 109
    low intensity activity requirement, 155
    skeletal muscle metabolism, 108
    sudden death, 270
    utilization during physical activity, 369
    weight loss diets, 132–3
'fat utopia', 61
feeding formula, obesity risk, 97
fenfluramine–fluoxetine, 388
fertility, 281–282
fetal macrosomia, *285*, 286, 289–290
fetal origins of obesity, 93–101
  appetite programming, 99
  climate at birth, 98, *98*
  maternal nutrition, 96, 97
  overnutrition, 96
  smoking, maternal, 96–97
  undernutrition, 96
    Asian populations, 439
  see also infant origins of obesity
fetus, 'metabolic programming', 97
fibre consumption
  dietary interventions, 340
  high consumption diets, 133
Fighting the Obesity Epidemic (FOE), 451
Finnish diabetes prevention study, 263
first law of thermodynamics, 67–68
fitness centres, 451
fixed-energy diets, 328
flat feet in children, 240
flavanol, 153
FLEX HR method, 150
fluoxetine, **382**, 383, 388
FOE (Fighting the Obesity Epidemic), 451
food
  behaviour, 68
  choice, 145
  distribution and pricing, 466
  guide pyramid, 352
  labeling
    nutrition content, 464
    obesity prevention, 466
  manufacturers, 125
  marketing, 466–467
  pattern monitoring, 128
  role in aetiology of obesity, 47
  supply transformation, 124–125

food diaries, 337–339
  food pattern monitoring, 128
  weight management, 324
    diabetes, 261
    maintenance role, 416
food intake
  assessment in childhood obesity, 226
  changes in Asia, 438–439
  control, 71–75, 79
    adjustments with weight gain,
      131–134
    dietary factors, 127–128
    hunger, 71–72
    hunger-satiety control centres in brain,
      72
    hunger-satiety signals from the
      periphery, 72–74
    integrated models, 74–75
    normal in relation to dietary
      macronutrients, 126–127
    satiety, 71–72
  daily, energy density impact, 125–126
  diabetes, 261
  dietary composition *see* dietary
    composition
  energy density, 125–126, 125–128, *126*
  evolutionary perspective, 124
  integration with expenditure, 78–79, *79*
  patterns, 68–69
  resting energy expenditure, 152–153
  risk factor, 5
'food security' hypothesis, 50, **51**
foot pronation, 240
foot-to-foot bioelectrical impedance analysis
  (BIA), 17
forced expiratory volume (FEV), 277
forced vital capacity (FVC), 277
formula diets, 132
four-compartment model
  body composition measurement,
    15–16
  children, 19
fragile X syndrome, 84
frame size/proportions, Asian populations,
  436
Framingham Heart Study
  congestive heart failure in obesity, 276
  IQ, 31
fraternal interest groups hypothesis, 50, **51**
free fatty acids (FFAs), 184–186, *185*, *186*, 257,
  258
fructosans
  dietary composition, evolutionary
    perspective, 125
  weight loss diets, 133
fructose, 153
fructose-rich diets, 133
fruit, free/subsidized in schools, 466
Fucus vesiculosus kelp, **448**

galanin, 99
gall bladder disease, 241
gastric banding, adjustable, **445**
gastric bypass, **445**
gastric inhibitory peptide (GIP), 73
gastroesophageal reflux
  children, 240, 241
  surgery for obesity effect, 398
gastrointestinal tract
  appetite control, 139
  complications in childhood obesity, **237**,
    240–241
  hunger-satiety signals from, 72–73
gastroplasty, 395, 399
  non-adjustable, **445**
  vertical-banded, 395, *395*
gender
  body mass ratio determination, 69
  employment, 29–30
  fat oxidation, 371
  metabolic efficiency, 130
  prevalence, 6, *6*, **7**
  risk factor, 5, *5*
  visceral adipose tissue, 165–166
gene–environment interaction, 81–82
gene polymorphisms, 154
gene therapy, 381, 387
genetic defects, 24
  childhood obesity, 241
  leptin deficiency, 74
  metabolic syndrome, 174–175
genetics, 81–92
  of appetite control, 142–144
    drive for food defect, 143
    ghrelin and hunger drive, 144
    leptin deficiency, *140*, 142–143
    melanocortin system mutations, 143
    satiety defect, 143
  childhood obesity, 225
  common obesity basis, 83
  energy expenditure genes, 89–90
  energy homeostasis, molecular
    mechanisms, 85–86
  gene-environment interaction, 81–82
  gene map, 83
  heritability of fat mass, 82
  historical perspective, 81
  monogenic obesity syndromes, 86–89, 90
  perspectives, 90
  pleiotropic obesity syndromes, **83**, 83–85
  role in aetiology of obesity, 47
  susceptibility to weight gain, 457
  testing, 208–209
  see also specific syndromes
genitalia, small, 236
gestational diabetes mellitus (GDM), 97, 286,
  287
  infant adipocyte mass, 98
gestodene, 291

ghrelin, 356
  endocrine testing, 208
  gastrointestinal hunger-satiety signals, 73
  hunger drive, 144
  obesity cause, 202
  Prader–Willi syndrome, 84
  weight regain role, 356
Gimello v. *Agency Rent-A-Car systems, Inc.,*
  1991, 30
Gingko biloba EGb761, **448**
ginseng, 449
global comparisons
  active transport infrastructure, 465
  childhood obesity, 222, **222**
  obesity prevalence, 184, 432, *432*
  obesity problem, 431
glucagon-like peptide 1 (GLP-1), 386, **387**
  appetite control, 140–141
  gastrointestinal hunger-satiety signals, 73
glucocorticoids
  asthma treatment, increased obesity risk,
    238
  weight gain role, 259
gluconeogenesis
  insulin resistance, 185, *186*
  the liver, 255
glucose
  disposal rate, 106–107
  homeostasis, 255, *256*
  metabolism
    energy expenditure measurement, **150**
    inhibition by free fatty acids, 257
    white adipose tissue, 111
  post-absorptive state, 104
  postprandial state, 107
  production, insulin resistance, 185, *186*
  skeletal muscle uptake, *105*
  tolerance impairment in childhood obesity,
    225
glucose clamp, 106
α-glucosidase inhibitors, pharmacotherapy in
  the obese diabetic patient, 262
glucostatic signals, 73
'gluttony experiments', 76
glycaemic control, weight loss benefits, 260
glycaemic index (GI), 332, 332–333
  food classification, **333**
  insulinaemic index correlation, *333*
  weight loss diets, 133
glycogen
  skeletal muscle, 102, 105, **105**
  utilization during physical activity, 106,
    370, *371*
glycogenostatic signals, 73
'glycogenostatic theory,' 74–75
glycolysis, anaerobic, ATP synthesis energy
  source, 105
'gold standard' definition of adiposity,
  222–223

Goldstein meta-analysis (1992), 407
gonadotrophins, endocrine testing, 207
Gothenburg Swedish Obese Subjects study
　　see Swedish Obese Subjects (SOS)
　　study
gout, 332
government role, obesity prevention, 459, *459,*
　　460
grapeseed extract, **448**
green tea extract, 449
gross body composition measurement,
　　13–24
group interventions, 355
　　'closed group approach', 355
growth
　　adult body weight association, *95,* 95–96
　　obesity association, *95, 95*
　　resting energy expenditure, 153
growth hormone-binding protein (GHBP),
　　202
growth hormone (GH), 386, **387**
　　deficiency
　　　childhood obesity, 225
　　　endocrine testing, 208
　　　obesity cause, 201–202
　　　Prader–Willi syndrome, 84
growth hormone-insulin-like growth factor
　　1-axis, **201,** 201–202
growth hormone-releasing hormone
　　(GHRH), 202
guarana, 447
GutBusters programme, 450
gymnasiums, 451
gymnema sylvestre, 449
gynaecomastia, children, 236
gynoid obesity, 165, *166*
　　diabetes risk, 253

'habitual' food (energy) intake, 68–69
'H@AS (health at any size)' system, 334–335
health
　　of childhood obesity, 225
　　following obesity surgery, 397–399
　　obesity prevention, 458–459, *459*
　　stigma consequences, 39, **40**
health care, 30–31, 35
　　childhood obesity disadvantages, 234
　　equipment, 321, **321**
　　examination reluctance, 31
　　hesitancy in seeking, 30–31, 38
　　professionals' attitudes, 30, 35
　　　to childhood obesity, 227, 242
　　　improvement in, 39
　　quality of care, 35
　　underutilization, 31
'health foods'
　　claims by food manufacturers, 466
　　weight loss claims, 337
health insurance denial, 30

health professionals, education/training *see*
　　professional education/training
Health Professionals Study, 437–438
Health Promoting Schools model, 463
health risk assessment, body composition
　　analysis, 23
Health Survey for England (2003), 252
'healthy narcissism', 412, 415, 416
heart failure *see* cardiac failure
heart rate
　　childhood obesity, 237
　　energy expenditure measurement,
　　　150–151
　　physical activity intensity classification,
　　　375
heart remodeling, cardiac hypertrophy, 274,
　　274
heat intolerance, childhood obesity, 235
heat loss, 68
　　energy expenditure measurement, 149
heat production, skeletal muscle, 69
heat rash, childhood obesity, 235
hedonic processes, appetite control, 144–146
height, children, 217
height-for-age percentiles, children, 223
height–weight index, 227
hepatic steatosis (fatty liver), children, 240,
　　241
herbal preparations, 386, **386, 446**
heritability of fat mass, 82
　　see also genetics
high-density lipoprotein (HDL) cholesterol
　　coronary heart disease risk, 165
　　dyslipidaemic state of abdominal obesity,
　　　172
　　physical activity, 156, 373
　　visceral adipose tissue effect, 166, *168*
　　weight loss effects, 260
high-density lipoprotein(s) (HDLs)
　　dyslipidaemia, 163
　　hypertriglyceridaemia, 165
　　weight loss effects, 261
high-fat diets, 108
high-fibre diets, 133
high-monounsaturated fatty acid diets, **445**
high-protein diets, 331–332
high-salt diets, 133–134
hirsutism
　　pituitary–gonadal axis abnormalities in
　　　obesity, 203
　　polycystic ovary syndrome, 190, 204, 281
HIV infection
　　epidemic reduction, 458
　　treatment, weight gain association,
　　　259–260
homeostasis model assessment (HOMA),
　　256
homeostatic processes, appetite control, *138,*
　　140, 144–146

homes, obesity prevention, 462–463
hormones, 198–212
　　endocrine functions of adipose tissue, *205,*
　　　205, 205–206
　　endocrine testing *see* endocrine testing
　　growth hormone-insulin-like growth
　　　factor 1-axis, **201,** 201–202
　　insulin resistance, 258
　　pituitary–adrenal axis, *200,* **200,** 200–201
　　pituitary–gonadal axis, 202–204
　　pituitary–thyroid axis, 204–205
　　primary endocrine disease, 198–200, *199*
　　resting energy expenditure, 153–154
　　see also individual hormones
hormone-sensitive lipase (HSL), 111–112
　　role in obesity development, 113–114
horse chestnut, **448**
Human Relations Area Files, 50
hunger
　　definition, 71
　　food intake control, 71–72
　　ghrelin, 144
hunger–pleasure interaction, 144–145
hunger–satiety control centres in brain, 72
'Hunger Winter' (Dutch famine 1944–1945)
　　infant feeding, 97
　　maternal starvation, 96
hunter-gatherers, 47
hydrodensitometry, children, 216, **216**
hydroxycitric acid, 447, **448,** 449
11β-hydroxysteroid dehydrogenase, 258
hyperandrogenism
　　pituitary-gonadal axis abnormalities in
　　　obesity, 203
　　polycystic ovary syndrome, 281
hypercapnia, 297
　　obese hypoventilation syndrome, 299
hyperglycaemia
　　pathogenesis of diabetes mellitus type 2,
　　　255
　　during pregnancy, 97
hyperinsulinaemia
　　childhood obesity, 234, *234*
　　coronary heart disease, 171
　　fetal, 289
　　glucose disposal rate, 107
　　glucose uptake reduction, 111
　　infant origins of obesity, 99
　　insulin resistance, 258
　　metabolic syndrome *see* metabolic
　　　syndrome
　　polycystic ovary syndrome, 190, 204,
　　　282
　　sex hormone binding globulin, 203
hyperinsulinaemic clamp, 106, 109
hyperinsulinaemic–euglycaemic clamp
　　technique, 169, 184
hyperleptinaemia, 206
　　insulin resistance, 258

hyperlipidaemia
  high-protein diets, 336
  orlistat therapy, 384
hyperphagia (over-feeding), 341
  appetite control risk factors, 146
  determination of, 75
  following food deprivation, 75
  Prader–Willi syndrome, 84
  during pregnancy, 284
  pro-opiomelanocortin deficiency, 88
  see also overeating
hypertension, 272–273, 275, 276
  body mass index association, ethnic
    differences, 434, *434*
  childhood obesity, 236–237, 272–273
  following surgery for obesity, 398
  insulin resistance, 257
  metabolic syndrome *see* metabolic
    syndrome
  obstructive sleep apnoea, 278, 302, *304*,
    304–305
  oral contraceptives, 291
  physical activity effect, 373
  pregnancy, 286–287, **287**
  pulmonary *see* pulmonary hypertension
  salt intake, 133
Hypertension Control Programme (HCP), 260
hyperthyroidism, endocrine testing, 208
hypertriglyceridaemia
  carbohydrate induced, 133
  coronary artery disease, 256
  dyslipidaemic state of abdominal obesity,
    172
  HDL metabolism, 165
  ischaemic heart disease, 171
hypertrophy, cardiac, *274*, 274–275
hypnosis, 449–450
  weight loss maintenance role, 417
hypocortisolaemia, insulin resistance, 258
hypogonadism, 203
  diagnosis, 198
hypokalaemia, long QT syndrome, 270
hypomagnesaemia, long QT syndrome, 270
hypopnoea, **297**
  see also obstructive sleep apnoea (OSA)
hypothalamic arcuate nucleus, 85
hypothalamic-pituitary-adrenal axis (HPA)
  insulin resistance, 258
  metabolic syndrome, 257
hypothalamus
  appetite suppression, 99
  dysfunction in obesity, 199, *199*
  energy homeostasis involvement, 85
  fetal development, nutritional need, 96
  hunger-satiety control, 72
  leptin, 206
  tumours, childhood obesity, 225
hypothyroidism, 301
  childhood obesity, 225

endocrine testing, 208
  low resting energy expenditure, 157
  weight gain presentation, 198, 204
hypoventilation, **297**

'ideal body shape', female, 50–52, **51**
idiopathic hypersomnolence (IHS), **300**
idiopathic tibia vara in children, 240
impaired glucose tolerance (IGT), diabetes
    mellitus type 2, 256
implanon, 291
income, risk factor, 5
incremental approach to weight loss, 321
industrial revolution, 47
infant origins of obesity, 93–101
  adult body weight, *95*, 95–96
    birth size, 93–95, *94*
  adult obesity, 93–96
  environmental influences, 98–99
    climate at birth, 98, *98*
    feeding method, 97–98
  hyperinsulinaemia, 99
  leptin resistance, 99
  nutritional excess, 97
  socioeconomic status, 96
  see also fetal origins of obesity
infertility, 398
inflammation, 272
information sources, 348–349
  for weight management, 461, *461*
infrared spectrophotometry
  children, 19
  total body water measurement, 14
injury risk, 374
inositol, **448**
insulin
  adiposity signal, 74
  energy intake adaption to energy
    expenditure, 369
  hunger-satiety signals, 73–74, *74*
  hypertension, 273
  metabolic effects, 255, *255*
  postprandial state, 107
  resistance *see below*
  secretion, 254, *254*
    abnormalities, 258
    diabetes mellitus, 188
  sensitivity
    low GI food effects, 333
    physical activity effects, 156
  synthesis, 254
  visceral adipose tissue effect, 167–168, *169*
insulinaemic index (II), *333*
insulin-like growth factor-binding proteins
    (IGFBP), 202
insulin-like growth factors (IGFs), 386, **387**
  endocrine testing, 208
insulin resistance, 184–188, 256–258
  adipokines, 186, 257–258

adiponectin, 186–187
adipose tissue, *114*, 114–115, 174
  appetite regulation, 98
  carbohydrate metabolism, effect on, 255,
    256
  causes, acquired, 256
  diabetes mellitus type 2 pathogenesis,
    255–256
  etiology, 184–188
  free fatty acids, 184–186, *185*, *186*, 257, *258*
    oxidation, 108
  hormones, 258
  hypertension, 257
  induction, 133
  interleukin-1, 258
  interleukin 6, 187
  leptin, 187–188, *188*
  lipid metabolism, 255, *256*, 256–257
  neurotransmitters, 258
  obstructive sleep apnoea association,
    305–306
  ovarian function effects, 282
  physical activity effect, 373
  polycystic ovary syndrome, 190–191, 204,
    240
  pregnancy, 284–285, *285*, 286, 289–290
  prothombotic state, 257
  during puberty, 238
  Randle cycle, 257, *258*
  resistin, 186
  skeletal muscle metabolism, 109, 110, *110*
  tumour necrosis factor-α, 186
  visceral adipose tissue, 169
  see also metabolic syndrome
insulin resistance syndrome *see* metabolic
    syndrome
intelligence quotient (IQ), 31–32
interleukin-1 (IL-1), insulin resistance, 258
interleukin-6 (IL-6)
  adipose tissue release, 205, 272
  insulin resistance, 187, 258
  obesity, 206
    vascular disease, 272
intermediate-density lipoproteins (IDLs), 163
internalization of negative views, 34
  children, 227, 243
International Agency for Research on Cancer
    (IARC), 348
International Association for the Study of
    Obesity
  Asian body mass index cut-off points, **439**,
    440
  physical activity in diabetes, 261
International Classification of Diseases
  classification, 58
International Obesity Task Force (IOTF), 348,
    349
  body mass index centile curves, 222
  growth standards in child obesity, 227

Internet resources
  weight loss interventions, 358, **446**, 450
  weight loss maintenance, 417
interpersonal relationships, 32–33
intra-abdominal pressure in obesity, 276–277
intra-abdominal region
  dual energy X-ray absorptiometry, 20
  fat distribution measurement, 20
intraoral orthodontic devices, 308
intrauterine devices (IUDs), 291–292
intravenous glucose tolerance test, 284
in vitro neutron activation analysis (IVNAA),
  23
involuntary energy expenditure, 70
IOTF *see* International Obesity Task Force
  (IOTF)
ischaemic heart disease
  metabolic abnormalities, 170–171, *171*
  visceral adiposity, therapeutic implications,
  176
islet amyloid polypeptide (IAPP), 259
  appetite control, 141
islets of Langerhans
  insulin synthesis/secretion, 254
  pathogenesis of diabetes mellitus type 2,
  255
isoflavine, **448**
isometric thermogenesis, 70

Japanese diets
  fat intake, 124
  sugars, 125
jejuno-ileal bypass (JIB), 394, *395*
'jolly fat' person hypothesis, 33

Karolinska Scale of Personality (KSP), 413
ketoacidosis, weight gain, 259
ketosis
  Atkins diet, 132–133
  carbohydrates intake restriction, 132
  pregnancy, 285, 289
Keys' Seven Country Study, 124
Khosla–Lowe index, 217
Kirch, Kuche, Kinder hypothesis, 50, **51**
Kraft Foods, portion size cap, 464

labour, induced, **287**
lactation, lower body fat mobilization, 48
land development patterns, obesity
  prevention, 465
laparoscopic adjustable gastric band (LAGB),
  326, 402–403
  asthma, 398
  body image effect, 399
  depression effect, 399
  diabetes mellitus type 2 effects, 397
  effects, 402–403, **403**
  evolution, 396, *396*
  female fertility following, 398

gastro–oesophageal reflux disease, 398
  hypertension effects, 398
  obstructive sleep apnoea effect, 399
  quality of life effect, 399
  side-effects, 402–403
  technical features, 402
  weight loss outcomes, 397
laparoscopic banded gastroplasty (LBG),
  pregnancy after, 289
large body size preference, 49
laser-assisted uvulopalatoplasty (LAUP),
  309
lateral hypothalamic (LH) region, 72
Laurence–Moon syndrome, 225
laxative use, long QT syndrome, 270
lean-fat tissue ratio, 22, *22*
  physical activity changes, 13, *13*
learned culture, 46
The Learn Program for Weight Management 2000,
  353
left ventricular hypertrophy, 274–275, 276
  children, 237
leg length, body mass index effect, 436
leipostatic theory, 73
leptin, 386, **387**
  adipose tissue, 205–206
  appetite control, 142
  deficiency, 24, *24*, 73–74
    appetite control, *140*, 142–143
    characteristics, 103
    childhood obesity, 225
    congenital, 86
    genetic defects, 74
    obesity, 206
    ob gene mutation, 85
    partial, 87–88
  energy intake adaption to energy
    expenditure, 369
  hunger-satiety signals, 73–74, *74*
  insulin resistance, 187–188, *188*, 258
  neuropeptide-Y interaction, 142
  obesity hypertension, 273
  ovulation role, 282
  pituitary-thyroid axis role in obesity, 204–205
  resistance
    appetite regulation, 98
    role in obesity development, 99, 114
  secretion from white adipose tissue, 103
  sleep-disordered breathing role, 300
  testing for, 322
  therapy, 86–87, *87*, *88*
  weight regain role, 356
leptin-melanocortin pathway, 85–86
leptin receptor
  childhood obesity, 225
  deficiency, 88
less restrictive approach, 333–335, *335*
levies on unhealthy food, 466
levonorgestrel intrauterine system, 291–292

lifestyle, 324, 354, *355*
  childhood obesity, 226
  diabetes mellitus type 2 in children, 239
  diet commencement, 325
  media role, 450
  obese diabetics, 261
  weight homeostasis changes, 78
limits of obesity, definition, 57
linkage analysis, 83
linoleic acid, conjugated, 386, **386**
lipid metabolism
  dyslipidaemia, 163
  insulin resistance effect, 255, *256*, 256–257
  skeletal muscle, 102, 107–109
Lipid Research Study, 269
lipids
  physical activity effect, 373
  weight loss benefits, 260–261
  see also fats
lipoapoptosis, diabetes mellitus, 188, *189*
lipodystrophy, drug induced, 259–260
lipoprotein lipase (LPL)
  adipose tissue metabolism, 112–113, *114*,
  114–115
  dyslipidaemia, 163
  role in obesity development, 113
  skeletal muscle metabolism, 107
  triacylglycerol clearance, 112–113
lipoprotein(s)
  dyslipidaemia, 163, *164*
  genetic abnormality in metabolic
  syndrome, 174
lipostatic mechanism
  appetite control, 142
  thermogenesis, 78
lipostatic signals, hunger-satiety, 73
liquid meal replacements, 340, 353
  effects, **445**, 452
  weight loss maintenance role, 357–358,
  358
liver
  gluconeogenesis, 255
    role in physical activity, 370
  glycogenolysis, 370
  nutrient metabolism, 74
  volume measurement, 20
loneliness, 33
long-chain acyl CoA (LCACoA), 185
long QT syndrome, 270
long-term food intake control, 75
low birth weight, 439
low-carbohydrate diets, 353, *353*
low-density lipoprotein (LDL)-cholesterol
  coronary heart disease risk, 165
  ischaemic heart disease, 171
  physical activity effect, 373
  visceral adipose tissue effect, 166–167
  weight loss effects, 260, 261
  see also cholesterol levels

low-density lipoproteins (LDLs)
  coronary heart disease risk, 164–165
  dyslipidaemia, 163, 172
  ischaemic heart disease risk, 170–171
low-energy density diets, 353–354
low-energy diets (LEDs), 325, 328, **329**, 352
  combined with physical activity, 365
  effects, **445**
  inappropriateness, 131
lower body fat accumulation
  evolution, 48
  during pregnancy and lactation, 48
low-fat diets, 134, 324, 330–331, *331*, *353*
low-glycaemic diets, **445**
low-income families, 463
lung disease *see* respiratory
  diseases/disorders
lung function in obesity, 277–278
'luxusconsumption', 70

macroenvironments, 459, *459*
macronutrient composition of diet, **130**,
  130–131
macronutrients, 23
  oxidation, 150, **150**
magnesium stearate, 449
magnetic resonance imaging (MRI), 24
  children, 216, **216**, 225
  fat distribution measurement, 19–20, *20*
  visceral adipose tissue measurement, 166
magnetic resonance spectroscopy (MRS), 20
Ma Huang, 447
maintenance programme, 324
malabsorptive agents
  acarbose, **382**, 385
  orlistat, **382**, 383–384
'male preference hypothesis', 50, **51**
management (of obesity)
  adjunctive therapies, 325
  aims, **320**, 320–321
  alternative therapies *see* alternative
    medicine
  appetite control, 137–138
  assessment of patients *see* assessment (of
    obesity)
  behavioural *see* behavioural therapy
  body composition analysis use, 22, *22*, 22–23
  body mass index use, 12
  diabetes mellitus type 2, 260, 261–263
    lifestyle modification, 261
    pharmacotherapy, 261–263
    physical activity/exercise, 261
    surgery, 263
    very low-calorie diets, 261
  dietary *see* dietary interventions
  effectiveness, 460
  gene therapy, 381
  information sources, 461, *461*
  long term follow-up, 324–325

low-calorie/energy diets, 325
  monitoring, 324–325
  National Heart, Lung, and Blood Institute
    guidance, 350, **351**
  non-dietary
    behavioural *see* behavioural therapy
    H@AS system, 334–335
    outcome measures, **325**, 325–326
    overview, 319–326
    pharmacotherapy *see* pharmacotherapy
    population approaches, environmental *see*
      environment
    professional education/training, 423
    programmes, **323**, 323–324
    shared care approach, 450
    'stepped-care' approach, *444*
    surgery *see* surgery
    target groups, 460
    traditional, 444–446
    weight loss amount, 319–320
mandibular advancement devices (MADs),
  308
Marfan's syndrome, 301
margarine, invention of, 124
marital quality, 33
marital status, 33
  risk factor, 5
Massa of West Africa, 50
mass-media campaigns, 450, 462–463, 467
mass spectrometry
  children, 19
  total body water measurement, 14
maternal influence on obesity *see entries under*
  parental; pregnancy
maximal oxygen uptake (VO$_{2max}$)
  energy expenditure through physical
    activity, 155
  substrate utilization during physical
    activity, 370–371
mazindol, **382**, **382**
McCune–Albright syndrome (MAS), 84
McDonald's, nutritional content
  communication, 464
McKusick–Kaufman syndrome, 85
meals
  frequency, 335–336
    irregularity, 152
  size, 152
  thermic effects, 152–153
  type, 152–153
measurement of obesity
  children *see* childhood/adolescent obesity
  see assessment (of obesity)
meat consumption, 340
mechanoreceptors
  appetite control, 139
  hunger-satiety signals, 72
medical assessment, childhood obesity,
  225–226

medical definitions, culture influence, 57–58
medical dieting, 57
medical history, childhood obesity, 225
medicalization of obesity, 58–59
Mediterranean diets
  fat intake, 124
  sugars, 125
medium-term food intake control, 74–75
medroxyprogesterone, 309
Mehmo's syndrome, **83**
melanin-concentrating hormone (MCH), 72,
  72
melanin-concentrating hormone (MCH)
  antagonists, **387**
melanocortin 4 receptor (Mc4r)
  appetite control, 143
  deficiency, 89
  feeding behaviour, 86
  mutation, 142
melanocortin system
  mutations, appetite control, 143
  prohormone convertase 1 deficiency, 89
α-melanocyte stimulating hormone
  appetite control, 143
  energy intake adaption to energy
    expenditure, 369
  feeding behaviour, 85–86
melanoma, epidemic reduction, 458
menstrual cycle
  basal metabolic rate effect, 127
  disturbances
    pituitary–gonadal axis abnormalities in
      obesity, 203
    polycystic ovary syndrome, 281
  energy intake control effects, 127
  resting metabolic rate effect, 154
mental health, physical activity effect, 374
mental health professionals' attitudes, 35
mental retardation, non-specific, 225
metabolic diseases, body mass index
  association, 13
metabolic efficiency
  gender differences, 130
  obese subjects, 129–130
'metabolic programming', fetus, 97
metabolic syndrome, 166–175, 189–190, *190*,
  251, 256
  Asian population, 437
  coronary heart disease risk, 170–172, *171*
  definition, 253, **253**
  diabetes mellitus type 2 association, 254,
    254
  epidemiological associations, **253**, 253–254,
    254
  genetic susceptibility, 174–175
  insulin resistance, 256
  low GI food benefits, 333
  physiopathology and causal relationships,
    172–174, *173*

prevalence, 170, 189, 253
very low-energy diets, 330
see also insulin resistance
metabolism, pregnancy effects, 284–285
metformin, **382**, 388
diabetes mellitus type 2, 262, *262*
polycystic ovary syndrome therapy, 282,
385
methamphetamine, 382, **382**
methylphenidate, 146
methylxanthines, 385, 386
microenvironments, 459
Micronesians, diabetes, 252
micropenis, children, 236
micturition difficulty, children, 236
Midtown Manhattan study, 52
Minnesota Multiphasic Personality Inventory
(MMPI), 413
Mirena, 291–292
mitochondrial 'proton' leak, thermogenesis,
77
MMPI (Minnesota Multiphasic Personality
Inventory), 413
modafinil, 309
moderate-fat diets, 331
moderate obesity, potential health benefits, 58
MONICA study *see* World Health
Organization (WHO)
monitoring, obesity prevention, 460, 468
monogenic obesity syndromes, 86–89, 90
genetic testing, 208–209
morbidity, 8–10
childhood obesity, 233, *233*–234, *234*
physical activity effect, 372–374
morbid obesity, 60
mortality, 4, *8*, 8–10
childhood obesity, 233–234
fitness and fatness as predictors, 269
physical activity effect, 364, 374
weight loss effect, 319
motion sensors, 151
motivational interviewing, 226
motivation to lose weight, assessment, 323
motor vehicle ownership, 439
movement-associated thermogenesis, 76
movement sensing, 150–151
multicompartment models, 15–16
children, 19
multimedia programmes, 450
multiple strategy approach to prevention, 458
muscle, skeletal *see* skeletal muscle
muscular contraction efficiency, 76
'muscular work', energy expenditure, 69–70
musculoskeletal discomfort, childhood
obesity, 236
musculoskeletal injuries, physical activity
risk, 376
myocardial infarction, physical activity risk,
376

NAAFA (National Association to Advance Fat
Acceptance), 59, 349
NAO (National Audit Office), 343, 349
narcolepsy, **300**
nasal continuous positive airway pressure
(nCPAP) treatment, 278
nasal dilator strips, 307
National Association to Advance Fat
Acceptance (NAAFA), 59, 349
National Audit Office (NAO), 343, 349
National Centre for Health Statistics (NCHS),
18
National China Health and Nutrition Survey
(CHNS)
energy intake and body mass index, 438–439
weight gain in Asian population, 438
National Cholesterol Education Program
Expert Panel on Detection, Evaluation
and Treatment of High Blood
Cholesterol in Adults
metabolic syndrome definition, 253, **253**
Step 1 and Step 2 programmes, 328
national communication campaigns, obesity
prevention, 460
National Health and Medical Research
Council of Australia, 343
National Health and Nutrition Examination
Survey (NHANES)
bioelectrical impedance analysis, 17
depression, 33
diabetes mellitus type 2 in children, 239
ethnic differences in size preference, 55
health risk analysis, 23
metabolic syndrome, 170
obesity prevalence, 252
prevalence, 6, *6*
puberty in females, 239
subscapular skinfold measurements, body
mass index percentile association, 223
National Health Interview Survey (1992), 31
National Heart, Lung, and Blood Institute
(NHLBI), 343
contact details, 348
treatment algorithm, 350, **351**
National Heart Foundation, 466
National Institute of Health (NIH), 374
National Longitudinal Study of Adolescent
Health in the USA, 61
National Longitudinal Survey Youth Cohort,
29–30, *30*
National Nutrition Survey 1998 (Thailand),
433
National Obesity Forum (NOF), 349
childhood obesity, 224
National Task Force on the Prevention and
Treatment of Obesity for adults, 227
National Weight Control Registry (USA), 342,
358
'successful dieters' definition, 342, *342*

'nature–nurture', 60
Nauruan fattening practices, 50
NCHS (National Centre for Health Statistics),
18
NEAT *see* non-exercise activity thermogenesis
(NEAT)
neck circumference
obstructive sleep apnoea role, 298–299
patient assessment, 321
Nedder v. *Rivier College*, 1995, 30
negative energy balance, 68
negative stereotypes, of obese children, 36
neighbourhoods, active, 463–464
neonates
adrenal crisis, 88
Prader–Willi syndrome, 84
Netherlands
obesity prevalence, 8
obesity prevention, 459, *459*, *460*
neural tube defects, 290
neurological complications, childhood
obesity, **237**, 241
neuropeptide-Y (NPY)
antagonists, **387**
energy intake adaption to energy
expenditure, 369
leptin, 85, 142
neurotensin, 386, **387**
neurotransmitters
appetite control, 138, *138*, 144
insulin resistance, 258
'Newton's special diet plan', 337
'New World syndrome', Asian populations,
438
NHANES *see* National Health and Nutrition
Examination Survey (NHANES)
NHLBI *see* National Heart, Lung, and Blood
Institute (NHLBI)
nicotine, **382**, 386
drug-induced thermogenesis, 70
NIH (National Institute of Health), 374
nitrogen balance, 23
NOF *see* National Obesity Forum (NOF)
non-adjustable gastroplasty, **445**
non-alcoholic fatty liver disease (NAFLD),
251, 263–264, *264*
non-alcoholic steatohepatitis (NASH), 251, 264
childhood obesity, 225
testing for, 322
non-dietary management
behavioural *see* behavioural therapy
H@AS system, 334–335
non-esterified fatty acids (NEFAs)
adipose tissue, 103, 104, *105*, 111–112, 114–115
lipotoxicity, 259
oxidative metabolism contribution, 106
physical activity, 108, 370
pregnancy, 284
skeletal muscle, 102, 107–109

non-exercise activity thermogenesis (NEAT),
    70–71
    obesity susceptibility predictor, 76–77
    resting energy expenditure, 154
non-invasive positive pressure ventilation
    (NIPPV), 310
non-resting energy expenditure, 70–71
non-shivering thermogenesis, 70, 153
non-weight-bearing activity, 375
noradrenaline (NA)
    energy expenditure, 156, 157
    insulin resistance, 257
    thermogenesis mechanism, 77
'normal' weight perception, 57
NPY-AGRP pathway, leptin regulation, 206
nucleoside reverse transcriptase inhibitors,
    259
Nurses Health Study, 438
nutrient balance theory, 75
nutrient-induced thermogenesis, 156
nutrition
    claims by food manufacturers, 466
    excess, early infancy, 97
    fast food, 464
    information panels, 466
    maternal *see* pregnancy
    nutrient intake
        familial resemblance, 82
        World Health Organization
            recommendations, **130**, 130–131
    'signposts' (logos), 466
'nutrition transition', 124

obese hypoventilation syndrome (OHS), 278,
    297, *299*, 299–300
    management, 309–310, *310*
The Obesity Awareness and Solutions Trust
    (TOAST), 349
obesity hypoventilation syndrome (OHS)
    childhood obesity, 238
    lung function in obesity, 278
ob gene mutation, 85
    congenital leptin deficiency, 86
obligatory diet-induced thermogenesis, 70
ob/ob mice
    appetite control, 142
    congenital leptin deficiency, 86
    insulin resistance, 187–188
    model of obesity, 85
ob protein *see* leptin
obstructive sleep apnoea (OSA), 296–315
    cardiovascular risk, 272
    children, 235, 237–238
    congestive heart failure, 276
    with daytime respiratory failure *see*
        obesity hypoventilation syndrome
        (OHS)
    definition, 296–297
    diagnosis, *297*

epidemiology, 300–302, *301*
lung function, 278
obesity, 278
pathogenesis, 298–299, *299*
stroke, 275
sudden death in obesity, 269–270
treatment, **306**, 306–310, **307**
    CPAP *see* continuous positive airway
        pressure (CPAP)
    hypnotherapy, 449
    surgery, 399
oedema, 14
    bioelectrical impedance analysis, 17
    body fat overestimation, 16–17
oestradiol, 202–203
olanzapine, 259
olestra, 386, **386**
olfactory cues, energy intake control, 127
Online Mendelian Inheritance in Man
    (OMIM), 83
opportunistic eating, appetite control, 147
OPTIFAST, 353
orexin, hunger-satiety control, 72, *72*
organizations, patient-centred, 349
orlistat, 291, 325, **382**, 383–384, 388
    diabetes mellitus, 262, *262*
    effects, **445**
    non-alcoholic fatty liver disease, 264
    weight loss and diabetes prevention, 263
orthopaedic diseases/disorders, childhood
    obesity, 225, **237**, 240
ovarian dysfunction, 398
overeating
    appetite control risk factors, 146, *146*
    carbohydrates, 128
    experimental, 8
        adaptive thermogenesis role, 76
        appetite control, 144
        body weight control, 67
        hyperphagia, 75
    fat, thermogenesis increase, 128
    triggers, 339
    see also hyperphagia (over-feeding)
'overlap syndrome', 278, 305
overnight in-laboratory sleep studies,
    302–303, *303*, **303**
overweight
    body mass index classification, **4**, 215
    UK classification, 223
    USA classification, 223
ovulation
    failure in polycystic ovary syndrome,
        281–282
    leptin role, 282
    pituitary-gonadal axis abnormalities,
        203
oxygen consumption
    energy expenditure measurement, 149
    of skeletal muscle, 102–103

oxygen-18 isotope
    doubly labelled water , energy expenditure
        measurement, 150
    total body water measurement, 14
oxyntomodulin, 386, **387**

paediatric healthcare equipment, 234
palatability of food, 144–145
pancreas
    beta cells *see* beta-cells
    islets of Langerhans *see* islets of
        Langerhans
pancreatic polypeptide (PP), 386, **387**
panhypopituitarism, obesity cause, 198–199
paraventricular nucleus (PVN)
    appetite control, 143
    meal cessation initiation, 72
parents
    bias, 35, 36
    concern for child's weight, 223–224
    eating behaviours, 245
    influence in obesity prevention, 462–463
    obesity, 232
        childhood obesity association, 225–226
    perceptions, 242–243
parity, risk factor, 5
patient-centred organizations/charities, 349
patient management of stigma, 38–39
pectin, **446**, 447, **448**
Pederson hypothesis, *285*, 289
pedestrian-friendly street design, 465
pedometers, 354
    energy expenditure measurement, 151
    weight management, 324
peer relationships, 32
Pennington Biomedical Research Centre, 83
peppers, **448**
peptide YY3–36 (PYY3–36), 386, **387**
    appetite control, 141
    gastrointestinal hunger-satiety signals, 73
perilipin, 112
periodic breathing *see* Cheyne–Stokes
    respiration
periodic leg movement disorder (PLMS), **300**
peripheral hunger-satiety signals, 72–74,
    139–142
personality, weight regain association, 413,
    414–415
'personal weight coaches', 450
'pester power', 467
pet ownership, 451
pharmacotherapy, 325–326, **351**, 380–393
    adrenergic drugs, 382, **382**
    approved drugs, 381–384, **382**
    criteria and contraindications, 381, **381**
    diet supplements, 386
    drug combinations, 387–388
    effects, **445**
    herbal preparations, 386

non-approved drugs, 384–387, **386**, **387**
obese diabetics, 261–263
patient selection, 325–326
practical guidelines, 388
rationale, 380–381
serotonergic drugs, **382**, 383
sleep-disordered breathing, 309
weight loss maintenance role, 414, 417
see also specific drugs
phendimetrazine, 382, **382**
phenmetrazine, **382**
phentermine, 382, **382**
combinations, 387–388
in diabetes mellitus, 263
effects, **445**
phentermine–fenfluramine, 387
phenylalanine, hunger-satiety signals, 73
phenylpropanolamine–benzocaine, 387
phenylpropanolamine (PPA), 382, **382**
phosphoenol pyruvate carboxykinase
(PEPCK), insulin resistance, 185
physical activity, 354, 363–379, **445**, 452
Asian populations, 438–439
benefits
aerobic fitness, 374
congestive heart failure, 276
hypertension effect, 275
obese diabetics, 261
resting energy expenditure, 155
cardiovascular mortality risk predictor,
269
child activity patterns, obesity prevention,
462
childhood obesity assessment, 226
definition, 364
drop-out rates, 374, 376
predictors, 364
endurance training, 363, 364, 365
energy balance, 366–369
body weight, 156
energy expenditure, 68, 69–70, **154**, 154–156,
363, 366–367, *367*
daily energy expenditure, 367
definition, 154
diet-induced thermogenesis, 367
fuel utilization, 155
post-exercise, 367, **367**
resting metabolic rate, 367
training effect, 366, 367
type, 366, **366**
types, 155
energy intake, *368*, 368–369
acute post-exercise, 368–369
adaption to increased energy
expenditure, 364, 369, *369*
injury risk, 374
intensity
cardiovascular effects, 375
classification, 375, **375**

fat oxidation, 370
substrate utilization effects, 371
limited, 7
metabolism
carbohydrate, 107
lean–fat ratio changes, 13, *13*
lipids, 107–109
muscle glycogen utilization, 106
muscle-specific differences, 103
non-esterified fatty acid release from
adipose tissue, 112
oxygen consumption, 102–103
thermogenesis associated, 76–77
morbidity (obesity related) effect,
372–374
mortality (obesity related) effect, 364, 374
passive exercise devices, 449
patterns, 131
professional education/training, 425–426
programme, 324
promotion, 10
reduction, gene-environment interactions,
81–82
risk factor, 6
substrate utilization, 364, 369–372, *370*
daily, 371, 372
obesity, 371
training effect, 371–372, *372*
weight management, 324, 363, 374–376
body mass index changes, *13*
body weight, 364–366
children, 452
combined with dietary restriction, 365
composition influence, 23
exercise adherence, 376
exercise mode, 375
exercise prescription, **375**, 375–376
exercise risk, 376
gain prevention, 364–365
loss maintenance, 355, 357, *357*, 365–366,
410, 413
reduction, 365
see also exercise
physical activity level (PAL), 128–129
gender differences, 128–129
physical measurements in children, 19
Physicians' Health Study
cardiovascular disease, 272
stroke and body mass index, 275
'Pick the tick' symbol, 466
Pickwickian syndrome *see* obesity
hypoventilation syndrome (OHS)
Pierre Robin sequence, 301
Pima Indians
diabetes, 252
energy expenditure, 157
pituitary–adrenal axis, *200*, **200**, 200–201
female obesity, 203
pituitary function testing, 208

pituitary–gonadal axis, 202–204
female obesity, 203
pituitary–thyroid axis, obesity role, 204–205
plateau, weight loss, 409
plate model, 416
pleiotropic obesity syndromes, **83**, 83–85
plethysmography, 14, 19
plumpness preference, 49
politicians, obesity prevention, 467
polycystic ovary syndrome (PCOS), 190–191,
191
childhood obesity, 239–240
definition, 281
endocrine abnormalities, 203–204, **204**
energy expenditure in, 282
hyperinsulinaemia, 282
insulin resistance, 190–191, 204, 240
metformin therapy, 282, **283**, 385
ovarian function, 281–282
polygenic obesity, 90
Polynesians
bigness preference, 49
response to modernization, 55
ritual fattening, 50
polyphenols, 153
polysomnography (PSG), 302–303, *303*
polyunsaturated fatty acids (PUFAs), 270
ponderal index, children, 217
ponderstatic mechanism, appetite control, 142
population assessments, body mass index, 12
population-based obesity prevention, 461, 468
'portal vein theory', 172–173
portion sizes
behavioural therapy, 352–353, 355
food intake control, 128
positional therapy, 307
positive energy balance, 68
adaption inability, 89
agent of obesity, 457
prolonged periods, 157, **157**
post-exercise energy expenditure, 367, **367**
post-exercise energy intake, 368–369
post-exercise oxygen consumption (EPOC),
366, **367**
post-exercise stimulation of thermogenesis,
77
postgraduate training, 423
postpartum haemorrhage, **287**
postprandial state
fatty acid utilization, 108
glucose concentration, 107
insulin, 107, 254, *254*
skeletal muscle metabolism, 104
triacylglycerol clearance by adipose tissue,
112
postprandial thermogenesis (PPT)
polycystic ovary syndrome, 282
during pregnancy, 284
post-registration training, 423

post-SPA stimulation of thermogenesis, 77
poverty, 52–53
Prader–Willi syndrome, 24, 84, 225, 327, 341–342
  endocrine testing, 208
    children, 208
  genetic cause of obesity, 200
pramlintide, 141
'p' ratio, 130
precursor proopiomelanocortin (POMC), appetite control, 143
prediction techniques
  body composition measurement, 16–18
  index of normal food intake, *129*
pre-eclampsia, **287**
pregestational diabetes, 286
pregnancy, 283–289
  body weight control, 67
  diabetes mellitus, 97
  energy intake control, 127
  hyperglycaemia, 97
  lower body fat mobilization, 48
  maternal body composition, 283–284
  maternal complications, 286–289, **287**
  maternal hyperglycaemia, 97
  maternal smoking, 96–97
  maternal starvation, 96
  metabolism effects, 284–285
  nutrition
    effects on fetus, 96, 285, *285*, 289–290
    excess, 97
    excess nutrition, 97
    fetal origin of obesity, 96
  post-laparoscopic banded gastroplasty, 289
  prenatal care costs, 290–291
  surgery for obesity effect, 398
  weight gain associated, 288–289
preregistration training, 422–423
pre-schools, obesity prevention role, 463, **463**
prevalence (of obesity), 3, 6, *6*, 7, **8**
  Asian populations, **432**, 432–434, **433**, 438
  Baltic states, **8**
  children, 456
  Europe, 6, **7**
  gender, 6, *6*, **7**
  global comparisons, 184
  Netherlands, 8
  UK, 6, *6*
  USA, 6, *6*
prevention (of obesity), 10, 456–471
  active neighbourhoods, 463–464
  built environment, 465–466
  clinical management programme role in prevalence reduction, 460–461, *461*
  community-based action in Colac, 461–462, *462*
  community settings, 464–465
  comprehensive approach, 458–460, *459, 460*

environmental interventions, 356, 359
  epidemic approach, 456–458
  evidence of effectiveness of interventions, 467–468, *468*
  fast-food outlets, 464, *464, 465*
  food distribution and pricing, 466
  food-labeling interventions, 466
  food marketing targeting young children, 466–467
  future research requirements, 468–469
  influencing homes and parents, 462–463
  mass-media campaigns, 467
  monitoring role, 460, 468
  pre-schools, 463, **463**
  primary care role, 359
  schools, 463, **463**
  target groups, 460
  unpaid media, lobbying, 467
primary care, prevention and treatment role, 359
primary endocrine disease in obesity, 198–200, *199*
probucol, 264
professional education/training, 421–427
  continuing professional development, 423
  Core Curriculum, 422, 424–427
  obesity management, 423
  undergraduate/preregistration, 422–423
  weight loss maintenance, 424
progesterone-only contraceptive pills, 291
prohormone convertase 1 deficiency, 89
pro-opiomelanocortin deficiency, 88–89
proopiomelanocortin (POMC) neurons, 85
protease inhibitors, 259
protein
  animal, 123–125
  handling in obese people, 129
  normal intake, 134
  only diets, 132
  oxidation, 150, **150**
  quality, food intake effects, 126
  thermic effect of food, effect on, 153
  weight loss diets, 133
protein-sparing modified fasts (PSMF), 329
protein-static signals, 73
prothombotic state, insulin resistance, 257
protriptyline, 309
pseudogynaecomastia, 236
pseudopseudohypoparathyroidism, 84
psychological aspects (of obesity)
  appetite control, 138, *138*
  in children, 36–37, 225, 235
  dieting, 59, **59**
  outcome variables, 33–34, 235
    see also specific variables
  stigma, 39, **40**
psychosocial aspects (of obesity)
  in children, *242*, 242–245
  sleep-disordered breathing effects, 303

stigma, 39, **40**
  weight loss effects, 408
puberty
  childhood obesity complications, 236, 239
  insulin resistance, 238
  weight gain risk period, 232
pulmonary embolism, pregnancy, **287**
pulmonary hypertension, 278–279
  obstructive sleep apnoea association, 305
'puppy fat', 232
purging, childhood obesity, 245
purines, high-protein diets, 332
pyruvate, 386, **386**, 449
PYY (peptide YY(3–36)) *see* peptide YY3–36 (PYY3–36)

quality of life
  children, 37
  psychological outcome influence, 34
  surgery for obesity effect, 399
  weight loss effects, 408
Quebec Cardiovascular Study
  hyperinsulinaemia in CHD, 171
  ischaemic heart disease, 176
  low-density lipoproteins in IHD risk, 170–171
  metabolic abnormalities contributing to CHD, 170
Quebec Family Study, 82
Quebec overfeeding study, 457, *457*
Quetelet index, 327
  children, 217

Randle cycle, 257, *258*
rapid urbanization, Asian populations, 438–439
'readiness to change', 261
refeeding syndrome, 330
'reference adolescent', 18
'reference child', 18
'reference man', 102, 103
reference methods of body composition measurement, 13–15
'reference woman', 102, 103
religious institutions, obesity prevention, 465
renal disease, end-stage, 273
renin-angiotensin-aldosterone system, 273
renin-angiotensin system, 206
reproductive complications, childhood obesity, 239–240
resistance exercise training, 354, 365
  daily fat oxidation effect, 372
resistance to normalizing process of obesity, **59**, 59–60
resistin
  adipose tissue, 115, 205
  genetic abnormality in metabolic syndrome, 174

insulin resistance, 186, 257–258
   obesity, 206
respiratory diseases/disorders
   childhood obesity, **237**, 237–238
   obstructive sleep apnoea association, 305
   sleep related *see* obstructive sleep apnoea
      (OSA); sleep-disordered breathing
respiratory disturbance index (RDI), **297**
respiratory gas exchange, energy expenditure
      measurement, 149–150
respiratory quotient
   energy expenditure measurement, 150
   training effect, 372
resting energy expenditure (REE), 70, 152–154
   cold, 153
   diet induced thermogenesis, 152, 153
   fasting, resting metabolic rate, 152
   food ingestion, 152–153
   gene polymorphism, 154
   growth, 153
   hormonal factors, 153–154
   non-exercise activity thermogenesis
      (NEAT), 154
   physical activity, effect of, 155
   polycystic ovary syndrome, 282
   responses associated with weight regain,
      356
   thermic effect of food, 152–153
resting metabolic rate (RMR)
   appetite control, 143
   energy expenditure, 366, 367
   exercise training effect, 363
   fasting, 152
   prediction, energy expenditure, 151, **151**
   pregnancy effects, 283
right ventricular hypertrophy, children,
      237
rimonabant, 386, 387
risk factors, 5–6
   appetite control, 146, **146**
   behavioural, 5–6
   biological, 5
   demographic, 5
   sociocultural, 5
   see also individual risk factors
risperidone, 259
ritual fattening, 50
road traffic accidents/deaths, 458
rodent models of obesity, 85
Rohrer index, 217
romantic partnerships, 33
rosiglitazone, 264
Roux-en-Y gastric bypass (RYGB), 400–401,
      401, **401**
   dyslipidemia effects, 398
   evolution, 394–395, *395*
   mortality, 400
   patients with diabetes, 263
   side-effects, 401

SAD (seasonal affective disorder), 417
sagittal abdominal diameter, 4, 21
Salote, Queen of Tonga, 49
salt, weight loss diets, 133–134
saponins, **448**
satiety
   anti-obesity drugs in diabetes, 262
   defect, 143
   definition, 71, 139
   food intake control, 71–72
   signals, 139
satiety cascade
   appetite control, *138*, 138–139, *139*, *140*
   peptides, 141–142
saturated fats, 153
   intake reduction, 125
schools
   fruit, free/subsidized, 466
   obesity prevention role, 463, **463**
   peer harassment/rejection, 36
Scottish Intercollegiate Guidelines Network
      (SIGN), 343
   childhood obesity assessment, 223, 224
   contact details, 348
seasonal affective disorder (SAD), 417
second law of thermodynamics, 68
sedentary behaviour
   discouragement, 10
   food intake control bypass, 127
selective serotonin reuptake inhibitors
      (SSRIs), **382**, 383
   obstructive sleep apnoea treatment, 309
self-blame reduction, 39
self-esteem
   children, 36–37, 243
   psychological outcome influence, 34
self-help weight loss organizations, 58
self-limiting (*ad libitum*) diets, 328, **445**
self-monitoring (of food intake), 340, 351, 412
semistarvation, experimental, 131
sensitivity to reward (STR), 145
sensory specific satiety, 71
'Sentinel Site for Obesity Prevention', 462
serotonergic drugs, **382**, 383
sertraline, **382**, 383
sex hormone-binding globulin (SHBG)
   endocrine testing, 207
   obesity cause, 203
   polycystic ovary syndrome, 282
sex steroid secretion/action
   fat distribution differences, 201
   obesity cause, 202–204
SHBG *see* sex hormone-binding globulin
      (SHBG)
Sheldon's index, 217
shivering thermogenesis, 70, 153
short insulin tolerance test, 284
short-term food intake control, 74
shoulder dystocia, 290

sibutramine, 262, *262*, 325, **382**, 383, 388
   effects, **445**
   weight loss maintenance, 410, 417
SIGN *see* Scottish Intercollegiate Guidelines
      Network (SIGN)
Simpson–Golabi–Behmel, type 2 syndrome,
      83
single nucleotide polymorphisms (SNPs),
      90
single strategy approach to prevention, 458
Siri's equation, 16
size acceptance promotion, 38, 59
skeletal muscle, 105–111
   daily energy fluxes, role in, 104, *105*
   heat production, 69
   metabolism, 102–104
      ATP synthesis, **105**, 105–107, *106*
      carbohydrates, 107
      disturbance and obesity development,
         109–110
      lipids, 107–109
      obesity, 110–111
      oxygen consumption, 102–103
skin creams, 449
skin examination, patient assessment, 321
skinfold thickness
   body composition measurement, 16
   children, 217, 221, 224
   difficulties in obese subjects, 16–17
   fat distribution measurement, 21
skinfold thickness, children, 225
skin lesions, childhood obesity, 235
sleep apnoea, 278–279
   childhood obesity, 225
   heart failure coexistence, 276
sleep-disordered breathing, 278, 296–315
   childhood obesity, 225, 237–238
   consequences, 303–306, *304*
   definitions, 296–298, **297**
   diagnosis, 302–303, *303*, **303**
   epidemiology, 300–301, *301*
   obstructive sleep apnoea *see* obstructive
      sleep apnoea (OSA)
   pathogenesis, 296
   symptoms and signs, 302, **302**
   treatment, **306**, 306–310, **307**, *310*
Sleep Heart Health Study, 278, 304, 305
sleepiness
   causes, **300**
   excessive daytime, 302, 303
sleep studies, 302–303, *303*, **303**
SlimFast, 353
slim ideal emergence, 55, **56**, 57
slimming clubs, 336
Slimming World (UK), 336
slimness, as ideal body shape, 55
slipped capital femoral epiphysis, 240, *241*
small bowel bypass, 394
'small but healthy hypothesis', 50, **51**

small for gestational age (SGA) infants, 290
smallness preference, culture, 50
Smaw v. *Virginia Department of State Police*, 1994, 30
smoking
  cessation, 7
    weight gain, 70
  epidemic reduction, 458
  maternal, obesity of offspring, 96–97
  mortality at low body mass index, 8–9
  risk factor, 5
  time trend cause, 7–8
snoring, 296, 302
  nasal dilator strips, 307
  stroke association, 305
  sudden death in obesity, 269–270
  see also obstructive sleep apnoea (OSA)
social aspects, 29–45
  causes, 34–37
    see also specific causes
  clinical implications, 38–39
  culture, 52
  education, 31–32
  employment, 29–30
  health care, 30–31
  interpersonal relationships, 32–33
  IQ, 31–32
  isolation, 227
  orientation on obesity, 60
  psychological outcome variables, 33–34
    see also specific variables
  socioeconomic status, 32
  stigma, 39, **40**
social/biological body divide, 55
'social consensus theory', 38
social skill acquisition limitations, peer relationships, 32
social stratification emergence, 47
society differences, culture *see* culture
sociocultural risk factors, 5
socioeconomic status, 32, 52
  infant origins of obesity, 96
  predisposition to weight gain, 457
somatostatin, 202
somnoplasty, 309
soy lecithin, **448**
'specific dynamic action', 70
spirometric ratio, 277
spontaneous physical activity (SPA)
  associated thermogenesis, 76
  efficiency, 76
statins, vascular disease, 272
'stepped-care' approach, obesity management, *444*
stigma, 34–37
  causes, 37–38
  children, 35–37, 227
    by adults, 36
    negative stereotypes, 36

peer harassment and rejection at school, 36
  psychological sequelae, 36–37
  environmental improvement, 39
  health care professionals, reduction in, 39
  patient management of, 38–39
  reduction intervention research, 39–40, **40**
  research recommendations, 39–40, **40**
stimulus control, behavioural therapy, 339, 340–341, 352
St John's wort, **448**
stomach stapling, 326, 394–395, 397
STORM trial, 383, 410
stress, weight regain association, 412
stretch marks, children, 236
stretch-receptors, 72
strokes, 275
  snoring association, 305
  see also cerebrovascular disease
stunted growth
  animal protein effect, 124
  Asian populations and obesity, 439
  fat distribution, 95–96
subcutaneous fat deposits, 20
subscapular skinfold measurements, 223
subscapular-tricep skinfold ratio
  birth weight association, 95, **95**
  body composition measurement, 16
  children, 233
sudden death
  cardiovascular causes in obesity, 269–271
  physical activity risk, 376
sugar beet, 125
sugars
  consumption, 340
  dietary composition, evolutionary perspective, 125
  energy density, 125, *126*
  food intake control bypass, 127
suicide attempts/ideation, 34
  children, 37
sulphonylureas, 262
Sumo wrestlers, 50
'supersizing' meals, 464
suprailiac skinfold, 16
surgery, 326, **351**, 394–406, **445**
  evolution of techniques, 394–396
  ideal procedure characteristics, **400**, 400–403
  jejuno–ileal bypass, 394, *395*
  maxillofacial, obstructive sleep apnoea treatment, 309
  minimally invasive/adjustable procedures, 396
  obese diabetics, 263
  outcomes, 396–399
    health changes, 397–399
    weight loss, 397
  small bowel bypass, 394

stomach stapling, 394–395, 397
  vertical-banded gastroplasty, 395, *395*
  weight loss maintenance role, 414
  see also specific procedures
surveillance programmes, body mass index, 12
Swedish adjustable gastric band (SAGB®), 403, **403**
Swedish Obese Subjects (SOS) study, 326, 408, *409*
  sleep-disordered breathing, 300, 303
  surgery for obesity, 263, 399
  vascular disease risk, 271
sweet clover, **448**
sweet tastes, 125
sympathetic nervous system (SNS)
  diet response, 78, *78*
  insulin resistance, 258
  metabolic drive in obese people, 129
  metabolic syndrome, 257
  obesity hypertension, 273
  role in physical activity, 369, *370*
  sudden death in obesity, 270
  thermogenesis, 77, 156–157
  ventricular hypertrophy, 275
sympathomimetics, energy expenditure stimulation, 157
syndrome x *see* metabolic syndrome
'syndrome Z', **272**

t'ai chi, 449
tallness, desirability, 49
Tanner stages of pubertal development, 235
target groups, obesity prevention, 460
Task Force on Obesity, 10
taxing energy-dense foods, 469
taxing initiatives, 451
teacher attitudes, 35
teasing, 36
'technologies of power', 58
telephone-based interventions, 450
television advertising, *467*
  ban in Sweden, 467
  obesity causal factor, 466
temperature, environmental
  birth, body weight association, 98, *98*
  resting energy expenditure, 153
temperature-controlled radiofrequency ablation to the tongue base and palate (TCRFTA), 309
terpenes, **448**
testosterone
  endocrine testing, 207, 208
  obesity cause, 202–204
  polycystic ovary syndrome, 204
  testing for, 322
theobromine, 385
theophylline, 385
therapeutic overdosing, 234
therapeutic underdosing, 234

thermic effect of food (TEF)
  reduction in obesity, 157–158
  resting energy expenditure, 152–153
  sympathetic nervous system link, 157
thermodynamics, 67–68, *68*
  first law, 67–68
  second law, 68
thermogenesis
  adaptive *see* adaptive thermogenesis
  mechanisms for energy expenditure, 77–78,
    156–157
  physical activity associated, 76–77
  stimuli, 156
    energy expenditure response, 70
  sympathetic nervous system, 156–157
  thermogenic stimuli, 156
Thermoplasma acidophilum, 85
thiazolidinediones
  diabetes mellitus, 262
  non-alcoholic fatty liver disease, 264
thigh creams, 449
thirst, salt intake, 133
three-compartment model, 15, 16
  children, 19
Three Factor Eating Questionnaire (TFEQ), 411
  appetite control, 147
'thrifty genotype' hypothesis, 124
  diabetes mellitus type 2, 48
thromboembolic disease, pregnancy, 288
thyroid hormones
  resting metabolic rate effect, 153–154
  role in weight gain, 204
thyroid-stimulating hormone (TSH)
  endocrine testing, 208
  leptin therapy, 86
  role in weight gain, 204
  testing for, 322
thyrotrophin-releasing hormone (TRH), 86
thyroxine, 86
time trend causes, 7–8
tiredness, childhood obesity, 235–236
tonic signals, appetite control, 139–142, *140*,
  142
topiramate, **382**, 384–385, 388
total body potassium, 13
total body water
  body composition measurement, 13, 14
  chemical maturation in children, 18
total-body wrapping, 324
total fasting, 330
'toxic environments' role, 356, 359
tracheostomy, 308–309
trained athletes, skeletal muscle mass, 102
training programmes
  energy expenditure, 366, 367
  obesity prevention, 460
  physical activity substrate utilization,
    371–372, *372*
transcendental meditation, 417

transcutaneous electrical stimulation (TENS),
  449
transport investment, obesity prevention, 465
treatment *see* management (of obesity)
triacylglycerols
  adipose tissue clearance, 112–113
  energy fluxes, normal daily, 104
  intramuscular measurement, 106
  skeletal muscle, 102, 105, **105**, 107–109
  white adipose tissue, 103
triaxial monitors, 151
tricep skinfold, 16
triggers (for overeating), 339
  see also behavioural therapy
triglyceride(s)
  dyslipidaemia, 163
  oxidation, **150**
  physical activity, 156, 370, 373
  pregnancy, 284
  visceral adipose tissue effect, 166, *168*
  weight loss effects, 260
truncal fat deposition, 94–95
trunk-to-extremity skinfold ratio, 21
tryptophan, hunger-satiety signals, 73
tumour necrosis factor-α (TNF-α)
  adipose tissue, 115, 174, 205, 272
  insulin resistance, 186, 257
  non-alcoholic fatty liver disease, 264
  obesity, 206
  skeletal muscle, 111
twenty-four hour recall method, 128
twin studies, fat mass heritability, 82
two compartment model of body
    composition, 13
type 2 diabetes mellitus *see* diabetes mellitus
L-tyrosine, 449

UKPDS *see* United Kingdom Prospective
    Diabetes Study Group (UKPDS)
ulnar-mammary syndrome, **83**
uncoupling proteins (UCPs), 103
  resting metabolic rate effect, 154
  skeletal muscle metabolism disturbances in
    obesity, 110
  thermogenesis mechanism, 77
undergraduate training, 422–423
undernutrition, Asian populations, 434
underwater submergence, body volume
    measurement, 14
underwater weighing, children, 216, **216**
United Kingdom Prospective Diabetes Study
    Group (UKPDS), 256
  glycaemic control in weight loss, 260
  lipids in weight loss, 261
  pharmacotherapy in the obese diabetic
    patient, 262
United Kingdom Prospective Diabetes Study
    Group (UKPDS), b-cell dysfunction,
    258

United Kingdom (UK), prevalence, 6, *6*
United States Centres for Disease Control
    (CDC) 2000 growth charts, 217–218,
    220
  percentiles, 223
United States 1977 National Centre for Health
    Statistics growth charts, 217
United States of America (USA)
  prevalence, 6, *6*, 99
  prevention, 459, *460*
upper airway resistance syndrome, 297
upper airway surgery, 309
upper airway tone, 277–278
urbanization
  aetiology of obesity, 52
  Asian populations, 438
uric acid levels, 332
urinary tract infections (UTIs), **287**, 287–288
US Nurses Health Study
  coronary heart disease risk, 271, *271*
  sudden death in obesity, 270
uvulopalatopharyngoplasty (UPPP), 309

vascular diseases/disorders, *271*, 271–272
  childhood obesity, 237
vasopressin, 386, **387**
vending machines, ban in schools, 464
venous thromboembolic disease, pregnancy,
  291
ventromedial hypothalamus (VMH)
  energy homeostasis involvement, 85
  satiety control, 72
verbal abuse, 36
vertical-banded gastroplasty (VGB), 395,
  395
very low-calorie diets (VLCDs), 325
  combined with physical activity, 365
  obese diabetics, 261
very low-density lipoproteins (VLDLs)
  dyslipidaemia, 163
    abdominal obesity, 172
  hepatic synthesis, 172
  weight loss effects, 261
very low-energy diets (VLEDs), 328–330
  complications associated, 328–329
  contraindications, **330**
  effects, **445**
  Prader–Willi syndrome use, 342
  sudden death, 270
virtual reality devices, 452
visceral adipose tissue
  cardiovascular risk factor, 224–225
  children, 224–225
  dyslipidaemia, 165–166, *166*
  gender differences, 166, *167*
  metabolic syndrome *see* metabolic
    syndrome
  regulatory/secretory characteristics, 206
  risk assessment, 323, **323**

visceral obesity, 165, *166*, 381
  Asian population, **437**
  diabetes risk, 253
  endocrine causes, 200–201
  endocrine secretion, 206
  ethnicity, 437
  health risks, 165
  moderate weight loss effects, 176
  respiratory effects, 298–299
  rimonabant therapy, 387
visual cues, energy intake control, 127
voluntary energy expenditure, 70
vulnerable groups, 33

wage penalty, employment, 29
waist circumference, 4, **4**, 21, 321
  children, 217, 233
    abdominal adiposity, 225
    reference standards, 227
  diabetes risk, 253, *253*
  health risk assessment, 408
  ill health association, 434
  visceral adipose tissue measurement,
    176
waist–height ratio, 4
waist–hip ratio (WHR), 4, 21
  abdominal obesity, 165
    children, 225
  children, 225, 233

coronary heart disease risk, 271, *271*
  diabetes risk, 253
  health risk assessment, 408
  visceral adipose tissue measurement, 176
walking, 410, 451–452
'walking school buses', 452, 464
water consumption, dietary interventions,
  340
weight *see* body weight
'weight-clamping' experiments, 76
Weight Concern, 349
weight cycling, 411, 413, 416
weight-for-age percentiles, 223
weight-for-height indices, 217
weight-for-stature, 217
  percentiles, 217
Weight Watchers, 324, 336, 358–359, 445–446
Western cultures, 47
  concept of obesity, 59
  culture in 20th century, 55–59
  diabetes prevalence, 252
  epidemic of obesity, 456
  gene–environment interactions, 82
  process of, 53, 55
  slim ideal, supportive cultural context, 57
  slimness preference, 50
  stigmatism of obesity, 49
  typical diet, 104
white adipose tissue *see* adipose tissue

whole-body plethysmography, 19
Wilson–Turner syndrome, **83**
Wisconsin Sleep Cohort Study, 301, 304
women, 'ideal body shape', 50–52, **51**
World Health Organization (WHO)
  Expert Consultation on Appropriate Body
    Mass Index for Asian Populations,
    435–436, 440, *440*
  graded classification system for obesity, 431
  MONICA study
    European prevalence, 6, **7**
    vascular disease risk, 271
  nutrient intake goals, **130**, 130–131
  obesity definition, 408
  physical activity recommendations, 374
    diabetes, 261
  Task Force on Obesity, 10
  weight-for age classification, Asian
    population, 434

XENDOS study, 263
X-linked pleiotropic obesity syndromes, **83**

Yasmin, 291
yearly re-evaluation in children, 224
yoga, 449

zonisamide, **382**, 385, 388
z-scores, 221